# End Stage Renal Disease in Children

**Richard N. Fine, M.D.**
Professor of Pediatrics
UCLA School of Medicine
Head, Division of Pediatric Nephrology
UCLA Center for the Health Sciences
Los Angeles, California

**Alan B. Gruskin, M.D.**
Director of Pediatric Nephrology
St. Christopher's Hospital for Children
Philadelphia, Pennsylvania

**W. B. Saunders Company**     **1984**
**PHILADELPHIA / LONDON / TORONTO / MEXICO CITY / RIO DE JANEIRO / SYDNEY / TOKYO**

W. B. Saunders Company: West Washington Square
Philadelphia, PA 19105

1 St. Anne's Road
Eastbourne, East Sussex BN21 3UN, England

1 Goldthorne Avenue
Toronto, Ontario M8Z 5T9, Canada

Apartado 26370—Cedro 512
Mexico 4, D.F., Mexico

Rua Coronel Cabrita, 8
Sao Cristovao Caixa Postal 21176
Rio de Janeiro, Brazil

9 Waltham Street
Artarmon, N.S.W. 2064, Australia

Ichibancho, Central Bldg., 22-1 Ichibancho
Chiyoda-Ku, Tokyo 102, Japan

**Library of Congress Cataloging in Publication Data**

Fine, Richard N.

End stage renal disease in children.

1. Renal insufficiency.   2. Hemodialysis.   3. Pediatric
nephrology.   I. Gruskin, Alan B.   II. Title. [DNLM:
1. Kidney failure, Chronic—In infancy and childhood.
2. Kidney failure, Chronic—Therapy. WJ 342 F495e]

RJ476.K5F56 1984      618.92′61      83–6614

ISBN 0–7216–1025–0

End Stage Renal Disease in Children                    ISBN  0–7216–1025–0

Last digit is the print number:    9    8    7    6    5    4    3    2    1

# Dedicated to

our wives—Peachie and Shawney
our children—Glenn, Jeffrey, Joanne, Karen, Michael, and Robin

whose patience, tolerance, and support have given us the privilege and time to pursue end stage renal disease in children

and our colleagues, patients, and families who have helped us learn so that it might be easier for those who follow.

# Contributors

**STEVEN R. ALEXANDER, M.D.**

Associate Professor of Pediatrics, Oregon Health Sciences University, Portland; Medical Director, CAPD Training Program, Oregon Health Sciences University Hospital, Portland; Attending Pediatric Nephrologist, Oregon Health Sciences University Affiliated Hospitals, Portland, Oregon

*Treatment of Infants with ESRD; CAPD in Infants Less Than One Year of Age*

**JOEL M. ANDRES, M.D.**

Professor and Chief, Division of Pediatric Gastroenterology, University of Florida, Gainesville; Chief, Division of Pediatric Gastroenterology, Shands Teaching Hospital and Clinics, University of Florida, Gainesville, Florida

*Liver Problems Associated with ESRD in Children*

**GERALD S. ARBUS, M.D., F.R.C.P.(C)**

Associate Professor of Pediatrics, University of Toronto, Ontario; Chief, Division of Nephrology, The Hospital for Sick Children, Toronto, Ontario

*Immunosuppressive Therapy for Pediatric Renal Allograft Recipients*

**JAMES B. ATKINSON, M.D.**

Assistant Professor of Surgery (Pediatric), University of Southern California School of Medicine, Los Angeles, California; Attending Staff, Childrens Hospital of Los Angeles, California

*Vascular and Peritoneal Access: Technical Considerations*

**J. WILLIAMSON BALFE, M.D., F.R.C.P.(C)**

Associate Professor of Pediatrics, University of Toronto, Ontario; Senior Staff Physician, Director of CAPD Program, The Hospital for Sick Children, Toronto, Ontario

*Continuous Ambulatory Peritoneal Dialysis: Clinical Aspects*

**H. JORGE BALUARTE, M.D.**

Associate Professor of Pediatrics, Temple University School of Medicine/St. Christopher's Hospital for Children, Philadelphia, Pennsylvania; Staff Nephrologist, Director of Dialysis and Transplant Program, St. Christopher's Hospital for Children, Philadelphia, Pennsylvania

*Intermittent Peritoneal Dialysis: Technical and Clinical Aspects*

**FRANK G. BOINEAU, M.D.**

Associate Professor of Pediatrics, School of Medicine, Tulane University, New Orleans, Louisiana; Head, Section of Pediatric Nephrology, Tulane University Hospital, New Orleans, Louisiana

*Sexual Maturation in Children with Renal Insufficiency: Response to Dialysis and Transplantation; Anemia in Children with ESRD*

**JAKOB BRINER, M.D., PD**

Head of the Pediatric Pathology Section, Department of Pathology, University of Zurich, Switzerland

*Recurrence of the Primary Disease in the Transplanted Kidney*

**MICHEL BROYER, M.D.**

Professor of Paediatrics, Faculté de Médécine Necker, Paris, France; Director of Paediatric Nephrology Department, Hospital des Enfants Malades, Paris, France

*Incidence and Etiology of ESRD in Children*

**PHILIP L. CALCAGNO, M.D.**

Professor/Chairman, Department of Pediatrics, Division of Pediatric Hemodialysis, Georgetown University Medical Center, Washington, D.C.

*Hemoperfusion in Therapeutic Medicine*

**CYRIL CHANTLER, M.A., M.D., F.R.C.P.**

Professor of Paediatric Nephrology, Guy's Hospital and Medical School, London, England

*Nutritional Assessment and Management of Children with Renal Insufficiency*

**RUSSELL W. CHESNEY, M.D.**

Professor of Pediatrics, University of Wisconsin School of Medicine, Madison, Wisconsin; Director, Pediatric Nephrology, University of Wisconsin Hospitals, Madison, Wisconsin

*Treatment of Renal Osteodystrophy During Childhood*

**SHERMINE DABBAGH, M.D.**

Pediatric Renal Fellow, University of Wisconsin Clinical Science Center, Madison, Wisconsin

*Treatment of Renal Osteodystrophy During Childhood*

RAYMOND A. DONCKERWOLCKE, M.D.

University of Utrecht, The Netherlands; Director, Dialysis and Transplant Program, Wilhelmina Kinderzickenhuis, Children's Hospital, Utrecht, The Netherlands

*Survival on Renal Replacement Therapy*

ROBERT B. ETTENGER, M.D.

Associate Professor of Pediatrics, University of California, Los Angeles School of Medicine; Attending Physician, Department of Pediatrics, University of California, UCLA Center for the Health Sciences, Los Angeles, California

*The Role of Pretransplant Blood Transfusion in Renal Transplant Outcome; Immunology of Transplantation*

ROBERT S. FENNELL, III, M.D.

Associate Professor of Pediatrics, University of Florida College of Medicine, Gainesville; Medical Director, Dialysis and Transplant Units, University of Florida Shands Teaching Hospital and Clinics, Gainesville, Florida

*Liver Problems Associated with ESRD in Children*

RICHARD N. FINE, M.D.

Professor of Pediatrics, School of Medicine, Division of Pediatric Nephrology, UCLA Center for the Health Sciences, Los Angeles, California

*Historical Perspective of the Treatment of ESRD in Children*

SHAWNEY E. FINE, R.N.

Clinical Nurse Specialist, UCLA Center for the Health Sciences, Los Angeles, California; Division of Pediatric Nephrology, UCLA Center for the Health Sciences, Los Angeles, California

*The Clinical Nurse Specialist in Renal Transplantation*

CASIMIR F. FIRLIT, M.D., Ph.D.

Professor of Urology, Department of Urology, Northwestern University, Chicago, Illinois; Head, Division of Pediatric Urology and Transplantation, Children's Memorial Hospital, Chicago, Illinois

*Urologic Aspects of Transplantation in Children*

JAMES W. FISHER, Ph.D.

Professor of Pharmacology, Tulane University School of Medicine, New Orleans, Louisiana

*Anemia in Children with ESRD*

EDUARDO H. GARIN, M.D.

Associate Professor of Pediatrics, University of Florida College of Medicine, Gainesville; Attending Physician, Pediatric Nephrology, University of Florida Shands Teaching Hospital and Clinics, Gainesville, Florida

*Liver Problems Associated with ESRD in Children*

GIULIO GILLI, M.D.

Section of Pediatric Nephrology, Florence Nightingale Hospital, Düsseldorf, Federal Republic of Germany

*Growth in Children with Chronic Renal Insufficiency*

DORIT GRADUS (BEN-EZER), M.D.

Assistant Professor of Pediatrics, Ben-Gurion University School of Medicine, Bèer-Sheba, Israel; Staff Physician, Division of Pediatrics, Soroka Medical Center, Bèer-Sheba, Israel

*The Role of Pretransplant Blood Transfusion in Renal Transplant Outcome; Immunology of Transplantation*

THOMAS P. GREEN, M.D.

Assistant Professor, Departments of Pediatrics and Pharmacology, University of Minnesota, Minneapolis; Attending Physician, University of Minnesota Hospitals, Minneapolis, Minnesota

*Principles of Drug Therapy in Children with ESRD*

MICHAEL B. GROSSMAN, R.N., M.S.N.

Former Nephrology Program Coordinator, St. Christopher's Hospital for Children, Philadelphia, Pennsylvania

*The Role of the Pediatric Nephrology Nurse in the Dialysis Unit*

WARREN E. GRUPE, M.D.

Associate Professor of Pediatrics, Harvard Medical School, Boston, Massachusetts; Director, Pediatric Nephrology, The Children's Hospital, Boston, Massachusetts

*Urea Kinetics in the Clinical Management of Children on Chronic Hemodialysis*

ALAN B. GRUSKIN, M.D.

Professor of Pediatrics, Temple University School of Medicine, Philadelphia, Pennsylvania; Chief, Section of Nephrology, St. Christopher's Hospital for Children, Philadelphia, Pennsylvania

*Kinetics of Peritoneal Dialysis in Children*

TERESA L. HALL, R.N., M.S.

Head Nurse, Pediatric Dialysis, Pediatric and Adult Dialysis Home Training Programs, UCLA Center for the Health Sciences, Los Angeles, California

*Nursing Management of the Child Undergoing CAPD*

BRIAN E. HARDY, M.B., Ch.B., F.R.A.C.S.

Assistant Professor, University of Toronto, Ontario; Staff Urologist, Hospital for Sick Children; Chief, Renal Transplantation, Hospital for Sick Children, Toronto, Ontario

*Immunosuppressive Therapy for Pediatric Renal Allograft Recipients*

WILLIAM E. HARMON, M.D.

Assistant Professor of Pediatrics, Harvard Medical School, Boston, Massachusetts; Director, Dialysis Unit, The Children's Hospital, Boston, Massachusetts

*Urea Kinetics in the Clinical Management of Children on Chronic Hemodialysis*

IAN K. HEWITT, M.B.B.S., F.R.A.C.P.

Senior Registrar, Pediatric Nephrology, Princess Margaret Hospital for Children, Perth, Western Australia

*Continuous Ambulatory Peritoneal Dialysis: Clinical Aspects*

JULIE R. INGELFINGER, M.D.

Assistant Professor of Pediatrics, Harvard Medical School, Boston, Massachusetts; Associate in Pediatrics and Director of Special Renal Clinic, Children's Hospital, Boston, Massachusetts

*Hypertension in Children with ESRD*

ABDOLLAH IRAVANI, M.D.

Associate Professor, University of Florida College of Medicine, Gainesville; Attending Physician, Pediatric Nephrology, Shands Teaching Hospital and Clinics, University of Florida, Gainesville

*Liver Problems Associated with ESRD in Children*

ROBIN S. JOHNSON, M.A., M.S.S., A.C.S.W.

Clinical Social Worker, ESRD, St. Christopher's Hospital for Children, Philadelphia, Pennsylvania

*The Role of the Social Worker in the Management of the Child with ESRD*

STANLEY C. JORDAN, M.D.

Assistant Professor of Pediatrics, UCLA School of Medicine, Los Angeles, California; Attending Physician, Department of Pediatrics, UCLA Medical Center, Los Angeles, California

*Allograft Rejection: Types, Mechanisms, and Diagnosis*

BARBARA M. KORSCH, M.D.

Professor of Pediatrics, USC School of Medicine, Los Angeles, California; Head, Division of General Pediatrics, Childrens Hospital of Los Angeles, California

*Psychosocial Adaptation of Children with ESRD: Factors Affecting Rehabilitation*

JACQUES M. LEMIRE, M.D., F.R.C.P.(C)

Fellow, Department of Pediatrics, Division of Pediatric Nephrology, UCLA School of Medicine, Los Angeles, California; Fellow, Division of Pediatric Nephrology, UCLA Medical Center, Los Angeles, California

*Allograft Rejection: Types, Mechanisms, and Diagnosis*

MICHAEL R. LEONE, M.D.

Fellow, University of Cincinnati, Cincinnati, Ohio

*Infection in the Child Receiving Therapy for ESRD*

ERNST P. LEUMANN, M.D., PD

Head of the Section of Pediatric Nephrology, University Children's Hospital, Zurich, Switzerland

*Recurrence of the Primary Disease in the Transplanted Kidney*

JOHN E. LEWY, M.D.

Professor and Chairman, Department of Pediatrics, Tulane University School of Medicine, New Orleans, Louisiana; Chief of Pediatrics, Tulane Medical Center; Chief of Tulane Pediatrics, Charity Hospital of New Orleans, Louisiana

*Sexual Maturation in Children with Renal Insufficiency: Response to Dialysis and Transplantation; Anemia in Children with ESRD*

JO ANN MALONEY, R.N., B.S.A.

CAPD Home Training Instructor, St. Christopher's Hospital for Children, Philadelphia, Pennsylvania

*Nursing Management of the Child Undergoing CAPD*

LESTER W. MARTIN, M.D.

Professor of Surgery and Pediatrics, The College of Medicine, University of Cincinnati, Ohio; Director of Pediatric Surgery, The Childrens Hospital, Cincinnati, Ohio

*Surgical Aspects of Transplantation: Technique and Complications*

S. MICHAEL MAUER, M.D.

Professor of Pediatrics, University of Minnesota School of Medicine, Minneapolis, Minnesota

*Infant Hemodialysis*

PAUL T. McENERY, M.D.

Associate Professor, University of Cincinnati, Ohio; Attending Pediatric Nephrologist, Children's Hospital Research Foundation, Cincinnati, Ohio

*Infection in the Child Receiving Therapy for ESRD*

OTTO MEHLS, M.D.

Professor, Department of Pediatrics, University of Heidelberg, Federal Republic of Germany; Head, Pediatric Dialysis Unit, University Children's Hospital, Heidelberg, Federal Republic of Germany

*Renal Osteodystrophy in Children: Etiology and Clinical Aspects*

BRUCE Z. MORGENSTERN, M.D.

Fellow, Pediatric Nephrology, St. Christopher's Hospital for Children, Philadelphia, Pennsylvania

*Kinetics of Peritoneal Dialysis in Children*

VIDA FRANCIS-NEGRETE, P.H.N., M.S.

Research Consultant, Childrens Hospital of Los Angeles, Los Angeles, California

*Psychosocial Adaptation of Children with ESRD: Factors Affecting Rehabilitation*

PAULINE NELSON, R.D.

Pediatric Renal Dietitian, Division of Pediatric Nephrology, UCLA Center for the Health Sciences, Los Angeles, California

*Principles of Nutritional Assessment and Management of Child with ESRD*

**THOMAS E. NEVINS, M.D.**

Assistant Professor of Pediatrics, University of Minnesota School of Medicine, Minneapolis; University of Minnesota Hospitals, Minneapolis, Minnesota

*Infant Hemodialysis*


**JOHN NOSEWORTHY, M.D.**

Assistant Professor of Surgery and Urology, Department of Surgery, University of Cincinnati College of Medicine, Cincinnati, Ohio; Pediatric Surgery/Urology, Children's Hospital Medical Center, Cincinnati, Ohio

*Surgical Aspects of Transplantation: Technique and Complications*


**ANTONIA C. NOVELLO, M.D.**

Executive Secretary, General Medicine, B Study Section, Division of Research Grant, National Institutes of Health, Bethesda, Maryland

*Hemoperfusion in Therapeutic Medicine*


**PETER-JOACHIM OERTEL, M.D.**

Fellow in Pediatric Nephrology, University Children's Hospital, Heidelberg, Federal Republic of Germany

*Endocrine Function in Children with ESRD*


**SEAN O'REGAN, M.B., B.Ch., F.R.C.P.(C)**

Associate Professor, Department of Pediatrics, University of Montreal, Quebec; Pediatric Nephrologist, Hôpital Ste. Justine, Montreal, Quebec

*Cardiovascular Abnormalities in Pediatric Patients with ESRD*


**ZOE L. PAPADOPOULOU, M.D.**

Associate Professor, Department of Pediatrics, Division of Pediatric Hemodialysis, Georgetown University Medical Center, Washington, D.C.

*Hemoperfusion in Therapeutic Medicine*


**SHARON A. PERLMAN, M.D.**

Fellow, Pediatric Nephrology, St. Christopher's Hospital for Children, Philadelphia, Pennsylvania

*Kinetics of Peritoneal Dialysis in Children*


**MARTIN S. POLINSKY, M.D.**

Assistant Professor of Pediatrics, Temple University Medical School, Philadelphia, Pennsylvania; Attending Nephrologist, St. Christopher's Hospital for Children, Philadelphia, Pennsylvania

*Neurologic Complications of ESRD, Dialysis, and Transplantation*


**DONALD E. POTTER, M.D.**

Associate Clinical Professor of Pediatrics, University of California, San Francisco; Attending Pediatrician, University of California Medical Center, San Francisco, California

*Hemodialysis in Children with ESRD: Technical Aspects*


**WOLFGANG RAUH, M.D.**

Assistant Professor, University Children's Hospital, University of Heidelberg, Federal Republic of Germany; Head of Pediatrics, Kinderklinik St. Katharinen, Trier, Federal Republic of Germany

*Endocrine Function in Children with ESRD*


**GEORGE A. RICHARD, M.D.**

Professor and Chief, Pediatric Nephrology Division, University of Florida College of Medicine, Gainesville; Chief, Division of Pediatric Nephrology, University of Florida, Shands Teaching Hospital and Clinics, Gainesville, Florida

*Liver Problems Associated with ESRD in Children*


**KARL SCHARER, M.D.**

Professor of Pediatrics, Division of Nephrology, University Children's Hospital, Heidelberg, Federal Republic of Germany

*Growth in Children with Chronic Renal Insufficiency*


**DANIEL V. SCHIDLOW, M.D.**

Director, Pediatric Pulmonary and Cystic Fibrosis Center and Chief, Section of Pulmonary Medicine, St. Christopher's Hospital for Children, Philadelphia, Pennsylvania; Associate Professor of Pediatrics, Temple University School of Medicine, Philadelphia, Pennsylvania; Attending Pediatrician, St. Christopher's Hospital for Children, Philadelphia, Pennsylvania

*Pulmonary Function in ESRD*


**NEIL J. SHERMAN, M.D.**

Assistant Clinical Professor of Surgery (Pediatric), University of Southern California School of Medicine, Los Angeles, California; Attending Staff, Childrens Hospital of Los Angeles, Los Angeles, California

*Vascular and Peritoneal Access: Technical Considerations*


**ALAN R. SINAIKO, M.D.**

Associate Professor of Pediatrics and Pharmacology, Division of Clinical Pharmacology, University of Minnesota, Minneapolis, Minnesota

*Principles of Drug Therapy in Children with ESRD*


**BRIAN T. STEELE, M.B., B.Ch., M.R.C.P.(UK), F.R.C.P.(C)**

Assistant Professor of Pediatrics, McMaster University, Hamilton, Ontario; Director of Pediatric Nephrology at the McMaster University Medical Center, Hamilton, Ontario

*Continuous Ambulatory Peritoneal Dialysis: Clinical Aspects*


**CONSTANTINOS J. STEFANIDIS, M.D.**

"Aglaia Kyriakou" Children's Hospital, Athens, Greece

*Continuous Ambulatory Peritoneal Dialysis: Clinical Aspects*


**JEAN STOVER, R.D.**

Renal Nutritionist, St. Christopher's Hospital for Children, Philadelphia, Pennsylvania

*Principles of Nutritional Assessment and Management of Child with ESRD*

# Preface

The outlook for children afflicted with end stage renal disease (ESRD) has changed dramatically during the past quarter century. From utter despair the dual modalities of dialysis and transplantation now permit cautious optimism. Not only have the lives of many children been prolonged, but in the process of caring for these children intense investigative efforts have been stimulated to understand the consequences of uremia. Much has been learned about ESRD in children and it is now appropriate to bring together our collective knowledge.

Although many of the clinical problems confronting medical personnel caring for the child with ESRD are similar to those encountered in adult patients, unique differences primarily related to factors related to growth and development do exist. Optimal care requires that these characteristics be considered when rendering care to children with ESRD. It is these differences which have led to the development of this text.

Quality care for the child with ESRD is complex, extending across many of the classical boundaries involved in health care, and is best accomplished by a team approach. The care of the child with ESRD requires participation of professional personnel from many disciplines in order to adequately address the total needs of the child and members of his or her family. Such care also requires knowledge and experience ranging from the experimental to the practical and applied. This book contains information pertaining to all aspects of care required for the child with ESRD. Such a comprehensive approach is evident from the varied backgrounds of the individuals who have contributed.

The editors are exceedingly grateful to the contributors who have taken the time and effort to summarize available data as well as to relate their current experiences and thoughts in a rapidly changing medical specialty. Many have been pioneers in the development of ESRD care in children. We believe that all who share in the care of the child with ESRD will find the information helpful in caring for their patients.

Delivery of medical care to children is founded on helping individuals. The Talmud says that the act of saving one life is tantamount to saving the world. The information contained in this text will certainly not solve the multitude of problems that currently confronts this troubled world. But if one child suffers less and his or her life is made less onerous by the information in this text, then the effort expended by all those involved will have been justified.

RICHARD N. FINE, M.D.
ALAN B. GRUSKIN, M.D.

# Contents

# Historical Perspective of the Treatment of ESRD in Children

*Richard N. Fine, M.D.*

A historical perspective of the treatment of children afflicted with end stage renal disease (ESRD) encompasses not only the evolution of the therapeutic modalities of peritoneal dialysis, hemodialysis, and renal transplantation but also an analysis of the philosophical considerations prevalent during the past two decades regarding the desirability of prolonging life by extraordinary means in an otherwise fatal disease.

In 1964 Conrad M. Riley, M.D., in an editorial comment in the Journal of Pediatrics[1] thoughtfully reviewed the dilemma of utilizing the emerging treatment modality of renal transplantation for children with ESRD. Dr. Riley's insight was obtained primarily from the pioneering program initiated by Dr. Thomas Starzl at the University of Colorado.

Riley felt that the decision to offer such treatment should be "balanced" by two major judgments: "The length of prolongation of life" and "the expected totality of discomfort factors as seen through the eyes of the child." In regard to the latter, he emphasized the potential for continued growth retardation following successful transplantation, resulting in the kidney's being housed in a "healthy dwarf." At that time the life expectancy of pediatric allograft recipients could only be anticipated and the discomfort factors only estimated.

Six years later, John B. Reinhart, M.D., commented in the same journal on the initial reports from pediatric dialysis and transplant centers.[2] He "seriously questioned the value of chronic dialysis or renal transplantation" in children because of the "cost to the child in terms of physical and emotional discomfort." In addition, he felt that "progress of dialysis and renal transplantation for children should be carefully evaluated in terms, not of gross survival, but in parameters of meaningful growth and development—living."

These disquieting comments stimulated those involved in caring for children with ESRD to carefully evaluate the psychosocial and rehabilitative effects of such therapeutic intervention on the patients and their families. Reports from individual pediatric centers in the United States[3, 4] as well as cooperative studies in Europe[5] addressed the issue regarding the virtue of employing these new therapeutic modalities in children. The fact that children appeared to resume their premorbid level of functioning after one year of a successful transplant indicated that renal transplantation was the optimal therapeutic modality for the child with ESRD.[7] Therefore, although all the questions raised by Riley and Reinhart have not been definitively answered, there is currently general acceptance of the virtue of treating children and adolescents with ESRD by means of dialysis and transplantation in affluent countries.

## PERITONEAL DIALYSIS (PD)

In 1922, Putnam defined the peritoneum as a dialyzing membrane and extended previous studies initiated in the nineteenth century.[8] These studies established that solutes and water could be added to or removed from the body by placing solutions of appropriate composition in the peritoneal cavity. The peritoneal membrane was characterized as semipermeable and inert.

The first reported use of the peritoneal membrane to remove uremic substances in man was by Ganter in 1923.[9] He envisaged PD as a replacement for kidney function in individuals with chronic renal failure. During the subsequent three decades, minimal advances occurred because of inadequate peritoneal access devices, morbidity and mortality from peritonitis, and the limited availability of acceptable dialysis solutions. The widespread clinical use of PD was initiated by Maxwell et al. in 1959.[10] The authors described the use of commercially available dialysate solutions and disposable tubing sets. These technical advances facilitated the use of PD in acutely ill patients. The technique required opening the system to potential bacterial contamination during each dialysis pass, which obviated the use of PD for prolonged periods of time. In 1964, Boen et al. described a closed system which minimized the potential for bacterial contamination during repeated procedures.[11] This concept led to the development of automated PD machines. Such equipment utilized ordinary tap water and a concentrated dialysate solution to deliver large volumes of sterile dialysate. The automated equipment was a significant technical advance which facilitated repetitive PD by minimizing the incidence of peritonitis and by reducing the volume and therefore the cost of commercially sterilized dialysate. In conjunction with the permanently implantable peritoneal access catheter described by Tenckhoff and Schechter in 1968,[12] the automated equipment permitted the use of intermittent PD as a realistic alternative for patients with ESRD.

The actual use of intermittent peritoneal dialysis (IPD) as a primary treatment modality was minimal, however. Reduced efficiency of solute and water removal was a major disadvantage, compared to hemodialysis (HD). To achieve comparable results, the weekly dialysis time for IPD was almost three times that of HD. Consequently, IPD was impractical in the hospital setting primarily because of significantly increased personnel costs. It followed that, from a practical standpoint, family involvement was required in order to initiate IPD in the home. In addition, peritonitis remained an impediment.

These factors, along with the increased availability of HD, curtailed interest in IPD as a primary treatment modality. Nevertheless, certain centers for adults fostered the use of home IPD for selected patients. Meanwhile, experience with IPD in pediatric patients was limited, until the difficulties encountered with long-term hemodialysis in children stimulated renewed interest.[13–15]

In 1976 Popovich et al. described a "novel portable/wearable equilibrium, peritoneal dialysis technique."[16] This technique utilized instillation of dialysate in the peritoneal cavity four or five times daily for periods of four to eight hours and was labeled continuous ambulatory peritoneal dialysis (CAPD). The procedure alleviated the clinical consequences of uremia and led to a biochemical steady state. Excessive fluid removal was accomplished by increasing the osmolality of the dialysate solution. Conceptually, CAPD had a significant impact; however, the use of bottles containing dialysate solution necessitated "breaking" the system twice during each pass, or eight to ten times daily, leading to unacceptable high rates of peritonitis. In 1978 Oreopoulos et al. introduced the use of plastic bags filled with dialysate.[17] Following instillation of the dialysate solution, the bag could be attached to the body rather easily and utilized for efflux of dialysate four to eight hours later. The number of disconnections was reduced and the incidence of peritonitis decreased markedly to one episode every 10.5 patient-months. In July, 1980, the Food and Drug Administration approved the sale of 500 and 1000 ml of dialysate in plastic bags in the United States, and this permitted the potential widespread use of CAPD in pediatric patients. Preliminary reports from Canada,[18] the United States,[19] and Europe[20] indicate that CAPD is gaining acceptance as a primary treatment modality for children with ESRD, especially young children weighing less than 20 kg.

## HEMODIALYSIS

Although the modern use of an artificial kidney was introduced by Kolff and Berk in 1944,[21] successful hemodialysis in a child was not reported until 1955.[22] In 1958 Holliday reviewed the use of the artificial kidney in children.[23] Published experience at that time consisted of 10 patients described in two reports.[22, 24] Serious technical difficulties related to the size of pediatric patients and lack of experienced personnel were considered primary factors contributing to the meager use of hemodialysis in pediatric patients. Between 1958 and 1966 numerous reports appeared describing various modifications designed to overcome serious technical difficulties, thereby facilitating successful hemodialysis in children.[25-37] These reports dealt mainly with problems of vascular access and modifications of existing dialysis equipment to accommodate the smaller blood volume of younger patients who required acute hemodialysis. A majority of children received only one or two dialyses for acute renal insufficiency or accidental poisoning.

Kallen et al. in 1966 reviewed the subject of hemodialysis in children and was able to find reports of 62 patients in the pediatric age group treated with short-term hemodialysis for renal insufficiency.[37] These authors added 22 children from their experience. In addition, 27 children with accidental poisoning had been treated with hemodialysis by 1966.[38] Thus, the feasibility of utilizing an artificial kidney to treat children with acute disorders was established. However, at that time less than a dozen children with chronic renal insufficiency had undergone extended hemodialysis.[37, 39-42]

A disquieting note in the applicability of hemodialysis in treating children with chronic renal insufficiency was raised by a group at the University of Washington.[42] They related their experience with extended dialysis in a preadolescent girl over a period of 23 months. In addition to encountering cannula difficulties and a myriad of psychological problems, they were unable to demonstrate growth in this patient despite multiple manipulations of the dialysis regimen. Because of their unrewarding experience, especially the child's failure to grow, they proposed a concept that extended hemodialysis was not applicable to the pediatric age group.

Despite these reservations two pediatric programs were initiated in California in 1967 to treat children with ESRD. These centers, in addition to providing clinical care, demonstrated the feasibility of extended hemodialysis in children.[3, 4] Subsequent programs evolved in other parts of the United States,[43] Canada,[44] and Western Europe[44] to extend hemodialysis to children with ESRD.

In the United States, federal legislation was enacted in 1973 which entitled every citizen, regardless of age, to obtain Medicare reimbursement for dialysis and transplantation; this was a major impetus in extending care to all children with ESRD. However, financial constraints remain an impediment to the use of hemodialysis in children with ESRD in many areas of the world.

## TRANSPLANTATION

The concept of organ transplantation can be found in Greek mythology; however, one of the first bona fide considerations of organ transplantation was by Gaspare Tagliacozzi in 1597.[46] He was requested by a nobleman with a destroyed syphilitic nose to replace the nose with one from a slave. Tagliacozzi discarded the idea with the statement that "the singular character of the individual entirely dissuades us from attempting this work on another person."

Almost 400 years have passed since Tagliacozzi made the above statement, yet the singular character of the individual—i.e., the ability of the body to recognize foreign substances and call forth an immunologic reaction to eliminate them—remains the omnipresent impediment to successful organ transplantation today.

The first attempt at kidney transplantation in man was by Emmerich Ullmann in Vienna in 1902.[47] A pig kidney was unsuccessfully transplanted to the elbow of a uremic woman.

In 1906 Paul Ehrlich transplanted a mouse tumor into a rat.[48] He noted that the tumor would grow for approximately eight days and then regressed. Conceptually, Ehrlich proposed that each species synthesized a substance that was vital for survival and growth, and that the mouse tumor regressed because the rat could not provide the species-specific "vital substance." In actuality, the rat, in all probability, rejected the mouse tumor. The "immunity theory" of transplant rejection was initially proposed by James B. Murphy in 1912.[49] He advanced the concept that the small lymphocyte was primarily involved in tissue rejection. Seventy years hence the search for the specific small lymphocyte continues.

Marked advances in our understanding of the immunity theory were made by Medawar in 1943[50] and Billingham, Brent, and Medawar in 1953.[51] Medawar demonstrated that accelerated rejection or *second set reaction* occurred with repeated grafting from the same donor. The concept of *immunologic tolerance* was first demonstrated experimentally by Billingham, Brent, and Medawar. Inoculation of fetal mice or chick embryos with donor tissue resulted in permanent acceptance of such donor tissue following grafting after birth or hatching. Grafts from third-party donors were rejected. During the past 20 years, attempts to unlock the mechanism of immunologic tolerance in order to apply it to clinical organ transplantation as a means of specific immunosuppression have not come to fruition. Consequently, nonspecific immunosuppression remains the sole treatment modality currently utilized.

Slightly more than a quarter of a century ago, in 1954, the first successful clinical renal transplants in man were reported by Murray and colleagues from the Peter Bent Brigham Hospital in Boston.[52] These transplants were between identical twins and therefore obviated the immunologic phenomenon of rejection.

Subsequently, attention was directed toward methods of nonspecific immunosuppression in order to facilitate clinical renal transplantation using more immunologically disparate donors, living as well as cadaver.

In 1959 Hamburger et al. reported the use of whole body irradiation as a method of nonspecific immunosuppression.[53] The degree of bone marrow suppression and subsequent infection rate minimized enthusiasm for this method. Calne et al. in 1961 reported the successful prolongation of survival of canine renal allografts with an experimental drug which was subsequently named azathioprine (Imuran).[54] These studies led to the use of azathioprine in clinical renal transplantation. In 1962 Goodwin et al. demonstrated the efficiency of corticosteroids in reversing clinical rejection episodes.[55] For the past two decades azathioprine and corticosteroids have remained the primary immunosuppressive drugs used in clinical renal transplantation.

Because azathioprine and corticosteroids were not totally effective in suppressing rejection, alternative approaches were sought. In 1967 Starzl et al. introduced antilymphocyte serum as an immunosuppressive agent.[56] For about 15 years this agent in various forms has been used with equivocal results. Controlled studies in adults have both confirmed[57] and refuted its efficacy.[58] A recent controlled study utilizing antithymocyte globulin in pediatric recipients has not confirmed improvement in cadaver allograft survival

rates.[59] Therefore, although antithymocyte globulin is now available commercially for the treatment of rejection episodes, its prophylactic use in clinical renal transplantation to prevent rejection and increase allograft survival rates remains equivocal.

More recently, Borel et al. demonstrated potent immunosuppressive effects from an antifungal agent, cyclosporin A.[60] Initial enthusiastic reports are available utilizing cyclosporin A in adult[61] and pediatric allograft recipients[62]; however, the results of additional controlled studies are awaited before this new drug can be added with confidence to the immunosuppressive regimen for clinical renal transplantation.[63, 64]

In the early 1960's when clinical renal transplantation was just beginning to be utilized for patients with ESRD, a few children received allografts at major transplant centers.[65] Subsequently, in the late 1960's and early 1970's, numerous reports indicated the general acceptance of renal transplantation for children with ESRD. In fact, most pediatric nephrologists involved in the care of children with ESRD have concluded that a successful renal transplant is the optimal treatment modality.

The major impediment to successful renal transplantation in children remains immunologic. In addition, optimization of growth, as will be discussed in a subsequent chapter, is a major concern for those caring for pediatric recipients. The success of the procedure must be measured in the pediatric patient not only in terms of providing sufficient function to avoid the need for dialysis but also in terms of growth and development. In this regard, only an allograft which provides a glomerular filtrate rate in excess of 60 ml/min/1.73 m² should be considered a success.[66]

During the past quarter of a century, the lives of many children with ESRD have been prolonged. Many children and adolescents have reached adulthood and are engaged in productive lives. However, the disquieting comments of Riley and Reinhart regarding the virtue of treating children with ESRD need to be considered carefully each time we embark upon a treatment program for such a child.

## REFERENCES

1. Riley CM: Thoughts about kidney hemotransplantation in children. J. Pediatr 65:797, 1964.
2. Reinhart JB: The doctor's dilemma. J Pediatr 75:505, 1970.

3. Potter D, Larsen D, Leumann E, et al: Treatment of chronic uremia in childhood. II: Hemodialysis. Pediatrics 46:678, 1970.
4. Fine RN, DePalma JR, Lieberman E, et al: Extended hemodialysis in children with chronic renal failure. J Pediatr 73:706, 1968.
5. Scharer K, Brunner FR, von Dehn H, et al: Combined report on regular dialysis and transplantation of children in Europe, 1972. Proc Eur Dial Transplant Assoc 10:58, 1973.
6. Korsch BM, Fine RN, Grushkin CM, et al: Experiences with children and their families during extended hemodialysis and kidney transplantation. Pediatr Clin North Am 18:625, 1971.
7. Ettenger RB, Korsch BM, Maine ME, et al: Renal rehabilitation of children and adolescents with end-stage renal disease, Chyatte SB (ed). Baltimore, The Williams and Wilkins Co, 1979, p 115.
8. Putnam TJ: The living peritoneum as a dialyzing membrane. Am J Physiol 63:548, 1922.
9. Ganter G: Ueber die Beseitigung giftiger Stoffe aus Blute durch Dialyse. Munchen Med Wochenschr 70:1478, 1923.
10. Maxwell MH, Rockney RB, Kleeman CR, et al: Peritoneal dialysis. I. Technique and applications. JAMA 170:917, 1959.
11. Boen ST, Mion C, Curtis PK, et al: Periodic peritoneal dialysis using the repeated puncture technique and an automated cycling machine. Trans Am Soc Artif Intern Organs 10:409, 1964.
12. Tenckhoff H, Schecter H: A bacteriologically safe peritoneal access device. Trans Am Soc Intern Organs 14:181, 1968.
13. Counts S, Hickman R, Garbaccio A, et al: Chronic home peritoneal dialysis in children. Trans Am Soc Artif Intern Organs 19:157, 1973.
14. Brouhand BH, Berger M, Cunningham RJ, et al: Home peritoneal dialysis in children. Trans Am Soc Artif Intern Organs 25:90, 1979.
15. Gagnadoux MF, Henandez MA, Broyer M, et al: Alternative de l'hemodialyse interative chez l'enfant. Arch Fr Pediatr 34:860, 1977.
16. Popovich RP, Moncrief JW, Decherd JB, et al: The definition of a novel portable/wearable equilibrium peritoneal dialysis technique. Abstr Trans Am Soc Artif Intern Organs 5:64, 1976.
17. Oreopoulos DG, Robson M, Izatt S, et al: A simple and safe technique for continuous ambulatory peritoneal dialysis (CAPD). Trans Am Soc Artif Intern Organs 24:484, 1978.
18. Balfe JW, Vigneux A, Willumsen J, et al: The use of CAPD in the treatment of children with end-stage renal disease. Periton Dial Bull 1:35, 1981.
19. Kohaut EC: Continuous ambulatory peritoneal dialysis: A preliminary experience. Am J Dis Child 135:270, 1981.
20. Guillot M, Cleremont MJ, Gagnadoux MF, et al: Nineteen months experience with CAPD in children: Main clinical and biological results. Advances in Peritoneal Dialysis, Gahl GM, Kessel M, Nolph KD (eds). Excerpta Medica 1981, p 203.
21. Kolff WJ, Berk HTJ: Artificial kidney: dialyzer with great area. Acta Med Scand 117:121, 1944.
22. Mateer RM, Greenman L, Danowski TS: Hemodialysis of the uremic child. Am J Dis Child 89:645, 1955.
23. Holliday MS: Dialysis in pediatrics, including use of the artificial kidney. Pediatrics 22:418, 1958.
24. Carter FH, Aoyama S, Mercer RD, et al: Hemodialysis in children: report of five cases. J Pediatr 51:125, 1957.
25. Keleman WA, Kolff WJ: Use of artificial kidney in the very young, the very old and the very sick. JAMA 171:535, 1959.
26. Spritz N, Fakey TJ, Thompson DD, et al: Treatment of salicylate intoxication in a 2-year-old child. Pediatrics 24:540, 1959.
27. Breakey BA, Woodruff MA, Reus WF Jr: The adaptability of the Kolff twin coil artificial kidney for dialysis in infancy. J Urol 86:304, 1961.
28. Clapp WM, Holmes H, O'Brien D: Extracorporeal hemodialysis in children. Am J Dis Child 104:77, 1962.
29. Walker JG, Garsenstein M, Higgs B, et al: The use of hemodialysis in acute renal failure and overhydration in children. Arch Dis Child 37:578, 1962.
30. Hickman RO, Scribner BH: Application of the pumpless hemodialysis system to infants and children. Trans Am Soc Artif Intern Organs 8:309, 1962.
31. Nayman J: Use of arteriovenous shunt for hemodialysis in an 8 month old infant. Br Med J, 2:160, 1963.
32. Walker CHM, Wersberg JM, Simons SI, et al: Hemodialysis in infantile nephrotic syndrome. Am J Dis Child 106:479, 1963.
33. Mahoney CP, Manning GB, Hickman RO: Hemodialysis in a patient with cystinosis. Am J Dis Child 112:65, 1966.
34. Anderson J, Lee HA, Stroud CE: Hemodialysis in infants and small children. Br Med J 1:1405, 1965.
35. Moorhead JF, Edwards EC, Goldsmith HJ: Hemodialysis of three children and one infant with a haemolytic-uraemic-syndrome. Lancet 1:570, 1965.
36. Lee HA, Sharpstone P: Haemodialysis in pediatrics. Acta Pediatr Scand 55:529, 1966.
37. Kallen RJ, Zaltzman S, Coe FL, et al: Hemodialysis in children: technique, kinetic aspects related to varying body size and application to salicylate intoxication, acute renal failure and some other disorders. Medicine (Baltimore) 45:1, 1966.
38. Fine RN, Stiles Q, DePalma JR, et al: Hemodialysis in infants under 1 year of age for acute poisoning. Am J Dis Child 116:657, 1968.
39. Holmes JH, Ogden DA: The roles of hemodialysis in renal transplantation. Trans Am Soc Artif Intern Organs 10:256, 1964.
40. Maher JF, Freeman RB, Schreiner GE: Hemodialysis for chronic renal failure. II. Biochemical and clinical aspects. Ann Intern Med 62:535, 1965.
41. Curtis FK, Cole JJ, Fellows BJ, et al: Hemodialysis in the home. Trans Am Soc Artif Intern Organs 11:7, 1965.
42. Hutchings RH, Hickman R, Scribner BH: Chronic hemodialysis in a preadolescent. Pediatrics 37:68, 1966.
43. Kjellstrand CM, Shideman JR, Santiago EA, et al: Technical advances in hemodialysis of very small pediatric patients. Proc Dial Transplant Forum 1:124, 1971.
44. Borra S, Kaye M: Long term home hemodialysis in children. Can Med Assoc J 105:927, 1971.
45. Broyer M, Loirat C, Kleinknecht C, et al: Eighteen months experience with hemodialysis in children. Proc Eur Dial Transplant Assoc 7:261, 1970.
46. Tagliacozzi G: De curtorum chirugia per insitionem Venice, 1957, p 61, Translated by Gnudi MT, Webster JP, in The Life and Times of Gaspare Tagliacozzi. New York, Reichner, 1960, p 185.

47. Ullmann E: Experimentelle Nierentransplantation. Wien Klin Wschr 15:281, 1902.

48. Ehrlich P: Experimentelle karzinomstudien an mausen. Arb Inst Esp Ther Frankfurt 1:77, 1906.

49. Murphy JB: Transplantability of malignant tumors to the embryos of a foreign species. JAMA 59:874, 1912.

50. Medawar PB: The behavior and fate of skin autografts and skin homografts in rabbits. J Anat Lond 78:176, 1944.

51. Billingham RE, Brent L, Medawar PB: Quantitative studies in tissue transplantation immunity. III. Actively acquired tolerance. Philos Trans R Soc Lond 239:357, 1956.

52. Murray JE, Merrill JP, Harrison JH: Kidney transplantation between seven pairs of identical twins. Ann Surg 148:343, 1958.

53. Hamburger J, Vayasse J, Crosnier J, et al: Renal homotransplantation in man after radiation of the recipient. Am J Med 32:854, 1962.

54. Calne RY: Inhibition of the rejection of renal homografts in dogs by purine analogues. Transplant Bull 28:65, 1961.

55. Goodwin WE, Kaufman JJ, Mims MM, et al: Human renal transplantation. I. Clinical experience with 6 cases of renal homotransplantation. J Urol 89:13, 1963.

56. Starzl RE, Marchioro TL, Porter KA, et al: The use of heterologous antilymphoid agents in canine renal and liver homotransplantation and in human renal homotransplantation. Surg Gynecol Obstet 124:301, 1967.

57. Shell AG, Kelley GE, Storey BG, et al: Controlled clinical trial of antilymphocyte globulin in patients with renal allografts from cadaver donors. Lancet 1:359, 1971.

58. Turcotte JG, Feduska NH, Haines RF, et al: Antithymocyte globulin in renal transplant recipients. Arch Surg 106:484, 1973.

59. Uittenbogaart CH, Robinson BJ, Malekzadeh MH, et al: The use of antithymocyte globulin (dose by rosette protocol) in pediatric renal allograft recipients. Transplantation 28:291, 1979.

60. Borel JF, Feurer C, Magnee C, et al: Effects of the new antilymphocyte peptide cyclosporin A in animals. Immunology 32:1017, 1977.

61. Calne RY: Immunosuppression for organ grafting. Observations on cyclosporin A. Immunol Rev 46:113, 1979.

62. Starzl TE, Iwatsuki S, Malatack JJ, et al: Liver and kidney transplantation in children receiving cyclosporin A and steroids. J Pediatr 100:61, 1982.

63. Harder R, Loertscher R, Calne RY, et al: Cyclosporin A as sole immunosuppressive agent in recipients of kidney allografts from cadaver donors. Lancet 2:57, 1982.

64. Ferguson RM, Rynasiewicz JJ, Sutherland DE, et al: Cyclosporin A in renal transplantation: A prospective randomized trial. Surgery 92:175, 1982.

65. Starzl TE, Marchioro TL, Porter KA, et al: The role of organ transplantation in pediatrics. Pediatr Clin North Am 13:381, 1966.

66. Pennisi AJ, Costin G, Phillips LS, et al: Somatomedin and growth hormone studies. Am J Dis Child 133:950, 1979.

# I

# Dialysis

# 2

# Incidence and Etiology of ESRD in Children

*Michel Broyer, M.D.*

The incidence of ESRD in children is important in determining the need for specialized pediatric dialysis facilities in a given area and in identifying areas where preventative approaches might be developed. However, it is also important to consider that data concerning the incidence and etiology of ESRD in a specific area reflect the available diagnostic and therapeutic methodology available.

## INCIDENCE

Two sources have been used to determine the incidence of ESRD. First, data are derived from death certificates, and second, data are compiled from the number of patients accepted by dialysis programs. Both sources of information should be viewed with caution. Death certificates often include discrepancies between reversible and irreversible renal failure. The renal failure noted on the death certificate may be only one of several causes which resulted in death. The second source of information may be an underestimate, because some children with ESRD are not accepted for dialysis either for technical reasons or lack of facilities. Conversely, including foreign children from countries without dialysis facilities may result in an overestimate. The denominator used for calculating incidence data should reflect the population of children in the area studied and not the total population because large differences in age distribution from one area to another may exist.

McCrory et al published incidence data from New York City based upon death certificates.[1] This study, excluding renal malignancies, revealed an incidence of 9 deaths from renal failure per million child population (pmcp) for children 5 to 14 years of age and 49 deaths pmcp for infants and children 0 to 4 years old for the year 1965. A decrease in the number of deaths from glomerulonephritis was noted for both children and adults between the years 1959 and 1965.

Surveys based upon new cases accepted by dialysis programs are more revealing because the data permit one to calculate the need for providing appropriate facilities. Such surveys have shown that the incidence of ESRD in children varies from one country to another.

The study of Helin and Winberg reported an incidence in Sweden of 4.17 new cases per year pmcp at 1 to 15 years of age, for the years 1974–1977.[2] Leumann found a similar incidence of 5.6 new cases per year pmcp in Switzerland.[3] A study performed in Paris between 1978 and 1980 found an incidence of 10 new cases per year pmcp considering only the patients living within the catchment area.[4] These data can be compared to the 4.9 new cases per year pmcp accepted by dialysis programs throughout France during this time period. Such discrepancies indicate that important differences concerning the acceptance rate of children by dialysis facilities exist not only between countries but also within different areas in a given country.

Data from the European Dialysis and Transplant Association (EDTA) registry are interesting to consider. There were 3 new cases pmcp started on dialysis in Europe during 1981,[5] with a range of 0.2 to 12 new cases reported by the various participating countries. These differences may reflect differences in the economic development of the various countries. Noteworthy is the observation that the number of children with ESRD surviving pmcp is proportional to the number of specialized pediatric centers in a given area.[5] Thus, the availability of such centers appears to be a crucial factor for providing care for children with ESRD.

Limited data on the incidence of ESRD in children are available from the United States—8 new cases per year pmcp in northern California[6] and 20 pmcp in Virgina.[7] These figures are difficult to interpret and could be an overestimation because of the mobility of the population in the United States and the prominence of the centers involved in these two studies.

In Japan, 130 children under 15 years of age, or 4.8 new cases pmcp, were started on dialysis.[8]

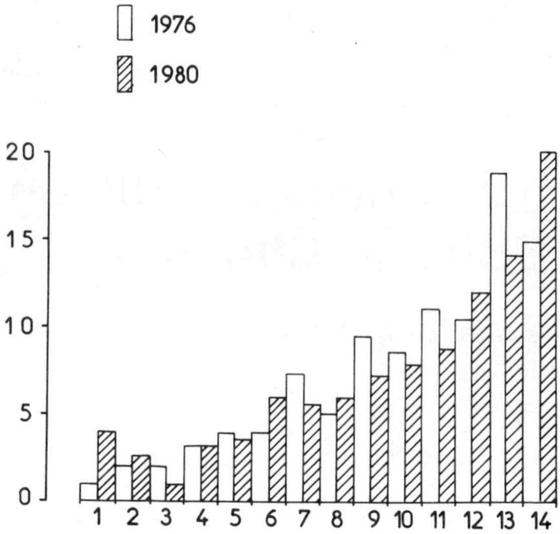

### Incidence According to Age

The incidence of children with ESRD accepted for dialysis increases with age when considering the age groups 0–5, 5–10, and 10–15 years. This is illustrated by the 1980 data of the EDTA (Fig. 2–1):[9] 67% of the patients were 10 to 15 years of age while only 8.3% were less than 5 years of age. In some countries children less than 5 years of age are not considered suitable candidates for dialysis. In France no such discrimination exists, and children less than 5 years of age constitute 17% of the pediatric dialysis population. Similarly, 19% of the children accepted for dialysis in northern California are in this younger age group.[6] Because many children are not accepted for dialysis for either ethical or technical reasons, the real incidence of ESRD in children less than 5 years is probably higher than is generally recognized.

### ETIOLOGY OF RENAL INSUFFICIENCY IN CHILDREN

Several studies defining the etiology of renal insufficiency in children are available.[2, 3, 6, 10] The distribution of disorders in children with chronic renal insufficiency is

**Figure 2–1.** Numbers of new patients according to age at onset of dialysis in the EDTA pediatric registry.[9]

different from that of adults with ESRD because of the variability of progression to ESRD, with some disease categories requiring dialysis only during adulthood.

### Chronic Renal Insufficiency

The distribution of the diseases causing progressive renal insufficiency in three pediatric centers is summarized in Table 2–1. The diseases are categorized into five groups: glomerulonephritis, malformations of the urinary tract with or without pyelonephritis, renal hypoplasia, hereditary diseases, and others. Differences in the incidence of the various categories between centers are probably related to the definition of renal insufficiency at the various centers and the time period during which the cases were collected. It is noteworthy that malformations of the

**Table 2–1.** CAUSES OF CHRONIC RENAL INSUFFICIENCY IN CHILDREN AT THE STAGE OF CONSERVATIVE TREATMENT

|  | France[10] (102 patients) | Sweden[2] (28 patients) | Switzerland[3] (36 patients) |
|---|---|---|---|
| Glomerulonephritis | 6% | 13.6% | — |
| Urinary tract malformations | 43% | 52.7% | 53.5% |
| Renal hypoplasia | 26% | — | 14.3% |
| Hereditary diseases | 20% | 8.3% | 17.9% |
| Miscellaneous | 5% | 14.1% | 14.3% |

urinary tract and renal hypoplasia represent 60 to 70% of childhood chronic renal insufficiency, while glomerulonephritis represents a smaller segment of the total. This is related primarily to the age of onset and the duration of the disease, which is shorter in patients with glomerulonephritis than in the groups with either renal hypoplasia or malformation. The mean duration of progression to ESRD of different disease categories in different studies is of limited value because individual patient variation is significant. Nevertheless the mean time interval between a given serum creatinine level (2 mg/dl) and the development of ESRD is similar in the studies of Habib et al[10] and Höhman et al[11]: $1\frac{4}{12}$ to 2 years for glomerulonephritis, $1\frac{10}{12}$ to 2 years for hereditary diseases, and 3 to $3\frac{8}{12}$ years for renal hypoplasia, respectively.

## ESRD

Knowledge concerning the etiology of the primary renal disease (PRD) is important in planning the treatment program of a child with ESRD for numerous reasons. Different disorders require different treatment regimens. For example, it may be necessary to give sodium supplements to a child with nephronophthisis even during maintenance dialysis therapy. The potential recurrence of the PRD after transplantation is another important consideration. Diseases which recur may dictate a strategy for transplantation which differs from one case to another. For example, transplantation may be delayed for one to two years in diseases which have rapidly destroyed the native kidneys. Finally, the preparation for transplantation and the follow-up are different according to the PRD.

The diagnosis of the PRD is generally best made during the phase of progressive renal failure; in some children referred with ESRD the PRD is often difficult to establish. Histologic diagnosis is most complete when the pathologic examination includes a combination of light microscopic immunofluorescence and electron microscopic studies of the native kidneys. It is usually possible by histologic techniques to determine the PRD in the majority of pediatric patients. Unclassified cases represent only 1.5 to 5% of the total number of affected children compared to the high percentage of adult cases with ESRD who are diagnosed as chronic renal failure of unknown etiology.

Several studies review the distribution of PRD in children. A study performed by a single pathologist from one center has been reported from France[4] (Table 2–2). Glomerulonephritis represented approximately one quarter of the cases; half the children with glomerular diseases had the nephrotic syndrome with focal segmental hyalinosis. Membranoproliferative glomerulonephritis was the second most common form of glomerulonephritis and represented 5.6% of the total cases. Hereditary nephropathies also represented one quarter of the cases. Nephronophthisis was the most important cause of ESRD in this group, accounting for 14.3% of the patients. Cystinosis, Alport's syndrome, and oxalosis completed this group. Malformations of the urinary tract accounted for nearly 20% of the total when the cases of "segmental hypoplasia" with reflux were included in this group. Renal hypoplasia and dysplasia represented 13.3% of the total. The most frequently observed vascular diseases were Henoch-Schönlein purpura (5% of total) and the hemolytic uremic syndrome (3.8% of total).

Data from a pediatric center in Southern California[12] were different for some disease categories and similar for others (Table 2–2). Glomerulonephritis occurred more frequently in California than in France (37% versus 26.4%). Other primary renal diseases occurred at similar rates: nephrotic syndrome with focal segmental sclerosis, membranoproliferative glomerulonephritis, and glomerulonephritis with anti–basement membrane antibodies. Hereditary nephropathies were seen less frequently in California. Recessively inherited diseases (nephronophthisis, cystinosis) occurred less frequently, while dominantly inherited diseases (Alport's syndrome, polycystic disease) had a similar or a higher incidence in California. Other differences observed in California were found for systemic diseases with a higher incidence of lupus and a lower incidence of Henoch-Schönlein purpura and of the hemolytic uremic syndrome. Urinary tract malformations were more frequent in California; the incidence of hypoplasia or dysplasia was similar.

A detailed analysis of ESRD caused by obstructive uropathy has been recently published by the California group.[13] Twenty-three of 54 patients had abnormalities of vesicoureteral junction (reflux or obstruction), 20 patients had posterior urethral valves, four had ureteropelvic junction obstruction, three had bladder neck obstruc-

Table 2–2. ETIOLOGY OF ESRD IN CHILDREN (Single-Center Reports)

| | France[4] | | Southern California[12] | |
| --- | --- | --- | --- | --- |
| | *Number* | *Percentage* | *Number* | *Percentage* |
| *Glomerulonephritis (GN)* | (103)* | (26.4) | (102) | (37.0) |
| Nephrotic syndrome with focal sclerosis | 46 | 11.7 | 27 | 9.7 |
| Mesangial sclerosis | 6 | 1.5 | | |
| Finnish congenital nephrotic syndrome | 4 | 1.0 | | |
| Membranoproliferative GN | | | | |
| Type I subendothelial deposits | 15 ⎱ | 5.6 | 16 | 5.7 |
| Type II dense deposits | 7 ⎰ | | | |
| GN with mesangial IgA deposits | 5 | 1.3 | | |
| GN with anti-basal membrane antibodies | 5 | 1.3 | 3 | 1.1 |
| Other types of GN or unclassified | 15 | 3.8 | 56 | 20.2 |
| *Pyelonephritis and urinary tract malformations* | (77) | (19.6) | (64) | (23.2) |
| Miscellaneous malformations | 61 | 15.6 | | |
| "Segmental hypoplasia" with reflux | 16 | 4.0 | | |
| *Renal dysplasia/hypoplasia* | (52) | (13.3) | (37) | (13.4) |
| *Hereditary diseases* | (101) | (25.8) | (36) | (13.0) |
| Nephronophthisis | 56 | 14.3 | 10 | 3.6 |
| Cystinosis | 21 | 5.3 | 7 | 2.5 |
| Alport's syndrome | 12 | 3.0 | 12 | 4.3 |
| Oxalosis | 6 | 1.5 | | |
| Polycystic disease | 2 | 0.5 | 6 | 2.1 |
| Nail-patella syndrome | 1 | | | |
| Acro-osteolysis with nephropathy | 1 | | | |
| Periodic disease with amyloidosis | 1 | | | |
| Bartter's syndrome | 1 | | 1 | |
| *Systemic diseases* | (37) | (9.4) | (23) | (8.3) |
| Henoch-Schönlein syndrome | 20 | 5.1 | 5 | 1.8 |
| Lupus erythematosus | 1 | | 14 | 5.0 |
| Periarteritis nodosa | 1 | | | |
| Hemolytic uremic syndrome | 15 | 3.8 | 5 | 1.8 |
| *Vascular disease* | (4) | (1.0) | (6) | (2.1) |
| Cortical necrosis | 2 | 0.5 | 3 | 1.0 |
| Renal vein thrombosis | 1 | | 1 | |
| Sickle cell nephropathy | | | 2 | |
| Others | 1 | | | |
| *Miscellaneous* | (11) | | (7) | (2.5) |
| Bilateral Wilms' tumor | 5 | 1.3 | 4 | 1.4 |
| Surgical loss | 3 | 0.75 | | |
| Spina bifida and neurologic disease | 3 | 0.75 | | |
| Others | | | 3 | |
| *Unclassified* | (6) | (1.5) | | |
| Totals | 391 | 100 | 276 | 100 |

*Each figure in parentheses represents a subtotal.

tion, three had neurogenic bladder, and one was undefined. This distribution is quite similar to that reported in another study,[10] although abnormalities of the ureterovesical junction were more frequent.

Differences between single-center reports may be related to differences in diagnostic practice but may also be related to differences in genetic or environmental factors.

Data from the EDTA pediatric registry for 1981 based on more than 3000 cases[5] are slightly different from data reported from the single centers (Table 2–3). Glomerulonephritis was the most common PRD (31.3%) followed by pyelonephritis and urinary tract malformations (22.5%), hereditary nephropathies (16.2%), and renal hypoplasia (12.1%).

The distribution of causes of PRD has changed over the years (Table 2–3). Data are based on the relative frequency of PRD reported before 1980 compared with that for the years 1980–1981. The incidence of glo-

**Table 2–3.** DISTRIBUTION OF PRIMARY RENAL DISEASES IN CHILDREN FROM THE EDTA REGISTRY[5]

| | Onset of Dialysis | | | Children Less Than 5 Years | | |
|---|---|---|---|---|---|---|
| **Total Cases** | *All* | *< 1980* | *1980–81* | *All* | *< 1980* | *1980–81* |
| | 3342 | 2541 | 801 | 263 | 159 | 104 |
| *Glomerulonephritis* | (31.3)* | (32.7) | (26.4) | (20.9) | (23.2) | (17.3) |
| *Pyelonephritis and malformation of urinary tract* | (22.5) | (22) | (23.9) | (15.2) | (10) | (23) |
| Malformations | 6.2 | 5.6 | 7.8 | 6.1 | 5.6 | 6.7 |
| Reflux | 6.9 | 6.2 | 9.3 | 3.4 | 0.7 | 7.6 |
| Pyelonephritis | 9.4 | 10.2 | 6.8 | 5.7 | 3.7 | 8.6 |
| *Renal hypoplasia* | (12.1) | (11.6) | (13.8) | (12.1) | (8.8) | (17) |
| Oligomeganephronia | 1.3 | 1.2 | 1.8 | 0.7 | 0.6 | 0.9 |
| Other hypoplasia | 10.8 | 10.4 | 12 | 11.4 | 8.2 | 16.3 |
| *Hereditary diseases* | (16.2) | (15.9) | (16.6) | (13.7) | (15.7) | (10.5) |
| Nephronophthisis | 6.1 | 6.2 | 5.5 | 4.1 | 6.3 | 0.9 |
| Polycystic kidneys | 1.9 | 1.9 | 1.8 | 3.8 | 2.5 | 5.7 |
| Cystinosis | 2.8 | 2.4 | 4.6 | 0.7 | — | 1.9 |
| Alport's syndrome | 1.5 | 1.4 | 1.5 | — | — | — |
| Oxalosis | 1.2 | 1 | 1.6 | 1.9 | 1.8 | 1.9 |
| Other hereditary diseases | 2.7 | 3 | 1.6 | 3.2 | 5.1 | — |
| *Systemic diseases* | (7.0) | (6.9) | (7.6) | (13.5) | (16.7) | (10.4) |
| Henoch-Schönlein syndrome | 2.4 | 2.6 | 2 | 0.3 | 0.6 | — |
| Hemolytic uremic syndrome | 3.1 | 2.8 | 4 | 10.2 | 11.3 | 8.6 |
| Other systemic diseases | 1.5 | 1.5 | 1.6 | 3 | 4.8 | 1.8 |
| *Vascular diseases* | (1.5) | (1.51) | (1.6) | (4.2) | (3.7) | (4.8) |
| *Other diagnoses* | (5.7) | (5.8) | (6.4) | (14.7) | (16.3) | (11.3) |
| *Diagnosis unknown* | (3.7) | (3.6) | (3.7) | (5.7) | (5.6) | (5.7) |
| Totals (%) | (100) | (100) | (100) | (100) | (100) | (100) |

*Each figure in parentheses represents a subtotal.

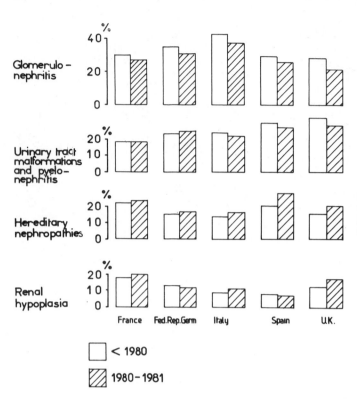

**Figure 2–2.** Principal causes of ESRD in children in several European countries and changes over the years.[5] Less common causes and uncertain diagnoses are not represented here.

merulonephritis decreased from 32.7 to 26.7%, whereas most other categories remained stable except for a slight increase in the incidence of urinary tract malformations with reflux and of renal hypoplasia.

Geographic differences both in the distribution of the PRD and in the change in the PRD over time (Fig. 2–2) were noted between countries in Europe. Glomerulonephritis was the most frequent cause in all European countries with the exception of United Kingdom, where the urinary tract malformation–pyelonephritis group was the most common. A clear decrease in the relative frequency of glomerulonephritis was observed in all countries in 1980–1981 compared to previous years. Pyelonephritis and urinary tract malformations decreased in Italy, Spain, and the United Kingdom, while hereditary nephropathies and renal hypoplasia increased. A decrease in glomerulonephritis had been noted in the past in the United States during the period of 1950–1970[14] and in the United Kingdom.[15] These changes may result from altered patient selection policies or changes in diagnostic practice, or they may be a true variation of incidence, perhaps related to better preventive approaches, including early

and effective treatment of pharyngeal and cutaneous infections.

Knowledge of the distribution of PRD in children with ESRD is limited in countries outside Europe and North America. Some information is available from Japan.[8] There, glomerulonephritis represented more than 75% of the causes of ESRD, of which 8.3% had rapidly progressive glomerulonephritis and 6.6% Henoch-Schönlein purpura. The group of children with hypoplasia, dysplasia, and pyelonephritis represented only 2.0% of the cases and the hemolytic uremic syndrome only 0.6%. More than 10% of cases remained unclassfied in Japan.

***Children Less than Five Years of Age.*** Renal failure in the neonate is usually related to bilateral renal agenesis or to bilateral multicystic kidneys with ureteral atresia. These abnormalities are associated with oligohydramnios and can be detected during fetal life by sonography. The incidence of both malformations has been estimated in France to be approximately 1 per 5000 births (Dr. Stroll, Strasbourg, personal communication).

***Children Less than Two Years of Age.*** Chronic renal failure in this age group occurs primarily in boys. The principal cause is a severe malformation of the urinary tract—posterior urethral valves—with bilateral hypoplasia or dysplasia of kidneys. Other causes include bilateral hypoplasia without any urinary tract abnormality, and oligomeganephronia. Sequelae of neonatal vascular accidents, bilateral renal vein thrombosis, and cortical and medullary necrosis also cause chronic renal failure in infants.

There are few reports detailing the etiology of ESRD in this age group. At the Enfants Malades 20 infants and children three months to two years of age reached ESRD between 1969 and 1982 (Table 2–4). The sex ratio in this series was 0.7 with an excess of males due to the fact that almost half of the patients had either a malformation of the urinary tract or severe hypoplasia. Another frequent cause was mesangial sclerosis, which represented almost a quarter of the cases. This disease was initially described by Habib and Bois[16] and is specific for this age group of children. Hemolytic uremic syndrome and bilateral Wilms' tumor accounted for some cases. Two cases were unusual, with a rapidly progressive renal failure and the histologic features of tubulointerstitial nephritis with unique microcysts. The etiology of ESRD in children under two years of age is significantly different from that observed in older children and adults. Conspicuously absent is glomerulonephritis and hereditary renal diseases.

***Children Two to Five Years of Age.*** The etiology of chronic renal failure in this age group is closer to that of the under-two age group than that of older children. Urinary tract abnormalities, hypoplastic/dysplastic kidneys, and sequelae of vascular diseases are the primary diseases encountered. When compared to the entire data in the EDTA registry, the distribution of causes of ESRD is different in children less than five years of age (Table 2–3). Glomerulonephritis and hereditary renal diseases occurred less frequently, but the hemolytic uremic syndrome was more frequent. Changes in the etiology of this age group noted during the past few years include a decrease of glomerulonephritis similar to that in the whole registry and an increase in the number of cases of renal hypoplasia. This increase is probably due to the inclusion of younger children into dialysis and transplant programs.

In examining the series of the Enfants Malades hospital (Table 2–4), the distribution of causes of ESRD is slightly different. In children two to five years of age glomerulonephropathies represented 36% of the total, whereas 20.9% of all children less than five

**Table 2–4.** ETIOLOGY OF ESRD IN CHILDREN LESS THAN FIVE YEARS OF AGE AT THE ENFANTS MALADES HOSPITAL (1969–1982)

| | Children Less Than 2 Years | | Children 2 to 5 Years | | |
| --- | --- | --- | --- | --- | --- |
| | *Males* | *Females* | *Males* | *Females* | *Total* |
| Glomerulonephropathies | | | | | |
|   Mesangial sclerosis | 2 | 2 | | | 4 |
|   Nephrotic syndrome with focal sclerosis | | | 5 | 5 | 10 |
|   Finnish congenital nephrotic syndrome | | | | 1 | 1 |
|   Idiopathic GN with diffuse crescents | | | 1 | 1 | 2 |
|   GN with anti–basal membrane antibodies | | | 2 | 1 | 3 |
| Urinary tract malformations with renal hypoplasia | 4 | 1 | 7 | | 12 |
| Bilateral renal dysplasia/hypoplasia | 4 | | 4 | | 8 |
| Hereditary diseases | | | | | |
|   Nephronophthisis | | | 4 | 2 | 6 |
|   Polycystic disease | | | 1 | | 1 |
|   Oxalosis | | | 1 | | 1 |
| Systemic diseases | | | | | |
|   Hemolytic uremic syndrome | 1 | 2 | | 4 | 7 |
|   Polyarteritis nodosa | | | | 1 | 1 |
| Miscellaneous | | | | | |
|   Wilms' tumor | 2 | | | 2 | 4 |
|   Tubulo-interstitial nephropathy | 2 | | | | 2 |
| Unclassified | | | 2 | | 2 |
| Totals | 15 | 5 | 27 | 17 | 64 |

years of age in the EDTA registry had some form of glomerulonephritis. Corticosteroid-resistant nephrotic syndrome with focal hyalinosis was the primary cause in those two to five years of age. Rapidly progressive glomerulonephritis with anti-TBM and GBM antibodies was also seen. The other causes of ESRD were similar to those of the EDTA registry: hemolytic uremic syndrome, 9% versus 10.2%; hypoplastic/dysplastic kidneys with or without urinary tract abnormalities, 25% versus 27%; and hereditary nephropathies, 18% versus 13.7%. Finally, bilateral Wilms' tumor occurred in approximately 5% of the children in this age group.

In conclusion, epidemiologic studies of ESRD in children are important in order to follow the variations in etiology over time and to detect differences between different geographic areas. It is hoped that such studies might identify methods of prevention. However, the available studies lead to the tentative conclusion that more than half of the cases of ESRD in children are related to congenital or hereditary diseases for which there is as yet no way to prevent the inevitable progression to ESRD.

*Acknowledgment:* I am grateful to Dr. Sakai, who provided information from Japan.

## REFERENCES

1. MacCrory WW, Shibuya M, Yano K: Recent trends in the mortality rate from renal disease in children and young adults in New York City. J Pediatr 87:928, 1975.
2. Helin I, Winberg J: Chronic renal failure in Swedish children. Acta Paediatr Scand 69:607, 1980.
3. Leumann EP: Die chronische Niereninsuffizienz in Kindesalter. Schweiz Med Wochenschr 106:244, 1976.
4. Donckerwolcke R, Chantler C, Broyer M: Pediatric dialysis. *In*: Drukker W, Parsons F, and Maher J: Replacement of renal function by dialysis, 2nd Ed The Hague, Martinus Nijhoft Medical Division, 1982, p. 514.
5. Donckerwolcke R, Broyer M, Brunner F, et al: Combined report on regular dialysis and transplantation in Europe, 1981. Proc Eur Dial Transplant Assoc 19:16, 1982.
6. Potter D, Holliday M, Diel C, et al: Treatment of end stage renal disease in children: a 15-year experience. Kidney Int 18:105, 1980.
7. Chan JC, Mendez-Picon GJ, Landwehr DM: A 3-year survey of referral pattern and case material in pediatric nephrology. Int J Pediatr Nephrol 2:109, 1981.
8. Ito K, et al: Children with chronic renal failure in Japan. Kidney and Dialysis 9:475, 1980 (in Japanese).
9. Broyer M, Donckerwolcke R, Brunner F, et al: Combined report on regular dialysis and transplantation in Europe, 1980. Proc Eur Dial Transplant Assoc 18:59, 1981.
10. Habib R, Broyer M, Benmaiz H: Chronic renal failure in children. Causes, rate of deterioration and survival data. Nephron 11:209, 1973.
11. Höhman B, Scharer K, Schuler HW, et al: Atiologie und Verlauf der chronischen Niereninsuffizienz in Kindesalter. Mschr Kinderheilk 123:415, 1975.
12. Fine RN: Renal transplantation in children. *In*: Organ Transplantation, SN Chaterjee (Ed) Boston, John Wright 1982, p. 243.
13. Warshaw B, Edelbrock H, Ettenger R, et al: Progression to end stage renal disease in children with obstruction uropathy. J Pediatr 100:183, 1982.
14. Florey C, Kessner DM, Kashgarian M, Senter MG: Mortality trends for chronic nephritis and infections of the kidney—a clinical and statistical comparison between mortality of New Haven, Connecticut and the United States, 1950–1960. J Chron Dis 24:71, 1971.
15. Waters WE: Trends in mortality from nephritis and infection of the kidney in England and Wales. Lancet 1:241, 1968.
16. Habib R, Bois E: Hétérogénéité des syndromes néphrotiques á début précoce du nourrisson (syndrome néphrotique "infantile"). Helv Paediatr Acta 28:91, 1973.

# 3

# Treatment of Infants with ESRD

*Steven R. Alexander, M.D.*

As recently as twenty years ago children who suffered irreversible renal failure rarely survived. It is a tribute to the spectacular advances in renal replacement therapy which have come about during the past two decades that today children with end-stage renal disease (ESRD) survive routinely, the majority living for many years on dialysis or with renal allografts.[1,2] Early efforts to treat pediatric ESRD patients aroused controversy despite impressive technical achievements. It was argued that children paid too great a price in physical and emotional discomfort for the limited extension of life afforded them by treatment with dialysis and renal transplantation.[3,4] While never fully resolved, these concerns have faded during the past 15 years as dialysis and transplantation have become accepted therapies for adult and pediatric patients alike.[5]

There remains, however, a group of children for whom successful renal replacement therapy has not been well established: those children who develop irreversible renal failure as young infants, particularly during the first year of life. There is little information available on the outcome of treatment in this age group, and what is available is generally discouraging. Technical difficulties, largely resolved for the older pediatric dialysis or transplant recipient, continue to complicate the therapy of young infants. It is not surprising that treatment for young infants is as controversial today as was the treatment of older children 10 to 15 years ago, for many of the same issues are involved.[6] Until very recently pediatric dialysis and transplantation programs routinely excluded infants less than one year of age,[5,7] reasoning with Hur-

ley that ". . . although it is technically possible to perform hemodialysis and transplantation in these children, the myriad of well-known problems . . . should contraindicate such therapy except under the most unusual circumstances. . . ."[8] During a period in which advances in ESRD therapy have pushed the upper age limits for successful renal replacement therapy well into the eighth decade, the youngest ESRD patients have remained "therapeutic orphans," considered by many to have severely limited chances for survival.[9,10]

This situation may now be changing as a result of recent developments in chronic peritoneal dialysis. The advent of continuous ambulatory peritoneal dialysis (CAPD)[11] and its subsequent adaptation for use in infants and small children[12,13] have stimulated renewed interest in the treatment of these youngest ESRD patients. CAPD has much to recommend it to the infant with chronic renal failure. The simplicity and safety of the method are striking. Because no elaborate technology nor machinery is required, CAPD can be offered by most pediatric dialysis programs and taught to most families, who can then perform dialysis on their infants at home. The convenience and safety inherent in the CAPD technique, along with a number of theoretical advantages,[14] have made CAPD an attractive treatment for very young infants who might not otherwise be treated at all.[15]

This chapter will examine current approaches to the treatment of infants whose irreversible renal failure occurs during the first year of life. The use of hemodialysis (HD), intermittent peritoneal dialysis (IPD), and renal transplantation in this age group will be reviewed briefly. The use of CAPD is presented in detail in a separate chapter. Suggestions for the clinical management of these tiny patients are included, but only with trepidation. These suggestions should be considered to reflect primarily the author's current approach to specific clinical problems.

## THE INCIDENCE OF ESRD IN INFANTS

The incidence of ESRD in children less than 16 years of age is estimated to be from 1.0 to 3.5 per million total population per year.[16, 17] The lowest estimates have been derived from sequential surveys of nephrology units within well-defined catchment areas. Results from four such surveys are summarized in Table 3–1.[5, 18, 19, 20]

Unfortunately these studies contain little information on the incidence of ESRD among infants less than one year of age. Infants under one year of age were excluded from two of the studies listed in Table 3–1;[5, 18] in a third, children only as young as six months of age were considered.[19] In the latter study the incidence of ESRD in infants 6 to 12 months of age was found to be 0.19 per million total population per year. Only the European survey attempted to obtain data on children from birth to 16 years of age, reporting an incidence of ESRD in children 0 to 5 years of age of 0.31 per million total population per year.[20] The same incidence figure was reported for children 1 to 5 years of age by the survey from the United States.[5] While this is likely to be coincidence, it may also reflect the difficulties inherent in attempts to identify the youngest ESRD victims.

**Table 3–1.** INCIDENCE OF ESRD IN CHILDREN UNDER 16

| Region (Ref.) | Age Ranges (Years) | ESRD Incidence* |
|---|---|---|
| Sweden (18) | 1–16 | 0.94 |
| Switzerland (19) | 0.5–16 | 1.36 |
| | 0.5–1.0 | 0.19 |
| Europe (20) | 0–16 | 1.54 |
| | 0–5 | 0.31 |
| N. California/N. | 1–16 | 1.58 |
| Nevada (15) | 1–5 | 0.31 |
| Oregon | 0–16 | 1.49 |
| (present study) | 0–1 | 0.20 |

*Per million total population per year.

Surveys of nephrology units provide valuable information on current ESRD patient profiles, but, to the extent that decisions to refer children for dialysis and transplantation reflect contemporary medical and social judgments, incidence figures may underestimate actual ESRD occurrence. This may be particularly true of young infants for whom treatment has not been routinely recommended in the past.

Beginning in January, 1979, we have attempted to obtain information on all children with ESRD who live in the state of Oregon. This process has been facilitated by several factors: ESRD services for children are available in only one medical center in Oregon; region-wide pediatric nephrology referral patterns are well-established; active neonatal and pediatric transport systems have been effectively used to bring infants requiring acute and chronic dialysis to the pediatric dialysis center; early treatment of young infants using CAPD was widely publicized throughout the state.

From 1979 through 1982, 15 Oregon children, ages 12 days to 15.7 years, developed irreversible renal failure and survived to begin dialysis or receive a renal transplant. Ten additional children received primary ESRD care in Oregon during this same period but were excluded from the survey because their homes were in other states. The incidence of ESRD in Oregon children 0 to 16 years of age was 1.49 per million total population per year during the 4-year survey period. Two infants less than one year of age were identified, yielding an incidence of ESRD in this age group of 0.2 per million total population per year.

Extrapolation from the Oregon experience would predict that, in the United States alone, 40 infants less than one year of age could be referred for ESRD therapy each year. The relatively short duration of the Oregon study, the small number of patients involved, and demographic characteristics which may be unique to this region severely limit the reliability of such predictions.

## ETIOLOGY

The etiology of chronic renal failure in children has been shown to vary according to the age of the child at the time of presentation.[21] There is little information available on the causes of ESRD in young infants.

**Table 3–2.** CAUSES OF ESRD IN INFANTS LESS THAN ONE YEAR OF AGE*

| Diagnosis | Cases According to Age at Presentation | | |
|---|---|---|---|
| | *< 4 Weeks* | *1 to 12 Months* | *Totals* |
| Glomerulonephritis | 1 | 1 | 2 |
| Cortical necrosis | 1 | 1 | 2 |
| Obstructive uropathy | 2 | 2 | 4 |
| Congenital hypoplasia-dysplasia | 2 | 2 | 4 |
| Wilms' tumor | – | 6 | 6 |
| Infantile polycystic kidneys | 2 | – | 2 |
| Congenital nephrotic syndrome | – | 1 | 1 |
| Hemolytic-uremic syndrome | – | 1 | 1 |
| Oxalosis | – | 1 | 1 |
| Totals | 8 | 15 | 23 |

*References: 22 to 37.

A review of the medical literature published since 1969 identified only 23 infants less than one year of age at presentation of ESRD who were described in sufficient detail to allow classification according to ESRD etiology.[22–37] (Table 3–2.) Infants treated with chronic dialysis or transplantation and those who appeared likely to have survived to receive chronic treatment, had it been offered, were included in this analysis. The predominance of urologic disorders (urinary tract malformations with and without obstruction, bilateral Wilms' tumor) and congenital diseases (infantile polycystic kidney disease, congenital nephrotic syndrome, oxalosis) is noted.

The relative infrequency of acute renal failure (ARF) at presentation was somewhat unexpected. Up to 6% of admissions to a Neontal Intensive Care Unit have been shown to develop ARF,[38] yet only one neonate and no older infants listed in Table 3–2 presented with ARF. This finding is ac-

tually consistent with the findings of several large surveys of ARF in infants which failed to demonstrate a common association between ARF and ESRD.[27, 39, 40] It appears that infants who develop ARF, similarly to older children and adults, usually either die or recover with renal function largely intact.

Bilateral renal agenesis (Potter's syndrome) is also missing from Table 3–2 despite a reported incidence of 2 per million total population per year.[41] These infants are unlikely candidates for renal replacement therapy, because they usually present with other lethal congenital malformations (e.g., pulmonary hypoplasia).[41]

The causes of ESRD seen in 154 children one to 16 years of age reported by Potter and associates are summarized in Table 3–3.[5] For comparison with these children the 23 infants less than one year of age described in Table 3–2 are also listed in Table 3–3. Except for a high incidence of Wilms' tumor,

**Table 3–3.** CAUSES OF ESRD IN CHILDREN AT VARIOUS AGES

| Diagnosis | Incidence by Age Group (Years)* | | | |
|---|---|---|---|---|
| | *< 1†* *(n = 23)* | *1–5‡* *(n = 26)* | *6–10‡* *(n = 24)* | *11–16‡* *(n = 84)* |
| Glomerulonephritis | 9% | 27% | 34% | 39% |
| Cortical necrosis | 9% | – | – | – |
| Obstructive uropathy | 17% | 4% | 5% | 20% |
| Congenital hypoplasia-dysplasia | 17% | 8% | 20% | 6% |
| Wilms' tumor | 26% | 35% | – | – |
| Infantile polycystic kidneys | 9% | – | 2% | 1% |
| Hemolytic-uremic syndrome | 4% | 8% | 14% | 1% |
| Oxalosis | 4% | – | – | – |
| Congenital nephrosis | 4% | 12% | – | – |
| Pyelonephritis | – | 4% | 9% | 7% |
| Cystinosis | – | – | 7% | – |
| Medullary cystic disease | – | – | 2% | 10% |
| Other | – | 2% | 7% | 16% |

*Expressed as a percentage of total cases in each age group.
†Table 3–2.
‡Potter and associates.[5]

common causes of ESRD seen in young infants were different from those seen in even the youngest age group (1 to 5 years) reported by Potter and associates. Obstructive uropathy appears to be a frequent cause of ESRD at opposite extremes of childhood, occurring relatively infrequently between 1 and 10 years of age. A peak incidence of obstructive uropathy in late childhood is consistent with the findings of Krieger and associates, who noted that renal failure from obstructive uropathy requires an average of 8.1 years to progress from diagnosis of urologic diease in early childhood to ESRD.[31] A severe form of obstructive uropathy presenting in the first month of life has also been previously described.[42]

## SPECIAL CONCERNS IN THE YOUNG INFANT WITH RENAL FAILURE

### Progressive Encephalopathy of Renal Insufficiency

Pediatric nephrologists have been aware for some time that young children with mild to moderate renal insufficiency often develop seizure disorders and other neurologic abnormalities. Scattered reports called attention to the apparent association between this encephalopathy and very early onset of chronic renal insufficiency.[43, 44] It was the report by Rotundo and associates which demonstrated the magnitude of this alarming syndrome.[45] These investigators performed a retrospective analysis of the courses of 23 infants whose diagnosis of chronic renal insufficiency was made during the first year of life. In 20 of 23 patients, a syndrome of serious neurologic dysfuntion was identified, which typically consisted of decreased head growth followed by seizures, dyskinesia, hypotonia, and developmental delay. Electroencephalograms were abnormal in 17 of 18 patients evaluated, and sequential EEGs obtained in eight of these patients showed progressive deterioration. EEG abnormalities were said to be similar to those described in adults with dialysis dementia thought to be related to aluminum intoxication; however, none of the 20 children reported by Rotundo, et al.[45] had been dialyzed prior to the appearance of encephalopathy, and four had received no oral aluminum when their central nervous system (CNS) dysfunction appeared. Similar efforts

to relate the presence of encephalopathy to abnormalities in parathyroid hormone, serum electrolytes, acid-base status, and degree and duration of renal insufficiency were unsuccessful.

All but two of the 20 encephalopathic children had either renal dysplasia or hypoplasia with or without associated obstruction as the cause of renal failure, but none had evidence of congenital CNS abnormalities or perinatal insults. Head circumference was normal at birth in all patients.

Rotundo and associates were struck by the consistency with which the encephalopathy was preceded by a dramatic reduction in overall growth rate, most apparent in the serial head circumference measurements, which fell below normal in 15 of 20 patients.[45] CT scans showed mild to moderate cortical atrophy in five of 12 children so studied. Brain weights obtained in autopsies of four patients were more than 2 S.D. below the mean for age or height. Detailed information on nutritional therapy was not given, but the authors conceded that these children undoubtedly had suboptimal nutrition for variable periods following diagnosis and prior to development of progressive encephalopathy. The authors were reluctant to attribute the encephalopathy seen in these children solely to deleterious influences of chronic malnutrition on the developing brain. The authors postulated that the developing brain may be uniquely vulnerable to some unknown neurotoxic effect of mild to moderate renal insufficiency.

Their report concludes with the comment: "Earlier renal transplantation may be necessary to protect or stabilize the developing brain, and we are presently pursuing this strategy."[45] Unfortunately, the value of renal transplantation as a therapeutic tactic in this syndrome is not apparent from the courses of the seven children in this series who received renal transplants. All had evidence of encephalopathy prior to transplantation. Three recipients died of complications related to rejection or immunosuppression. Of the four who survived with functioning grafts, one had worsening of encephalopathy, one had improvement, and two were unchanged. From this experience it would seem that, for transplantation to be an effective treatment for this condition, it probably should be done prior to or very soon after the onset of CNS dysfunction. However, in 10 of the 20 encephalopathic children described by Rotundo et al, such a strategy would have dictated renal transplantation prior to one year of age when the serum creatinine level averaged less than 3 mg/dl.

Clearly much more information is needed to fully elucidate this syndrome. The apparent prevalence of progressive encephalopathy in children whose renal insufficiency presents in infancy provides further impetus for a reassessment of current approaches to management of such patients. It would also seem reasonable to regard decreased head growth in an infant with chronic renal failure as a particularly ominous finding.

## Early Loss of Growth Potential

The prevalence of severe growth retardation among young children with chronic renal failure has been recognized for over 25 years,[46] yet remains poorly understood. Several different conditions arising from inadequate kidney function may interfere with normal growth, either independently or in conjunction with other problems. Protein-calorie malnutrition (PCM), renal osteodystrophy, and acidosis are most often listed as possible causes of growth failure in these children, but other less well-defined factors may also be involved.[47, 48]

The potential impact of growth retardation suffered during infancy can be appreciated when normal infant growth rates are considered. Table 3–4 lists average growth rates for head circumference, weight, and height seen in normal male infants during the first three years of life.[49] While incremental changes in weight (birth weight is doubled by 5 months, tripled by 12 months) and height (statural growth rate in the first six months is 3 to 5 times greater than will be seen again prior to puberty) are impressive, the most striking feature of growth in early infancy is the growth of the brain, as reflected in increasing head circumference.

The relative magnitude of early growth is further considered in Figure 3–1. By the end of the first year of life over 85% of ultimate growth in head circumference and 50% of ultimate height potential has been attained by the normal infant.[50] It is not surprising then that when renal disease interferes with normal growth during the first year or two of life, the loss of ultimate growth potential is more severe than when growth retardation begins later in childhood.

This early loss of growth potential has been best described in children with congenital renal anomalies whose renal disease typically presents during the first few months of life. Renal function is usually only moderately impaired in such infants, with progression to ESRD occurring slowly over a number of years.[31] Betts and Magrath first defined the pattern of growth typically exhibited by these

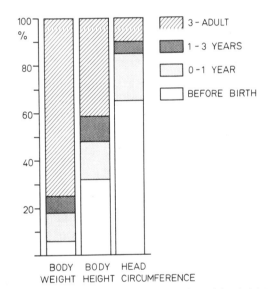

**Figure 3–1.** Proportional increase in weight, height, and head circumference during the four periods of normal growth and development. (From: Vahlquist B: The young child: normal. *In*: Human Nutrition. Nutrition and Growth, Jelliffe, DB, Jelliffe, EFP [Eds]. New York, Plenum Press, 1979, p 157. Reprinted by permission.)

**Table 3–4.** NORMAL GROWTH RATES DURING THE FIRST THREE YEARS OF LIFE (MALE)*

| Age Interval (months) | Head Circumference (cm/month) | Weight (kg/month) | Height (cm/month) |
|---|---|---|---|
| 0–1 | 3.6 | 0.93 | 3.53 |
| 1–3 | 1.7 | 0.93 | 3.53 |
| 3–6 | 1.0 | 0.63 | 2.2 |
| 6–9 | 0.6 | 0.47 | 1.5 |
| 9–12 | 0.4 | 0.37 | 1.3 |
| 12–24 | 0.2 | – | – |
| 24–36 | 0.08 | 0.17 | 0.7 |

*Adapted from Fomon SJ: Infant Nutrition. Philadelphia, W. B. Saunders Company, 1974, pp 34–94

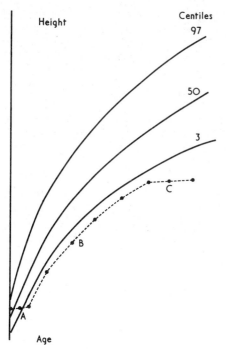

**Figure 3–2.** Schematic representation of growth of children with renal insufficiency dating from infancy. (From: Betts PR, Magrath G: Growth pattern and dietary intake of children with chronic renal insufficiency. Br Med J 2:189, 1974.)

children, documenting the profound effects on growth potential of growth failure in infancy.[51] Figure 3–2 presents a linear growth chart for a typical child described by Betts and Magrath. Despite normal length at birth, linear growth throughout the first two years of life is extremely poor (Growth Curve Segment A, Fig. 3–2); height for chronologic age is seen to rapidly fall away from normal values. During childhood (Growth Curve Segment B, Fig. 3–2) growth rate may return to normal with increases in height paralleling the normal growth curve. However, ground lost during infancy is not regained (i.e., catch-up growth does not occur).

Final progression to ESRD with development of renal bone disease frequently occurs during the adolescent years of such children. The blunted pubertal growth spurt (Growth Curve Segment C, Fig. 3–2) compounds the lost growth potential which occurred in infancy, resulting in a final height which is well below normal.

While growth in some of these children may continue beyond adolescence, ultimate growth potential is most often irretrievably lost owing to an apparent (and as yet unexplained) inability to achieve catch-up growth

rates prior to skeletal maturity.[52] Permanent loss of ultimate growth potential at some finite point following early onset of renal failure is also suggested by observations on growth rates of pediatric recipients of successful renal transplants. Skeletal maturity probably plays a role in limiting growth potential in these patients. In one large study growth was uniformly poor when bone age exceeded 12 years at the time of transplantation.[53] The potential to achieve catch-up growth may be even more limited. In a recent report Ingelfinger and associates documented accelerated linear growth in all eight children who received successful renal transplants prior to their fifth birthdays but in only one of 19 children 5 to 11 years of age at the time of transplantation.[54] These authors could not identify the factors responsible for the catch-up growth exhibited by their younger patients; neither steroid dose, degree of bone age retardation, original renal disease, nor degree of renal osteodystrophy could explain the differences in growth potential seen in the two groups.

The mechanisms involved are probably more complex than can be explained on the basis of skeletal maturity alone. Jones and associates recently reported detailed studies on body composition in 21 children with onset of renal insufficiency during the first year of life, which provide an intriguing glimpse of what may be adaptive physiologic mechanisms serving to limit the potential for catch-up growth in these children.[55] Fourteen patients were under three years of age at the time of study (Group I), while seven were between 5 and 11.9 years of age (Group II). All were below normal in height for chronologic age and exhibited growth patterns similar to those reported by Betts and Magrath for such children.[51]

Weight-for-height ratios were different for the two groups. Children in Group I had substantially reduced weight-for-height ratios, a condition seen commonly in children suffering from acute protein-calorie malnutrition (PCM).[56] Children in Group II were found by Jones et al to have near normal weight-for-height ratios.[55] Children with PCM whose height is below normal for chronologic age but whose weight for height is appropriate are said to be stunted (nutritional or hypocaloric dwarfs).[56] This stunting is thought to be an adaptive response to chronic malnutrition in which growth is limited to allow the subnormal energy and protein intakes to suffice for basic metabolic processes.[57, 58]

Studies of body composition in the 21 children reported by Jones et al supported this analogy with children suffering from PCM.[55] For example, the ratio of observed to predicted intracellular water (ICW O/P) is considered to be an index of body cell mass and is often diminished in acutely malnourished children.[59] Children in Group I were found to have ICW O/P levels which were significantly reduced when compared to normal (Fig. 3–3). Children in Group II had near normal ICW O/P values, suggesting an increased body cell mass consistent with their normal weight-for-height ratios. Moreover, when seven Group I children were studied again six to ten months later, six were found to have significantly increased ICW O/P values during the interstudy period (Fig. 3–3), suggesting to the authors that some process of metabolic adaptation to chronic PCM was already underway in these children.

The authors of this study noted that caloric intake in both patient groups was generally low (<80% of RDA in most patients) and protein intake was also below the RDA for children in Group I. They suggest that their younger patients demonstrated acute undernutrition with depleted body protein stores. As inadequate nutrition ( and renal insufficiency) persisted beyond three years of age, the authors postulate that these children demonstrated metabolic adaptation to

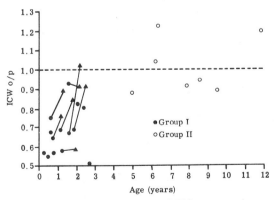

**Figure 3–3.** Intracellular water (ICW) expressed as a ratio of observed:predicted (O/P), plotted against age. Repeat studies in six Group I children are shown (●–▲). The increase in ICW O/P ratio toward unity (as shown by the broken line) through early childhood is evident. See text. (From: Jones RWA, Rigden SP, Barratt TM, Chantler C: The effects of chronic renal failure in infancy on growth, nutritional status and body composition. Pediatr Res 16:784, 1982.)

chronic malnutrition which was reflected in normal ICW O/P values and weight-for-height ratios along with profound stunting: in effect the "normalization" of body *cell mass* for height. Jones et al speculate that catch-up growth may not be possible in response to nutritional supplementation once body cell mass has been normalized for height by virtue of these adaptive processes.[55] Their study does not examine, however, the possible role of aggressive nutritional supplementation in reversing these processes, and it provides only circumstantial (albeit impressive) evidence that chronic malnutrition is responsible for the loss of growth potential seen in these children.

Although the mechanisms involved remain obscure, renal insufficiency severe enough to interfere with growth during infancy clearly exacts a heavy price in terms of lost growth potential which may not be recoverable. Treatment strategies designed for the young infant with ESRD must reflect the importance of establishing normal growth rates during this critical period.

## TREATMENT OPTIONS FOR INFANTS WITH ONSET OF ESRD DURING THE FIRST YEAR OF LIFE

### Hemodialysis

Although hemodialysis (HD) can be performed on infants and children of almost any size and age,[60] including premature newborns,[61] reports of successful long-term HD in infants less than one year of age are rare.[23, 26, 62] Serious technical problems (e.g., difficulty in achieving and maintaining vascular access, limitations on tolerable extracorporeal blood volume and ultrafiltration rates)[63] have discouraged most pediatric dialysis programs from attempting chronic HD in very young infants.[7] Hemodialysis has not been found to be suitable for use as a home dialysis technique for very young children.[16] Thus treatment of the infant with chronic HD is likely to require disruption or relocation of the family to the few metropolitan areas where HD is available for infants or, at best, long commuting trips to and from the dialysis center for most patients.

Chapter 5 contains a complete review of current approaches to the use of HD in infants and young children. Despite the recent advances, the use of HD in contrast to peritoneal dialysis[63] as a modality for the chronic care of infants less than one year of age is likely to remain extremely limited in the forseeable future.

## Transplantation

Reported experience with renal transplantation in very young infants is quite limited; the few published cases span a period of over 20 years during which medical and surgical methods underwent many changes. Transplantation programs traditionally have been reluctant to accept very young children owing to the technical difficulties inherent in the treatment of these small patients.[5, 7] Of those programs attempting transplantation in infants, most relied on cadaveric grafts from pediatric donors,[32, 64] including anencephalic infants.[16, 65] While there have been some notable successes,[25, 35] overall experience with renal transplantation in very young infants has been discouraging.[32, 64, 66]

Only 18 transplants performed in 16 infants less than one year of age have been reported in sufficient detail to allow analysis.[22, 25, 28, 35, 64, 67–70] These reports are summarized in Table 3–5. All but three of the 18 allografts were from pediatric cadaveric donors, including four from anencephalics. At the time they were reported, only four of 18 allografts were functioning. Even more disturbing, 11 of the 16 infant recipients had died, including all four of the infants who received kidneys from anencephalic donors.

Table 3–5 also summarizes reported experience with 28 transplants in 25 slightly older infants, 13 to 24 months of age at the time of first transplantation.[22, 32, 35, 64, 70–73]

Overall results in this age group are somewhat better: 12 of 28 grafts were functional at the time they were reported and only eight of 25 infants had died. Ten of the 28 allografts in this group came from living related donors, a parent in all cases.

Closer inspection of results in this older group (13–24 months of age) shows a marked difference in outcome when living related and cadaveric donor kidneys are compared. Seven of the eight deaths occurred among recipients of cadaveric grafts, and nine of the 12 functional grafts were from living related donors.

These differences are more clearly seen when outcome is expressed in terms of the actuarial patient survival rates at 1 and 2 years post transplantation. Table 3–6 presents calculated actuarial patient survival rates for the two age groups discussed above, and includes results from two series of older children for comparison.[1, 66] In the youngest children (less than 1 year of age) 1- and 2-year actuarial patient survival rate was only 41%. Children between 13 months and 24 months of age had a somewhat better overall patient survival rate (70% and 57% at 1 and 2 years, respectively). However, when donor source is considered in this older group, a difference in outcome is seen. Patient survival was 89% at 1 and 2 years among 13- to 24-month-old infants receiving grafts from their parents; survival rates among infants of the same age receiving cadaveric grafts was 64% and 39% at 1 and 2 years, resembling that seen in the infants less than 1 year of age. It will be recalled that over three-fourths of this youngest group received cadaveric grafts.

The results of living related donor transplantation in a group of older children, 2 to

**Table 3–5.** RENAL TRANSPLANTATION IN INFANTS LESS THAN TWO YEARS OF AGE

| | | Donor Source | | | Outcome | | |
|---|---|---|---|---|---|---|---|
| *Recipient Age* | *No. of Patients* | *Anencephalic* | *Cadaver* | *Live-Related* | *Died* | *Non-Functioning* | *Normal Function* |
| 6 Days to 1 Year* | 16 | 4 | | | 4 | 0 | 0 |
| | | | 11 | | 6 | 3 | 2 |
| | | | | 3 | 1 | 0 | 2 |
| Totals | | | | | 11 | 3 | 4 |
| 13 Months to 2 Years** | 25 | 5 | | | 1 | 4 | 0 |
| | | | 13 | | 6 | 4 | 3 |
| | | | | 10 | 1 | 0 | 9 |
| Totals | | | | | 8 | 8 | 12 |

*References: 22, 25, 28, 32, 35, 64, 67–70
**References: 22, 32, 35, 64, 70–73

**Table 3–6.** ACTUARIAL PATIENT SURVIVAL IN PEDIATRIC RENAL TRANSPLANTATION

| Recipient Age | Donor Source | | | Actuarial Patient Survival | |
| --- | --- | --- | --- | --- | --- |
| | *Cadaver* | *Live-Related* | *Total* | *1 Year (n)* | *2 Years (n)* |
| 6 Days to 1 Year* | 15 | 3 | 18 | 41% (10) | 41% (6) |
| 13 Months to 2 Years** | 18 | | | 64% (5) | 39% (3) |
| | | 10 | | 89% (7) | 89% (5) |
| | | | 28 | 70% (12) | 57% (8) |
| 11 Months to 5 Years[66] | 27 | 4 | 31 | 83% | 75% |
| 2 Years to 22 Years[1] | 36 | | | 85% (28) | 85% (16) |
| | | 82 | | 92% (61) | 92% (53) |

*References: 22, 25, 28, 32, 35, 64, 67–70
**References: 22, 32, 35, 64, 70–73

22 years of age[1] were similar to the patient survival rates seen in 13- to 24-month-old recipients of a parent's kidney (Table 3–6). Striking differences are noted, however, between the results of cadaveric transplantation in older children[66] and the outcome seen in both groups of younger infants receiving cadaveric grafts. Actuarial patient survival rates at 2 years after cadaveric transplantation in infants under 24 months of age was only about half of that seen in older age groups.

It is not clear why younger infants should fare so poorly following cadaveric transplantation. The negative influence of anencephalic donors on outcome does not entirely account for the observed differences in patient survival. These observations are based on relatively small numbers of patients treated in many different centers and must be accepted with caution. However, Rizzoni and associates also noted unexplainably inferior results obtained with cadaveric transplantation in a larger group of infants and children (less than 5 years of age) when compared to older children, all of whom received their cadaver grafts in the same center.[66] We presently consider cadaveric transplantation particularly hazardous for infants less than 1 year of age. Without a substantial breakthrough in anti-rejection therapy, this impression will be difficult to alter.

Experience with living related donor (LRD) transplantation in infants less than 1 to 2 years of age is extremely limited. Considering the generally dismal outcome following cadaveric transplantation in this age group, it is not difficult to understand the reluctance of some programs to risk a parent's kidney in these infants,[32, 35] although the "catch 22" created by this approach is obvious. For most programs, parental kidney size has been the limiting factor, restricting LRD transplantation to those infants weighing at least 8 to 10 kg.[32] It would appear, however, that outcome following LRD transplantation may be the same, irrespective of the age of the recipient. Thus, a dialysis method is needed by which the smallest infants can be safely maintained while they grow to a size at which LRD transplantation is technically more suitable.

## Peritoneal Dialysis

**History.** The successful use of peritoneal dialysis (PD) in the treatment of infants and young children with renal failure was first reported by Swan and Gordon in a remarkable paper published in 1949.[74] These investigators described three acutely anuric children, 9 months, 3 years, and 8 years of age, who were treated with a technique known as continuous peritoneal lavage. Developed by Seligman and others,[75, 76] continuous peritoneal lavage required surgical placement of two rigid peritoneal sumps, one above, the other below the umbilicus. A continuous infusion of fresh dialysate through one sump and drainage from the other resulted in sustained unidirectional dialysate flow through the peritoneal cavity. The three children treated by Swan and Gordon received an average of 33 liters of dialysate each day during continuous treatment periods ranging from 5 to 12 consecutive days.

Despite impressive obstacles, outcome in these three children was generally favorable. Peritonitis occurred only once and responded promptly to antibiotics. Two of the children recovered normal renal function after peritoneal lavage for periods of 5 and 12 days. The 9-month-old infant was sustained for 28 days but eventually died of obscure complications. Acknowledging the complexity, expense, and intense effort involved, the authors noted that their technique could be life-saving in properly selected cases, and recommended further evaluation.[74]

The use of PD in infants next appeared in the medical literature over a decade later, long after continuous peritoneal lavage had been abandoned. In 1960 Segar described the use of PD to treat three neonates with boric acid poisoning.[77] Subsequent reports documented the effectiveness of short term PD in the treatment of acute renal failure in neonates and older infants.[78–81] The manual PD technique used throughout the 1960's required reinsertion of the dialysis catheter at the beginning of each treatment, which made prolonged use in infants and small children exceedingly difficult. It was the development of a permanent peritoneal catheter by Palmer, Quinton, and Gray[82] and its successful modification by Tenckhoff and Schecter[83] which made chronic intermittent peritoneal dialysis (IPD) an acceptable form of treatment for infants and children. The concomitant development of automated peritoneal dialysate delivery devices led in 1968 to the establishment of the first chronic home IPD program for children.[84] Unfortunately the automated equipment could not be modified to deliver the small exchange volumes required by infants who weighed less than 8 to 10 kg[33] (a problem which persisted until 1982!). Thus, prior to the advent of CAPD, the only chronic treatment option available for infants was manual IPD performed either in the hospital (usually a pediatric outpatient dialysis center) or at home.

## Intermittent Peritoneal Dialysis (IPD)

Although there have been no reports detailing the use of chronic IPD in infants who were treated in the hospital or dialysis center, it is likely that this method was favored by many pediatric dialysis programs for those infants thought to be too small to be safely managed on hemodialysis.[63] Home use of chronic IPD in infants has been reported only by Lorentz and associates, who treated two infants, five months and nine months of age at the onset of dialysis.[33] Parents were taught to perform dialysis using bottled dialysate and standard hospital tubing sets for a minimum of three 12-hour treatments each week. This regimen sustained these infants for 10 and 13 months until cadaveric transplantation could be performed.

There were many problems: the smaller infant required 11 hospitalizations in 13 months of dialysis for treatment of such problems as catheter failures, peritonitis, dehydration, hypocalcemia, and anemia. Neither infant grew well (Fig. 3–4). Linear growth was less than 33% of expected for chronologic age in both patients. Weight gain was less than 20% of expected in one infant and about 60% of expected in the other. Head circumference data were not reported. Dietary goals of 1.5 gm/kg/day of protein and at least 67% of the RDA for energy were thought to have been achieved. Both infants had radiographic evidence of renal osteodys-

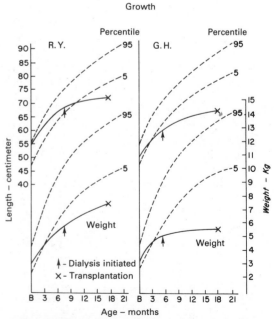

**Figure 3–4.** Growth data on two infants maintained on chronic home manual IPD during the first year of life. (From: Lorentz WB Jr., Hamilton RW, Disher B, Crater C: Home peritoneal dialysis during infancy. Clin Nephrol 15:191, 1981.)

trophy, which persisted throughout the period on dialysis. Breaks in sterile technique were exhibited by the mother of one infant who had repeated episodes of peritonitis. This family was apparently under severe stress, and the characteristic features of "parent fatigue"[13] seemed to the authors to be related to the full responsibility for dialysis falling on only one parent.

Despite these problems, the authors point out that manual IPD was the only treatment available for these infants in their center while awaiting cadaveric transplantation, and home treatment was preferable to in-center treatment for financial, logistic, and psychosocial reasons.

### Continuous Ambulatory Peritoneal Dialysis (CAPD)

CAPD has been used in the treatment of pediatric ESRD patients only since 1978. In this brief period CAPD has been found to be particularly well suited to the needs of infants, in contrast to the other dialysis techniques currently available. At present, CAPD is considered by many to be the dialysis treatment of choice for the infant ESRD patient while awaiting transplantation. A detailed discussion of the use of CAPD in infants less than one year of age will be found in Chapter 13.

## REFERENCES

1. Avner ED, Harmon WE, Grupe WE, et al: Mortality of chronic hemodialysis and renal transplantation in pediatric end-stage renal disease. Pediatrics 67:412, 1981.
2. Chantler C, Carter JE, Bewick M, et al: Ten years' experience with regular hemodialysis and renal transplantation. Arch Dis Child 55:435, 1980.
3. Riley CM: Thoughts about kidney homotransplantation in children. J Pediatr 65:797, 1964.
4. Reinhart JB: The doctor's dilemma: whether or not to recommend continuous renal dialysis or renal homotransplantation for the child with end-stage renal disease. J Pediatr 77:505, 1970.
5. Potter DE, Holliday MA, Piel CF, et al: Treatment of end-stage renal disease in children: a 15-year experience. Kidney Int 18:103, 1980.
6. Fine RN: Renal transplantation in children. J Pediatr 100:754, 1982.
7. Arbus GS, DeMaria JE, Galivango J, et al: The first 10 years of the dialysis-transplantation program at The Hospital for Sick Children, Toronto. 1: Predialysis and dialysis. Can Med Assoc J 120:655, 1980.
8. Hurley JK: Kidney transplantation in infants (Letter). J Pediatr 93:538, 1978.
9. Dialysis and transplantation in young children (Editorial). Br Med J 2:1033, 1979.
10. Renal transplantation in very young children (Editorial). Lancet 2:367, 1982.
11. Popovich RP, Moncrief JW, Decherd JW, et al: The definition of a novel portable/wearable equilibrium peritoneal dialysis technique. Trans Am Soc Artif Intern Organs 5:64, 1976.
12. Balfe JW, Vigneux A, Willumsen J, Hardy BE: The use of CAPD in the treatment of children with end-stage renal disease. Perit Dial Bull 1:35, 1981.
13. Alexander SR, Tseng CH, Maksym KA, et al: Clinical parameters in continuous ambulatory peritoneal dialysis for infants and children. In: CAPD Update: Continuous Ambulatory Peritoneal Dialysis, Moncrief JW, Popovich RP (Eds). New York, Masson, 1981, p 195.
14. Popovich RP, Pyle WK, Rosenthal DA, et al: Kinetics of peritoneal dialysis in children. In: CAPD Update: Continuous Ambulatory Peritoneal Dialysis, Moncrief JW, Popovich RP (Eds). New York, Masson, 1981, p 227.
15. Oreopoulos DG, Katirtzoglou A, Arbus G, Cordy P: Dialysis and transplantation in young children (Letter), Br Med J 1:1628, 1979.
16. Cameron JS: The treatment of chronic renal failure in children by regular dialysis and by transplantation. Nephron 11:221, 1973.
17. Novello AC, Fine RN: Renal transplantation in children—a review. Int J Pediatr Nephrol 3:87, 1982.
18. Helin I, Winberg J: Chronic renal failure in Swedish children. Acta Paediatr Scand 69:607, 1980.
19. Leumann E: Die chronische Nierenin suffizienz in Kindesalter. Schweiz Med Wochenschr 106:244, 1976.
20. Scharer K: Incidence and causes of chronic renal failure in childhood. Proc Eur Dial Transplant Assoc 7:211, 1971.
21. Habib R, Broyer M, Benmaiz H: Chronic renal failure in children. Nephron 11:209, 1973.
22. LaPlante MP, Kaufman JJ, Goldman R, et al: Kidney transplantation in children. Pediatrics 46:665, 1970.
23. Makela P, Ahola T, Bjorkman H, et al: Infant dialysis. Proc Eur Dial Transplant Assoc 9:187, 1972.
24. Meadow SR, Cameron JS, Ogg CS, Saxton HM: Children referred for acute dialysis. Arch Dis Child 46:221, 1971.
25. Cerilli GJ, Nelsen C, Dorfman L: Renal homotransplantation in infants and children with the hemolytic uremic syndrome. Surgery 71:66, 1972.
26. Mauer SM, Shideman JR, Buselmeier TJ, Kjellstrand CM: Long-term hemodialysis in the neonatal period. Am J Dis Child 125:269, 1973.
27. Griffin NK, McElnea J, Barratt TM: Acute renal failure in early life. Arch Dis Child 51:459, 1976.
28. Kwun YA, Butt KMH, Kim KH, et al: Successful renal transplantation in a 3-month old infant. J Pediatr, 92:426, 1978.
29. Penn I: Renal transplantation for Wilms' tumor: report of 20 cases. J Urol 122:793, 1979.
30. DeMaria JE, Hardy BE, Brezinski A, Churchill BM: Renal transplantation in patients with bilateral Wilms' tumor. J Pediat Surg 14:577, 1979.
31. Krieger JN, Stubenbord WT, Vaughan ED Jr: Transplantation in children with end-stage renal disease of urologic origin. J Urol 124:508, 1980.
32. Moel DI, Butt KMH: Renal transplantation in children less than 2 years of age. J Pediatr 99:535, 1981.
33. Lorentz WB, Hamilton RW, Disher B, Crater C:

Home peritoneal dialysis during infancy. Clin Nephrol 15:194, 1981.

34. Balfe JW, Irwin M-A, Oreopoulos DG: An assessment of continuous ambulatory peritoneal dialysis (CAPD) in children. *In*: CAPD Update: Continuous Ambulatory Peritoneal Dialysis, Moncrief JW, Popovich RP (eds). New York, Masson, 1981, p 211.

35. Miller LC, Bock GH, Lum CT, Mauer SM: Transplantation of the adult kidney into the very small child: long-term outcome. J Pediatr 100:675, 1982.

36. Alexander SR, Lubischer JT: Continuous ambulatory peritoneal dialysis in pediatrics: three years' experience at one center. Nefrologia (Madrid) 11(Suppl) 2:53, 1982.

37. Alkalay A, Mogilner BM, Nissim F, Edelstein S: Production of the hydroxylated metabolites of vitamin D in a neonate with a single hypoplastic-dysplastic kidney. Arch Dis Child 58:66, 1983.

38. Norman ME, Asadi FK: A prospective study of acute renal failure in the newborn infant. Pediatrics 63:475, 1979.

39. Hodson EM, Kjellstrand CM, Mauer SM: Acute renal failure in infants and children: outcome of 53 patients requiring hemodialysis treatment. J Pediatr 93:756, 1978.

40. Counahan J, Cameron JS, Ogg LS, et al: Presentation, management, complication, and outcome of acute renal failure in childhood: five years' experience. Br Med J 1:599, 1977.

41. Barratt TM: Renal failure in children. Proc Roy Soc Med 64:1045, 1971.

42. Tsingoglou S, Dickson JAS: Lower urinary obstruction in infancy: a review of lesions and symptoms in 165 cases. Arch Dis Child 47:215, 1972.

43. Baluarte HJ, Gruskin AB, Hiner L, et al: Encephalopathy in children with chronic renal failure (abstract). Pediatr Res: 11:547, 1977.

44. Bale JF, Siegler RL, Bray PF: Encephalopathy in young children with moderate chronic renal failure. Am J Dis Child 134:581, 1980.

45. Rotundo A, Nevins TE, Lipton M, et al: Progressive encephalopathy in children with chronic renal insufficiency in infancy. Kidney Int 21:486, 1982.

46. West CD, Smith WC: An attempt to elucidate the cause of growth retardation in renal disease. Am J Dis Child 91:460, 1956.

47. Stickler GB: Growth failure in renal disease. Pediatr Clin North Am 23:885, 1976.

48. Broyer M: Growth in children with renal insufficiency. Pediatr Clin North Am 29:991, 1982.

49. Fomon SJ: Normal growth, failure to thrive and obesity. *In*: Infant Nutrition, Fomon SJ (Ed). Philadelphia, WB Saunders, 1974, p 34.

50. Vahlquist B: The young child: normal. *In*: Human Nutrition: Nutrition and Growth. Jelliffe DB, Jelliffe EFP (Eds). New York, Plenum, 1979, p 157.

51. Betts PR, Magrath G: Growth pattern and dietary intake of children with chronic renal insufficiency. Br Med J 2:189, 1974.

52. Ingelfinger JR: Factors affecting growth following renal transplantation in childhood. Dial Transplant 11:1075, 1982.

53. Grushkin CM, Fine RN: Growth in children following renal transplantation. Am J Dis Child 125:514, 1973.

54. Ingelfinger JR, Grupe WE, Harmon WE, et al: Growth acceleration following renal transplanta-

tion in children less than 7 years of age. Pediatrics 68:255, 1981.

55. Jones RWA, Rigden SP, Barratt TM, Chantler C: The effects of chronic renal failure in infancy on growth, nutritional status and body composition. Pediatr Res 16:784, 1982.

56. Waterlow JC: Classification and definition of protein-calorie malnutrition. Br Med J 2:566, 1972.

57. Jelliffe DB: Protein-calorie malnutrition in tropical preschool children (a review of recent knowledge). J Pediatr 54:227, 1959.

58. Downs EF: Nutritional dwarfing: a syndrome of early protein-calorie malnutrition. Am J Clin Nutr 15:275, 1964.

59. Cheek DB, Habicht JP, Berall J, Hold AB: Protein-calorie malnutrition and the significance of cell mass relative to body length. Am J Clin Nutr 30:851, 1977.

60. Mauer SM, Lynch RE: Hemodialysis technique for infants and children. Pediatr Clin North Am 23:843, 1976.

61. Bock GH, Campos A, Thompson T, et al: Hemodialysis in the premature infant. Am J Dis Child 135:178, 1981.

62. Gagnadoux MF, Pascal B, Bronstein M, et al: Arteriovenous fistulae in small children. Dial Transplant 9:318, 1980.

63. Fine RN: Peritoneal dialysis update. J Pediatr 100:1, 1982.

64. DeShazo CV, Simmons RL, Bernstein DM, et al: Results of renal transplantation in 100 children. Surgery 76:461, 1974.

65. Iitaka K, Martin LW, Cox JA, et al: Transplantation of cadaver kidneys from anencephalic donors. J Pediatr 93:216, 1978.

66. Rizzoni G, Malekzadeh M, Pennisi AJ, et al: Renal transplantation in children less than 5 years of age. Arch Dis Child 55:532, 1980.

67. Cerilli J, Evans WE, Sotos JF: Renal transplantation in infants and children. Transplant Proc 4:633, 1972.

68. Lawson RK, Talwalkar YB, Musgrave JE, et al: Renal transplantation in pediatric patients. J Urol 113:225, 1975.

69. Lum CT, Fryd DS, Najarian JS: Kidney transplantation in children zero to 10 years of age. Curr Surg 39:27, 1982.

70. Harmon WE, Levey RH: Successful living related donor (LRD) renal transplantation (RTx) as treatment for very young children with chronic renal failure (Abstract). Program and Abstracts, National Kidney Foundation Twelfth Annual Clinical Dialysis and Transplant Forum, Chicago, Illinois, December 8–13, 1982, p 14.

71. Hodson EM, Najarian JS, Kjellstrand CM, et al: Renal transplantation in children ages 1 to 5 years. Pediatrics 61:458, 1978.

72. Fine RN, Korsch BM, Brennan LP, et al: Renal transplantation in young children. Am J Surg 125:599, 1973.

73. Salvatierra O Jr, Belzer FO: Pediatric cadaver kidneys. Their use in renal transplantation. Arch Surg 110:181, 1975.

74. Swan H, Gordon HH: Peritoneal lavage in the treatment of anuria in children. Pediatrics 4:586:1949.

75. Seligman AM, Frank HA, Fine J: Treatment of experimental uremia by means of peritoneal irrigation. J Clin Invest 25:211, 1946.

76. Frank HA, Seligman AM, Fine J: Treatment of uremia after acute renal failure by peritoneal irrigation. JAMA 130:703, 1946.
77. Segar WE: Peritoneal dialysis in the treatment of boric acid poisoning. N Engl J Med 282:798, 1960.
78. Manley GL, Collipp PJ: Renal failure in the newborn: Treatment with peritoneal dialysis. Am J Dis Child 115:107, 1968.
79. Lugo G, Ceballos R, Brown W, et al: Acute renal failure in the neonate managed by peritoneal dialysis. Am J Dis Child 118:655, 1969.
80. Segar WE, Gibson RK, Rhanz R: Peritoneal dialysis in infants and small children. Pediatrics 27:603, 1961.

81. Etteldorf JN, Dobbins WT, Sweeney MJ, et al: Intermittent peritoneal dialysis in the management of acute renal failure in children. J Pediatr 60:327, 1962.
82. Palmer RA, Quinton WE, Gray JE: Prolonged peritoneal dialysis for chronic renal failure. Lancet 1:700, 1964.
83. Tenckhoff H, Schechter H: A bacteriologically safe peritoneal access device. Trans Am Soc Artif Intern Organs 14:181, 1968.
84. Counts S, Hickman R, Garbaccio A, Tenckhoff H: Chronic home peritoneal dialysis in children. Trans Am Soc Artif Intern Organs 19:157, 1973.

# 4

# Hemodialysis in Children with ESRD: Technical Aspects

*Donald E. Potter, M.D.*

Chronic hemodialysis has been performed in children for two decades, and several pediatric centers have accumulated experience extending for more than 15 years. The kinetics and technical aspects of dialysis in children have been described and the short-term results and complications of treatment have been documented. Because pediatric nephrologists have generally considered renal transplantation to be a better long-term form of treatment for children with ESRD, the average duration of dialysis in many centers prior to transplantation is less than a year. There is, therefore, little experience with long-term dialysis in children. In addition, since children are transferred out of pediatric units when they reach adulthood, the outcome and medical and psychosocial consequences of extended dialysis in patients who started treatment as children are unknown.

## GENERAL CONSIDERATIONS

Hemodialysis is a process in which blood comes into contact with a balanced salt solution (dialysate) across a semipermeable membrane. Solutes pass across the membrane by diffusion along a concentration gradient, usually from blood to dialysate. In addition, water and solutes (extracellular fluid) can be removed from the blood by ultrafiltration, which involves the creation of a hydrostatic pressure gradient across the membrane. A variation of hemodialysis, hemofiltration, utilizes rapid ultrafiltration across a highly permeable membrane to remove both solutes and water; most of the ultrafiltrate, 60 to 120 ml/min, is replaced by a balanced salt solution.[1]

The rate of removal of solutes from the blood by an artificial kidney is defined by their clearance measurement. This is analogous to the clearance of solutes by the human kidney and is defined as the amount of blood cleared of solute per unit time. The formula is $C = Q_B \times \dfrac{C_{Bi} - C_{Bo}}{C_{Bi}}$, where $Q_B$ is blood flow in ml per minute, $C_{Bi}$ is the concentration of the solute in the blood flowing into the dialyzer and $C_{Bo}$ is the concentration of the solute in the blood flowing from the dialyzer.

The clearance of solutes by a dialyzer is governed by the laws of mass transfer as they apply to fluid systems in motion. A consideration of these laws is beyond the scope of this chapter, and the reader is referred elsewhere.[2] The characteristics of dialyzers which affect clearance are the geometry of the blood and dialysate paths, the type of membrane, and membrane surface area. A variety of dialyzers with different characteristics and clearance capabilities are available.

The clearance of different solutes by a dialyzer is determined by their physicochemical properties in the blood, including molecular size, electrical charge, protein binding, and water solubility. Typical clearances obtained during dialysis in an adult using a dialyzer with a membrane surface area of 1.0 m$^2$ and a blood flow of 200 ml/min are related to solute molecular weight in Table 4–1. The

**Table 4–1.** CLEARANCE AS A FUNCTION OF MOLECULAR WEIGHT

| Solute | Mol. Wt. (daltons) | Clearance* (ml/min) |
|---|---|---|
| Urea | 60 | 150 |
| Creatinine | 113 | 120 |
| Uric acid | 165 | 100 |
| Sucrose | 342 | 65 |
| Vitamin B$_{12}$ | 1355 | 30 |
| Inulin | 5200 | 6 |
| Albumin | 69,000 | 0 |

*Representative clearances achieved with standard dialyzers in adult patients.

end-products of protein metabolism are small molecules, whereas substances in the molecular weight range of 300 to 2000 daltons have been designated as middle molecules. Although clearance increases with increasing blood flow through the dialyzer up to a blood flow of approximately 300 ml/min, the clearance of small molecules is much more flow-dependent than that of middle molecules. The efficiency of a dialyzer is usually defined by its urea clearance, and dialyzers with urea clearances of 140 to 175 ml/min are most commonly used in adult patients.

The adequacy of dialysis as a therapeutic tool is judged by its ability to lower blood levels of uremic toxins, to ameliorate uremic signs and symptoms, and to improve tests of organ system function which are abnormal in uremia. Traditionally, urea has been considered to be the most important uremic toxin, and there is considerable in vitro and in vivo evidence to support this belief. There is a poor correlation between BUN levels and some of the toxic manifestations of uremia, however, and chronic dialysis patients with well-controlled BUN levels are still subject to uremic complications such as neuropathy. To account for these discrepancies, more recently it has been postulated that middle molecules, which are more poorly dialyzed than urea, also contribute to uremic toxicity.[3] Middle molecules which exhibit in vitro toxicity have been isolated in the plasma and urine of uremic patients,[4] but studies of dialysis regimens which enhance the clearance of middle molecules, but not urea, have yielded conflicting results.[5-7]

Although dialysis relieves the overt signs of uremia—drowsiness, nausea and vomiting, asterixis, myoclonus—dialysis patients may still be subject to problems such as inability to concentrate, weakness, anorexia, and decreased taste acuity. These symptoms are subjective, however, and it is difficult to assess their response to changes in the dialysis regimen. Similarly, although tests of nervous system function, such as EEG power analysis and motor nerve conduction time, show improvement when uremic patients are dialyzed, the ability of these tests to detect physiologic variations in response to changes in dialysis efficiency has not been proved. There is little agreement, therefore, as to what constitutes adequate dialysis, and the criterion most often used is simply the patient's sense of well-being.

Although firm criteria for assessing the adequacy of dialysis have not been established, several techniques for prescribing quantitatively the amount of dialysis necessary to achieve arbitrary goals have been proposed. The dialysis index[8] compares the weekly clearance of a middle molecule, vitamin B$_{12}$, achieved with a given dialyzer (plus the patient's residual renal function) to a reference standard, 29 liters per week per 1.73 m$^2$, thought to represent adequate dialysis. A pediatric dialysis index,[9] relating dialyzer surface area × weekly hours of dialysis/body surface area to values derived from adult dialysis experience, has been formulated. Kinetic modeling of urea[10] makes use of computer calculations of the urea generation rate to predict the dialyzer clearance and time which will produce a desired predialysis BUN, usually 80 mg/dl. This technique has been validated in children.[11] In most pediatric centers, however, both the initial prescription of dialyzer clearance and time and changes made in response to altered BUN and creatinine levels are determined empirically (see below).

## DIALYZERS AND DIALYSIS PRESCRIPTION FOR CHILDREN

There are three types of dialyzers: parallel plate, hollow fiber, and coil. The parallel plate type is composed of multiple layers, each of which is composed of two layers of cellophane sandwiched between plastic boards. The hollow fiber type is composed of thousands of minute cellulose capillary fibers running longitudinally in a plastic case. The coil type consists of a flattened roll of cellophane tubing with a plastic mesh support wound concentrically on a central core and positioned at the top of a large tank of dialysate.

Children are usually dialyzed with parallel

**Table 4–2.** CHARACTERISTICS OF PEDIATRIC DIALYZERS

| | Surface area ($m^2$) | Volume (ml) | Urea Clearance (ml/min) at $Q_B$ (ml/min) | | Ultrafiltration rate (ml/hr/ mm Hg) | Residual Blood Volume (ml) |
|---|---|---|---|---|---|---|
| | | | **100** | **200** | | |
| Gambro mini-minor* | 0.24 | 20 | 51 | 61 | 0.6 | 0.5 |
| Gambro minor* | 0.41 | 33 | – | 100 | 1.4 | 0.6 |
| Cordis Dow 0.6[12, 13] | 0.60 | 60 | 83 | 118 | 0.6 | 3.9 |
| Meltec[14] | 0.61 | 102 | 80 | 116 | 1.7 | 1.0 |
| Rhone-Poulenc RP5–6[15, 16] | | | | | | |
| 2 layers | 0.12 | 18 | 21† | – | 0.2 | – |
| 5 layers | 0.30 | 45 | 50 | – | 0.6 | 4.8 |
| 8 layers | 0.48 | 72 | 65 | – | 1.0 | 7.0 |

*Data from manufacturer. Clearances are in vitro.
†At $Q_B$ 36 ml/min.

plate or hollow fiber dialyzers. Pediatric dialyzers are generally designed for children in either the 10-to-20-kg weight range or in the 20-to-40-kg weight range. Children who weigh more than 40 kg can usually be dialyzed with adult dialyzers. Dialyzer characteristics which have to be adapted to the needs of children of varying size are volume and compliance, ultrafiltration rate, and urea clearance. Pediatric dialyzers with their values for these characteristics are listed in Table 4–2.

The volume of the dialyzer and blood lines should be as small as possible and should not exceed 8 to 10% of the patient's blood volume. Otherwise, hypotension is likely to occur during dialysis and hypertension at the end of dialysis when blood is returned to the patient. The degree to which the volume expands when the transmembrane pressure gradient between the blood compartment and the dialysate compartment increases, the compliance, must be considered in the calculation of the volume. The volume of adult blood lines is 150 ml and the volume of pediatric blood lines is 75 ml.

The ultrafiltration rate is defined as milliliters of ultrafiltrate formed per millimeter of transmembrane pressure per hour. In pediatric dialyzers this figure varies from 0.5 to 1.5. Since transmembrane pressure gradients greater than 500 mm are seldom used, maximum filtration rates vary from 250 to 750 ml per hour or one to three liters during a four-hour dialysis. Since children rarely retain more than 6 to 8% of their body weight as fluid between dialyses, these rates are usually sufficient to remove accumulated fluid and maintain stable body weight.

The most important clinical characteristic of a dialyzer is its urea clearance. This must

be high enough to maintain the BUN, and other blood solute levels, in an acceptable range but not so high as to induce dialysis dysequilibrium (see below). The empiric formulation of Kjellstrand and associates[16, 17] that urea clearance should be three times the child's weight in kilograms has gained general acceptance, and dialyzers for children are usually chosen on the basis of this criterion. When this formulation is used and dialysis is performed for four hours, the patient's BUN level decreases by approximately 65%.[18] This amount of dialysis, performed three times a week will usually maintain a child's predialysis BUN at less than 100 mg/dl.

## INDICATIONS FOR DIALYSIS

The indications for starting dialysis in children with chronic renal failure are the severity of the signs and symptoms and biochemical abnormalities of uremia. The indications often are not clear-cut and the timing of the decision is frequently arbitrary. Hyperkalemia and metabolic acidosis, unresponsive to diet or medications, are usually late manifestations of uremia and are uncommon indications for dialysis. Salt and water retention resulting in severe hypertension or pulmonary edema are more common indications, especially in children whose renal function deteriorates rapidly. The need for dialysis is usually determined by the evolution of uremic symptoms, however, which may be quite gradual. Decreased exercise tolerance is an early symptom, followed by a worsening school performance and the willingness of a previously active child to take daily naps, and, finally, the development of morning nausea and vomiting. The latter symptoms usually correlate with a BUN level of 120–150 mg/ dl, a serum creatinine level of 6–8 mg/dl in younger children and 10–12 mg/dl in older children, and a GFR of 5–10 ml/min/1.73m². There is considerable variability among patients, however. Dialysis should be initiated before children become severely symptomatic.

## TECHNIQUE AND COMPLICATIONS OF THE DIALYSIS PROCEDURE

A variety of signs and symptoms may occur in patients during and after a dialysis procedure. These include nausea and vomiting, headache, backache, chest pain, dizziness, tachycardia, hypotension, hypertension, confusion, and postdialysis fatigue. Convulsions can occasionally occur and, rarely, stupor, coma, and even death. The signs and symptoms are usually attributed to either dialysis dysequilibrium or plasma volume depletion, but both of these entities can occur simultaneously and many of the signs and symptoms are common to both. Other factors may also contribute to morbidity and it is often difficult to identify the precise cause.

Although the pathogenesis of dialysis dysequilibrium is controversial,[19-21] it occurs in the setting of highly efficient dialysis when there is a more rapid decrease in extracellular fluid osmolality than intracellular fluid osmolality and cell swelling results. A rise in intracranial pressure is accompanied by signs of central nervous system involvement— headache, nausea and vomiting, hypertension and, in severe cases, convulsions and changes in consciousness. Patients with high BUN levels, especially those undergoing their first or second dialysis treatment, are at greatest risk. Dysequilibrium is prevented by decreasing the efficiency of dialysis—a dialyzer urea clearance of 1.0 to 1.5 ml/min/kg—or by infusing 25% mannitol, 1 g/kg, over the course of dialysis, thus maintaining extracellular fluid osmolality.[17, 22]

The signs of plasma volume depletion are restlessness, nausea and vomiting, dizziness, tachycardia, and hypotension. Headache can also occur. During ultrafiltration, fluid removed from the plasma is replaced by fluid equilibrated from the expanded interstitial space (edema). Although equilibration is rapid, signs of plasma volume depletion frequently occur when there is still evidence of edema, indicating either an excessive rate of ultrafiltration, a low plasma oncotic pressure, or vascular instability. Bergstrom[23] has shown that ultrafiltration performed alone is associated with fewer signs of volume depletion than ultrafiltration and dialysis performed simultaneously, suggesting that the changes of osmolality that occur with dialysis are one cause of vascular instability. The technique of sequential ultrafiltration and dialysis has proved useful in treating both adult and pediatric[24] patients who gain excessive weight between dialyses.

Intolerance to acetate may be another cause of vascular instability during dialysis.[25] When high efficiency dialyzers are used, the rate of transfer of acetate into the blood may exceed the rate of metabolism of acetate to bicarbonate, resulting in elevated serum acetate levels and decreased serum bicarbonate levels. This has been associated with symptoms of nausea, vomiting, and hypotension in both children and adults.[26, 27] Although this problem can be solved by using dialysate containing bicarbonate instead of acetate,[28] a simpler solution is to avoid the use of dialyzers with clearance inappropriately high for children. Bicarbonate dialysis, which involves special equipment, is probably unnecessary except in special circumstances, such as patients with lactic acidosis.

Several techniques can be used to minimize symptoms of volume depletion during ultrafiltration. It is important to calculate and apply the ultrafiltration rate which will remove the desired quantity of fluid evenly during the course of dialysis. The use of a bed or chair scale with a continuous readout will facilitate this process. If hypotension occurs, the intravenous administration of small amounts of 5% saline, 1 to 2 ml/kg, will usually restore the circulation and obviate the need for larger amounts of isotonic saline. The infusion of 20% human albumin, 5 ml/kg, during the course of dialysis may sustain blood pressure and facilitate ultrafiltration in patients with low serum albumin levels. Vasopressors, e.g., metaramine, can also be used.[16] Mannitol infusions and sequential ultrafiltration and dialysis, both noted above, are other methods which can be used to enhance the success of ultrafiltration.

## ORGANIZATION OF CARE

The incidence of end stage renal disease in children is approximately 1.5 to 3.0 cases per million total population per year.[29-32] In

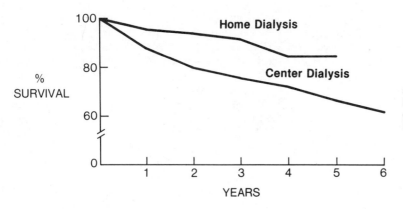

**Figure 4–1.** Actuarial patient survival of 252 children undergoing home dialysis and 1886 children undergoing center dialysis in Europe.[33]

most European countries[33] with well-developed dialysis and transplant facilities, less than one child per million total population is accepted for treatment each year although larger numbers have been accepted for treatment in Israel[33] and northern California.[32] Because few children develop ESRD and treatment is complex and costly, regional pediatric centers that provide or coordinate the care of all children within large geographic areas have been developed.

Most children who receive chronic hemodialyses are dialyzed in the center. Only 19% of patients in Europe[33] and 4%[34] and 8%[32] of patients in two programs in the United States were dialyzed in the home. Two pediatric programs in London,[35] however, have treated most of their patients, including children as young as four years, in the home with good results.

The cost of center dialysis in 11 Children's Hospitals in the United States varied from $217 to $401 per procedure, with an average of $309.[36]

## RESULTS

The most objective measurement of the results of dialysis is patient survival. Statistics accumulated by the European Dialysis and Transplant Association (EDTA) indicate that survival in children is influenced by age,[33] location of dialysis (center vs. home),[33] and type of facility,[37] and demonstrate that survival has increased in the last decade.[38] Actuarial survival curves from 1979[33] (Fig. 4–1) show that five-year pateint survival is 85% with home dialysis and 66% with center dialysis. The two-year survival of patients on center dialysis in three age groups, 0 to 4, 5 to 9, and 10 to 14 years, was 73%, 74%, and

82%, respectively.[33] The two-year survival of children treated in specialized pediatric facilities was 87% and the survival of children treated in general facilities without specialized pediatric care was 81%.[37] The two-year survival of children started on center dialysis in 1978–1980 was 81% and the two-year survival of all children started on center dialysis since 1965 was 68%.[38] The survival of children was similar to that of young adults but greater than that of adults older than 34 years. Twenty-seven children were identified who had survived on dialysis for more than eight years.[39]

In the United States the report of the National Dialysis Registry in 1975[40] showed a one-year survival rate of children 0–19 years of 89%. In an individual program[34] actuarial survival calculated on 98 courses of dialysis in 81 patients was 95% at five years. All but three of the patients were dialyzed in the center, and the only two deaths were caused by liver failure and a brain tumor. The most frequent causes of death in children dialyzed in Europe[41] were cerebrovascular accident, 17%; hypertensive heart failure, 10%; hyperkalemia, 10%, and infections, 8%.

## COMPLICATIONS

The complications of chronic dialysis are primarily related to vascular access and to uremia. Dialysis provides patients with only 10 to 15% of the normal weekly renal clearance of small molecules, is even less efficient in the clearance of larger molecules, and performs none of the metabolic and endocrine functions of the kidney. In addition, substances important to the body, such as vitamins and amino acids, which are not excreted by the kidneys, are removed by dialysis. It is not surprising, therefore, that dialysis patients are subject to many of the complications of chronic renal failure.

The manifestations of uremia that are most commonly encountered in children undergoing dialysis are anemia, hypertension, osteodystrophy, and retardation of growth and sexual development. These are all considered elsewhere in this volume. Less common complications of dialysis or uremia, also considered elsewhere, are heart failure, pericarditis, neurologic disorders, and hepatitis.

A number of metabolic, endocrine, and nutritional abnormalities are present in uremic patients and those undergoing dialysis. Hyperlipidemia is common and probably contributes to the greatly increased risk of death from cardiovascular disease in adult dialysis patients. Hypertriglyceridemia[42-46] and an increased serum fraction of very low density lipoproteins[43-46] are the most common abnormalities noted in children, although hypercholesterolemia[42-44] and an increased serum fraction of low density lipoproteins[44, 46] also occur. The high density lipoprotein fraction is decreased.[46] At autopsy there were no plaques in the coronary arteries of children treated with dialysis and transplantation, but collagenization of the intima, which is thought to be a preatheromatous change, was noted more frequently than in a control group of children.[42]

Serum triglyceride levels in children have been positively correlated with both calorie intake[43] and carbohydrate intake as a percentage of total calories.[42-44] Blood glucose and insulin levels are elevated in children,[44, 47] and a positive correlation between insulin and triglyceride levels was found in one study,[44] but not in another.[47] Patterns of plasma amino acids show low levels of branched-chain amino acids, a low tyrosine-to-phenylalanine ratio, and normal or high levels of nonessential amino acids.[48]

Serum levels of growth hormone are high in children undergoing dialysis.[47, 49] Somatomedin levels measured by bioassay are low,[50, 51] but somatomedin levels measured by radioreceptor assay are high.[52] Studies of thyroid function in children in two centers revealed low normal or low plasma levels of $T_3$ and $T_4$ and normal levels of TSH,[53, 54] which did not respond to stimulation with TRF.[53] The children in one of the centers[54] were clinically euthyroid, however, and the relationship of the function tests to clinical thyroid disease is unclear.

Deficiency of vitamins C,[55] B$_6$,[56] and folic acid[57] and high blood levels of vitamin A[58] have been reported in adult dialysis patients. Children undergoing dialysis should probably receive 1 mg of folic acid after each dialysis and 5 mg of B$_6$ and 100 mg of ascorbic acid daily. Zinc deficiency has also been documented in dialysis patients.[59]

Among a variety of other complications described in dialysis patients are gynecomastia,[60] hypermenorrhea,[61] sexual dysfunction,[62] immune deficiency,[63] ascites,[64] hypersplenism,[65] clotting abnormalities,[66] subdural hematoma,[67] anti-N antibodies,[68] and embolization of silicone from dialysis tubing.[69]

## VASCULAR ACCESS

Techniques of vascular access in children continue to evolve. Arteriovenous fistulas are used in most children, but in children who weigh less than 15 kg the construction of fistulas can be difficult, and the use of shunts is sometimes necessary. Although the creation of primary fistulas in the forearm (Brescia-Cimino) of children was described in 1970,[70] the blood vessels in this area are often small, and other techniques using saphenous vein,[71, 72] bovine carotid artery,[73] or polytetrafluoroethylene (PTFE)[73] grafts between the radial artery and cephalic vein in the elbow have been used. Primary fistulas have also been created in the elbow.[74] More recently microsurgical techniques for creating primary forearm fistulas in infants as small as 5 kg have been described.[75] These fistulas could not be used for a period of six months, however.

The immediate success rate of forearm fistulas was 70% in children greater than 20 kg but only 54% in smaller children in one center.[73] The cumulative one-year survival of fistulas which functioned was 84% for forearm fistulas, 78% for fistulas in the elbow, and 43% for saphenous, bovine, and PTFE grafts. In another center[76] the immediate success rate of forearm fistulas was 85%, and only one of 28 failed over periods of dialysis as long as 48 months.

Thrombosis is the commonest complication of shunt and fistula use. Mild hypertrophy of the leg in a child with a groin fistula[76] and ischemic damage of the leg of a child with a groin shunt[77] have been reported. Detrimental effects of fistula flow on cardiac contractility have been noted.[78] Systolic hypertension as a consequence of high flow through an upper-arm fistula and congestive heart failure as a consequence of high flow through a thigh shunt[79] have each been observed in a single child in the author's center.

## REHABILITATION

A number of factors affect the rehabilitation of children undergoing chronic dialysis. These include the location of dialysis—center or home[38]—the time of day and the number of hours dialysis is performed,[35] the complications and the time spent in hospital, and the success of the child's psychosocial adjustment. The latter is considered in Chapters 39 and 40.

School attendance is the usual criterion used to assess rehabilitation. In children undergoing dialysis in specialized programs in Europe,[38] 31% on center dialysis and 89% on home dialysis were enrolled in school full-time. In children on home dialysis in London[35] the attendance rate of those enrolled was only 65%, however. Slightly more than 50% of children on center dialysis in Europe[37] were considered to be fully rehabilitated, and more than 50% of the children had spent some time in the hospital during the previous year. A hospitalization rate of 18.5 days per patient-year has been reported.[80] A study[39] of the rehabilitation of 26 adolescents and young adults who had started dialysis as children more than eight years previously revealed that 54% were employed full- or part-time, 27% were unemployed, 4% received a pension, and 15% were incapacitated.

## CONCLUSIONS

It has been amply demonstrated that hemodialysis can successfully prolong the lives of uremic children for extended periods of time. Mortality rates are low in selected groups of patients, e.g., patients on home dialysis, but are higher, approximately 7% per year during the first five years of dialysis, in unselected patients on center dialysis. Dialysis provides only a fraction of normal kidney function and children undergoing treatment are subject to a variety of uremic complications as well as the psychosocial problems associated with a chronic illness. Although dialysis is often regarded as a temporary expedient until a successful transplant can be performed, in reality there are many children who have rejected transplants and developed cytotoxic antibodies and who face indefinite dialysis. It is important for pediatric nephrologists to accept the concept of dialysis as a way of life so that they can help their patients and families plan realistically for the future and, hopefully, ameliorate some of the medical and psychosocial problems associated with chronic treatment. Dialysis has been aptly described as a "half-way technology."[81] It is hoped that the next decade will see advances toward a more complete form of therapy which will allow children to lead healthier lives.

## REFERENCES

1. Henderson LW, Cotton CK, Ford C: Kinetics of hemodiafiltration. II. Clinical characterization of a new blood cleansing modality. J Lab Clin Med 85:372, 1975.
2. Cotton CK, Lowrie EG: Hemodialysis: Physical principles and technical considerations, In: Brenner BM, Rector FC (Eds), The Kidney. Philadelphia, WB Saunders, 1981, pp 2425–2489.
3. Babb AL, Farrell PC, Uvelli DA, Scribner BH: Hemodialyzer evaluation by examination of solute molecular spectra. Trans Am Soc Artif Intern Organs 18:98, 1972.
4. Funck-Brentano J-L, Mann NK, Sausse A, et al: Characterization of a 1100–1300 MW uremic neurotoxin. Trans Am Soc Artif Intern Organs 22:163, 1976.
5. Funck-Brentano J-L, Mann NK, Sausse A: Effect of more porous dialysis membranes on neuropathic toxins. Kidney Int (Suppl) 2:S552, 1975.
6. Kjellstrand CM, Evans RL, Petersen RJ, et al: The "unphysiology" of dialysis: a major cause of dialysis side effects? Kidney Int (Suppl) 2:S30, 1975.
7. Lowrie EG, Steinberg SM, Galen MA, et al: Factors in the dialysis regimen which contribute to alterations in the abnormalities of uremia. Kidney Int 10:409, 1976.
8. Babb AL, Strand MJ, Uvelli DA, et al: Quantitative description of dialysis treatment: a dialysis index. Kidney Int (Suppl) 2:S23, 1975.
9. Gardiner AOP, Sawyer AN, Donckerwolcke RA, et al: Assessment of dialysis requirement for children on regular dialysis. Dial Transplant 11:754, 1982.
10. Gotch FA, Sargent JA, Keen M, et al: Clinical results of intermittent dialysis therapy (IDT) guided by ongoing kinetic analysis of urea metabolism. Trans Am Soc Artif Intern Organs 22:175, 1976.
11. Harmon WE, Spinozzi N, Meyer A, Grupe WE: Use of protein catabolic rate to monitor pediatric dialysis. Dial Transplant 10:324, 1981.
12. Scharer K, Chantler C, Donckerwolcke RA: Paediatric dialysis. In: Drukker W, Parsons FM, Maher JF (Eds), Replacement of Renal Function by Dialysis. The Hague, Martinus Nijhoff, 1978, pp 444–461.
13. Shideman JR, Meyer RM, Streifel AJ, et al: The

evaluation and applications of hemodialyzers for pediatric patients. J Dial 2:217, 1978.

14. von Hartitzsch B, Hoenich NA: Meltec multipoint haemodialyzer. Br Med J 1:237, 1972.

15. von Hartitzsch B, Bosl R, Meyer R, et al.: Safe efficient pediatric dialysis using a new variable size disposable dialyzer. Proc Clin Dial Transplant Forum 4:115, 1974.

16. Kjellstrand CM: Hemodialysis for children. In: Friedman EA (Ed), Strategy in Renal Failure. New York, John Wiley and Sons, 1978, pp 149–174.

17. Kjellstrand CM, Shideman JR, Santiago EA: Technical advances in hemodialysis of very small pediatric patients. Proc Clin Dial Transplant Forum 1:124, 1971.

18. Kjellstrand CM, Mauer SM, Buselmeier TJ, et al: Hemodialysis of premature and newborn babies. Proc Eur Dial Transplant Assoc 10:349, 1973.

19. Kennedy AC, Linton AL, Eaton JC: Urea levels in cerebrospinal fluid after hemodialysis. Lancet 1:410, 1962.

20. Wakim KG: Predominance of hyponatremia over hypoosmolality in simulation of the dialysis dysequilibrium syndrome. Mayo Clin Proc 44:433, 1969.

21. Arieff AI, Massry SG, Barrientos A, Kleeman CR: Brain water and electrolyte metabolism in uremia: effects of slow and rapid hemodialysis. Kidney Int 4:177, 1973.

22. Rodrigo F, Shideman JR, McHugh R, et al: Osmolality changes during hemodialysis: natural history, clinical correlations and influence of glucose and mannitol. Ann Intern Med 86:554, 1977.

23. Bergstrom J, Asaka H, Furst P, Oules R: Dialysis ultrafiltration and blood pressure. Proc Eur Dial Transplant Assoc 13:293, 1976.

24. McMann BJ, deLeon LB, Weiss LS, Moore ES: Negative-pressure hydrostatic ultrafiltration in children. Dial Transplant 7:1170, 1978.

25. Novello A, Kelsch RC, Easterling RE: Acetate intolerance during dialysis. Clin Nephrol 5:29, 1976.

26. Tolchin N, Roberts JL, Hayashi J, Lewis EJ: Metabolic consequences of high mass-transfer hemodialysis. Kidney Int 11:366, 1977.

27. Kaiser BA, Potter DE, Bryant RE, et al: Acid-base changes and acetate metabolism during routine and high-efficiency hemodialysis in children. Kidney Int 19:70, 1981.

28. Graefe U, Milutinovich J, Follette WC, et al: Less dialysis-induced morbidity and vascular instability with bicarbonate in dialysate. Ann Intern Med 88:332, 1978.

29. Meadow R, Cameron JS, Ogg C: Regional service for acute and chronic dialysis of children. Lancet 2:707, 1970.

30. Pendreigh DM, Heasman MA, Howitt LF, et al: Survey of chronic renal failure in Scotland. Lancet 1:304, 1972.

31. Leumann EP: Die chronische niereninsuffizienz im kindesalter: ergebnisse einer Schweizerischen rundfrage. Schweiz Med Wochenschr 106:244, 1976.

32. Potter DE, Holliday MA, Piel CF, et al: Treatment of end-stage renal disease in children: a 15 year experience. Kidney Int 18:103, 1980.

33. Donckerwolcke RA, Chantler C, Broyer M, et al: Combined report on regular dialysis and transplantation of children in Europe, 1979. Proc Eur Dial Transplant Assoc 17:87, 1980.

34. Avner ED, Harmon WE, Grupe WE, et al: Mortality

of chronic hemodialysis and renal transplantation in pediatric end-stage renal disease. Pediatrics 67:412, 1981.

35. Wass VJ, Barratt TM, Howarth RV, et al: Home haemodialysis in children: report of the London Children's Home Dialysis Group. Lancet 1:242, 1977.

36. McEnery PT: Personal communication.

37. Donckerwolcke RA, Chantler C, Brunner FP, et al: Combined report on regular dialysis and transplantation of children in Europe, 1978. Proc Eur Dial Transplant Assoc 18:74, 1979.

38. Broyer M, Donckerwolcke RA, Brunner FP, et al: Combined report on regular dialysis and transplantation of children in Europe, 1980. Proc Eur Dial Transplant Assoc 18:59, 1981.

39. Chantler C, Broyer M, Donckerwolcke RA, et al: Growth and rehabilitation of long-term survivors of treatment for end-stage renal failure in children. Proc Eur Dial Transplant Assoc 18:329, 1981.

40. Bryan FA: The National Dialysis Registry, Seventh Annual Progress Report. Report #AK-7–1387, North Carolina, Research Triangle Park, October, 1975.

41. Scharer K, Chantler C, Brunner FP, et al: Combined report on regular dialysis and transplantation of children in Europe, 1975. Proc Eur Dial Transplant Assoc 13:59, 1976.

42. Pennisi AJ, Heuser ET, Mickey MR, et al: Hyperlipidemia in pediatric hemodialysis and renal transplant patients. Am J Dis Child 130:975, 1976.

43. Broyer M, Tete MJ, Laudat MH, Dartois AM: Plasma lipid abnormalities in children on chronic hemodialysis: relationship to dietary intake. Proc Eur Dial Transplant Assoc 13:385, 1976.

44. El-Bishti M, Counahan R, Jarrett RJ, et al: Hyperlipidemia in children on regular haemodialysis. Arch Dis Child 52:932, 1977.

45. Berger M, James GP, Davis ER, et al: Hyperlipidemia in uremic children: response to peritoneal dialysis and hemodialysis. Clin Nephrol 9:19, 1978.

46. Papadopoulou ZL, Sandler P, Tina LU, et al: Hyperlipidemia in children with chronic renal insufficiency. Pediatr Res 15:887, 1981.

47. Broyer M, Czernichow P, Tete M-J, et al: Insulin and growth hormone secretion in dialyzed children: influence of dietary manipulation. Am J Clin Nutr 31:1876, 1978.

48. Counahan R, El-Bishti M, Cox BD, et al: Plasma amino acids in children and adolescents on hemodialysis. Kidney Int 10:471, 1976.

49. El-Bishti MM, Counahan R, Bloom SR, Chantler C: Hormonal and metabolic responses to intravenous glucose in children on regular dialysis. Am J Clin Nutr 31:1865, 1978.

50. Saenger P, Wiedermann E, Schwartz E, et al: Somatomedin and growth after renal transplantation. Pediatr Res 8:163, 1974.

51. Phillips LS, Pennisi AJ, Belosky C, et al: Somatomedin activity and inorganic sulfate in children undergoing hemodialysis. J Clin Endocrinol Metab 46:165, 1978.

52. Schiffrin A, Guyda H, Robitaille P, Posner B: Increased plasma somatomedin reactivity in chronic renal failure as determined by acid gel filtration and radioreceptor assay. J Clin Endocrinol Metab 46:511, 1977.

53. Czernichow P, Dauzet MC, Broyer M, Rappaport

R: Abnormal TSH, PRL and GH response to TSH releasing factor in chronic renal failure. J Clin Endocrinol Metab 43:630, 1976.

54. Wassner SJ, Buckingham BA, Kershnar AJ, et al: Thyroid function in children with chronic renal failure. Nephron 19:236, 1977.

55. Sullivan JF, Eisenstein AB: Ascorbic acid depletion in patients undergoing chronic hemodialysis. Am J Clin Nutr 23:1339, 1970.

56. Dobbelstein H, Korner WF, Mempel W, et al: Vitamin $B_6$ deficiency in uremia and its implications for the depression of immune responses. Kidney Int 5:233, 1974.

57. Hampers CL, Streiff R, Nathan DG, et al: Megaloblastic hematopoiesis in uremia and in patients on long-term hemodialysis. N Engl J Med 276:557, 1967.

58. Smith FR, Goodman OS: The effects of diseases of liver, thyroid and kidneys on the transport of vitamin A in human plasma. J Clin Invest 50:2426, 1971.

59. Mansouri K, Halsted J, Gombos EA: Zinc, copper, magnesium and calcium in dialyzed and nondialyzed uremic patients. Arch Intern Med 125:88, 1970.

60. Lindsey RM, Briggs JD, Luke RB, et al: Gynecomastia in chronic renal failure. Br Med J 4:779, 1967.

61. Rice GG: Hypermenorrhea in the young hemodialysis patient. Am J Obstet Gynecol 116:539, 1973.

62. Levy NB: Sexual adjustment to maintenance hemodialysis and renal transplantation: national survey by questionnaire: preliminary report. Trans Am Soc Artif Intern Organs 19:138, 1973.

63. Byron PR, Mallick NP, Taylor G: Immune potential in human uremia. 2. Changes after regular haemodialysis therapy. J Clin Pathol 29:770, 1976.

64. Eknoyan G, Dichoso C, Hyde S, Yium J: "Overflow ascites"—the safety valve of the volume-expanded patient on dialysis. Proc Clin Dial Transplant Forum 3:156, 1973.

65. Berne TV, Bischel MD, Payne JW, Barbour BH: Selective splenectomy in chronic renal failure. Am J Surg 126:271, 1973.

66. Stewart JH, Castaldi PA: Uraemic bleeding: a reversible platelet defect corrected by dialysis. Quart J Med 36:409, 1967.

67. Leonard CD, Weil E, Scribner BH: Subdural hematomas in patients undergoing hemodialysis. Lancet 2:239, 1969.

68. Harrison PB, Jansson K, Kronenberg H, et al: Cold agglutinin formation in patients undergoing hemodialysis. A possible relationship to dialyser reuse. Aust N Z J Med 5:195, 1975.

69. Leong S-Y, Disney APS, Gove DW: Spallation and migration of silicone from blood-pump tubing in patients on hemodialysis. N Engl J Med 306:135, 1982.

70. Wander JW, Moore EJ, Jonasson O: Internal arteriovenous fistulae for dialysis in children. J Pediatr Surg 5:553, 1970.

71. Perez-Alvarez JJ, Vargas-Rosendo R, Gutierrez-Bosque R, et al: A new type of subcutaneous arteriovenous fistula for chronic hemodialysis in children. Surgery 67:355, 1970.

72. D'Apuzzo VG, Grushkin CM, Brennan LP, et al: Saphenous vein autograft arteriovenous fistula for extended hemodialysis in children. Acta Pediatr Scand 62:28, 1973.

73. Gagnodoux MF, Pascal B, Bronstein M, et al: Arteriovenous fistulae in small children. Dial Transplant 9:318, 1980.

74. Kinnaert P, Jannssen F, Hall M, van Geertruyden J: Hemodialysis techniques in young children. Surgery 86:906, 1979.

75. Bourquelot P, Wolfeler L, Lamy L: Microsurgery for haemodialysis distal arteriovenous fistulae in children weighing less than 10 kg. Proc Eur Dial Transplant Assoc 18:537, 1981.

76. Sicard GA, Merrell RC, Etheredge EE, Anderson CB: Subcutaneous arteriovenous fistulas in pediatric patients. Trans Am Soc Artif Intern Organs 24:695, 1978.

77. Belzer FO, Kountz SL: Arteriovenous Quinton-Scribner shunt with the profunda femoris artery and saphenous vein. Surgery 70:443, 1971.

78. O'Regan S, Villemant D, Ducharme G, et al: Effects of Brescia-Cimino fistulae on myocardial function in pediatric patients. Dial Transplant 10:202, 1981.

79. Potter D, Larsen D, Leumann E, et al: Treatment of chronic uremia in childhood. II. Hemodialysis. Pediatrics 46:678, 1970.

80. Baum M, Powell D, Calvin S, et al: Continuous ambulatory peritoneal dialysis in children: comparison with hemodialysis. N Engl J Med 307:1537, 1982.

81. Thomas L: Notes of a biology-watcher. The technology of medicine. N Engl J Med 285:1366, 1971.

# Infant Hemodialysis

*Thomas E. Nevins, M.D.*
*S. Michael Mauer, M.D.*

In the mid-1940s, adults were first successfully hemodialyzed in Europe.[1] Initially, the techniques were primitive, cumbersome, and dangerous. The technology rapidly evolved, and within 10 years, although still difficult, adult hemodialysis was considerably more reliable. In the next decade older children with acute and chronic renal failure were treated in adult dialysis centers.[2, 3] As pediatric dialysis equipment became available, younger and smaller children were treated with hemodialysis.[4–6] In the last decade smaller children and infants have been the direct beneficiaries of improvements in equipment, technology, and clinical experience.[7–9] Originally, hemodialysis was seen only as a temporizing measure for small children with acute renal failure. However, as the feasibility of renal transplantation in infants and young children was clearly demonstrated,[10, 11] the indications for hemodialysis in infancy have broadened. Today it is possible to safely and reliably treat infants with chronic hemodialysis.[12] An absolute lower limit in size and weight for hemodialysis patients has not been precisely defined; however, we have hemodialyzed premature infants as small as 1500 grams for several weeks with only modest difficulties.

Since the general principles of hemodialysis in children have already been reviewed (Chapter 4), here we will focus almost exclusively on the technique of hemodialysis as applied to infants and young children who, although chronologically older, have the body mass of an infant. The discussion will include both the technical aspects of hemodialysis and, where appropriate, the clinical principles which have direct application to infant dialysis.

## INDICATIONS FOR HEMODIALYSIS

The indications for hemodialysis in infancy tend to be similar to those in older children and adults. A difficulty that logically arises in discussing these indications is that there are few specific biochemical values which can be viewed as absolute. For example, a small child with hemolytic-uremic syndrome may be anuric with a serum potassium in the upper normal range and a hemoglobin count of 3 grams. Although neither value mandates dialysis, it is clear that this child will not be able to be safely transfused without careful attention to intravascular volume status and that the serum potassium will further increase in proportion to the severity of the continuing hemolysis and the amount of potassium in the transfused blood. It is logical in this setting to hemodialyze the child to allow rapid and safe restoration of the circulating red cell mass while avoiding the serious complications of volume expansion and hyperkalemia. At the same time, hemodialysis offers the secondary benefits of correcting pre-existing fluid overload, hypocalcemia, hyperphosphatemia, and acidosis. With this background, the general risk factors constituting indications for dialysis may be discussed.

Fluid overload in the presence of oliguria or anuria is a relative indication for dialysis. Patients with evolving acute renal failure or fixed chronic renal failure may initially appear to be euvolemic. In spite of this, the requirement for parenteral fluids, sodium bicarbonate, or blood products, as well as the fluid intake required to maintain adequate nutrition, means that the patient will shortly develop significant volume expansion with resultant edema and ascites. Particularly dangerous with fluid overload is the development of hypertension, congestive heart failure, and pulmonary edema. In this setting, in view of the patient's need for additional fluid therapy, hemodialysis is an appropriate method to restore or maintain the patient's euvolemic status. Recognition of this clinical situation avoids significant nutritional impairment due to prolonged periods of severe fluid restriction.

Along these lines, it is our experience that small children with severe congenital nephrotic syndrome may suffer profound failure to thrive despite aggressive efforts to maximize nutrition and the administration of parenteral albumin, potent diuretics, and prophylactic antibiotics. In this situation, bilateral nephrectomy effectively substitutes chronic uremia and hemodialysis for profound proteinuria and is frequently associated with a significant improvement in both the patient's well-being and nutrition.

Still other patients, following cardiovascular surgery, may receive excessive fluids to maintain an appropriate cardiac output, but their decreased renal perfusion leads to fluid overload. In some of these patients it may be necessary to undertake emergency dialysis to control both the peripheral and pulmonary edema that results from hypervolemia. In several instances, we have witnessed a marked improvement in both cardiac function and tissue perfusion following aggressive ultrafiltration in patients with severe postoperative fluid overload. Other children have had persistent and severe hypotension which restricted ultrafiltration despite the administration of cardiotonic drugs. In general, this is a poor prognostic sign, although continued and intensive support has occasionally been rewarded with a decreased colloid requirement, improved myocardial function, and greatly increased tolerance for dialysis and ultrafiltration.

Hyperkalemia is universally recognized as a critical indication for the initiation of dialysis. Most clinicians would agree that potassium values above 6 to 6.5 meq/L constitute an indication for immediate therapy. In evaluating the individual patient's serum potas-

sium level, it is also important to examine the electrocardiogram for evidence of hyperkalemic effects on the myocardium. Again, the numerical value for an infant's serum potassium must be considered in the context of several factors. First, infants have a range of normal serum potassium which is slightly higher than that of older children. A more important consideration is the rate at which the serum potassium is changing, since patients with serum potassium levels that are rising at a rate of more than 2 meq in 24 hours[13] should certainly be considered at greater risk than stable patients. In situations with renal impairment and ongoing tissue catabolism with cell injury due to hemolysis, anoxia, infection, infarction, or significant tumor lysis, "earlier" dialysis must be considered. As 98% of total body potassium is intracellular, shifts in serum pH may abruptly present increased amounts of potassium to the extracellular space and acutely raise serum potassium. Since calcium counteracts the effect of potassium on the myocardial cell membrane, hypocalcemia, frequently seen in infants and in children with acute renal failure, may seriously aggravate the cardiotoxicity of a moderate elevation in serum potassium.

Acute measures to control hyperkalemia include the intravenous administration of calcium and sodium bicarbonate, as well as glucose and insulin, and the use of sodium polystyrene resin orally and rectally. Generally, these therapies are temporary in effect, and in patients with serious renal impairment dialysis is usually necessary to finally restore appropriate potassium balance.

Severe acidosis per se is not usually an indication for dialysis; however, in patients with extensive tissue injury or profound systemic hypoperfusion and associated lactate accumulation, the severity of acidosis may constitute an indication for dialysis. Further, in the presence of associated renal impairment, the administration of sodium bicarbonate in the required quantities may result in severe hypernatremia and fluid overload. In this situation emergency dialysis with a bicarbonate dialysate provides effective therapy. However, peritoneal dialysis may potentially further complicate the situation by its effects on lung capacity and cardiac output.[14, 15]

Uremia per se is often an indication for dialysis. Again, there is no specific critical level of BUN or creatinine. Rather, the recognition of a rising BUN and creatinine level that could lead to pericarditis, uremic coagulopathy, gastrointestinal bleeding, and neurobehavioral dysfunction should stimulate earlier intervention. Additional caveats are necessary when considering dialysis therapy in uremic infants and small children. Since creatinine is a metabolite of muscle, its serum level is a composite reflection of total muscle mass and renal function. Therefore, an infant with a relatively small muscle mass will normally have a low serum creatinine. The normal serum creatinine in a child between 18 months and two years is about 0.4 mg/dl.[16] It is slightly lower in the first year of life. Normal values reflect ongoing maturation of renal function during the first year.[17] Consequently, a serum creatinine level of 3 or 4 mg/dl in the first year of life, though not an alarming value in older children or adults, probably reflects a loss of more than 80 to 90% of the normal renal function for an infant. A second concern involves the rapidity of change; that is, a child with a serum creatinine level rising at a rate of more than 1 mg/dl/day is more likely to need dialysis in the near future than a child who has a higher but stable serum creatinine level. Urea values in infants and young children are much more widely variable and reflect dietary composition, glomerular filtration rate (GFR), and catabolic stresses (surgery, infection, gastrointestinal bleeding, steroid therapy, etc.).

A final caution in this area concerns the fact that many children with renal failure in the first year of life will maintain a significant solute diuresis. Usually, the solutes are BUN, sodium, and non-reabsorbed ions. If such a child has an abrupt decrease in oral intake secondary to an intercurrent illness with vomiting and diarrhea, or if the child enters the hospital and is inappropriately placed on a sodium restricted diet because of the diagnosis of renal disease, one may be faced with a situation in which the solute diuresis leads to volume depletion with a rapid fall in GFR and compromise of the remaining renal function. Similarly, an abrupt solute load, as a result of changing from infant formula to cow's milk or the administration of intravenous contrast media, may also lead to additional diuresis, volume depletion, and reduced GFR. A careful physical examination with particular attention to signs of fluid overload or fluid depletion as well as a review of serial weight, blood pressure, heart rate, and records of daily fluid intake and output will usually lead the clinician to the correct diagnosis. If the patient is found to be clinically volume-depleted, a trial of fluid replacement is appropriate since this cause of decreased GFR is frequently reversible. If this trial is unsuccessful, then the availability of hemodialysis offers an opportunity to rapidly restore normal fluid balance.

Finally, a few unique situations arise in the newborn in which initiation of emergency hemodialysis may be life-saving. Poisonings or drug overdoses may dramatically reverse with hemodialysis or hemoperfusion (discussed below). Hyperammonemia in the newborn period represents a rare form of endogenous intoxication. It has been shown that hemodialysis removes approximately ten times as much ammonia as peritoneal dialysis.[18] Emergency hemodialysis allows the immediate treatment of unstable patients in coma and provides time for less efficient peritoneal dialysis treatments to be instituted as well as therapy with parenteral arginine, sodium benzoate, and the nitrogen-free analogs of essential amino acids.[19]

As is often the case in clinical medicine, the decision regarding institution of dialysis is not solely dependent on laboratory values but more often an admixture of clinical findings and judgments. On one hand, for example, the child who has rapidly developed acute renal failure is likely initially to have serious problems with fluid balance, acidosis, and hyperkalemia while maintaining BUN and creatinine values that are not markedly abnormal. On the other hand, many children with chronic renal failure will gradually develop significant elevations of BUN and serum creatinine levels, while often not having severe problems with hypertension, fluid overload, or hyperkalemia and at the same time developing appropriate respiratory compensation for their metabolic acidosis. Finally, the decision will depend on a balance of the risks of the patient's disorder versus the risk of dialysis therapy. As the individual dialysis center gains experience and ability in the hemodialysis of infants, the indications for this therapy will broaden.

Very often a major indication for the institution of dialysis therapy in infants and tiny children with chronic renal insufficiency is complete failure to thrive despite aggressive efforts at optimizing more conservative medical management, including nutrition, blood pressure regulation, adjustment of fluid balance, and treatment of acidosis, hyperphosphatemia, and bone disease. It is our view that dialysis in these children is only preparative for renal transplantation,[20] and, therefore, prolonged dialysis with attendant problems of blood access, nutritional limitations, and bone disease, as well as emotional and financial stresses, represents an unwise treatment plan. This presents the responsible physician with difficult moral, ethical, and medical dilemmas. It is clear that infants reaching a weight of 5.5 to 6 kg and 6 to 8 months of age can undergo successful living related adult donor renal transplantation[21] with patient and graft survival results essentially identical to those of older children or adults. It is equally clear that, to date, success with the transplantation of pediatric cadaver kidneys into smaller and younger babies has been spotty,[22, 23] and awaiting such donors obligates the patient to long-term dialysis. It is not too difficult, based on these results, to decide that a trial of dialysis therapy may be worthwhile for a 5-month-old baby weighing 5 kg since it is reasonable to hope that, following one or two months of treatment, the child may be big and strong enough to undergo transplantation. Is this a reasonable plan for the 2-month-old baby weighing 3.5 kg with terminal uremia? Does the time, effort, expense, and family stress as well as the potential for failure justify aggressive treatment? Is one form of dialysis treatment more likely successful than another in these circumstances? At present these questions remain unanswered.

Finally, it is clear that children uremic from birth are delayed in psychomotor as well as physical development and often manifest serious neurologic abnormalities.[24] Should these children receive dialysis and transplant therapy? Will earlier treatment positively influence the developmental outcome of uremic infants? Data addressing these issues are sparse. Although provocative and gratifying improvements in neurologic status have been seen in successfully transplanted small children,[20] much more work in this area is required before meaningful guidelines for infant dialysis and transplantation can be provided.

## EQUIPMENT

The equipment used for infant hemodialysis is similar to that used in older children. However, owing to the smaller body mass and blood volume of an infant, special dialyzers, blood lines, and monitoring procedures are required.

In any form of dialysis, access is the most fragile link in the chain. Infant blood access presents some unique situations. Although the blood flowing to the dialyzer per minute is reduced proportionally to the child's size, the problem of obtaining and maintaining access to the vascular space of a small child is 'disproportionately difficult. Standard hemodialysis access with a Scribner shunt is technically feasible even in infants,[25] and appropriate size Silastic shunt tubing and Teflon vessel tips are available. Generally, the shunt sites are limited to four prime areas including the superficial femoral artery and the saphenous vein as well as the brachial artery and cephalic or basilic vein bilaterally. As with the construction of any shunt, meticulous care and attention to detail are rewarded with success. In small children with reduced subcutaneous tissue, bulky shunt materials are avoided and care must be taken to avoid tension or torsion at the site of insertion of the shunt tips. As is true for any shunt, it is best to use the largest vessel tips which can be accommodated to ensure good blood flow, while avoiding excessively large vessel tips that create obstructing intimal flaps.

Unique to the perinatal period, infants have large umbilical vessels available for cannulation. The flow from these vessels is more than adequate for hemodialysis. Standard Silastic or polyvinyl chloride umbilical vessel catheters may be inserted and connected directly to hemodialysis equipment. Between dialysis treatments, the umbilical catheters may be used for infusion of fluids and medications and for monitoring arterial blood gases.

Percutaneous vascular access by means of the Seldinger technique has been used in infants for cardiac catheterization and placement of central lines[26] and may also be used for hemodialysis access. Standard femoral vein (Shaldon) catheters are too large for safe use in children less than 10 kg. However, once a guide wire has been positioned intravascularly, a number of smaller catheters (polyethylene tubing–190 or 240) are available which can be safely inserted, with the aid of vein dilators, and maintained for a period of time in femoral vessels. In addition, direct surgical placement of catheters is possible in the femoral vessels and the larger vessels of the neck. Polyvinyl chloride catheters in these sites may serve as temporary vascular access. The advantage of using these catheters is that they are frequently already present in critically ill children or may be placed utilizing only local anesthesia on a relatively acute basis.

A modification of this technique which has been very successful is the use of a silicone rubber (Silastic) right atrial catheter (Hickman catheter),[27] which will be discussed later. It may be used short term (weeks to several months) until the need for dialysis resolves or a more permanent access is available. Extensive experience with Silastic catheters exists in oncology patients and in patients requiring long-term hyperalimentation.[28, 29] Based on this experience, the catheter appears less thrombogenic and less subject to infection than other catheters. A further advantage of the Hickman catheter is that its placement does not require the same level of technical expertise required for the creation of a Scribner shunt in patients of the same size. The Broviac catheter is unsuited to hemodialysis since its internal diameter (1.0 mm) is too small to permit adequate blood flow.

Finally, it has been possible, utilizing microsurgical technique, to create arteriovenous fistulae in children weighing less than 10 kg.[30] There is also some experience with the use of polytetrafluoroethylene grafts to create fistulae in smaller children.[31] It is obvious that this approach in the first year of life is technically very demanding; however, in expert hands, success rates with 90% patency have been achieved. In general, however, the technique is not useful for infant dialysis since the need is usually more immediate, and relatively long periods of maturation are required for the fistulae to be usable. But in selected cases these approaches may have important applications.

## Dialyzers

As will be discussed, the choice of equipment must be made with conscious attention to the size and blood volume of the patient. In the past a number of pediatric dialyzers have been examined.[32] Only one currently available dialyzer is suited, however, to the needs of an infant or small child weighing less than 10 kg, and that is the Gambro Mini-Minor (Gambro USA, Barrington, IL 60010).

This dialyzer is constructed with five parallel plates of 13.5 micron thick Cuprophan and has an effective surface area of 0.23 m². The static priming volume of the dialyzer is approximately 19 ml, and the volume increases 6 ml for every 100 mm Hg of transmembrane pressure. The combination of a relatively small priming volume and low compliance makes this dialyzer particularly useful in smaller children. At the same time, the dialyzer has appropriate clearance and ultrafiltration characteristics at clinically achievable blood flows and transmembrane pressures (Fig. 5–1, A and B).

If a larger dialyzer is required, we use the Gambro Lundia Minor. This dialyzer has a total blood volume of 29 ml and a compliance of 10 ml/100 mm Hg. Although too large for routine use in a child of less than 8 to 10 kg, certain clinical situations may warrant use of the Lundia Minor when improved clearance or ultrafiltration characteristics are necessary. In these instances the dialyzer could be adapted to the small child by priming the entire system with donor red blood cells or 5% albumin prior to initiating dialysis, thereby minimizing the contribution of the patient's own blood volume to the extracorporeal circuit.

The final components of the dialysis system are the blood lines used to connect the infant to the blood pump and dialyzer. Because of the special constraints imposed by dialysis of very small children, we routinely use "neonatal" blood lines with a volume of approximately 15 ml manufactured by Extracorporeal (King of Prussia, PA). If longer lines are required, pediatric blood lines (Extracorporeal, King of Prussia, PA) with a volume of 52 ml may be used and the entire system primed with blood or colloid. For critically ill infants the pediatric blood lines are recommended since their extra length allows easier patient access for manipulation or resuscitation.

In defining safe volume relationships for infant dialysis, it is necessary to follow the general principle used in older children and adults, that the extracorporeal circuit should not contain more than 10% of the patient's blood volume. In estimating an infant's blood volume a factor of about 8% of total body dry weight may be used. Therefore, to safely dialyze a 10 kg child, the dialysis circuit should be less than 80 ml. In a 3 kg child that volume should not exceed 24 ml. In the circuit described above, the combination of

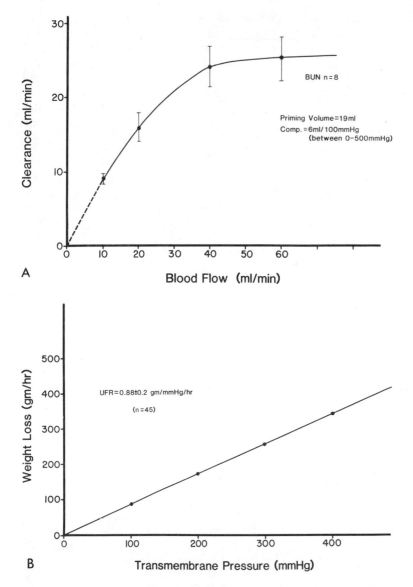

**Figure 5–1.** *A,* The in vivo BUN clearance data for the Gambro Mini-Minor as a function of blood flow. *B,* The in vivo rate of ultrafiltration for the Gambro Mini-Minor at various total transmembrane pressures. (Data kindly supplied by Mr. James Ebben, Regional Kidney Disease Program, Minneapolis.)

the Gambro Mini-Minor and neonatal blood lines is approximately 40 ml, and again volume may be expected to increase by 6 ml for every additional 100 mm Hg of transmembrane pressure. That system then should be appropriate for a child weighing 5 kg or more, but for the child less than 5 kg additional care and concern are necessary.

In practice, children under 5 kg receive a "blood prime" for the first several dialyses. When these small children have proved to be stable on chronic dialysis it is possible to prime the system with 5% albumin and have additional blood available in the blood bank to transfuse the patient if a technical problem leads to unexpected blood loss. At the end of each dialysis when a "blood prime" has

been used, a clinical judgment must be made to transfuse the extra blood back into the patient. If this risks inappropriate volume expansion and hypertension, the blood pump may be shut off and the blood lines clamped, thereby nullifying the volume effect of the "blood prime." Note that priming with packed red blood cells (hematocrit > 60%) will lead to a predictable net increase in the patient's red cell mass even if the lines are clamped.

## Other Equipment

While the guidelines for infant dialysis parallel those for older children and adults, the patients must be monitored more closely, and critical attention must be paid to maintaining homeostasis. In order to do this, additional equipment which is not generally required for adults may be needed.

First, the infants' vital signs must be followed closely. Pulse is continuously monitored with a cardiac monitor. Blood pressure is followed using either a direct arterial transducer in the most critically ill patients or, more routinely, a standard sphygmomanometer or a Doppler equipped blood pressure cuff.

Critically ill infants are at risk for hypothermia. Transportation to the dialysis unit, handling, and the hemodialysis treatment itself may all be complicating factors which lead to further loss of body heat. In the small infant, core temperature is continuously measured with a rectal probe during the dialysis treatment. A free-standing infrared heater may be necessary to warm the child, even if the dialysate is heated to 40–41° C (the highest temperature compatible with avoiding hemolysis). If ultrafiltration alone is performed, the absence of warm dialysate leads to a marked cooling of the patient's blood and hypothermia. For this reason, an overhead heater is mandatory during the ultrafiltration.

Finally, it is of critical importance in small children and infants to continuously and accurately record their body weight during hemodialysis.[33] We use a special electronic bed scale attached to a crib (James Addison Potter Co., West Hartford, CT). This equipment permits the detection of weight changes in the range of 5 to 10 grams, even when weights in excess of 75 kg are in the crib. This degree of precision is necessary if one is to safely dialyze a small child. In order to take full advantage of this equipment, several precautions are necessary. Before beginning the dialysis treatment, all necessary equipment is placed within the crib. Dialyzer blood lines, respirator tubing, intravenous tubing, electrical cables for monitoring equipment, and any other equipment attached to the child is then secured to the railing of the bed with tape in order not to alter the weight of the bed by repositioning of equipment. These lines are then taped a second time to a free-standing platform adjacent to the bed which is attached to the non-weighing frame of the scale, so that traction on the lines does not produce traction on the bed scale (Fig. 5–2). Finally, since some damping is inherent in the system, especially with double taping, the bed scale is maintained at a zero value continuously during the dialysis by the addition of small weights to the bed, compensating for patient weight loss.

When this system is properly operating, the addition or removal of 5-gram weights to or from the bed should be readily detected by the scale. Unless this level of accuracy is present and can be maintained, there are very real risks in attempting to dialyze a small child. Sudden changes in pressure within the dialysis system will alter both the ultrafiltration rate and the blood volume of the dialyzer, leading to unexpected weight loss fol-

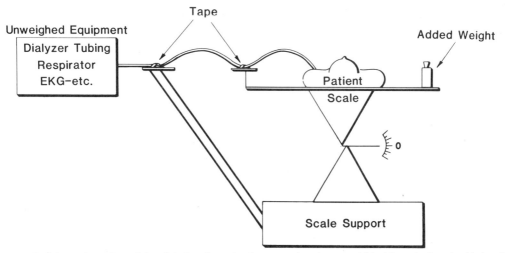

**Figure 5–2.** Schematic outline of the dialysis crib-scale, demonstrating the use of "double taping" and added weights to maximize scale sensitivity. (From Kjellstrand CM, et al., Proc Clin Dial Transplant Forum, 1:124, 1971.)

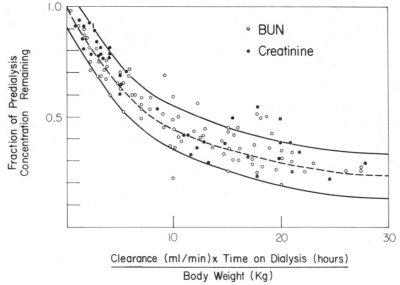

**Figure 5–3.** The curve depicts the decline in serum BUN and creatinine in small children as a function of clearance per kilogram and hours of dialysis. The dashed line is the best fit curve for these data. This curve is an invaluable guide to the hemodialysis prescription for children. (From Kjellstrand CM, et al., Proc Eur Dial Transplant Assoc, 10:349, 1973.)

lowed by hypotension. If one is unable to identify these volume shifts, hemodialysis of the critically ill infant will not only be unsuccessful but will pose a serious hazard to the child.

## DIALYSIS TECHNIQUE

As alluded to above, hemodialysis is actually a composite of two separable operations: dialysis per se and ultrafiltration. Since the ultrafiltration and dialysis characteristics of individual dialyzers are already known, the physician can predict and control both the timing and magnitude of each operation.

Earlier workers have described the variables which determine the magnitude of solute removal by dialysis. They include blood flow rate, dialysate flow rate, concentration, molecular size, protein or lipid binding of the solute, clearance characteristics of the individual dialyzer, and the duration of dialysis. Grouping some of these terms and measuring actual blood values have produced curves which predict the fractional disappearance rate for BUN and creatinine as a function of clearance and time (Fig. 5–3).[8] An examination of these curves reveals a rapid disappearance rate at the time when the serum concentration of each solute is the highest. Using the available clearance curves for a

dialyzer it is possible to prescribe a blood flow rate proportional to a clearance rate which will result in a gradual and well-tolerated fall in serum osmolality. Initially, our patients are dialyzed at a clearance rate equal to 1.5 ml to 2.0 ml/kg/min. Stable patients will tolerate clearance values of 3 ml/kg/min.[34] The usual duration of individual dialysis treatments is 4 to 6 hours. These treatments regularly lead to the removal of approximately 2/3 of the predialysis BUN and creatinine and result in minimal symptoms associated with osmolar flux.

Further, if the patient is subject to significant osmotic changes during dialysis (a decrease of more than 20 mOsm as with BUN greater than 100 mg/dl or sodium over 140 meq/L), mannitol should be administered at a rate of 1 gm/kg of body weight during the dialysis treatment in order to moderate the osmotic shift.[35] The most important practical lesson is that children with significant elevations of their serum osmolality should receive frequent (daily) dialyses at lower clearances for shorter periods (3 to 5 hours). Once the risk of sudden osmotic shifts with disequilibration, seizures, and even death is reduced, a chronic (thrice weekly) dialysis schedule may begin. Also, since dialysis removes a number of medications, particularly antibiotics and anticonvulsants, it is necessary to determine if the patient should receive additional doses, either during the dialysis treatment or immediately afterward.[36]

In evaluating the infant for dialysis a number of decisions are made prior to the initiation of the actual hemodialysis. The composition of the dialysate bath with regard to sodium, calcium, phosphorus, and potassium may all be varied according to the individual patient. Also, in patients with lactic acidosis, evidence of severe circulatory problems, or hepatic dysfunction, a decision to substitute sodium bicarbonate for acetate in the dialysate may be appropriate. As noted earlier, since it is important to maintain normothermia, the dialysate should be warmed to 40° C unless the infant is febrile.

A final decision regards the need for ultrafiltration and is based on the patient's cardiovascular status, blood pressure, and clinical examination. An ideal "dry weight" goal is set and total transmembrane pressures during the dialysis treatment are adjusted to produce the required weight loss gradually. If hypotension limits ultrafiltration, mannitol, albumin, packed red blood cells, or other appropriate colloids may be used to achieve the desired weight loss.

The infant, on reaching the hemodialysis unit, is transferred into the dialysis crib, and the various monitoring devices previously described are attached. Initially, the child is evaluated and, if necessary, stabilized before the actual dialysis treatment is begun. During this time measuring the patient's level of arterial oxygenation may be important, since it is well recognized that the patient is likely to experience some hypoxemia at the beginning of hemodialysis,[37] and additional inspired oxygen may be necessary. When the patient is ready, the necessary vascular connections are made and hemodialysis begins. Initially, the blood pump operates at a minimal rate in order to verify that the entire circuit is open and functioning. Then every 5 or 10 minutes the blood flow is increased stepwise until the prescribed flow is reached.

During dialysis, patients are systemically anticoagulated with heparin, infused initially at a rate of 0.6–0.8 units/kg/min over the first 15 to 30 minutes; the infusion rate is subsequently adjusted according to the Lee-White clotting time, and monitored throughout the dialysis at frequent intervals.[38] An effort is made to maintain the clotting time no greater than 150% of the predialysis value. In patients who are considered to be at risk for bleeding, protamine may be infused at the

end of dialysis in an amount calculated to counteract one-half of the total administered heparin dose (approximately 1 mg of protamine per 200 units of heparin). Regional heparinization has been used in some older children with active bleeding. However, the technique is cumbersome, requires frequent coagulation testing, and carries with it the additional risk of rebound heparinization 2 to 3 hours after dialysis is completed.[39]

To repeat, throughout the dialysis treatment itself, the patient's temperature, vital signs, and weight loss are continuously observed. Blood flow rate, venous resistance, total transmembrane pressure, and dialysate flow rate are also recorded. Combining these data, it is possible to closely follow the patient's status and adjust the dialysis technique to meet the patient's requirements.

In general, infant hemodialysis should not be seen as onerous, but rather as an opportunity to correct a number of significant metabolic derangements over a fairly short period of time. Some critically ill infants may derive the greatest benefit from the rapidity with which hemodialysis can restore them to a more normal fluid and electrolyte balance. Furthermore, during dialysis patients may receive supplements of sodium bicarbonate, calcium, parenteral nutrition, and blood products at rates and in quantities not usually practical or safe on the ward. Generally, it is not useful to measure serum electrolyte concentrations during dialysis because these values are not in equilibrium and rather tend to reflect the composition of the dialysate. However, in patients with critical hyperkalemia, hypocalcemia, hypoglycemia, or hyperammonemia frequent determinations of these values may be of practical assistance in specific directing or adjusting of the dialysis treatment.

## SPECIAL SITUATIONS

As noted earlier, hemodialysis may be of particular benefit to infants suffering from an intoxication or neonatal hyperammonemia. In these children, as with adults, major therapeutic benefits may be obtained by dramatically augmenting the removal of the offending agent from the patient's blood. To this end, much higher clearance rates than are customarily used for uremic infants may be appropriate, provided that the serum osmolality and electrolyte values are near normal. In these situations, it is possible to gradually increase the patient's blood flow, as tolerated, to obtain clearances in the range of 10 to 12 ml/kg/min with corresponding improvement in the toxin removal. Anticipating this special situation for an individual patient, it is useful to select a dialyzer capable of higher clearance rates and compensate for the increased dialyzer volume by priming the system with donor blood. At these very high clearance rates, particular attention must be paid to the dialysate composition since the use of dialysate without potassium or phosphorus in a nonuremic patient will rapidly produce clinically important hypokalemia or hypophosphatemia.

Hemodialysis should be considered in a variety of circumstances. Recently, at this institution, a 3.5 kg infant could not be taken off cardiopulmonary bypass because of hyperkalemia (11 meq/L). Hemodialysis was instituted in the operating room by means of blood directly from the bypass apparatus. High clearance rates brought the potassium to 8 meq/L within 30 minutes, allowing resumption of a normal cardiac rhythm.

In other clinical situations, fluid removal may be the major goal of treatment. As with adults,[40] this can be accomplished most efficiently by maintaining appropriate transmembrane pressures while not circulating dialysate through the dialyzer. Since this technique removes an ultrafiltrate of plasma, oncotic pressure rises in the vascular space, speeding the mobilization of interstitial fluid, and supporting the patient's vascular volume and blood pressure. In some patients who require dialysis as well, ultrafiltration can be performed for 1 to 3 hours followed by dialysis for an appropriate length of time. In others, ultrafiltration may be the only treatment required.

With ultrafiltration, some special concerns may arise. First, ultrafiltration will remove some buffer-base, and pre-existent hyperkalemia may be aggravated. This situation may be further complicated by transient hypoxemia. If the patient's potassium is over 5.5 meq/L, we would choose to begin hemodialysis and perform the necessary ultrafiltration during the dialysis treatment. A second and consistent problem is hypothermia. As noted above, the patient's blood is cooled as it flows through the circuit, and since there is no warmed dialysate in contact with the dialysis membrane, the cooled blood is returned to the patient. Even with the use of a radiant warmer over the patient, ultrafiltration alone may lower the small patient's temperature and thus limit the duration of ultrafiltration. Finally, if the dialyzer membrane develops a blood leak, there may be a delay in recognition owing to the reduced flow of fluid through the dialysate compartment. Nevertheless, for a small child such a leak can rapidly lead to serious volume loss, especially in an infant with a large percentage of the blood volume already in the extracorporeal circuit. During ultrafiltration the patient requires constant observation. Blood should be available if transfusion is required, and a total transmembrane pressure of 400 mm Hg should not be exceeded, since membrane rupture is a frequent problem above this level.

The technique of exchange transfusion may also be incorporated into hemodialysis when it is indicated. It may be beneficial to do so in disseminated intravascular coagulation or severe anemia complicating the course of acute renal failure. Exchange transfusion and dialysis may be useful in combined liver and renal failure, although at present its efficacy is unproved. The equipment to perform the exchange transfusion is spliced into the arterial blood line as it comes from the patient (Fig. 5–4), and the exchange transfusion is performed in the usual manner, withdrawing patient blood and replacing it with an equal volume of donor blood. An exchange transfusion during hemodialysis has the added benefit of dialyzing the exchanged blood, thereby reducing the administered load of citrate, potassium, and hydrogen ions. If the patient has a "single-needle" access, the exchange circuit is interposed between the patient and the unipuncture clamp, and the exchange cycles are synchronized to the blood pump so that blood is withdrawn from the patient with minimal venous admixture and exchanged blood is infused into the dialyzer when the blood pump is on.

It is also possible to treat infants with charcoal hemoperfusion[41] if this treatment is necessary to remove specific toxins or if it is thought to be a potential benefit for a patient with liver failure. Again, the extracorporeal circuit is arranged in exactly the same manner as for adults and older children (Fig. 5–5). The larger volumes required will necessitate priming the circuit with donor red cells, and the marked fall of platelets, calcium, and glucose which may occur re-

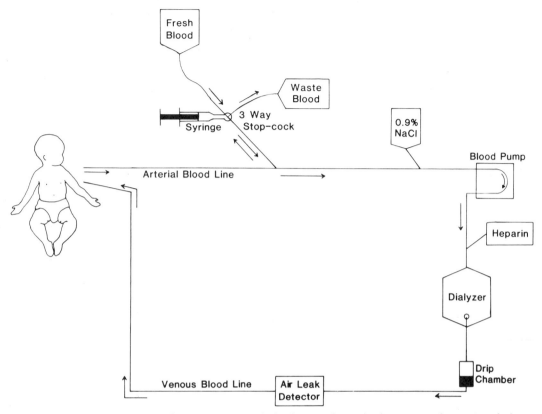

**Figure 5–4.** Schematic outline of the extracorporeal circuit to perform simultaneous exchange transfusion and hemodialysis in an infant.

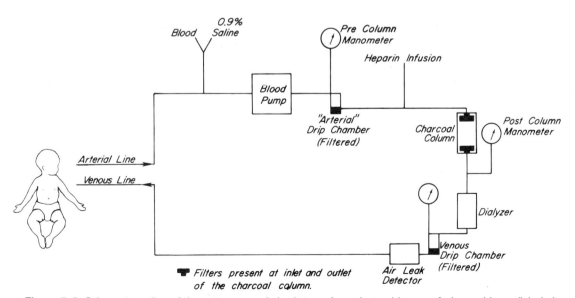

**Figure 5–5.** Schematic outline of the extracorporeal circuit to perform charcoal hemoperfusion and hemodialysis in an infant. Note the three manometers in the circuit to detect increasing pressure gradients associated with progressive clotting of the column, the dialyser, or the drip chambers. (Adapted from Chavers et al.; Reprinted from Kidney International 18:386–389, 1980 with permission.)

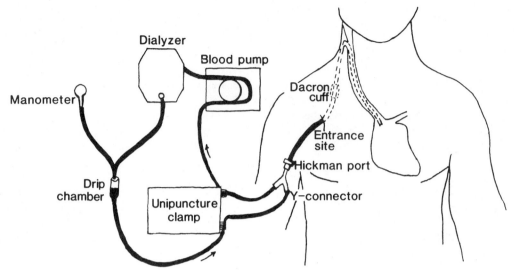

**Figure 5–6.** Outline of the "single needle" circuit used with a Hickman catheter as blood access to allow hemodialysis of an infant. The subcutaneous and intravascular portions of the catheter are illustrated with dashed lines.

quires careful monitoring and supplementation as necessary. Recent animal studies confirm the clinical impression that charcoal hemoperfusion carries significant risks. Infant pigs treated only with hemoperfusion developed fatal electrolyte disturbances and hypothermia (Chavers, personal communication). These problems are possibly reduced in human infants by the addition of hemodialysis.

Small, critically ill infants generally tolerate changes in their circulating blood volume relatively poorly. For this reason, an approach to hemodialysis in these children should generally utilize two separate blood cannulae, one for the arterial circuit removing blood from the patient and the other for the venous circuit returning the dialyzed blood to the patient. The advantage of this situation is that the blood pump runs continuously and there is minimal oscillation in the patient's circulating blood volume. Also, as noted earlier, the entire system may be filled with blood prior to initiating hemodialysis, so that no substantial change in the child's circulating blood volume occurs when dialysis is initiated or concluded. However, maintenance of such dual blood accesses in an infant may be difficult in the long term. Stable infants (up to 12 kg in weight) requiring dialysis have been satisfactorily dialyzed with a Silastic right atrial catheter (Hickman catheter, Evermed Co., Medina, WA).[42] This system is schematically outlined in Figure 5–6.

To surgically place the catheter, a neck incision is made, and the appropriate vein (facial, internal or external jugular) is isolated. The catheter is cut to the correct length, and the catheter tip is positioned in the mid-right atrium through a venotomy. While still in the operating room, the catheter position is verified by x-ray, and the surgeon demonstrates adequate blood flow through the catheter. Then the catheter is tunneled subcutaneously to exit on the anterior chest wall. Although the surgery is not complex, the success rate is increased if these procedures are done by a single surgeon who is interested and understands the problems of uremia and dialysis. Postoperatively, the catheter exit site is cleansed and sterilely dressed with Op-site (ACME United Corp., Bridgeport, CT) every other day in the dialysis unit. Between dialyses catheter patency is assured by instillation of 2 ml of heparin solution (100 units/ml) every 12 hours.

Presently, the complication rate for 26 patients with 28 Hickman catheters in place for over 1800 days and used for more than 600 dialyses is lower than in our previous experience with other types of access. There has only been one episode of catheter-related sepsis, no recognized thrombotic complications, and two superficial skin infections which were successfully treated without catheter removal.

One problem is that the blood flow may be reduced by the patient's position without x-ray evidence of a change in the catheter position. This problem is usually intermittent and, in general, is managed by putting the patient in a prone or left decubitus position and temporarily reducing the blood pump speed.

With single-needle dialysis, during the first part of the cycle, blood is pumped from the patient into the dialyzer, thereby increasing the patient's volume loss into the extracorporeal circuit and increasing the total transmembrane pressure in the dialyzer (not to exceed 400 mm Hg). During the second part of the cycle, the venous side of the system is unclamped and dialyzed blood is returned, propelled by the head of pressure within the dialyzer.[43] As with exchange transfusion, there is a fraction of the blood in the system which is "recirculated." This volume of recirculated blood must be calculated and controlled since it reduces the efficiency of solute clearance by the dialysis treatment. The volume of a standard Hickman catheter is determined by the actual catheter length in each individual patient; however, it is generally 1 ml or less. The stroke volume of each cycle is determined by the blood pump flow rate and the number of seconds during which the blood pump runs in each cycle. A stroke volume of 6 or 7 ml is sufficiently large to reduce the percentage of recirculation to something less than 15% (1 ml of recirculation per 6 ml cycle). The actual recirculation may be measured by obtaining blood samples for BUN and creatinine from the arterial line (A), the venous line (V), and a peripheral (P) site on the patient. The percentage of recirculation is then calculated[44] according to the formula $P - A/P - V \times 100$. If necessary, stroke volume to the dialyzer may be increased by a percentage proportionate to the recirculation in order to minimize this effect. Simply increasing the number of cycles per minute will not alter the percentage of recirculation.

As the patient increases in size, the problem of recirculation is diminished. Since the dead space is constant as each stroke volume increases (up to the maximal volume fluctuation that the drip chamber will contain), the percentage recirculated will decrease. For example, a 5 kg infant will require 15 ml of blood flow to the dialyzer each minute. With 10-second arterial and venous cycles, each stroke volume will be 5 ml, and a 1 ml "dead space" will result in 20% recirculation. However, an 8 kg child requiring 40 ml of blood flow per minute with 6-second cycles for arterial flow and 6-second venous cycles will have an 8 ml stroke volume but with the same volume of "dead space" only about 12% recirculation. If clinically appropriate, a larger drip chamber accommodating up to 15 ml (DX-228; Extracorporeal, King of Prussia, PA) may be substituted into the circuit. This will permit an increased stroke volume and further reduce recirculation.

## ORGANIZATIONAL CONSIDERATIONS

The hemodialysis of infants and small children cannot be performed safely without a cadre of highly motivated and experienced dialysis nurses and technicians. We recommend that new pediatric hemodialysis units or established units with experience only in the treatment of older and larger children evolve toward infant dialysis by taking responsibility for successively smaller and smaller children, increasing the unit's skill and experience level. A leap from the care of a 20 kg child to that of a 5 kg child is discouraged since it may be fraught with unanticipated difficulties for the dialysis staff. Frequent group discussions, reviews of protocols and procedure manuals, and dissemination of experience throughout the staff is vital to avoid unnecessary complications. It cannot be overstressed that rigid adherence to safety protocols, including frequent checks of equipment function and ongoing staff education, is critical to the development of safe hemodialysis procedures for babies. The development of a unit can be accelerated by staff educational visits to another unit with experience in infant dialysis. Such sharing of information will minimize the "reinvention of the wheel" phenomenon which otherwise may occur. Infant hemodialysis represents a major commitment of time and resources and should involve constant staff exposure to patients, with a resultant improvement in skill levels. Infant hemodialysis should not be undertaken on an occasional basis.

## CONCLUSION

Hemodialysis can be a safe and reliable therapy for acute and chronic renal failure occurring in infants and small children. In addition to being a practical therapy, it has direct clinical advantages in those situations in which the patient will particularly benefit by the rapid and safe correction of fluid or electrolyte imbalances or the removal of a toxin. While infant dialysis requires meticulous attention to detail and an in-depth understanding of hemodialysis, its evolution is a valuable and direct extension of dialysis therapy in adults and older children with ESRD.

# REFERENCES

1. Drukker W: Haemodialysis: A historical review. *In*: Replacement of Renal Function by Dialysis, Drukker W, Parsons FM, Maher JF (eds). Hague, Martinus Nijhoff Medical Division, 1978.
2. Kallen RJ, Zaltzman S, Coe FL, et al: Hemodialysis in children: Technique, kinetic aspects related to varying body size, and application to salicylate intoxication, acute renal failure and some other disorders. Medicine 45:1, 1966.
3. Mateer FM, Greenman L, Danowski TS: Hemodialysis of the uremic child. Am J Dis Child 89:645, 1955.
4. Broyer M, Loirat C, Kleinknecht C: Technical aspects and results of regular hemodialysis in children. Acta Paediatr Scand 61:677, 1972.
5. Fine RN, Korsch BM, Grushkin CM, et al: Hemodialysis in children. Am J Dis Child 119:498, 1970.
6. Potter D, Larsen D, Leumann E, et al: Treatment of chronic uremia in childhood. II. Hemodialysis. Pediatrics 46:678, 1970.
7. Ahola T, Bjorkman H, Makela P, et al: The low-weight groups and haemodialysis. Acta Paediatr Scand 61:1, 1972.
8. Kjellstrand CM, Mauer SM, Buselmeier TJ, et al: Haemodialysis of premature and newborn babies. Proc Eur Dial Transplant Assoc 10:349, 1973.
9. Kjellstrand CM, Shideman JR, Santiago EA, et al: Technical advances in hemodialysis of very small pediatric patients. Proc Dial Transplant Forum 1:124, 1971.
10. Hodson EM, Najarian JS, Kjellstrand CM, et al: Renal transplantation in children ages 1 to 5 years. Pediatrics 61:458, 1978.
11. Miller LC, Bock GH, Lum CT, et al: Transplantation of the adult kidney into the very small child: Long-term outcome. J Pediatr 100:675, 1982.
12. Bock GH, Campos A, Thompson T, et al: Hemodialysis in the premature infant. Am J Dis Child 135:178, 1981.
13. Schrier RW: Acute renal failure. Kidney Int 15:205, 1979.
14. Gotloib L, Mines M, Garmizo L, et al: Hemodynamic effects of increasing intra-abdominal pressure in peritoneal dialysis. Peritoneal Dial Bull 1:41, 1981.
15. Gotloib L, Garmizo L, Varak I, et al: Reduction of vital capacity due to increased intra-abdominal pressure during peritoneal dialysis. Peritoneal Dial Bull 1:63, 1981.
16. Schwartz GJ, Haycock GB, Spitzer A: Plasma creatinine and urea concentration in children: Normal values for age and sex. J Pediatr 88:828, 1976.
17. Winberg J: The 24-hour true endogenous creatinine clearance in infants and children without renal disease. Acta Paediatr 48:443, 1959.
18. Wiegand C, Thompson T, Bock GH, et al: The management of life-threatening hyperammonemia: A comparison of several therapeutic modalities. J Pediatr 96:142, 1980.
19. Batshaw ML, Thomas GH, Brusilow SW: New approaches to the diagnosis and treatment of inborn errors of urea synthesis. Pediatrics 68:290, 1981.
20. Nevins TE, Chang PN, Mauer SM: Renal transplantation in the very young child. *In*: Contemporary Issues in Nephrology, Vol 12, Brenner BM, Stein J (eds). In press.
21. Miller LC, Lum CT, Bock GH, et al: Transplantation of the adult kidney into the very small child: Technical considerations. Am J Surg 145:243, 1983.
22. Rizzoni G, Malekzadeh MH, Pennisi AJ, et al: Renal transplantation in children less than 5 years of age. Arch Dis Child 55:532, 1980.
23. Trompeter RS, Bewick M, Haycock GB, et al: Renal transplantation in very young children. Lancet 1:373, 1983.
24. Rotundo A, Nevins TE, Lipton M, et al: Progressive encephalopathy in children with chronic renal insufficiency in infancy. Kidney Int 21:486, 1982.
25. Buselmeier TJ, Santiago EA, Simmons RL, et al: Arteriovenous shunts for pediatric hemodialysis. Surgery 70:638, 1971.
26. Takahashi M, Petry EL, Lurie PR, et al: Percutaneous heart catheterization in infants and children. I. Catheter placement and manipulation with guide wires. Circulation 42:1037, 1970.
27. Hickman RO, Buckner CD, Clift RA, et al: A modified right atrial catheter for access to the venous system in marrow transplant recipients. Surg Gynecol Obstet 148:871, 1979.
28. Pollack PF, Kadden M, Byrne WJ, et al: 100 patient years' experience with the Broviac silastic catheter for central venous nutrition. J Parenteral Enteral Nutr 5:32, 1981.
29. Riella MC, Scribner BH: Five years' experience with a right atrial catheter for prolonged parenteral nutrition at home. Surg Gynecol Obstet 143:205, 1976.
30. Bourquelot P, Wolfeler L, Lamy L: Microsurgery for haemodialysis distal arteriovenous fistulae in children weighing less than 10 kg. Proc Eur Dial Transplant Assoc 18:537, 1981.
31. Applebaum H, Shashikumar VL, Somers LA, et al: Improved hemodialysis access in children. J Pediatr Surg 15:764, 1980.
32. Shideman JR, Meyer RM, Streifel AJ, et al: The evaluation and applications of hemodialyzers for pediatric patients. J Dialysis 2:217, 1978.
33. Kjellstrand CM, Mauer SM, Shideman JR, et al: Accurate weight monitoring during pediatric hemodialysis. Nephron 10:302, 1973.
34. Mauer SM, Lynch RE: Hemodialysis techniques for infants and children. Pediatr Clin North Am 23:843, 1976.
35. Rosa AA, Shideman J, McHugh R, et al: The importance of osmolality fall and ultrafiltration rate on hemodialysis side effects. Nephron 27:134, 1981.
36. Bennett WM, Muther RS, Parker RA, et al: Drug therapy in renal failure: Dosing guidelines for adults. Ann Intern Med 93:62, 286, 1980.

37. Aurigemma NM, Feldman NT, Gottlieb M, et al: Arterial oxygenation during hemodialysis. N Engl J Med 297:871, 1977.

38. Kjellstrand CM, Buselmeier TJ: A simple method for anticoagulation during pre- and post-operative hemodialysis, avoiding rebound phenomenon. Surgery 72:630, 1972.

39. Hampers CL, Blaufox MD, Merrill JP: Anticoagulation rebound after hemodialysis. N Engl J Med 275:776, 1966.

40. Bergstrom J, Asaba H, Furst P, et al: Dialysis, ultrafiltration, and blood pressure. Proc Eur Dial Transplant Assoc 13:293, 1976.

41. Chavers BM, Kjellstrand CM, Wiegand C, et al: Techniques for use of charcoal hemoperfusion in infants: Experience in two patients. Kidney Int 18:386, 1980.

42. Mahan JD, Mauer SM, Nevins TE: The Hickman catheter: A new hemodialysis access device for infants and small children. Kidney Int, 24:694, 1983.

43. Hocken AG: Modular single-needle haemodialysis; Ultrafiltrational characteristics. Nephron 22:342, 1978.

44. Lazarus JM: Complications in hemodialysis: An overview. Kidney Int 18:783, 1980.

# 6

# Urea Kinetics in the Clinical Management of Children on Chronic Hemodialysis

*William E. Harmon, M.D.*
*Warren E. Grupe, M.D.*

The loss of renal function produces a state of profound and diverse metabolic chaos. Uremia results not only from the loss of control of body fluid spaces and electrolyte concentrations but also from the accumulation of identified and suspected toxins, and even from the imbalance of endocrinologic function. Thus, it is not surprising that hemodialysis, in its present state, is only an imperfect treatment for renal failure. It should be equally apparent that the appropriate application of this treatment is controversial.

The precise application of a mathematical model to the prescription of dialysis therapy would presuppose that the elements of uremic toxicity are both known and quantifiable. This is not the case. Thus, any method of determining the adequacy of dialysis therapy must depend upon a reduced model of uremia in which the elements monitored are identified and quantifiable. In addition, to be clinically useful, these elements should be (1) easily measured by available laboratory methods, (2) significantly affected by the dialysis procedure, (3) related to as wide a range of uremic toxicity as possible, (4) descriptive of both the rates of solute generation and removal, and (5) simultaneously indicative of metabolic status and dialysis adequacy. Given

these parameters, it is conceivable that a satisfactory method of both quantifying and prescribing dialysis therapy can be constructed.

## HISTORICAL PERSPECTIVE

Despite the fact that the kinetic aspects of hemodialysis in children have been known for a long time,[1] most descriptions of pediatric dialysis have been limited to the technical aspects of performing the procedure in small patients or to defining what is necessary in order to reduce mortality.[2-8] These techniques, of course, have been quite successful since the mortality of children on dialysis is quite low.[9, 10] Nonetheless, techniques designed to reduce morbidity and to optimize therapy are not as well defined.

The principal models of dialysis therapy include: "The Dialysis Index" (middle molecule); the "Nephroid Clearance"; and "Urea Kinetics." A brief discussion of the first two of these models and of some of the recommendations concerning "adequate" pediatric dialysis techniques follows. (See list of abbreviations used in following text and tables).

**The Dialysis Index.** It has been suggested that relatively large molecular weight (1000–2000 dalton) uremic toxins, which have been called "Middle Molecules" (MM), contributed to the continuing morbidity of chronically

Supported by AM 16392 from the National Institutes of Health and the Margaret Laurie Rehill Fund.

## ABBREVIATIONS USED

| | |
|---|---|
| β | Rate of change of volume |
| BUN | Blood Urea Nitrogen |
| BSA | Body Surface Area |
| C | Concentration |
| Cr | Creatinine |
| $C_0TAR$ | Targeted Predialysis Concentration |
| DI | Dialysis Index |
| G | Generation rate |
| K | Clearance |
| $K_D$ | Dialyzer Clearance |
| KoA | Dialyzer Permeability—Surface Area Product |
| $K_R$ | Residual Native Renal Clearance |
| L | Liter |
| MM | Middle Molecule |
| MNCV | Median Nerve Conduction Velocity |
| PCR | Protein Catabolic Rate |
| $Q_B$ | Blood Flow Rate |
| $Q_D$ | Dialysate Flow Rate |
| $t_D$ | Duration of Dialysis |
| TAC | Time-Averaged Concentration |
| TBW | Total Body Water |
| θ | Interdialytic Interval |
| U | Urea |
| UGR | Urea Generation Rate |
| V | Volume of Distribution |

dialyzed patients.[11] This hypothesis evolved from the clinical observation of crippling neuropathy which developed in patients despite apparently adequate control of measurable metabolic abnormalities as determined by periodic assessment of blood levels. Scribner and Babb correctly suggested that the patient's residual native renal function could account for relatively large clearance of these MM toxins. They retrospectively correlated the magnitude of the neuropathy to the patient's residual renal clearance. Subsequently they proposed the use of a "Dialysis Index" (DI) as a basis of comparing overall clearance of various molecular weight molecules in any individual patient to that which had been demonstrated "historically" to be adequate for an anephric 1.73 $M^2$ patient.[12] The calculation of DI is shown in equation 1:

$$DI = \frac{\text{prescribed } K_D t_D + K_R CrTwk}{(D1Kiil \text{ reference value}) (BSA/1.73)} \quad (1)$$

where the D1Kiil reference value was given for each of three solutes: 29 L/wk for a 1355 dalton molecule, 31 L/wk for a 1000 dalton molecule or 77.4 L/wk for creatinine. The ultimate dialysis prescription ($K_D \times t_D$) was

determined as the greatest of the three calculated values for each of the reference solutes. "Adequate dialysis" was said to have been achieved when DI was greater than or equal to 1. Although some early results suggested that there was a correlation between DI and evidence of neuropathy as measured by Median Nerve Conduction Velocity (MNCV),[13] subsequent studies have failed to demonstrate any correlation between the DI or the concentration of MM and MNCV or any other outcome variable.[14, 15] Thus, the use of the DI to prescribe dialysis therapy appears to have little practical value. Furthermore, subsequent analysis of the original data has suggested that any improvement in outcome variables can be better correlated with control of small molecules than with the MM.[16] Additionally, there is, as yet, no consensus as to the identity of any of the MM toxins.[17] Also, the hypothesis is based upon comparing dialysis requirements to historically derived controls, and, thus, it is generally insensitive to individual variations in metabolic requirements. Finally, it has not been rigorously applied in a pediatric setting. Thus, the use of DI does not appear to be a satisfactory method of prospectively prescribing individual dialysis therapy for pediatric patients.

**Nephroid Clearance.** A similar attempt to quantify dialysis therapy based solely on solute removal was proposed by Ginn and Teschan.[18] They once again noted the importance of residual renal function and proposed the use of the index shown below:

$$NC = (K_D U + K_R Cr)/TBW \quad (2)$$

where NC is the nephroid clearance, $K_D U$ the dialyzer urea clearance (ml/week), $K_R Cr$ the residual renal creatinine clearance (ml/week), and TBW the total body water (liters). Historical evidence demonstrated that uremic symptoms appeared when NC was less than 2000 ml/week/L (equivalent to a residual creatinine clearance of about 8 ml/min/1.73 $M^2$). Further, the evidence suggested that "adequate" dialysis resulted from a total NC greater than 3000 ml/week/L. While this model does provide certain broad guidelines concerning the need for initiating and providing sufficient dialysis, as conceived it is not sensitive to changes in metabolic requirements, nor does it provide sufficient insight into the relationship between nutritional intake and subsequent solute removal in the patients. Additionally, it has not been applied rigorously in a pediatric setting.

**Descriptive Studies of Pediatric Dialysis.** Numerous studies have demonstrated that both acute and chronic hemodialysis can be achieved in children and even infants. Yet, most of these reports are largely experiential or descriptive and few address the concept of optimizing therapy. There are generally accepted criteria for selection of the dialyzer size based upon the fraction of the patient's total blood volume contained in the extracorporeal circuit of the dialyzer and blood lines (not to exceed 8–10%).[19]

The determination of dialysis prescription (clearance, duration, and interval) is less well-established. Some reports suggest that the dialyzer urea clearance should not exceed 2–3 ml/min/kg body weight[20] and that the duration of dialysis should be determined by multiplying that clearance/kg by the number of hours of dialysis to give an "arbitrary" number which is predictive of changes in the BUN.[7] While this method is descriptive of the changes in BUN which occur during a dialysis treatment, it has not been used to determine what the best parameters should be. Other reports have suggested that merely dividing the dialyzer surface area by the patient's body surface area and multiplying the result by the number of hours of dialysis per week produces an approximate index of "adequacy" of dialysis for a given patient, based upon historical controls of values obtained in adult patients.[8]

In many dialysis units the adequacy of the dialysis prescription is assessed through the periodic evaluation of predialysis blood levels of BUN, creatinine, and other solutes. While these methods do provide certain guidelines for prescribing dialysis treatments, none addresses the question of the balance which should be achieved between an individual's solute generation, as determined by the nutritional intake and metabolic status, and the removal of that solute by dialyzer clearance. They all presuppose that all patients of similar size will be adequately treated by the same dialysis prescriptions. Furthermore, none of these techniques considers the varying proportional amount of total body water nor the actual dialysis kinetics, which are particularly important in the pediatric patient. In addition, the inadequacy of monitoring only periodic predialysis laboratory determinations should be obvious and has been described elsewhere.[21]

## RATIONALE OF UREA KINETIC MODELING

The concept of adequate removal of waste products and toxins by dialysis must be coupled with an appreciation of their rate of accumulation and their distribution within the body spaces. The identified and proposed abnormalities of solute concentration in renal failure and their proposed relationship to uremic toxicity are shown in Table 6–1. A mathematical model designed to control all these elements within optimal ranges by dialysis therapy would be unwieldy, difficult to apply to a dynamic clinical situation, and perhaps conceptually impossible to construct because of the interrelationships between toxicities. For these reasons, a reasonable model of dialysis prescription must be based on a smaller scale.

The uremic state is related to the products of protein metabolism. Indeed, the blood levels of urea, the major metabolic end-product of protein nitrogen, have themselves been related to toxic manifestations in dialysis patients.[22, 23] Also, since the urea generation rate (UGR) is directly proportional to the catabolic rate of protein, urea may serve as a probe molecule for other uremic toxicities.[24–26] In a large group of stable dialysis patients, both dietary phosphorus and potassium intake have been shown to be related directly to the protein intake,[27] and net hydrogen ion generation was similarly directly proportional to protein catabolism.[28] Thus, a model of dialysis therapy based upon the measurement of the generation and removal rates of urea should, correspondingly, be informative in assessing adequacy of control of the products of protein catabolism, potassium, phosphorus, and acid-base control.

The conceptual basis of urea kinetic modeling is based upon the analysis of the rates of accumulation and removal of urea. Urea is generated at a constant rate, which in turn is proportional to the protein catabolic rate.[24–25] The urea is distributed into a single body pool, which is equivalent to the total body water,[29, 30] and thus the concentration of urea can be described by a single pool mathematical model.[31–32] The rate of removal of urea is determined by the sum of the dialyzer urea clearance and the residual renal urea clearance. The relationship among generation, removal, and accumulation is shown in Figure 6–1. The overall mass balance relationship is given by:

**Table 6–1.** RELATIONSHIP OF ABNORMALITIES OF SOLUTE CONCENTRATION AND ELEMENTS OF UREMIC TOXICITY

| Element | Chronic Toxicity | | Control by | | Treatment-Related Toxicity |
| | *Established* | *Proposed* | *Hemodialysis* | *Diet + Med* | |
| --- | --- | --- | --- | --- | --- |
| Water | Hypertension; CHF; hyponatremia | | Good | Necessary | Shock, Cramps |
| Sodium | Hypertension; CHF; hyponatremia | | Good | Necessary | Cramps, ? Shock |
| Potassium | Arrhythmias | | Fair | Primary | Arrhythmias with rapid flux |
| Acid-Base | Metabolism; bone mineralization | | Good | Secondary | ? Shock |
| Calcium | Bone mineralization; muscle metabolism; hyperparathyroidism | ?CHF | Good | Primary OH-vit. D | |
| Phosphorus | Bone mineralization; hyperparathyroidism | Muscle | Poor | Primary Al-OH | |
| Urea | Hyperosmolarity; altered hemoglobin structure; coma | Altered protein metab.; altered taste; bleeding tendencies; GI + neurologic changes | Good | Necessary | Dysequilibrium |
| Uric acid | Gout | | Good | | |
| Aluminum | | Dialysis dementia; bone mineralization | Poor | | ? Source in $H_2O$ |
| Glucose | | Acid generation; protein catabolism | Poor | | AA loss |
| Creatinine | None | | Good | None | |
| Middle molecules | | Neuropathy | Variable | None | |

$$\frac{d(VC)}{dt} = G - KC \quad (3)$$

If there is no volume change,* equation 3 can be solved to yield:

$$C_T = C_0 e^{-\frac{Kt}{V}} + \frac{G}{K}\left[1 - e^{-\frac{Kt}{V}}\right] \quad (4)$$

where $C_T$ and $C_0$ are concentrations at times T and 0, K is the overall dialyzer and residual renal clearance of the solute, t is the time interval between 0 and T, G is the generation rate, and V is the volume of distribution of the solute. If K and t are known and successive solute concentrations ($C_T$ and $C_0$) are measured, unique solutions for V and G can be calculated from equation 2 by using an iterative technique.[31, 32] The measurement of the volume distribution of urea (V) is pri-

marily based upon the pharmacologic principle of negative infusion. That is, knowing the change in concentration of urea during a dialysis treatment, the overall clearance rate, and the duration of the treatment, the volume cleared is easily calculated. Subsequently, using that calculated V, the change in concentration during the interdialytic period is used to calculate the generation rate. The calculated G is used then to recalculate the V more precisely and the same process is continued until the most accurate solutions for both V and G are obtained.

The schematic representation of the change in the concentration of urea during and between dialyzer treatments is shown in Figure 6–2. It should be noted that during the period of dialysis, the concentration of urea is a function of five variables, V, G, $K_D$, $K_R$, and $t_D$, whereas during the interdialytic period, the concentration is a function of V, G, $K_R$, and $\theta$.

*The more general solution is:

$$C_T = C_0\left(\frac{V_0+\beta t}{V_0}\right)^{-\frac{K+\beta}{\beta}} + (G/K+\beta)\left[1 - \left(\frac{V_0+\beta t}{V_0}\right)^{-\frac{K+\beta}{\beta}}\right]$$

where $\beta$ is the rate of change of the volume.

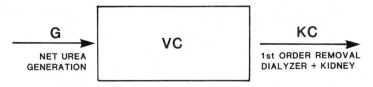

Accumulation = Input − Output

(Change in urea content) = (Generation) − (Removal)

$$\frac{d(V \cdot C)}{dT} = G - K \cdot C$$

**Figure 6–1.** Diagram of the urea model in the dialyzed patient including the mass balance equation. (From Kidney International 18:S2–S10, 1980, with permission.)

Thus, by obtaining three BUN determinations (pre- and postdialysis and predialysis for the subsequent treatment), equation 4 can be used to determine both G and V for that period. By obtaining the repetitive determinations, the average urea volume can be determined with excellent accuracy.[25] Subsequently, the controllable variables ($K_D$, $t_D$, θ, G) can be manipulated to "set" the variation of the BUN within predetermined limits.[27, 33]

## CLINICAL METHOD OF UREA KINETIC MODELING

The use of urea kinetic modeling to guide or study hemodialysis therapy is based upon the knowledge that the concentration of urea is a function of only six variables:

$$C = f(t_D, \theta, K_R, K_D, V, G) \qquad (5)$$

Thus, the variation of concentration can be fixed by adjusting the variables; and, conversely, knowledge of the changes in concentration can be used to calculate some of the variables. Consideration of the measured and calculated values follows:

**Dialysis Time, $t_D$.** The actual length of dialysis can be very reliably determined. It must be stressed, however, that the time recorded must be the actual time of the treatment, not the planned time. While small errors of $t_D$ will result in negligible errors in the resultant calculations, the dimension of the errors is inversely proportional to the dialyzer clearance, so that the accuracy is particularly important in pediatric patients. For example, whereas a 12% error in $t_D$ will result in a 4% error in calculating concentration change for a $K_D$ of 160 ml/min, there will be a 9% error for a $K_D$ of 50 ml/min.[31]

**Interdialytic Interval, θ.** Again, the interdialytic interval can be accurately measured. It must be noted, however, that because of the difficulty in evenly spacing treatments within a weekly interval, interdialytic intervals will not be equal. The magnitude of error in the calculations in assuming evenly spaced treatment times rather than using the actual times can approach 20%.[31]

**Figure 6–2.** Single pool model of the change in urea concentration (BUN) during a dialysis treatment (t) and between treatments (θ).

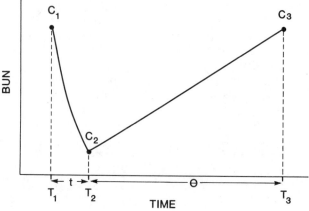

**Residual Renal Function, $K_R$.** The contribution of the $K_R$ in removing solutes is inversely proportional to the clearance of that solute by the dialyzer and is of particular importance during the interdialytic interval. Accurate determinations of $K_R$ are usually performed during the largest possible interval between dialyses. Practically, the $K_R$ measurement can be assumed to be stable over a long period of time.

**Dialyzer Clearance, $K_D$.** The dialyzer clearance for any solute is a function of the overall permeability–surface area product (KoA), the blood ($Q_B$) and dialysate ($Q_D$) flow rates, and the flow geometry of the dialyzer.* Thus, dialyzer clearance is easily calculated. Nonetheless, the actual dialyzer clearance may vary owing to unequal distribution or flow of blood and dialysate within the dialyzer, clotting or obstruction of the blood compartment, variable blood or dialysate flow rates, inaccuracies of blood flow measurement, or even to blood recirculation due to poor vascular access performance. Scrupulous attention to the details of determining prescribed dialyzer clearance will minimize any errors, and comparison of the achieved (effective) clearance to the prescribed clearance should identify the source of any errors.[31]

**Volume of Distribution (V) and Generation Rate (G) of Urea.** If $K_R$, $K_D$, $t_D$, and $\theta$ are known, and three urea concentrations ($C_{01}$, $C_T$, $C_{02}$) are measured, equation 4 can be used to calculate unique solutions for V and G during the two intervals, $t_D$ and $\theta$. Since a single equation cannot be solved for two unknowns, an iterative technique must be used. Practically, the rate of fall in concentration during the dialysis period, $t_D$, is used to calculate V. The calculated V and the rate of rise in concentration during $\theta$ is used to calculate G. Then the calculated G is used to calculate V during $t_D$ more precisely and the process is repeated until the solutions of both V and G converge, resulting in accurate solutions of both values.[31, 32] Because of the repetitive nature of the solution, a computer is necessary in order to achieve reasonable efficiency.

---

*For countercurrent flow,

$$K_D = Q_B \left[ \frac{e^{\left( \frac{KoA}{Q_B} - \frac{KoA}{Q_D} \right)} - 1}{e^{\left( \frac{KoA}{Q_B} - \frac{KoA}{Q_D} \right)} - \frac{Q_B}{Q_D}} \right]$$

**Overall Use of Urea Kinetic Modeling.** By measuring $K_D$, $K_R$, $t_D$, $\theta$, and pre-, post-, and pre-subsequent dialysis blood urea concentrations, assessments of V and G can be made. By repeating these measurements during several dialysis sessions, a very accurate evaluation of the mean urea volume can be determined. Additionally, these data can be used to assess variations in G. Alternatively, knowledge of V and G can be used to set $K_D$, $t_D$, and $\theta$ in order to achieve predetermined levels of $C_0$ or $C_T$.

## VERIFICATION OF UREA KINETIC MODELING TECHNIQUES

**Accuracy of Urea Volume (V) Measurements.** The calculation of the urea space by the modeling techniques described above has been shown to correspond closely to the urea space independently determined by urea infusions.[25] In addition, the reproducibility of the calculation of V by the urea kinetic modeling technique has been shown to be highly accurate. The coefficient of variation of repetitive measurements in the same patients in two separate studies averaged 7%.[25, 32]

The urea space is equivalent to the total body water.[29, 30] It is important to note, however, that the total body water, even in normal children, may vary between 40 and 80% of body weight, depending upon the distribution of body fat. The ratio of measured urea space to the mean dry weight in 26 chronic dialysis patients treated at Children's Hospital Medical Center during 1981 is shown in Figure 6–3. Each of the patients was studied for a three-month interval during which at least three determinations of V were made. The coefficient of variation of V for each of the patients was less than 6%. While the mean volume/weight ratio for all of the patients is 0.57, the variation is quite wide. The variation in the ratio is not predictable from the patients' age, from the weight or from the urea volume. Calculations based upon the assumption of urea space being equivalent to a fixed proportion (for example, 60%) of body weight, therefore, would be prone to large inaccuracies. Thus, it is clear that the urea space should be determined for each individual patient if further calculations are to be made on the basis of those data.

**Relationship of UGR to Protein Catabolism.** Since urea is the primary nitrogenous

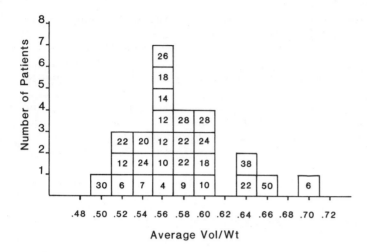

**Figure 6–3.** Distribution of the ratio of measured urea space (liters) to mean dry weight (kg) in 26 pediatric chronic dialysis patients. The number inside each box is the urea space in liters.

metabolic product of protein catabolism, there should be a direct relationship between the net protein catabolic rate (PCR) and the rate of generation of urea nitrogen. An early study of the relationship between the independently determined PCR and the calculated UGR in stable dialyzed patients resulted in:

$$UGR = 0.154 \ PCR - 1.7 \qquad (6)$$

(R = 0.96, n = 26) where UGR and PCR were expressed in gm/24 hours.[24] This result is similar to one previously determined for stable, nondialyzed uremic adults (UGR = 0.149 PCR − 1.2, R = 0.99, n = 12).[34] The relationship correlated very closely with expected results since it indicated that each 100 grams of protein catabolized gave rise to 15.4 grams of urea nitrogen, quite close to the 16 grams expected if urea were the sole end-product. Further, the negative intercept when PCR was extrapolated to zero indicated that some nitrogen was excreted by non-urea routes such as creatinine, uric acid, and stool. The value of the obligatory non-urea nitrogen excretion from these two studies, 1.2–1.7 gm/day, agrees favorably with findings of other studies.[35] Neither of these results, however, was directly applicable to children since the quantity of non-urea nitrogen excretion should have been proportional to body size. Thus, further studies in hemodialyzed children weighing 9–37 kg were undertaken to determine the appropriate relationship. These studies yielded the relationship:

$$UGR = 0.15 \ PCR - 0.0264 \ wt \qquad (7)$$

(R = 0.96, n = 14) where wt is given in kg.[36]

Rearranging the expression for the prediction of PCR, the correct relationship for all patients is now given by:

$$PCR = 6.50 \ UGR + 0.17 \ wt. \qquad (8)$$

**Sensitivity of PCR to Dietary Changes.** Although previous studies had demonstrated that the PCR derived from urea–kinetic modeling was closely correlated with an independently measured PCR, the question remained whether the PCR would reflect a change in the dietary strategy for an individual patient. To answer this question, two stable chronically hemodialyzed patients were studied.[37] The clinical data is shown in Table 6–2. The first patient (#1) was given both increased calories and protein. As expected, the PCR increased by 43%, but because of the proportionally greater protein intake, the net nitrogen balance was improved by 70%. The second patient (#2) was receiving sufficient protein, thus only the caloric intake was increased. As expected, the PCR decreased, reflecting improved protein utilization, once again leading to a significant improvement in the net nitrogen balance. Similar results in both stable and unstable adult patients have been reported.[25]

**Studies of Changes in Dialysis Morbidity with Individual Dialysis Prescription.** A large multicenter cooperative study designed to evaluate the clinical effects of different dialysis prescriptions, based upon urea kinetic modeling, has been undertaken.[32] A total of 151 patients from eight dialysis centers were studied. They were prospectively randomized into one of four possible treatment groups, divided along two dimensions:

**Table 6–2.** THE EFFECT OF CHANGING NUTRITIONAL PRESCRIPTION ON PROTEIN CATABOLIC RATE AND NET NITROGEN BALANCE IN TWO PEDIATRIC HEMODIALYSIS PATIENTS

| Patient | Period | Weight (kg) | Dietary | | UGR* (mg/min) | PCR† (gm/day) | $\Delta N_t$‡ (gm/day) |
| | | | KCal | Protein | | | |
|---|---|---|---|---|---|---|---|
| #1 | Control | 19.8 | 800 | 30 | 1.40 | 16 | +14 |
| | Experimental | 20.4 | 1325 | 48 | 2.11 | 23 | +25 |
| | Change | | +66% | +60% | | +43% | +78% |
| #2 | Control | 46.4 | 2400 | 64 | 5.25 | 57 | + 7 |
| | Experimental | 47.9 | 3300 | 64 | 3.34 | 39 | +25 |
| | Change | | +41% | 0% | | −32% | +257% |

*UGR = Urea Generation Rate, †PCR = Protein Catabolic Rate, ‡$\Delta N_t$ = Protein Balance

dialysis treatment time (short = 2.5 to 3.5 hours, long = 4.5 to 5 hours) and BUN averaged with respect to time ($TAC_{urea}$) (high = 100 mg/dl, low = 50 mg/dl). The dialyzer clearance was adjusted to control the BUN at the predetermined levels within the four groups. Dietary protein was not restricted.

Overall, the use of urea kinetic modeling techniques led to excellent control of the $TAC_{urea}$ within the predetermined boundaries: the mean BUN concentrations for the high and low groups were 89 and 52 mg/dl respectively.[38] Dialysis treatment time had no significant effects on patient morbidity. However, the occurrence of morbid events, including hospitalization or removal from the study because of pericarditis, anorexia, and so forth, was significantly greater in the high BUN group than in the low BUN group.[39] These results demonstrated that the occurrence of morbid events was affected by the individual dialysis prescription. Morbidity was decreased by prescriptions associated with more efficient removal of urea, leading to relatively low $TAC_{urea}$ if dietary protein and other nutrients were adequate. Similar studies in growing children have not yet been performed.

## CLINICAL USE OF UREA KINETIC MODELING

The determination of the appropriate "dose" of dialysis treatment is a particularly important concern for pediatric hemodialysis. The use of urea kinetic modeling permits the prescription to be based not only on the patient's size but also on the metabolic status and residual renal function.

For example, the clinical data for two children undergoing chronic hemodialysis is shown in Table 6–3. Both patients had been on dialysis for six months and both were

dialyzed with a 0.6M² hollow fiber dialyzer (KoA urea = 165 ml/min). Neither patient was restricted in dietary protein; patient A was receiving about 2 gm/kg/day of protein whereas patient B was taking 1.5 gm/kg/day.

Several possibilities of altering the dialysis prescription in order to achieve several different levels of midweek predialysis concentration of BUN are shown in the table. The adjustments of the prescriptions were made by changing the dialysis duration, the frequency of dialysis and/or the dialyzer clearance through the blood flow rate. To achieve a midweek predialysis BUN of 80 mg/dl (equivalent to a $TAC_{urea}$ of about 50 mg/dl) for patient A, there are at least 2 options:

**Table 6–3.** DIALYSIS PRESCRIPTIONS (BLOOD FLOW, FREQUENCY, AND DURATION) NECESSARY TO MAINTAIN $C_0TAR$ AT VARIOUS LEVELS FOR TWO PEDIATRIC PATIENTS OF SIMILAR SIZE BUT DIFFERENT RESIDUAL KIDNEY FUNCTION AND PROTEIN CATABOLIC RATES.

| Patient A | | | Patient B | | |
|---|---|---|---|---|---|
| Age: 6 Yr | | | Age: 7 Yr | | |
| Dry Wt: 16.2 Kg | | | Dry Wt: 17.1 Kg | | |
| Urea Vol: 9.8 L | | | Urea Vol: 10.66 L | | |
| Residual Urea | | | Residual Urea | | |
| Clearance: 0 ml/min | | | Clearance: 0.94 ml/min | | |
| PCR: 1.55 Gm/Kg/d | | | PCR: 1.07 Gm/Kg/d | | |
| **Dialysis Rx:** | | | | | |
| **HFK 0.6M²†** | | | | | |
| $Q_B$ (cc/min) | 100 | 150 | 100 | 100 | 150 |
| Frequency^X | 3 | 3 | 3 | 2 | 2 |
| $C_0TAR$ (mgm BUN/dl) | $t_D$* | $t_D$ | $t_D$ | $t_D$ | $t_D$ |
| 60 | 11.2 | 6.5 | 2.9 | 7.6 | 6.7 |
| 80 | 4.9 | 3.1 | 1.6 | 2.8 | 2.4 |
| 100 | 3.2 | 2.1 | 1.0 | 1.6 | 1.3 |

†0.6M² hollow fiber dialyzer with a urea KoA = 165 ml/min

^X Frequency of dialysis = treatments/week

* $t_D$ = Duration of dialysis (hours)

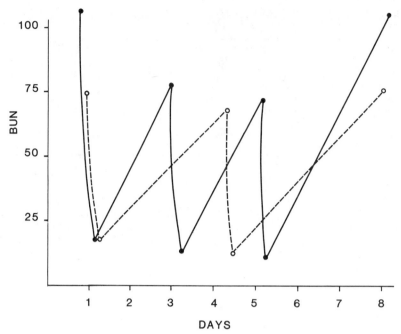

**Figure 6–4.** Change in BUN during a one-week cycle of intermittent hemodialysis treatments for two patients. The clinical details of the patients are shown in Table 6–3. Patient A (●——●) was dialyzed with an 0.6 M² dialyzer at a blood flow of 150 cc/min for 3 hours three times per week, while patient B (○— —○) was dialyzed with the same dialyzer and blood flow rate for 2.5 hours twice per week.

either 4.9 hours of dialysis at a blood flow of 100 ml/min ($K_D$ = 77 ml/min) or 3.1 hours at 150 ml/min ($K_D$ = 94 ml/min) will be required three times per week. For patient B, who has a nearly equivalent urea volume but who has a lower PCR and some residual renal function, much less time is required at the same clearance to achieve an equivalent $C_0TAR$. Additionally, it should be noted that satisfactory overall urea clearance can be achieved by twice per week dialysis for that patient. The overall changes in BUN concentrations over a one-week interval for patient A (dialyzed three times per week for three hours, $Q_B$ = 150 ml/min) and patient B (dialyzed twice per week for 2.5 hours, $Q_B$ = 150 ml/min) are shown in Figure 6–4. As can be seen, equivalent control of BUN has been achieved in both patients by individually prescribing the dialysis parameters.

Data concerning a third patient (C), who presents a different problem, is shown in Table 6–4. Because of the patient's small size, only a very small parallel plate dialyzer, (KoA urea = 67 ml/min) with a low blood flow rate (50 ml/min) could be used. This patient was receiving intravenous hyperalimentation providing 80 Cal/kg and 1.5 gm/kg protein per day. Because a relatively large amount of

fluid was required to provide these nutrients (600–700 ml/day), at least three hours of ultrafiltration three times per week was necessary. Thus, at least minimum levels of the dialysis variables were established without considering solute clearance. In order to determine whether satisfactory urea clearance could be achieved by this dialysis prescription, the projected $TAC_{urea}$ was calculated as shown in Table 6–4. As can be seen, three hours of dialysis three times per week pro-

**Table 6–4.** EFFECT OF CHANGING DURATION OF DIALYSIS ON $TAC_{urea}$ OF A PEDIATRIC DIALYSIS PATIENT

| Patient C | |
|---|---|
| Age: 1 year | |
| Dry Wt: 9.5 kg | Urea Vol: 5.4 L |
| Residual Urea Clearance: 0 ml/min | |
| PCR: 0.84 Gm/kg/d | |
| Dialysis Rx: 0.25M² Flat-Plate Dialyzer (KoA | |
| Urea = 67 ml/min) | |
| $Q_B$ = 50 ml/min | |
| Frequency: 3x/week | |
| $t_D$ (Hours) | $TAC_{urea}$ (mg BUN/dl) |
| 2 | 52 |
| 3 | 36 |
| 4 | 29 |
| 5 | 25 |

vided sufficient clearance ($TAC_{urea}$ = 36 mg/dl); whereas increasing the amount of time would only lead to a rapidly diminishing increase in overall clearance. Using the above prescription, the patient sustained positive nitrogen balance for three months and grew satisfactorily while awaiting transplantation.

In addition to providing guidelines for individualizing dialysis treatment, urea kinetic modeling has been used to assess and guide nutritional protocols.[25, 39, 40] As previously noted, the model provides a calculation of the urea generation rate which is closely correlated with the overall protein catabolic rate. By comparing the PCR with dietary protein intake, an immediate assessment of nitrogen balance can be made without need for tedious collection protocols.

A further example of the long-term clinical utility of urea kinetic modeling is shown in Table 6–5. The figure is an example of one data-output format available from the urea kinetic modeling computer program and summarizes some of the data for a 10-month period for patient D, a six-year-old girl who had been treated with chronic dialysis for over two years. It should be noted that during the ten months her postdialysis weight (dry weight) and her total body water both increased proportionally, signifying a true increase in lean body mass. Also, the low vol/

wt ratio suggests that the patient had a relatively large volume of body fat. Additionally, her actual (achieved) pre- and postdialysis BUN concentrations were generally close to the prescribed levels. Two of the monthly values, however, were aberrant and are indicative of the clinical value of the urea kinetic technique. The predialysis BUN on 3/2/82 was only 36 mg/dl. The PCR at that time was only 0.54 gm/kg/day and questioning of the patient's parents revealed that her nutritional intake had decreased markedly. Adjustments in her diet were undertaken, and, three months later, her predialysis BUN was 112 mg/dl. This higher value could have been due to a decreased effective dialyzer clearance (wrong prescription or fistula recirculation), a significant increase in urea volume without sufficient increase in the clearance, or a significant increase in PCR. Review of the data revealed that her dialyzer clearance was satisfactory and appropriate for her V (post-BUN = 21 mg/dl) but that her PCR had risen to 1.62 gm/kg/d. Dietary evaluation revealed a protein intake of over 2 gm/kg/day. Adjustment of the diet to provide 1.5 gm/kg/day of protein led to a lowering of the pre-dialysis BUN. More importantly, the PCR decreased to 1.05 gm/kg/day with this new diet, indicating that she remained in positive nitrogen balance at the lower protein

**Table 6–5.** UREA KINETIC MODELING DATA-OUTPUT FOR A PEDIATRIC DIALYSIS PATIENT

| PATIENT: D LISTING DATE: 11/05/82 | CONFERENCE DATE: _____ Printed: 11/24/82 | | | | | | | | |
|---|---|---|---|---|---|---|---|---|---|
| Record: Date: | TUE 1/05/82 | TUE 2/02/82 | TUE 3/02/82 | TUE 4/06/82 | TUE 5/04/82 | TUE 6/01/82 | TUE 6/29/82 | TUE 8/31/82 | TUE 10/05/82 | TUE 11/02/82 |
| **PATIENT DATA** | | | | | | | | | | |
| Kidney urea clearance, ml/min: | 0.13 | 0.13 | 0.13 | 0.13 | 0.13 | 0.13 | 0.13 | 0.13 | 0.13 | 0.13 |
| Weight (post treatment): | 13.5 | 13.7 | 13.9 | 14.1 | 14.1 | 14.3 | 14.5 | 15.2 | 15.2 | 15.8 |
| Volume (total body water): | 6.24 | 6.53 | 6.55 | 6.32 | 6.10 | 6.84 | 6.40 | 6.55 | 7.28 | 7.29 |
| Volume/Post Weight: | 0.46 | 0.48 | 0.47 | 0.45 | 0.43 | 0.48 | 0.44 | 0.43 | 0.48 | 0.46 |
| **TREATMENT DATA** | | | | | | | | | | |
| Dialysis Frequency (Rx/wk): | 3 | 3 | 3 | 3 | 3 | 3 | 3 | 3 | 3 | 3 |
| Dialysis Time (minutes): | 180 | 180 | 180 | 180 | 180 | 180 | 180 | 180 | 180 | 180 |
| Dialyzer used: | MOD6 | MOD6 | MOD6 | MOD6 | MOD6 | MOD6 | MOD6 | MOD6 | FRO6 | FRO6 |
| Blood Flow (ml/min): | 95 | 99 | 100 | 96 | 111 | 96 | 93 | 101 | 106 | 96 |
| Dialysate Flow (ml/min): | 500 | 500 | 500 | 500 | 500 | 500 | 500 | 500 | 500 | 500 |
| Urea Clearance (ml/min): | 77 | 78 | 78 | 77 | 83 | 77 | 75 | 79 | 90 | 84 |
| **NUTRITION** | | | | | | | | | | |
| Gm Protein Catabolism/kg: | 1.30 | 1.58 | 0.54 | 1.29 | 1.47 | 1.62 | 1.31 | 1.35 | 1.06 | 1.05 |
| Est Weekend Catabolism: | 1.17 | 1.25 | 0.62 | 1.42 | 1.51 | 1.78 | 1.24 | 1.21 | 1.16 | 1.11 |
| Weight gain between Rx (kg): | 1.2 | 0.9 | 0.2 | 0.7 | 0.7 | 0.3 | 0.5 | 0.9 | 0.3 | 0.1 |
| Weight loss during Rx (kg): | 1.3 | 0.7 | 0.6 | 0.9 | 0.5 | 0.9 | 0.6 | 0.6 | 0.4 | 0.4 |
| Ultrafiltration (kg/hr): | 0.43 | 0.23 | 0.20 | 0.30 | 0.17 | 0.30 | 0.20 | 0.20 | 0.13 | 0.13 |
| **BUN DATA** | | | | | | | | | | |
| 1st pre (target 78): | 71 | 77 | 36 | 89 | 93 | 112 | 79 | 78 | 72 | 70 |
| 1st post (target 13): | 13 | 13 | 6 | 15 | 14 | 21 | 12 | 12 | 11 | 11 |
| 2nd pre (target 60): | 58 | 72 | 23 | 63 | 70 | 86 | 63 | 61 | 51 | 52 |

intake (protein balance = protein intake −
PCR = 1.5 − 1.05 = + 0.45 gm/kg/day).

## UREA KINETICS IN STUDIES OF PROTEIN AND ENERGY UTILIZATION

Urea kinetics have been applied successfully to several ambiguous areas in the nutritional management of uremic children on
hemodialysis. In this arena also, the technique has several advantages. Firstly, it is not
cumbersome or additionally invasive, thus
allowing multiple measurements in the same
child under actual field conditions without
collection errors (Table 6–5). Secondly, the
capability of quantitative control of dialysis
eliminates metabolic variables introduced by
the dialysis treatment itself. Both these advantages allow a quantitative measure of protein metabolism, while standardization of the
dialysis conditions permits the appropriate
investigation of the optimal relationship between protein and energy, the effect of excess
energy intake on the interpretation of protein requirement, and the efficiency of protein utilization.

Using urea kinetics to define the urea generation rate, and, thus, the protein catabolic
rate, protein balance can be determined by
subtracting the net protein catabolic rate
from the measured dietary protein in-
take.[24, 27, 36] With this technique, a linear relationship has been demonstrated between
protein balance and energy intake in a study
of 45 balance periods in 15 children.[41, 42]
Neutral balance occurred at 10 kcal/cm of
height/day; the energy intake which accompanied positive balance varied between 6.4
and 21.2 kcal/cm/day. These data also revealed that 3 mg of nitrogen was retained
for each kilocalorie increase in energy. This
slope is similar to a 2–4 mg change noted in
normal adults on a marginal protein intake
comparable to that often prescribed for
uremic patients. In the same study, a linear
relationship between protein balance and
protein intake was demonstrated, with neutral balance occurring at 0.3 gm/cm/day. The
protein intake during positive balance varied
between 0.2 and 0.5 gm/cm/day. In this study,
all data were standardized for statural height
in centimeters since height is known to correlate with both creatinine production and
lean body mass, can be accurately and re-
producibly assessed in children, does not vary

from dialysis to dialysis, and is independent
of variations in total body water.

Further studies demonstrated an inverse
relationship between protein catabolic rate
and protein balance. Previous balance studies
have noted a decline in protein catabolic rate
associated with increasing energy intake and
a rise with increasing protein intake. However, when evaluation was made over a broad
range of protein and energy intake, in which
the amount of total energy represented by
protein remained constant, the proportional
changes in protein catabolic rate were offset
so that no correlation between the net protein
catabolic rate and either protein intake or
energy intake existed. That the protein catabolic rate diminished as protein balance increased suggested that the production of positive protein balance, despite increasing
protein intake, reduced urea generation.
This was further supported when it was
noted that for any given protein intake the
protein catabolic rate, and hence the urea
generation rate, was uniformly lower in those
children in positive protein balance. This
demonstrated that the patients in positive
nitrogen balance did not require additional
dialysis for nitrogen removal despite their
higher protein intake.

Although protein intake was closely correlated with energy intake in these studies,
multiple regression analysis indicated that
protein intake was a better predictor of protein balance than energy intake when both
variables were considered simultaneously. In
addition, a trend developed suggesting that
the energy intake needed to attain neutral
nitrogen balance when protein intake was
below 0.3 gm/cm/day could be as much as
20% higher than when higher protein intakes
were given. Of concern, this requirement for
excess energy could exceed the appetite capability of an appreciable proportion of
uremic children.

Nutrient intake was not the only determinant of protein catabolic rate. Factors other
than protein and energy altered protein catabolism sufficiently in 10 of 45 balance periods to reverse the expected protein balance
results. Although the factors contributing to
protein catabolism have not been defined in
these studies, it must be remembered that
dialysis itself is a catabolic event.[24] For the
child's management, therefore, these data
demonstrate that isolated knowledge of the
net protein catabolic rate or of nutrient intake alone is insufficient to predict the pro-

tein balance status of the patient. Nor can manipulation of nutrient intake alone assure a change in either the protein catabolic rate or the protein balance that will be regularly appropriate for or beneficial to the patient.

The controlled nature of the technique allows studies in the individual patient to determine whether positive protein balance can be maintained and whether improved protein balance is synonymous with improved protein synthesis or increased lean body mass (Table 6–5). Likewise, the ability of the individual child to adapt to changes in the diet can be measured; that which appears adequate by short-term analysis in the depleted child, for example, may underestimate the long-term need in the repleted child. Thus, urea kinetic evaluation, coupled with an accurately determined dietary intake, is a convenient and accurate tool to monitor protein metabolism, to define nutrient needs, and to derive nitrogen balance in the child on hemodialysis.

## CONCLUSION

Urea kinetic modeling is a mathematical model of dialysis therapy that is based upon the assessment of the changes in urea concentrations during and between dialysis treatments. The model has been shown to be a clinically useful tool, which provides accurate information about an individual dialysis patient's urea space, urea generation rate, and protein catabolic rate. Additionally, the model has been used for individual patients as the basis of prescribing the variables of dialysis treatments, including duration, clearance, and frequency. Appropriate application of these individual prescriptions has been associated with decreased patient morbidity. Also, the model has been used to guide and assess the nutritional management of individual dialysis patients and to provide insight into the efficiency of protein utilization.

Since the mortality of chronic hemodialysis is low, and since the technical aspects of providing this treatment are no longer a major hurdle, future research should be directed at lessening morbidity. Thus, studies to assess or optimize such things as nutritional status, cognitive functions, growth, orthopedic status, or erythropoiesis need to be carefully designed. In order to remove any bias introduced by the dialysis treatment itself on the outcome variables, it is essential that the "dose" of dialysis be standardized and measurable. Urea kinetic modeling is a well-established method of prescribing and measuring dialysis therapy and can be used for this purpose.

## REFERENCES

1. Kallen RJ, Zaltzman S, Coe FL, Metcoff J: Hemodialysis in children: Technique, kinetic aspects related to varying body size, and application to salicylate intoxication, acute renal failure and some other disorders. Medicine 45:1, 1966.
2. Grushkin CM, Korsch B, Fine RN: Hemodialysis in small children. JAMA 221:869, 1972.
3. Fine RN, Grushkin CM: Hemodialysis and renal transplantation in children. Clin Nephrol 1:243, 1973.
4. Lee HA, Sharpstone P: Haemodialysis in paediatrics. Acta Paediatr Scand 55:529, 1966.
5. Potter D, Larsen D, Leumann E., et al: Treatment of chronic uremia in childhood. II. Hemodialysis. Pediatrics 46:678, 1970.
6. Mauer SM, Shideman JR, Buselmeier TJ, Kjellstrand CM: Long-term hemodialysis in the neonatal period. Am J Dis Child 125:269, 1973.
7. Mauer SM, Lynch RE: Hemodialysis techniques for infants and children. Pediatr Clin North Am 23:843, 1976.
8. Gardiner AOP, Sawyer AN, Donckerwolcke RA, et al: Assessment of dialysis requirement for children on regular hemodialysis. Dial Transplant 11:754, 1982.
9. Avner ED, Harmon WE, Grupe WE, et al: Mortality of chronic hemodialysis and renal transplantation in pediatric end-stage renal disease. Pediatrics 67:412, 1981.
10. Potter DE, Holliday MA, Piel CF, et al: Treatment of end-stage renal disease in children: A 15-year experience. Kidney Int 18:103, 1980.
11. Babb AL, Popovich RP, Christopher TG, Scribner BH: The genesis of the square meter–hour hypothesis. Trans Am Soc Artif Intern Organs 17:81, 1971.
12. Babb AL, Strand MJ, Uvelli DA, et al: Quantitative description of dialysis treatment: A dialysis index. Kidney Int 7 (Suppl 2):S23, 1975.
13. Ginn HE, Bugel HJ, James L, Hopkins P: Clinical experience with small surface area dialyzers. Proc Dial Transplant Forum 1:53, 1971.
14. Kjellstrand CM, Petersen RJ, Evans RL, et al: Considerations of the middle molecule hypothesis. II: Neuropathy in nephrectomized patients. Trans Am Soc Artif Intern Organs 19:325, 1973.
15. Raja RM, Kramer MS, Rosenbaum JL: Long-term short hemodialysis—Implications to dialysis index. Trans Am Soc Artif Intern Organs 24:367, 1978.
16. Gotch FA: A quantitative evaluation of small and middle molecule toxicity in therapy of uremia. Dial Transplant 9:183, 1980.
17. Cantreras P, Later R, Navarro J, et al: Molecules in the middle molecular weight range. Nephron 32:193, 1982.

18. Ginn HE, Teschan PE, Bourne JR, et al: Neurobehavioral and clinical responses to hemodialysis. Trans Am Soc Artif Intern Organs 24:376, 1978.

19. Kjellstrand CM, Mauer SM, Buselmeier TJ, et al: Haemodialysis of premature and newborn babies. Proc Eur Dial Transplant Assoc 10:349, 1973.

20. Kjellstrand CM, Shideman JR, Santiago EA, et al: Technical advances in hemodialysis of very small pediatric patients. Proc Dial Transplant Forum 1:124, 1971.

21. Johnson WJ, Schniepp BJ: Comparison of urea kinetic modeling with other approaches to dialysis prescription. Dial Transplant 10:280, 1981.

22. Johnson WJ, Hagge WW, Wagoner RD, et al: Toxicity arising from urea. Kidney Int 7 (Suppl 3):S288, 1975.

23. Cohen BD, Handelsman DG, Pai BN: Toxicity arising from the urea cycle. Kidney Int 7 (Suppl 3):S285, 1975.

24. Borah MF, Schoenfeld PY, Gotch FA, et al: Nitrogen balance during intermittent dialysis therapy of uremia. Kidney Int 14:491, 1978.

25. Sargent J, Gotch F, Borah M, et al: Urea kinetics: A guide to nutritional management of renal failure. Am J Clin Nutr 31:1696, 1978.

26. Blumenkrantz MJ, Kopple JD, Moran JK, et al: Nitrogen and urea metabolism during continuous ambulatory peritoneal dialysis. Kidney Int 20:78, 1981.

27. Sargent JA, Lowrie EG: Which mathematical model to study uremic toxicity? Clin Nephrol 17:303, 1982.

28. Gotch F, Sargent JA: Measurement of H+ balance during acetate and bicarbonate dialysis therapy (Abs). Kidney Int 16:887, 1979.

29. San Pietro A, Rittenberg D: A study of the rate of protein synthesis in humans: I. Measurement of the urea pool and urea space. J Biol Chem 201:445, 1953.

30. Walser M, Bodenlos LJ: Urea metabolism in man. J Clin Invest 38:1617, 1959.

31. Sargent JA, Gotch FA: The analysis of concentration dependence of uremic lesions in clinical studies. Kidney Int 7(Suppl 2):S35, 1975.

32. Lowrie EG, Sargent JA: Clinical example of pharmacokinetic and metabolic modeling: Quantitative and individualized prescription of dialysis therapy. Kidney Int 18 (Suppl 10):S11, 1980.

33. Sargent JA, Gotch FA: Mathematical modeling of dialysis therapy. Kidney Int 18 (Suppl 10):S2, 1980.

34. Cottini EP, Gallina DL, Dominguez JM: Urea excretion in adult humans with varying degrees of kidney malfunction fed milk, egg, or an amino acid mixture: Assessment of nitrogen balance. J Nutr 103:11, 1973.

35. Mitch WE, Walser M: Effects of oral neomycin and kanamycin in chronic uremic patients: II. Nitrogen balance. Kidney Int 11:123, 1977.

36. Harmon WE, Spinozzi NS, Sargent JA, Grupe WE: Determination of protein catabolic rate in children on hemodialysis by urea kinetic modeling. Pediatr Res 13:513, 1979.

37. Harmon WE, Spinozzi, N, Meyer A, Grupe WE: Use of protein catabolic rate to monitor pediatric hemodialysis. Dial Transplant 10:324, 1981.

38. Lowrie EG, Laird NM, Parker TF, Sargent JA: Effect of the hemodialysis prescription on patient morbidity. N Engl J Med 305:1176, 1981.

39. Bennett N: Urea kinetics: A dietitian's clinical tool in the nutritional management of patients with end-stage renal disease. Dial Transplant 10:332, 1981.

40. Cogan MG, Sargent JA, Yarbrough S, et al: Prevention of prednisone-induced negative nitrogen balance. Ann Intern Med 95:158, 1981.

41. Grupe WE, Spinozzi NS, Harmon WE: Protein balance more dependent on protein intake than on energy intake in hemodialysed children. Kidney Int 23:149, 1983.

42. Grupe WE, Harmon WE, Spinozzi NS: Protein and energy requirements in children receiving chronic hemodialysis. Kidney Int 1983 (In Press).

# 7

# The Role of the Pediatric Nephrology Nurse in the Dialysis Unit

*Michael B. Grossman, R.N., M.S.N.*

The role of nursing in the care of children with ESRD has gone through a process of role expansion and redefinition in response to changes in the complex technology of treatment modalities. The nursing role has also been affected by psychosocial phenomena, expanding roles of health team members, and an expanding population of children requiring the specialized care provided by pediatric nephrology programs. The role of the hemodialysis nurse has correspondingly expanded in terms of technological knowledge and skills. Hemodialysis nurses currently utilize a variety of skills in cannulation, operate a variety of types of hemodialysis machines, monitor the effectiveness of dialyzer clearances, ultrafiltration, and heparinization, and use specific techniques and medications to identify and relieve symptoms occurring during hemodialysis treatments. While these issues are within the scope of nursing practice in a hemodialysis unit, the principles and body of knowledge involved can be drawn from other professions and have been addressed by authors in this and other texts,[1-9] and will not be considered here.

This chapter will focus on the current role of pediatric nephrology nurses in the hemodialysis unit, the expansion of the role from that of a hemodialysis nurse to that of a nephrology nurse with skills in a variety of hemodialysis and peritoneal dialysis treatment modalities as well as self-care concepts, the environment of the dialysis unit, and

nursing processes in the care of children with ESRD.

Children with ESRD receive care in a variety of settings including inpatient facilities, outpatient facilities, exclusive pediatric units, and units which primarily care for adults. Our own experience has been that nursing care can effectively be administered in any setting if attention is paid to the specific technical guidelines involved in pediatric dialysis, as well as to the unique psychosocial aspects of the care of children with ESRD. The factors which need to be considered in designing a program for the care of children with ESRD are summarized in Table 7–1.

## NURSING PHILOSOPHY

Nursing has been defined as the diagnosis and treatment of human responses to actual or potential health problems.[10] Nursing focuses on human responses as opposed to the disease, its character, and medical treatment. Such a goal is the key element defining nurs-

**Table 7–1.** FACTORS IN DEVELOPING A PEDIATRIC NEPHROLOGY PROGRAM

1. Program philosophy
2. Defined roles (job descriptions)
3. Documentation process
4. Policy procedure manual
5. Environment of dialysis unit
6. Support services
7. Formal interdisciplinary meetings

ing practice and establishes the boundaries of nursing practice in relation to the practice of physicians and other members of the health care team.

In order for nurses to function optimally in providing care for children with ESRD, they must develop specific knowledge and skills in pediatric nephrology, but, equally important, they need to work in an environment conducive to the utilization of their expertise. The pediatric nephrology program should have a philosophy of practice which clearly defines the program's goals, organization, framework, role of its members, boundaries of their practice, and theories of care. These theories have goals, including the changing dynamics of the developing child, actions to meet those goals, methodology for ongoing evaluation, and the redefinition at intervals of the nature of care based upon the program's overall effectiveness.

The field of pediatric nephrology has seen considerable change and improvement in the past 20 years in preventive and primary care. Improvements in conservative management, dialysis treatment technology, development of new treatment modalities and improved success with kidney transplantation, in many cases, have arrested the progress of the primary renal disease or relieved the biophysical symptoms of the condition. It is the human response of the child to the disease itself or the condition brought about by the medical treatment of the disease which remains perhaps the most overwhelming challenge to the various members of the nephrology team. Delayed physical growth, as well as limited emotional and psychological development, is widely seen in pediatric ESRD programs.[1, 4, 6, 8, 9, 11, 12, 13] In an attempt to address these issues, nephrology programs have solicited the input of various health professionals, including psychiatrists, psychologists, clinical social workers, educational specialists, and child life (play therapy) workers. While the input of these professionals is known to be essential in improving the child's response to illness, the effectiveness of their recommendations has often been restricted by the limitations of medical and nursing care.

Although nurses appreciate the primary importance of relief of symptoms of the disease and improvement of the child's physical state, they also recognize that, unless there is a resultant resumption of developmentally appropriate activities of daily living, the success of these treatments is limited. Nursing's

focus on human responses requires that individual nephrology nurses do not blindly accept traditional care practices in their program. Instead, they should use their imaginations and knowledge to design care and utilize treatment measures which enable the child to respond optimally in all areas of his or her life. The nurse has the unique knowledge base which allows her or him to see the value of medical measures, while also keeping in perspective the secondary limitations which these measures may impose upon the child on both a short-term and long-term basis. Nursing's goal is to design care which optimizes the child's response to illness, while minimizing the limitations imposed by the medical and nursing measures.

The choice of treatment modality and design of nursing care should reflect an emphasis on the child's psychosocial development by allowing the child to have developmentally appropriate participation and responsibility for his or her care. While all treatment modalities have specific limitations, there should be an emphasis on optimizing the child's interactions with family and peers and especially on encouraging the participation of the child in a formal school program, with supplemental tutoring only if needed.

## PARTICIPATORY CARE AND HOME HEMODIALYSIS •

The literature has shown considerable improvement in patient outcome in adult and pediatric programs when treatment modalities which encourage patient participation are used.[14–24] While the literature has reported improved patient rehabilitation with self-dialysis and various forms of home dialysis, there have been limited reports of improved patient responses through the use of in-center dependent care hemodialysis treatments. Home dialysis was an early form of treatment of children with ESRD which involved parents as the primary care agents. The use of home hemodialysis subsequently diminished because of the increase in funding and availability of in-center hemodialysis facilities. Also, many centers found it more convenient to perform in-center hemodialysis than to develop or maintain time-consuming home hemodialysis training programs.[24–27]

While home hemodialysis was often an overwhelming experience for the entire family, the alternative of in-center care has its own limitations and effects on the child. The key to success or failure of any treatment modality lies not only in its medical effectiveness but in the extent that it allows the developing child to continue with normal "activities" and life style. While various forms of home dialysis offer advantages to families who must travel great distances, there may be serious psychosocial consequences if the child is placed in a dependent, passive overprotected role.

The success of various forms of self-hemodialysis has been reported in the literature of adult nephrology.[1, 11, 13, 16, 20, 23, 26] Despite claims of success with self-dialysis, the use of in-center dependent care hemodialysis continued to rise through the 1970's in adult and pediatric programs, while the use of self-care dialysis (in-center self-dialysis, home hemodialysis, intermittent peritoneal dialysis, continuous ambulatory dialysis) did not show a commensurate rise until quite recently.[28] It is encouraging to see a return to the use of self-care modalities and a shift in the focus of nephrology teams toward treatment modalities which best optimize the child's response. Claims that home dialysis is the ideal treatment modality for children are irresponsible, for they lack insight into the multiple issues which make these modalities unavailable to all children and families and imply that children and their families are failures unless they perform certain forms of home dialysis. The key to the success of home dialysis is the participation of the child and family in the patient's care and the resultant benefits in terms of improved self-esteem and ability to maintain a more usual life style.

While home dialysis may not be an option for all children owing to physical limitations, programmatic limitations, psychosocial limitations, or child and family preference, many of the benefits of home dialysis can be achieved in an in-center hemodialysis unit through the incorporation of a self-care model by the nursing staff. Dorothea Orem introduced self-care as a model for the practice of nursing throughout the health-care system.[29] The adaptation of this self-care model in pediatric nephrology has obvious application to home dialysis programs. It is perhaps equally important and necessary in the in-center environment, where children who receive dependent hemodialysis treatments often exhibit depression, impaired psychosocial development, noncompliant be-

havior, and other alterations in behavior as compared to their behavior prior to the initiation of treatments.

## ACUTE CARE MODEL

Health care members who work in hospitals, especially those working on pediatric services, are routinely faced with acute care situations and are tempted to apply these models of care in the chronic hemodialysis unit. Acute care models have a natural focus toward early resolution of the child's disease process. Short-term care plans enable a child to remain in a dependent role and then return to developmentally appropriate activities after recovery from the illness. Conversely, a dependent role on a long-term basis can have serious repercussions for the child with ESRD, if it does not allow him or her to make age-appropriate developmental progress over time. While the primary goal must be to alter the disease process, it is equally important that children continue to grow, develop, attend school, and relate normally to peers and families.

The predominant use of acute care models in the care of children with ESRD has been a major factor in the development of serious psychosocial complications, including regression, dependency, delayed development, social deprivation, poor school attendance, and lack of vocational goals. Acute care models which presuppose that the child's developmental progress can be safely postponed until he overcomes his illness are inappropriate in the child with ESRD because of the nature of treatment of the child's renal disease, his or her response to treatment modalities, and the uncertainty of when, if ever, the child will receive a "successful" kidney transplant which will allow him or her to resume "a normal life." Health care professionals often find it easier on themselves and better accepted by parents if they utilize an acute care approach which presents an optimistic, though often unrealistic, scenario of short-term hemodialysis followed by early transplantation and return to the child's previous health status. It is the responsibility of nephrology nurses to share their knowledge and experience in the care of children with ESRD, to design care which is realistic, to encourage developmentally appropriate involvement of the child from the onset and throughout his or her involvement in the program, and to act as a role model to parents through the nurse's own nursing interaction with the child.

## SELF-CARE

Self-care has been defined as deliberate actions performed by oneself in order to meet needs as a human being.[29] Humans have natural capacity to care for themselves. The goal of child rearing is for growing children to achieve changing levels of maturity at which they can develop an expanding set of skills in caring for themselves and, eventually, enabling them to become independently functioning adults. In caring for children with ESRD, self-care requisites are addressed through medical treatment of the child's renal disease while also providing a humane environment and approach that is supportive (Table 7–2).

In order to optimize the child's developmental progress, nurses in a pediatric nephrology program must first consider the routine self-care activities that the child has had responsibility for in his life prior to the onset of illness, and strive to have the child not only maintain but continue to develop ongoing responsibility for various factors in his life.

The environment of a pediatric dialysis unit should reflect a design, philosophy, and standard of care with these goals: (1) to enable the child to maintain his previous level of involvement in meeting daily, routine self-care needs; (2) to provide for ongoing developmentally appropriate involvement of the child as he matures; and (3) to promote ongoing developmentally appropriate involvement of the child in addressing new self-care demands imposed by the disease and its treatment. The pediatric nephrology nurse must address the long-term develop-

**Table 7–2.** GOALS IN SELF-CARE ENVIRONMENT[29]

1. Support the life process
2. Maintain human structures and human functioning within a normal range
3. Support development in accordance with human potential
4. Prevent injury and pathological states
5. Contribute to the regulation or control of the effects of injury and pathology
6. Contribute to the cure or regulation of pathological processes.

**Table 7–3.** DESIRABLE FEATURES IN COMPARISON OF TREATMENT MODALITIES

1. Medically effective in safely controlling symptoms of ESRD
2. Allows for ongoing appropriate developmental progress of the child
3. Maintains child's ability to physically function in activities of daily living
4. Minimizes distortion of body image
5. Minimizes time expenditure devoted to treatments
6. Is accessible
7. Allows for appropriate social interactions with family and peers
8. Provides opportunity for formal educational and vocational needs
9. Provides ongoing support to child and family

mental needs of the child during her or his initial contacts and subsequent care plans for the child must reflect these needs.

The successful outcome of self-care activities is dependent upon the acceptance of this concept by the child and family. Dependent care is traditionally practiced throughout the health-care system, and self-care is not a goal which members of our society consciously value. It is important that all members of the nephrology team value the concept of self-care and support nurses in their actions. In addition to explaining the medical implications of the child's renal disease, physicians must explain the program's philosophy, recommendations, and expectations for the child and family. Physicians, clinical social workers, nurses, and other health professionals who orient families to an ESRD program should address self-care issues in their initial discussions with the child and family, as well as in their initial acts of care. Early introductory meetings with families, by conveying a realistic presentation of the current state of the art of medical care for children with ESRD, can help avoid the temptation by staff members to apply an acute care model despite encouragement by the parents. The child and family should be assisted in choosing a treatment modality based upon a variety of factors, which are summarized in Table 7–3.

The child and family should be active participants in the decision-making process of choosing a treatment modality. The nurse provides knowledge and expertise in assisting the child and family to develop a rational basis for choosing a treatment modality which, from the child and family's perspective, best optimizes the above factors. Patients and families should be allowed flexibility in choosing a treatment modality which best meets their needs at a point in time and the nurse should avoid imposing her or his own values upon the family. The child and family should be assured that they will receive equal nursing attention and quality of care regardless of their choice of treatment modality. The option to change treatment modalities should be offered, and nurses should not convey a sense of failure if the child or family desires to change to a different form of treatment modality because of a change in attitude or situation in the future.

The literature has shown that self-dialysis is better accepted by patients if training is performed early in their care, and they are not exposed to dependent care in an in-center hemodialysis unit.[13, 14, 23] We have found that when self-care issues are addressed in initial meetings with families, and when self-care is encouraged in the hemodialysis unit, there is a greater tendency for children and families to initially choose or later attempt self-care treatment modalities which best optimize their life style.

## PHYSICAL DESIGN

The physical design of the dialysis unit should reflect the self-care philosophy and should be an environment which is conducive to the child's participation in his or her care. The atmosphere should not be visually overwhelming to the child and family despite the high level of technology required in performing hemodialysis. Bright colors, pictures, toys, mobiles, and other decorations can deemphasize the machinery and create a comfortable, relaxed, humanized atmosphere. Chronic hemodialysis should be performed with children in chairs with a capacity to recline if necessary. It is preferable to perform acute hemodialysis in a separate area from that of children receiving routine maintenance hemodialysis on a chronic basis. Areas should be designed where nurses can work with children and families in privacy for educational instruction or periodic review of care plans, work on projects, and meet privately with other health care professionals.

Emergency equipment should be readily available but placed in a concealed area where the child does not have to be exposed to it on a routine basis. Acute care equipment such as beds, elaborate monitors, suctioning equipment, oxygen, and so on should be limited in their use if the child is expected to perceive that he or she is capable of participating in his or her own care. Nurses may need to sacrifice their own needs for control, personal gratification, and convenience in order to create an environment in which the child and family do not perceive that routine hemodialysis is a highly technical treatment to be performed only by skilled professionals.

It is preferable to use hemodialysis machines which are esthetically pleasing to the child and designed for ease of function. Highly technical machinery should be available but utilized in the acute area only. (Children who require acute dialysis owing to noncompliance should be encouraged to alter their behavior rather than altering the parameters of routine dialysis.) The arrangement of chairs should facilitate the child's access to the machine for monitoring and adjustments. Seating arrangements should also facilitate interactions between children receiving treatments while allowing the flexibility to rearrange equipment and chairs in order to provide privacy for children who are doing school work or require isolation. Sinks, scales, and supplies should be accessible to small children if they are expected to participate in preparations for their treatment.

The input of child life (play therapy) workers and educational specialists is valuable in creating an environment where children learn recreational skills and supplement their formal schooling. Nurses working in collaboration with these members of the team can facilitate activities which encourage appropriate development, peer interactions, and constructive use of time. The child learns to set priorities for his care, education, and recreation, and through ongoing interactions and review is encouraged to optimize his life outside the dialysis unit.

## DIALYSIS UNIT ORGANIZATION

The Table of Organization (Table 7–4) shows the Nephrology Program Coordinator at the highest level of nursing supervision within the Nephrology Program. The Coordinator is responsible for overseeing the care of children throughout the program and works in close collaboration with the Executive Director of the ESRD Program, Medical Director of the Dialysis Unit, and the Head Nurses of the Dialysis Inpatient and Intensive Care Units. The Coordinator has the respon-

**Table 7–4.** TABLE OF ORGANIZATION OF PEDIATRIC DIALYSIS UNIT

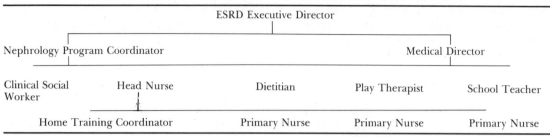

sibility of working with nurses to establish a nursing philosophy within the program and oversees nursing care to assure that it is implemented in a manner which is consistent with that philosophy of care. The Coordinator maintains liaison with those individuals who are administratively responsible for the Nephrology Program and collaborates with physicians and other members of the nephrology team. The Coordinator acts as a nephrology nursing clinical specialist, lends nursing expertise, and coordinates care for children in collaboration with health care professionals in other departments, including the transplant clinic, inpatient acute care areas, intensive care unit, nursing department, other specialty nurses, and other nephrology programs which provide partial care to children with ESRD.

The Head Nurse of the dialysis unit is directly responsible for supervision of care provided by nurses in the hemodialysis unit as well as for those children who receive ongoing home dialysis care.

The Home Training Coordinator (HTC) has responsibility, in collaboration with the child's primary nurse, for overseeing the education of children and families involved with home dialysis. The HTC is also responsible for providing consistent, ongoing refinement of the training program and manual, while supplying nursing expertise through collaboration with other primary nurses, physicians, and members of the nephrology team. The HTC solicits the assistance of the primary nurse throughout the training program and encourages the child and family to maintain their ongoing relationship with their primary nurse throughout training and subsequent follow-up care.

We have developed and implemented a primary nursing system in which one nurse is directly responsible for the ongoing care of a particular child and family. The primary nurse collaborates with all members (Fig. 7–1) of the nephrology team and utilizes the

nursing process to assess, plan, implement, and evaluate the child's care. The primary nurse is *not* responsible for providing all direct care to the child but is responsible for designing care plans and providing ongoing evaluation of the medical effectiveness of care as well as addressing the self-care requisites of the child.

While the hemodialysis unit may have as its primary focus providing in-center hemodialysis treatments, it is advantageous for the nurses to also be responsible for the care of children receiving home dialysis treatments (hemodialysis, CAPD, IPD). It may initially appear easier to have one or two nurses responsible for all home dialysis patients, but it is also beneficial, especially in units with limited numbers of patients, to have primary nurses formally oriented and educated as nephrology nurses, who have knowledge and skills in all aspects of nephrology care. The nurse who has expertise in all treatment modalities has a knowledge base which facilitates interactions with children and families to initially choose an appropriate treatment modality. Continuity of care is best provided through a continued primary nurse relationship regardless of the treatment modality which her primary patient has chosen to receive at any particular point in time.

The role and responsibilities of the pediatric nephrology primary nurse are quite extensive and require a commitment by the nurse to ongoing personal education in order to initially obtain expertise and to maintain that expertise in the rapidly changing field of nephrology. Recruitment of nurses to work in pediatric nephrology should involve specific attention to the nurses' commitment to ongoing education, a willingness to reexamine one's values on an ongoing basis, experience or desire to work with a multidisciplinary professional team, and a philosophy of nursing which values patient independence utilizing self-care theory. Recruitment of nurses who have values consistent with the

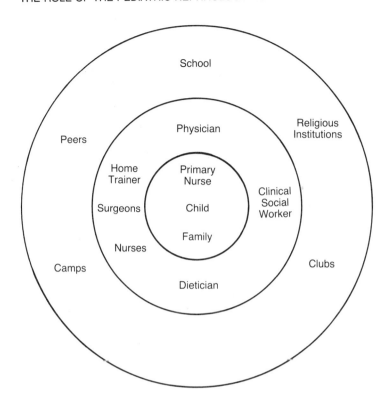

**Figure 7–1.** Graphic description of the relationship of the child's interaction with a variety of individuals. The child's relationships with family and primary nurse facilitate interactions with other individuals.

program's philosophy of care aids in their adjustment to the role of a primary nurse and reduces the level of future "burn out" and turnover.

## NURSING PROCESS

The primary nurse in the hemodialysis unit utilizes the nursing process as a foundation for her or his practice as follows:

**Assessment.** The primary nurse establishes a relationship as early as possible with the child and family in order to develop trust but also to begin initial assessment of their self-care needs and capabilities, in addition to traditional physical assessments. Assessment of the child is often difficult if he or she is acutely ill or has CNS manifestations of renal disease, which often distorts the character of the child's personality and behavior. It is not uncommon for families to report that their child was "normal," but in the past few years has been doing poorly in school, has become a behavior problem, and has reduced his interactions with peers and family. The parents' input should be solicited in attempting to assess the child's behavior, personality, and capabilities prior to the onset of illness.

It is important that the primary nurse not accept the child's behavior during an acute crisis as being the norm but instead set higher expectations for the child and reinforce to parents that the child's behavior will probably change once treatment begins and he or she is less uremic. While unrealistically high expectations should be avoided, for they may frustrate the child, it is also important that nurses do not establish for the child too low a set of expectations, which discourage ongoing development and maturity of the child. The first assessments and expectations of the child in initial care situations are often the most influential in terms of the child and family's acceptance of themselves as capable, productive members of society who have mastered the illness by caring for themselves as opposed to being dependent on society because of illness.

Assessment of the child requires the input of the child and family as well as other professional members of the nephrology team. The primary nurse develops a formal nursing assessment of the medical status of the child as well as a baseline of routine self-care requisites that the child has established in his daily care prior to his or her illness. The primary nurse should consider a variety of factors in assessing the child, including

**Table 7–5.** SELF-CARE ASSESSMENT
OF PATIENT

1. Chronologic age
2. Developmental age
3. Family background, roles, interactions, dynamics
4. Personality
5. Physical and social environment
6. Child/family response to stress situations
7. Home routines
8. Schooling/vocational training
9. Peer interactions
10. Special interests
11. Health status, needs, limitations

**Table 7–6.** GOALS OF SHORT-TERM
TREATMENT PLANS

1. Set treatment parameters
2. Encourage appropriate parent participation
3. Allow dependency to develop trust, but encourage development of the child's independence
4. Set specific goals for child's participation in self-care activities
5. Provide therapeutic use of recreation time
6. Allow time for formal school or vocational training
7. Encourage appropriate peer interactions
8. Encourage normalcy of life style

but not limited to those listed in Table 7–5. The nursing assessment is shared with other members of the nephrology team and utilized to develop care plans on a short-term and long-term basis.

**Planning.** Planning of care is based upon the nurse's assessment of the child and family as well as previous experience and knowledge of the nephrology team in caring for children with ESRD. It is crucial that the child and parents be involved in the planning of care, for unless they understand and accept the primary nurse's expectations for the child they will not support or comply with care as planned. It is unrealistic for nurses to design care to meet their (the nurse's or the team's) expectations unless the child and family have simultaneously committed themselves to achieving those goals. Formal periodic meetings with child and family should include a review of care plans and, in some cases, the signing of a written contract explaining what is expected of child, family, and staff. Written contracts are valuable in clarifying and documenting the expectations of staff and families as well as in identifying the roles of all parties, including the child.

Plans for involvement of parents and significant others in the care of children are important to reduce separation anxiety, lessen parental guilt and feelings of helplessness, provide the opportunity for professionals to assess the family's understanding and implementation of information, and to provide the opportunity for nurses and other team members to view family interactions and aid in the development of appropriate parent-child relationships. While involvement of parents is essential to a successful outcome for the child, it is the primary nurse's responsibility to constantly re-evaluate care plans and to adjust them so that the parents are not overly involved and so that the child increasingly participates actively in

his or her care, at a developmentally appropriate level. It has been stated that acting for another is appropriate in infant and child care situations, but other methods should be added as soon as the child is ready for it.[30] The primary nurse must view the child as a growing, developing human being and should serve as a role model to parents by designing and implementing care which continually presents new challenges to the child in meeting his or her self-care demands.

The planning of care should involve formal documentation so that other nurses are aware of the primary nurse's expectations for the child. A Kardex or other file should include the short-term plans listed in Table 7–6.

**Implementation.** Implementation of nursing care plans may be performed by the primary nurse or any nurse in the dialysis unit. The nurse's role in a self-care environment is summarized in Table 7–7. The child should be encouraged to view himself as a responsible self-care agent by gradually learning to perform care measures through which self-care requisites are met.[29] The nurse caring for the child during an individual treatment should follow the primary nurse's care plan and encourage the child to participate in self-care activities as developmentally appropriate, including hand washing, cleaning the cannulation site, placing plastic adhesive strips on needle sites, charting, recording vital signs, setting up supplies, and eventually progressing to calculation of

**Table 7–7.** NURSING ACTS IN SELF-CARE
PROGRAM[29]

1. Acting for or doing for another
2. Guiding another
3. Supporting another (physically or psychologically)
4. Providing an environment that promotes personal development in preparation for becoming able to meet present or future demands for action
5. Teaching another

ultrafiltration requirements, machine setup, and monitoring and treatment of symptoms during the hemodialysis treatment. The nurse oversees the child's actions to avoid any dangerous situations; however, he or she encourages the child toward achieving a goal of being his own agent in performing self-care acts.

**Evaluation.** Evaluation is a two-fold process of ongoing assessment of care plans for effectiveness of their actions. Evaluation of care should be performed by the primary nurse on a daily basis, with particular attention to medical effectiveness of hemodialysis treatments as well as attention to ongoing self-care expectations for the child. While the child may be responsible for his or her daily treatment record, the nurse oversees the treatment and makes evaluative comments on treatment records and progress notes. The formal monthly summary written by the primary nurse should include a review of the child's status (Table 7–8).

The monthly summary is reviewed with the attending physician at a formal meeting outside the dialysis unit. This meeting provides an opportunity for the primary nurse and physician to evaluate the child's care and also serves as an educational experience and forum for sharing knowledge, expertise, judgments, and opinions. Primary nurses are also responsible for presenting their care plans at nursing rounds and team conferences where others are made aware of the child's status and can offer input and help to readjust care plans. Interdisciplinary nephrology team meetings are conducted on a regular basis in order for members of the team to share information and evaluate patient care and offer suggestions for further care. Peer review, in these meetings, helps the nurse to evaluate herself or himself and is a subtle way of exploring one's attitudes and the extent to which they are incorporated into care plans.

**Nurse Stress.** It is often overwhelming for nurses to deal with the complexities of caring for chronically ill children who may exhibit noncompliance or behavior disorders or who do not respond as favorably to medical treatment as the professional staff may have hoped. These issues, as well as the nurses' attitudes, beliefs, values, and personal growth needs, can best be addressed through separate formal discussions held outside the dialysis unit and are facilitated by input from a clinical social worker, psychologist, psychiatrist, psychiatric nurse specialist, or nursing

**Table 7–8.** MONTHLY SUMMARY OF PROGRESS

1. Medical status
2. Dialysis treatment parameters
3. Vascular access condition
4. Body chemistries
5. Medications prescribed and compliance
6. Self-care requisites
7. Nutrition
8. Education
9. Psychosocial progress
10. Transplant status
11. Short-term and long-term goals

coordinator. Such meetings often serve as valuable experience for nurses to evaluate their own professional progress, aid in the establishment of realistic goals, provide relief from anxiety and frustration, and permit nurses to interact with co-workers in non-stressful, supportive situations which ease interactional difficulties in the stressful environment of the dialysis unit. Nursing "burn-out" and turnover are minimized through these self-evaluation activities as well as through recruitment of nurses with values consistent with the program and the development of a program in which nurses have autonomy, a variety of educational and practical experiences, a supportive team of professionals, and a flexible work schedule that allows them the freedom to participate in patient-related or special projects outside the dialysis unit.

## CONCLUSION

The role of nursing in the care of children with ESRD has been continually expanded over time. The role of the pediatric hemodialysis nurse has been expanded to that of a nephrology nurse, who has the knowledge and skills to care for children who receive a variety of different treatment modalities. The nephrology nurse focuses his or her practice on the child's human response to renal disease and the limitations imposed by the treatment of the disease. As a primary nurse, the nephrology nurse assesses, plans, implements, and evaluates the care of children, utilizing a self-care model in which the child is encouraged to have increasing responsibility through participation in his or her own care. The environment of the dialysis unit, philosophy of the nephrology program, and systems of care are reflective of the self-care theory.

While further nursing research is needed to isolate the actions which best optimize self-care acceptance by children, it has been shown that self-care activities can reduce the limitations imposed by dialysis treatments, improve the child's self-esteem, meet the needs of parents, promote patient compliance, and help to establish a more normal life style for children with ESRD. Self-care hemodialysis offers children a chance to see themselves as productive, capable members of society. The unique role of pediatric nephrology nurses in designing a self-care model which focuses on optimizing the child's human response to his or her disease has become a valuable contribution to the management of the child with ESRD. Most importantly, it provides an alternative for those children and families who cannot or do not wish to receive a transplant or perform home dialysis and gives them the opportunity to successfully master their disease and to live as normal a life as possible.

## REFERENCES

1. Freidman EA: Strategy in Renal Failure. New York, John Wiley and Sons, 1978.
2. Hekalman FP, Ostendarp CA: Nephrology Nursing Perspectives of Care. New York, McGraw-Hill Book Co., 1979.
3. Lancaster LE: The Patient with End Stage Renal Disease. New York, John Wiley and Sons, 1979.
4. Lewy JE, Poter DE: The management of dialysis and transplantation in children. J Dial 1:75, 1976.
5. Leonard MO: Current nursing practice in dialysis care: A summary. J Dial 1:181, 1977.
6. Lewy JE: The management of dialysis and transplantation in children. J Dial 1:75, 1977.
7. Mauer SM, Lynch RE: Hemodialysis techniques for infants and children. Pediat Clin North Am 23:4, 1976.
8. McDaid TK: Chronic hemodialysis in children. Issues of Comprehensive Pediatric Nursing 2:53, 1978.
9. Topor M: Symposium on chronic renal failure: Chronic renal disease in children. Nurs Clin North Am 16:587, 1981.
10. Lang N, Argondizzo NT, Barnard K, et al: Nursing: A Social Policy Statement. American Nurses Association, Kansas City, Missouri, 1980, p 9.
11. Chyate SB: Rehabilitation in Chronic Renal Failure. Baltimore, Maryland, Williams and Wilkins Co, 1979.
12. Lansing L: Back to school for the child on long term hemodialysis. J Am Assoc Nephrol Nurses Technicians 8:13, 1981.
13. Grossman MB: Self-care for children and adolescents on dialysis. J Am Assoc Nephrol Nurses Technicians 8:36, 1981.
14. Blagg C: Home dialysis. Dial Transplant 6:10, 1977.
15. Hekelman FP, Phillips JA: Teaching and learning for self-care dialysis. Nephrol Nurse 3:12, 1981.
16. Jenkins PG, Guttman FD, Riesselback RE: Self hemodialysis: The optimal mode of dialytic therapy. Arch Intern Med 3:357, 1976.
17. Leinweber BA: The hemodialysis client: nursing focus on self-care. Nephrol Nurse 3:8, 1981.
18. Levy NB: Self-dialysis: A psychological two-edged sword. Dial Transplant 6:10, 1977.
19. Nebeck B: A view of self-care as seen by patients. . . the dialysis program. Nephrol Nurse 2:27, 1980.
20. Rhodes V: Promoting patient independence: Self-care dialysis. Nephrol Nurse 1:36, 1979.
21. Rusk GH: Psychological aspects of self-care and home dialysis. J Dial 2:165, 1978.
22. Self Dialysis: A Monograph. J Am Assoc Nephrol Nurses Technicians (Supplemental Edition), 1977.
23. Sullivan JF, Sullivan MT, Bryant D, et al: Two years experience with an in-center self-care program. Dial Transplant 6:10, 1977.
24. Tenckhoff H: Home peritoneal dialysis. Dial Transplant 6:10, 1977.
25. Delano BG: Whatever happended to home hemodialysis? J Dial 1:465, 1977.
26. Friedman EA, Delano BG, and Butt KM: Pragmatic realities in uremia therapy. N Engl J Med 298:368, 1978.
27. Blagg CR: Incidence and prevalence of home dialysis. J Dial 1:475, 1977.
28. Sorrels PAJ: Peritoneal dialysis: A rediscovery. Nurs Clin North Am 16:511, 1981.
29. Orem DE: Nursing: Concepts of Practice. New York, McGraw-Hill Book Co., 1980, p. 64.

# 8

# Hemoperfusion in Therapeutic Medicine

Zoe L. Papadopoulou, M.D.
Antonia C. Novello, M.D.
Philip L. Calcagno, M.D.

Hemoperfusion is an elective extracorporeal detoxification technique used for the removal of endogenous or exogenous toxins from the blood stream. In this technique blood is passed through adsorbent materials such as activated charcoal or resin for the removal of toxic compounds from the circulatory system. It has been used over the past several years either experimentally or therapeutically for the treatment of uremia,[1-10] in cases of abnormal ingestion of drugs and toxins,[11-20] reversal of coma and hepatic failure,[21-26] and enhancement of clearance of various other noxious substances.[27, 28]

The first clinical experiments of blood detoxification by extracorporeal circulation through columns of activated carbon were performed in 1964 by Yatzidis et al.[29] It was demonstrated that 200 gm of activated charcoal particles could absorb from the plasma 1 to 2 gm of short- and long-acting barbiturates as well as glutethimide and salicylic acid. These findings were later used to support a clinical trial in which two patients with barbiturate poisoning were successfully treated by charcoal hemoperfusion.[20]

The pioneer work by Yatzidis brought significant interest in the development of sorbent hemoperfusion. Additional studies, however, demonstrated that charcoal hemoperfusion utilizing uncoated or poorly washed carbon granules was often associated with significant complications. These complications included the possibility of embolization of charcoal particles from the hemoperfusion device, as well as significant platelet loss.[30] Subsequently, various efforts were made to develop safe and effective hemoperfusion systems. Chang, in pioneering work, demonstrated that by encapsulating the charcoal particles in albumin or albumin-collodion, he enhanced the biocompatibility of the sorbent and prevented the possibility of embolization of the charcoal material.[31]

## HEMOPERFUSION SYSTEMS USED CLINICALLY

Following Chang's important work utilizing the albumin-collodion-coated activated charcoal (ACAC) hemoperfusion system, various other microencapsulating materials for activated charcoal have been investigated by using different polymers with the purpose of enhancing biocompatibility and preventing embolization of charcoal. These encapsulated charcoal systems have evolved into the Smith and Nephew Hemacol device (acrylic hydrogel encapsulated charcoal), the Gambro Hemoadsorba device (cellulose acetate encapsulated charcoal), and other commercial systems (Table 8–1). The fixed-bed charcoal system (B-D Hemodetoxifier) is an uncoated charcoal sorbent device in which the granular charcoal is fixed to a polyethylene backing and wound into a spiral.

**Table 8–1.** TYPES OF CHARCOAL HEMOPERFUSION SYSTEMS AVAILABLE

| Hemoperfusion Device | Composition | Membrane Thickness |
| --- | --- | --- |
| ACAC | Albumin-cellulose nitrate encapsulated charcoal (300 gm) | 0.02–0.05 micron |
| Hemacol (Smith & Nephew/Warner-Lambert) | Acrylic hydrogel encapsulated charcoal (300 gm) | 3–5 micron |
| Adsorba 300C (Gambro) | Cellulose acetate encapsulated charcoal (300 gm) | 3–5 micron |
| B-D Hemodetoxifier (Becton-Dickinson) | Fixed-bed charcoal chlorosulfonated polyethylene (100 gm) | Fixed-bed |

All these systems are effective in minimizing particulate embolism. Unfortunately, the various types of polymer membranes used to coat the carbon have different permeability characteristics, which affect the rate of drug adsorption or blood clearance by the adsorbent column. In addition, during hemoperfusion there is a progressive decrease in the clearance of drugs with time because of competitive utilization of adsorptive sites by various blood solutes.

Besides the charcoal, other adsorbing agents employed involve the use of a non-ionic microporous resin such as the XAD-2 and XAD-4 materials. These polystyrene Amberlite series sorbents have been demonstrated to be very effective in the removal of lipid-soluble drugs from the blood. In addition to their specific adsorptive attraction for lipid-soluble solutes, they have a large adsorptive capacity and clearance rate, thereby avoiding a progressive decrease in column clearance with time.

## SAFETY OF HEMOPERFUSION DEVICES

Most of the industrial hemoperfusion models available have been developed with emphasis on the safety of the large-scale production. This necessitated the use of thicker membranes, resulting in low clearances for creatinine, uric acid, and other molecules. Some systems are very blood-compatible whereas others are not. Those which are not blood compatible may deplete platelets or cause platelet aggregates within the circulation, perhaps as a result of the release of platelet-aggregating factors on contact with some sorbents. Thus, the severity of thrombocytopenia induced during hemoperfusion depends primarily on the type of col-

umn used. The ACAC and Adsorba 300C[32] hemoperfusion columns, which are very blood compatible, are associated with only a 10% reduction in platelet count. On the other hand, the use of either the Hemacol or the B-D Hemodetoxifier[32] hemoperfusion columns results in a reduction in the platelet count of 30% and 53% respectively. Similar degrees of platelet reduction have been reported with the use of Amberlite (uncoated XAD-4 nonionic polystyrene resin).[33]

In order to prevent fibrin-induced clotting of the column, significant doses of heparin, which may be dangerous to patients with preexisting clotting abnormalities or existing sites of bleeding, are often required. Hemolysis of red cells, although potentially a problem, does not appear to be a significant problem, especially when hemoperfusion is used in short-term situations, such as the treatment of drug intoxication. Most of the hemoperfusion columns have been demonstrated to have no significant release of particulate material. However, particulate embolism may occur with some of the available hemoperfusion systems, especially when high blood flow rates are used (particularly early in the procedure) or when high pressures are allowed to be generated within the system (e.g., clotting or venous outlet obstruction). Finally, since the adsorptive capacity of most charcoal hemoperfusion systems decreases with time, they become ineffective when used longer than 6 hours.

## USE OF HEMOPERFUSION IN THERAPEUTIC MEDICINE

Investigators continue to seek a positive role for carbon hemoperfusion in therapeutic medicine. Hemoperfusion has been widely explored for the treatment of drug poisoning, hepatic encephalopathy, and uremia. It has also been considered as a possible mode of treatment for psoriasis, rheumatism, chronic schizophrenia, and for various uremic problems such as uremic pericarditis, pruritus, and neuropathy.

## Hemoperfusion in Acute Intoxication

The main goal in the treatment of acute poisoning is the fast removal of the poison from body tissues. Charcoal and resin sorbent systems have been demonstrated to be quite effective in the removal of significant amounts of various drugs. In the majority of cases, the XAD-4 resin system appears to be somewhat superior to charcoal systems, but in general both are highly efficient in remov-

ing drugs. Hemoperfusion is particularly effective in the removal of substances which are lipid-soluble, highly protein bound, and poorly distributed in plasma water. Such substances are not significantly removed by hemodialysis or peritoneal dialysis. Compounds which are shown to be amenable to charcoal or resin hemoperfusion are listed in Table 8–2. Under appropriate conditions, therefore, there is little doubt that hemoperfusion is very effective in removing a large number of toxins from the blood.

In terms of rate of drug clearance, it has been shown that hemoperfusion is superior to dialysis. When comparable blood flow rates are used, hemoperfusion achieves higher total body clearance than hemodialysis and is considered to be the treatment of choice in patients with severe overdosage with certain commonly abused compounds, such as bar-

**Table 8–2.** COMPOUNDS REMOVED BY CHARCOAL OR RESIN HEMOPERFUSION*

| | | |
|---|---|---|
| Analgesics | Nonbarbiturate | Endogenous Toxins |
| Acetyl salicylic acid | Hypnotics, Sedatives & | Amino acids |
| Methyl salicylate | Tranquilizers | Uric acid |
| Acetaminophen | Ethchlorvynol | Creatinine |
| (Paracetamol) | Glutethimide | Cholic acid |
| | Methyprylon | Polyamino acids |
| Alcohols | Methaqualone | Polypeptides |
| Ethyl alcohol (Ethanol) | (Diazepam) | Uremic toxins |
| | Chloral hydrate | Indicans |
| Antiasthmatics | Carbromal | Phenolic compounds |
| Theophylline | Chlorpromazine | Organic acids |
| | Promazine | Middle molecules |
| Antimicrobials | Promethazine | Thyroxine |
| Chloramphenicol | Meprobamate | Triiodothyronine |
| Gentamycin | | Immune proteins |
| Isoniazid | Cardiovascular Agents | |
| | Digoxin | Metals/Inorganics |
| Anticancer Agents | Procainamide | Mercury |
| Adriamycin | N-Acetylprocainamide | |
| Methotrexate | | Miscellaneous |
| | Plant/Animal Toxins, | Cimetidine |
| Anticonvulsants | Herbicides/Insecticides | Epinephrine |
| Carbamazepine | *Amanita phalloides* | Norepinephrine |
| Phenytoin | Amanitin | Phenylbutazone |
| | Phalloidin | L-Dopamine |
| Antidepressants | Chlorinated insecticides | Methoxamine |
| Amitryptiline | Polychlorinated | Serotonin |
| Clomipramine | biphenyls | Nucleotides |
| Desipramine | Methyl parathion | Cholic Acid |
| | Demeton-S-methyl | Vitamin $B_{12}$ |
| Barbiturates | sulfoxide | Folic acid |
| Amobarbital | Dimethoate | Bromosulphthalein |
| Butabarbital | Nitrostigmine | Inulin |
| Medinal (Russian) | Paraquat, Diquat | Sucrose dilaurate |
| Pentobarbital | | |
| Phenobarbital | Solvents/Gases | |
| Quinalbital | Carbon tetrachloride | |
| Secobarbital | Ethylene oxide | |

*Adapted from Winchester JF, Gelfand MC, Knepshield JH, Schreiner GE: Dialysis and hemoperfusion of poisons and drugs—Update. Trans Am Soc Artif Intern Organs 23:762, 1977. (By permission.)

**Table 8–3.** MEASURED CLEARANCES (ml/min) OF DRUGS FREQUENTLY INVOLVED IN POISONING*

| Drug | Hemodialysis | Charcoal Hemoperfusion | Resin Hemoperfusion |
|---|---|---|---|
| *Barbiturates* | | | |
| Phenobarbital | 22,[54] 27[53] | 60[53] (50–72)[54] | 80[53] |
| Amobarbital | 26[53] | 66[53] | 88[53] |
| Pentobarbital | 35[54] | 63–80[54] | |
| Secobarbital | 15[54] | 30–75[54] | |
| | | | |
| *Nonbarbiturates, Hypnotics* | | | |
| Ethchlorvynol | 64[54] | 36–114[54] | |
| Glutethimide | 16, 24–149[54] | 72,135.4 ± 50.8[54] | 83[53] |
| Methaqualone | 23[53] | 56[53] | 100[53] |
| *Other Drugs* | | | |
| Phenothiazines | Poor | 20–30[53] | |
| Meprobamate | 62[53] | 172–186[53] | |
| Acetaminophen | 120[54] | 190–315[54] | |
| Paraquat | 0–8.5[54] | 109 ± 28.6[54] | |
| Digoxin | 10[53] | 90–40 falling to 50–25[53] | 45[53] |

*Figures obtained from various data compiled and reported by Winchester JF, Gelfand MC, Knepshield JH, Schreiner GE: Dialysis and hemoperfusion of poisons and drugs—Update. Trans Am Soc Artif Intern Organs 23:762, 1977.[53] Also reported in part by Gelfand MC: Charcoal hemoperfusion in treatment of drug overdosage. Dial Transplant 6:8, 1977.[54]

biturates (especially short- and medium-acting), glutethimide, and acetaminophen. (Table 8–3).

A special situation wherein other forms of facilitated drug removal, such as hemodialysis or peritoneal dialysis, may be superior to hemoperfusion includes instances in which the ingested drug has resulted in the development of severe acid-base derangements (as for example in the case of salicylate, methanol, and ethylene glycol poisoning). Under these circumstances hemodialysis may be the preferred mode of therapy, since it is effective in the simultaneous treatment of the acidosis. Several other factors mitigating against the use of hemoperfusion in acute poisoning include drugs with very rapid action such as cyanide, or drugs whose metabolic elimination rates exceed hemoperfusion removal rates.[34, 35] In addition the value of hemoperfusion for the treatment of ingestion of drugs which have large volumes of distribution and slow intercompartmental transfer rates (for example, tricyclic antidepressants) has not been clearly established.[34, 35]

There is still a controversy as to the effectiveness of hemoperfusion in reducing morbidity or increasing survival in patients with acute poisoning. Hemoperfusion has been shown to reduce coma time in laboratory animals as well as in man, and to enhance the rate of drug elimination.[13, 36, 37] It has been argued that the duration of time a patient remains in coma directly affects his probability of survival, and, therefore, any methods which are effective in reducing the duration of coma, as, for example, hemoperfusion, should also be effective in reducing morbidity and mortality.[38] At the International Workshop on Hemoperfusion held in Haifa, Israel, certain criteria were established for the use of charcoal or resin hemoperfusion in patients with serious intoxications[39] (Table 8–4). It is in patients fulfilling these criteria that hemoperfusion may play a significant role as an adjunct to expert, intensive supportive therapy.

## Hemoperfusion in Hepatic Failure

The efficacy of hemoperfusion in the treatment of hepatic failure and the coma associated with hepatic failure has not yet been clearly established. Although it remains unclear as to which toxin or toxins are responsible for the coma associated with hepatic failure, hemoperfusion is potentially capable of removing a variety of toxins which have been implicated in the pathogenesis of hepatic coma. These toxins include ammonia, false neurotransmitters, short-chain fatty acids, phenols, mercaptans, aromatic amino

**Table 8–4.** INDICATIONS FOR CHARCOAL OR RESIN HEMOPERFUSION IN PATIENTS WITH SERIOUS INTOXICATIONS*

1. Severe clinical intoxication leading to hypoventilation, hypothermia, hypotension, and nonresponsiveness despite supportive clinical measures.
2. Lethal blood concentration of one or more potentially adsorbable drugs.
3. Prolonged coma associated with pneumonitis or known severe chronic pulmonary disease.

*From International Workshop on Hemoperfusion, Haifa, Israel.[39]

acids, and others. Reversal of hepatic coma might allow time for the regeneration of hepatic tissue to sustain life.[35]

Ever since Chang's report[21] on the successful use of hemoperfusion in reversing hepatic coma, other investigators have obtained variable results, especially pertaining to patient survival. Hemoperfusion resulted in 38% and 40% survival respectively in a group of patients with stage IV hepatic coma.[24, 25] However, less encouraging results have been reported by others.[40] In the absence of controlled clinical trials it is not yet certain that hemoperfusion is, in fact, superior to any other form of treatment, including conservative medical management. Although most of the available data are suggestive that hemoperfusion is able to reverse hepatic coma, its overall ability to enhance patient survival has not yet been clearly established.[35] Moreover, the currently available hemoperfusion devices are not completely satisfactory in terms of efficacy and severity of complications. Some of the complications, already present in patients with hepatic failure, include thrombocytopenia and deficiencies in circulating clotting factors. In order to prevent hemorrhagic complications, platelet and coagulation factor infusates should be used routinely at the end of each hemoperfusion procedure. Other systems which would be more biocompatible are currently under investigation.[41, 42]

## Hemoperfusion in Uremia

The hypothesis that uremic symptoms in dialysis patients may result from the retention of middle molecular weight substances has prompted the use of hemoperfusion as an alternative method for the treatment of uremia. Since hemodialysis does not completely reverse the metabolic and endocrine consequences of uremia, the choice of hemoperfusion appeared to be a logical one since the uremia "toxins" may be adsorbable on solutes such as charcoal.

Various studies have indicated that hemoperfusion alone does not remove urea, electrolytes, or water. A comparative analysis of hemoperfusion and standard hemodialysis was performed by Chang et al,[4] utilizing comparable blood flows. It was concluded that with the commercial charcoal devices available in the market, hemoperfusion is not superior to hemodialysis in the removal of known uremic "toxins."

Two present developments that are of interest include the use of hemoperfusion in series with hemodialysis, and the inclusion of activated charcoal within hemodialysis membranes (sorbent membrane dialysis). Large-scale studies comparing the use of hemoperfusion in series with hemodialysis have indicated that this technique is very effective in enhanced removal of creatinine and uric acid and reduces considerably other symptoms of uremia such as pruritus, pericarditis, and abnormal nerve conduction velocities.[3, 9, 43] However, most of these studies have been of "open" design. More controlled clinical trials (in a double blind fashion) are needed before such cumbersome and costly procedures become applicable in clinical medicine.

Similarly, the use of sorbent membrane dialysis for the treatment of uremia has been disappointing so far. Various studies have shown that this procedure is less effective than conventional hemodialysis in controlling metabolite levels in uremia and appears to offer no advantages over hemodialysis.[44] This is due to the fact that the charcoal content of the sorbent membrane dialyzer is too small to effect any advantages over conventional dialysis.[44] It is hoped that newer sorbents with greater specificity and superiority for removal of creatinine and middle molecules will become available in the near future.

## THE USE OF HEMOPERFUSION IN CHILDREN

The application of hemoperfusion technique in children has not been adequately explored in the past. A significant limitation for its use has been the large dead space present in the commercially available devices. With few modifications in the technique to account for the child's small circulating blood volume, we, and others, have not encountered any technical difficulties by using the standard columns presently available.[45–49] A full description of the hemoperfusion technique has been given elsewhere.[50]

In general, the use of hemoperfusion in infants and children has been limited to the treatment of drug intoxication or in the management of hepatic coma. Considering a mortality rate of 5%[51] to 38%[38] in hospitalized poisoned patients in stage IV coma managed conservatively, other therapeutic measures such as hemoperfusion should be seriously considered in the management of such patients. Our experience, as well as that of others, shows that hemoperfusion may be of considerable value in the treatment of patients with life-threatening intoxications causing deep coma with associated depression of the respiratory or circulatory systems.

Of the children with drug ingestion treated at our center, one patient was in stage IV coma with shallow respirations requiring intubation with respiratory assistance and three patients were in stage I coma. One patient had multiple drug ingestion following ingestion of alcohol and marijuana; one had ingested acetaminophen, and two had paraquat poisoning. All the patients recovered following hemoperfusion.[49] In addition, hemoperfusion has been used successfully by other investigators for the treatment of severe theophylline intoxication in a three-year-old patient[45] and for the treatment of severe chloramphenicol intoxication in one infant.[38, 46]

There are only a few reports in the literature which deal with the use of hemoperfusion for the treatment of hepatic coma in children. In our own experience, of four children with stage IV hepatic coma treated with this technique, only one patient with severe halothane hepatitis recovered completely.[49] Interestingly the three children with hepatic decompensation in whom hemoperfusion had no beneficial effect also had associated cerebral edema. Although hemoperfusion may be a logical approach to the management of patients with hepatic decompensation, the various devices currently available in the market are not completely satisfactory in terms of efficiency and severity of complications. Because certain complications such as platelet destruction and depletion of coagulation factors may be especially severe

in patients with hepatic failure,[52] care should be taken to use hemoperfusion devices which are blood-compatible. Until more efficient devices become available for clinical use, hemoperfusion should be used only in carefully selected patients with acute and potentially reversible hepatic failure.

In conclusion, it is our belief that hemoperfusion can be performed safely in children without the development of serious complications, provided meticulous attention is given to technical details. Overall, the indications for hemoperfusion in children are the same as those in adults, and it should be considered for children with severe poisonings or drug overdosages who meet the criteria suggested at the International Workshop On Hemoperfusion[39] (see Table 8–4).

## REFERENCES

1. Chang TMS, Gonda A, Dirks JH, et al: ACAC microcapsule artificial kidney for the long term and short term management of eleven patients with chronic renal failure. Trans Am Soc Artif Intern Organs 18:465, 1972.
2. Chang TMS: Hemoperfusion alone and in series with ultrafiltration or dialysis for uremia, poisoning, and liver failure. Kidney Int 10:S-305, 1976.
3. Chang TMS, Chirito E, Barre B. et al: Clinical performance characteristics of a new combined system for simultaneous hemoperfusion-hemodialysis-ultrafiltration in series. Trans Am Soc Artif Intern Organs 21:502, 1976.
4. Chang TMS, Chirito E, Barre P, et al: Long-term clinical assessment of combined ACAC hemoperfusion-ultrafiltration in uremia. Artif Organs 3:127, 1979.
5. Gelfand MC, Winchester JF: Hemoperfusion results in uremia. Clin Nephrol 11:107, 1979.
6. Henderson LW, Sanfelippo ML: Newer approaches to solute removal in chronic renal failure. Adv Intern Med 25:303, 1980.
7. Siemsen AW, Dunea G, Mandani BH, Guruprakash G: Charcoal hemoperfusion for chronic renal failure. Nephron 22:386, 1978.
8. Stefoni S, Feliciangelli G, Coli L, Bonomini V: Evaluation of a new coated charcoal for hemoperfusion in uremia. Int J Artif Organs 2:320, 1979.
9. Winchester JF, Apliga MT, Kennedy AC: Short-term evaluation of charcoal hemoperfusion combined with dialysis in uremic patients. Kidney Int 10:5–315, 1976.
10. Yatzidis H, Yulis G, Digentis P: Hemocarboperfusion-hemodialysis treatment in terminal renal failure. Kidney Int 10:S-312, 1976.
11. Crome P, Hampel G, Widdop B, Goulding R: Experience with cellulose acetate-coated activated charcoal haemoperfusion in the treatment of severe drug intoxication. Postgrad Med J 56:763, 1980.

12. De-Broe ME, Verpooten GA, Christiaens MA, et al: Clinical experience with prolonged combined hemoperfusion-hemodialysis treatment of severe poisoning. Artif Organs 5:59, 1981.

13. Gelfand MC, Winchester JF, Knepshield JH, et al: Treatment of severe drug overdosage with charcoal hemoperfusion. Trans Am Soc Artif Intern Organs 23:599, 1977.

14. Heath A, Delin K, Eden E, et al: Hemoperfusion with Amberlite resin in the treatment of self-poisoning. Acta Med Scand 207:455, 1980.

15. Lorch JA, Garella S: Hemoperfusion to treat intoxication. Ann Intern Med 91:301, 1979.

16. Pond S, Rosenberg J, Benowitz NL, Takki S: Pharmacokinetics of hemoperfusion for drug overdose. Clin Pharmacokinet 4:329, 1979.

17. Rosenbaum JL, Kramer MS, Raja RM: Amberlite hemoperfusion in the treatment of acute drug intoxication. Int J Artif Organs 2:316, 1979.

18. Rosenbaum JL: Hemoperfusion for acute drug intoxication. Kidney Int 10:106, 1980.

19. Trafford A, Horn C, Sharpstone P, et al: Hemoperfusion in acute drug toxicity. Clin Toxicol 17:547, 1980.

20. Yatzidis H, Voudiclari S, Oreopoulos D, et al: Treatment of severe barbiturate poisoning. Lancet 2:216, 1965.

21. Chang TMS: Hemoperfusion over microencapsulated adsorbent in a patient with hepatic coma. Lancet 2:1371, 1972.

22. Chang TMS, Lister C: Analysis of possible toxins in hepatic coma including the removal of mercaptan by albumin-collodion charcoal. Int J Artif Organs 3:108, 1980.

23. Chirito E, Reiter B, Lister C, Chang TMS: Artificial liver: The effect of ACAC microencapsulated charcoal hemoperfusion on fulminant hepatic failure. Artif Organs 1:76, 1977.

24. Gelfand MC, Winchester JF, Knepshield JH, et al: Biochemical correlates of reversal of hepatic coma coated with charcoal hemoperfusion. Trans Am Soc Artif Intern Organs 24:239, 1978.

25. Gazzard BG, Portmann B, Weston MJ, et al: Charcoal hemoperfusion in the treatment of fulminant hepatic failure. Lancet 1:1301, 1974.

26. Krumlovsky FA, Del-Greco F, Niederman M: Prolonged hemoperfusion and hemodialysis in management of hepatic failure and hepatorenal syndrome. Trans Am Soc Artif Intern Organs 24:235, 1978.

27. Hermann J, Rudorff KH, Gockenjan G, et al: Charcoal hemoperfusion in thyroid storm. Lancet 1:248, 1977.

28. Lauterburg BH, Pineda AA, Burgstaler EA, et al: Treatment of pruritus of cholestasis by plasma perfusion through USP-charcoal-coated glass beads. Lancet 2:53, 1980.

29. Yatzidis H: A convenient hemoperfusion microapparatus over charcoal for the treatment of endogenous and exogenous intoxications: Its use as an effective artificial kidney. Proc Eur Dial Transplant Assoc 1:83, 1964.

30. De Myttenaere MH, Maher JF, Schreiner GE: Hemoperfusion through a charcoal column for glutethimide poisoning. Trans Am Soc Artif Intern Organs 13:190, 1967.

31. Chang TMS: Removal of endogenous and exogenous toxins by microencapsulated adsorbent. Can J Physiol Pharmacol 47:1043, 1969.

32. Chang TMS: Criteria, evaluation, and perspectives of various microencapsulated charcoal hemoperfusion systems. Dial Transplant 6:50, 1977.

33. Sangster B, Van Heijst Ad NP, Sixma JJ: The influence of haemoperfusion on hemostasis and cellular constituents of the blood in the treatment of intoxications. Arch Toxicol 47:269, 1981.

34. Farrell PC: Acute drug intoxication and extracorporeal intervention. Trans Am Soc Artif Intern Organs 3:39, 1980.

35. Gelfand MC: Hemoperfusion in toxic ingestions and hepatic encephalopathy: Have the expectations been achieved? Contrib Nephrol 29:101, 1982.

36. Medd RK, Widdop B, Braitwaite RD, et al: Comparison of hemoperfusion and haemodialysis in the therapy of barbiturate intoxication in dogs. Arch Toxicol 31:163, 1973.

37. Rosenbaum JL, Kramer MS, Raja R: Resin hemoperfusion for acute drug intoxication. Arch Intern Med 136:263, 1976.

38. Arieff AI, Friedman EA: Coma following non-narcotic drug overdosage: Management of 208 adult patients. Am J Med Sci 266:405, 1973.

39. Better OS, Brunner G, Chang TMS, et al: Controlled trials of hemoperfusion for intoxications. Ann Intern Med 91:925, 1979.

40. Silk DBA, Williams R: Treatment of fulminant hepatic failure by charcoal haemoperfusion and polyacrylonitrite haemodialysis. In: Artificial Kidney, Artificial Liver, and Artificial Cells, Chang TMS (Ed). New York, Plenum Press, 1977, p. 125.

41. Brunner G: Microsomal enzymes bound to artificial carriers. A new approach towards an extracorporeal detoxification in liver failure. In: Artificial Liver Support, Williams R, Murray-Lyon IM (Eds). London, Pitman Medical Publishing. 1975, p 153.

42. Wolf CFW, Munkelt BE: Bilirubin conjugation by an artificial liver composed of cultured cells and synthetic capillaries. Trans Am Soc Artif Intern Organs 21:16, 1975.

43. Stefoni S, Coli L, Feliciangelli G, et al: Regular hemoperfusion in regular dialysis treatment: A long-term study. J Artif Organs 3:348, 1980.

44. Randerson DH, Gurland HJ, Schmidt B, et al: Sorbent membrane dialysis in uremia. Contrib Nephrol 29:53, 1982.

45. Chang TMS, Espinosa-Melendez E, Francoeur TE, Eada NR: Albumin-collodion activated coated characoal hemoperfusion in the treatment of severe theophylline intoxication in a 3 year old patient. Pediatrics 65:811, 1980.

46. Chavers BM, Kjellstrand CM, Wiegand C, et al: Techniques for use of charcoal hemoperfusion in infants: Experience in two patients. Kidney Int. 18:386, 1980.

47. Gelfand MC, Colon AR, Knepshield JH, et al: Successful management of stage IV hepatic coma in a child by haemocarboperfusion. In: Artificial Organs, Kenedi RM, Courtney JM, Gaylor, JDS, Gilchrist T (Eds). London, Macmillan Press, 1977, p 425.

48. Mauer SM, Chavers BM, Kjellstrand CM: Treat-

ment of an infant with severe chloramphenicol intoxication using charcoal-column hemoperfusion. J Pediatr 96:136, 1980.

49. Papadopoulou ZL, Novello AC, Gelfand MC, et al: The use of charcoal hemoperfusion in children. Int J Pediatr Nephrol 1:187, 1980.

50. Papadopoulou ZL, Novello AC: The use of hemoperfusion in children. Pediatr Clin North Am 29:1039, 1982.

51. Matthew H, Lawson AAH: *In:* Treatment of Common Acute Poisoning, Edinburgh, Churchill Livingstone, 1970.

52. Engle WD, Jacobs JF, Swartz RD, et al: Severe coagulopathy complicating charcoal hemoperfusion in children with Reye syndrome. J Pediatr 93:972, 1978.

53. Winchester JF, Gelfand MC, Knepsheild JH, Schreiner GE: Dialysis and hemoperfusion of poisons and drugs—update. Trans Am Soc Artif Intern Organs 23:762, 1977.

54. Gelfand MC: Charcoal hemoperfusion in treatment of drug overdosage. Dial Transplant 6:8, 1977.

# 9

# Vascular and Peritoneal Access: Technical Considerations

*Neil J. Sherman, M.D.*
*James B. Atkinson, M.D.*

The advances of the past few decades in both knowledge and manipulation of body fluids in renal failure are dependent upon a safe and reliable access to these fluids, regardless of the type of dialysis used. The earliest commercial artificial kidney required access through repeated surgical vascular exposures and sacrificing of these vessels.[1] The cornerstone of vascular access for the patient with ESRD was provided by Quinton, Dillard, and Scribner, who collaborated to develop the first semipermanent vascular access technique.[2] Subsequent refinements have essentially eliminated these external devices, except for acute dialysis situations. Chronic vascular access is presently provided by the use of vascular surgical techniques, either by direct arteriovenous anastomosis, use of autologous or homologous vessels, or use of synthetic vascular substitutes.[3]

Substantial knowledge of the uses and function of the peritoneum as a dialyzing membrane predated the use of the artificial kidney. Peritoneal dialysis for acute renal failure has been an available clinical tool for 60 years.[4] Only recently have techniques for chronic peritoneal dialysis been achieved successfully, and these are dependent on a satisfactory peritoneal catheter which will resist intraluminal occlusion, intra-abdominal irritation, and infection. Siliconized rubber catheters (Silastic) are soft enough to avoid erosion of any intra-abdominal structures, yet resist kinking and collapse. Their hydrophobic properties tend to prevent occlusion. The placing of a dacron cuff around the catheter and implanting this cuff within the tissue, as introduced by Tenckhoff,[5] has been the most recent refinement as an effective barrier to infection and dislodgment.

Both of the above modalities were originally developed for use in adults and have been modified for use in the pediatric patient with ESRD. While most techniques are applicable to pediatric patients by utilizing smaller-sized equipment and material, refinements in the technique of both vascular and peritoneal access are necessary, especially in the very small child. Significant differences in approach will always exist, such as the widespread use of general anesthesia for these procedures in children, as contrasted to local anesthesia for adults. As the increasing worldwide experience in the pediatric aspects of vascular and peritoneal access continues to grow, the techniques described herein which are presently used will surely undergo further modifications.

## PERITONEAL ACCESS

Since the early 1920's, it has been recognized that the peritoneum is a semipermeable membrane which can be used for exchange of solutes and fluids.[4] Peritoneal dialysis has been used successfully for decades in patients with acute renal failure, but its effectiveness in the treatment of ESRD awaited the development of a reliable permanent catheter. This modality is particularly useful, and almost a necessity, for children under 10 kilograms, in whom long-term vascular access and repeated hemodialysis presents many technical problems. The standard catheter, with minimal modifications, can be used in patients of any size. Contraindications to chronic peritoneal dialysis, from a technical viewpoint, include previous peritonitis with extensive adhesions, and an ongoing abdominal wall infection. These conditions represent only relative contraindications and may not be applicable, depending on the clinical situation.

**Catheter.** Numerous implantable valves, ports, and catheters have been devised for chronic peritoneal access.[5] None have equaled the reliability of the Tenckhoff catheter, and it is currently our recommendation that this type be used exclusively for chronic peritoneal access.[6] The catheters are made of siliconized rubber with one or two bonded dacron cuffs for tissue fixation. The catheters are commercially available* in adult and pediatric lengths (15 and 12.5 inches respectively). Because of the shorter subcutaneous and peritoneal distances in small infants and children, catheters are available with only the peritoneal cuff bonded. The second cuff may be placed and bonded at the time of implantation. This allows proper positioning of the cuffs regardless of patient size.

**Surgical Technique.** The catheters are inserted in the operating room under general anesthesia, with careful attention to sterile technique. In severely ill patients with uremic symptoms, a temporary peritoneal catheter can be inserted percutaneously, with local anesthesia, in an intensive care unit. The technique described herein should probably be reserved for the operating room.

Following induction of adequate general anesthesia, the abdomen is prepared and draped in a sterile field. The site for implantation of the catheter is selected based on previous surgery and catheter insertion sites. An infraumbilical midline or an oblique lateral incision may be used to position the catheter in the pelvis. A right subcostal incision is used to place the catheter in the suprahepatic space (Fig. 9–1). The lateral incisions are preferred in that a stronger peritoneal and multiple layer muscle closure may be accomplished.

Following opening of the peritoneal cavity, a brief exploration is performed. Adhesions are divided and as much of an omentectomy

---

*Life Med Inc., Compton, CA.

is performed as possible to prevent subsequent occlusion of the catheter. The catheter is then brought through the tunnel so that one cuff will lie at the peritoneal closure and the second cuff midway in the subcutaneous tunnel. The tunnel should be at least 5 cm in length because erosion or exposure of the proximal cuff through the skin or exit site must be avoided. When placed suprahepatically, a single nonreactive, nonabsorbable suture is placed in the lower diaphragmatic peritoneum anteriorly and tied around the catheter to secure it in the suprahepatic space. A pursestring nonabsorbable suture is then placed in the peritoneum and tied around the catheter at the cuff. The remaining fascial layers are then reapproximated to assure a watertight closure of the wound. These operative steps are depicted in Figure 9–1. During closure the catheter is periodically flushed and drained with dialysate containing 1000 units of heparin in 500 ml of saline to prevent any clot formation in the immediate postoperative period. Continuous flow in the catheter is initiated immediately after surgery, and continued for two to three days to prevent plugging. The patient is observed in the hospital for several days. Antibiotics are recommended perioperatively for 48 to 72 hours. Although intraoperative peritoneography has been recommended to determine catheter position and to diagnose occult hernia, we have found this to be an unnecessary and cumbersome procedure.[7]

## Complications and Management

**Nonfunction.** Prior to adding partial omentectomy and placing some catheters in the suprahepatic space, plugging was a common cause of early and late catheter failure. If the catheter inflow is adequate but the outflow impaired, the catheter can occasionally be salvaged by gentle irrigation with heparin or a fibrinolytic agent. High pressures must be avoided to prevent rupture of the catheter in an attempt to dislodge stubborn fibrin plugs. If these methods are unsuccessful, then the catheter must be surgically revised or replaced. The incidence of acute plugging may be greatly reduced by maintaining continuous flow of heparinized dialysate for two to three days postoperatively.

**Catheter Extrusion.** The catheter is considered to have extruded when the dacron cuff is visible either through the catheter exit site

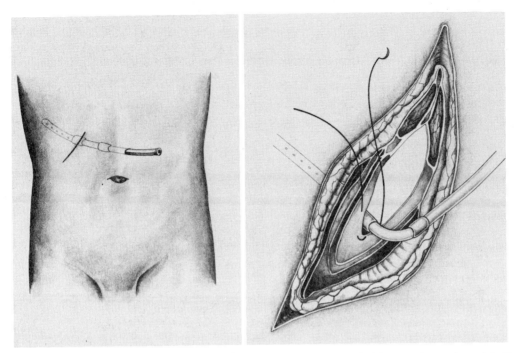

**Figure 9–1.** The position of the catheter and its relationship to the abdominal incision are shown above, left. On the right, the location of the two cuffs is seen in relation to the peritoneum and tunnel. When a single cuff is used, it should be placed in the subcutaneous tunnel.

or by erosion of the overlying skin. This complication results from placing the dacron cuff too close to the catheter exit site or making the subcutaneous tunnel too superficial. If not accompanied by an infection, this problem may be managed by rerouting the catheter through a new subcutaneous tunnel after a careful antiseptic scrub of the extruded cuff. This procedure should be accompanied by antibiotic therapy started before surgery and continued for five to seven days postoperatively.

**Infection.** This complication is both the most common and most difficult to treat. Infection may involve the peritoneum or the subcutaneous catheter alone, or both may be involved. While these problems may present separately or concurrently, they are more easily discussed individually.

Infection in the subcutaneous tunnel with or without peritonitis has a worse prognosis than simple peritonitis, in regard to salvage of the catheter. Non-removal therapy may be tried, including drainage of any local purulent collections, and treatment with local, intraperitoneal and/or systemic antibiotics. When this is not successful, an attempt may be made to reposition only the subcutaneous portion of the catheter, although this has only occasionally been successful. If the peritoneal fluid cannot be sterilized with intraperitoneal and systemic antibiotics, then the catheter must be removed, and the patient may require hemodialysis until the infection is completely under control. Subsequently, another catheter can be placed and peritoneal dialysis resumed.

Simple peritonitis unaccompanied by inflammation or external evidence of catheter infection is initially managed with intraperitoneal antibiotics and, if severe systemic symptoms are present, parenteral antibiotics. When culture results are available, antibiotic therapy is altered appropriately. Infections of this type are a result of errors in technique while handling the catheter, and are occasionally resistant to any medical treatment, short of removal of the catheter.

The incidence of infection has been reported as developing in from 1 to 40% of catheters at one-year follow-up.[8, 9] The wide variation clearly relates to the care exercised in maintaining aseptic technique when manipulating the catheter. Prevention is clearly the most desirable aspect of care. Time and effort spent in preventing infection is much more rewarding than the treatment of an established infection.

## VASCULAR ACCESS

Surgery for vascular access is one of the most common operations performed today.[10] There continues to be rapidly increasing experience in the use of vascular accesses described in the literature, but reports are limited in children, since less than 2% of patients reported are in the pediatric age group.[11-13] Fortunately, the need for vascular access in children is usually for a significantly shorter period of time than in adults, because of the incidence of successful transplantation. Certain problems arise that are unique to infants and small children, such as the technical challenge of maintaining vessel patency in the small child, the effect of growth on the vascular access, and the effect of the underlying disease peculiar to the pediatric population. With careful attention to detail and planning in the insertion and care of these accesses, most children can be managed with a minimal amount of morbidity.

### External Shunts

Since 1960 various external shunts have been utilized for chronic hemodialysis in children. Basically, these consist of a vessel tip, a connecting shunt tubing constructed of soft Silastic and of various configurations, and a rigid connector. The two types most frequently used are the Kjellstrand modification of the Scribner shunt and the Ramirez shunt.[14] The Scribner shunt is commercially available in pediatric sizes with right and left bends and incorporates a 180-degree gentle turn and a stepped cannula. These features allow the surgeon to select a cannula of proper configuration for any given anatomic region. The Ramirez shunt is straight and stepped, but adds a Silastic wing to prevent dislodgment, rotation, or kinking. While the latter is available complete with vessel tips in small, medium, and large sizes, frequently infants and children are encountered for whom even the small shunt is too large for distal vessels.

Separate vessel tips are available in sizes 13 to 18, with the larger number having a smaller tip diameter. Special pediatric tips are commercially available* in sizes 17 to 19 which have thinner cannula walls with a larger functional internal diameter. The out-

---

*Life Med. Inc., Compton, California.

side diameter of these vessel tips measures from 1.14 mm to 2.75 mm. The cannula tip is selected after the vessel is visualized and then secured into the shunt tubing with two nonabsorbable ties.

In small infants and children (less than 20 kg) the site for shunt placement is usually proximal, such as the midbrachial or the superficial femoral vessels. While the groin sites contain larger vessels, in our experience, they have an unacceptably short functional life owing to difficulties with dislodgment and infection. It has been our practice to cannulate the midbrachial artery, ligating the vessel distally, and placing the venous cannula in a brachial, antecubital, or low axillary vein.

Children weighing more than 20 kg may have Scribner or Ramirez shunts placed in the radial artery-cephalic/basilic vein or posterior tibial artery/saphenous vein sites. The technique is similar in both groups of patients, although special precautions are advised in the smaller children, because of the delicacy of the tissues and the size of the vessels.

The artery and vein are isolated through small incisions, allowing space for a subcutaneous pocket and a separate incision for the cannula exit site. Care must be exercised to avoid trauma to the small vessels with clamps and vessel tips during insertion of the cannula. A useful technique, particularly in arterial cannulation, is the utilization of fine stay sutures placed in the proximal arteriotomy flap at 9, 12, and 3 o'clock, to aid in visualization and introduction of the cannula tip. Prior to insertion of the cannula tip, dilators are frequently helpful so that a slightly larger tip may be utilized. Particular caution is necessary in flushing the arterial limb to avoid cerebral embolism; injection of 2 ml or more of contrast medium into the radial artery has been shown to reflux into the cephalic circulation in small children and could easily produce embolism.[15] Care must be taken during the exposure and manipulation of the brachial artery to avoid injury to the median nerve, which lies posterior and medial to the vessel in the arm. In spite of reports in the adult literature suggesting a 50 to 75% limb loss with ligation of the brachial artery, we have not encountered any serious sequelae with this procedure in children.[16]

Advantages of external shunts include the ease of insertion, simplicity, immediacy of access, and the avoidance of needle punctures. The undesirable aspects are that they seriously limit activity in older children and, most significantly, the expected patency rate is only 2.2 to 15.6 months.[17] Since the shunts are unacceptable on a long-term basis, they are used primarily as a temporizing measure to correct the initial uremic problems and to provide access until a permanent internal fistula can be constructed and allowed to mature. This applies both to new patients and to those in whom a previous access has failed.

When the external shunts are removed, they can occasionally be pulled out with traction, although in children this is not only uncomfortable but may produce significant bleeding. We prefer to remove the shunt under general anesthesia. The brachial shunts should be removed surgically under anesthesia to avoid the risk of injury to the adjacent median nerve. Occasionally a secondary procedure may be performed at the same site to create an autogenous arteriovenous fistula, taking advantage of the veins which have already dilated and thickened from the previous flow through the shunt.

## Chronic Vascular Access

Chronic vascular access implies construction of arteriovenous fistulae, either direct, autogenous or synthetic, which can be expected to sustain the patient for a prolonged period of time. They will be discussed in order of our preference, recognizing the regional differences; individual surgeons might arrange them otherwise.

**Cimino-Brescia Fistula.** Dissatisfaction with the Scribner shunt for long-term use led to the development of an arteriovenous fistula at the wrist by Cimino, Brescia, et al in 1966.[18] The fistula is constructed by direct anastomosis between the radial artery and cephalic vein using a 7–0 vascular suture. All variations of the anastomosis have been tried; the anastomosis that is technically easiest should be selected, most frequently the end of the vein to the side of the artery. The anastomosis will predictably function satisfactorily as long as the anastomotic diameter is 70% or more of the arterial diameter.[19] This anastomosis has been used in children weighing 20 kg or more with a three-year patency rate of 80%.[20] Direct fistulae may be constructed at the wrist, using the radial artery and cephalic vein, or in the upper arm, using the brachial artery and cephalic or basilic vein. Site selection is based upon the size of the child and the sites of previous access surgery. Venography may be helpful in locating vessels of adequate size in adults but is rarely used in children. A recent description of a new location, the anatomic snuffbox in the hand,[21] has been described in adults, but there has been no experience with this in children.

Technically the vessels are exposed through a single incision, and side branches of the vessels are divided as necessary, mobilizing 3 cm of vein and artery. The anastomosis is performed utilizing a running and interrupted technique with 7–0 sutures. If at least 50% of the anastomosis is interrupted, then it should enlarge as the vessel grows. Upon completion of the anastomosis, a thrill should be palpable. Usually four to six weeks is allowed for "arterialization" of the vein before initial use of the access for hemodialysis can be accomplished. Flows of 100 to 200 ml per minute can be expected even when the vessels are quite small. While flow measurements have been used in adults for determining adequacy of the fistula in the operating room, this technique has not been utilized in children.

Principal advantages of the Cimino-Brescia fistula are the ease of construction, high long-term patency rate, and low infectious complications. Disadvantages include limitations as to sites and vessels available, failure to mature (particularly in obese patients), long maturation period, and in some cases, development of large aneurysmal veins which are cosmetically unacceptable to many adolescents. Interestingly, many children complain of pain in the arm during dialysis with an arteriovenous fistula, but not when a graft is used. While the mechanism is unclear, this fact has decreased the construction of these direct arteriovenous fistulas in our unit.

**Polytetrafluoroethylene Bridge Grafts.** The availability of expanded polytetrafluoroethylene* (PTFE) grafts since 1975 has greatly increased the sites which may be used for vascular access.[13] Virtually any artery and vein of sufficient size may be bridged by such grafts. These grafts are particularly useful in pediatric patients in whom more proximal vessels must be used to obtain vessels of adequate size.

---

*W. L. Gore & Associates, Newark, Delaware.

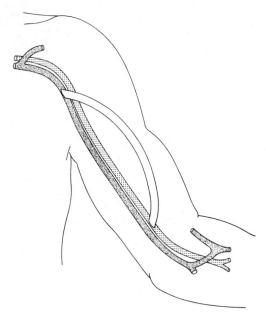

**Figure 9–2.** The preferred location and orientation of the Goretex graft in the upper arm.

The usual sites of implantation are pictured in Figures 9–2 and 9–3. These applications must be modified by the surgeon when previous procedures or thrombosis of the vessels has occurred. In children we favor the use of the brachial artery with a loop in the forearm, or a straight graft with anastomosis to the low axillary vein in the upper arm.

Lower extremity fistulae tend to have higher flow rates and lower thrombosis rates. In addition, they allow the patient to have

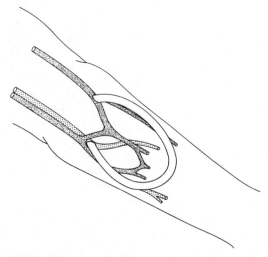

**Figure 9–3.** The preferred site for a loop graft in the forearm; in some patients it extends more distal than shown above.

both hands free during dialysis. Disadvantages of lower extremity fistulae are a higher infection rate as well as a theoretically increased risk of venous hypertension and arterial steal. In addition, infectious complications and thrombosis of the parent vessel are much greater problems in the lower extremity than in the arm. At the present time lower extremity fistulae are being used only as the last resort.

The technique of implantation involves incisions overlying the artery and vein. A 3 to 4 cm length of vessel is mobilized and flow controlled atraumatically with vessel loops. A subcutaneous tunnel is created using a Hegar dilator or aneurysm clamp, making counter incisions as necessary to avoid undue trauma to the subcutaneous tissue. The tunnel should be slightly larger than the graft and lie in a gentle curve to avoid kinking. Systemic heparinization (100 units/kg) is used during surgery and heparin is continued postoperatively in patients in whom the initial flow is considered marginal. Aspirin is administered chronically in patients with a history of recurrent thrombosis.

A Goretex graft is selected, using a 7 mm to 4 mm tapered or a straight 6 mm tube. We prefer the tapered graft and suture the smaller end at the arterial side. This is because the initial venous outflow will predictably be much less than the arterial inflow, and postoperative extremity edema and blistering have been avoided with the use of the tapered graft. The graft is cut obliquely and anastomosed at a 30 to 45 degree angle to the previously mobilized artery in an end-to-side fashion, using continuous suture technique. The anastomosis is constructed such that the lumen is 1½ to 2 times the diameter of the graft. The graft is then clamped and gently distended as it is drawn through the previously constructed subcutaneous tunnel. A longitudinal mark on the graft, made with a marking pen, is particularly useful for orientation and to avoid twisting or kinking. The graft is then cut to the proper length and anastomosed obliquely to the vein in a similar end-to-side fashion.

Implantation is preferred at the most distal site feasible. We no longer use the distal radial artery and proximal antecubital vein owing to the high incidence of clotting.

**Autogenous Vein Bridge Grafts.** Various fistulae using transposed or reversed basilic or saphenous veins have been employed successfully.[22–24] These techniques are applicable only to larger children (greater than

25 kg) and have limited usefulness because of thrombosis, aneurysm formation, and greater technical difficulties in construction. We would restrict this technique to older children who repeatedly develop infection in their synthetic grafts but technically cannot have a direct arteriovenous anastomosis.

**Heterologous Bridge Grafts.** Bovine carotid artery and human umbilical vein have been used in the past for bridge grafts.[25, 26] Both have higher failure rates and are no longer recommended for pediatric patients.[20]

## Complications

Some types of complications are unique to the type of access employed while others are universal.

**External Shunts.** These shunts have a patency of from two to 15 months, as previously noted. A common acute complication is bleeding, which is usually arterial from an inadequately secured ligature around the vessel tip. Additional problems include thrombosis, infection, and erosion of the Silastic wings or tubing through the skin. Thrombosis may be relieved by gentle aspiration and irrigation or catheter embolectomy with a #2 or #3 Fogarty catheter. If thrombosis recurs, then the shunt is declotted and a shuntogram is obtained to define the cause (either residual clot, inadequate inflow, or venous stenosis). Minimal infection may be managed locally, with the shunt tubing acting as a surgical drain. More severe infection or exposure of the native vessels by skin erosion usually requires revision or removal of the shunt and the use of systemic antibiotic therapy.

**Cimino-Brescia Fistula.** This access carries an 80% three-year patency rate, once established, and is relatively free of complications.[20] Early failure may occur as a result of technical error at the anastomotic site or, more commonly, from unsuspected stenosis in the artery or vein. Angiography is useful in evaluating the need to revise a fistula that has not matured satisfactorily in 4 to 6 weeks.

Occasionally flow will be large enough through the fistula to result in arterial steal from the distal extremity. This is usually the result of reversal of flow in the distal artery and may be corrected by simply ligating the distal artery. Flow may also be decreased by banding the vein to increase resistance to the outflow. These are unusual complications in pediatric patients.

Late infection almost always occurs at the site of repeated needle punctures. Local therapy, systemic antibiotics, and drainage may be successful, but commonly the infected vein must be excised, either partially or totally. Repeated punctures at the same site may also produce stenosis and subsequent thrombosis. Declotting and angioplasty may be successful occasionally, but adequacy of function cannot be predicted after this complication. The best treatment is prevention by avoiding repeated punctures at the same site, and careful treatment of the puncture site following dialysis.

**Bridge Fistulae.** Complications with these grafts may occur acutely or in a delayed manner. Acute thrombosis of these grafts results from technical problems with the anastomosis or an unsuspected venous stenosis. The graft must be surgically exposed and incised; after the clot is extracted with the use of a Fogarty balloon catheter, angiography is performed. A #8 Foley catheter is

**Table 9–1.** HEMODIALYSIS: CUMULATIVE PATENCY FOR GORETEX

| First Author | Number Implanted | Percent Cumulative Patency | | | | |
|---|---|---|---|---|---|---|
| | | *Early* | *6 Months* | *1 Year* | *2 Years* | *3 Years* |
| Anderson | 100 | 97 | 88 | 87 | 73 | – |
| Sabanayagam | 225 | 98 | 94 | 90 | 84 | – |
| Morgan | 112 | 90 | 82 | 61 | 33 | – |
| Chatterjee | 36 | 95 | 84 | 84 | 84 | – |
| Overall | 473 | 96 | 89 | 82 | 70 | – |
| Tellis | 66 | 90 | 68 | 62 | – | – |
| Goretex Vascular Graft Registry | 2,296 | 94 | 85 | 76 | 67 | 51 |
| (Data from 31 surgeons, each with at least 25 procedures) | (Standard Error) | (0.5) | (1.0) | (1.4) | (2.1) | (4.2) |

This table summarizes the patency rate of the Goretex Arteriovenous Fistula for hemodialysis: published or presented 1966–1980.[20]

**Table 9–2.** HEMODIALYSIS: INCIDENCE OF COMPLICATIONS
SUMMARY OF PUBLISHED/PRESENTED DATA: 1966–1980

| Procedures | First Author or Source | Graft Months of Followup | Incidence per 100 Graft Months of Follow-up | | | | | | | | | |
| --- | --- | --- | --- | --- | --- | --- | --- | --- | --- | --- | --- | --- |
| | | | Infections* | Pseudo-aneurysm | Arterial Steal | Hemor-rhage | Hema-toma | High Output Failure | Edema Swelling | Erosion of Skin | Other** | Total |
| Cimino-Brescia Fistulae | Higgins Zerbino Limet | 6,332 | 0.13 | 0.08 | 0.08 | 0.05 | — | 0.08 | — | — | 0.27 | 0.69 |
| Bovine Hetero-Grafts | Butt VanderWerf Kumar Oakes Sannella Rolley Butler Anderson Morgan | 8,012 | 1.37 | 0.37 | 0.16 | 0.07 | 0.04 | 0.05 | 0.04 | 0.02 | 0.32 | 2.44 |
| Goretex Vascular Grafts | Goretex Vascular Graft Registry | 9,179 | 0.76 | 0.22 | 0.11 | 0.09 | 0.07 | — | 0.17 | 0.03 | 0.08 | 1.53 |

*Most infections were *Staphylococcus aureus* or *S. epidermidis.*
**"Other" included unspecified category, embolectomy, reduced orifice, poor flow and cardiac arrhythmia.
(Courtesy of W. L. Gore & Associates, Technical Note #236).

introduced through the arteriotomy. The Foley balloon prevents reflux of dye during injection of contrast material. The angiogram confirms whether all clots have been extracted and will demonstrate any venous stenosis that may have caused the thrombosis. Similarly, a retrograde study may be done to visualize the arterial limb and anastomosis of the graft, using the Foley balloon catheter. Corrective measures based on angiographic findings may then be taken, and we advise that the patients requiring these procedures be heparinized for 72 hours following thrombectomy.

Late thrombosis of a graft is managed surgically in a similar fashion with embolectomy and intraoperative angiography. Late thrombosis usually occurs as a result of hyperplastic neo-intima at the venous anastomosis or from a hematoma at a needle puncture site. This obstruction may be corrected by patch angioplasty or by jump grafting to a different vein or proximally on the same vein.

Infection is by far the most common complication associated with a vascular prosthesis. Owing to the presence of a foreign body, the infection can rarely be managed with antibiotics alone. The infection may be indolent, introduced at the time of implantation, or it may be suppurative and virulent from an infected hematoma at a needle puncture site. The management may require removal of all or part of the graft if local drainage and systemic antibiotics are insufficient. Infections localized in a portion of the subcutaneous tunnel may allow excision of that area with rerouting of the graft through uninvolved tissue. Continuity is established by end-to-end graft-graft anastomosis. Breakdown of the skin overlying the graft may occasionally be managed in a similar manner or by moving a flap of well-vascularized skin and subcutaneous tissue over the graft. Infection in these and most other types of vascular access is usually due to *Staphylococcus aureus* or *Staphylococcus epidermidis*.

The patency rate for Gortex AV fistulae in large cumulative adult series is 70% at two years (Table 9–1). In children the statistics are difficult to measure owing to the frequency of transplantation; however, in our experience it is similar to that reported in adults. Table 9–2 is a compendium from the Gortex registry summarizing the complication rate in a large number of adult patients.[20]

While these figures are not directly comparable to those of the pediatric patient on chronic hemodialysis, they do provide the best guide at present.

## REFERENCES

1. Kolff WJ: The first clinical experience with the artificial kidney. Ann Intern Med 62:608, 1965.
2. Quinton WE, Dillard D, Scribner BH: Cannulation of blood vessels for prolonged hemodialysis. Trans Am Soc Artif Intern Organs 6:104, 1960.
3. Brescia MJ, Cimino JE, Appel K, et al: Chronic hemodialysis using venipuncture and a surgically created arteriovenous fistula. N Engl J Med 275:1089, 1966.
4. Putnam TH: The living peritoneum as a dialyzing membrane. Am J Physiol 64:548, 1922.
5. Vidt DG, Somerville J, Schult RW: A safe peritoneal access device for repeated peritoneal dialysis. JAMA 214:2293, 1970.
6. Strikerm GE, Tenckhoff HAM: A transcutaneous prosthesis for prolonged access to the peritoneal cavity. Surgery 69:70, 1971.
7. Alexander SR, Tank ES: Surgical aspects of continuous ambulatory peritoneal dialysis in infants, children and adolescents. J Urol 127:501, 1982.
8. Brewer TE, Caldwell FT, Patterson R, Flannigan WJ: Indwelling peritoneal dialysis catheter. JAMA 219:1011, 1972.
9. Devine H, Oreopoulos DJ, Izatt S, et al: The permanent Tenckhoff catheter for chronic peritoneal dialysis. Can Med Assoc J 113:219, 1975.
10. Mandel S: Vascular access in a transplant and dialysis program: results, costs and manpower implications in vascular access surgery. Wilson SE, Owens M (Eds). Chicago, Year Book Medical Publishers, pp 337–344, 1980.
11. Applebaum H, Shashikumar VL, Somers LA, et al: Improved hemodialysis access in children. J Pediatr Surg 15:764, 1981.
12. Mauer SM, Lynch RE: Hemodialysis techniques for infants and children. Pediatr Clin North Am 23:843, 1976.
13. Geis PW, Giacchino J: A game plan for vascular access for hemodialysis. Surg Rounds 62:62, 1980.
14. Buselmeier TJ, Santiago EA, Simmons RL, et al: Arteriovenous shunts for pediatric hemodialysis. Surg, 70:638, 1971.
15. Gaan D, Brewis RAL, et al: Cerebral damage from declotting Scribner shunts. Lancet, July 12, 1969, p. 77.
16. Debakey M, Simeone F: Battle injuries of the arteries in WW II. Ann Surg 123:534, 1946.
17. Foran RF, Golding AL, Treiman RL, DePalma JR: Quinton Scribner cannulas for hemodialysis: Review of four years experience. Cal Med 112:18, 1970.
18. Brescia MJ, Cimino JE, Appel K, Hurwich B: Chronic hemodialysis using venipuncture and a surgically created arteriovenous fistula. N Engl J Med 275:1089, 1966.
19. Owens ML, Bower RW: Physiology of arteriovenous fistula in vascular access surgery. Wilson SE, Owens ML (Eds). Chicago, Year Book Medical Publishers, 1980, pp 101–113.

20. Mehta S: A Statistical Summary of the Results of Vascular Access Procedures for Hemodialysis Published 1966–1980. Technical Publication No. 236. Newark, Delaware, WL Gore & Associates, 1981.

21. Mehigan JT, McAlexander RA: Snuffbox arteriovenous fistula for hemodialysis. Am J Surg 143:252, 1982.

22. D'Apuzzo VG, Grushkin C, Brennan LP, et al: Saphenous vein autograft arteriovenous fistula for extended hemodialysis in children. Acta Paediat Scand 62:28, 1973.

23. Pérez Alvarez JJ, Vargas-Rosenda R, Gutiérrez-Bosque R, et al: A new type subcutaneous arteriovenous fistula for chronic hemodialysis in children. Surgery 67:355, 1970.

24. Lo Gerfo FW, Menzoian JO, Kumaki, DJ, et al: Transposed basilic vein-brachial arteriovenous fistula. Arch Surg 113:1008, 1978.

25. Lefrak EA, Noon GP: Surgical technique for creation of an arteriovenous fistula using a looped bovine graft. Ann Surg 182:782, 1975.

26. Bone GE, Pomajel MJ: Prospective comparison of polytetrafluoroethylene and bovine grafts for dialysis. J Surg Res 29:223, 1980.

# 10

# Kinetics of Peritoneal Dialysis in Children

*Alan B. Gruskin, M.D.*
*Bruce Z. Morgenstern, M.D.*
*Sharon A. Perlman, M.D.*

Peritoneal dialysis has assumed increasing importance as a therapeutic alternative for children with renal failure.[1, 2] An understanding of the movement of solute and water through the peritoneal membrane, the kinetics of peritoneal transport, is central to the clinical application of peritoneal dialysis. When treating children, it is also necessary to know how differences in body size and age impact upon these transport processes. This chapter will initially consider the anatomy of the peritoneal membrane and the descriptive terms and formulae used to characterize the transperitoneal movement of solute and water. It is not intended to provide derivations of these formulae but to consider their meaning and clinical application; a number of excellent reviews of the mathematics and formulae used to describe peritoneal dialysis have appeared in the past few years.[3-7] Subsequently, the relevant experimental and clinical studies of the peritoneal membrane focusing on data pertinent to pediatric populations will be discussed.

## ANATOMY OF THE PERITONEAL MEMBRANE

The peritoneal cavity, which normally exists as a potential space, is lined by the parietal peritoneum which overlies the abdominal musculature, and by the visceral peritoneum which covers the organs within the abdominal cavity. Few direct measurements of the actual surface area of the peritoneum are available. The precise proportion of the peritoneal membrane, or the functional peritoneal surface area, which participates in the exchange process is unknown. Between 0.2 and 0.6% of the total peritoneal surface area has been estimated to participate in the exchange process in rabbits.[8] The ratio of peritoneal surface area to body weight varies with age, and in the neonate is approximately twice that found in adults[9, 10] (Table 10–1). The relationship between body weight and peritoneal surface area (in square centimeters) has been estimated to be equal to (weight in kg)$^{0.7}$ × 1000.[11]

The manner in which the peritoneal cavity accommodates dialysate is not clear. It is not known whether fluid introduced into the peritoneal cavity fills it like an empty container, or whether the potential space functions as a balloon, with small amounts of fluid contacting the entire surface available for exchange and subsequently distending as more fluid is added.[12]

The process of exchange between blood and dialysate requires that solvent and solute be delivered to the exchange site, that transmembrane movement occur, and that the peritoneal cavity be drained. The circulatory systems participating in the transperitoneal exchange process include:[13]

Supported in part by NIH General Research Center Grants RR-75, HL 23511, and HL 19869.

**Table 10–1.** RELATIONSHIP OF MEASURED PERITONEAL SURFACE AREA TO BODY SIZE

| Number of Patients | Body Size | Peritoneal Surface Area (cm²) | Weight (kg) | Surface Area per kg Weight | Reference No. |
|---|---|---|---|---|---|
| 1 | Infant | 1,512.44 | 2.900 | 522 | 59 |
| 6 | Infant | 1065[a] | 2.743[a] | 383[a] | |
| | | 476–1860[b] | 1.74–4.48[b] | 281–488[b] | 9 |
| 1 | Adult | 20,781.94 | 70.0[c] | 281 | 59 |
| NA | Adult | 22,000 | 70.0[c] | 314 | 10 |
| 6 | Adult | 10,379[a] | 59.3[a] | 177[a] | 9 |
| | | 8798–11,650[b] | 46.9–68.1[b] | 131–206[b] | |

[a]—mean, [b]—range, [c]—assumed weight, NA–not available

1. The vasculature of the visceral peritoneum derived from the mesenteric and celiac arteries and drained primarily by the portal venous system.

2. The vasculature of the parietal peritoneum derived from iliac, lumbar, intercostal, and epigastric arteries and drained by the systemic venous system.

At the level of the microcirculation, six sites of resistance to the movement of solute and water exist between blood and dialysate:[14, 15] the stagnant fluid film within the capillary, the capillary endothelium, the capillary basement membrane, the peritoneal interstitium, the mesothelium, and the stagnant fluid film within the peritoneal cavity. Chemical and anatomic structure as well as the thickness of the interstitium and fluid films, rather than the rate of blood flow through the peritoneal capillaries,[10, 14] are the major factors influencing the transperitoneal movement of small molecular weight compounds such as urea.[11] The rate of movement of larger molecular solutes such as protein[16] and inulin is related primarily to the degree of vascular permeability.

The possible anatomic pathways for transport include endothelial fenestrae (pores), intercellular channels (gaps), and vesicles (pinocytosis) located in small, thin-walled vessels. The microanatomy of the small vessels through which solute and water pass varies. Venous capillaries have up to 12 times more fenestrae and a total fenestrae area to gap area ratio 15 times greater than that found in arteriolar capillaries.[17] It has been suggested that ultrafiltration occurs primarily across the proximal segment of the capillary while solute diffusion occurs predominantly in the distal segment of the capillary.[17] Solutes with molecular weight less than 3400 daltons pass primarily through arterioles, capillaries, and venules, whereas transport of solutes with a higher molecular weight occurs primarily across venules. It is believed that most of the movement of solute with molecular weights greater than 30,000 daltons is through intercellular channels.[18]

Although the transcellular movement of solute and water would greatly enhance the effective peritoneal surface area available for exchange, most data argue against such transcellular movement.[19, 20] The lymphatic system does not appear to be significantly involved in the movement of solute into the peritoneal cavity.[20] Since the mesentery does not contain many capillaries, it has been suggested that most of the capillaries participating in the exchange are located where the peritoneum reflects over the bowel.[14, 21]

## TRANSPORT CHARACTERISTICS OF THE PERITONEAL MEMBRANE

Active transport is not a major characteristic of the peritoneal membrane. Solute and water move by passive processes in both directions across the peritoneal membrane. Two types of passive transport occur across the semipermeable peritoneal membrane— diffusive and convective.[22] Diffusive transport is the transport of solute down a concentration gradient in the absence of any osmotic gradient or of ultrafiltration. In clinical practice glucose is added to dialysate, creating an osmotic gradient between dialysate and blood. This results in ultrafiltration of water with convective transport of solute, which is the passive entrainment of solute with the ultrafiltrate through a semipermeable membrane in the absence of a concentration gradient. The overall transperitoneal movement of solute or overall mass transfer of solute, therefore, equals the sum of solute transported by both diffusive and convective transport. Although the primary objective of peritoneal dialysis is the removal of excess solute and water from the body, movement of solutes from dialysate to blood also occurs. Although this may cause hyperglycemia,[23] the same process may be used beneficially to provide nutrients such as amino acids.[24]

Factors influencing the movement of solute across the peritoneal membrane include: (1) the size of the membrane through which transport can occur (functional peritoneal surface area); (2) the rate of delivery of solute and water to the exchange site (peritoneal blood flow); (3) the size (molecular weight) and configuration of solute (charge, etc.); (4) the size and number of fenestrae (pores) and intercellular channels (gaps) in the capillary system; (5) the solute concentration (diffusion gradient) and osmotic gradients (convective gradient) between blood and dialysate; and (6) dialysis mechanics, including the volume of dialysate, the duration of inflow, dwell, and outflow phases of the exchange, and dialysate temperature.

## Peritoneal Membrane Transport— Descriptive Terms

Four measurements have been used to describe the transport characteristics of peritoneal membrane: peritoneal clearances, peritoneal dialysances, mass transfer area coefficients (MTAC), and ultrafiltration rates including convective coefficients.

### Peritoneal Clearances

The most widely used, but least precise, method to characterize solute transport has been the measurement of peritoneal clearances.[3, 25, 26] The formula for clearance is:

$$C = \frac{C_D Q_D}{C_B}$$

where
  $C$ = peritoneal clearance (ml/min)
  $C_B$ = midpoint plasma solute concentration (mg/dl)
  $C_D$ = final dialysate solute concentration
  $Q_D$ = rate of flow of dialysate (ml/min), (which is the dialysate volume drained divided by the time elapsed from the beginning of inflow to the end of outflow of an exchange).

The term peritoneal clearance expresses the average amount of plasma cleared of solute per unit time. Although an easily obtained value, the measurement of clearance reflects a time-averaged as opposed to an instantaneous rate of transport of solute across the membrane.[3] This permits neither the permeability nor surface area characteristics of the peritoneal membrane involved in instantaneous exchange to be critically examined.[27] Clearance measurements do not reflect the constantly changing concentration gradient between dialysate and blood and are not performed with the aim of distinguishing between the inflow, dwell, and outflow phases of an exchange.[3] The drainage phase of an exchange imposes most of the limitation on the use of clearances as a technique to critically evaluate solute transport across the peritoneal membrane.[28] Clearance studies are usually performed in a clinical setting, using hypertonic dialysate, and the relative contributions of diffusive and convective transport are indistinguishable. Clearance studies can be used, however, for obtaining simple comparative data when dialysis mechanics are held constant in a given patient or are identical in different patients.[2, 29–33]

### Peritoneal Dialysance

A more precise description of solute transport is given by the measurement of peritoneal dialysance.[3, 34] Peritoneal dialysance may be defined as: (1) the product of the effective peritoneal surface area times the membrane permeability; (2) the peritoneal clearance at time zero of an exchange when the dialysate concentration equals zero; (3) the peritoneal clearance at infinite dialysate flow rates (assuming maximal peritoneal blood flow), or (4) the net rate of solute exchange per unit concentration difference between blood and dialysate. Dialysance measurements are used primarily to quantitatively estimate the rate of transfer of solute across the peritoneal membrane and to evaluate the relative contribution of peritoneal membrane surface area and/or permeability to the exchange process.

The performance of dialysance measurements assumes that certain factors remain unchanged throughout the exchange cycle. One factor is the peritoneal blood flow. Another absolute requirement is that no ultrafiltration occur so that convective transport is noncontributory. The volume of distribution within the body for a given solute is also assumed to remain constant throughout the exchange cycle. Comparative studies require that dialysis mechanics be held rigidly constant. If the area of the peritoneal membrane in contact with dialysate during any of the phases of an exchange varies, transfer rates will be different and the peritoneal dialysance will be altered. Any such differences, however, will be systematic and reproducible if the time of each phase of the exchange cycle is constant. Dialysance values obtained from exchanges conducted with different time sequences cannot be compared.[34]

When the above parameters are held constant, the measurement of dialysance reflects two factors: (1) the functional surface area of the peritoneum; and (2) the permeability of the membrane. Thus, dialysance can be viewed as an area-permeability product with units of $cm^3/min$.

The formula for dialysance follows:

$$D = \frac{-V_B V_D}{t(V_B + V_D)} \times \ln \left[ 1 - \frac{C_D(V_B + V_D)}{C_B V_B} \right]$$

$D$ = Peritoneal dialysance (ml/min) of whole blood

$V_B$ = The volume of distribution of solute throughout the body and outside the peritoneal space (ml)

$V_D$ = The volume of dialysis fluid returned at the end of an exchange (ml). This should be within 5% of the volume infused

$C_B$ = Solute concentration measured in whole blood (whole blood dialysance) or plasma (plasma dialysance) at the midpoint of the exchange

$C_D$ = Solute concentration measured in the drained dialysate

$t$ = Time in minutes for the completion of the exchange

During a single exchange, it is possible to measure the dialysance of a single solute or several solutes of differing molecular weights. A relative, as opposed to an absolute, permeability index can be determined by measuring simultaneously the dialysance of two solutes of widely differing molecular weights, such as urea and inulin. The formula for estimating relative permeability is:[3, 27, 35-38]

Because the functional peritoneal surface area involved in the exchange of both solutes is thought to be identical, the membrane area term equals unity. Thus, the permeability index represents a value which is dimensionless and is indicative of the overall permeability characteristics of the peritoneal membrane. If studies of the dialysance of two solutes of widely differing molecular weights are made, examination of the direction and magnitude of exchange of one solute compared to the other permits the relative contribution of surface area and/or permeability to the overall transperitoneal diffusive movement of solute to be critically evaluated. It is the opportunity to determine these contributions to the transperitoneal movement of solute which is the major application of dialysance measurements. Perturbations and the interpretation of changes in the permeability index are tabulated in Table 10–2.

What is the relationship between peritoneal clearance and dialysance? In the absence of ultrafiltration, it has been shown that clearances approximate the overall permeability—surface area product (dialysance)—when studies involve large molecular weight solutes and short dwell times. The values for clearance and dialysance become disparate when long dwell times are used to study highly permeable solutes.[3]

### Ultrafiltration and Convective Transport

Although dialysance determinations can characterize the contribution of diffusive transport to total solute transport, the measurement of either peritoneal clearance or dialysance does not permit critical evaluation of the role of ultrafiltration and its attendant convective transport in the process. The contribution of convective solute transport to total solute transfer is influenced by three factors:[39] the degree of peritoneal permeability, the rate of ultrafiltration, and the weighted average transperitoneal membrane solute concentration gradient which existed throughout the exchange. The latter reflects the net dialysate to blood ratio of solute as affected by both convective and diffusive transport. Convective transport involves two components: water (solvent) movement across the semipermeable peritoneal membrane and solute movement (entrainment) within a solvent stream.

$$\text{Permeability Index} = \frac{\text{Dialysance solute X}}{\text{Dialysance solute Y}} = \frac{\text{Permeability X}}{\text{Permeability Y}} \times \frac{\text{membrane area for exchange of X}}{\text{membrane area for exchange of Y}}$$

**Table 10–2.** THEORETICAL CHANGES AND INTERPRETATION OF DIRECTIONAL DIFFERENCES IN PERITONEAL DIALYSANCE OF UREA AND INULIN

| Dialysance Urea | Dialysance Inulin | Permeability Index | Interpretation | |
|---|---|---|---|---|
| | | | *Surface area* | *Permeability* |
| ↑ | ↑↑ | → | ↑ or → | → or ↑ |
| ↑ | ↓ | ↓ | ↑ | ↑ |
| → | ↑ | ↑ | → | ↑ |
| → | → | → | → | → |
| → | ↓ | ↓ | → | ↓ |
| ↓ | ↓ | → | ↓ or → | → or ↓ |
| ↓ | ↑ | ↓ | ↓ | ↑ |
| ↓ | ↓↓ | ↑ | ↓ | ↑ |

Arrow indicates directional change following a maneuver, such as addition of a drug to the dialysate.

The amount of water ultrafiltrated during an exchange is related to the duration of inflow, dwell, and outflow phases, and to the magnitude of the osmotic gradient (assuming surface area, peritoneal blood flow, nonglucose solute concentration gradients, and permeability remain constant). The magnitude and overall rate of ultrafiltration is clinically determined as the difference in measured volume between inflow and outflow divided by the time from the beginning of inflow to the end of outflow. This may be inaccurate owing to fluid which does not easily drain and may give a falsely low value. A more precise technique has been used to measure ultrafiltration as changes in intraperitoneal volume by adding a relatively impermeable solute to the dialysate and measuring its dilution by removing small aliquots of dialysate at specific intervals. Isotope-labeled albumin, dextran, or inulin has been used in this manner to measure instantaneous ultrafiltration rates and volumes in both children and adults.[3, 5, 37, 38, 40, 41]

The major solute responsible for the transperitoneal osmotic gradient and for driving ultrafiltration is glucose, which has a molecular weight of 180 daltons and diffuses from dialysate to blood in accordance with its concentration gradient. A hydrostatic pressure of 19 mm Hg is generated across an ideal semipermeable membrane by an osmotic gradient of one milliosmole which contains $6.02 \times 10^{20}$ osmotically active particles of solute per kg of water.[39] When the glucose concentration in dialysate is 1.5 gm/dl or 4.25 gm/dl and the plasma glucose concentration is 100 mg/dl, the maximum transperitoneal hydrostatic gradient for ultrafiltration is 1481 mm Hg (78 mOsm) and 4391 mm Hg (231 mOsm) respectively.[39]

The initial osmotic gradient for ultrafiltration does not persist throughout the exchange cycle for two reasons: glucose moves into blood, and water moves into the peritoneal cavity. These two factors reduce the dialysate concentration of glucose and the osmotic gradient between blood and dialysate. The gradient generated by the difference in urea concentration between blood and dialysate simultaneously generates an osmotic force in the opposite direction (dialysate to blood). Each solute present, either in dialysate or blood, contributes to the net osmotic force. It is the minute-to-minute net osmotic difference created by the solutes which ultimately determines the rate of ultrafiltration as well as quantity of solute moved by convective transport.[42, 43]

An appreciation of the ultrafiltration profile of an exchange can help plan a more efficient dialysis prescription. A reproducible pattern follows the infusion of hypertonic dialysate into the peritoneal cavity (Fig. 10–1). The ultrafiltration volume and rate rapidly rise and reach a maximum after which dialysate begins to be reabsorbed as the osmotic gradient dissipates.[5] The higher the intraperitoneal osmolality, the more rapid the rate of ultrafiltration, the greater the volume of ultrafiltrate formed, and the longer period of time over which ultrafiltration occurs. Once the osmotic gradient has dissipated, reabsorption of peritoneal fluid occurs at a rate independent of the initial concentrations of glucose.[5, 6] Large variations in the transperitoneal movement of water and solute have been observed in most studies.

The peritoneal membrane does not behave as an ideal semipermeable membrane in the usual clinical setting. Physical and chemical factors oblige solute to move together with solvent when ultrafiltration occurs.[44] Solutes of varying size and configuration existing in blood move in the solvent stream in propor-

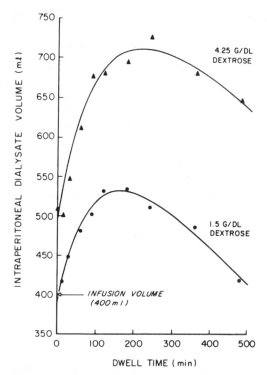

**Figure 10–1.** Intraperitoneal volume profile in a child following instillation of 1.5 and 4.25% dextrose-containing dialysate. (From Popovich RP, Pyle WK, Rosenthal DA, et al: Kinetics of Peritoneal Dialysis in Children. *In* [Eds.] Moncrief JW, Popovich RP: CAPD Update. Masson Publishing, NY, 1981, p. 239.)

tion to their concentration in blood. A factor known as the Staverman reflection coefficient (σ) for the solute adjusts for the intrinsic degree of permeability of the peritoneal membrane.[22] The reflection coefficient may be viewed as the percent of solute reflected at the peritoneal membrane and, therefore, not convected through the membrane. The reflection coefficient for solutes varies from 1.0 to 0.0.[22, 39] When the peritoneal membrane exhibits no permeability to a given solute (σ = 1 = 100% reflection or no convection) no entrainment occurs, and the ultrafiltrate will not contain that solute. Conversely, if a solute has a reflection coefficient of 0.0, the solute concentration of the ultrafiltrate will not change as fluid crosses the peritoneal membrane, and the concentration of solute in the ultrafiltrate will equal that of blood.

Because direct measurements of reflection coefficients for the peritoneal membrane are difficult to perform, solute sieving coefficients (S) have been measured clinically. The sieving coefficient (S) may be defined as the concentration ratio of solute in ultrafiltrate to that in plasma water.[39]

$$S = \frac{\text{Concentration of solute in ultrafiltrate}}{\text{Concentration of solute in plasma water}}$$

Measurement of an individual solute sieving coefficient is performed by infusing hypertonic dialysate which contains that solute in a concentration equal to that of plasma.

The sieving coefficient can be viewed as the complement of the reflection coefficient, S = 1-σ, and, therefore, represents the percentage of solute sieved, or not reflected at the membrane. The reflected molecules help generate a transperitoneal solute concentration difference and osmotic force across the membrane. Solute sieving and/or reflection coefficients available for the peritoneal membrane are summarized in Table 10–3. Measurements of sieving coefficients are unavailable in children. The lower the molecular weight of a solute the lower the reflection coefficient and the higher its sieving coefficient, and vice versa. This relationship can be expressed by the formula[5]

$$\sigma = 1 - \exp[-0.0609(mw)^{1/3}].$$

The overall convective transport is equal to the weighted average concentration difference between blood and dialysate ($\overline{C}$) times the ultrafiltration rate (Qu) times the sieving coefficient (S):

Convective transport = $\overline{C} \cdot Qu \cdot S$, or $[Qu (1-\sigma)\overline{C}]$[39]

Convective transport may be more important for high molecular weight solutes than diffusive transport. To illustrate, consider protein transport in a long dwell exchange containing 4.25% glucose. The high initial ultrafiltration rate rapidly convects protein by entrainment, and by 80 minutes the dialysate concentration of protein reaches 30 mg/dl. As the convective process slows it takes an additional 240 minutes for the dialysate concentration of protein to double. Convective transport is less important for lower molecular weight compounds such as urea, which, although readily transported by convection, are removed to a much greater extent by diffusive transport. Thus, convective transport accounts for a small fraction of the total transport of low molecular weight solutes, whereas it has a major impact on the total quantity of high molecular weight solute removed.

**Table 10–3.** CHEMICAL FEATURES, SIEVING COEFFICIENTS AND REFLECTION COEFFICIENT ($\sigma$) INDIRECTLY OBTAINED AND EXPRESSED AS 1-$\sigma$ OF SOLUTES ACROSS THE HUMAN PERITONEAL MEMBRANE*

| Solute | Mol. Wt. (daltons) | Hydrated Radius (angstroms) | Sieving Coefficient (measured $\overline{X} \pm$ SEM) | Reflection Coefficient ($1 - \sigma \overline{X} +$ range) |
|---|---|---|---|---|
| Sodium | 23 | 5.12 | 0.54 ± 0.2 | NA |
| Chloride | 35 | 3.86 | 0.78 ± 0.2 | NA |
| Potassium | 37 | 3.97 | 0.36 ± 0.2 | NA |
| Urea | 60 | 2.7 | 0.81 ± 0.03 | 0.82(0.73—0.91) |
| Creatinine | 113 | NA | NA | 0.67(0.51—0.83) |
| Uric Acid | 168 | NA | NA | 0.63(0.54—0.83) |
| Glucose | 180 | 4.4 | NA | 0.62(0.57—0.82) |
| Inulin | 5200 | 12 | 0.83 ± 0.04 | 0.63(0.30—0.91) |
| Albumin | 69,000 | 35.5 | 0.02 | NA |
| Dextran | 70,000 | NA | NA | 0.14 |
| Plasma Protein | 340,000 | NA | 0.01 | 0.016 |

*Modified from Reference 39.
NA—not available, SEM—standard error of the mean.

## Overall Mass Transfer of Solute and the Mass Transfer Area Coefficient (MTAC)

Our basic understanding of the complex interrelations involved in diffusive and convective transport of solute and water across the peritoneal membrane has been enhanced by the use of mathematical models and computer programs.[5, 45–48] The most extensive applications of mathematical modeling to clinical studies evaluating peritoneal dialysis kinetics have been undertaken by Popovich, Pyle, and Moncrief.[5, 48] They have examined simultaneously the contribution of the diffusive and convective components of an exchange by determining the time-related diffusion curves (dialysate to blood ratio of solutes) for prolonged dwells of hypo-, iso- and hypertonic dialysate, and by simultaneously measuring instantaneous rates of ultrafiltration. Computer models and equations defining the overall mass transfer of solute have been developed for the usual dialysate volumes and dwell times used in the clinical setting in adults[6] and in a few children.[41]

The mathematical models used to derive dialysance and the MTAC differ. In their initial derivation of the dialysance expression, Henderson and Nolph used a first-order rate constant (K) which incorporated such factors as temperature gradient (patient to dialysate), total membrane surface area, the cyclic patterns of the exchange, the volumes of distribution of solute, and membrane permeability.[34] By experimentally controlling all variables except surface area and permeability, a description of the membrane, i.e., dialysance, was obtained.

In the MTAC model, Pyle et al sought to characterize the concentration of solute in the system directly in terms of membrane parameters.[12, 48] When using a model based on concentrations and factoring out fluid transfer with its attendant solvent drag, the MTAC reflects the membrane area and permeability in the typical clinical situation, i.e., one in which solutes are generated and fluid is ultrafiltrated. The MTAC by design is also independent of dialysis mechanics and such other factors as temperature and volumes of distribution.

In an ideal isotonic dialysis exchange, solute transfer would occur by diffusion alone. In the absence of fluid transfer and solvent drag, the rate of mass accumulated in the peritoneal cavity should equal the product of the MTAC times the transperitoneal concentration gradient of solute, $MTAC(C_B - C_D)$, where $C_B$ and $C_D$ equal the concentration of solute in blood and dialysate respectively. This latter product describes membrane transport in accordance with either pore theory or homogeneous membrane theory. Although this equality should make direct measurement of the MTAC relatively easy, ultrafiltration is practically unavoidable in clinical practice. Therefore, in order to obtain the MTAC, the diffusive and convective components of mass transfer are measured simultaneously and the MTAC obtained using a complex computer program.

The law of conservation of mass is another principle underlying the overall transfer of mass as developed by Pyle. Mass can neither be created nor lost; therefore, the intrinsic renal clearance and solute generation rate are also factors involved in the computer solution.

The contribution of convective transport to the total transperitoneal movement of solute is separated by the computer and the MTAC determined. Inasmuch as the actual calculation of the MTAC is complex, nomograms have been designed from which the MTAC may be estimated from the time-related dialysate-to-blood concentration ratio, if the exchange has been performed in a manner similar to that used to directly measure MTAC.[5]

It has been shown mathematically that MTAC does not equal dialysance.[12] Certain simplifying assumptions can be made after which it can be demonstrated that MTAC may be linearly related to dialysance. No experimental evidence has been produced to verify or disprove these assumptions. It should be noted that theoretically both MTAC and dialysance are reflective of the surface area and permeability of the peritoneum, despite the mathematical disparity or the linear relationship which may exist. Both may be viewed as representing the maximal clearance of the peritoneal membrane, either at infinite dialysate flow rates or at time zero of an exchange when the dialysate concentration is zero.

The overall mass transfer of solute (OMTS) occurring during peritoneal dialysis is equal to the combined contributions of diffusive and convective transport. Diffusive transfer has been shown to equal KA $(C_B - C_D)$, where K equals the overall mass transfer coefficient for a given solute, A equals the functional peritoneal transfer area, which is of indeterminate size, and $C_D$ and $C_B$ equal the concentration of solute in dialysate and blood respectively.[5, 45] The product of K times A equals the mass transfer area coefficient, MTAC.[5] As already discussed, the term $S \cdot Qu \cdot \overline{C}_B$ represents the contribution of convective transport to transperitoneal solute movement.[5, 39] Therefore, OMTS (mg/min) $= KA(C_B - C_D) + SQu\overline{C} = KA(C_B - C_D) + (1 - \sigma)Qu\overline{C}$.

## PRINCIPLES OF INTERMITTENT AND CONTINUOUS PERITONEAL DIALYSIS

Two types of peritoneal dialysis are used clinically: intermittent (IPD) and continuous ambulatory peritoneal dialysis (CAPD). The five primary factors influencing the dialysis prescription for any form of chronic peritoneal dialysis include: (1) the generation rate of the metabolites, influenced by type of diet, size of patient, and intrinsic metabolic rate; (2) the MTAC or dialysance for various solutes; (3) vascular status, including peritoneal blood flow, degree of tonicity of peritoneal capillaries, hydraulic and osmotic pressures within the capillaries, and presence or absence of peritonitis; (4) the ultrafiltration rate required to maintain water balance as influenced by water intake, and (5) the residual renal clearance with its contribution to solute and water removal and its change over time.

The theoretical basis for the IPD prescription will be considered first. Intermittent dialysis is based on the principle that one's internal milieu can be satisfactorily maintained by a number of exchanges lasting from 30 to 60 minutes that remove metabolites and water faster than they accumulate. Thereafter the dialysis procedure is stopped, metabolites are allowed to accumulate, and the process is repeated. The process may be easily understood by an example. Assume that a 25 kg anephric child on IPD has a urea generation rate of 3.6 mg/min[49], a quantity of body water equal to 60% of weight, and gains 1 kg during the 36 hours between dialysis treatments. The goal of each treatment is to have a BUN of about 60 mg/dl at the end of dialysis as well as achieving the patient's "dry weight." Between dialysis treatments the child will generate 10,368 mg of urea (3.6 mg/min × 2880 min), assuming that urea generation continues at the same rate during both the intra- and interdialytic periods. Between dialyses total body water will increase one kg from 15 to 16 liters. The BUN would increase by 65 mg/dl (10,368/16 = 648 mg/liter or 64.8 mg/dl), and the pre-second dialysis BUN would be 125 mg/dl. Using the standard formula for simple diffusion kinetics

$$C_t = C_o e^{-Kt/V}$$

where

$C_t$ = BUN at the end of dialysis (60 mg/dl)

$C_o$ = BUN at onset of dialysis (125 mg/dl)

$K$ = MTAC for urea (assumed to be 30 ml/min)

$t$ = time in minutes of dialysis (720 min or 12 hours)

$V$ = volume of dialysate

the volume of dialysate required can be easily estimated. (This approach views solute movement quite simply. More complex definitions of solute movement during IPD require computer solutions of simultaneous equations.) Solving for V the expression becomes

$$V = -Kt/\ln \frac{C_t}{C_o} \quad \text{or}$$

the volume of dialysate required,

$$(V) \text{ would equal } \frac{-(30)(720)}{\ln 60/125}$$

or approximately 30,000 ml. A dialysis prescription of 30,000/12/2 ml (two exchanges per hour) or an exchange volume of 1250 cc (50 cc/kg) with half-hour cycles should be adequate. The estimated volume can be modified downward because of the anticipated solute removal due to convective transport. The required dialysate volume might also be reduced by the quantity of solute and water excreted by the patient's remaining kidney function, i.e., residual GFR, as discussed below. In practice each patient, of course, should initially have pre- and postdialysis chemistries and weights monitored to ensure that the dialysis is adequate.

The technique of continuous ambulatory peritoneal dialysis (CAPD) is one which aims to maintain constant serum levels of metabolites by providing a continuous source of dialysate into which solute and excess water can move at a rate equal to their production.[46, 50–52] The theoretical basis of solute removal during CAPD follows:[5]

In order to maintain a steady blood concentration ($C_B$) of a solute, its rate of removal via residual renal function and dialysis must equal its metabolic generation rate (G)

$$C_B K_R + C_B K_D = C_B K_T = G$$

where
$C_B$ = blood concentration
G = metabolic generation rate
$K_R, K_D$ & $K_T$ = residual renal, peritoneal, and total or combined clearance respectively.

Once again the process may be understood most easily by giving a specific example. Assume that the clinical objective in a child undergoing CAPD is to maintain his BUN at 60 mg/dl (0.6 mg/ml) and that his urea gen-

eration equals 3.6 mg/min.[49] The total clearance necessary to maintain a stable blood level of urea would be:

$$K_R + K_D = K_T = \frac{G}{C_B} = \frac{3.6 \text{ mg/min}}{0.6 \text{ mg/ml}}$$
$$= 6.0 \text{ ml/min}$$

To simplify the calculation, assume the child to be anephric (GFR = 0, $K_R$ = 0) and $K_T$ = $K_D$. The daily required urea clearance to maintain a stable BUN would equal K × 1440, the number of minutes in a day, or 6 × 1440 = 8640 ml/day.

The peritoneal dialysis clearance equals

$$K = \frac{V_D \cdot C_D}{t \cdot C_B}$$

The term $C_D/C_B$ approaches unity because the dwell time is sufficiently long in the usual CAPD exchange to permit almost complete equilibration between blood and dialysate of small molecular weight solutes.[53] Thus

$$K_D = \frac{V_D}{t}$$

where $V_D$ equals the drained volume of dialysate and t equals the total time of the exchange in minutes. In long-dwell exchanges the term $V_D/t$, which is the dialysate flow rate, virtually equals the solute clearance.

In summary, a peritoneal clearance, or dialysate flow rate of 8640 ml/day would be needed in order for the level of BUN to remain at 60 mg/dl. The required 8640 ml could be provided by doing six exchanges of 1.5 liters with each exchange lasting 240 minutes or by a combination of four 2-liter exchanges, each lasting for four hours, and a single 1-liter exchange lasting eight hours. As with IPD, the entire 8640 ml does not have to be infused in view of ultrafiltration and convective transport. The required amount of infusate could be reduced by the amount of ultrafiltrate formed.

The relationship between dialysate flow rate and urea clearance during CAPD or IPD exchanges is illustrated in Figure 10–2. IPD capitalizes upon the concept of maximizing solute exchange by utilizing as high a dialysate flow rate as possible. Transmembrane solute transfer is therefore limited by the intrinsic nature of the peritoneal membrane, i.e., the MTAC. Conversely, in the long-dwell

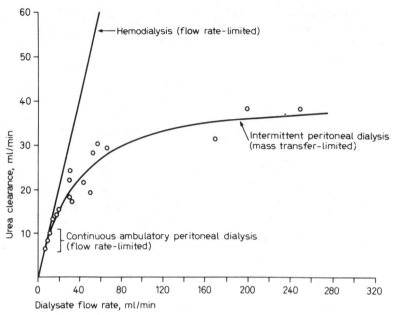

**Figure 10–2.** Urea clearance as a function of dialysate flow rate. (From Popovich RP, Moncrief JW: Kinetic modeling of peritoneal transport. Cont. Nephrology 17:59, 1979, Kargel, Basel.)

exchanges of CAPD, solute movement is flow-rate limited.

The volume of dialysate required for either IPD or CAPD can also be reduced by the contribution of any residual renal function. A child with an uncorrected GFR of 1.0, 1.5, and 2.0 ml/min will clear BUN from 1440, 2160, and 2880 ml/day (GFR ml/min times minutes per day) of plasma respectively, and the quantity of dialysate needed can theoretically be reduced by an equivalent amount. Nomograms based on the above considerations but using the serum creatine as the indicator of adequate control of uremia have been developed with the aim of defining the required volume per CAPD exchange at given levels of residual renal function and a stable creatinine generation rate (Fig. 10–3). It has been shown that a CAPD regimen consisting of four to five exchanges per day at volumes of 20 to 35 ml/kg per exchange will permit satisfactory chemical and water balance to occur.[54]

Because of the variability of the transport characteristics of the peritoneal membrane in patients, it is clinically helpful to estimate a peritoneal clearance and/or MTAC for each patient. Guidelines for determining the $C_D/C_B$ ratio for given exchange volumes, dialysate glucose concentrations, and MTAC, have been developed by Popovich and co-workers for adults undergoing CAPD. Overall adequacy of solute transport can be estimated in adult-sized patients as follows:[5, 55]

1. 30 ml/kg of 1.5% Dianeal is infused intraperitoneally and permitted to dwell for four hours;

2. The exchange is drained and a blood sample obtained and the $C_D/C_B$ creatinine ratio between dialysate and plasma obtained;

3. The MTAC for creatinine is estimated

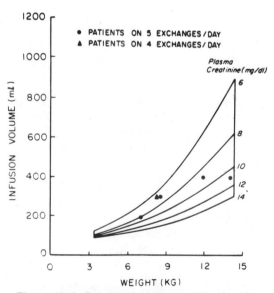

**Figure 10–3.** Relationship between dialysate volume per CAPD exchange and body weight in kilograms required to maintain plasma creatinine at various levels. (From Popovich RP, Pyle WK, Rosenthal DA, et al: Kinetics of peritoneal dialysis in children. In [Eds.] Moncrief JW, Popovich RP: CAPD Update. Masson Publishing, NY, 1981, p. 233.)

using a previously developed MTAC to equilibration curve for creatinine.

The $C_D/C_B$ creatinine ratio, which corresponds in adult patients to an MTAC for creatinine of 20 to 25 ml/min after a four-hour dwell time, usually exceeds 0.8. If the MTAC is reduced as reflected by a $C_D/C_B$ creatinine ratio of less than 0.5, adequate peritoneal dialysis will probably not occur unless additional exchanges are planned. Although similar data have not yet been developed for children, it is probable that similar $C_D/C_B$ creatinine ratios can be used as criteria for adequate dialysis for children beyond the immediate neonatal period, and when the exchange volume approaches 30 to 40 ml/kg. This suggestion is based on the fact that peritoneal diffusion curves in children are not substantially different from those reported in adults.[2, 26, 32, 33, 56–58] Also, peritoneal clearances and MTAC scaled for body weight are not significantly different between children and adults.[5, 41]

## DEVELOPMENTAL ASPECTS OF PERITONEAL DIALYSIS

Although much remains to be learned, a fund of developmental information on the subject of peritoneal dialysis kinetics in pediatric populations is now available. The data available on the topics of peritoneal anatomy, diffusive and convective transport in children, and the corresponding information in the experimental animal will be sequentially considered.

Relatively little is known about changes which occur in the gross anatomy of the peritoneal membrane during maturation. Developmental data on the ultrastructural characteristics of the peritoneal membrane are conspicuously absent. Information defining the fractional areas of parietal and visceral peritoneum is also lacking. Although the grossly measured total surface area of the peritoneum is, as expected, less in newborns than in adults, the ratio of peritoneal surface area to body mass in neonates is approximately twice that found in adults.[9, 59] Although the time during development at which the ratio of peritoneal surface area to body weight becomes constant is unknown, the relative size of the peritoneal cavity apparently changes during infancy and then grows in parallel with body size.

The maximal volume of dialysate per kg tolerated without clinical problems such as pain or respiratory compromise is greater in the neonate and young child than in adults. Clinically tolerated dialysate volumes range from 20 to 100 ml/kg in neonates, 20 to 50 ml/kg in children,[2, 9, 32, 33, 40, 56, 60–70] and up to 3000 ml in adults[25, 26, 71] (35–43 ml/kg/70 kg). The usual volume of dialysate used in adults is 2000 ml or 28.5 ml/kg for an (ideal) adult weighing 70 kg.

Limited numbers of peritoneal clearance determinations have been reported in children.[2, 9, 56, 63, 66, 72, 72a] The available data suggest that in the very young there is rapid or "efficient" transperitoneal transport of urea and creatinine, based on the observation that peritoneal urea clearances scaled for either 70 kg body weight or 1.73 m² are higher in neonates than in adult populations.[9] Comparisons between the reported studies are difficult, however, because the dialysis mechanics have varied significantly and the use of scaling factors to compare individuals of widely varying size has not been routine.

Prior to the advent of CAPD most peritoneal clearance studies in adults used two liters per exchange, with the cycle lasting 30 to 70 minutes. Clearance values in adults have been reported simply in ml/min, not corrected for body size. It is well known that if the volume of dialysate is altered in a patient while maintaining the same exchange times, peritoneal clearances are altered.[56, 73–75] When the dialysate volume was held constant at 2000 ml in a group of adults of varying weight, the fractional change in BUN was greatest in the smaller patients, suggesting that they had higher clearances.[75a] Thus, it is possible that some of the widely varying peritoneal clearances reported in adults might become more comparable if dialysate volumes and peritoneal clearances were to be scaled for weight in adult patients.

The most convenient manner of expressing clearance and dialysance values for comparison among individuals of varying body size appears to be in ml/min/kg or ml/min/70 kg, rather than as actual values or values scaled for surface area, as illustrated by the sets of theoretical calculations in Tables 10–4 and 10–5. When dialysis mechanics are kept constant in children beyond the neonatal period, weight-scaled peritoneal clearances are similar (Table 10–4). If the length of the exchange cycle and/or the volume of dialysate is varied the resulting peritoneal clearance is altered significantly (Table 10–5). Also, changes in either the peritoneal surface area or permeability will alter peritoneal clearances (Table 10–5).

**Table 10–4.** RELATIONSHIP OF PERITONEAL UREA CLEARANCE TO BODY SIZE*

| Weight (kg) | SA† | SACF‡ | $C_D/C_B$ Ratio | Dialysate Volume Drained Actual | ml/kg | Time | Dialysate Flow Rate $\frac{V}{T}$ | Peritoneal Urea Clearance¶ ml/min | ml/min/kg | ml/min/70 kg | ml/min/1.73 |
|---|---|---|---|---|---|---|---|---|---|---|---|
| 1  | .12  | 14.4 | .55 | 30   | 30 | 30 | 1  | .55  | .55  | 38.5 | 7.92  |
| 10 | .47  | 3.68 | .43 | 300  | 30 | 30 | 10 | 4.3  | 0.43 | 30.1 | 15.82 |
| 30 | 1.06 | 1.63 | .43 | 900  | 30 | 30 | 30 | 12.9 | 0.43 | 30.1 | 20.0  |
| 50 | 1.48 | 1.17 | .43 | 1500 | 30 | 30 | 50 | 21.5 | 0.43 | 30.1 | 25.2  |
| 70 | 1.79 | 0.97 | .43 | 2100 | 30 | 30 | 70 | 30.1 | 0.43 | 30.1 | 29.2  |

*Values for peritoneal urea clearances were calculated for individuals for varying weights assuming exchange cycle of 30 minutes, and infused and drained dialysate volume of 30 ml/kg. The $C_D/C_B$ ratio is greater in the neonate than in the older child.

†SA = $\dfrac{4(\text{wt kg}) + 7}{90 + \text{wt kg}}$ ,   ‡SCAF = $1.73 \div$ SA,   ¶Peritoneal Urea Clearance = $\dfrac{C_D}{C_B} \cdot \dfrac{V_D}{T}$ .

**Table 10-5.** PERTURBATIONS OF THE PERITONEAL CLEARANCE FORMULA*

| Example Number | Factor Altered | Wt (kg) | SA† (m²) | Ratio $C_D/C_B$ | T (Minutes) | Dialysate Volume (V) | | Peritoneal Clearance (ml/min) |
| --- | --- | --- | --- | --- | --- | --- | --- | --- |
| | | | | | | Actual | ml/kg | |
| *Child* | | | | | | | | |
| 1 | Control | 10 | 0.47 | 0.6 | 60 | 400 | 40 | 3.99 |
| 2 | Permeability | 10 | 0.47 | 0.5‡ | 60 | 400 | 40 | 3.33 |
| 3 | Permeability or surface area | 10 | 0.47 | 0.4‡ | 60 | 400 | 40 | 2.66 |
| 4 | Permeability and Time | 10 | 0.47 | 0.4‡ | 30‡ | 400 | 40 | 5.33 |
| 5 | Time | 10 | 0.47 | 0.6 | 30‡ | 400 | 40 | 7.99 |
| 6 | Dialysate Volume | 10 | 0.47 | 0.6 | 60 | 300‡ | 30‡ | 3.00 |
| 7 | Dialysate Volume | 10 | 0.47 | 0.6 | 60 | 200‡ | 20‡ | 1.99 |
| *Adult* | | | | | | | | |
| 8 | Control ideal | 70 | 1.73 | 0.6 | 60 | 2000 | 28.6 | 19.99 |
| 9 | Control (SA Formula)+ | 70 | 1.79 | 0.6 | 60 | 2800‡ | 40 | 27.99 |
| 10 | Permeability or surface area | 70 | 1.79 | 0.4‡ | 60 | 2800 | 40 | 18.66 |

*Effect of changes in permeability ($C_D/C_B$), dwell times, and exchange volumes on theoretical urea clearances in a child and an adult. Values for the concentration of dialysate urea have been obtained from diffusion curves performed in children and adults. Dwell times and dialysate volumes are those used when performing intermittent dialysis.

†SA $= \dfrac{4(wt\ kg) + 7^+}{90 + wt\ kg}$  From Costeff H: A simple empirical formula for calculating approximate surface area in children. Arch Dis Child 41:681, 1966.

‡Parameter altered.

The initial suggestion that peritoneal clearances are higher in the neonate was based on peritoneal clearance studies obtained in neonatal and adult dogs and one infant 11 days of age.[9] Although the peritoneal clearance of urea expressed in ml/min/70 kg was higher in the neonatal animals, dialysis mechanics were not similar in both groups. More recent studies in which dialysis mechanics have been held constant provide critical support for the original suggestion that the peritoneal membrane of the newborn functions differently.[37, 38, 76] Dialysate ratios ($C_D/C_B$) of urea and creatinine were higher during the neonatal period than in older children in exchanges performed with similar dialysis mechanics. All other factors being equal, a higher $C_D/C_B$ ratio is indicative of a greater clearance.

The age at which the transperitoneal movement of solute approaches that of adults is probably between the latter half of the first year and the second year of age.[56] This suggestion is supported by the results of peritoneal diffusion curves performed in a group of children of differing age and body size.[49] When the dialysate to blood ratios of a number of solutes were systematically evaluated in a group of children, they were similar among three children ages 4–18 months and among four children 11–18 years of age[56, 57] (Fig. 10–4). The corrected peritoneal clearances of urea, creatinine, phosphate, and uric acid expressed in ml/min/kg or ml/min/70 kg were similar in all the children (Table 10–6). Thus, the peritoneal clearance of solutes with molecular weights up to 168 daltons appears to be similar throughout most of childhood.

Clearances are higher in the neonate and similar among individuals of other size when expressed in relation to body weight, yet quite different when corrected for surface area.[56] The discrepancy between values scaled for weight vs. surface area can be explained by the fact that surface area is not linearly related to body weight. This is supported by dialysance studies in the experimental animal[37, 38] and by measurements of peritoneal clearances and/or MTAC[5, 42] in children. The better fit occurring when clearances are scaled for weight, however, may reflect the fact that they were derived by using dialysate volumes based on body weight rather than surface area. It remains to be established whether clearances scaled for surface area will be similar when the volume of dialysate infused is also related to surface area.

The relationship between peritoneal permeability, functional peritoneal surface area, and development has been critically examined by measuring dialysance in dogs.[37, 38] The dialysance of urea and inulin as well as the dialysance ratio, i.e., permeability index, was found to be significantly higher in puppies less than one month of age than in adult dogs[37, 38] (Table 10–7). Such data demonstrate that both the effective peritoneal surface area and permeability are greater during the neonatal period. Thus, the movement of solute is more rapid or efficient in the neonatal period in the exper-

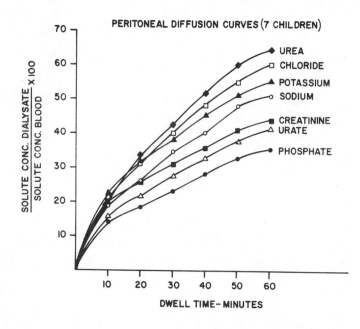

**Figure 10–4.** Peritoneal diffusion curves in seven children ages 4 months to 18 years. (Adapted from Gruskin AB, Cote ML, Baluarte HJ: Peritoneal diffusion curves, peritoneal clearances and scaling factors in children of differing age. Int J Pediatr Nephrol 3:271, 1982.)

**Table 10–6.** PERITONEAL SOLUTE CLEARANCE*—ML/MIN/70 KG IN CHILDREN†

| Age | Number | Urea | Creatinine | Urate | Phosphate |
|-----|--------|------|-----------|-------|-----------|
| 4–18 mos | 3 | 29.4 ± 4.7 | 24.8 ± 5.3 | 22.9 ± 6.3 | 14.9 ± 6.0 |
| 11–18 yrs | 4 | 25.6 ± 8.7 | 17.5 ± 5.9 | 19.1 ± 8.4 | 15.2 ± 6.0 |
| P | | 0.36 | 0.046 | 0.40 | 0.92 |

*X ± S.D.
†Dialysate volume used per exchange was 40 ml/kg.

imental animal. The finding of elevated urea and creatinine dialysate to blood ratios ($C_D/C_B$) obtained in human neonates[63] supports the suggestion that the peritoneal membrane is also more permeable and/or relatively larger in the human neonate.

## CLINICAL AND EXPERIMENTAL OBSERVATIONS

Although dialysance studies have not yet been reported in children, the results of studies of the MTAC performed in four children using an unspecified infused volume of 1.5 and 4.25% dextrose are available (Table 10–8). Mean values for MTAC in children scaled for surface area differed by more than two standard deviations from the adult references, yet were similar when scaled for weight.[5, 41] The MTAC is designed to be theoretically independent of the dialysate volume. The observation that values for MTAC of various size solutes are similar to adult values when scaled for body weight independently supports the concept that the effective peritoneal surface area and permeability are similar after the neonatal period.

Data which define the contribution of convective solute transport to the total transport of solute in children are not yet available. Although sieving coefficients have not yet been determined in children, they might be expected to be similar to those reported in adults, because diffusion curves (i.e., time-related $C_D/C_B$ ratio including both diffusive and convective components) for multiple solutes are similar in adults and children beyond the neonatal period.

Studies of ultrafiltration rates and patterns performed by measuring either actual drainage volumes or intraperitoneal dilution of chemicals or isotopes have revealed a wide range of values. The general shape of the intraperitoneal volume vs. dwell time curve is similar in children[40] and adults.[5] Ultrafiltration rates and volumes scaled for weight (ml/kg) rather than surface area in children beyond the neonatal period give values similar to those obtained in adults.[5, 40] Maximum ultrafiltration rates range between 0.136–0.167 and 0.237–0.254 ml/min/kg for infusates containing 1.5 and 4.25% dextrose respectively (Table 10–9).[5, 41] The mean duration of ultrafiltration following instillation of these solutions is 140 and 247 minutes respectively. The rate of reabsorption of dialysate once it begins ranges from 0.0097 to 0.0124 ml/min/kg.

In older children undergoing four-hour exchange cycles with 4.25% dextrose solution, drainage volumes usually exceed infused volumes by 10 to 20%. The net water balance (the difference between infused and drained dialysate) often is close to zero in children less than three years undergoing four-hour exchanges with 1.5% dextrose solution.[40] The wide differences in ultrafiltration rates and volume probably reflect the differences in the time-related transmembrane glucose concentration gradient. The large variability observed in ultrafiltration patterns between patients mandates that individual patient information be obtained whenever volume regulation is a problem.

Although the shape of the glucose concentration vs. time curve after instillation of 1.5 or 4.25% dextrose solution in children over three years of age is similar to that found in adults, the curve for children shows a slightly faster but not statistically significant drop in the glucose concentration.[40] The number of patients examined, however, is small and the differences are not sufficient to suggest that major differences in ultrafiltration exist between older children and adults. Additional support for such a conclusion is provided by the measurement of the MTAC for glucose which when scaled for weight (Table 10–8) is similar in children and adults.

When four-hour exchanges are performed in neonates, adequate ultrafiltration using either 1.5% or 4.25% dextrose solution is difficult to achieve. The difference in ultrafiltration between neonates and older children can be explained by the reported dif-

**Table 10-7.** COMPARATIVE STUDY OF DIALYSANCE OF UREA AND INULIN IN NEONATAL VS. ADULT DOGS*

| | Wt. range (kg) | Number | Urea | | Inulin | | Dialysance Ratio |
|---|---|---|---|---|---|---|---|
| | | | $C_D/C_B$ | Dialysance Urea, ml/kg | $C_D/C_B$ | Dialysance Inulin, ml/kg | $D_I/D_u$ |
| Puppy | 1.8–3.15 | 6 | $0.405 \pm 0.023$ | $0.765 \pm 0.054$ | $.095 \pm 0.013$ | $0.146 \pm 0.023$ | $0.187 \pm 0.026$ |
| Adult | 19–24 | 5 | $0.29 \pm 0.027$† | $0.462 \pm 0.059$† | $0.036 \pm 0.007$† | $0.052 \pm 0.010$† | $0.110 \pm 0.015$† |

*Adapted from Reference 37.
† = p<0.05 (comparison of adult to puppy).

**Table 10–8.** MASS TRANSFER AREA COEFFICIENTS FOR SOLUTES IN CHILDREN†

| Solute | Mol. Wt. | Children*—MTAC—ml/min | | | Adults—MTAC | | Ratio Child: adult |
| | | per 1.73m² | per 70 kg | per kg | ml/min | per kg | |
|--------|----------|------------|-----------|--------|--------|--------|-------|
| Urea | 60 | 21.9±5.4 | 40.2±9.5 | 0.574 | 33.6 | 0.480 | 1.20 |
| Creatinine | 113 | 9.2±2.0 | 16.9±3.1 | 0.241 | 23.5 | 0.336 | 0.72 |
| Uric Acid | 168 | 10.7±3.7 | 19.5±6.4 | 0.279 | 19.5 | 0.279 | 1.0 |
| Glucose | 180 | 11.8±2.9 | 21.7±5.1 | 0.31 | 18.1 | 0.259 | 1.20 |

*Data derived from four children weighing 7.0, 8.2, 11.7 and 14.7 kilograms. The data in the children were obtained during exchanges containing 1.5% and/or 4.25% dextrose; the exchange volume was not specified.

†Corrected for surface area and body weight and compared to values obtained in adults undergoing dialysis with 4.25% dextrose. Note the similarity of values between adults and children when values are expressed in ml/min/kg. Adult values per kg were obtained by dividing the actual MTAC by 70. Adapted from Reference 41.

ference in the shape of the time-related dialysate glucose curve.[40] Dialysate glucose concentration falls significantly more rapidly in the neonatal period,[40] and after a dwell of 45 to 60 minutes is often low enough to enable dialysate to be reabsorbed. Ultrafiltration can be achieved in the very young when exchange cycles of 30 to 45 minutes are used. The more rapid fall in dialysate sugar in neonates may reflect the greater effective peritoneal membrane area, increased membrane permeability, or differences in the rate of utilization of glucose. During CAPD five children less than two years of age absorbed dextrose at a mean rate of 2.74 ± 1.06 gm/kg/day versus a rate of 1.79 ± 0.87 gm/kg/day in four children over six years of age.[77] In seven adults undergoing CAPD net glucose absorption averaged 182 ± 61 gm/day or approximately 2.3 gm/kg/day.[78]

Successful chronic peritoneal dialysis requires the removal of a volume of water equal to that resulting from the combined intake of liquids, water content of food, and the water of oxidation. The usual quantities of water ingested and that formed via metabolic processes are both inversely related to body weight, and are relatively greater in the smaller child.[79] Therefore, a greater amount of ultrafiltration (expressed in ml/kg) is re-quired in smaller sized children in order to achieve water balance.

Measured ultrafiltration volumes in adults undergoing one-hour exchange cycles with 2000 ml of dialysis solutions containing 1.5 and 4.25% glucose average 150–200 (5–10%) and 200–400 (10–20%) ml respectively. In adults, the measured ultrafiltrated volumes after a 4 to 8 hour dwell of such solutions averaged 200–300 ml and 400–800 ml respectively.[63, 80] Mean measured drainage volumes in six children dialyzed with 30-minute exchanges of 30 ml/kg of 1.5% and 4.25% (standard) dialysate exceeded input volumes by 6 and 15% respectively.[81]

Because of the nature of the peritoneal membrane, peritoneal dialysis is associated with losses of larger quantities of protein, especially albumin, than is hemodialysis. An inverse relationship exists between the molecular weights of plasma proteins and their peritoneal clearances.[82] Albumin losses averaged 0.30 ± 0.66 gm/kg/day in five children on CAPD below two years of age compared to an average loss of 0.16 ± 0.02 gm/kg/day in four children older than six years of age.[77] It is not possible to ascertain whether these reported differences reflect dialysis mechanics, or age-related differences in the peritoneal membrane.[77]

**Table 10–9.** MAXIMUM ULTRAFILTRATION RATES IN CHILDREN UNDERGOING HYPERTONIC DIALYSIS*

| Dextrose Concentration | Ultrafiltration Rate ml/min (Children) | | | Ultrafiltration Rate ml/min (Adult) | |
| | per 1.73m² | per 70 kg | per kg | Actual | per kg |
|------------------------|------------|-----------|--------|--------|--------|
| 1.5% single study | 5.3* | 9.5 | 0.136 | 11.7 | 0.167 |
| 4.25% | 9.6±1.7 | 17.8±3.5 | 0.254 | 16.6 | 0.237 |

*The reported adult values have been divided by 70 to obtain an ultrafiltrate rate per kg of body weight. Adapted from References 5 and 41.

# CLINICAL APPLICATIONS

During the past few years peritoneal dialysis, both intermittent and continuous, has been increasingly used as a therapeutic alternative for children being dialyzed in hospital and especially at home.[1, 77, 83–85] It is helpful to perform certain studies in each child to individually characterize his or her peritoneal membrane. Such studies might include a dialysate-to-blood ratio of urea and creatinine, and perhaps potassium and phosphate, at 30, 60, and 240 minutes if CAPD is to be used. Peritoneal clearances or the MTAC can be estimated on the basis of the data obtained, and an overall assessment made of the transperitoneal movement of solute and control of the uremic process. These studies may also provide an indication of how quickly potassium can be removed if necessary, and the impact of dialysis on calcium and phosphorus balance.

Because of the large variability in ultrafiltration among patients, determinations of the average quantity of fluid ultrafiltrated in response to the varying concentrations of dextrose containing dialysate should be made so that individual basal rates of ultrafiltration are known. When it is necessary to remove larger quantities of water, cycles with short dwell (20–30 minutes) and short drain times are most effective because a greater transperitoneal osmotic gradient is maintained. It is not necessary to wait for complete drainage to occur before starting another exchange; however, drainage volumes should be measured to ensure that significant ultrafiltration has occurred with each exchange cycle.

Problems achieving adequate ultrafiltration may occur in patients who develop peritonitis because peritoneal inflammation is associated with an increased rate of transport of glucose from dialysate to blood.[86] Peritoneal clearances of urea and creatinine and transmembrane losses of protein are also increased in patients with peritonitis.[87] Clearances have been reported to return to normal within one week after beginning treatment for the infection.[88]

It is important to determine whether changes in the transperitoneal movement of solute occur over time. Peritoneal clearances of urea and creatinine have been noted by some to decrease over a ten-month period in patients undergoing IPD.[87, 89] Others have observed that the clearance of urea, creatinine, and inulin do not change significantly in patients undergoing CAPD[88, 90] for up to one year despite multiple episodes of peritonitis. We have found borderline decreases in the clearance of inulin, but not urea or creatinine, after six months of home peritoneal dialysis in a small group of children. Progressive increases in BUN or creatinine routinely obtained at monthly intervals may be the earliest signs of diminished peritoneal clearances.

Periodic determinations of blood glucose through the course of dialysis are helpful in ensuring that hyperglycemia with its attendant problems has not developed. Sequential exchanges of hypertonic dialysate may result in hyperglycemia, thus eliminating the transperitoneal osmotic gradient and significantly reducing ultrafiltration. Rates of metabolism of glucose may change as children become older or after their nutritional status improves if they had been either malnourished or hypercatabolic when dialysis was initiated. When the blood sugar exceeds 400 mg/dl maneuvers designed to lower the blood sugar should be taken. These include the use of dialysate containing lower concentrations of glucose and/or the use of insulin either systemically or added to the dialysate.[91] Most patients develop a hyper-insulinemic state in response to prolonged continuous peritoneal dialysis with high concentrations of glucose; thus, acute hypoglycemia may develop when dialysis is abruptly discontinued. If an interruption in dialysis is anticipated, the dialysate glucose concentration should be reduced and adequate time should elapse to allow recovery of insulin-glucose homeostasis.

Hypernatremia and hyperchloremia can develop when large quantities of fluid are rapidly ultrafiltrated because the sieving coefficients for these solutes are such that their removal from the extracellular compartment is retarded.[31, 92] The use of dialysate containing a sodium concentration less than that of plasma can somewhat alleviate this problem.[93] Potassium concentrations in dialysate approach Gibbs-Donnan equilibrium with serum.[94] Hypertonic exchanges may help to reduce serum levels of potassium in hyperkalemic patients more rapidly than iso-osmotic exchanges by the enhancement of convective transport. Hyperkalemia rarely occurs clinically because potassium, unlike sodium, is infrequently added to dialysate, and the diffusive component of the total transport is usually rapid enough to offset the effect of membrane reflection. However, if potassium is added to dialysate and the dialysate-to-blood diffusive gradient for potassium reduced, hypertonic dialysis can cause hyperkalemia.

Changes in the temperature[95] of the dialysate can alter solute transport across the peritoneum. An increase in clearances of 30 to 35% occurs when dialysate is warmed from a room temperature of 20°C to body temperature of 37°C.[95] Patient comfort and improved clearances mandate the use of warmed dialysate.

All of the commercially available solutions used for peritoneal dialysis are initially acidic and have a pH that ranges from 5.0 to 5.8.[96] Evidence that the pH of the dialysate alters peritoneal clearances has been mixed.[96] Changes in the pH of dialysate have been shown to influence the rate of diffusion of barbiturates and uric acid.

Attempts have been made to increase the efficiency of peritoneal dialysis by the addition to dialysate of pharmaceutical agents such as isoproterenol[30] and nitroprusside.[29] The mechanism for increased transport varies, depending upon the agent used. Changes in membrane area, permeability, and capillary blood flow have been documented.[97, 98] Lipid added to dialysate has been shown to enhance the transperitoneal movement of salicylate[99] and glutethimide[100] respectively. Intraperitoneal albumin and lipids trap solute which has diffused across the membrane and help sustain a maximal gradient for diffusion. Albumin has also been used in copper poisoning.[100a] Systematically collected data on the enhancement of solute movement is not available in children.

Of interest is the report that protein losses per week in adults were similar in patients undergoing acute or maintenance IPD and CAPD.[101] It has been shown that amino acids can be absorbed from dialysate and that positive nitrogen balance can be obtained.[102] There have been attempts to improve nitrogen balance in children by adding amino acids to dialysate, to counteract the large losses of protein and amino acids occurring during peritoneal dialysis. We have observed a dramatic increase in serum triglycerides in a child when amino acids were added to the dialysate. The bidirectional movement of amino acids as evaluated by diffusion curves is complex and cannot be readily explained by their size, charge, or hydrophobic or hydrophilic properties.[103, 104]

Despite the importance of divalent ion metabolism in growth, little is known about the transperitoneal movement of divalent ions in children. Peritoneal diffusion curves of phosphate in children beyond the neonatal period are similar to those reported in adults.[49] It has been shown that calcium moves across the peritoneal membrane in both directions, that calcium clearances are inversely related to the serum protein concentration, and that net calcium balance in adults on CAPD with dialysate containing calcium at a concentration of 3.5 mEq/L is positive.[105, 106] Calcium absorption is lower when hypertonic exchanges which involve convective transport are performed. The net absorption of calcium may be of help in treating renal osteodystrophy but may also lead to hypercalcemia. Conversely, calcium-free dialysate has been successfully used to treat hypercalcemia.[107] CAPD exchanges containing magnesium at a concentration of 1.5 mEq/L may elevate serum magnesium levels.[79]

In addition to its use to treat renal failure, peritoneal dialysis has been used with variable degrees of success in neonates and infants to treat metabolic disorders such as maple syrup urine disease,[108] inborn errors of urea cycle synthesis,[109–111] latic acidosis,[112] hypernatremia,[113] congestive heart failure,[114] drug ingestion, hepatic failure,[115] the Reye syndrome,[116] and hyaline membrane disease.[117, 118]

Virtually all children on dialysis receive various medications, yet little definitive information is available on drug usage in children with renal insufficiency and the rate of removal of such agents.[119–120] It is probable that the kinetics of drug removal scaled for body weight in older children are similar to those reported in adults.[121, 122] The peritoneal clearance of gentamicin of $4.0 \pm 2.6$ ml/min/m$^2$ observed in five children ages 8 to 15 years was similar to values reported in adults.[123] Although usable guidelines for the use of drugs in children with renal insufficiency are available, the large variations observed in the peritoneal clearances of drugs suggest that drug levels be monitored when possible and individualized therapy be provided.

## CONCLUSION

The major theories describing the movement of solutes and water across the peritoneal membrane have been reviewed, their contribution to the basis of CAPD and IPD discussed, and their clinical effects analyzed. Despite some significant advances in the understanding of dialysis kinetics, especially as they relate to children, gaps in our knowledge persist. Why is peritoneal dialysis more efficient in the neonate? Can pharmaceutical manipulations be useful in the routine dialysis of children? How will long-term maintenance peritoneal dialysis affect the peritoneum as a dialyzer? In the future, we hope to have greater insight into these and other questions. The institution of peritoneal dialysis in the child should be viewed as an opportunity to enhance our understanding of dialysis kinetics.

## REFERENCES

1. Fine RH: Peritoneal dialysis update—medical progress. J Pediatr *100*:1, 1982.
2. Gruskin AB, Elzouki AY, Baluarte HJ, et al: Peritoneal dialysis kinetics—pediatric perspective. *In*: Pediatric Nephrology Vol VI, Strauss J (Ed). New York, Plenum Press, 1981, p 439.
3. Henderson LW: Peritoneal dialysis. *In*: Clinical Aspects of Uremia and Dialysis, Massry SG, Sellers AL (Eds). Springfield, Illinois, Charles C Thomas, 1976, p 555.
4. Popovich RP, Moncrief JW: Kinetic modeling of peritoneal transport. Cont Nephrol *17*:58, 1979.
5. Popovich RP, Pyle WK, Moncrief JW: Kinetics of peritoneal transport. *In*: Peritoneal Dialysis, Nolph KD (Ed). Developments in Nephrology, Vol. 2, The Hague, Martinus Nijhoff, 1981, p 79.
6. Pyle WK, Moncrief JW, Popovich RP: Peritoneal transport evaluation in CAPD. *In*: CAPD Update, Moncrief JW, Popovich RP (Eds). New York, Masson Publishing, 1981, p 35.
7. Popovich RP, Pyle WK, Hiatt MP, et al: Metabolite transport kinetics in peritoneal dialysis. Proceedings of International CAPD Symposium, Paris, Nov. 2–3, 1979. Excerpta Medica, pp 28–33.
8. Gosselin RE, Berndt WO: Diffusional transport of solutes through mesentery and peritoneum. J Theor Biol *3*:487, 1962.
9. Esperanca MJ, Collins DL: Peritoneal dialysis efficiency in relation to body weight. J Pediatr Surg *1*:162, 1966.
10. Odel HM, Ferris DO, Power MH: Clinical consideration of the problem of external excretion: Peritoneal lavage. Med Clin North Am *32*:989, 1948.
11. Kallen RJ: A method for approximating the efficacy of peritoneal dialysis for uremia. Am J Dis Child *111*:156, 1966.
12. Pyle WK: Personal communication.
13. Miller FN: The peritoneal microcirculation. *In*: Peritoneal Dialysis, Nolph KD (Ed). Developments in Nephrology, Vol. 2. The Hague, Martinus Nijhoff, 1981, p 42.
14. Nolph KD, Sorkin MI: The peritoneal dialysis system. *In*: Peritoneal Dialysis, Nolph KD (Ed). Developments in Nephrology, Vol. 2. The Hague, Martinus Nijhoff, 1981, p 21.
15. McGary TJ, Nolph KD, Rubin J: In vitro simulation of peritoneal dialysis: A technique for demonstrating limitations on solute clearance. J Lab Clin Med *96*:1, 148, 1980.
16. Giordano C, DeSanto NG: Dietary management of patients on peritoneal dialysis (Vol 17 of Contrib Nephrol). *In*: Today's Art of Peritoneal Dialysis, Trevino-Becerra A, Boen F (Eds). Basel, Karger, 1979, p 77.
17. Nolph KD: An hypothesis to explain the ultrafiltration characteristics of peritoneal dialysis. Kidney Int *20*:543, 1981.
18. Nolph KD, Popovich RP, Ghods AJ, Twardowski A: Determinants of low clearances of small solutes during peritoneal dialysis. Kidney Int *13*:117, 1978.
19. Kelton JG, Vlan R, Stiller C, Holmes E: Comparison of chemical composition of peritoneal fluid and serum. Ann Intern Med *89*:67, 1978.
20. Henderson LW, Nolph KD: Altered permeability of peritoneal membrane after using hypertonic peritoneal dialysis fluid. J Clin Invest *48*:992, 1969.
21. Barbour GL: The kinetics of peritoneal dialysis. Dialysis Transplant *8*:1055, 1979.
22. Bresler EH, Groome LJ: On equations for combined convective and diffusive transport of neutral solute across porous membranes. Am J Physiol *10*:469, 1981.
23. Nolph KD, Rosenfield PS, Powell JT, Danforth E: Peritoneal glucose transport and hyperglycemia during peritoneal dialysis. Am J Med Sci *259*:272, 1970.
24. Giordano C, DeSanto NG, Capodicasa G: Peritoneal nutrition in children. Preliminary results in renal failure. *In*: Developments in Nephrology, Vol. 3, Proceedings Fifth International Pediatric Nephrology Symposium, Gruskin AB, Norman ME (Eds). The Hague, Martinus Nijhoff, 1981, p 303.
25. Boen ST: Peritoneal Dialysis in Clinical Medicine. Springfield, Illinois: Charles C Thomas, Publisher, 1964.
26. Boen ST: Kinetics of peritoneal dialysis. Medicine *40*:243, 1961.
27. Henderson LW: The problem of peritoneal membrane area and permeability. Kidney Int *3*:409, 1973.
28. Penzotti SC, Mattocks AM: Effects of dwell time, volume of dialysis fluid, and added accelerators on peritoneal dialysis of urea. J Pharm Sci *60*:1520, 1971.
29. Nolph KD, Ghods AJ, Brown PA: Effects of intraperitoneal nitroprusside on peritoneal clearances in man with variations of dose, frequency of administration and dwell times. Nephron *24*:114, 1979.
30. Nolph KD, Miller L, Husted FC, Hirszel P: Effects of intraperitoneal isoproterenol on reduced peritoneal clearances in patients with systemic vascular disease. J Int Urol Nephrol *8*:161, 1976.
31. Nolph KD, Hano JE, Teschan PE: Peritoneal sodium transport during hypertonic peritoneal dialysis: Physiologic mechanisms and clinical implications. Ann Intern Med *70*:931, 1969.
32. Gruskin AB, Cote ML: Kinetics of peritoneal dialysis in children. Abst Soc Pediatr Res, May, 1970.
33. Gruskin AB: Peritoneal dialysis in acute renal failure: Indications and technical considerations. Proc Int Cong Pediatr, Nephrology Issue, Vienna, Aug-Sept, 1971, p 261.
34. Henderson LW, Nolph KD: Altered permeability

of the peritoneal membrane after using hypertonic peritoneal dialysis fluid. J Clin Invest 48:992, 1969.

35. Henderson LW, Kintzel JE: Influence of antidiuretic hormone on peritoneal membrane area and permeability. J Clin Invest 50:2437, 1971.

36. Elzouki AY, Gruskin AB, Baluarte, HJ, et al: Age-related changes in peritoneal dialysis (PD) kinetics. Pediatr Res 14:618, 1980.

37. Elzouki AY, Gruskin AB, Baluarte HJ, et al: Developmental changes in peritoneal dialysis kinetics in dogs. Pediatr Res 15:853, 1981.

38. Elzouki AY, Gruskin AB, Baluarte HJ, et al: Developmental aspects of peritoneal dialysis. In: Developments in Nephrology, Vol. 3, Proceedings Fifth International Pediatric Nephrology Symposium, Gruskin AB, Norman ME (Eds). The Hague, Martinus Nijhoff, 1981, p 517.

39. Henderson L: Ultrafiltration with peritoneal dialysis. In: Peritoneal Dialysis, Nolph, KD (Ed). Developments in Nephrology, Vol. 2, The Hague, Martinus Nijhoff, 1981, p 124.

40. Kohaut EC, Alexander S: Ultrafiltration in the young patient on CAPD. In: CAPD Update, Moncrief JW, Popovich RP (Eds). New York, Masson Publishing, 1981, p 221.

41. Popovich RP, Pyle WK, Rosenthal DA, et al: Kinetics of peritoneal dialysis in children. In:CAPD Update, Moncrief JW, Popovich RP (Eds). New York, Masson Publishing, 1981, p 227.

42. Kiil F: Mechanism of osmosis. Kidney Int 21:303, 1982.

43. Aune S: Transperitoneal exchange: IV. The effect of transperitoneal fluid transport on the transfer of solutes. Scand J Gastroenterol 5:241, 1970.

44. Henderson LW: Peritoneal ultrafiltration dialysis: Enhanced urea transfer using hypertonic peritoneal dialysis fluid. J Clin Invest 45:950, 1966.

45. Moncrief JW, Popovich RP, Okutan M, Decherd JF: A model of the peritoneal dialysis system. Proceedings of 25th Annual Conference on Engineering in Medicine and Biology. 14:172, 1976.

46. Popovich RP, Moncrief JW: Clinical development of the low dialysis clearance hypothesis via equilibrium peritoneal dialysis. 1st Ann Rep No N01–AM–6–2211, AK–CUP, NIAMDD, NIH, Bethesda, Md, 1977, p 123.

47. Babb AL, Johansen PJ, Strand MJ, et al: Bi-directional permeability of the human peritoneum to middle molecules. Proc 10th Cong Eur Dial Transplant Assoc, Vienna, 10:247, 1973.

48. Pyle WK: Mass transfer in peritoneal dialysis. Ph D Dissertation, University of Texas, 1981.

49. Sargent J, Gotch F, Borah M, et al: Urea kinetics: A guide to nutritional management of renal failure. Am J Clin Nutr 31:1696, 1978.

50. Popovich RP, Pyle WK, Moncrief JW, et al: Preliminary verification of the low dialysis clearance hypothesis via a novel equilibrium peritoneal dialysis technique. Proc 2nd Austral Conf Heat Mass Transfer 2:217, 1977.

51. Popovich RP, Moncrief JW, Decherd JF, et al: Preliminary verification of low dialysis clearance hypotheses via a novel equilibrium peritoneal dialysis technique (Abst) Am Soc Artif Intern Organs 5:64, 1976.

52. Moncrief JW: Continuous ambulatory peritoneal dialysis. Dial Transplant 8:1077, 1979.

53. Nolph KD, Twardowski ZJ, Popovich RP, Rubin J: Equilibration of peritoneal dialysis solutions during long-dwell exchanges. J Lab Clin Med 93:246, 1979.

54. Alexander S, Tseng CH, Maksym RA, et al: Clinical parameters in CAPD for infants and children. In: CAPD Update, Moncrief JW, Popovich RP (Eds). New York, Masson Publishing, 1981, p 195.

55. Popovich RP, Hiatt MP, Moncrief JW, Pyle WK: Mathematical modeling and minimum treatment requirements in peritoneal dialysis. Proc 3rd Capri Conf on Chronic Uremia (in press), 1980.

56. Gruskin AB, Cote ML, Baluarte HJ: Peritoneal diffusion curves, peritoneal clearances and scaling factors in children of differing age. Int J Pediatr Nephrol 3:271, 1982.

57. Gruskin AB, Rosenblum H, Baluarte HJ, et al: Transperitoneal solute movement in a pediatric population (Abst). International Workshop on Recent Advances in Diagnosis and Treatment of Children with Chronic Renal Failure. Heidelberg, Federal Republic of Germany, May 21–22, 1982.

58. Maxwell NW, Rockney RE, Kleeman CR, Twiss MR: Peritoneal dialysis. 1. Technique and application. JAMA 170:917, 1959.

59. Putiloff PV: Materials for the study of the laws of growth of the human body in relation to the surface areas of different systems; the trial on Russian subjects of planigraphic anatomy as a means for exact anthropometry—one of the problems of anthropology. Presented at the Meeting of the Siberian Branch of the Russian Geographic Society, October 29, 1884, Omsk, 1886.

60. Day RE, White RHR: Peritoneal dialysis in children. Preview of 8 years of experience. Arch Dis Child 52:56, 1977.

61. Donn SM, Swartz RD, Thoene JG: Comparison of exchange transfusion, peritoneal dialysis and hemodialysis for the treatment of hyperammonemia in an anuric newborn infant. J Pediatr 95:67, 1979.

62. Etteldorf JN, Dobbins WT, Summit RL, et al: Intermittent peritoneal dialysis using 5% albumin in the treatment of salicylate intoxication in children. J Pediatr 58:226, 1961.

63. Gruskin AB, Elzouki AY, Baluarte HJ, et al: The peritoneal membrane—developmental consideratons. In: The Kidney during Development: Morphology and Function, Spitzer A (Ed). New York, Masson Publishing, p 315.

64. Lee HA: Evaluation of peritoneal dialysis and haemodialysis in paediatrics. Isr J Med Sci 3(1):28, 1967.

65. Lloyd-Still JD, Atwell JD: Renal failure in infancy with special reference to the use of peritoneal dialysis. J Pediatr Surg 1(5):466, 1966.

66. Siegel NJ, Brown RS: Peritoneal clearance of ammonia and creatinine in a neonate. J Pediatr 82:1044, 1973.

67. Segar WE, Gibson RK, Rhomy R: Peritoneal dialysis in infants and small children. Pediatrics 27:603, 1961.

68. Wiggelinkhuizen J: Peritoneal dialysis in children. S Afr Med J 45:1047, 1971.

69. Lorentz WB: Acute hydrothorax during peritoneal dialysis. J Pediatr 94:417, 1979.

70. Lugo G, Ceballos R, Brown W, et al: Acute renal failure in the neonate managed by peritoneal dialysis. Am J Dis Child 118:655, 1969.

71. Nolph KD, Stoltz M, Maher JF: Altered peritoneal

permeability in patients with systemic vasculitis. Ann Intern Med 75:753, 1971.

72. Feldman W, Beilah T, Drummond KN: Intermittent peritoneal dialysis in the management of chronic renal failure in children. Am J Dis Child 116:30, 1968.

72a. Baum M, Powell D, Calvin S, et al: Continuous ambulatory peritoneal dialysis in children—comparison with hemodialysis. N Engl J Med 307:1537, 1982.

73. Robson M, Oreopoulos DG, Izatt S, et al: Influence of exchange volume and dialysate flow rate on solute clearance in peritoneal dialysis. Kidney Int 14:486, 1978.

74. Goldschmidt ZH, Pote HH, Katz MA, Shear L: Effect of dialysate volume on peritoneal dialysis kinetics. Kidney Int 5:240, 1974.

75. Tenckhoff H, Ward G, Boen ST: The influence of dialysate volume and flow rate on peritoneal clearance. Proc Eur Dial Transplant Assoc 2:113, 1965.

75a. Nolph KD, Whitcomb ME, Schrier RW: Mechanisms for inefficient peritoneal dialysis in acute renal failure associated with heat stress and exercise. Ann Intern Med 71:317, 1969.

76. Elzouki A, Gruskin A, Prebis J, et al: Age-related changes in peritoneal dialysance. Proc Nat Kidney Fdn, 9th Annual Clinical Dialysis and Transplant Forum, November 16–19, 1979, p 37.

77. Balfe JW, Irwin MA, Oreopoulos DG: An assessment of continuous ambulatory peritoneal dialysis in children. In: CAPD Update, Moncrief JW, Popovich RP (Eds). New York, Masson Publishing, 1981, p 211.

78. Grodstein GP, Blumenkrantz J, Kopple JD, et al: Glucose absorption during CAPD. Kidney Int 19:564, 1981.

79. Gruskin A: Parenteral fluid therapy and treatment for electrolyte disorders in children and genitourinary disorders. In: Practice of Surgery-Urology, Kendall AR, Karafin L (Eds). Hagerstown, MD, Harper & Row Publishers, 1981.

80. Rubin J, Nolph KD, Popovich RP, et al: Drainage volumes during continuous ambulatory peritoneal dialysis. Trans Am Soc Artif Intern Organs 2(2):54, 1979.

81. Gruskin AB: Unpublished observation.

82. Bonomini V, Zucchelli P, Mioli V: Selective and unselective protein loss in peritoneal dialysis. Proc Eur Dial Transplant Assoc 4:146, 1967.

83. Baluarte HJ, Grossman M, Polinsky MS, et al: Home peritoneal dialysis in children: In: Pediatric Nephrology, Strauss J (Ed). Vol VII, In Press.

84. Baluarte HJ, Grossman MB, Polinsky MS, et al: Experience with intermittent home peritoneal dialysis (IHPD) in children. Pediatr Res 14:994, 1980.

85. Brouhard BH, Berger M, Cunningham RJ, et al: Home peritoneal dialysis in children. Trans Am Soc Artif Intern Organs 25:90, 1979.

86. Farrell PC, Schindhelm K, Roberts CG: Mass transfer characteristics of plasma filtration membranes. Trans Am Soc Artif Intern Organs 27:554, 1981.

87. Rubin J, McFarland S, Hellems EW, Bower JD: Peritoneal dialysis during peritonitis. Kidney Int 19:460, 1981.

88. Rubin J, Nolph K, Arfania D, et al: Follow-up of peritoneal clearances in patients undergoing continuous ambulatory peritoneal dialysis. Kidney Int 16:619, 1979.

89. Finkelstein FO, Kliger AS, Bastl C, Yap P: Sequential clearance and dialysance measurements in chronic peritoneal dialysis patients. Nephron 18:342, 1977.

90. Rubin J, Arfania D, Nolph KD, et al: Peritoneal clearances after 6–12 months on continuous ambulatory peritoneal dialysis. Trans Am Soc Artif Intern Organs 25:104, 1979.

91. Moncrief JW, Pyle WK, Simon P, Popovich RP: Hypertriglyceridemia, diabetes mellitus and insulin administration in patients undergoing continuous ambulatory peritoneal dialysis. In: CAPD Update, Moncrief JW, Popovich RP (Eds). New York, Masson Publishing, 1981, p 143.

92. Raja RM, Cantor RE, Boreyko C, et al: Sodium transport during ultrafiltration peritoneal dialysis. Trans Am Soc Artif Intern Organs 18:429, 1972.

93. Raja R, Kramer MS, Rosenbaum JL, et al: Evaluation of hypertonic peritoneal dialysis solutions with low sodium. Nephron 11:342, 1973

94. Brown ST, Ahearn DJ, Nolph KD: Potassium removal with peritoneal dialysis. Kidney Int 4:67, 1973.

95. Gross M, McDonald HP: Effect of dialysate temperature and flow rate on peritoneal clearance. JAMA 202:363, 1967.

96. Nolph KD, Rubin J, Wiegman DL, et al: Peritoneal clearances with three types of commercially available peritoneal dialysis solutions. Effects of pH adjustments and intraperitoneal nitroprusside. Nephron 24:35, 1979.

97. Maher JF: Pharmacologic manipulation of peritoneal transport. In: Peritoneal Dialysis Developments in Nephrology, Vol. 2. Nolph KD (Ed). The Hague, Martinus Nijhoff, 1981, p 213.

98. Miller FN, Wiegman DL, Joshua IG, et al: Effects of vasodilators and peritoneal dialysis solution on the microcirculation of the rat cecum. Proc Soc Exp Biol 161:695, 1979.

99. Mattocks AM: Accelerated removal of salicylate by additive in peritoneal dialysis fluid. J Pharm Sci 58:595, 1969.

100. Shinaberger JH, Shear L, Clayton LE, et al: Dialysis for intoxication with lipid soluble drugs: enhancement of glutethimide extraction with lipid dialysate. Trans Am Soc Artif Intern Organs 11:173, 1965.

100a. Cole DEC, Lirenman D: Role of albumin enriched peritoneal dialysate in acute copper poisoning. J Pediatr 92:955, 1978.

101. Blumenkrantz MJ, Ghal GM, Kopple JD, et al: Protein losses during peritoneal dialysis. Kidney Int 19:593, 1981.

102. DeSanto NG, Capodicasa G, Pluvio D, et al: Protein-energy requirements of children and adolescents on CAPD. Preliminary results of nitrogen balance studies. In: Developments in Nephrology, Vol. 3, Proc Fifth Int Ped Neph Symp, Gruskin AB, Norman ME (Eds). The Hague, Martinus Nijhoff, 1981, p 199.

103. DeSanto NG, Capodicasa G, DiLeo VA, et al: Kinetics of amino acid equilibration in the dialysate during CAPD. Int J Artif Intern Organs 4:23, 1981.

104. Girodano C, DeSanto NG, Capodicasa G, et al: Amino acid losses during CAPD. Clin Nephrol 14:230, 1980.

105. Stoltz ML, Nolph KD, Maher JF: Factors affecting calcium removal with calcium free peritoneal dialysis. J Lab Clin Med 78:389, 1971.

106. Parker A, Nolph KD: Magnesium and calcium

mass transfer during continuous ambulatory peritoneal dialysis. Trans Am Soc Artif Intern Organs 26:194, 1980.

107. Hamilton JW, Lasrich M, Hirszel P: Peritoneal dialysis in the treatment of severe hypercalcemia. J Dial 4(2, 3):129, 1980.

108. Rettig KR, DiGeorge AM, Rezvani I, et al: Peritoneal dialysis in the initial treatment of maple syrup urine disease (MSUD). Pediatr Res 9:354, 1975.

109. Batshaw ML, Brusilow SW: Treatment of hyperammonemic coma caused by inborn errors of urea synthesis. J Pediatr 97:893, 1980.

110. Francois B, Cornu G, deMeyer R: Peritoneal dialysis and exchange transfusion in a neonate with arginino-succinic aciduria. Arch Dis Child 51:228, 1976.

111. Wiegand C, Thompson T, Bock GH, et al: The management of life-threatening hyperammonemia: A comparison of several therapeutic modalities. J Pediatr 96:142, 1980.

112. Nash MA, Russo JL: Neonatal lactic acidosis and renal failure: the role of peritoneal dialysis. J Pediatr 91:101, 1977.

113. Miller NL, Finberg L: Peritoneal dialysis for salt poisoning. N Engl J Med 263:1347, 1960.

114. Nora JJ, Trygstad CW, Mangos JA, et al: Peritoneal dialysis in the treatment of intractable congestive heart failure of infancy and childhood. J. Pediatr 68:693, 1966.

115. Krebs R, Flynn M: Treatment of hepatic coma with exchange transfusion and peritoneal dialysis. JAMA 199:430, 1967.

116. Pross DC, Bradford WD, Krueger RP: Reye's syndrome treated by peritoneal dialysis. Pediatrics 45:845, 1970.

117. Boda D, Muryani L, Altorjay I, Veress I: Peritoneal dialysis in the treatment of hyaline membrane disease of the newborn premature infants. Acta Pediatr Scand 60:90, 1971.

118. Boda D: Demonstrations of the accumulation of metabolites in hypoxic conditions of premature infants: Therapeutical trials with peritoneal dialysis. Pediatr Res 1:111, 1967.

119. Gruskin AB, Baluarte HJ, Polinsky MS, et al: Usage of antibiotics in children with renal insufficiency. In: Pediatric Nephrology, Vol VI, Strauss J (Ed). New York, Plenum Press, 1981, p 391.

120. Hiner LB, Baluarte HJ, Polinsky MS, Gruskin AB: Cefazolin in children with renal insufficiency. J Pediatr 96:335, 1980.

121. Cutler RE, Christopher TE: Drug therapy during renal insufficiency and dialytic treatment. In: Clinical Aspects of Uremia and Dialysis, Massry SG, Sellers AL (Eds). Springfield, Illinois, Charles C Thomas, 1976, p 427.

122. Anderson RJ, Bennett WM, Gambertoglio JG, Schrier RW: Fate of drugs in renal failure. In: The Kidney, Brenner BM, Rector FC Jr (Eds), Vol. II. Philadelphia, WB Saunders, 1981, p 2659.

123. Jusko WJ, Baliah T, Kim KH, et al: Pharmacokinetics of gentamicin during peritoneal dialysis in children. Kidney Int 9:430, 1976.

# 11

# Intermittent Peritoneal Dialysis: Technical and Clinical Aspects

*H. Jorge Baluarte, M.D.*

Intermittent peritoneal dialysis (IPD) is the oldest form of peritoneal dialysis used chronically to replace kidney function. This chapter will review the development of IPD as a therapeutic modality for children, consider pertinent technical aspects of manual automated IPD, and conclude by comparing our clinical experience with that of other centers and with the newer technique of continuous ambulatory peritoneal dialysis (CAPD).

## HISTORICAL REVIEW

Significant historic events related to peritoneal dialysis (Table 11–1) start as early as 1923 with Ganter[1] who was the first to describe the use of the peritoneal membrane in a human to remove uremic substances. During the three decades following the report of Ganter, peritoneal dialysis was widely used, but doubts about its efficacy existed because of insufficient knowledge of peritoneal clearances and the inflow volume to be used. Maxwell et al in 1959[2] first described their technique of inserting a catheter into the peritoneum through a large trocar which permitted the infusion of commercial dialysis solution. The development of the Teflon Silastic external fistula for hemodialysis in 1960,[3] followed by the rapid technologic advances, the proliferation of treatment facilities, and the successful employment of renal homotransplantation, relegated peritoneal dialysis to a secondary role. Boen in 1964[4] described the first closed system for peritoneal dialysis, which solved one of the two major problems posed by long-term peritoneal dialysis. Tenckhoff and Schechter[5] modified the permanent implanted Silastic catheter described by Palmer,[6] reducing the repeated access to the peritoneal cavity. Finally, the development in 1970 of automated equipment, to be used in conjunction with the permanent peritoneal catheter, enabled IPD to develop as a realistic therapeutic alternative.

Although neither peritoneal dialysis nor hemodialysis is optimal in the treatment of children with end stage renal disease (ESRD),[7] renewed interest in chronic peritoneal dialysis has developed partly as a result of the difficulties encountered with long-term hemodialysis. Programs of infrequent peritoneal dialysis in children were reported with limited success.[8, 9] The first chronic home peritoneal dialysis program for children in the United States was started in Seattle in 1968.[10] Several other centers have subsequently described limited experience with hospital[11, 12] or home peritoneal dialysis.[13–15] In 1976 Moncrief and Popovich[16] described CAPD, which has had a significant impact in the treatment of irreversible renal failure and further stimulated the interest in peritoneal dialysis. These technical improvements have occurred concurrently with increased government support for chronic dialysis. Increasing numbers of pediatric dialysis programs are treating uremic children with CAPD.[17–20] The ESRD program at St. Christoper's Hospital for Children currently offers two modalities of home peritoneal dialysis: IPD (cycler) and CAPD.

**Table 11-1.** HISTORY OF PERITONEAL DIALYSIS (PD)

| | | |
|---|---|---|
| 1923 | Ganter[1] | Use of peritoneal lavage in man to remove uremic substances |
| 1950's | | PD used for acute or chronic renal failure |
| 1959 | Maxwell[2] | Commercial dialysis solution and tubing led to widespread use of PD |
| 1964 | Boen[4] | Closed system dialysis cycler |
| 1965 | | Advent of stylet catheters |
| 1968 | Tenckhoff[5] | Permanent PD catheters |
| 1970 | | Automated PD equipment |
| 1970's, 1980's | | Pediatric centers for IPD |
| 1976 | Moncrief[16] | Continuous ambulatory peritoneal dialysis (CAPD) |
| 1978 | | FDA approval of plastic bags used in CAPD |
| 1979 | | Medicare approval for use of CAPD for patients with ESRD |

## METHODS OF PERITONEAL DIALYSIS

### Manual Method

Conventional IPD is well accepted as a treatment for both adults and children with acute renal failure.[4, 21, 22] This technique is simple, requires minimal equipment, can be performed in the most remote hospital on an emergency basis, and can be used to chemically sustain children, if necessary.

**Technique.**[9, 23, 24] The technique for manual peritoneal dialysis is as follows:

1. From 30 to 60 minutes before inserting the catheter sedation is established with meperidine HCl 2 mg/kg, promethazine HCl 1–2 mg/kg, and chlorpromazine 1 mg/kg.

2. Empty bladder: have patient void, or catheterize the bladder with a No. 5 or No. 8 feeding tube.

3. Keep the dialysis solution (bottles or plastic bags) warmed to 37° to 38° C in a water bath. The administration set should be attached to the bottle(s) and the tubing must be completely cleared of air bubbles so as to minimize the occurrence of an air lock and loss of siphon effect.

4. The preferred site for the insertion of the catheter is along the linea alba at a point approximately one third of the way from the umbilicus to the symphysis.

5. Using sterile technique, anesthetize the skin and subcutaneous tissue with a local anesthetic at the proposed site of the insertion of the peritoneal catheter.

6. If ascites is not present infuse 25 ml/kg of dialysis solution via a 16- or 18-gauge lumbar puncture needle (or a soft angiocath) into the peritoneal cavity prior to insertion of the catheter. The purpose of this is to distend the anterior abdominal wall and minimize the possibility of accidental perforation of bowel or a major blood vessel.

7. Two types of catheters can be used: stiff (Trocath peritoneal dialysis catheter, McGaw Laboratories, Inc., Irvine Calfornia) or soft.[5] The stylet catheter is then inserted through the same tract made by the lumbar puncture needle. Be sure that the catheter perforations have been advanced completely into the peritoneal cavity so as to avoid subcutaneous fluid infiltration of the abdominal wall. After the stylet has been partially withdrawn, the tip of the catheter is directed gently into the right or left pelvic gutter. The main disadvantage of this catheter is the repeated insertion needed for each dialysis, which is uncomfortable, sometimes painful, and usually frightening to the patient. Often one is tempted to leave stiff catheters in place for subsequent dialysis, but prolonged dialysis with a single stiff catheter is associated with a high risk of peritonitis. The duration of dialysis in most instances should not exceed 48 hours before the catheter is removed. Stiff catheters frequently cause discomfort, make mobilization of the patient difficult, and often require manipulation or repositioning to maintain adequate abdominal drainage. With the aid of the Deane method[25] a conventional stylet catheter is employed for initiation of dialysis. When the catheter is removed, a prosthesis consisting of a Teflon rod fused to a retainer disc is inserted into the sinus tract. For subsequent dialysis the prosthesis is removed and a new stylet catheter is inserted.

The Tenckhoff catheter used for acute dialysis has a single felt cuff, placed subcutaneously below the catheter exit site, which is somewhat easier to insert and remove than the two-cuff catheters used for chronic dialysis.

8. The initial dialysate bottles should be prepared with appropriate additives. Heparin (1000 units/L) is added to the first set of bottles. When the fluid drained from the peritoneal cavity ceases to be bloody, heparin may be discontinued. Potassium chloride should be added to the bottles according to the predialysis blood concentration. When the serum potassium is more than 6 mEq/L or there are signs of potassium toxicity, potassium should be omitted from the dialysis for the first eight to ten exchanges. Once the serum potassium has fallen to the normal range, potassium should not be omitted from the dialysate for an extended period of time or potassium depletion may develop. If the serum potassium concentration is 4 to 6 mEq/L, KCl should be added at a concentration of 2 mEq/L for the first ten exchanges, and 4 mEq/L subsequently.

9. The selection of glucose concentration (1.5%, 2.5%, 4.25%) depends on the state of fluid balance of the patient. In most instances these concentrations are satisfactorily tolerated; but in the event that marked hyperglycemia occurs (>200 mg/dl), short-acting insulin (regular), 0.1–0.2 u/kg, should be given intravenously.

10. Dialysis cycle:

a. *Inflow*, the dialysis solution (40 to 50 ml/kg, up to 2 liters) is allowed to run in rapidly, over a period of 5 to 10 minutes. It is important that the inflow be stopped and the tubing clamped before the drip chamber completely empties of solution to avoid the trapping of air in the tubing with the consequent loss of the siphon effect.

b. *Equilibration (dwell)*, the dialysis fluid should be allowed to equilibrate for 20 to 30 minutes before beginning the outflow phase. Although equilibration at 30 minutes is less than complete,[26] the bulk of exchange-diffusion occurs during this time, and the most efficient dialysis results from exploiting this fact.[23]

c. *Outflow*, dialysis fluid is allowed to drain "wide open" over 10 to 15 minutes. With each cycle the peritoneal cavity should be drained completely. This may require repositioning of the patient.

11. Accurate cumulative records of fluid balance must be kept. The first exchange is often partially absorbed. If a progressive positive balance develops, a solution with higher dextrose concentration may be used. If an excessive negative balance develops, the abdominal cavity should still be drained completely each cycle. Replacement of the deficit may be given by mouth or by the intravenous administration of a solution similar in composition to Ringer's lactate, depending upon the condition of the patient and the state of fluid and electrolyte balance.

12. Vital signs: temperature, pulse and blood pressure should be recorded at the end of each exchange (or more often if needed) and the patient's weight should always be obtained in a uniform fashion two to three times a day.

13. The dialysis fluid should be cultured at least twice daily by aspirating outflow fluid via the side-arm injection site into a sterile plastic syringe. To avoid problems indicate on the laboratory slip the time and the number of the particular exchange during which the culture was obtained. Whenever cloudy fluid appears, or undue abdominal pain or fever develops, obtain blood and dialysate fluid cultures immediately and begin administration of antibiotics systemically and/or intraperitoneally.

14. Laboratory monitoring: CBC, BUN, serum creatinine, potassium, sodium, total $CO_2$, glucose, and total protein levels should be obtained prior to and at the end of dialysis to assess therapy and to prevent complications. Manual peritoneal dialysis is usually recommended for the treatment of acute renal failure, whether it is performed with a stiff catheter and multiple punctures, the Deane prosthesis, or the Tenckhoff catheter. If the patient requires prolonged dialysis (more than four weeks), the family and patient should be systematically introduced or referred (if a program is not available at local facility) to the appropriate pediatric medical center.

## Automated Systems

Although intermittent manual peritoneal dialysis, as discussed above, can be used as an alternative form of chronic peritoneal dialysis,[9] automated systems of dialysis are more convenient and efficient.[26] Currently, there are two major types of automated peritoneal dialysis machines used in the United States, the Lasker automatic peritoneal cycler[27, 28] and the reverse osmosis (RO) machine designed by Tenckhoff.[29]

**Cycler Dialysis.** The cycling device (AMP 80/2 peritoneal dialysis system, American Medical Products Corporation, Freehold,

New Jersey) utilizes premixed commercially available dialysis solution bottles, which are suspended from an eight-pronged hanger at the top of the adjustable central pole (Fig. 11–1). The peritoneal cycler has two time controls on its front: one determines the duration of the "fill-dwell cycle" (time for the inflow and equilibration) and the other the duration of the "drain cycle" (time for outflow). One side of the cycler has a special metal bar with four holders that accept an equal number of tubes. Two motor-driven T-shaped plungers control the dialysate flow by pressing and releasing the four tubes in pairs. On the other side of the cycler, a counterbalanced scale monitors the volume of fluid draining from the peritoneal cavity. Disposable equipment used in performing each dialysis includes special tubing which has an eight-pronged connector, a weighing bag that is hung from the side scale, and a heater bag (Fig. 11–2).

The heater cabinet performs two functions, temperature control and fluid volume control. The inflow volume is determined by the distance between the heater plates inside the heater cabinet and ranges from 1000 to

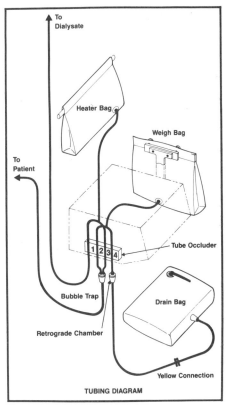

**Figure 11–2.** Tubing diagram of the AMP 80/2 cycler. (Reproduced from Service Manual.)

2000 cc in the standard model or 250 to 750 cc in the pediatric model. The dialysis fluid leaves the bottles or plastic containers, which partially empty simultaneously, and fills the heater bag (tube 1). The fluid stays in the heater bag for a period preset by the drain timer and is warmed to body temperature.

From the heater bag, the fluid empties into the peritoneal cavity (tube 3), where it stays for a period controlled by the fill-dwell timer. At the end of this period, the fluid drains out into the weighing bag (tube 2), which sounds an alarm (patient drain alarm) and stops the dialysis if the patient has not drained 75% of the preset volume in 75% of the preset drain time. From the weighing bag the fluid drains into the final drainage set (tube 4) and an alarm (system drain alarm) will go off if the weigh bag has not drained in 75% of the preset fill-dwell time.

During the "fill-dwell cycle" the two tubes that are open allow warm dialysate to run into the peritoneal cavity from the heater bag (tube 3) and from the weighing bag into the drainage bag (tube 4). During this time, tubes 1 and 2 are closed. At the end of the drain cycle, tubes 3 and 4 will be closed and tubes

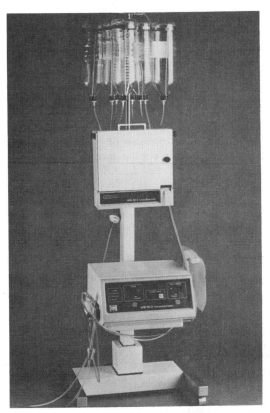

**Figure 11–1.** The AMP 80/2 peritoneal dialysis system. (Reproduced from Service Manual.)

1 and 2 will open, allowing fluid to run from the containers into the heater bag (tube 1) and from the patient into the weighing bag (tube 2) (Fig. 11–2).

To commence dialysis, the Beta-cap II obturator is removed from the permanently placed peritoneal catheter and discarded. The catheter is then connected to the dialysis tubing with strict aseptic technique. The patient, parent, or helper wears a mask and, after a thorough hand scrubbing, puts on sterile gloves. Following removal of the cover Air Strip and gauze, the exit site is carefully scrubbed with Betadine solution (Fig. 11–3). The entire area except for the cleaned catheter is covered by a fenestrated drape.

At the completion of dialysis, again using aseptic technique, the patient line is disconnected from the catheter. Then the Beta-cap II adapter is filled with Betadine solution, and a new obturator is secured in place.

The cycler is operated by gravity and retains the simplicity of the manual peritoneal dialysis technique. After surgical implantation of the Tenckhoff catheter, the patient, parent, or helper can begin the home training program, which is usually accomplished in 10 to 12 dialysis days. Satisfactory dialysis is generally achieved with an exchange volume of 40 to 50 ml/kg (maximum 2 liters) and short dialysis cycles of about 30 minutes each with 20 minutes for filling and dwelling and 10 minutes for drainage. The exchange volume is usually determined by the weight of the patient, but the appropriate amount will depend on the patient's tolerance of the calculated volume, and the volume range of the cycler model in use. Each dialysis treatment lasts 10 to 14 hours and is done three to four times a week. Home peritoneal dialysis using the cycler is usually performed at night while the patient is asleep and unattended. Performing dialysis in this fashion offsets the major disadvantage of the long dialysis time required to perform IPD.

The AMP peritoneal dialysis system was originally designed to provide IPD. Recently, with minor modifications, this system has been used to provide continuous cycling peritoneal dialysis (CCPD). This dialysis method utilizes the medical advantage of longer dwells combined with the convenience of machine delivery. As the name implies, the treatment is on a continuous 24-hour basis lasting five to seven days per week and offers an alternative to CAPD. Automated cycles of three to four hours are performed at night

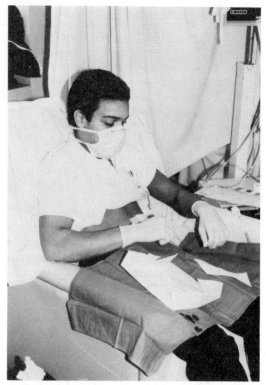

**Figure 11–3.** Patient performing catheter care.

by the cycler. After the last exchange the peritoneal cavity is allowed to fill for a long dwell and the catheter is disconnected. The process is started again in the evening.

**Reverse Osmosis Machine.** This type of automated peritoneal dialysis equipment sterilizes and deionizes tap water by passage through a reverse osmosis (RO) membrane. If the tap water has a high content of impurities and/or calcium, it is unsuitable for direct use and has to be pretreated with a deionizer or other appropriate filters. The integrity of the RO membrane is monitored by comparing the conductivity of the water before and after passage through the membrane. Two automated peritoneal dialysis machines are presently commercially available: one is manufactured by Drake-Willock Co., Portland, Oregon, and the other by Physio-Control Corporation, Redmond, Washington (Fig. 11–4).

Beyond the RO membrane, the water (sterile and deionized) is passed over long tubes of ultraviolet (UV) light, which provide "back-up" sterilization. The water is then warmed to body temperature and mixed with concentrated peritoneal dialysate in a ratio of 10 to 1 by proportioning pumps. The dialysate concentrate is available in two dif-

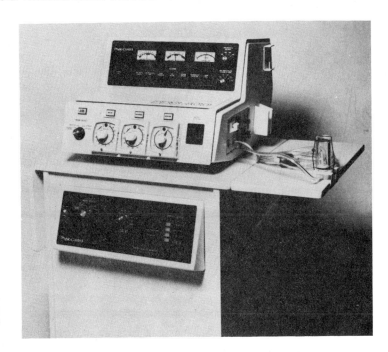

**Figure 11–4.** Peritoneal dialysis system manufactured by Physio-Control (PDS 400). (Reproduced from Service Manual.)

ferent dextrose concentrations, providing a final concentration of 1.5% or 2.5%. In the event that additional dextrose is required, it can be pumped into the final dialysate through extra tubing connected to a 50% dextrose container. The solution is pumped into the peritoneal cavity through a permanently placed catheter at a flow rate of 200 or 400 ml/min. Three timers at the front of the machine control the infusion time, dwell time, and drain time. Drainage is passive to a sump tank and from there to the floor drain.

Once a week the machine is sterilized, being filled with 30% formaldehyde solution for 2 1/2 hours, then rinsed twice with tap water and tested with Clinitest tablets to ensure that the formaldehyde has been removed. The integrity of the RO membrane is tested monthly by use of a dye.

### Comparison of Automated Systems of Dialysis

The peritoneal cycler is simple, noiseless, easy to operate, small, and mobile. Recent modifications in the heater cabinet of the cycler have overcome the serious complication of overheating of the dialysis fluid. The greater range of the inflow volume from 2000 ml down to 250 ml has allowed the application of this mode of IPD to small children. The initial cost of the cycler is low, but its yearly operating costs are high, mainly owing to the cost of premixed dialysate and the special disposable tubing required for its operation.

The RO machine is complex and only a limited fraction (40 to 50%) of patients can master its operation.[30] The device cannot be moved, so, for example, a patient who wishes to use the bathroom during dialysis must use a bedside commode. Offsetting these disadvantages is the annual operating cost, which is two to three thousand dollars less than that of the cycler.

### PERMANENT PERITONEAL CATHETERS AND CONNECTING DEVICES

The introduction of a permanent catheter by Tenckhoff[5] eliminated the need for repeated peritoneal puncture for each dialysis, thus reducing the risk of bowel perforation and permitting relatively infection-free long-term access to the peritoneum.[31] Until recently most indwelling peritoneal catheters have been inserted with two attached cuffs (Fig. 11–5). Tissue grows into the cuffs and acts as a barrier to prevent bacterial movement along the catheter tract.

The Tenckhoff catheter is commercially available from several manufacturing companies and it has been subjected to various modifications. Catheters are available in var-

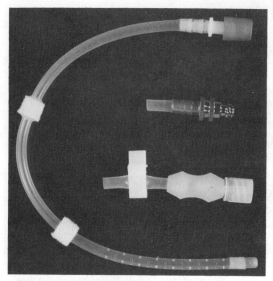

**Figure 11–5.** Tenckhoff's double-cuffed catheter and connecting devices (titanium adapter and Beta-cap system).

ious lengths: adult size (42 cm), pediatric (27 cm), and neonatal (21 cm). The standard catheter is clear. Impregnation with barium sulfate (shadow cath or shadow stripe by Quinton Instrument Co.) makes the catheter radiopaque and easy to localize radiographically. At our hospital, we use the adult catheter for all children except neonates, in whom we prefer to use the neonatal catheter. The catheter is trimmed to the desired length by the surgeon at the time of implantation. We prefer a custom-made catheter with one loose cuff which is cemented in the appropriate place for the patient's size prior to surgical insertion. This single-cuff catheter avoids the complication of distal cuff extrusion from the exit site and subsequent infection.

Available modifications of the Tenckhoff catheter include a Silastic catheter with an inflatable saline-filled balloon at the end[32] or the addition to the end of the catheter of two plastic discs.[33, 34] The purpose of these modifications is to prevent the omentum from occluding the drainage holes and prevent catheter tip displacement. The Tenckhoff catheter insertion technique is discussed elsewhere in this text (Chap. 9 by Sherman and Atkinson).

Proper connection and disconnection techniques should decrease or eliminate infectious complications from chronic peritoneal dialysis. The standard adapter and rubber cap used to close the Tenckhoff catheter at

the completion of IPD has been replaced in the majority of centers by the Beta-cap.[35] The Beta-cap is a new system consisting of an adapter which is permanently fixed to the end of the catheter, a cap which is designed as a reservoir for povidone-iodine, a clamp, and a finger grip (Fig. 11–5). This system is a useful advance because it allows for a shorter connection time and lower infection rate.[35] Iodine toxicity has been a matter of concern with the use of the Beta-cap system, although recent data[36] have failed to show any clinical relevance. The titanium adapter (Fig. 11–5) is a metal device used primarily by patients on CAPD, but it can also be used temporarily in patients undergoing IPD.

## Catheter Complications

Problems related to catheter malfunction are considerably more common in centers which have recently initiated a peritoneal dialysis program and with a staff inexperienced with its use.

**Leakage.** If leakage at the catheter exit site occurs during the initial cycle performed in the operating room, it should be surgically corrected, thus reducing the need for repeated catheter insertion. A leak noted on return to the ward is usually corrected by using smaller volumes of dialysate, although sometimes it is necessary to stop dialysis for up to 72 hours to allow the development of a tissue seal around the cuff. The risk of external leakage is high in patients who have had previous abdominal surgery for multiple catheter insertions[24, 37–39] and in debilitated patients who have lax abdominal walls. Fluid may dissect into the abdominal wall as a result of tears in the peritoneum or the infusion of dialysate into the potential space between the layers of abdominal wall. This dissection of fluid may spread to the scrotum or labia, thighs, or up to the chest wall, causing some discomfort and necessitating discontinuation of dialysis in order to give any peritoneal tear time to heal. Such patients may need hemodialysis for a few days through an acute subclavian vascular access,[40] unless a chronic vascular access is available. Uncommonly, dialysate enters the pleural cavity[41–45] through a congenital defect in the diaphragm. In such cases of acute hydrothorax, peritoneal dialysis is usually discontinued and the patients switched to hemodialysis therapy.

**Obstruction.** Outflow obstruction is a frequent complication and has multiple causes. Fibrin or blood clots may be trapped in the catheter and block the terminal holes, especially when dialysis is complicated by peritonitis or significant hemorrhage. Large amounts of heparin (2500–5000 units) in a small volume of dialysis solution is used to irrigate the catheter in an attempt to expel the fibrin or clot. Mechanical manipulations using an obturator may be employed in certain cases, but extreme caution must be taken to prevent perforation of the catheter and possible injury to the bowel. Passage of a Fogarty catheter is often successful in removing fibrin or blood clots and is generally considered to be a safer method of manipulation. If poor drainage still persists, the surgeon should insert a new catheter. Inadequate drainage due to loss of the siphon effect is more of a problem with acute dialysis, and the air bubbles can be expelled from the system by running in a small amount of dialysate.

Catheter tip displacement is a common cause of catheter malfunction, especially when the surgeon does not appreciate the importance of placing the catheter in the desired caudal direction. Constipation may be associated with dialysate inflow problems and it may also contribute to catheter tip displacement. Effective evacuation of the bowel may help the catheter to return to its original position. Posturing sometimes helps to correct catheter displacement, but usually the patient needs to return to the operating room. Catheter displacement can also be minimized by using the Toronto Western catheter,[33, 34] and in recurrent cases of this problem the tip of the catheter should be sutured with nonabsorbable sutures to the pelvic peritoneum.[39]

Combined inflow-outflow obstruction is due to entrapment of omental tissue in the catheter lumen and usually develops within a few days of implantation. The patient may experience localized or diffuse abdominal discomfort. Injection of contrast material during a peritoneogram may show the displaced catheter and the internal obstruction as one or multiple round shadows within the lumen.[46] Temporary success may occasionally be achieved by the use of the "Italian corkscrew."[47] Catheter replacement is eventually necessary if an attempt to reposition the catheter proves ineffective. A partial omentectomy may be helpful when this is a recurrent problem. Intra-abdominal adhesions or fibrosis around the catheter tip produces loculation of fluid, increased resistance to dialysate inflow, and abdominal pain. The performance of a peritoneogram with contrast material will make this diagnosis. Surgical intervention with lysis of adhesions may solve the problem.

Deep pelvic pain, usually felt during the inflow phase, is an early complication experienced by a few patients and is presumably caused by the catheter's pressing on bowel or peritoneum. It often improves after the patient has a bowel movement. The use of the Fogarty catheter for repositioning of the tip is advised before an exploratory laparotomy is considered.

**Dacron Cuff Extrusion.** Cuff extrusion is usually a late complication when the placement of the cuff has been too close to the skin at the exit site. It is usually an indolent process unless accompanied by an exit site infection or subcutaneous tunnel abscess. If the cuff extrusion is not complete, surgical exposure will be necessary with subsequent "shaving" of the cuff to prevent further maceration of the skin and the development of a tunnel infection.

Other complications observed in children include unilateral or bilateral hydroceles due to dialysate accumulation, necessitating the ligation of a patent processus vaginalis. Abdominal hernias (inguinal, periumbilical, and incisional) become more prominent and symptomatic owing to the increased intra-abdominal pressure from the dialysis fluid, and require elective surgical correction. The infusion of contrast materal and performance of a peritoneogram at the time of the initial insertion of a catheter will enable the surgeon to identify and correct any hernias at the same time.[48]

## DIALYSIS SOLUTIONS

Maxwell et al[2] in 1959 introduced the use of commercially prepared solutions, which encouraged the widespread use of peritoneal dialysis. The composition of three commercially available dialysis solutions is tabulated in Table 11–2. Automatic peritoneal dialysis systems mix RO purified and sterilized water with a concentrated dialysate solution, so that the final solution is similar in electrolyte composition to that used for manual dialysis.

**Table 11–2.** COMPOSITION OF DIALYSATE SOLUTION

|  | McGaw | Dianeal 137 (Travenol) | Inpersol (Abbott) |
|---|---|---|---|
| Glucose (gm/L) | 15 | 15 | 15 |
| Sodium (mEq/L) | 141 | 132 | 132 |
| Calcium (mEq/L) | 4.0 | 3.5 | 3.5 |
| Magnesium (mEq/L) | 1.5 | 1.5 | 1.5 |
| Chloride (mEq/L) | 103 | 102 | 102 |
| Potassium (mEq/L) | — | — | — |
| Lactate (mEq/L) | — | 35 | 35 |
| Acetate (mEq/L) | 45 | — | — |
| Bisulfate (mEq/L) | 1 | 1 | 2.9 |
| Osmolality (mOsm/kg $H_2O$) | 353 | 347 | 347 |
| pH | 5.8 | 5.5 | 5.2 |

Dialysate sodium concentration affects the amount of sodium removed as well as the ultimate serum sodium level. When dialysis is performed in patients with hypernatremia, it is recommended to use dialysate solution with a sodium concentration of 130 mEq/L, instead of the customary 140 mEq/L.[49, 50]

The rate and amount of water removed from the patient depends upon the osmotic pressure generated by the dextrose. Solutions with 1.5%, 2.5% and 4.25% are commonly available. They can be mixed or alternated to obtain the desired effect. Solutions containing 7% dextrose are no longer available because their misuse has led to rapid volume reduction with hypovolemia, hypernatremia, hyperglycemia, abdominal pain due to peritoneal irritation, and hyperosmolar coma.[51] The shorter the dwell time, the greater the amount of free water removed per minute. Prolonging the time the dialysate remains in the abdomen will increase solute removal until osmotic and diffusive equilibriums have been reached after 2 to 4 hours. Dialysate does not contain sodium bicarbonate because it is unstable. Base is provided by alkalinizing substances like acetate or lactate. Acetate appears to have an advantage over lactate because it seems to be bacteriostatic.[52]

The provision of a dialysate with a lower magnesium concentration may achieve greater magnesium removal and prevent or delay hypermagnesemia.[30] A potassium-free dialysate is used in the dialysis of most renal failure patients because the peritoneal membrane clears potassium slowly[53] and severe dietary potassium restriction is difficult to achieve.

## CLINICAL EXPERIENCE WITH IPD

Because of the limited number of reports on IPD in children, our clinical experience with IPD will be reviewed and compared to that available from other pediatric centers. Our experience can be viewed as being typical for children undergoing IPD.

## Patients and Methods

We have treated 24 children (Table 11–3), 12 boys and 12 girls, ranging in age from 1.7 to 17.3 years at the onset of dialysis (mean age 10.5 years), with maintenance cycler IPD from 2 to 62 months (mean duration of dialysis 13 months).[15, 20, 54] Seventeen patients were initially treated with cycler IPD. Prior to starting IPD 6 patients were on hemodialysis from 2 weeks to 12 months and one patient was on CAPD for 11 months. Indications for starting IPD included the distance from the dialysis unit (12 patients), preference by the family or the medical staff (8 patients), lack of adequate vascular access because of the small size of the patient (2 patients) or the duration of time on hemodialysis (3 patients). Inadequate ultrafiltration on CAPD was the deciding factor for considering IPD in one patient.

Access to the peritoneal cavity between 1977 and 1981 was established by surgical implantation of a double dacron cuff Tenckhoff catheter. Because of frequent episodes of cuff extrusion we switched to a single dacron cuff catheter in 1981. After catheter function was assured, the parents and patient began their home training, which was accomplished in 10 to 12 dialysis days. Commercially available dialysate supplied in 2-liter bottles was used (McGaw, Irvine, California). Initially, dialysis was performed with an automatic peritoneal cycler LJ300 Series II; subsequently the AMP 80/2 was used (American Medical Products Corp., Freehold, New Jersey). Each dialysis treatment lasted an average of 10 to 12 hours, for a total of 30 to

**Table 11–3. CLINICAL DATA**

| Patient | Age (yr) | Sex | Diagnosis | Duration of IPD (mos) | Previous ESRD Therapy | Urine output | Residual GFR (ml/min/1.73 m²) | Outcome of Dialysis |
|---|---|---|---|---|---|---|---|---|
| 1 (AW) | 6 | F | WT | 62 | HD | 0 | Anephric | Expired |
| 2 (SW) | 5 | F | CGN | 22 | None | 0 | 0 | TR(C) |
| 3 (MS) | 10.5 | M | RPGN | 8 | None | | Anephric | TR(C) |
| 4 (SW) | 9 | F | CGN | 3.5 | None | <100 | 0 | TR(LR) |
| 5 (SM) | 12.6 | M | N | 14 | None | 1600 | 6.2 | CAPD |
| 6 (PD) | 9.5 | F | D | 5 | HD | 0 | Anephric | TR/Expired |
| 7 (WB) | 10.7 | F | CGN | 9 | None | 600 | 3.1 | TR(LR) |
| 8 (MK) | 13 | F | CP | 28 | HD | 1800 | 6.0 | TR(C) |
| 9 (LM) | 13.3 | F | D/CP | 3 | HD | 0 | Anephric | TR(LR) IPD |
| 10 (RB) | 7.6 | M | MPGN | 23 | None | 750 | 4.6 | HD |
| 11 (TR) | 11.7 | M | D/CP | 29 | None | 350 | — | IPD |
| 12 (MM) | 9.4 | F | D | 15 | None | <100 | — | TR(C) |
| 13 (JS) | 10.1 | M | CGN | 20 | None | <100 | 0 | TR(LR) |
| 14 (JM) | 2 | M | WT | 3 | None | | — | IPD |
| 15 (DH) | 10.1 | F | CGN | 13 | HD | 300 | 0 | CAPD TR(C) |
| 16 (TL) | 11.7 | M | CY | 9 | None | 0 | 0 | IPD |
| 17 (DL) | 17.3 | M | CGN | 4 | None | 0 | 0 | CAPD TR(LR) |
| 18 (MZ) | 7.8 | M | D | 2 | None | <100 | — | TR(LR) |
| 19 (NS) | 15 | M | D | 11 | HD | <100 | — | TR(LR) IPD Expired |
| 20 (PF) | 9 | F | HUS | 8 | None | 0 | Anephric | TR(C) |
| 21 (SS) | 14.6 | M | AS | 4 | None | 1450 | 3.0 | TR(C) |
| 22 (KL) | 17.3 | F | CGN | 5 | None | 600 | 2.1 | IPD |
| 23 (KH) | 17.1 | M | CGN | 7 | None | 1400 | 4.1 | IPD |
| 24 (CB) | 1.7 | F | HUS | 5 | CAPD | 0 | 0 | IPD |

Code: CGN = Chronic glomerulonephritis
RPGN = Rapidly progressive glomerulonephritis
N = Nephronophthisis
D = Dysplasia
MPGN = Membranoproliferative glomerulonephritis
CY = Cystinosis
WT = Wilms' tumor
HUS = Hemolytic uremic syndrome
AS = Alport's syndrome

HD = Hemodialysis
TR = Transplant
C = Cadaver
LR = Live related
IPD = Intermittent peritoneal dialysis
CAPD = Continuous ambulatory peritoneal dialysis
CP = Chronic pyelonephritis
GFR = Glomerular filtration rate

40 hours per week. Patient 24 (CB) underwent daily overnight dialysis. An exchange volume of 40 to 50 ml/kg (maximum 2 liters) was used with an inflow and dwell time of 20 minutes and an outflow time of 10 minutes. The daily urine output in 9 patients ranged between 300 and 1800 ml and their residual GFR ranged between 2.1 and 6.2 ml/min/1.73 $m^2$. The remaining patients were anephric or had a urinary output of less than 100 ml/day. A "dry weight" was estimated during the period of training and all the patients were encouraged to attain this weight after each dialysis. Variable dextrose concentrations (1.5% to 4.25%) were used, depending on the amount of fluid to be removed. All patients were instructed in a basic high protein (2 to 3 gm/kg), low sodium (800 to 2000 mg), low potassium (1500 mg), and low phosphate (400 to 800 mg) diet, which was modified on the basis of individual needs and degree of residual renal function. The fluid limit prescribed depended upon the existence of hypertension and the urine output. Laboratory studies were obtained at monthly intervals during clinic visits, and blood transfusions were arranged at local hospitals or at our dialysis center. Back-up hemodialysis and in-center peritoneal dialysis was provided as needed.

## Long-term Results of IPD

Children maintained on IPD encountered many of the medical problems seen in children maintained on hemodialysis: growth failure, malnutrition, hypertension, anemia, and bone disease.

**Growth.** Linear growth was evaluated in 9 patients who had a bone age less than 12 years and who were dialyzed longer than 12 months, an age and time period adequate for assessment using the whole-year growth velocity standards for height.[55] Their linear growth rate ranged from 0.09 to 0.98 cm/month with a mean growth rate of 0.32 cm/month. Similar linear growth rates were observed in Seattle (0.31 cm/month)[10] and San Francisco (0.35 cm/month).[56] The group in Galveston[14] reported that the linear growth analyzed in 7 patients on dialysis for more than 6 months averaged 37% of that expected.

**Protein.** The mean serum protein level was 6.10 gm/dl and the serum albumin was 3.65 gm/dl. Protein losses in the dialysate in the San Francisco series ranged from 0.27 to 0.47 gm/kg per treatment.[56] Protein concentration in the dialysate is greatest in the first cycle, dropping rapidly in the next three to four cycles, followed by stable low levels throughout the rest of the dialysis.[57] Protein losses are constant as long as the dialysis technique is constant. A steady state of serum protein is reached by increased synthesis and decreased catabolism, and the patient is free of peritonitis.

**Hypertension and Volume Status.** Hypertension is usually a manifestation of fluid overload and thus inadequate dialysis. The "dry weight" representing a state of euvolemia was determined for all patients during the course of their home training period. Their actual weights fluctuated from 0 to 12.5% above their dry weight, requiring various combinations of dextrose concentration and/or additional treatments, depending on the amount of fluid to be removed. Hypertension, defined as diastolic pressures exceeding 95% confidence limits, was present in 19 of the 24 patients prior to maintenance IPD; 4 became normotensive and antihypertensive medications were discontinued; 4 became normotensive with antihypertensive therapy; 8 were better controlled and 3 required bilateral nephrectomy. Blood pressure was satisfactorily controlled in 58% of the hypertensive patients. Nephrectomy for renin-dependent hypertension will improve the patient's well-being and eliminate the need for antihypertensive medications; however, nephrectomy should not be lightly undertaken since preservation of residual renal function and renal mass per se is desirable. Nephrectomy is likely to be associated with a more rapid evolution of bone disease, worsening of the anemia,[10] and the need for a more severe fluid restriction.

**Anemia.** All patients had hypoproliferative anemia, and blood transfusions with leukocyte-poor packed red cells were given to maintain their hematocrits above 18% or when symptoms developed. The average interval between blood transfusions was 6.8 weeks, which is longer than that observed in children on maintenance hemodialysis in our unit.

**Calcium, Phosphorus, and Renal Osteodystrophy.** Bone disease remains a significant problem in children maintained on IPD, despite adequate control of the serum calcium and phosphorus levels with the use of calcium supplements, phosphate binders, and vitamin

D therapy.[10, 14, 56] The mean value for serum calcium was 8.9 mg/dl, for serum phosphorus 5.0 mg/dl, and for alkaline phosphatase 340 IU. Serum parathyroid hormone levels were elevated in 14 patients. Radiographic evidence of hyperparathyroidism was present at the onset of dialysis in 15 patients, and considerable progression occurred in 4 patients. No patient underwent parathyroidectomy. Patient 1 (AW) had severe renal osteodystrophy characterized by bone pain, multiple fractures and skeletal deformities, despite a normal or slightly elevated serum calcium level with small doses of 1, $25(OH)_2D_3$, a normal serum phosphorus with phosphate binders, and serum parathyroid hormone levels which were low to normal. This patient represents a case of the so-called "osteomalacia of dialysis."

**Control of Azotemia and Electrolytes.** The BUN ranged between 65 and 93 mg/dl and the serum creatinine level between 8 and 10.7 mg/dl. The daily ingestion of 2 to 3 gm/kg of protein to compensate for the peritoneal losses of albumin may contribute to a greater degree of azotemia, although a predialysis BUN in the range of 80 to 110 mg/dl is not detrimental[27] if the patient feels well. Peritoneal urea clearance and calculated total clearance per week in the San Francisco series[56] averaged 16.8 ml/min and 1.1 liter/kg/wk respectively. The mean postdialysis values in our patients for serum potassium and serum bicarbonate were 4.6 mEq/l and 24 mEq/l, respectively.

## Outcome

Of the 24 patients maintained on IPD, 21 are alive, one died following a cadaveric kidney transplant, of causes unrelated to dialysis, one died after septicemia and systemic candidiasis, and one died following an episode of aspiration pneumonia. Six patients remain on IPD, 3 changed to CAPD, and one was changed to hemodialysis after developing fungal peritonitis. Twelve patients had a kidney transplant: 10 continue to function satisfactorily, and 2 are now on hemodialysis after chronic irreversible rejection.

Intermittent peritoneal dialysis is easily performed in children and is well accepted by the child and parents. While IPD has been considered a promising alternative for the treatment of children with ESRD, one report has shown that fewer than 10% of pediatric

patients remained on long-term peritoneal dialysis.[14] The specific role of IPD in pediatric ESRD programs, in which transplantation is the ultimate goal of treatment, remains to be identified.

## INFECTIONS

### Peritonitis

Peritonitis is one of the major complications of peritoneal dialysis.[58] The incidence has been reduced by improvements in aseptic technique, and the development of the Tenckhoff catheter and closed system automated equipment.

**Diagnosis and Incidence.** The symptoms and signs of peritonitis are abdominal pain with tenderness, cloudy effluent (drainage), fever, less commonly nausea and vomiting and, rarely, paralytic ileus. To ascertain the organism responsible for the episode of peritonitis, gram stains and cultures of the dialysis fluid should be obtained. The dialysate white cell count in IPD is not as helpful as with CAPD in making the diagnosis of peritonitis.[59] Antibiotic therapy should be initiated immediately after recognition of the above symptoms in order to prevent critical illness and to preserve patency of the catheter. Experience suggests it is wiser to start treatment rather than wait for positive cultures. An appropriately obtained gram stain may assist the physician in the choice of antibiotics until the results of the culture and sensitivities are obtained. Fourteen of 24 patients in our program had a total of 34 episodes of peritonitis during 313 dialysis months, an overall incidence of one episode per 9.2 patient-month[5]. Our experience with peritonitis is compared with that of three other centers in Table 11–4. Of importance is the fact that 56% of all episodes of peritonitis were attributable to recurrent infections in 4 patients (Table 11–5). Patient #1 (AW), who experienced the greatest number of episodes (7), experienced only 3 infections during the first 50 months of IPD therapy; during the final 12 months prior to her death, she experienced four additional episodes in association with increasing nutritional and physical debility. Patient #11 (TR) had five episodes of peritonitis over 28 months of dialysis therapy. The last three episodes were in association with a subcutaneous tunnel infection, which was unsuccess-

**Table 11–4.** COMPARISON OF PERITONITIS DATA IN HOME IPD IN CHILDREN

| Center | Number of Patients | Duration (mos) | Catheter Survival (mos) | Peritonitis Incidence/mo | Death | Outcome (Tx) |
|---|---|---|---|---|---|---|
| Seattle | | | | | | |
| (Counts '73) | 29 | 16 | 16.8 | 10.7 | 4 | — |
| (Hickman '79) | 12 | 14.5 | 7.16 | 12.8 | 1 | 3 |
| Galveston | | | | | | |
| (Brouhard '79) | 19 | 11 | 11.3 | 10.2 | 3 | 9 |
| San Francisco | | | | | | |
| (Potter '81) | 7 | 13.3 | 9.2 | 10.2 | 0 | 3 |
| Philadelphia | | | | | | |
| (Baluarte '82) | 24 | 13 | 8.4 | 9.2 | 3 | 12 |

fully treated with oral and parenteral antibiotics. Removal of the catheter, temporary hemodialysis, and replacement of a catheter allowed the patient to resume home IPD.

The life span of catheters at our center averaged 8.4 months. Replacement of catheters was required for tunnel infections, malposition of the catheter (tip displacement), obstruction by fibrin or blood clots, and omental entrapment. Since 15 of the 24 patients had functioning catheters at the time of transplantation or at the time of death, we feel that the average life span of the catheter is considerably longer than 8.4 months, in concurrence with the opinion of other pediatric centers.[56]

**Etiology and Sources of Infection.** Peritonitis is caused by contamination of fluid or equipment and almost always can be identified as a failure in technique. Peritonitis can also be caused by infection of the exit site, resulting in a tunnel infection with subsequent cuff erosion. In our experience, 63% of the episodes of peritonitis occurred after a documented break in sterility, and 25% were associated with an exit site infection. If infections at the catheter exit site are detected and treated promptly, the incidence of peritonitis can be reduced. As in other series, staphylococci were responsible for a large proportion of the cases[10, 14, 56] and in our series accounted for over 70% of all episodes. Gram-negative bacteria were responsible for 10% of the episodes, and fungal peritonitis occurred in 5% of our cases. We were unable to isolate an organism in 15% of our cases. These patients do not necessarily represent cases of aseptic peritonitis, since they presented with signs of peritonitis and appeared to respond to antibiotic therapy.

Aseptic peritonitis is reported to occur in 15% to 30% of patients.[60] The exact etiology of aseptic peritonitis is unknown, but possible causes include endotoxins or endotoxin-like substances, the presence of formaldehyde or other peritoneal irritants, and infection with slow-growing organisms.

**Treatment.** During our first few years of experience with IPD, over 70% of patients with peritonitis were hospitalized for treatment; however, home treatment was instituted 2½ years ago.

The following is the protocol used in cases of suspected peritonitis at St. Christopher's Hospital for children:

Continuous peritoneal lavage with antibiotics is begun for 2 days, followed by daily dialysis for 3 days. With inpatient treatment a systemic priming dose of antibiotic is given (gentamicin, 1.5 to 2.5 mg/kg/dose). Gentamicin, 5 mg/liter, or cephalothin, 250 mg/

**Table 11–5.** INFECTIONS ON IPD

| Patient | Peritoneal | Tunnel | Exit Site | No. catheters |
|---|---|---|---|---|
| 1 (AW) | 7 | 0 | 2 | 2 |
| 2 (SW) | 2 | 0 | 1 | 2 |
| 3 (MS) | 0 | 0 | 0 | 1 |
| 4 (SW) | 1 | 0 | 1 | 1 |
| 5 (SM) | 4 | 0 | 1 | 1 |
| 6 (PD) | 0 | 0 | 0 | 1 |
| 7 (WB) | 0 | 0 | 0 | 1 |
| 8 (MK) | 3 | 1 | 2 | 2 |
| 9 (LM) | 0 | 0 | 1 | 1 |
| 10 (RB) | 1 | 0 | 2 | 3 |
| 11 (TR) | 5 | 1 | 2 | 3 |
| 12 (MM) | 0 | 0 | 1 | 3 |
| 13 (JS) | 2 | 0 | 3 | 4 |
| 14 (JM) | 1 | 0 | 1 | 1 |
| 15 (DH) | 2 | 1 | 2 | 2 |
| 16 (TL) | 2 | 0 | 0 | 3 |
| 17 (DL) | 0 | 0 | 0 | 1 |
| 18 (MZ) | 0 | 0 | 0 | 1 |
| 19 (NS) | 0 | 0 | 0 | 1 |
| 20 (PF) | 0 | 0 | 0 | 1 |
| 21 (SS) | 1 | 0 | 2 | 2 |
| 22 (KL) | 0 | 0 | 1 | 1 |
| 23 (KH) | 2 | 0 | 0 | 1 |
| 24 (CB) | 1 | 0 | 1 | 1 |

liter, and heparin, 1000 units/liter, are added to the dialysate. An oral antibiotic (cloxacillin, 50-100 mg/kg/day) is given when gentamicin is the intraperitoneal antibiotic. Adjustment of antibiotics is made within 24 to 48 hours according to the antimicrobial sensitivities. Antibiotics are continued both orally and in the dialysis bath for 2 weeks.

Symptoms usually diminish after the first 12 to 24 hours of treatment and usually disappear within 48 hours. The patient is admitted to the hospital if the condition worsens or does not improve after 12 to 24 hours of antibiotic therapy.

Additional points to consider during the treatment of peritonitis are:

1. If patients cannot tolerate gentamicin or cephalosporin, other antibiotics can be used in the doses shown in Table 11–6.

2. The oral protein intake should be increased to compensate for the greater protein losses during peritonitis. Parenteral nutrition may be required if patients cannot increase their oral protein intake.

3. Drugs containing aluminum hydroxide may need to be temporarily discontinued to avoid aggravation of the constipation so common in patients with peritonitis.

4. The patient's weight and blood pressure should be monitored closely and the dialysate glucose concentration lowered to avoid hypovolemia.

5. Consider removal of the Tenckhoff catheter (a) if the infection persists for more than 4 to 5 days despite the use of appropriate antibiotics, (b) in the presence of a tunnel abscess, (c) in patients in whom fecal peritonitis has developed,[36, 61] and (d) in the presence of tuberculous or fungal peritonitis.

The best approach in treating fungal peritonitis is the removal of the catheter.[61] We have been singularly unsuccessful in our attempts to treat children with systemic and intraperitoneal antifungal agents. After removing the catheter, the children need to be maintained on hemodialysis for 2 to 3 weeks, during which time the patient is usually treated with oral or systemic antifungal agents. The latter may not be necessary, because in the absence of the permanent catheter the immune system can handle the fungi very well.[61] After treatment of the fungal peritonitis a new permanent catheter can be implanted and IPD resumed.

### Exit Site Infection and Tunnel Abscess (Table 11–5)

Exit site infections are potentially serious because they may lead to tunnel infection and peritonitis. Parents or patients should be trained to inspect the catheter routinely during catheter care for local erythema, discharge, or tenderness, and a culture should be taken upon suspicion of an infection. Exit site infections occurred one or more times in 63% of our patients. Staphylococcus was isolated in the majority of cases and the treatment consisted of scrubbing with Betadine solution, frequent dressing changes, and oral antibiotics (cloxacillin). Tunnel infection occurred in 3 patients and the infection was not cured until the catheter was removed.

### INDICATIONS FOR INTERMITTENT PERITONEAL DIALYSIS

The indications at our center for selecting patients for IPD are not rigid. We initially selected patients referred to us from adult-oriented dialysis units not willing to accept children in their programs or from geographic areas where home or in-center hemodialysis was not readily available. Small children were considered for IPD because of the difficulty in maintaining an adequate vascular access and the inadequate size of existing lines and dialyzers. Other children in need of prolonged dialysis prior to renal transplantation with either high titers of preformed cytotoxic antibodies or the presence of malignancy, such as Wilms' tumor, were selected for IPD. The recent availability of the low-volume pediatric cycler machine has made IPD possible in small children weighing as little as 4 to 5 kilograms. These small

**Table 11–6.** RECOMMENDED MAINTENANCE DOSES OF INTRAPERITONEAL ANTIBIOTICS FOR THE TREATMENT OF PERITONITIS

| | | |
|---|---|---|
| Amikacin | 50 | mg/L |
| Amphotericin B | 5 | mg/L |
| Ampicillin | 50 | mg/L |
| Cephalothin | 250 | mg/L |
| Clindamycin | 50 | mg/L |
| Cloxacillin | 100 | mg/L |
| 5 Fluorocytosine | 100 | mg/L |
| Gentamicin | 5 | mg/L |
| Penicillin | 50,000 | u/L |
| Septra | SMZ 25 | mg/L |
| | TMP 5 | mg/L |
| Ticarcillin | 100 | mg/L |
| Tobramycin | 8 | mg/L |
| Vancomycin | 30 | mg/L |

children, although some may be able to live without dialysis, sometimes suffered from irreparable consequences of uremia such as growth failure and renal osteodystrophy. These patients are certainly candidates for CAPD, but the schedule involved made its integration into the life style of single or working parents very difficult. The availability of IPD enables these parents to carry on with their usual daily activities and still be able to perform overnight unassisted dialysis. In our opinion, home IPD has been less stressful than CAPD or in-center hemodialysis for many families and patients, and gives them greater autonomy and control over the treatment of their disease. IPD makes rehabilitation a more realistic goal by allowing the family and patient to maintain more normal relationships with relatives, peers, and friends in school, work, and their neighbors.

## COMPARISON OF IPD WITH CAPD IN CHILDREN

The outlook for children with ESRD has changed dramatically during the past decade because of the technical and medical advances in the therapeutic modalities of dialysis and transplantation. Although renal transplantation remains the preferred treatment in most pediatric centers, and offers the best hope for a child to obtain full rehabilitation and a reasonably normal life, periods of dialysis of varying lengths are essential.

Only a few pediatric centers have published their experience in the use of IPD[10, 14, 15, 56] prior to the introduction of CAPD in the management of children with ESRD. The initial enthusiasm among the staff and patients in our program with this newer technique of CAPD has relegated IPD (cycler) to a secondary role, but its use is again increasing as the medical and psychosocial problems as well as the benefits of both CAPD and IPD are delineated.

We have used IPD and CAPD to treat 47 children with ESRD at St. Christopher's Hospital for Children.[20] Twenty-four children, ages 1.7 to 17.3 years, received IPD (cycler) for 2 to 62 months (312.5 dialysis months) and 23 children, ages 0.8 to 17.8 years, were on CAPD for 1 to 19 months (150 patient months). Biochemical comparisons of serum potassium, calcium, phosphorus, total pro-

tein, and albumin levels were not significantly different between IPD and CAPD, although patients receiving CAPD had lower levels of BUN (49 mg/dl) and creatinine (7.8 mg/dl) than patients on IPD (BUN 78 mg/dl, creatinine 9.9 mg/dl). The linear growth rate of 9 patients on IPD for more than 12 months ranged from 0.09 to 0.98 cm/month (mean 0.32) and in 5 patients on CAPD for more than 6 months, ranged from 0.06 to 0.47 cm/month (mean 0.32). Hypertension was controlled or improved in 80% of patients in both groups. The incidence of peritonitis in patients on IPD was one episode per 9.2 patient-month, compared to one episode per 4.6 patient-month in patients on CAPD. Six patients (75%) are presently on IPD; 10 underwent successful renal transplants, while 11 patients (48%) are still on CAPD. Our impression is that both forms of dialysis therapy are equally effective in children beyond the period of infancy.

Despite the rate of infectious complications, CAPD in our program as well as in other centers[17, 18, 19, 56] has had subjective and objective benefits, and families and children have welcomed the freedom from a machine and the chance to pursue a more normal life. Others have found the switch to IPD from CAPD equally satisfactory.[56] The relative merits and problems of each mode of dialysis in children will become clearer in the next few years.

## REFERENCES

1. Ganter G: Ueber die beseitigung giftiger stoffe aus blute durch dialyse. Munchen Med Wochenschr 70:1478, 1923.
2. Maxwell MH, Rockney RB, Kleeman CR, et al: Peritoneal dialysis. I. Technique and applications. JAMA 170:917, 1959.
3. Quinton W, Dillard D, Scribner BH: Cannulation of blood vessels for prolonged hemodialysis. Trans Am Soc Artif Intern Organs 6:104, 1960.
4. Boen ST, Mulinari AS, Dillard DH, Scribner BH: Periodic peritoneal dialysis in the management of chronic uremia. Trans Am Soc Artif Intern Organs 8:256, 1962.
5. Tenckhoff H, Schechter H: A bacteriologically safe peritoneal access device. Trans Am Soc Artif Intern Organs 14:181, 1968.
6. Palmer RA, Newell JE, Gray JE, Quinton WE: Treatment of chronic renal failure by prolonged peritoneal dialysis. N Engl J Med 274:248, 1966.
7. Khan AV, Herndon CH, Ahmadian SY: Social and emotional adaptations of children with transplanted kidneys and chronic hemodialysis. Am J Psychiatry 128:1194, 1971.
8. Levin S, Winkelstein, JA: Diet and infrequent peri-

toneal dialysis in chronic anuric uremia. N Engl J Med 277:619, 1967.

9. Feldman W, Baliah T, Drummond KN: Intermittent peritoneal dialysis in the management of chronic renal failure in children. Am J Dis Child 116:30, 1968.

10. Counts S, Hickman R, Garbaccio A, Tenckhoff H: Chronic home peritoneal dialysis in children. Trans Am Soc Artif Intern Organs 19:157, 1973.

11. Sakai T, Kasai N, Shinagawa I: Treatment of chronic renal failure by peritoneal dialysis with Tenckhoff indwelling catheter in childhood. Proceedings of Third International Symposium of Pediatric Nephrology, Washington, DC, September, 1974, p 19 (Abst).

12. Gagnadoux MF, Hernandez MA, Broyer M, et al: La dialyse peritoneale chronique: Alternative de L'hemodialyse interative chez l'enfant. Arch Fr Pediatr 34:860, 1977.

13. Potter DE: Comparison of peritoneal dialysis and hemodialysis in children. Dial Transplant 7:800, 1978.

14. Brouhard GH, Berger M, Cunningham RJ, et al: Home peritoneal dialysis in children. Trans Am Soc Artif Intern Organs 25:90, 1979.

15. Baluarte HJ, Grossman MB, Polinsky MS, et al: Experience with intermittent home peritoneal dialysis in children. Pediatr Res 14:994, 1980.

16. Popovich RP, Moncrief JW, Decherd JB, et al: The definition of a novel portable/wearable equilibrium peritoneal dialysis technique. (Abstr) Trans Am Soc Artif Intern Organs 5:64, 1976.

17. Balfe JW, Vigneux A, Willumsen J et al: The use of CAPD in the treatment of children with end stage renal disease. Perit Dial Bull 1:35, 1981.

18. Alexander SR, Talwalkar YB: Continuous ambulatory peritoneal dialysis (CAPD) for infants and children. (Abstr) Clin Dial Transplant Forum, Nov, 1981.

19. Fine RN: Peritoneal dialysis update. J Pediatr 100:1, 1982.

20. Baluarte HJ, Gruskin AB, Polinsky MS, et al: Comparison of chronic intermittent (IPD) and continuous ambulatory (CAPD) peritoneal dialysis in children. (Abstr) Pediatr Res 16:318A, 1982.

21. Weston RE, Roberts M: Clinical use of stylet-catheter for peritoneal dialysis. Arch Intern Med 115:659, 1965.

22. Chan JCM, Campbell RA: Peritoneal dialysis in children: A survey of its indications and applications. Clin Pediatr 12:131, 1973.

23. Kallen CJ, Zaltzman S, Coe FL, et al: Hemodialysis in children: technique, kinetic aspects related to varying body size, and application to salicylate intoxication, acute renal failure and some other disorders. Medicine 45:1, 1966.

24. Miller RB, Tassistro CR: Peritoneal dialysis. N Engl J Med 281:945, 1969.

25. Jacob GB, Deane N: Repeated peritoneal dialysis by the catheter replacement method: Description of technique and a replaceable prosthesis for chronic access to the peritoneal cavity. Proc Eur Dial Transplant Assoc 4:136, 1967.

26. Boen ST: Kinetics of peritoneal dialysis; A comparison with the artificial kidney. Medicine (Baltimore) 40:243, 1961.

27. Lasker N: Chronic peritoneal dialysis. Pa Med 74:67, 1971.

28. Lasker N, Shalhoub R, Habibe O, et al: Management of end-stage kidney disease with intermittent peritoneal dialysis. Ann Intern Med 62:1147, 1965.

29. Tenckhoff H, Meston B, Shilipetar G: A simplified automatic peritoneal dialysis system. Trans Am Soc Artif Inter Organs 18:436, 1972.

30. Oreopoulos DG: Maintenance peritoneal dialysis. In: Strategy in Renal Failure, Friedman EA (Ed). New York, John Wiley and Sons, 1978, pp 393–414.

31. Tenckhoff H: Peritoneal dialysis today: a new look. Nephron 12:420, 1974.

32. Goldberg EM, Hill W: A new peritoneal access prosthesis. Proc Dial Trans Forum 3:122, 1973.

33. Oreopoulos DG, Izatt S, Zellerman G, et al: A prospective study of the effectiveness of three permanent catheters. Proc Dial Trans Forum 6:96, 1976.

34. Ponce SP, Pierratos A, Izatt S, et al: Comparison of the survival and complications of three permanent peritoneal dialysis catheters. Perit Dial Bull 2(2):82, 1982.

35. Sherman RA, Longnecker RE, Davis V: Initial experience with a quick connect/disconnect device for chronic peritoneal dialysis. Dial Transplant 9(7):665, 1980.

36. Ott S, Haas L, Scollard D, Sherrard DJ: Long term results in patients using a povidone-iodine connection device in peritoneal dialysis. Dial Transplant 11(4):275, 1982.

37. Maher JF, Scheiher GE: Hazards and complications of dialysis. N Engl J Med 273:370, 1965.

38. Barry KG, Schwartz FD: Peritoneal dialysis: current status and future applications. Pediatr Clin North Am 11:593, 1964.

39. Scott DF, Marshall VC: Insertion and complications of Tenckhoff catheters—surgical aspects. In: Atkins et al (Eds): Peritoneal Dialysis. New York, Longman, Inc 1981, pp 61–72.

40. Uldall PR, Dyck RF, Woods F, et al: A subclavian cannula for temporary vascular access for hemodialysis or plasmaphoresis. Dial Transplant 8:963, 1979.

41. Berlyne GM, et al: Pulmonary complications of peritoneal dialysis. Lancet 2:75, 1966.

42. Edwards SR, Unger AM: Acute hydrothorax: a new complication of peritoneal dialysis. JAMA 199:853, 1967.

43. Finn R, Jowett EW: Acute hydrothorax: complication of peritoneal dialysis. Br Med J 2:94, 1970.

44. Holm, J, Lieden B, Lindqrist B: Unilateral pleural effusion—a rare complication of peritoneal dialysis. Scand J Urol Nephrol 5:84, 1971.

45. Rudnick MR, Coyle JF, Beck H, McCurdy DK: Acute massive hydrothorax complicating peritoneal dialysis; report of 2 cases and a review of the literature. Clin Nephrol 12:38, 1980.

46. Oreopoulos DG, Khanna R: Complications of peritoneal dialysis other than peritonitis. In: Nolph KD (Ed): Developments in Nephrology: Peritoneal Dialysis. The Hague, Martinus Nijhoff Publishers, 1981, pp 309–343.

47. Haberstrob PB, Uniyal B, Trivedi H: A clot screw. Dial Transplant Dec/Jan:27, 1974.

48. Alexander SR, Tank ES: Surgical aspects of continuous ambulatory peritoneal dialysis in infants, children and adolescents. J Urol 127:501, 1982.

49. Tenckhoff H: Choice of peritoneal dialysis solutions. Ann Intern Med 75(2):313, 1971.

50. Nolph KD, Sorkin MI, Gloor HJ: Considerations

for dialysis solutions modifications. *In*: Atkins et al (Eds): Peritoneal Dialysis. New York, Longman, Inc 1981, pp 236–244.

51. Bhattacharjee N, Sharma BK, et al: Blood glucose changes and hazards of hyperosmolar coma during and after peritoneal dialysis. J Assoc. Physicians India 21(6):505, 1973.

52. Richardson JA, Borchardt KA: Adverse effect on bacteria of peritoneal dialysis solutions that contain acetate. Br Med J 3:794, 1969.

53. Brown ST, Ahearn DJ, Nolph KD: Potassium removal with peritoneal dialysis. Kidney Int 4:67, 1973.

54. Baluarte HJ, Grossman MB, Polinsky MS, et al: Experience with intermittent home peritoneal dialysis in children. *In*: Pediatric Nephrology, Vol. VII, Strauss J. (Ed), In Press.

55. Tanner JM, Whitehouse RH, Takaishi M: Standards from birth to maturity for height, weight, height velocity and weight velocity; British Children, 1965. Arch Dis Child 41:454, 613, 1966.

56. Potter DE, McDaid TK, Ramirez JA: Peritoneal dialysis in children. *In*: Atkins et al (Eds): Peritoneal Dialysis. New York, Longman, Inc., 1981, pp 356–367.

57. Scarpioni L, Poisetti PG, Ballocchi S, Bergonzi G: Follow-up of plasma proteins during long-term peritoneal dialysis. Effect of protein loss (abst). The First International Symposium on Peritoneal Dialysis, June 25–28, 1978, Chapala, Mexico. J Dial 2(5, 6):421, 1978.

58. Boen ST: Overview and history of peritoneal dialysis. Dial Transplant 6(2):14, 1977.

59. Polinsky MS: Personal communication.

60. Gandhi VC, Kamadana MR, Ing TS, et al: Aseptic peritoneal dialysis. Nephron 24:257, 1979.

61. Vas SI, Low DE, Oreopoulos DG: Peritonitis *In*: Nolph KD (Ed); Developments in Nephrology: Peritoneal Dialysis. The Hague, Martinus Nijhoff Publishers, 1981, pp 344–365

# 12

# Continuous Ambulatory Peritoneal Dialysis: Clinical Aspects

*J. Williamson Balfe, M.D., F.R.C.P. (C)*
*Constantinos J. Stefanidis, M.D.*
*Brian T. Steele, M.B., B.Ch., M.R.C.P. (UK), F.R.C.P. (C)*
*Ian K. Hewitt, M.B.B.S., F.R.A.C.P.*

## THE EVOLUTION OF PERITONEAL DIALYSIS

The evolution of peritoneal dialysis (PD) can be divided into three stages: (a) the early years (1923–1962), when PD was used basically for the treatment of acute renal failure; (b) the period of chronic intermittent PD (1962 until the present); and (c) the recent years of CAPD (1978 until the present).

**The Early Years of Peritoneal Dialysis.** In 1923 Ganter reported that a guinea pig with uremia from ureteral ligation showed improvement with intermittent infusion and removal of a saline solution from the peritoneal cavity. In addition, he noticed an improvement in the condition of a patient with uremia when this technique was applied.[1]

Two publications of importance preceded Ganter's observations. In 1894 Starling and Tubby studied the transfer of substances in both directions across the peritoneal membrane[2] and Putnam in 1922 described the transfer characteristics of the peritoneal membrane.[3] Both these reports had an impact on the development of peritoneal dialysis.

The early use of peritoneal dialysis was limited because peritonitis was a frequent complication. In 1948 Odel et al collected the data of all 101 patients treated with PD. Sixty-three had reversible renal disease and 32 of them recovered. In 6 cases (15%), peritonitis was the primary cause of death.[4]

The catheters used for PD usually were modifications from available tubing. Wear et al used a gallbladder trocar for the inflow and another type of trocar with many small holes in its distal segment for the outflow.[5] Boen used rubber gastric tubing with side holes.[6] Doolan et al initially used nasal oxygen tubes and later developed a polyvinyl chloride catheter with transverse ridges to prevent kinking and blockage by omentum.[7] In 1959 Maxwell et al described a nylon catheter, which is still used for PD in patients with acute renal failure.[8]

In the pioneer days of PD, normal saline or 5% glucose was used as the dialysate. In 1938 Wear et al used lactated Ringer's solution (Hartmann's solution) to which they added dextrose.[5] Abbott and Shea in 1946 modified Hartmann's solution by adding bicarbonate.[9] The ingredients of the various PD solutions used over the years have remained similar to those in the Abbott and Shea dialysate except that potassium has been omitted and bicarbonate has been replaced by acetate or lactate. Commercial solution developed by Maxwell et al became available in 1959. Using a V connection, two bottles of fluid were infused simultaneously and the same bottles were used to receive the drained dialysis effluent.[8]

Early publications were unable to document improvement of the patients' blood chemistry with PD. However, it was noted that the "dwell time" of the dialysate was frequently too short or the amount of fluid was too small. In 1959, Boen demonstrated that PD could achieve the same improvement in blood chemistry seen with hemodialysis provided a large volume of dialysate was used and the duration of dialysis was prolonged.[6] However, the clearance obtained with PD was lower than that of hemodialysis. The peritoneal urea clearance was 12 ml/min when one liter of dialysate was cycled per hour. Later, Tenckhoff et al showed that urea clearance could be increased to 40 ml/min at a dialysate flow rate of 10 L/day;[10] this is the limit which can be achieved with PD.

**The Period of Chronic Intermittent PD.** The reduction in the incidence of peritonitis was the prerequisite for the long-term applications of PD. The primary cause of peritonitis was either contamination of the catheter or of the dialysate. To avoid this contamination, Boen et al abandoned the indwelling catheter and used repeated peritoneal punctures for each dialysis procedure. In addition, Boen et al used a closed sterile system with a 40 liter carboy during the entire 10 hours of dialysis.[11] These carboys facilitated the later development of an automatic cycler.

In 1965, Tenckhoff et al demonstrated that the repeated puncture technique and an automatic machine facilitated PD in a home setting.[12] The repeated puncture technique was a major impetus for the success of chronic PD. However, this method was uncomfortable for the patient and time-consuming for the physician. In 1964, Palmer et al devised a silicon PD catheter.[13] This 84-cm catheter had a coiled intraperitoneal portion with perforations. Halfway along the tube there was a tri-flanged step for seating the tube between the deep fascia and peritoneum. The rest of the tube was placed in a long spiral, subcutaneous tunnel which exited from the skin in the left upper quadrant of the abdomen. The purpose of the long subcutaneous tunnel was to prevent infectious agents from entering the peritoneum via the catheter exit site.

Tenckhoff and his colleagues modified this catheter by making it shorter and by using two dacron cuffs, one placed outside the peritoneum and the other below the skin.[14] The purpose of the two cuffs was to close the sinus tract or tunnel around the catheter. The 10-cm subcutaneous part was placed in a curvilinear fashion and the 20-cm intra-abdominal part was straight and had many holes in the 15-cm distal portion. This cath-eter made chronic PD more readily available and since 1977 161 patients in the Seattle area have undergone chronic PD, many of them for over four years.[15] The second largest patient population receiving intermittent peritoneal dialysis (IPD) was in Toronto; Oreopoulos reported satisfactory results with IPD in 150 patients.[16]

During this period IPD was used in children. In 1968 Feldman et al reported that IPD was effective when used for 1.5 to 8 months in children 6 to 14 years of age who were awaiting transplantation.[17]

In 1973, Counts et al described their experience with 12 children treated with an automated system and permanent catheters. Only one child died and the incidence of peritonitis was less than one episode for every 12 patient-months.[18] Similar results with the use of home IPD in 19 children were reported by Brouchard et al.[19]

When the dialysis and transplantation program at The Hospital for Sick Children in Toronto was started in 1967, all children were treated with in-center IPD—repeated puncture technique—and were dialysed for 24 to 48 hours every 11 days. This technique was simple, effective, and well accepted by the children and their parents. However, because of the popularity of hemodialysis the children were converted gradually to in-center hemodialysis.

**The Period of CAPD.** In 1976, Popovich et al described an equilibrium PD technique.[20] Two liters of dialysate were infused intraperitoneally and allowed to equilibrate for four hours while the patient continued normal activities. The spent dialysate was then replaced with fresh solution. The continuous presence of dialysate in the peritoneal cavity provided greater weekly clearances than that obtained with IPD. A cooperative study was initiated in 1977 by the Austin Diagnostic Clinic (Dr. Moncrief) the University of Missouri (Dr. Nolph) and the Bio-Medical engineering department of the University of Texas (Dr. Popovich). Data derived from nine patients confirmed that CAPD could control the consequences of uremia. However, the incidence of peritonitis was high (one episode every 8 to 10 patient-weeks) and was related to the number of connections and disconnections required to change the dialysate solution.[21]

In 1978 a major advance was reported by Oreopoulos et al.[22] A modification of the technique using peritoneal dialysis solutions in plastic bags was described. Following instillation of fluid, the bag could be rolled up and carried easily under the patient's clothing. The number of disconnections was reduced and the incidence of peritonitis decreased markedly to one episode every 10.5 patient-months.[22] The popularity of CAPD increased subsequently[23] and by January, 1982, 4400 patients in the United States were being treated with CAPD.[24]

In 1978 CAPD using bags was applied to children in Toronto. The initial children treated were those whose vascular access sites were exhausted and who required prolonged dialysis because of the presence of high titers of preformed cytotoxic antibodies. The initial success with children stimulated the use of CAPD in small children because of the inherent difficulties encountered with hemodialysis in the young. Subsequently, CAPD was established as our preferred mode of dialysis in the young.[25] Similar satisfactory results were reported recently by Alexander[26] and by Fine.[27]

## DEVELOPING A PEDIATRIC CAPD PROGRAM

As with most aspects of renal medicine, a well-organized and smoothly functioning CAPD program is a team effort. It requires a physician who is technically aware of all aspects of PD and who is readily available to the team when problems arise. The CAPD nurse is the vital link between the CAPD team and the patient. Without a functioning catheter CAPD is not possible, and consequently an experienced surgeon is required for insertion of the peritoneal catheter. The dietitian plays a vital role in adjusting dietary intake to the dialysis regimen. Finally, the social worker provides valuable support to the family and advises the team on how well the family is coping with the unrelenting stress of CAPD.

The catheter is inserted using a general anesthetic. Preoperatively, the patient is given prophylactic antibiotics one hour before surgery (tobramycin, 1.5 mg/kg; cephalothin, 20 mg/kg intravenously). Proper insertion of the chronic peritoneal catheter requires special attention in children of less than 20 kg body weight. We have preferred a catheter with a single dacron cuff fixed 5 cm from the first drainage holes.[28] A pediatric and a neonatal catheter have been pre-

pared according to our specifications by Cardiomed, Stouffville, Ontario. Because of our preference for the single cuff, we have not had the problem of distal cuff erosion. In addition, exit site and tunnel infections have been minimal. On occasion we have used the Oreopoulos-Zellerman catheter, which has Silastic discs in the intra-abdominal part of the catheter to prevent obstruction by the omentum. The omentum does not seem to cause problems in young children, but this may not be the case for older children or adults. The proper positioning of the catheter in an infant is demonstrated in Figure 12–1. Note that the single cuff is buried between the peritoneum and the rectus abdominis muscle. A prolene pursestring suture secures the peritoneum around the catheter. Before the patient leaves the operating room, the catheter position is checked with a radiograph, and catheter function is ensured using irrigation and gravity drainage.

Dialysis is started immediately, following catheter placement, using a volume of 25 ml/kg body weight and no dwell time for 10 hours. Then, for the next 20 hours, the small volume exchange is continued but using a 10-minute dwell time (Table 12–1). More recently, because of the availability of pediatric automatic cyclers, the dialysis is continued for a number of days, gradually increas-

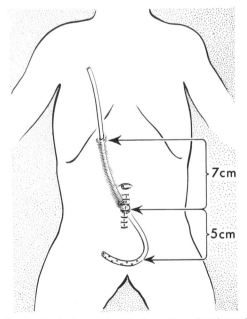

**Figure 12–1.** A chronic Silastic peritoneal catheter in an infant. The single cuff is positioned at the peritoneal entrance site (the middle arrow). Note that a vertical tunnel is preferred for infants.

**Table 12–1.** DIALYSIS PROTOCOL
IMMEDIATELY AFTER CATHETER
IMPLANTATION

1. IPD* with no dwell time for 10 hours.
2. IPD with 10 minutes' dwell time for 20 hours.
3. Daily IPD (4–6 hours/day) for 7 days.
4. Commence CAPD training.

*IPD = Intermittent Peritoneal Dialysis.

ing the dwell time and the volume. The initial "break-in" period takes about four days. Subsequently, the actual CAPD training, which takes two weeks, commences. During the first week of CAPD training, the exchange technique is taught and eventually performed by the patient or the parent but under close supervision. During the second week, at our institution, the CAPD training is done in a hostel, which is a separate building adjacent to the hospital. At this time the procedure is performed totally by the parent. One nurse is assigned to teach the parent or patient such aspects as bag change, tube change, dressing change (for those who are not using the "shower technique"), practical physiological aspects of dialysis, and recognition of the signs of peritonitis and early treatment. The Airstrip dressing may be more appropriate for the small child, whereas older children prefer no bandage, and utilize the "shower technique."

Once the patient is discharged from the hospital, close contact is maintained by telephone. Initially the patient is seen every two weeks and eventually every four weeks. During the routine monthly clinic visit, the patient is seen by various members of the team. The physician reviews the daily record sheet, noting the blood pressure and weight changes. The physical examination includes special attention to the state of hydration and the catheter exit site. Advice is given concerning the patient's correct "dry weight" and the type of dialysate required. The nurse changes the connecting tube and supervises the bag-changing technique. The dietitian indicates appropriate food intake, especially protein and energy intake. Every four or eight weeks, four-day home records are undertaken by the patient/parent. Blood tests are performed every two weeks for most patients. If hospital follow-up is inconvenient because of distance from the hospital, the family physician is invited to join in the care, obtaining appropriate blood tests and bacteriologic testing. For patients living a significant distance from our center the family

physician assumes total care of the patient and center personnel are available for advice. Such patients remain at home and return to the center only for major problems or to receive a renal transplant.

## INDICATIONS AND CONTRAINDICATIONS OF CAPD

Currently the proportion of children with ESRD who are treated with CAPD varies between pediatric centers, depending upon the enthusiasm and experience of the nephrology team and the availability of kidneys for transplantation. When a child is approaching ESRD, we believe it is still appropriate to create a fistula for vascular access. If an active transplantation program is available, such patients may then receive a successful renal transplant either before or after a short period of hemodialysis. Over the last few years at our center, relatively few children with ESRD have been treated with long-term hemodialysis, and for at least three groups of children, CAPD is a better alternative:

1. Children who live a long distance from a regional nephrology center and thus traveling or relocating for hemodialysis would be a significant problem.

2. Children, often on hemodialysis, with high levels of preformed cytotoxic antibodies, who can anticipate a long waiting time for a renal transplant. In such patients long-term hemodialysis is often accompanied by increasing problems with vascular access, and schooling.

3. Young children and infants in whom hemodialysis is technically difficult.

A large proportion of children with ESRD belong to one of these three groups. Other children will often choose CAPD over hemodialysis, hoping for better health and greater independence. The rare pediatric diabetic patient with end-stage renal disease is probably best managed with CAPD and intraperitoneal insulin.[29]

There are few real contraindications to CAPD in children. Our "drop-out" rate, excluding renal transplantation, has been negligible. Children who are regarded as unsuitable for CAPD are usually those whose parents either fear the responsibility of performing bag changes or are unwilling to jeopardize their own life style. Unwilling parents are unlikely to be successful and should not be unduly pressured or made to feel guilty for their decision. Children 10 to 12 years of age and older are usually able to learn the technique themselves, and even those with poor personal hygiene or a poor socioeconomic background can be taught to perform CAPD successfully. Children who have had multiple abdominal operations with subsequent adhesions and those with ileal conduits probably should not be treated with CAPD. Immunosuppression, which is being tapered following an unsuccessful renal transplant, is not a contraindication to CAPD. We have had three immunosuppressed patients do well on CAPD.

## BIOCHEMICAL CONTROL

Several publications have established that CAPD provides acceptable biochemical control of the consequences of uremia.[11, 21, 25, 30] The transperitoneal movement of solute and water during CAPD is considered in detail in Chapter 10. The removal of solutes over short periods of time with efficient hemodialysis causes rapid fluctuations of solute concentrations in body fluids with resultant fluid shifts within body water compartments, causing symptoms such as headache, nausea, and malaise. In contrast, because CAPD mimics the "steady state" control of body fluid chemistries, it is not associated with symptoms of dysequilibrium.[31]

Blood pH and serum bicarbonate, sodium, potassium, and chloride concentrations were acceptable in all our patients. Patients with hyperkalemia between hemodialysis treatments should do better with CAPD.[32] The good control of potassium with CAPD can be explained by the fact that CAPD patients lose a relatively large amount of potassium in

stool. In addition, as the serum potassium level increases, dialysate losses also increase.[31]

Biochemical values before and after 12 months of CAPD treatment are shown in Table 12–2. BUN decreased significantly with CAPD (Fig. 12–2). However, BUN alone can be a misleading index of the efficiency of small solute removal. The control of BUN may appear better than the prediction from weekly clearances because of a low protein intake and reduced urea generation rates.[33] The weekly clearance of small solutes such as urea with CAPD is comparable to that obtained with IPD, but worse than that seen with hemodialysis.[21] Gotch recently reported that dialysis of small solutes is important, because the retention of such toxic molecules may cause anorexia.[33]

Several studies have shown that substances with large molecular weights (middle molecules, 500 to 5000 daltons) may be toxic. The continuous nature of CAPD and the permeability characteristics of the peritoneal membrane make CAPD uniquely efficient for the elimination of middle molecules.[34] In fact, middle molecule clearance may be a better indicator of the adequacy of dialysis than the clearance of small molecules.

With CAPD, the serum creatinine level decreased significantly in children younger than six years of age, but a similar effect was not observed in the older children (Fig. 12–3). The serum magnesium level was consistently elevated during CAPD. Although balance studies would be more conclusive, it appears that the magnesium concentration in current commercially available dialysate solution should be reduced.

The serum albumin level has been used as an indicator of nutritional status.[35, 36] However, the serum albumin level is determined

**Table 12–2.** THE EFFECT OF DIALYSIS ON BIOCHEMICAL CONTROL IN 13 CHILDREN UNDERGOING CAPD FOR MORE THAN ONE YEAR (MEAN LEVEL ± SD)

|  | Before CAPD | On CAPD | P value |
|---|---|---|---|
| BUN (mg/dl) | 101 ± 19 | 68 ± 20 | 0.0002 |
| Creatinine (mg/dl) |  |  |  |
| < 6 years | 7.9 ± 2.2 | 4.8 ± 1.3 | 0.006 |
| > 6 years | 11.8 ± 2.3 | 10.2 ± 2.8 | NS* |
| Uric acid (mg/dl) | 7.2 ± 0.4 | 5.5 ± 0.8 | < 0.0005 |
| Magnesium (mg/dl) | 2.1 ± 0.3 | 2.7 ± 0.3 | < 0.005 |
| Calcium (mg/dl) | 8.6 ± 0.7 | 9.5 ± 1.0 | < 0.05 |
| Phosphorus (mg/dl) | 5.0 ± 2.1 | 4.7 ± 1.6 | NS |
| Alkaline phosphatase (IU/L) | 352 ± 356 | 227 ± 236 | NS |
| Parathormone (ng/ml) | 0.85 ± 0.5 | 0.71 ± 0.4 | < 0.05 |
| Albumin (g/dl) | 3.4 ± 0.7 | 3.8 ± 0.8 | NS |
| Triglycerides (mg/dl) | 215 ± 44 | 298 ± 52 | 0.002 |

*NS = not significant at the p < 0.05 level.

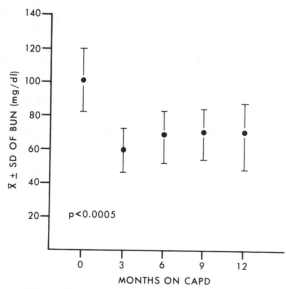

**Figure 12–2.** Changes in mean blood urea nitrogen (BUN) level during 12 months of CAPD.

by several factors, including rates of synthesis and catabolism, plasma volume, and compartmentalization of albumin.[37] Uremia per se seems to affect albumin metabolism.[38] The serum albumin level is not always sensitive to changes in the nutritional status of patients and often fails to correlate with fluctuations in other nutritional parameters.[37] In our patients the serum albumin level in 10 of 13 children increased after one year on CPAD, but this increase was not significant.

Our patients had a significant increase in their serum triglyceride concentration with

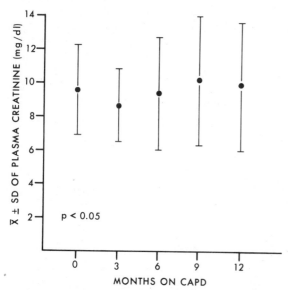

**Figure 12–3.** Changes in mean plasma creatinine level during 12 months of CAPD.

CAPD. Continuous glucose absorption may be responsible for the hypertriglyceridemia found frequently among CAPD patients.[24]

## RENAL OSTEODYSTROPHY

An important and sometimes incapacitating complication of chronic renal insufficiency is renal osteodystrophy. Children appear particularly susceptible to the striking biochemical and endocrine disturbances seen in uremia, leading to disturbed growth and remodeling of bones.

It is a generally accepted practice to consider childhood renal osteodystrophy to be divided into two components radiologically. Hyperparathyroid bone disease is characterized by subperiosteal erosions of the long bones and phalanges, and rickets is characterized by increased thickness and fraying of the radiolucent zone in the region of the growth plate. Mechanisms invoked have included phosphate retention;[39, 40] skeletal resistance to parathyroid hormone[41] and intestinal malabsorption of calcium[42] leading to hypocalcemia and secondary hyperparathyroidism; and defective vitamin D metabolism with impaired renal 1-hydroxylation of 25-hydroxy vitamin D.[43] Recent histologic evidence makes this separation less clear-cut. The growth zone lesions of "renal rickets" differ morphologically from lesions seen in vitamin D deficiency states and incorporate some features of hyperparathyroidism, including fibrosis and increased chondroclastic and osteoclastic activity.[44, 45] In addition, defective mineralization of osteoid has been found in patients with chronic renal failure in whom the blood levels of the active vitamin D metabolite, 1,25-hydroxy vitamin D, were either normal or mildly elevated.[46] Administration of 1,25-dihydroxy vitamin D does not always reverse or prevent the development of the different components of renal osteodystrophy.[47, 48] Other disturbances such as acidosis, malnutrition, and vitamin D resistance may also contribute toward development of bone disease in patients with renal insufficiency, and, as such, no single therapy should be expected to control the process.

CAPD prolongs the state of chronic renal insufficiency and increases the propensity to develop advanced bone disease; CAPD may offer some advantage over hemodialysis and IPD by providing a steady state control of the biochemical and hormonal parameters.

The loss of parathyroid hormone into the dialysate may reduce the degree of hyperparathyroidism.[49]

Sixteen children undergoing CAPD at our facility were evaluated for the prevalence and severity of renal osteodystrophy. All children received aluminum hydroxide with meals in a dosage adjusted to maintain the plasma phosphorus level within the normal range for age. Each child received 1,25-dihydroxy vitamin $D_3$ and 9 children were given supplemental calcium when hypocalcemia occurred. In general, the biochemical indices of mineral metabolism improved on CAPD (see Table 12–2). Plasma calcium levels tended to rise, and elevated alkaline phosphatase and immunoreactive parathyroid hormone levels tended to fall. Plasma phosphate values showed no significant change with CAPD; however, infants tended to develop hypophosphatemia early in the course of CAPD while adolescents were prone to display persistent hyperphosphatemia. Summarizing the radiographic data, 10 children had subperiosteal erosions, which was considered evidence of hyperparathyroid bone disease, at onset of CAPD, and three of these patients had concurrent growth zone lesions. The hyperparathyroid changes improved in seven and worsened in three, while all three children with growth zone lesions showed improvement. Two patients developed hyperparathyroid bone changes and a further two developed growth zone lesions during CAPD despite receiving supplemental 1,25 dihydroxy vitamin $D_3$.

Obvious skeletal deformities, including genu valgum, genu varum, and lateral bowing of the radii, were observed in four children, all of whom had chronic renal insufficiency since birth. Other features of bone disease, including slipped femoral epiphyses, fractures, and metastatic calcifications, were not seen in our patients while on CAPD. Both hyperparathyroid bone disease and growth zone lesions occurred in all age groups studied; however, both lesions had a tendency to involve infants and young children with greater frequency and severity.

## TRANSFUSION REQUIREMENTS

Increases in hemoglobin concentration are seen in CAPD patients.[50–53] Twenty of our patients were on CAPD for more than three months. The mean hemoglobin before CAPD was 6.2 gm/dl and by the end of the follow-up period had increased to 7.49 gm/dl.

Three of the 20 children with their native kidneys in situ did not require a transfusion during CAPD. Children with native kidneys required fewer transfusions than did children who had bilateral nephrectomies (1 transfusion per 6.2 versus 3.5 patient-months). When the transfusion requirements of 64 children on hemodialysis were compared with the CAPD patients, it was obvious that children on CAPD were transfused less frequently (1 transfusion per 1.5 patient months versus 5.2 patient months). This can be explained by the fact that CAPD patients have no blood loss with dialysis and possibly because a bone marrow inhibitor of erythropoiesis is removed more efficiently with CAPD.[31]

## GROWTH AND NUTRITION

Growth retardation is a common problem among children with chronic renal failure,[54–58] especially when the disease starts early in life.[59] As the survival rate of young patients with ESRD increased during the past decade, it became clear that growth which was usually poor during hemodialysis[60–63] improved after transplantation.[64–66]

The majority of children in our program wait only a few months for a transplant[67] and consequently growth is not adversely affected by the short dialysis period. However, in some patients, including very young children, dialysis may be prolonged. For these young children, CAPD seems to be the treatment of choice; consequently, growth is a major concern.

The growth velocity index for bone age (GVI) was used to evaluate the growth of 13 children (1.6–18 years of age) undergoing CAPD for 13 to 40 months. GVI was calculated as follows:

$$GVI\,\% = \frac{Observed\ height\ gain}{Expected\ height\ gain} \times 100$$

GVI was defined as satisfactory (type 1) when it was > 80%, fair (type 2) when between 50 and 80% and poor (type 3) when < 50%.[68]

None of our patients undergoing CAPD for more than one year had poor growth. Five children had fair growth, and the GVI of the remaining eight patients was satisfactory. The growth of our patients (Fig. 12–4, group 2) was somewhat better than that reported by Alexander[26] (Fig. 12–4, group 3); however, it was not as good as that reported by Kohaut[69] (Fig. 12–4, group 1).

When the data of the 36 children treated with CAPD from all three centers were analyzed as a group, it became obvious that 10 children had a GVI greater than 100% (27%) and 23 (64%) grew more than the 80% expected for their bone age. Only two children had poor growth, and the remaining 11 (30%) had fair growth.

The growth data of eight children (3 to 13 years of age) treated with CAPD for more than one year in Paris were similar. Seven of eight grew normally, while one child lost one SD in one year. However, no child demonstrated catch-up growth.[70]

Eleven of the 36 children in the three series were younger than four years of age; of these one grew poorly, four had fair growth, and six grew satisfactorily. Similarly, Conley et al reported that the growth of four infants (3 to 11 months of age) treated with continuous PD was normal. These patients received 6 to 9 daily exchanges of 30 to 50 ml/kg and had a high calorie (120 to 140 Kcal/kg/day) and a normal protein intake (2 gm/kg/day); only one infant required nasogastric tube feeding to achieve this intake.[71]

On the other hand, in a recent report from France, the growth of three children treated with hemodialysis and followed for at least one year before the age of three was severely reduced.[72] In such patients it is known that a prolonged period of dialysis usually leads to permanently short stature. In addition, hemodialysis is associated with many technical problems in very young children, especially creation and maintenance of an adequate

vascular access. For all these reasons, CAPD seems to be a more favorable form of dialytic treatment for the young child.

The caloric and protein intake of 11 children undergoing CAPD in our program was assessed from four-day home food records. Three children had an energy intake of less than 80% of that recommended, and three children had an intake slightly higher than 80% for their age group. The GVIs of the three children with an energy intake of less than 80% were lower compared to the rest of the patients. Only four of the 11 children had a protein intake of more than 1.5 gm/kg/day; however, all the patients had a positive nitrogen balance. Protein and amino acid losses into the dialysate represented approximately 70% of their protein intake.

Using linear regression analysis of the urea nitrogen appearance compared to estimated protein intake, we found a significant correlation in our patients which validates the reliability of the protein intake calculated from home food records.[80] Similar data were reported recently by Fine;[27] only three of the 12 children had an energy intake less than the 75% of that recommended. Poor energy and protein intake has been associated with abnormal growth.[73–75] However, an appropriate nutritional intake does not necessarily correct growth problems.[76, 77]

Renal osteodystrophy (ROD) has been associated with growth retardation.[77, 78] The growth of two of our very young patients improved significantly when their ROD lesions began to heal with high doses of 1,25-dihydroxy vitamin $D_3$. In addition, children with a PTH level < 0.5 ng/ml show better growth compared with patients with a PTH level higher than 0.5 ng/ml. Kohaut recently reported that patients with a PTH level less than double normal values (0.3 ng/ml) had better growth.[69]

Uremia,[54, 59] acidosis,[79] and anemia[80, 81] may affect growth. However, blood pH, BUN, plasma creatinine, bicarbonate, and hemoglobin levels in our CAPD patients did not differ significantly between those who had satisfactory GVIs and those with impaired growth.[82]

Most children undergoing CAPD show satisfactory growth.[85] Nutritional support should be considered essential for children with inappropriate energy and/or protein intake. Nasogastric tube feeding as used by Guillot et al[84] or the addition of amino acids to the dialysate[85] may improve the nutritional status of children undergoing CAPD. Our philosophy is to change the dialysis to suit

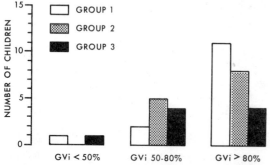

**Figure 12–4.** Comparison of growth velocity indices (GVI) in children on CAPD from Birmingham, Alabama (group 1), Toronto, Canada (group 2), and Portland, Oregon (group 3).

the diet rather than to manipulate the diet. In addition, the control of secondary hyperparathyroidism seems to be important. The measurement of serum parathormone concentration on a routine basis is essential for surveillance.

## RENAL TRANSPLANTATION

The ultimate goal for all children with ESRD is a successful renal allograft. Therefore, the effect of dialysis on graft function is of vital importance.

During the last four years, 23 children at The Hospital for Sick Children, Toronto, were treated with CAPD prior to transplantation. Seven of these patients developed ascites in the first few days after transplantation. In four, the ascites was mild and resolved spontaneously in a few days, but the remaining three children required drainage of the ascitic fluid. This complication resolved eventually in all the patients. The actuarial graft survival rates of children with and without ascites were similar. The cause of the ascites was not apparent; there was no correlation with the original renal disease; however, the children with ascites were younger than those without this complication.[86] Because of the aggressive nature of our current mode of fluid administration, most children develop fluid retention in the immediate postoperative period. This fluid administration, in combination with an immature or "leaky" peritoneal membrane, may lead to transudation of fluid. The fact that ascites was more common in the youngest patients supports this hypothesis.

Only one of the CAPD patients developed peritonitis after transplantation. This patient had candida peritonitis which could not be eradicated using intraperitoneal amphotericin, but quickly resolved with removal of the catheter. All 23 children had a retroperitoneal allograft, and thus the low incidence of peritonitis might be related to this surgical approach.

Our data indicate that children on CAPD can be given transplants safely. Similar results in adults were reported by Cardella.[87] Our current policy is to leave the peritoneal catheter in place after the transplant for dialysis if needed or drainage of ascitic fluid and remove it approximately two weeks posttransplant; however, Oreopoulos suggests catheter removal at three months.

## COMPLICATIONS

**Peritonitis.** Peritonitis is the most significant complication of CAPD. At least one episode of peritonitis has occurred in 16 of the first 30 children trained for CAPD in Toronto. A total of 29 episodes have occurred during 304 patient-months for an overall rate of one episode for 10.5 patient-months. Only four children have had more than two episodes of peritonitis. One teenager has had five episodes over the 28-month period with CAPD before receiving a successful renal transplant. A seven-year-old girl who has been treated with CAPD for almost four years has never had peritonitis. Approximately 3/4 of the organisms responsible for peritonitis are either *Staphylococcus aureus*, *Staphylococcus epidermidis*, or *Streptococcus viridans*. These three organisms are also the commonest in adult patients treated with CAPD. Peritonitis can be caused by a variety of other skin contaminants, and we have seen one patient who developed peritonitis with *Candida albicans* seven days after transplantation. In this patient and in two others with recurrent episodes of *Staphylococcus epidermidis* peritonitis, the catheter had to be removed because of persistent infection. The Candida infection was cured and after allograft rejection CAPD was successfully resumed six weeks later. In one patient with recurrent *Staphylococcus epidermidis* peritonitis, the organism was cultured from a clean-appearing Tenckhoff catheter which was electively removed and the peritonitis resolved, whereas the other child with no bacterial growth from the removed catheter developed peritonitis with the same organism two weeks later.

Abdominal pain and cloudy dialysate are the earliest and most consistent signs of peritonitis. Examination of dialysate is mandatory with the appearance of these signs alone, rather than waiting for classic features of peritonitis such as fever, vomiting, and rebound tenderness. The patient or parent is taught to initiate early treatment unless they can reach the hospital quickly. After obtaining a sample of dialysate for gram stain, cell count, and culture, three quick exchanges are immediately performed (Table 12–3). CAPD then is resumed on a six-hour schedule, with antibiotics added to each bag of dialysate. If no organism is found on gram stain or if the result is not available, a loading dose of 500 mg of cephalothin per liter of

**Table 12–3.** TREATMENT OF PERITONITIS FOR PATIENTS UNDERGOING CAPD

When peritonitis is suspected:
  Cloudy dialysate
  Signs of peritonitis
  Fever

1. Obtain a 10 ml specimen of dialysate for gram stain, culture, and sensitivity test on centrifuged sample and cell count and differential on uncentrifuged sample.
2. Three exchanges of dialysate without antibiotic (flushes)—no dwell time.
3. Then resume CAPD on a schedule of every 6 hours. If a *gram-positive organism* is reported add 500 mg cephalothin per liter of dialysate to first exchange, and to following exchanges add 250 mg cephalothin per liter of dialysate.
4. If *gram-negative organism* is present, then add tobramycin, 1.7 mg per kg body weight, to the first dialysate exchange, and to following exchanges 10 mg tobramycin per liter of dialysate.
5. If *no organism* is found on gram stain, then add 500 mg of cephalothin per liter of dialysate plus 1.7 mg tobramycin per kg body weight for the first exchange after the 3 flushes, and then 250 mg Cephalothin and 10 mg tobramycin per liter of dialysate.
6. Heparin (500 to 1000 units per liter) is added to the dialysate containing antibiotic until the fluid is clear in color and/or no fibrin clots are present.
7. Repeat cell count and differential 14 days after onset of peritonitis.

dialysate plus 1.7 mg/kg body weight of tobramycin is added to the first exchange after the three "flushes." Thereafter, 250 mg of cephalothin per liter and 10 mg of tobramycin per liter are added to the dialysate. If a gram-positive organism is identified, cephalothin alone is used, and if a gram-negative organism is identified, tobramycin alone is used. Because most infections are caused by gram-positive organisms, many patients probably do not require tobramycin. Consequently in selected patients, routine tobramycin could be withheld in view of its potential toxicity. Heparin (500 units per liter) is added to the dialysate containing antibiotic until the fluid is clear and free of fibrin clots. The duration of treatment depends upon the response to antibiotics but is usually seven days. Prior to stopping antibiotic treatment, a repeat culture and cell count of the dialysate is performed. Once the sensitivity of the reported organism is known, the appropriate antibiotic is used. In patients who cannot tolerate either tobramycin or cephalothin, other drugs can be used in the dosage shown in Table 12–4. No patient deaths have resulted from peritonitis and the majority of patients improve after 24 hours of treatment. Nonetheless some patients, particularly those

with *Staphylococcus aureus* and *Streptococcus viridans* can become critically ill with a concomitant bacteriemia. We have not encountered pseudomonas infections; however, this organism may produce serious infections and result in abscess formation. Therefore, follow-up with abdominal ultrasound assessment should be done. It is emphasized during the CAPD training period that accidental spike contamination may lead to peritonitis. In the event of such a contamination, the spike should be soaked in povidone-iodine solution for 10 minutes, and in some cases an antibiotic is added to the next dialysate bag. In the past we performed a tube change for spike contamination.

**Catheters.** Proper catheter placement is necessary to achieve good drainage. A radiograph in the operating room will ensure that the distal tip of the catheter lies in the pelvis. The catheter cuff should be embedded under the rectus fascia, just outside the peritoneum, and leakage is minimized by using a proline pursestring suture around the catheter. Erosion of the cuff through the skin is common if the single cuff or proximal cuff is embedded too close to the skin surface. We have not had any tunnel infections even though we have used only single-cuffed catheters.[28] Catheter exit site infections have not been a serious problem. The latter is possibly a predisposing cause of peritonitis and therefore

**Table 12–4.** RECOMMENDED DOSES OF INTRAPERITONEAL ANTIBIOTICS IN THE TREATMENT OF PERITONITIS IN CAPD PATIENTS*

| | Loading Dose | Maintenance Dose |
|---|---|---|
| *First Line Drugs* | | |
| Cephalothin | 500 | 250 |
| Tobramycin | 1.7 (mg/kg/bag) | 8 |
| *Second Line Drugs* | | |
| Ampicillin | 500 | 50 |
| Cloxacillin | 1000 | 100 |
| Ticarcillin | 1000 | 100 |
| Septra SMZ/TMP | 400/80 | 25/5 |
| Clindamycin | 300 | 50 |
| Amikacin | 250 | 50 |
| Penicillin | 1,000,000 (units/L) | 50,000 (units/L) |
| Vancomycin | 1000 mg or (10 mg/kg) (Intravenously) | 30 |

*(In mg/L dialysate, if not indicated otherwise) From Williams P, Vas S, Layne S, et al: The treatment of peritonitis in patients on CAPD: To Lavage or Not? Peritoneal Dialysis Bulletin 1:14, 1980, and Williams P: Loading doses of antibiotics for the treatment of peritonitis. Perit Dial Bull 1:45, 1981.

prevention and treatment of exit site infections are important. We favor air exposure and daily showering. Currently most of our older patients do not have a catheter dressing but clean the exit site daily in a shower with a Betadine sponge and peroxide rinse. If an exit site infection persists despite this routine, a course of antibiotics, appropriate for the organism, is prescribed. Even though the "shower technique" is preferred, certain patients may do better with an Airstrip dressing (e.g., infants, those with poor hygiene).

**Blood Pressure Control.** The blood pressure in CAPD patients is usually well controlled.[30, 50–52] Nine of the 20 children required antihypertensive management before the initiation of CAPD. Antihypertensive medications were discontinued in six and reduced in two. Hypertension was difficult to control in a five-year-old boy with the hemolytic uremic syndrome who was severely hypertensive for a long time prior to the initiation of CAPD. His blood pressure was elevated even though hydration was normal. It is possible that removal of salt and water by dialysis activated the renin-angiotensin system, resulting in more vasoconstriction. It has been reported that such patients on hemodialysis can have good blood pressure control using angiotensin II blockers.[88] Eventually this child's blood pressure was controlled with low dose captopril.

Our data are in agreement with a recent report by Fine stating that 13 of his 26 patients had hypertension before CAPD and only one child continued to require antihypertensive medications during CAPD.[27] Obviously most hypertension can be controlled with fluid removal, and one must weigh the burden of more dialysis against the risk of medications. It has been suggested that the dialysate of CAPD patients contains considerable amounts of catecholamine metabolites and renin substrate and the removal of such substances may possibly be related to the better control of the hypertension.[31]

**Anorexia.** A considerable amount of glucose is absorbed during CAPD. The energy from glucose absorption accounted for an average of 17% of the total energy intake in 12 of our children. Excessive weight gain, which is frequently encountered in adult CAPD patients, was attributed to this extra energy intake. However, the increase in weight among CAPD patients may be the result of the rise of the total body water, which may be due predominantly to an increase in intracellular fluid volume.[89] In addition, because of the adverse effect on appetite, glucose absorption via the peritoneal route[90] may be responsible for the fact that CAPD patients frequently have an inadequate nutritional status.[89]

The diets of our CAPD patients are based on the daily nutrient intake recommendations (RDNI) reported by the Dietary Standards of Canada.[91] The mean energy intake of 12 children undergoing CAPD was calculated from four-day home food records and was found to be 86% of the RDNI. Similarly, Fine reported that the mean energy intake of children undergoing CAPD was 82 per cent.[27]

Even though the clinical impression is that small children eat poorly, there was no difference between the intake of the younger children and that of the older patients.[83] Some children did require nasogastric tube feeding.

The use of glucose as the osmotic agent may be the cause of anorexia among our patients. Currently we are assessing the possibility of reversing the nutritional disturbances of our CAPD patients by using a dialysate containing amino acids.

## THE FUTURE FOR CAPD IN CHILDREN

CAPD is a useful tool for the management of children with chronic renal failure. Because it is simple to initiate and maintain compared to hemodialysis, more children, especially young patients, are able to be dialysed. The availability of CAPD raises new questions. Should CAPD be offered to children or infants with chronic renal failure who have a growth impairment despite significant residual renal function? Similar questions arise concerning the timing of renal transplantation. In considering growth one should also consider brain growth. Rotundo et al reported serious neurologic sequelae in children who had chronic renal insufficiency as infants.[92] Whether earlier initiation of dialysis and/or renal transplantation for such infants would prevent neurologic abnormalities cannot be answered at present.

For most children, the ultimate treatment goal of ESRD is a successful renal transplant. However, while awaiting a transplant optimal medical care must be provided. It appears that conservative management of chronic renal failure will not enable the child to grow normally and consequently there is a need to improve CAPD. The incidence of peritonitis should continue to fall with improved techniques and connectors to prevent contamination of the tubing or dialysate. The composition of the dialysate will need modifications. The concentration of sodium, lactate, magnesium, and calcium is being modified. The use of amino acids in the dialysate is currently being investigated. Amino acids can act as an osmotic agent to replace glucose in the dialysate and thus preclude the complications of glucose. Also amino acids may improve the nutritional status of children. It may be possible that the amino acid formulae prepared for adults on CAPD may not be acceptable for small children, a fact born out from data on total parenteral nutrition for children.[93] At present most patients require four exchanges per day, especially those who have no native kidney function. Three exchanges or less would prevent the fatigue or "burn out" so often observed in parents or children after a period of time. Ways to regenerate the dialysate and thus reduce the burden of numerous bag changes would be useful.

In conclusion, it would appear that CAPD has been accepted as a useful mode of chronic dialysis treatment for children. It is by no means a solution for ESRD, but it has improved the quality of life for children waiting for a renal transplant.

## REFERENCES

1. Ganter G: Über die Beseitigung giftiger Stoffe aus dem Blute durch Dialyse. Münch Med Wschr 70:478, 1923.
2. Starling AH, Tubby AH: On absorption from and secretion into the serous cavities. J. Physiol (Lond) 16:140, 1894.
3. Putnam PJ: The living peritoneum as a dialyzing membrane. Am J Physiol 63:548, 1922.
4. Odel HM, Ferris DO, Power MH: Peritoneal lavage as an effective means of extrarenal excretion. Am J Med 9:63, 1950.
5. Wear JB, Sisk IR, Trinkle AJ: Peritoneal lavage in the treatment of uremia. J Urol 39:53, 1938.
6. Boen ST: Kinetics of peritoneal dialysis. Medicine 40:243, 1961.
7. Doolan PD, Murphy WP, Wiggins RA, et al: An evaluation of intermittent peritoneal lavage. Am J Med 26:831, 1959.
8. Maxwell MH, Kleeman CA, Twiss MR: Peritoneal dialysis. JAMA 170:917, 1959.
9. Abbott WE, Shea P: The treatment of temporary renal failure by peritoneal lavage. Am J Med Sci 211:312, 1946.

10. Tenckhoff H, Ward G, Boen ST: The influence of dialysate volume and flow rate on peritoneal clearance. Proc Eur Dial Transplant Assoc 2:113, 1965.
11. Boen ST, Mion CM, Curtis FK, Shilipetar G: Periodic peritoneal dialysis using the repeated puncture technique and an automatic cycling machine. Trans Am Soc Artif Intern Organs 10:409, 1964.
12. Tenckhoff H, Shilipetar G, Boen, ST: One year's experience with home peritoneal dialysis. Trans Am Soc Artif Intern Organs 11:11, 1965.
13. Palmer RA, Quinton WE, Gray JF: Prolonged peritoneal dialysis for chronic renal failure. Lancet 1:700, 1964.
14. Tenckhoff H, Schecter H: A bacteriologically safe peritoneal access device. Trans Am Soc Artif Intern Organs 14:181, 1968.
15. Tenckhoff H: Advantages and shortcomings of peritoneal dialysis in the management of chronic renal failure. Séminar uro-Néphrologie Hopital Pitie, 1977, p 107.
16. Oreopoulos DG: Home peritoneal dialysis. Proc Eur Dial Transplant Assoc 12:139, 1975.
17. Feldman W, Baliah, T, Drummond K: Intermittent peritoneal dialysis in the management of chronic renal failure in children. Am J Dis Child 116:30, 1968.
18. Counts S, Hickman R, Garbaccio A, Tenckhoff H: Chronic home peritoneal dialysis in children. Trans Am Soc Artif Intern Organs 19:157, 1973.
19. Brouchard BH, Berger M, Cunningham RJ, et al: Home peritoneal dialysis in children. Trans Am Soc Artif Intern Organs 25:90, 1979.
20. Popovich RP, Moncrief JW, Decherd JF, et al: The definition of a novel portable/wearable equilibrium dialysis technique. Am Soc Artif Intern Organs 5:64, 1976.
21. Popovich RP, Moncrief JW, Nolph KD, et al: Continuous ambulatory peritoneal dialysis. Ann Intern Med 88:449, 1978.
22. Oreopoulos DG, Robson M, Batt S, et al: A simple and safe technique for continuous ambulatory peritoneal dialysis (CAPD). Trans Am Soc Artif Intern Organs 24:484, 1978.
23. Nolph KD, Twardowski ZJ: Clinical management and complications of the CAPD patient. Proceedings of 2nd Annual National Conference on CAPD, 1982, p 210.
24. Khanna R, Oreopoulos DG, Dombros N, et al: Continuous ambulatory peritoneal dialysis (CAPD) after three years: Still a promising treatment. Perit Dial Bull 4:24, 1981.
25. Balfe JW, Vigneux A, Willumsen J, Hardy BE: The use of CAPD in the treatment of children with end-stage renal disease. Perit Dial Bull 4:35, 1981.
26. Alexander SR: Pediatric CAPD: Three years' experience at one center. Proceedings of 2nd Annual National Conference on CAPD, 1982, p 345.
27. Fine RN: Metabolism and growth in pediatric CAPD. Proceedings of 2nd Annual National Conference on CAPD, 1982, p 349.
28. Vigneux A, Hardy BE, Balfe JW: Chronic peritoneal catheter in children—one or two dacron cuffs? Perit Dial Bull 1:151, 1981.
29. Amair P, Khanna R, Leibel B, et al: Continuous ambulatory peritoneal dialysis in diabetics with end-stage renal disease. N Engl J Med 306:625, 1982.
30. Nolph KD, Sorkin MI, Arfania D, et al: Continuous ambulatory peritoneal dialysis: Three years' ex-

perience at a single center. Ann Intern Med 92:609, 1980.

31. Nolph KD: Continuous ambulatory peritoneal dialysis. Am J Nephrol 1:1, 1981.

32. Nolph KD, Sorkin MI, Moore H: Autoregulation of sodium and potassium removal during continuous ambulatory peritoneal dialysis. Trans Am Soc Artif Intern Organs 26:334, 1980.

33. Gotch FA: A quantitative evaluation of small and middle molecules in therapy of uremia. Dial Transplant 9:183, 1980.

34. Popovich RP, Moncrief JW: Kinetic modeling of peritoneal transport. Contrib Nephrol 17:59, 1979.

35. James WPT, Hay AM: Albumin metabolism: effect of the nutritional state and the dietary protein intake. J Clin Invest 47:1958, 1968.

36. Rothschild MA, Oratz AM, Schreiber SS: Albumin metabolism. Gastroenterology 64:324, 1973.

37. Blumenkrantz MJ, Kopple JD, Gutman RA, et al: Methods for assessing nutritional status of patients with renal failure. Am J Clin Nutr 33:1567, 1980.

38. Bianchi R, Mariani G, Giuseppina M, Carmassi F: The metabolism of human serum albumin in renal failure on conservative and dialysis therapy. Am J Clin Nutr 31:1615, 1978.

39. Slatopolsky E, Caglar S, Penell JP, et al: On the pathogenesis of hyperparathyroidism in chronic experimental insufficiency in the dog. J Clin Invest 50:492, 1971.

40. Reiss E, Canterbury MJ, Bercovitz MA, et al: The role of phosphate in the secretion of parathyroid hormone in man. J Clin Invest 49:2146, 1970.

41. Massry SG, Coburn JW, Lee DBN, et al: Skeletal resistance to parathyroid hormone in renal failure: Study in 105 human subjects. Ann Intern Med 78:357, 1973.

42. Hartenbower DL, Coburn JW, Reddy CR, et al: Calciferol metabolism and intestinal calcium transport in the chick with reduced renal function. J Lab Clin Med 83:38, 1974.

43. Mawer EB, Backhouse J, Taylor CM: Failure of formation of 1,25-dihydroxy-cholecalciferol in chronic renal insufficiency. Lancet 1:626, 1973.

44. Avioli LV, Teitelbaum SL: Renal Osteodystrophy. *In*: Pediatric Kidney Disease, Vol. 1. Boston, Little, Brown, 1978, p 366.

45. Mehls O, Ritz E, Kreusser W, et al: Renal osteodystrophy in uraemic children. Clin Endocrinol Metab 9:151, 1980.

46. Slatopolsky E, Gray R, Adams ND, et al: Low serum levels of 1,25(OH)2 D3 are not responsible for the development of secondary hyperparathyroidism in early renal failure. Proceedings of 11th Annual Meeting of American Society of Nephrology 11:99A, 1978.

47. Coburn JW, Brickman AS, Sherrard DJ, et al: Clinical efficacy of 1,25-dihydroxy vitamin D3 in renal osteodystrophy. *In*: Vitamin D: Biochemical, Chemical and Clinical Aspects Related to Calcium Metabolism. Berlin, de Gruyter, 1977, p 657.

48. Kanis JA, Russell RGG, Cundy T, et al: An evaluation of 1-alpha-hydroxy and 1,25 dihydroxy vitamin D3 in the treatment of renal bone disease. Contrib Nephrol 18:12, 1980.

49. Delmez JA, Slatopolsky E, Martin KJ, et al: Minerals, vitamin D, and parathyroid hormone in continuous ambulatory peritoneal dialysis. Kidney Int 21:862, 1982.

50. Moncrief JW: Continuous peritoneal ambulatory dialysis. Dial Transplant 8:1077, 1979.

51. Oreopoulos DG, Robson M, Faller B, et al: Continuous ambulatory peritoneal dialysis. A new era in the treatment of chronic renal failure. Clin Nephrol 11:125, 1979.

52. Goldsmith HJ, Forbes A, Gyde OHB, Summerfield, GL: Hematologic aspects of CAPD. Proceedings of 1st International Symposium on CAPD. Amsterdam, Excerpta Medica, 1979.

53. Dorn D: Clinical observations with CAPD. Nieren-Hochdruckkrankh 5:188, 1979.

54. West CD, Smith WC: An attempt to elucidate the cause of growth retardation in renal disease. Am J Dis Child 91:460, 1956.

55. Bergstrom WH, De Leon AS, Van Gemund JJ: Growth aberrations in renal disease. Pediatr Clin North Am 11:563, 1964.

56. Stickler GB, Bergen BJ: A review: Short stature in renal disease. Pediatr Res 7:978, 1973.

57. Betts PR, Magrath G: Growth pattern and dietary intake of children with chronic renal insufficiency. Br Med J 1:189, 1974.

58. Schärer K, Chantler C, Brunner FP, et al: Combined report on regular dialysis and transplantation of children in Europe, 1974. Proc Eur Dial Transplant Assoc 12:334, 1978.

59. Potter DE, Greifer I: Statural growth of children with renal disease. Kidney Int 14:334, 1978.

60. Wass VJ, Barratt JM, Howarth RV, et al: Home hemodialysis in children. Lancet 1:242, 1977.

61. Cameron JS: The treatment of chronic renal failure in children by regular dialysis and by transplantation. Nephron 11:221, 1973.

62. Borra S, Kaye M: Long-term home hemodialysis in children. Can Med Assoc J 105:927, 1971.

63. Potter D, Larsen D, Leumann E, et al: Treatment of chronic uremia in childhood. II. Hemodialysis. Pediatrics 46:678, 1970.

64. McEnery PT, Gonzalez LL, Martin LW, West CD: Growth and development of children with renal transplants: Use of alternate day steroid therapy. J Pediatr 83:806, 1973.

65. Arbus GS, Wolff E, Williams V, et al: Ongoing protocols in end stage renal disease. 1. Height growth following renal transplantation. 2. Zinc supplementation in predialysis patients. 3. Renal transplants in children less than 6 years of age. Fifth International Pediatric Nephrology Symposium, Philadelphia, Pennsylvania, Oct. 6–10, 1980. *In*: Developments in Nephrology, Volume 3, Pediatric Nephrology. The Hague, Martinus Nijhoff, Publishers, 1981, p 494.

66. Ingelfinger JR, Grupe WE, Harmon WE, et al: Growth acceleration following renal transplantation in children less than 7 years of age. Pediatrics 68:225, 1981.

67. Arbus GS, DeMaria JG, Galiwango T, et al: The first 10 years of the dialysis-transplantation program at the Hospital for Sick Children, Toronto, II. Transplantation. Can Med Assoc J 122:659, 1980.

68. Broyer M, Kleinknecht C, Loirat C, et al: Growth in children treated with long term hemodialysis. J Pediatr 84:642, 1974.

69. Kohaut EC: Growth in children with end-stage renal disease treated with continuous ambulatory peritoneal dialysis for at least one year. Perit Dial Bull 4:159, 1982.

70. Guillot MG, Clermont MJ, Gagnadoux MF, Broyer M: Nineteen months' experience with CAPD in children: main clinical and biological results. Proceedings of the Second International Symposium on Peritoneal Dialysis' Berlin (West), June, 1981, p 203.

71. Conley SB, Brewer ED, Gandy S, Payne W: Chronic continuous peritoneal dialysis in infancy; successful treatment of end-stage renal disease with achievement of normal growth rates. Am J Kidney Dis (Suppl)1:9, 1981.

72. Kleinknecht C, Broyer M, Gagnadoux MF, et al: Growth in children treated with long-term dialysis. A study of 76 patients. Adv Nephrol 9:133, 1980.

73. Simmons JM, Wilson CJ, Potter DE, Holliday MA: Relation of calorie deficiency to growth failure in children on hemodialysis and the growth response to calorie supplementation. N Engl J Med 285:653, 1971.

74. Chantler C, Holliday MA: Growth in children with renal disease with particular reference to the effects of caloric malnutrition: A review. Clin Nephrol 1:230, 1973.

75. Friedman J, Lewy JE: Failure to thrive associated with renal disease. Pediatr Ann 7:11, 1978.

76. Mehls O, Ritz E, Gilli G, Kreusser W: Growth in renal failure. Nephron 21:237, 1978.

77. Betts PR, Magrath G, White RHR: Role of dietary energy supplementation in growth of children with chronic renal insufficiency. Br Med J 1:416, 1977.

78. Hsu AC, Kooh SW, Fraser D, et al: Renal osteodystrophy in children with chronic renal failure: An unexpectedly common and incapacitating complication. Pediatrics 70:742, 1982.

79. Cooke RE, Boyden DG, Haller E: The relationship of acidosis and growth retardation. J. Pediatr 57:326, 1960.

80. Brook CGD, Thompson EN, Marshall WC, Whitehouse RH: Growth of children with thalassaemia major and effect of two different transfusion regimens. Arch Dis Child 44:612, 1969.

81. Kattamis C, Touliatos N, Haidas S, Matsaniotis N: Growth of children with thalassaemia: effect of different transfusion regimens. Arch Dis Child 45:502, 1970.

82. Stefanidis CJ, Hanning R, Hewitt IK, et al: Nutritional status of children managed by continuous ambulatory peritonal dialysis (CAPD). Abstract from Third International Congress on Nutrition and Metabolism in Renal Disease, Sept. 1–4, 1982, Marseille, France. Kidney Int Oct. 1983.

83. Stefanidis CJ, Vigneux AM, Steele BT, et al: Comparison of growth in children treated with continuous ambulatory peritoneal dialysis (CAPD), hemodialysis (HD) and renal transplantation (Tx). Pediatr Res 16:328A, 1982.

84. Guillot M, Broyer M, Chatelineau L: Continuous enteral feeding in pediatric nephrology. Long-term results in children with congenital nephrotic syndrome, severe cystinosis and renal failure. Arch Fr Pediatr 37:497, 1980.

85. Oreopoulos DG, Balfe JW, Khana R, et al: Further experience with the use of amino acid containing dialysate in peritoneal dialysis. *In:* CAPD Update, Moncrief JW, Popovich RP (eds). New York, Masson Publishing Inc, 1981, p. 109.

86. Stefanidis CJ, Balfe JW, Arbus GS, et al: Renal transplantation in children treated with peritoneal dialysis. Perit Dial Bull 3:5, 1983.

87. Cardella CJ: Renal transplantation in patients on peritoneal dialysis. Perit Dial Bull 1:12, 1980.

88. Wauters JP, Waeber B, Brunner HR, et al: Uncontrollable hypertension in patients on hemodialysis: long-term treatment with captopril and salt subtraction. Clin Nephrol 16:86, 1981.

89. Williams P, Kay R, Harrison J, et al: Nutritional and anthropometric assessment of patients on CAPD over one year: contrasting changes in total body nitrogen and potassium. Perit Dial Bull 6:82, 1981.

90. Gahl GM, Baeyer HV, Auerdunk R, et al: Outpatient evaluation of dietary intake and nitrogen removal in continuous ambulatory peritoneal dialysis. Ann Intern Med 94:643, 1981.

91. Canada Department of National Health and Welfare: Dietary standards of Canada, revised, Ottawa, Ont., 1975.

92. Rotundo A, Nevins TE, Lipton M, et al: Progressive encephalopathy in children with chronic renal insufficiency in infancy. Kidney Int 21:486, 1982.

93. Anderson GH, Bryan MH, Jeejeebhoy KN, Corey P: Dose response relationships between amino acid intake and blood levels in newborn infants. Am J Clin Nutr 30:1110, 1977.

# 13

# CAPD in Infants Less Than One Year of Age

*Steven R. Alexander, M.D.*

## HISTORICAL BACKGROUND

The description of continuous ambulatory peritoneal dialysis (CAPD) by Popovich and associates in 1976[1] heralded a period of renewed interest in the treatment of very young infants with irreversible renal failure. As early experience with CAPD in adults was analyzed, it became apparent that this modality offered a number of theoretical advantages to infants and young children when compared to hemodialysis and intermittent peritoneal dialysis: greatly reduced dietary restrictions, simplicity of operation, elimination of need for blood access, and continuous biochemical and fluid control.[2] As first described, however, CAPD was poorly suited for use in infants and young children; with dialysate available only in 2-liter glass bottles it was difficult to reconcile the technique with the needs of infants, whose peritoneal capacities were only a fraction of that volume.

The introduction of dialysate in plastic containers in Canada led to the treatment of the first child with CAPD in Toronto in 1978.[3] The early availability of dialysate in small containers in Canada facilitated the CAPD treatment of infants and young children in that country. In the United States only 2-liter containers were available until July, 1980, and this presented serious obstacles to the care of smaller patients. Pediatric CAPD programs approached these problems in several ways: At first parents simply discarded most of the fluid from a 2-liter bag prior to infusing the remainder, a wasteful procedure which increased infection risks.[4] In some centers small-volume bags were prepared in hospital pharmacies and shipped periodically to individual patients. This process was expensive and beyond the scope of normal hospital pharmacy practices.[5]

In Oregon we taught families to prepare supplies of small-volume bags at home, using empty blood bank transfer packs filled to appropriate volumes from 2-liter bags.[6] Parents usually prepared a one-week supply of small bags at a single sitting, storing them in freezers or refrigerators until needed. This method offered some advantages: as children grew, exchange volumes could be increased in increments; dextrose concentrations could also be modified by the addition of prescribed amounts of 50% dextrose to modulate ultrafiltration, a particularly helpful capability prior to the introduction of the 2.5% dextrose solution. This home-preparation technique was inexpensive and easily adaptable to infants of any size, but its use contributed to problems of "parent fatigue" and theoretically increased the risk of peritonitis.

Recently the home-preparation technique has been replaced by the addition of 250 cc dialysate containers and the development of a "custom-fill" service* for infants who cannot be managed using standard sizes. The ability to prescribe patient-specific exchange volumes has now removed the last purely logistic obstacles hindering extension of CAPD to infants at any age and size.

---

*Travenol Laboratories, Inc., Deerfield, Illinois 60015.

## PATIENT SELECTION FOR CAPD

The only absolute contraindication to the use of CAPD in an infant is the absence of a sufficient peritoneal cavity (e.g., oomphalocele, gastroschisis, or diaphragmatic hernia).[7] During the first four years of pediatric CAPD experience in Oregon we have found the following conditions compatible with management on CAPD: prematurity; obstructive uropathy with cutaneous ureterostomies and vesicostomy; prune-belly syndrome; bilateral Wilms' tumor; recent abdominal surgery; radiotherapy involving the peritoneum; concurrent cancer chemotherapy; and extensive intra-abdominal adhesions requiring lysis to create an adequate peritoneal cavity. In our experience, and that of others, prior ESRD therapy, primary renal disease, and renal transplantation status have had no apparent influence on CAPD outcome in infants and children.[4, 7–9]

With such broad clinical applicability, the selection of infants for treatment with CAPD is likely to be determined by largely subjective factors. Before seriously considering an infant for CAPD, several basic questions should be answered affirmatively:

1. Is it possible that this infant will regain renal function or, failing that, is the infant an eventual candidate for renal transplantation?

2. Is this family sufficiently motivated to learn and to comply with a rigorous home dialysis and chronic care program?

3. Is this facility able to provide the multidisciplinary training and intensive on-going care and support this infant and family will require?

Parent motivation may be the most important determinant of CAPD success.[10] At this time, however, there are no generally accepted criteria by which parental motivation may be reliably assessed. In our experience single parents (with the help of "extended family" members), and parents with limited intelligence and those with nontraditional lifestyles have performed CAPD successfully when sufficiently motivated. In the past four years we have so often seen a motivated parent overcome seemingly insurmountable obstacles that we are now reluctant to deny a trial of CAPD to any family who requests it, regardless of the family's circumstances.

On the other hand, those parents who refuse dialysis or transplantation for their infant children should receive our compassionate support. Legal proceedings by the state to obtain custody of such infants over the objections of their parents are unwarranted at this time.[11]

Temporary medical foster care is an alternative which could be explored when parents desire treatment for their infant, but are unable to provide it themselves. Voluntary relinquishment of custody by the parent(s) and the infant's eventual return to them should be paramount in such arrangements.

## PERITONEAL ACCESS

A reliable peritoneal catheter is the cornerstone of successful CAPD. Surgical placement techniques suitable for use in infants have been suggested by several investigators.[12–14] There is general agreement on a few points: single-cuff catheters are preferred; the single deep cuff must be securely sutured to the peritoneum at the entry site; relatively short straight subcutaneous tunnels are generally recommended; the intraperitoneal portion of the catheter must be trimmed to fit the individual infant.

Most infants have been managed with Tenckhoff catheters. Vigneux and associates have suggested using catheters of different dimensions according to the size of the patient.[14] They propose a "pediatric" catheter for patients weighing 5 to 30 kg and a "neonatal" catheter for infants weighing less than 5 kg. In Oregon we have not found smaller catheters necessary, even in very small infants. Figure 13–1A, shows a standard adult-size Tenckhoff catheter in use in a 2.5 kg neonate. Figure 13–1B, is an abdominal radiograph of this same infant showing the position of the short intraperitoneal portion, which was trimmed to fit this infant intraoperatively.

The catheter placement procedure we currently use in infants is summarized below.[13–15] We now have the manufacturer glue a single dacron cuff at a point 3 cm above the first side hole of a standard adult Tenckhoff catheter. Preoperatively, surgeon and CAPD staff agree on the most desirable location for the tunnel and exit site. This is more important in older children where belt lines and body image concerns are more pertinent.

Intraoperative procedures begin with a 2.0 cm incision at least 1.0 cm below the umbilicus in the midline. The linea alba and peri-

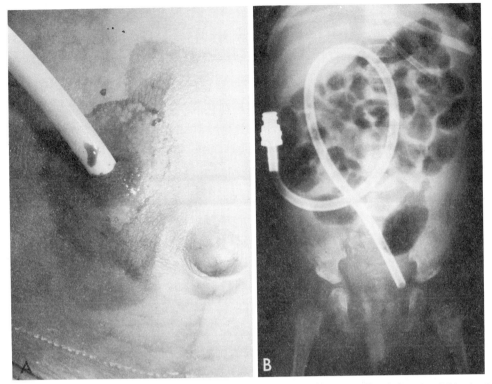

**Figure 13–1.** *A*, Close-up of standard adult Tenckhoff catheter with single deep cuff and short, straight subcutaneous tunnel in use in a 2.5 kg infant. *B*, Abdominal radiograph of this infant showing short intraperitoneal portion of the catheter.

toneum are incised and the peritoneum fixed by two temporary sutures (Fig. 13–2). Digital examination assures that no adhesions of the bowel to the peritoneum are present. A small patch of omentum is then delivered through the 2.0 cm incision in the peritoneum and resected. In our experience the omentum so removed should not exceed an area approximately 10 cm × 10 cm.

The Tenckhoff catheter is threaded over a lubricated catheter guide with a gentle distal curve. The guide and catheter are passed just behind the anterior abdominal wall for several cm, then turned 90° to allow a gentle curve in the deep pelvis on either side. The guide is removed as the catheter is advanced into position. At this point care is taken to trim the distal intraperitoneal portion to allow free movement within the peritoneal cavity. Catheters are better too short than too long. The catheter which is too long can result in painful infusion, poor drainage, and migration under the liver.

The peritoneum is now closed with a permanent purse string suture which is secured at one or more points to the bottom 0.1 cm of the cuff substance (Fig. 13–2). When this

suture is tightened, a "collar" of peritoneum is drawn snugly around the base of the cuff, creating a watertight seal and securely anchoring the catheter in position. Correct positioning of the catheter is confirmed by intraoperative radiographs which should be obtained prior to the construction of the subcutaneous tunnel.

Peritoneography can now be done to look for evidence of an inguinal hernia.[13] A short, straight subcutaneous tunnel is now constructed, usually passing at a slight angle from the midline (Fig. 13–1A). Before the skin incision is closed, continuous low volume dialysis exchanges (15 cc/kg) are instituted to ensure that the catheter is functional and that the peritoneal closure is watertight.

## MECHANICS OF DIALYSIS

CAPD was first proposed for adult patients on the basis of a knowledge of metabolite generation rates and the transport characteristics of the adult peritoneum.[16] Subsequent studies have refined these concepts,[17] leading to the development of guidelines by which

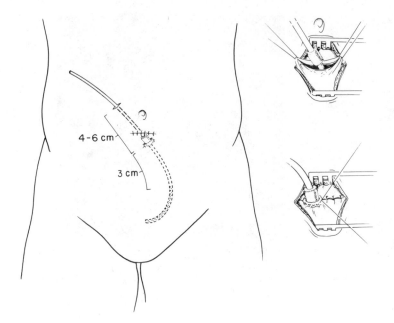

**Figure 13–2.** Schematic drawing of the technique of peritoneal catheter placement used in infants. (See text for details.) (Adapted from Alexander SR, et al, in CAPD update: Continuous Ambulatory Peritoneal Dialysis, Moncrief JW, Popovich RP [Eds]. New York, Masson, 1981.)

CAPD regimens (i.e., exchange volume and frequency) may be reliably prescribed to meet the needs of individual adult patients.[18]

A theoretical framework for CAPD in children has not been well defined. Much less is known about the transport characteristics of the child's peritoneum. Early observations were interpreted as demonstrating increased peritoneal transport capabilities in young patients;[19] this led to the commonly held belief that the peritoneum of the child is in some way more efficient than that of the adult.[20] Recent studies have clarified and limited this concept. It appears now that beyond the neonatal period transport properties are similar in adult and pediatric CAPD patients and can be related on a weight basis.[2, 21]

Not enough is known, however, to allow prescription of CAPD regimens for pediatric patients according to theoretical concepts similar to those used in adults. Current practice relies on guidelines which have largely evolved from empiric observations. Despite somewhat different patient populations, many pediatric CAPD programs have developed similar approaches to prescribing CAPD regimens. Table 13–1 lists CAPD guidelines used in three different pediatric CAPD programs.[4, 7, 9] Note the similarities in protein intake, total daily urea clearance, and average SUN among the three pediatric regimens.

Current practice in Oregon consists of adjusting exchange volumes and frequency for each patient to achieve a total urea clearance of from 210 to 250 cc/kg/day. Total daily urea clearance is the sum of dialysate and urinary urea clearances. In patients on CAPD, dialysate urea clearance is equal to the total drained dialysate volume. Residual renal function can proportionally reduce the amount of dialysis prescribed, although we have been reluctant to prescribe fewer than four exchanges per day. Individual exchange volumes have varied in our patients from 35 to 45 cc/kg. Infants who are not yet "ambulatory" are more tolerant of larger exchange volumes than older infants and children in

**Table 13–1.** REPRESENTATIVE PEDIATRIC CAPD REGIMENS

| Reference | Exchange Volume (cc/kg) | Total Daily Urea Clearance (cc/kg) | Average Daily Protein Intake (gm/kg) | Average SUN (mg/dl) |
|---|---|---|---|---|
| Salusky et al[9] | 43 | 238 | 2.4 | 77 |
| Potter et al[4] | 33–50 | 164–224* | 2.0 | 70 |
| Alexander et al[7] | 35–45 | 211 | 2.3 | 77 |
| Adult Reference[17] | 25 | 138 | 1.4 | 89 |

*Estimated from data in Reference 4.

whom abdominal distension may limit physical activity at exchange volumes approaching 50 cc/kg.

Careful nitrogen balance studies in stable adults on CAPD have shown that when total urea clearance is 138 cc/kg/day and protein intake is 1.4 grams/kg/day SUN averages 89 mg/dl and nitrogen balance is slightly positive.[17] (Adult reference values are included in Table 13–1). Similar studies have not been done in children. What has been shown is that on a CAPD regimen which provides a daily total urea clearance of at least 210 cc/kg a child who ingests up to 2.3 grams/kg/day of protein and 80 to 100% of the RDA for calories will maintain an average SUN of less than 80 mg/dl.[7, 9] These observations are at least reasonable. Considering the child's ability to retain nitrogen for growth, it might be expected that a protein intake 64% greater than that of an average adult patient when considered on a weight basis would be well tolerated when the child's CAPD regimen represented a 52% increase in total daily urea clearance over that of the adult.

A proper understanding of these relationships must await the appropriate metabolic balance studies in children on CAPD. In addition, no claims can be made for the adequacy of the dialysis provided by the regimens described above. Until this extraordinarily complex issue is better understood, guidelines for prescribing CAPD for infants will remain largely empiric.

## ULTRAFILTRATION (UF) AND WATER BALANCE

Early observations suggested that ultrafiltration (UF) was more difficult in infants and younger children on CAPD owing to more avid dextrose absorption from the dialysate.[12] In one study children under three years of age showed more rapid declines in dialysate dextrose concentration and osmolality when compared to older children and adults.[22] However, this study did not control for relative differences in exchange volumes. Very low exchange volumes (20 cc/kg) were used in the youngest patients, who also had the worst UF. Recent studies have confirmed a correlation between exchange volume and UF rate in young infants.[23] In another study, maximum ultrafiltration rates determined in four young children were found to be similar to adult values when scaled by body weight.[2] Thus, while the impression remains that younger infants require higher dialysate dextrose concentrations to achieve adequate UF, this phenomenon has yet to be rigorously demonstrated, and there is some evidence to suggest that, beyond the newborn period, factors other than patient age may be more important.

CAPD regimens are designed to maintain body water homeostasis by balancing output (insensible, stool, residual renal, and UF losses) with intake. Water requirements for growth (4.3 to 1.3 cc/kg/day at 1 and 4 months of age respectively) and the water produced by specific dynamic action when food is metabolized may be ignored for practical purposes.[24] The water content of solid foods commonly fed to infants is substantial, however, and may be a factor in determining daily fluid balance.

The normal infant weighing <10 kg requires 45 cc/kg/day to replace insensible losses and about 5 to 10 cc/kg/day to replace water lost in the stool.[24] At least another 50 cc/kg/day is usually provided to allow the kidneys to excrete solutes in a near isotonic urine. The infant with negligible urine output managed on CAPD requires similar insensible and stool water loss replacements. Total fluid requirement will equal insensible water losses plus stool water losses plus UF.

UF rate can normally be influenced by adjustment of:

1. Dialysate dextrose concentration,
2. Duration of exchange,
3. Exchange volume.

There are probably other physiologic processes involved. Reported daily net UF in children on CAPD has ranged from 24 to 35 cc/kg.[4, 7] We and others have attempted to match the CAPD regimen to the spontaneous intake of the child, prescribing a diet which is not limited in any way.[7, 25] Ad lib fluid intake in our youngest patients has rarely exceeded 80 to 90 cc/kg/day, and most require encouragement to drink even that much. Thus we have elected to use 35 cc/kg/day as a reasonable, though arbitrary, net UF for infants without residual urine output. Total daily fluid turnover in these patients then averages 85 to 90 cc/kg/day, although there are wide fluctuations.

Control of UF must also be used to guard body fluid homeostasis. Whenever there are increased body fluid losses, as with diarrhea, emesis, fever, etc., or diminished intake, as is often seen with peritonitis or almost any intercurrent illness,[25] the CAPD regimen must be promptly adjusted if serious dehydration is to be avoided. In our experience UF is not significantly reduced even in the face of up to 10% dehydration. Dialysate solutions containing 1.5% dextrose and prolonged dwell periods may be used to deliver fluids to the dehydrated infant.

The further impact of nutritional goals on UF requirements will be considered in the following sections.

## NUTRITION AND GROWTH IN INFANTS ON CAPD

### Energy

Energy requirements during the first year of life are enormous. The three-month-old needs nearly three times more energy per unit body mass than the adult for normal metabolic processes and to fuel normal growth.[26] Growth occurs in the normal infant only when energy (and protein) intakes are sufficiently in excess of requirements for basal metabolism and physical activity. In the first few months of life when activity is limited and growth rate is spectacular, up to 35% of consumed calories are expended for growth.[27] Considered another way, each gram of tissue gained requires 5 kcal over and above basal energy requirements. For infants gaining almost 30 gm/day during the first four months of life, daily energy requirements for normal growth may be as much as 30 to 40 kcal/kg over basal requirements.[27]

Growth has been used as the critical variable in determining energy requirements for healthy infants. Breast-fed male infants growing normally ingest from 100 to 131 kcal/kg/day during the first year of life.[27] Daily requirements for energy during the first year of life have been estimated as 115 kcal/kg from birth to six months and 105 kcal/kg from 6 to 12 months of age.[28] The critical nature of these levels of intake is suggested not only by the observation of subnormal growth on lower intakes but by the observation that infants who ingest more calories/kg/day do not increase statural growth, but do gain weight, presumably by addition of adipose tissue.[29]

In a series of classic experiments Fomon and associates further demonstrated the homeostatic importance of consistent daily energy intake.[30] Infants beyond 40 days of age were found to regulate ad lib feeding such that total daily energy intake was kept nearly constant, despite ingestion of formulas of differing caloric density. Infants spontaneously consumed less high-calorie formula (100 kcal/100 cc) than standard formula (67 kcal/100 cc), such that total daily energy intake on the two formulas remained nearly identical. Infants fed a more dilute formula (53 kcal/100 cc) consumed vast quantities in an apparent attempt to achieve the same total daily energy intake observed when they were fed standard formula. Infants were also observed to abruptly reduce intake of a high calorie formula (133 kcal/100 cc) at the first feeding when switched from standard formula. The mechanisms underlying these remarkably precise regulatory behaviors (which constitute "appetite" in perhaps its most basic form) are unknown.

Energy requirements for normal growth in infants with renal failure have not been established. It has been difficult to achieve levels of energy intake in such infants which would be considered adequate for normal growth in healthy infants.[31] Spontaneous intake, so well regulated in the healthy infant, is markedly reduced in the child with renal failure for reasons which are not clear.[32] For the child on CAPD the difficulties encountered in feeding are particularly frustrating since diet is essentially unlimited.

Energy requirements for catch-up growth are also unknown. Spontaneous energy intake observed in children recovering from protein-calorie malnutrition is often as high as 200 kcal/kg/day during the period of most dramatic catch-up growth.[39] Protein intake in these children is proportionally increased to 4 to 5 gm/kg/day.[33] There may be unique factors at work in children with ESRD which limit the effectiveness of supernormal energy intake in promoting catch-up growth, some of which have been discussed in Chapter 3. However, it seems reasonable to postulate that catch-up growth in such infants cannot be expected in the absence of energy intake which exceeds to some unknown degree 100% of the RDA for a child of the same height and sex.

In an earlier section, guidelines for CAPD were given which yielded an average daily fluid intake of 85 to 90 cc/kg in very young infants with negligible urine output. If energy requirement is set at 115 kcal/kg/day and dialysate dextrose absorption provides 8 kcal/kg/day,[4, 9] feedings must have a caloric density of 1.2 kcal/cc (Table 13–2) to achieve total energy goals. Augmentation of standard formulas with glucose polymers and medium chain triglycerides has been used to achieve these goals.[7, 25]

## Protein

Dietary protein is required by the normal infant to provide essential amino acids and nitrogen for metabolism, to replace obligatory losses, and to support growth. During the first year of life protein requirements are increased in proportion to energy requirements since the human diet must contain a relatively constant composition of protein to available energy from fat and carbohydrate to ensure proper utilization.[34] As with energy, dietary protein requirements have been estimated by determining the intake which is compatible with a satisfactory rate of growth.

Healthy breast-fed infants grow normally with a protein intake of 1.6 gm/100 kcal energy ingested.* When protein sources other than human milk are used, the dietary protein requirement is arbitrarily increased to 1.9 gm/100 kcal for the first four months of life.[34] Thus the infant required to ingest about 115 kcal/kg/day must also ingest about 2.2 gm/kg/day of protein. This requirement is reduced during the latter half of the first year of life to 1.7 gm/100 kcal or 2.0 gm/kg/day.[34]

The infant on CAPD must also replace dialysate protein losses, which in younger patients have been found to average 0.3 gm/kg/day.[7, 12] Protein losses are substantially greater during episodes of peritonitis.†

Suggested *minimal* daily intakes of energy and calories for infants less than one year of age on CAPD are given in Table 13–2. Intakes at these levels are theoretically sufficient to meet protein-calorie requirements for normal growth.[27, 28] There are as yet no data to support the adequacy of intakes at these levels for infants with ESRD, and catch-up growth may not occur unless both protein and energy intakes exceed the recommendations in Table 13–2. Of course, if nutri-

tional therapy and CAPD are instituted prior to the appearance of severe growth failure, catch-up growth may not be needed.

Although the dietary goals listed in Table 13–2 should be considered minimum requirements, it is unlikely that infants with ESRD will spontaneously ingest sufficient energy and protein to meet even those requirements. Chronic nasogastric tube feeding should be considered in all such infants when their spontaneous intake falls below 100% of the recommendations in Table 13–2. It should be recalled that intakes of 100% of the RDA may suffice only to permit (promote) normal growth and may be insufficient to yield catch-up growth.

## Amino Acids

Requirements for the nine essential amino acids are easily met by healthy infants when protein intake is adequate and of high quality. Estimated daily requirements for essential amino acids in infants less than one year of age are listed in Table 13–3.[34] Nearly one-third of the dietary protein requirement in growing infants must be supplied as essential amino acids. The high quality of human milk can be seen from the fact that 45% of its protein is supplied as essential amino acids (Table 13–3).

Minimum daily requirements for essential amino acids are increased in patients on CAPD at least by an amount sufficient to replace dialysate losses. Stable adult CAPD patients in slightly positive nitrogen balance were found to lose amino acids (essential plus nonessential) into the dialysate at a rate of 46 mg/kg body weight/day.[17] Adult requirements for essential amino acids are quite low when compared to infant requirements (Table 13–3).[28] Thus even if a majority of the measured dialysate amino acid losses were essential amino acids, total daily requirements in adults on CAPD would remain below 125 mg/kg body weight. This requirement should be easily met by ingestion of proteins of even marginal biologic value, although high-quality proteins are to be preferred for all ESRD patients.

The magnitude of dialysate amino acid losses in infants on CAPD has not been reported previously. We measured amino acids in 24-hour collections of dialysate drained from two infants who began CAPD during the first year of life. Samples were obtained

---

*Based on human milk in which 100 cc contains 1.1 gm protein and provides 75 kcal.

†We measure 24-hour dialysate protein losses periodically and adjust dietary guidelines accordingly. During episodes of peritonitis, dietary protein requirements probably are increased by an additional 0.5 to 1.0 gm/kg/day.

**Table 13–2.** MINIMUM DAILY DIETARY INTAKES AND CAPD GUIDELINES FOR YOUNG INFANTS*

| Height Age[1] (months) | Total Energy Requirement[2] (kcal/kg) | Average Energy from Dialysate[3] (kcal/kg) | Net Energy Requirement from Diet (kcal/kg) | Protein Requirement[4] (gm/100 kcal) | Average Dialysate Protein Losses[5] (gm/kg) | Total Dietary Protein Requirement (gm/kg/day) | Allowable Fluid Intake[6] (cc/kg/day) | Caloric Density and Protein Content of Feedings (kcal/cc) | (gm/100 kcal) |
|---|---|---|---|---|---|---|---|---|---|
| 0–4 | 115 | 8 | 107 | 1.9 | 0.3 | 2.5 | 90 | 1.2 | 2.2 |
| 4–6 | 115 | 8 | 107 | 1.7 | 0.3 | 2.3 | 90 | 1.2 | 2.0 |
| 6–12 | 105 | 8 | 97 | 1.7 | 0.3 | 2.1 | 90 | 1.1 | 1.8 |

*Based on requirements to sustain normal growth rates in healthy infants. Requirements for catch-up growth cannot be determined from present data, but are likely to be somewhat higher.
[1]Chronologic age of normal child (50th centile curve) of same sex and equivalent height.
[2]Reference 28.
[3]References 10, 12.
[4]References 28, 34.
[5]References 7, 12.
[6]Assumes negligible urine output, insensible and stool water loss = 55 cc/kg/day, ultrafiltration of 35 cc/kg/day. (See text.)

**Table 13–3.** MINIMUM DAILY REQUIREMENTS FOR THE ESSENTIAL AMINO ACIDS

| Amino Acid | Infants < 12 months[a] (mg/100 kcal) | Adults[b] (mg/kg body wt) | Amount Provided by Human Milk[c] (mg/100 kcal) |
|---|---|---|---|
| Histidine | 26 | ? | 33 |
| Isoleucine | 66 | 12 | 102 |
| Leucine | 132 | 16 | 150 |
| Lysine | 101 | 12 | 109.5 |
| Phenylalanine | 57 | 16[d] | 72 |
| Methionine | 24 | 10[e] | 37.5 |
| Threonine | 59 | 8 | 75 |
| Tryptophan | 16 | 3 | 27 |
| Valine | 83 | 14 | 105 |
| Total | 564 | 91 | 711 |

[a]Reference 34.

[b]Reference 28.

[c]Adapted from: Foman SJ, Filer LJ Jr: Milks and formulas. *In:* Fomon SJ (Ed), Infant Nutrition. Philadelphia, W. B. Saunders Company, 1974, p 362.

[d]Phenylalanine and tyrosine.

[e]Methionine and cystine.

once from Patient #1 (at age 16 months) and three times from Patient #2 (at ages 3, 7.5, and 10 months). Results of these assays are summarized in Table 13–4, where data on Patient #2 are shown as the average of three separate determinations. Total daily essential amino acid losses in these infants did not exceed 10 to 13 mg/kg/day, representing an increase over normal dietary essential amino acid requirements of less than 3%.

Amino acids were first added to peritoneal dialysate as a nutritional supplement by Gjessing.[35] More recently, Balfe and associates described the addition of amino acids to peritoneal dialysate in an infant on CAPD.[12] Balfe used a preparation which contained a mixture of amino acids* in only the overnight exchange; more frequent use resulted in an unacceptably high SUN (Balfe JW: personal communication).

Poor growth and inadequate dietary protein intake exhibited by our Patient #1 prompted us to begin intraperitoneal amino acid supplementation during this infant's thirteenth month on CAPD. We used an amino acid preparation which contained only essential amino acids,† adding it to every exchange to achieve a final concentration of approximately 0.5 gm essential amino acids/ 100 cc of dialysate. SUN remained stable or decreased slightly after addition of amino acids in this concentration.

**Table 13–4.** DIALYSATE AMINO ACID LOSSES IN TWO INFANTS ON CAPD (mg/kg/24 HOURS)

| | Patient #1* | Patient #2** |
|---|---|---|
| Histidine | 1.9 | 1.7 |
| Isoleucine | 0.8 | 1.1 |
| Leucine | 1.3 | 1.5 |
| Lysine | 2.0 | 2.3 |
| Phenylalanine | 0.9 | 1.5 |
| Methionine | 0.3 | 0.6 |
| Threonine | 0.9 | 2.0 |
| Tryptophan | NA | NA |
| Valine | 1.9 | 2.3 |
| Total Essential Amino Acids | 10.0 | 13.0 |
| Serine | 1.2 | 2.0 |
| Glutamine | 16.8 | 12.4 |
| Glutamic Acid | 2.3 | 5.7 |
| Glycine | 2.2 | 4.3 |
| Alanine | 4.9 | 5.8 |
| Tyrosine | 0.6 | 1.2 |
| Ornithine | 0.7 | 0.9 |
| Arginine | 1.0 | 1.8 |
| ½ Cystine | 1.5 | 1.0 |
| Asp. Acid | NA | 0.5 |
| Hydroxyproline | NA | 0.6 |
| Asparagine | NA | 0.7 |
| Proline | NA | 6.2 |
| Citrulline | NA | 1.9 |
| Total Non-Essential Amino Acids | 31.2 | 45.0 |
| Grand Total Dialysate Amino Acids | 41.2 | 58.0 |

NA = Not assayed

*Single determination, age 16 months.

**Average of three determinations, ages 3, 7.5, and 10 months.

*Travasol, Baxter Travenol Laboratories, Inc.

†Nephrimine, McGaw Laboratories, Inc.

**Table 13–5.** PLASMA AMINO ACID LEVELS WITH AND WITHOUT INTRAPERITONEAL ESSENTIAL AMINO ACID SUPPLEMENTATION IN AN INFANT ON CAPD

| Time on CAPD (Months) | Amino Acid Supplement Used?* | Avg. Dietary Protein Intake (gm/kg/day) | Total Essential Amino Acids (μM/L) | Total Non-Essential Amino Acids (μM/L) | Essential/ Non-Essential |
|---|---|---|---|---|---|
| Normal Reference** | | 2.0 | 626 | 1265 | 0.49 |
| 1 | No | 0.6 | 465 | 1776 | 0.26 |
| 8 | No | 1.0 | 824 | 2313 | 0.36 |
| 12 | Yes (Day #4 of Supplementation) | 1.9 | 1048 | 2865 | 0.37 |
| 15 | Yes (Month #3 of Supplementation) | 1.7 | 1390 | 3290 | 0.42 |
| 32 | No (Supplement discontinued for 1 month) | 2.9 | 1074 | 2851 | 0.38 |
| 37 | No (Supplement discontinued for 6 months) | 1.0 | 687 | 2305 | 0.30 |

*Nephrimine (McGaw) 0.25 to 0.5 gm/100 cc dialysate in all 5 daily exchanges.
**Adapted from Delaporte C, Jean G, Broyer M: Free plasma and muscle amino acids in uremic children. Am J Clin Nutr 31:1647, 1978.

We could document absorption of from 70% to 96% (mean = 85%) of administered essential amino acids, resulting in a net gain of nearly 650 mg/kg body weight/day of essential amino acids in this infant. Treatment continued for a total of 14 months. Plasma amino acid concentrations* were followed and are summarized in Table 13–5. Note that total essential amino acid concentration was diminished prior to starting intraperitoneal amino acid supplements and then rose and remained above normal during supplementation. The ratio of essential to nonessential amino acids also increased, yet remained below normal despite supplementation with only essential amino acids.

While requirements for essential amino acids were exceeded in this infant by amounts absorbed from the dialysate during supplementation, total protein intake remained suboptimal and growth was not improved. There were no adverse effects seen, but it could be argued that oral supplementation with high-quality dietary protein (via nasogastric tube feeding) could yield a similar intake of essential amino acids at a fraction of the cost of intraperitoneal supplements. Further studies are needed to define the potential role for intraperitoneal amino acid supplements in infants on CAPD.

**Fat**

Fat serves primarily as a source of energy in the diets of normal infants, routinely providing from 30% to 55% of total caloric intake.[36] While essential fatty acids have been identified (primarily linoleic acid and its derivatives), requirements are relatively small and are easily met. Only 3% of an infant's total daily calories (5% to 8% of dietary fat) need be provided as essential fatty acids to ensure normal growth and prevent clinical fatty acid deficiency disorders.[37]

Human milk and formulas containing one of a number of vegetable oils are rich in essential fatty acids and are well tolerated by infants; cow milk may not be as well tolerated, largely because butterfat is poorly absorbed from the infant's gastrointestinal tract when ingested in moderate to large quantities.[38] Thus when butterfat accounts for more than 35% of total caloric content of the diet, substantial fecal fat losses may occur.[38]

Formulas with increased caloric density often contain large concentrations of supplemental fat, usually as corn oil or medium chain triglycerides. As long as fat provides no more than 55% of total calories, such formulas can probably be safely used for periods of many months.[33]

Long-term use of diets high in fats in infants on CAPD may not be desirable. Pe-

---

*Guidelines for obtaining plasma amino acid levels in children on CAPD in a near fasting state have been suggested by I. Salusky, M.D. (personal communication) and were followed in most instances in our patients: a 1.5% exchange is used for at least eight hours overnight, during which the child is kept NPO. In the morning the overnight exchange is drained and a plasma sample for amino acid assay is drawn prior to infusing the next exchange.

diatric CAPD patients have been reported to develop hypertriglyceridemia, thought to be a consequence of constant dextrose absorption from the dialysate.[4, 9] Serum cholesterol levels, however, remain within normal limits in most children on CAPD.[4, 6, 9] Our two youngest CAPD patients described earlier in this chapter showed consistently high-normal serum cholesterol levels (mean = 230 ± 26 mg/dl) and mild to moderate elevations of serum triglycerides (mean = 307 ± 128 mg/dl) over many months of CAPD (Alexander SR, unpublished data).

The potential importance of altered lipid metabolism in infants on CAPD is unknown. Concerns have been raised regarding the possible acceleration of atherosclerosis in patients with hyperlipidemia.[9] Similar concerns have been raised over diets high in fat content.[28] While these concerns remain theoretical at this time, it would seem prudent to closely monitor lipid metabolism in infants on CAPD, and to avoid feeding these infants excessively, especially if their diet is high in fat content. Obesity and hyperlipidemia would seem questionable substitutes for undernutrition in such infants who are already at substantial risk for early onset of vascular disease by virtue of their renal failure. (One must hasten to add that, if forced to choose between obesity and undernutrition, one or the other, obesity is unquestionably the better choice!)

## Sodium

Throughout the first year of life the recommended daily intake of sodium for normal infants is only 6 to 8 mEq.[28] Infants eating solids and fed formulas based on cow milk may exceed these recommendations tenfold.[28] However, when intake consists entirely of breast milk or a proprietary formula with a similarly low sodium content (human milk sodium concentration averages 7 mEq/liter), sodium depletion is avoided by younger infants only because absolute sodium requirements are actually about one-third of the recommended daily allowance.[36]

When an infant is maintained on CAPD, dietary sodium intake must be substantially increased to replace dialysate sodium losses. When serum sodium is greater than 132 mEq/liter (the concentration of sodium in peritoneal dialysate routinely available in the United States), sodium will be removed from the blood by virtue of both diffusion and

ultrafiltration. Eventual dialysate sodium concentration approaches that of serum, and if the amount of ultrafiltrate is known the daily sodium loss can be predicted.

Both infants described earlier in this chapter required supplemental sodium to avoid hyponatremia. Patient #1 experienced a rapid fall in serum sodium from 136 mEq/L to 118 mEq/L before a method could be developed by which sodium supplementation could be accomplished in an exclusively breast-fed infant. Eventually, feeding at the breast was abandoned, although breast milk, supplemented with sodium, protein, carbohydrate, and fat, remained the basis for this infant's formulas for a number of months thereafter.

We now measure dialysate sodium losses early in an infant's course on CAPD and supplement the diet accordingly. This is not always easy, as in the case of Patient #2 who did not tolerate the addition of 40 mEq of NaCl per liter of formula (hypotonic saline can be a potent emetic!). Sodium depletion was prevented temporarily in this infant by increasing dialysate sodium concentration to 140 mEq/L while advancing the dietary sodium supplement at a rate which did not cause vomiting.

## Potassium

The normal infant requires only 2.3 mEq/day of potassium during the first year of life.[28] Dietary intake often greatly exceeds this amount when formulas are based on cow milk. Infants on CAPD usually maintain normal serum [K⁺] despite limited ability to remove potassium via dialysis.[4, 7, 9, 12]

In our experience, infants on CAPD do not tolerate wide swings in potassium intake. Hyperkalemia has occurred when infants were allowed to limit intake to foods high in potassium (fruit juices, applesauce, etc.). Hypokalemia should also be suspected when stool losses are increased by diarrhea or when dietary intake falters.

Hypokalemia may be forestalled by the addition of KCl to the dialysate. We add 4 mEq KCl/L of dialysate when serum [K⁺] is ≤ 3.5 mEq/L until dietary K can be increased to restore normal serum levels. Hypokalemia cannot be treated by adding KCl in higher concentrations to the dialysate. Dialysate containing KCl in higher concentrations is painful and may damage the peritoneum. Similarly, hyperkalemia is poorly treated with CAPD; cation exchange resins and IPD must be used.

## Vitamins

In the absence of any published data on vitamin metabolism in children on CAPD, only the vitamin requirements of normal infants can be used as a rough guide. These are listed in Table 13–6[28]

Studies of vitamin A metabolism in adults[39] and children[40] with chronic renal failure have demonstrated increased plasma levels and increased total body stores of this fat-soluble vitamin. A pathologic role for the excessive amounts of vitamin A seen in these patients has been proposed;[41] it is currently recom-

mended that adults with renal insufficiency avoid vitamin A supplementation in any form.[41]

It is interesting to note that vitamin A toxicity is manifested in infants and children as anorexia, irritability, increased intracranial pressure, desquamation of the skin and characteristic skeletal abnormalities.[42] Daily requirements for vitamin A do not exceed 2000 IU throughout the first year of life;[28] almost all formulas and milks currently in use provide at least this minimum daily requirement for vitamin A and many provide two or three times this amount.

Plasma vitamin A levels have not been reported in infants and children on CAPD. Until more is known, it seems reasonable to avoid vitamin A supplementation in these infants if the diet provides 2000 IU/day.

**Table 13–6.** RECOMMENDED DIETARY ALLOWANCES FOR VITAMINS AND CERTAIN MINERALS DURING THE FIRST YEAR OF LIFE†

| | Age | | |
| --- | --- | --- | --- |
| | <6 Months | 6–12 Months | Unit of Measure |
| *Vitamins* | | | |
| A* | 420 | 400 | μg retinol equivalents (1 retinol equivalent = 3.33 IU vitamin A activity from retinol or 10 IU vitamin A activity from β-carotene.) |
| D** | 10 | 10 | μg cholecalciferol (10 μg cholecalciferol = 400 IU of vitamin D) |
| K* | 12 | 10–20 | μg |
| E | 3 | 4 | mg *d*-α-tocopherol equivalents |
| C | 35 | 35 | mg |
| Thiamin | 0.3 | 0.5 | mg |
| Riboflavin | 0.4 | 0.6 | mg |
| Niacin | 6 | 8 | mg |
| B-6** | 0.3 | 0.6 | mg |
| Folacin** | 30 | 45 | μg |
| B-12 | 0.5 | 1.5 | μg |
| Biotin | 35 | 50 | μg |
| Pantothenic Acid | 2 | 3 | mg |
| *Minerals* | | | |
| Calcium** | 360 | 540 | mg |
| Phosphorus | 240 | 360 | mg |
| Magnesium* | 50 | 70 | mg |
| Iron | 10 | 15 | mg |
| Zinc | 3 | 5 | mg |
| Iodine | 40 | 50 | μg |
| Copper* | 0.5–0.7 | 0.7–1.0 | mg |
| Manganese | 0.5–0.7 | 0.7–1.0 | mg |
| Fluoride | 0.1–0.5 | 0.2–1.0 | mg |
| Chromium | 0.01–0.04 | 0.02–0.06 | mg |
| Selenium | 0.01–0.04 | 0.02–0.06 | mg |
| Molybdenum | 0.03–0.06 | 0.04–0.08 | mg |

*Supplements containing these nutrients should probably be avoided by infants on peritoneal dialysis (see text).
†Adapted from Reference 28.
**Requirements for these nutrients may be substantially greater in infants on peritoneal dialysis (see text).

There is general agreement that folic acid and pyridoxine are required by uremic adults in amounts greater than the recommended daily allowances.[43] A daily supplement of 1 mg of folic acid (2.5 × RDA), and 10 to 20 mg of pyridoxine (5 to 10 × RDA) is currently recommended for uremic adults.[41] Similar adjustments are probably indicated in uremic infants. Thus at least 0.25 mg of folic acid and 3 to 6 mg of pyridoxine should probably be given daily to infants on CAPD.

The status of the water-soluble vitamins in infants on CAPD is unknown. Supplementation of these compounds to ensure that at least the RDA for normal infants is received each day seems appropriate. If water-soluble vitamins are lost into the dialysate to the same degree as most other water-soluble nutrients, infants on CAPD may require several times the RDA for these substances.

## Minerals and Trace Elements

Current recommended dietary allowances for minerals and trace elements are listed in Table 13–6[28] Little is known about requirements in infants on CAPD.

**Zinc.** The identification of a syndrome of nutritional zinc deficiency characterized by anorexia, poor growth, delayed skeletal maturation, delayed puberty, mental depression and lethargy, increased susceptibility to infection, delayed wound healing, hypogeusia and dysgeusia, alopecia, and various skin lesions was certain to draw the attention of those caring for children with ESRD.[44] Moreover, dietary zinc requirements are relatively large and not as easily met as those for other trace elements.[44] Attempts to find evidence of zinc deficiency in dialysis patients have been complicated by difficulties inherent in its measurement and the problems with interpretation of plasma versus tissue levels.[44]

We measured plasma zinc levels in the two infants on CAPD described throughout this chapter. Patient #1 was two years of age at the time zinc levels were first obtained. Average plasma zinc was within the normal range at 145 μgm/dl in this patient receiving no zinc supplements.[40] Patient #2 had plasma zinc determined only once, when she was six months of age. Her plasma zinc level of 67 μgm/dl is below the normal range for older children[40] but may be acceptable in a young infant for whom normal ranges of plasma levels have not been established.[44]

Others have found normal plasma zinc levels in older children on hemodialysis.[40] Normal plasma levels probably do not rule out zinc deficiency in the absence of data on zinc in the tissues. It seems reasonable then to ensure the RDA for zinc with supplementation, but unlikely that zinc deficiency is of major importance in the pathophysiology of the anorexic syndrome seen in these children. At least in our patients daily zinc supplementation has not produced the surge of appetite seen in otherwise normal, zinc-deficient children when their diet is supplemented.[44]

**Copper.** Copper deficiency produces a characteristic syndrome of anemia, neutropenia, and osteoporosis.[44] Chronic copper toxicity is extremely rare, except as seen with Wilson's disease. Accumulation of copper in liver, brain, kidneys, and cornea characterizes the response to chronic copper intoxication by normal individuals.[44]

Serum copper levels remain mildly to moderately elevated during CAPD treatment in Patients #1 and #2 (serum copper: mean = 185 ± 28 μgm/dl, normal = 27 to 153 μgm/dl).[40] Normal serum copper levels in children on hemodialysis have been reported previously.[40]

Until more is known, copper supplementation is probably to be avoided in children on CAPD unless diets are deficient.

## GROWTH IN INFANTS TREATED WITH CAPD

CAPD offers children several theoretical advantages over existing dialysis methods, differences which were hoped would lead to improved growth.[6, 12] These potential advantages were largely nutritional: essentially unrestricted diets and absorption of a continuous carbohydrate energy boost from the dialysate. Steady state biochemical and fluid control was considered more likely to facilitate growth than the fluctuations seen with hemodialysis.[2]

Growth in children on CAPD, while better than that seen in hemodialyzed children,[46] has not met early expectations in most instances. Statural growth averaged 50% to 68% of expected in early reports,[7, 9, 10, 12] although near normal growth was seen in a few children.[45] Because of the small numbers of patients and relatively short observation

**Table 13–7.** CORRELATION OF PTH CONTROL AND PROTEIN AND CALORIE INTAKE WITH GROWTH (RDA = RECOMMENDED DIETARY ALLOWANCE)*

| No. of Patients | Growth | Aver. PTH <2 × Normal | Aver. Protein Intake >2 gm/kg/day | Aver. Caloric Intake >100% RDA |
|---|---|---|---|---|
| 5 | >100% of expected | 5/5 | 4/5 | 4/5 |
| 3 | 80–100% of expected | 2/3 | 1/3 | 2/3 |
| 3 | <80% of expected | 1/3 | 1/3 | 0/3 |

*From: Kohaut EC: Growth in children with end-stage renal disease treated with CAPD for at least one year. Perit Dial Bull 2:159, 1982.

periods on CAPD, interpretation of these findings is difficult.

Improved growth was recently reported by Kohaut in a group of 11 children, 3 months to 16 years of age at onset of CAPD, each of whom had been treated with CAPD for at least 12 months when studied.[25] Five of the 11 children exhibited growth rates in excess of 100% of expected and three others grew at rates ≥ 88% of expected. There were three infants less than one year of age in this group whose growth rates were 94%, 108%, and 67% of expected.

Kohaut analyzed the pattern of growth seen in these 11 children in relation to energy and protein intake and control of hyperparathyroidism. Table 13–7 shows that of the five children whose growth exceeded 100% of expected, all had average serum PTH levels below twice normal, while four of five had daily protein intakes of > 2 gm/kg/day and energy intakes >100% of the RDA for children of the same height and sex. Of the children who grew less well, three had similar control of hyperparathyroidism but only two had equivalent intake of either energy or protein.

These encouraging preliminary results suggest that when meticulous attention to protein and energy intake is combined with aggressive treatment of renal bone disease, normal or near normal growth is indeed

possible in a majority of children treated with CAPD; catch-up growth may also be possible for many of them.[25]

Unfortunately, growth observed in the youngest CAPD patients in Oregon has not resembled that of Dr. Kohaut's patients in Alabama. Statural growth data on the five infants who were less than two years of age at the onset of CAPD in Oregon are presented in Table 13–8. Observed growth is expressed as the percentage of expected growth which it represents. Expected growth is the height increment achieved by a child of the same sex and bone age growing along the 50th centile curve for normal children. In only one of the five children listed in Table 13–8 was observed growth greater than 50% of expected growth, and this boy (Patient #5) had a residual creatinine clearance of 6 ml/min/1.73 m$^2$.

More complete growth and nutrition data for the two Oregon infants less than one year of age at onset of CAPD (Patients #1 and #2, Table 13–8) are presented below in a brief overview of the CAPD treatment courses received by these infants.

Patient #1 was in good health, growing and developing normally on a diet limited exclusively to breast milk, when at the age of 9 months she became anuric following an upper respiratory infection. Renal biopsy was consistent with severe rapidly progressive

**Table 13–8.** STATURAL GROWTH OF THE FIVE YOUNGEST CHILDREN TREATED WITH CAPD IN OREGON FOR AT LEAST ONE YEAR

| Patient | Sex | Bone Age at Onset CAPD (months) | Residual Renal Function ($C_{CR}$ in cc/min/1.73 m$^2$) | Duration of CAPD (months) | Statural Growth* |
|---|---|---|---|---|---|
| 1 | F | 9 | 0 | 42 | 50% |
| 2 | F | 0 | 0 | 10.5 | 50% |
| 3 | M | 15 | 0 | 46 | 42% |
| 4 | F | 18 | <0.5 | 23 | 44% |
| 5 | M | 18 | 6 | 12 | 80% |

*Expressed as % of expected growth. Expected growth is height increment attained during equivalent time interval by normal child of same bone age and sex growing along the 50th centile curve of standard growth charts.

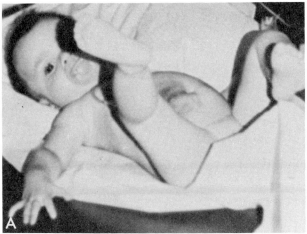
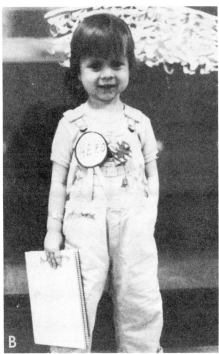

**Figure 13–3.** *A,* Patient #1 (see text) at age 12 months after 3 months on CAPD. *B,* Same patient after 42 months on CAPD.

glomerulonephritis with extensive scarring. When urine output failed to return, she was started on CAPD. Figure 13–3*A,* shows this infant on her first birthday after three months of CAPD. Figure 13–3*B,* is the same child in the fall of 1982 after 42 months on CAPD. Her course has been most notable for the discovery and resection of bilateral Wilms' tumor after 24 months on CAPD and subsequent completion of 15 months of chemotherapy and radiotherapy for this disorder. She has had four episodes of peritonitis. Other complications have included hyponatremia, anemia, renal osteodystrophy, hypertension, poor appetite, and growth retardation. Hospitalizations have averaged 22 days/year. Figure 13–4 depicts growth in head circumference, height, and weight and includes average intakes of energy and protein and average parathyroid hormone levels observed at various times during CAPD.

Despite statural and ponderal growth retardation, intellectual and psychosocial development have been normal. At four years of age performance on school readiness tests is at the first-grade level. Fine motor skills are normal; gross motor skills are not as well developed. This child is a friendly, articulate, and refreshingly self-reliant little girl who attends preschool regularly and in many important ways has a nearly normal home life. Renal transplantation from one of her par-

ents is to be considered if she continues free of metastatic disease.

In stark contrast is the course of Patient #2 who began CAPD at 12 days of age and died 10 months later of gram-negative sepsis. This infant was delivered at 36 weeks' gestation at another medical facility following an apparently traumatic amniocentesis which resulted in bloody amniotic fluid and diminished fetal heart tones. At birth the infant was in profound hypovolemic shock with a hemotocrit of 22%; there was no sign of trauma to the infant, but a placental vessel may have been lacerated. Birth weight was 2.8 kg. Resuscitation was successful, with Apgar scores of 5 and 7 at 1 and 5 minutes. When she failed to void by 48 hours of life acute renal failure was suspected and she was transferred to our institution for acute peritoneal dialysis.

For the next 10 days we managed this infant's renal failure conservatively. Studies showed two normally configured, nonfunctioning, poorly perfused kidneys. Renal vein thrombosis and/or renal cortical necrosis was suspected. Central nervous system and cardiopulmonary function were normal. Following extensive discussions, chronic peritoneal dialysis (CAPD) leading to renal transplantation in 3 to 4 years was chosen by her parents and the medical team. An adult Tenckhoff catheter was placed and CAPD

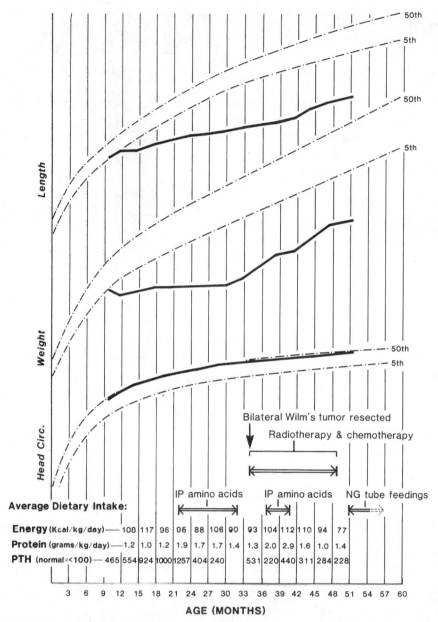

**Figure 13–4.** Growth in height, weight, and head circumference in Patient #1, who began CAPD at 9 months of age. Average dietary intake of energy and protein and average parathyroid hormone levels are given for most 3-month periods during CAPD treatment. Intraperitoneal (IP) amino acid supplementation and Wilms' tumor therapy periods are also noted. Dietary intake was estimated from 3-day diet histories. C-terminal parathormone assay was done by Nichols Institute. (See text for details.)

begun (Figs. 13–1*A* and *B*). Stabilization on CAPD required four weeks, after which she was discharged on a CAPD regimen of five exchanges/day, 45 cc/kg/exchange.

For the first two months at home the infant and her young parents did extremely well. Initial feedings used breast milk as the base with added fat, protein, sodium, vitamins, and minerals. During her third month at home she abruptly stopped feeding. In ret-

rospect, the formula base had been changed to a proprietary formula in the two weeks prior to the onset of anorexia. No other precipitating factor could be identified.

Figure 13–5 depicts growth in head circumference, height, and weight exhibited by this infant, along with data on nutrition. The rapid decline in growth rates is apparent once nutrition faltered. Adjustment of dialysis regimen, feeding technique, and formula composition did not improve intake substantially. During the sixth month on CAPD she had her first generalized seizure. Two episodes of peritonitis followed shortly thereafter.

Nasogastric tube feeding was considered at six months of age, but was rejected by parents and most CAPD team members, all of whom expressed concern over the disruptive effects of tube feedings on the development of the infant-parent bond. (In retrospect the naiveté of this concern is painfully obvious.)

After two more months of poor nutrition, chronic nasogastric tube feedings were begun. Ten weeks later, while hospitalized for evaluation of diarrhea and adjustment of her tube feedings, she became septic, probably from an infiltrated IV site which had become necrotic (peritoneal fluid was sterile), and died. Blood cultures and cultures of the exudate from the necrotic IV site grew *Pseudomonas aeruginosa*.

There is little doubt that poor nutrition was a major component of this infant's down-

hill course after three good months at the outset of CAPD (see Fig. 13–5). A more aggressive approach to nutritional support based on early institution of intermittent and continuous nasogastric tube feedings would seem advisable for infants whose spontaneous intakes fall below target levels. A similar approach to nutritional therapy has been highly successful in the treatment of infants with congenital nephrotic syndrome.[46] It is too soon to tell if aggressive nasogastric tube feedings will affect the growth rates of our youngest CAPD patients, but at least the potentially lethal impact of chronic malnutrition should be preventable in this manner.

## QUALITY OF LIFE OF THE INFANT AND FAMILY ON CAPD

There is little doubt that CAPD offers children and their families a better quality of life than hemodialysis. Praise for the benefi-

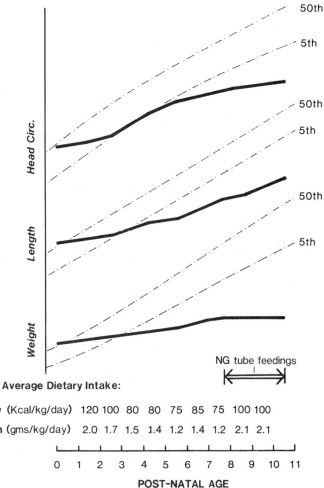

**Figure 13–5.** Growth in length, weight, and head circumference seen in Patient #2, who began CAPD at 12 days of age. Average dietary intake of energy and protein is given for each month of treatment, and institution of nasogastric (NG) feedings is noted. (See text for details.)

Average Dietary Intake:

Energy (Kcal/kg/day)  120 100 80  80  75  85  75  100 100
Protein (gms/kg/day)  2.0 1.7 1.5 1.4 1.2 1.4 1.2 2.1 2.1

0  1  2  3  4  5  6  7  8  9  10  11

POST-NATAL AGE

cial effects of CAPD on the emotional health of patients and families has been a consistent feature of published reports.[6–10, 12] Older children who have experienced both treatment modalities unanimously prefer CAPD over hemodialysis.[10] Greater freedom, absence of painful needle punctures, opportunities for regular school attendance and other peer group activities, in addition to a more normal family life, are obviously attractive features of CAPD.

Underlying this greater freedom of activity is the opportunity for the child to assume a large measure of responsibility for his own life. CAPD promotes independence and self-reliance in the older child and in families of children on CAPD. Successful families are strengthened by their ability to "take care of their own," relating to the medical team as full partners whose input is needed and respected.

As with other home therapies for serious illness, however, the advantages derived from the greater independence and self-reliance possible with CAPD are not achieved without cost. The stresses experienced by families of children on CAPD are substantial, especially during the first 12 months of therapy. We have identified a syndrome of "parent fatigue" which has been common to all the families we have seen to date, but which has been particularly evident in the families of young infants.

## Parent Fatigue

While recent examples of changing family roles have been widely publicized, the fact remains that in our culture the responsibility for the care of the infant falls almost entirely to the mother. Mothers are traditionally expected to devote an enormous amount of time and energy to the care of their infant children. Mothers of our CAPD patients typically assume total responsibility for the home care, quickly relegating the best-intentioned fathers to minor supporting roles. These fathers will soon lose confidence in their technical skills and tend to avoid CAPD procedures. When added to the usual burdens of caring for a small child, the CAPD procedures can seem overwhelming to any one individual.

Most parents find it difficult to acknowledge their fatigue and frustration. They will rarely spontaneously complain about the demands of the home dialysis regimen. In our experience, parent fatigue can lead directly to breaks in technique followed by repeated episodes of peritonitis.[6] The intense guilt experienced by parents when their child develops peritonitis further increases their tension and fatigue. This cycle of increased anxiety and perceived failure must be prevented or interrupted if CAPD is to continue.

## Parent Support

We have learned to look carefully for feelings of fatigue and frustration in the parents (particularly the mothers) of our young patients. The third through the ninth months on CAPD appear to be a critical period. We now insist that mothers allow other adults to share the regular CAPD care of their children. Fathers, grandparents, preschool teachers, visiting nurses, babysitters, and neighbors have all been trained by us to provide basic CAPD care in support of the primary care provided by the child's mother.

The importance of extensive involvement of the entire CAPD medical team in this supportive function cannot be overstated. Regular telephone contact (at least once each week) by CAPD nurses and social workers and frequent consultations with renal dietitians have been helpful; more frequent clinic follow-up visits are also important during the first year on CAPD.

In addition, we have found it important to be able to provide parents with a source of respite care for their children on CAPD so that they can confidently leave together for a day or two to focus on their feelings and needs as individuals and married partners. As our program has grown we have identified and trained several adults in our community who are capable of providing short-term respite care for infants and young children on CAPD and will do so for little or no remuneration. Such individuals should be cultivated by pediatric CAPD programs.

After the first year on CAPD we have observed a general reduction in the level of stress experienced by our families. Daily routines have by then accommodated the dialysis procedures, or, as most often occurs, the CAPD regimen has been adjusted to accommodate changing family activities. Parents have developed confidence in themselves and close ties to the medical team members. Vacations, an important time for most families, have taken place on schedule. (No other family event seems to be more reassuring to siblings of our patients.)

Underlying this more relaxed approach may be a fundamentally reduced fear of serious errors in the CAPD care of the child. It may take many months, but mothers as well as other family members eventually come to rely on the inherent safety of CAPD. Only the fear of peritonitis (which may in fact be a sublimation of the fear of death) continues to haunt these parents for as long as their child remains on CAPD.

## COMPLICATIONS

### Peritonitis

The incidence of peritonitis in pediatric CAPD patients has been reported to be 0.8,[9] 0.9,[12] 1.0,[46] 2.0,[10] 2.7[7] and 3.0[47] episodes per patient-year. Considered together, the data compiled from these reports yields an overall peritonitis incidence in children of 1.70 episodes per patient-year. This is similar to the incidence of peritonitis among the largely adult population included in the NIH CAPD Registry in 1982 (1.81 episodes per patient-year).[48]

Peritonitis seen in infants and children has not been found to differ in any important way from that seen in adults on CAPD. Commonly encountered organisms, signs and symptoms, approach to diagnosis, and response to treatment observed in pediatric patients have been much like the reported experience in adults.

### Anemia

Recent reports have called attention to the improvement in anemia observed in children treated with CAPD. Baum and associates noted that children on CAPD required 0.16 transfusions per month to maintain hematocrits at an average of 21.9%, whereas children treated with hemodialysis required almost five times as many transfusions to maintain hematocrits at 19.6%.[10] Salusky and associates called attention to the higher transfusion requirements of anephric children on CAPD compared to their pediatric CAPD patients who had native kidneys in situ.[9] However, both groups had substantially lower transfusion requirements than children treated with hemodialysis.

It has been our impression in Oregon that younger children have diminished energy and activity levels and eat even less well when hematocrits are allowed to approach 20%. Accordingly we have maintained hematocrits $\geq$ 23% in our younger patients. This has required an average of 0.33 transfusions (10/cc/kg packed red blood cells) per month.[7]

We elected to maintain the hematocrit of our youngest patient (Patient #2) at a higher level ($\geq$ 30%). Actual transfusion requiremets were the same for this infant (0.3 per month) as for the other children we followed.

We have previously noted that acute elevations in blood pressure were frequent complications of transfusions in infants and children whose blood pressures were normally well controlled.[7]

### Hypertension

Early reports described dramatic improvement in the control of hypertension when children were treated with CAPD.[47] Subsequent studies have confirmed these observations.[9]

CAPD does not result in resolution of hypertension in all children, however. For example, Patient #1 required substantial antihypertensive therapy for almost two years in order to maintain average blood pressures in the 110–120/70–80 mm Hg range. Following bilateral nephrectomies and resection of bilateral Wilms' tumor, blood pressure fell to 99/50 mm Hg and has remained at that level subsequently without antihypertensive medication.

### Renal Osteodystrophy

Persistence of renal osteodystrophy in children treated with CAPD has been a disturbing finding in several reports.[7, 12, 47] Hyperparathyroidism has been only minimally affected by the CAPD procedure itself and essentially all pediatric CAPD patients require vitamin D analogues.[12] Hyperphosphatemia has also been described in the absence of dietary phosphate binders.[49]

Therapy for renal bone disease in children on CAPD has occasionally been disappointing. Hewitt and associates recently described 16 children whom they followed on CAPD for a mean of 1.1 years.[50] Ten of 16 had radiographic evidence of renal osteodystrophy at the outset of CAPD; seven improved while three showed further skeletal deterioration. Moreover, of the six children who had no evidence of renal bone disease when CAPD was started, two developed x-ray evidence of osteodystrophy while being treated with CAPD.

Markedly elevated serum parathyroid hormone (PTH) levels have been reported in some children on CAPD.[10] Other investigators report successful control of PTH levels in a majority of patients.[25]

We were unable to prevent the development of renal bone disease in both of the infants described throughout this chapter (Patients #1 and #2). Severe rachitic changes were evident on the radiographs of Patient #2 (see Fig. 13–1B) after four months on CAPD, despite use of calcium supplements and calcitriol (Rocaltrol, Roche). Similar abnormalities developed in Patient #1 in association with elevated serum PTH levels (Fig. 13–4). Attempts to control hyperparathyroidism with increased calcitriol were often frustrated by the development of hypercalcemia. Calcitriol administration can be difficult in infants. Contents of each gelatin capsule provide 0.25 μg of calcitriol and can be expressed directly into the infant's mouth after puncturing the capsule with a pin or knife point. Doses must be increased cautiously, with frequent monitoring of serum calcium and phosphorus levels.

There is currently little agreement on the manner in which renal osteodystrophy may best be followed and treated in infants and children on CAPD. Skeletal growth occurs at such a rapid pace during the first year of life that it is not surprising that such infants can be so severely affected by renal bone disease. Normal ranges for PTH levels in growing infants have not been determined. Patient #2 developed radiologic evidence of renal osteodystrophy when C-terminal PTH levels were less than twice the mean value for adults.

Care must be taken to ensure an adequate calcium intake in infants who may be on special formulas, or who may have subnormal intakes. Similarly, adequate phosphate must be provided to allow normal growth. It is possible that dietary phosphate binders may not be required during periods of rapid growth in infants on CAPD.

## HOSPITALIZATION AND ACTUAL COSTS

There is little published information on the hospitalization rates of infants and children treated with CAPD. During the second and third years of the pediatric CAPD program in Oregon, hospitalization for complications of CAPD required an average of 22.8 and 24.2 days per patient-year respectively.[51] In addition, initial hospitalization was required by all children for peritoneal catheter placement and stabilization on CAPD. This stabilization period varied widely from patient to patient but averaged 27.5 days per new patient in 1981 and 17.5 days per new patient in 1982. Younger patients tended to require longer initial stabilization periods but did not differ substantially from older patients in subsequent hospitalization rates. Details of this analysis, including reasons for hospital admission, have been presented elsewhere.[51]

The cost of providing CAPD for children has been reported as $23,901/year in Alabama in 1979[5] and $19,600/year in San Francisco in 1981–82.[10] Both of these analyses excluded cost data from hospitalization for complications of CAPD, and the San Francisco study also excluded costs of laboratory tests and drugs.

Hatch and associates retrospectively compiled actual cost data on six small children who had been treated with CAPD for six months or more in Oregon prior to August 1982.[52] Complete accounting was made of all hospital charges, pharmacy and laboratory charges, physicians' fees, and the cost of dialysis supplies and equipment. Care was taken to separate costs related to routine outpatient management from costs incurred as a result of hospitalization.

Average annualized cost of the first two years on CAPD for infants and young children ($\leq$ 8 years of age) in Oregon prior to August, 1982, was found to be $34,910/year. Nearly 20% of this total ($13,143/patient) was attributable to costs of the initial hospitalization for catheter placement and stabilization on CAPD. Routine outpatient care, dialysis supplies, routine laboratory and pharmacy charges and medical supervision fees averaged $15,000/year. Average annualized costs incurred as a result of hospitalization for complications of CAPD ($13,335/year) nearly equaled the total cost of routine outpatient management.

It appears that in Oregon routine CAPD for infants and children would be relatively inexpensive once the child had been stabilized on dialysis if complications requiring hospital admissions could be minimized. These complications accounted for 38% of total CAPD costs for our young patients.

Hospitalization rates among these children were similar to those reported by others for children and adults on CAPD.[10, 48]

## CONTINUOUS PERITONEAL DIALYSIS (CPD)

Conley and associates recently proposed an intriguing chronic peritoneal dialysis regimen which they believe is particularly well suited to the infant with ESRD. These investigators have developed a Y-tubing apparatus* which allows "continuous peritoneal dialysis" (7 to 10 exchanges daily) while avoiding frequent bag changes. Infants managed in this way are thus accompanied at all times by up to 2 liters of dialysate apportioned between two bags containing either fresh or spent dialysate. Conley and co-workers described six infants less than two years of age whom they had maintained on CPD for one to 18 months.[53] All had been fed continously via nasogastric tubes with diets delivering 90 to 150 kcal/kg/day and 3.5 to 4.5 gm of protein/kg/day. Statural growth in three of the four infants who had been treated for at least one year was reported to be 100% of expected growth. A fourth infant grew at only 50% of expected; his caretakers were unable to meet the rigorous demands of the dialysis and feeding schedules. Ponderal growth was excellent to excessive in the three infants with normal linear growth.

Full interpretation of these findings must await publication of the complete report. However, it is encouraging to find that Conley and co-workers apparently obtained normal statural growth in a small group of infants by rather straightforward adjustment of diet and peritoneal dialysis mechanics. It is hoped that further experience with CPD in infants confirms these promising preliminary results.

## CONTINUOUS CYCLING PERITONEAL DIALYSIS (CCPD)

Until very recently automated peritoneal dialysis equipment could not be modified to deliver the small exchange volumes required by infants weighing less than 10 kg. New pediatric equipment† has now become available which allows use of an exchange volume as low as 250 cc. Further improvements in pediatric cyclers are certain to be forthcoming. It is likely that CCPD will soon be adaptable for use in very small infants in conjunction with chronic nasogastric tube feeding.

The advantages of a semi-automated dialysis technique like CCPD are particularly apparent when dialysis regimens composed of 7 to 10 daily exchanges are considered. Although there are a number of drawbacks to the use of CCPD (as it is currently configured) in very small infants, it would not be surprising if in only a few years CCPD in some form assumes an important role in the chronic dialysis of infants less than one year of age.

## REFERENCES

1. Popovich RP, Moncrief JW, Decherd JW, et al: The definition of a novel portable/wearable equilibrium peritoneal dialysis technique. Trans Am Soc Artif Intern Organs 5:64, 1976.
2. Popovich RP, Pyle WK, Rosenthal DA, et al: Kinetics of peritoneal dialysis in children. In:CAPD Update: Continuous Ambulatory Peritoneal Dialysis, Moncrief JW, Popovich RP (Eds). New York, Masson, 1981, p 227.
3. Oreopoulos DG, Katirtzoglou A, Arbus G, Cordy P: Dialysis and transplantation in young children (Letter). Br Med J 1:1628, 1979.
4. Potter DE, McDaid TK, McHenry K, Mar H: Continous ambulatory peritoneal dialysis CAPD) in children. Trans Am Soc Artif Intern Organs 27:64, 1981.
5. Shmerling J, Kohaut EC, Perry S: Cost and social benefits of CAPD in a pediatric population. In: CAPD Update: Continuous Ambulatory Peritoneal Dialysis, Moncrief JW, Popovich RP (Eds). New York, Masson, 1981, p 189.
6. Alexander SR, Tseng CH, Maksym KA, et al: Clinical parameters in continuous ambulatory peritoneal dialysis for infants and children. In: CAPD Update: Continous Ambulatory Peritoneal Dialysis, Moncrief JW, Popovich RP (Eds). New York, Masson, 1981, p 195.
7. Alexander SR, Lubischer JT: Continuous ambulatory peritoneal dialysis in pediatrics: three years' experience at one center. Nefrologia (Madrid) 11(Suppl) 2:53, 1982.
8. Balfe JW, Irwin M-A, Orepoulos DG: An assessment of continuous ambulatory peritoneal dialysis (CAPD) in children. In: CAPD Uptdate: Continous Ambulatory Peritoneal Dialysis, Moncrief JW, Popovich RP (Eds). New York, Masson, 1981, p 211.
9. Salusky IB, Lucullo L, Nelson P, Fine RN: Continous ambulatory peritoneal dialysis in children. Pediatr Clin North An 29:1005, 1982.
10. Baum M, Powell D, Calvin S, et al: Continuous ambulatory peritoneal dialysis in children: comparison with hemodialysis. N Engl J Med 307:1537, 1982.
11. Fine RN: Renal transplantation in children. J Pediatr 100:754, 1982.

*Travenol Laboratories, Deerfield, Illinois, 60015.

†American Medical Products Corporation, Freehold, NJ, 07728.

12. Balfe JW, Vigneux A, Willumsen J, Hardy BE: The use of CAPD in the treatment of children with end-stage renal disease. Perit Dial Bull 1:35, 1981.

13. Alexander SR, Tank ES: Surgical aspects of continuous ambulatory peritoneal dialysis in infants, children, and adolescents. J Urol 127:501, 1982.

14. Vigneux A, Hardy BE, Balfe JW: Chronic peritoneal catheter in children: one or two dacron cuffs? (Letter) Perit Dial Bull 1:151, 1981.

15. Alexander SR, Tank ES: Technical considerations in the implantation of Tenckhoff catheters for continuous ambulatory peritoneal dialysis in children. Nefrologia (Madrid) 11(Suppl) 2:49, 1982.

16. Nolph KD, Popovich RP, Moncrief JW: Theoretical and practical implications of continuous ambulatory peritoneal dialysis. Nephron 21:117, 1978.

17. Blumenkrantz MS, Kopple JD, Moran JK, et al: Nitrogen and urea metabolism during continuous ambulatory peritoneal dialysis. Kidney Int 20:78, 1981.

18. Blumenkrantz MS, Schmidt RW: Managing the nutritional concerns of the patient undergoing peritoneal dialysis. In: Peritoneal Dialysis, Nolph KD (Ed). Boston, Martins Nijhoff, 1981, p 181.

19. Esperanza MJ, Collins DL: Peritoneal dialysis efficiency in relation to body weight. J Pediatr Surg 1:162, 1962.

20. Lloyd-Still JD, Atwell JD: Renal failure in infancy: with special reference to the use of peritoneal dialysis. J Pediatr Surg 1:466, 1966.

21. Gruskin AB, Cole ML, Baluarte HJ: Peritoneal diffusion curves, peritoneal clearances and scaling factors in children of differing ages. Int J Pediatr Nephrol 3:271, 1982.

22. Kohaut EC, Alexander SR: Ultrafiltration in the young patient on CAPD: In: CAPD Update: Continuous Ambulatory Peritoneal Dialysis. Moncrief JW, Popovich RP (Eds). New York, Masson, 1981, p 221.

23. Kohaut EC: Effect of dialysate volume on ultrafiltration in small children (Abstract). Submitted to the Sixth International Symposium of Pediatric Nephrology, Hanover, West Germany, August 29–September 2, 1983.

24. Bergmann KE, Ziegler EE, Fomon SJ: Water and renal solute load. In: Infant Nutrition, Fomon SJ (Ed). Philadelphia, WB Saunders Company, 1974, p 246.

25. Kohaut EC: Growth in children with end-stage renal disease treated with CAPD for at least one year. Perit Dial Bull 2:159, 1982.

26. Gopalan C, Jaya Rao KS: Nutrient Needs. In: Human Nutrition: Nutrition and Growth. Jelliffe DB, Jelliffe EFP (Eds). New York, Plenum Press, 1979, p 7.

27. Fomon SJ: Normal growth, failure to thrive and obesity. In: Infant Nutrition, Fomon SJ (Ed). Philadelphia, WB Saunders Company, 1974, p 34.

28. Recommended Dietary Allowances, Ninth Edition. National Academy of Sciences, Washington, DC, 1980.

29. Fomon SJ, Thomas LN, Filer LJ Jr, et al: Food consumption and growth of normal infants fed milk-based forumulas. Acta Pediatr Scand (Suppl 223), 1971.

30. Fomon SJ: Volumtary food intake and its regulation.

31. Betts PR, Magrath G, White RHR: Role of dietary energy supplementation in growth of children with chronic renal insufficiency. Br Med J 1:416, 1977.

32. Holliday MA: Calorie deficiency in children with uremia: effect upon growth. Pediatrics 50:590, 1972.

33. Brooke OG, Wheeler EF: High energy feeding in protein-energy malnutrition. Arch Dis Child 51:968, 1976.

34. Fomon SJ, Thomas LN, Filer LJ Jr, et al: Requirements for protein and essential amino acids in early infancy. Studies with a soy-isolate formula. Acta Pediatr Scand 62:33, 1973.

35. Gjessing J: Addition of amino acids to peritoneal-dialysis fluid. Lancet 1:812, 1968.

36. Fomon SJ, Ziegler EE, O'Donnell AM: Infant feeding in health and disease. In: Infant Nutrition. Fomon SJ (Ed). Philadelphia, WB Saunders Company, 1974, p 472.

37. Commentary on breast feeding and infant formulas, including standards for formulas. Committee on Nutrition, American Academy of Pediatrics. Pediatrics 57:278, 1976.

38. Fomon SJ, Ziegler EE, Thomas LN, et al: Excretion of fat by normal full term infants fed various milk and formulas. Am J Clin Nutr 23:1299, 1970.

39. Yatzidis H, Digenis P, Fountas P: Hypervitaminosis A accompanying advanced chronic renal failure. Br Med J 3:352, 1975.

40. Casey CE, Moser MC, Hambidge KM, Lum GM: Zinc, copper, and vitamin A in pediatric dialysis. J Pediatr 98:434, 1981.

41. Mitch WE: Conservative management of chronic renal failure. In: Chronic Renal Failure, Contemporary Issues in Nephrology, Volume 7, Brenner BM, Stein JH (Eds). New York, Churchill Livingstone, 1981, p 143.

42. American Academy of Pediatrics: The use and abuse of vitamin A. Pediatrics 48:655, 1971.

43. Kopple JD, Swendseid ME: Vitamin nutrition in patients undergoing maintenance hemodialysis. Kidney Int 7:579, 1975.

44. Hambidge KM: Trace elements in pediatric nutrition. In: Advances in Pediatrics (Vol. 24), Barnes LA (Ed). Chicago, Year Book, 1977, p 191.

45. Guillot M, Broyer M, Cathelineau L: Nutrition entérale a débit constant en néphrologie pédiatrique. Arch Franc Pediatr 37:497, 1980.

46. Guillot M, Clarmont M-J, Gagnadoux M-F, Broyer M: Nineteen months' experience with continuous ambulatory peritoneal dialysis (CAPD) in children: main clinical and biological results. In: Advances in Peritoneal Dialysis: Proceedings of the Second International Symposium on Peritoneal Dialysis, Berlin (West), June 16–19, 1981, Gahl, GM, Kessel M, Nolph KD (Eds). Amsterdam, Excerpta Medica, 1981, p 203.

47. Kohaut EC: Continous ambulatory peritoneal dialysis: a preliminary pediatric experience. Am J Dis Child 135:270, 1981.

48. CAPD Patient Registry, National Institutes of Health, Report Number 82–3, July 1, 1982.

49. Eastham EJ, Kirplani H, Francis D, et al: Paediatric

continuous ambulatory peritoneal dialysis. Arch Dis Child 57:677, 1982.

50. Hewitt IK, Balfe JW, Reilly BJ, et al: Renal osteo-dystrophy in children on continuous ambulatory peritoneal dialysis (CAPD). (Abstract) Program and Abstracts, National Kidney Foundation Twelfth Annual Clinical Dialysis and Transplant Forum, Chicago, Illinois, December 8–13, 1982, p 14.

51. Alexander SR: Pediatric CAPD update: 1983. Perit Dial Bull 3:15, 1983.

52. Hatch DA, Tank ES, Millhollen MS, et al: Actual cost of pediatric CAPD in Oregon, 1980–1982. J Urol (in press).

53. Conley SB, Brewer ED, Gandy S, et al: Normal growth in very small children on peritoneal dialysis: 18 months' experience. (Abstract) Program and Abstracts, National Kidney Foundation Twelfth Annual Clinical Dialysis and Transplant Forum, Chicago, Illinois, December 8–13, 1982, p 8.

# 14

# Nursing Management of the Child Undergoing CAPD

*Teresa L. Hall, R.N., M.S.*
*Jo Ann Maloney, R.N., B.S.*

Despite advances in dialytic therapies for children with end stage renal disease (ESRD), a well-functioning kidney transplant remains the optimal solution for a child with irreversible renal failure. The goal, therefore, of dialysis programs for children is maximum biochemical and psychosocial management of the child's end stage disease until a kidney becomes available.

The development of continuous ambulatory peritoneal dialysis (CAPD) during the late 1970's provided pediatric dialysis centers with a new alternative in dialytic therapy for children. It was hoped that CAPD would permit greater biochemical equilibrium and psychosocial adjustment in children. The basis of CAPD and its clinical success in pediatric populations is discussed in detail in other chapters.

The role of the nurse in CAPD programs evolved from the need for someone to teach children and their families how to safely and successfully manage the CAPD regimen in their homes. Nurses, by the nature of their education, and functioning within an ESRD program, were logically sought to become the teachers. This chapter will discuss the role of the nurse in developing pediatric CAPD programs and in managing children undergoing CAPD.

## PROGRAM DESIGN AND THE MULTIDISCIPLINARY TEAM

The care of children undergoing CAPD requires a team approach. The primary members of this team must be each child and his or her family.[1]

The team of professionals who provide health care for these children and their families must include the pediatric nephrologist, the home training/management nurses, the renal dietitian, and the pediatric social worker. Other professionals who may contribute to the treatment and plan of care include the referring physician, surgeons, a child psychiatrist or psychologist, members of the child development or child life staff, transplant co-ordinator, school nurses, and school teachers, as well as the house staff and nursing staff in the acute care areas. Individual states or communities may also offer support services to these children and their families in the form of professional staff who contribute to the child's plan of care. Examples of such agencies include state crippled children's organizations, organizations which provide services to children with developmental disabilities, and public health nursing organizations.

The "core" multidisciplinary team within each facility, i.e., the pediatric nephrologist, nursing staff, dietitian, and social worker, determine the direction and design of the program. They generate the philosophy, policies, procedures, and operations format which guide the program. The assumptions which underlie the program design for a pediatric CAPD program vary with each facility according to the stated mission, goals, and objectives of the institution. We believe that the following assumptoms are critical to the successful operation of a pediatric CAPD program:

1. Parents maintain the ultimate authority and responsibility for their child.

2. CAPD is a successful treatment modality for maintenance of children with ESRD.

3. Children undergoing CAPD will have complications.

The first assumption, understood by the professional staff, allows the child and his family to be the primary members of the team, with the parents as the decision makers. The second assumption requires a belief in and commitment to CAPD by the professional staff. The third assumption that must be accepted is that the complications which later arise will not automatically be diagnosed as one team member's failure, i.e.: (1) failure of the child or his family to comply with the regimen; (2) failure of the physician to diagnose and prescribe adequately; (3) failure of the nursing staff to train appropriately; (4) failure of the dietitian to recommend and teach the dietary regimen; and (5) failure of the social worker to provide appropriate psychosocial support.

Within the program design, each professional team member's role and area of responsibility is defined. Careful program design, including definition of roles, promotes the co-ordinated effort of the team toward its stated goal. Each team member is granted the authority concomitant to the responsibility he or she accepts in order to fulfill the role. Careful definition of roles and mutual understanding of each professional team member's function provides for consistent and unified communication with the child and his family. Careful delineation of the boundaries of each individual's involvement also decreases the opportunities for misunderstanding and manipulation of staff by the clients. For example, if the dietitian *must* be consulted for changes in the dietary regimen, physicians, nurses, and social workers will be less likely to respond to a child's or parent's request for diet changes. The request will be referred to the dietitian.

Regular meetings of the team to discuss each child's current status and to make changes in the CAPD regimen need to be held to achieve this goal and maintain the team's communication and co-ordinated effort. The minimum number of meetings required is one a month. Minutes should be recorded.

Within this multiperson team, the CAPD nursing staff functions to provide the home training and co-ordinate the nursing management program.

## NURSING CARE DELIVERY IN CAPD PROGRAMS

Criteria for selection of nursing staff for CAPD programs is partially delineated by the law.[2] In addition, a minimum of one year's experience in pediatric nursing is an important requirement for pediatric CAPD nursing staff. The nature of pediatric nursing requires the nurse to have teaching skills, because when dealing with pediatric patients there are always at least two clients involved: the child and a parent or legal guardian. The pediatric nurse delivers care to children with the assistance and consent of the child's parents. All plans of nursing care for children include explanations to parents in order for care to be delivered satisfactorily and for medical and nursing regimens to be continued in the child's home.

In most instances, the institution will have to provide the nurse with extensive education. Because CAPD programs are relatively new, it is rare to find a nurse with CAPD experience, and finding a pediatric nurse with CAPD experience who is seeking a position is even rarer. Pediatric ESRD programs can provide education in CAPD, and an experienced pediatric nurse will in most instances readily adapt to the position.

Two other requirements contribute to a successful outcome for the pediatric CAPD nurse: (1) The nurse should be willing to commit to a minimum of one year's tenure in the position. This is important because of the extensive education which the institution will provide and because the relationship which the children and their families make with the primary training nurse is critical to their success, especially in the early months following training. (2) The pediatric CAPD nurse must have a strong sense of self and be flexible. These characteristics will allow the nurse to transfer the control of the dialysis regimen to the child and his family and then *assist* them in changing priorities and making appropriate alterations in their regimens.[3,4] In order for a child to undergo CAPD successfully, the dialysis regimen must be fitted into the lives of the child and his family, and not the reverse. The nurse with a strong sense of self and the ability to set priorities and then change them, make goals and modify them, is able to facilitate the addition of CAPD to a family's lifestyle.

The pediatric CAPD nursing staff should begin with *two* nurses who have been prepared to provide the training and management.[5] This allows for nursing procedures and training materials to be prepared without isolation. It allows for training and management activities to occur simultaneously, and provides for coverage during illness and vacations. Once the program is in full operation, a nurse-to-patient ratio of 1:10 has proved manageable.[6, 7] Planning for additions to nursing staff needs to include the education time needed by new nurses.

Two delivery systems for training and management of pediatric CAPD clients can be identified. In one system, a separate nursing staff provides both training and management for CAPD patients with the staffing ratio described above. In the other system, one nurse (who must have a qualified backup), provides the initial training, and other nurses within the pediatric ESRD program help complete training and provide on going management in a primary care model. That is, once training is started, patients are assigned to a primary nurse who initially shares and subsequently assumes the nursing management responsibilities.

During initial program design, each institution must establish a plan for providing a back-up dialysis system. Pediatric hemodialysis, intermittent peritoneal dialysis, and continuous peritoneal dialysis must be available when the child undergoing CAPD must be hospitalized or has complications. Once a child begins continuous peritoneal dialysis, unless his physiological complications dictate an intermittent form of dialytic therapy, the inpatient service institution must be prepared to provide for continuous peritoneal dialysis when the child is hospitalized. This further requires that only personnel *trained* in peritoneal dialysis techniques or trained family members perform the child's dialysis.

The institution's overall plan for pediatric CAPD must also include a 24 hour on-call nursing system. Home care, both from a technical and management standpoint, can be unpredictable, and the questions the families may have on "off hours" can be answered only by a qualified nurse well informed on the program's policies, procedures, and philosophies.

## THE ROLE OF THE NURSE IN A PEDIATRIC CAPD PROGRAM

The role of the nurse in a pediatric CAPD program is multifaceted. It can be divided into two components: (1) program development and management and (2) client training and nursing management.

Program development includes the nursing contributions to overall program design described earlier. It includes the writing of procedures and training materials which ultimately solidify into client training manuals, the CAPD nursing policy and procedure manual, and the CAPD program operations manual.

The nurse's role in CAPD program development has a major education component in training both nursing and medical staff in CAPD protocols, procedures, and techniques. Hospital nursing staff members and house staff need regular inservice education programs including such topics as : "What is CAPD?" "How does it work?" "What are the needs of hospitalized CAPD clients?" Because peritoneal dialysis techniques are continuing to change rapidly and because hospital staff turns over frequently, regular and on-going education and consultation are part of the program development responsibilities of CAPD nursing staff.

Providing for continuous peritoneal dialysis for hospitalized CAPD clients via trained personnel becomes either a direct care responsibility of the CAPD nursing staff or an educational responsibility of the CAPD nursing staff in training those personnel.

Program management aspects of the CAPD nurse's role include maintenance of records required by outside accrediting bodies and the institution. A comprehensive list of records and data which must be prepared and collected is provided in Appendix A. The CAPD nursing staff are responsible for ensuring that the program complies with the requirements of the law delineating "Conditions for Coverage of Suppliers of End Stage Renal Disease (ESRD) Service" as published in the Federal Register by the Department of Health, Education and Welfare.[2]

Depending upon a given institution's procedure, the CAPD nurses usually order dialysis supplies for the training program and regular outpatient clinics as well as initial supplies for delivery to each new CAPD client's home. The nursing staff may frequently meet with the representatives of dialysis product vendors as improvements in technology, the CAPD delivery system, commercially prepared training materials, and adaptive devices continue to occur on a frequent basis.

Because pediatric CAPD programs are primarily found in major university medical centers, research is an integral component of these programs. Part of the program management responsibility of the pediatric CAPD nursing staff will frequently include co-ordination of research protocols in which CAPD patients are participating.

The nursing staff participates in program evaluation with the other professional members of the multidisciplinary team. Periodic review of policies, procedures, and protocols is needed in order to make the changes which are necessary to keep the program and its design current. The nursing staff then translates the changes to the CAPD patients and their families and to the ancillary team members.

## The Training Program

Determining the approach for the CAPD training program begins with the selection of candidates. All dialysis modalities are presented to each family, and an explanation of the advantages and disadvantages of each modality are identified by the professional team members who have been given this responsibility by program design and operations format. The selection of candidates for CAPD will be determined by affirmative answers to the following questions:

1. Do the child and family wish to undertake CAPD?

2. Does the child have a functional peritoneal membrane?

3. Is there someone (the child or a family member) who is available to undergo the training and perform the dialysis on a daily basis after the training is completed?

If these questions are answered positively, potential candidates are interviewed by the CAPD nursing staff prior to final acceptance in the program. The interview may successfully be accomplished in conjunction with the licensed clinical social worker (LCSW), as there are several areas of mutual concern to the nurse and LCSW which require assessment. Combined interviews frequently yield for each professional more information than either could have obtained alone.

A negative answer to any of the above questions constitutes a basic contraindication to a child's undergoing CAPD. At the present time, the presence of an abdominal wall bowel ostomy is considered a relative contraindication for CAPD. (However, both authors have experienced success in training clients with abdominal wall urinary ostomies). Emotional disorders diagnosed by the LCSW, psychiatrist, or psychologist in the primary learner may prevent the successful completion of CAPD training. Also, unresolved hygiene problems in the home, e.g., lice, can be a contraindication. Other contraindications are based on the philosophies of individual programs.

## Assessment

The nursing assessment is performed to screen candidates and to provide information that will be used later to determine an individualized approach to training and designing a successful teaching plan.

During the interview the nurse should attempt to assess the following areas:

1. Knowledge of ESRD care and CAPD.

2. Functional style of the family and motivation of family members.

3. Cognitive functioning of the primary learner.

It is important to clarify the family's knowledge of the modality, including knowledge of body image changes. An informal referral to another child and family undergoing CAPD is beneficial in offering the personal and practical perspective experienced by other families. The camaraderie that can ensue is encouraged, if only for the support that it offers. This introduction to other families may be part of the presentation of all modalities of dialytic therapy.

Previous experiences with medical delivery systems may either help or hinder the training program. These experiences will influence the family's response and must be assessed. For example, a family who has experience with insulin-dependent diabetes mellitus may have a greater understanding of the value of compliance with diet, exercise, and medical therapy. Knowledge levels of ESRD care will vary greatly. The family whose child has gradually gone from chronic renal failure to ESRD will respond quite differently, with a much broader knowledge base, than the family whose child precipitously arrives at ESRD.

The reasons a family expresses for choosing CAPD may not be a reflection of true understanding of the modality. Many clarifications may be needed. Successful CAPD management is not easy. It should not facilitate the family's isolation from medical personnel. The experience should not be confined to one or two family members.

During assessment of the family's knowledge, the nurse can begin to "seed" the family with the following critical concepts:

1. CAPD procedures are simple, but the regimen is exacting.

2. The child and his family are the primary members of the team, who cooperate and collaborate to provide CAPD.

3. CAPD is a family process.

4. Maintaining regular contact with the team is essential, as well as advantageous.

Assessment of the family's functioning occurs concurrently with the knowledge assessment. Points to be considered include:

1. Which family member is dominant?

2. Which member is the decision maker?

3. What is the role of this child within the family?

4. What are the roles of other family members?

5. What is the stress level of individual family members?

6. What coping behaviors do family members exhibit?

7. Who and where and what are the family's support systems?

Assessing the stress level of each family member provides important insights into the outcome of training and home management. It is assumed that initiating CAPD will be a stressful and change-oriented phase in a family's life. The coping mechanisms used by the family to deal with this particular stress will most likely be used in future crises, e.g., peritonitis, failed catheter, inefficient dialysis. Understanding the family's coping behaviors will be helpful in determining the nurse's approach to dealing with the family's crises, one of which will be the crisis of training.

Support systems available to the family, may include extended family members, close friends of the family, other groups of professionals such as faculty of the school system, organizations to which family members belong, and associates from the work environment of family members. It is important to remember that all these potential support systems may also be sources of stress to the child and his family.

Critical to assessment during the selection process is a determination that all primary family members agree to the undertaking of CAPD. The long-term success of a child undergoing CAPD is proportionally decreased with the resistance of any family member.

The third area of assessment, cognitive functioning of the primary learner, helps in designing the teaching plan for the individual. Both adult and child learners may think only in concrete patterns; this affects how they will manage the home regimen. It is important to remember, also, that children and adults who have little difficulty with abstract thinking under usual conditions frequently regress under stress. Both adults and children can often identify how they learn most readily. It is important to remember to ask them about this and to use their suggestions in designing the teaching plan.

When the initial interviewing process is completed with positive answers to the selection questions by all members of the team—child, parents, physician, nurse, dietitian, and LCSW—the child and his family are accepted into the CAPD Home Training Program.

## Designing the Teaching Plan

After a child is accepted to the CAPD program and before the home training begins, two objectives must be achieved. One of these is the establishment of a functioning peritoneal dialysis catheter with appropriate catheter break-in. The other is the design of a teaching plan for the child and family.[1, 4, 8, 9]

Whether the CAPD nursing staff participates in catheter placement and break-in depends upon the overall plan for peritoneal dialysis in the institution. During this time period, the CAPD nursing staff must have contact with the family to establish dates for training, arrange for delivery of home dialysis supplies to the child's home, and continue to answer questions which arise. All these contacts are utilized for continued assessment and for reinforcement of the critical concepts "seeded" during the initial interview, i.e., (1) CAPD is simple, but it must be done exactly; (2) the child and his family are the primary members of a cooperative team; (3) CAPD is a family process; and (4) regular contact with the professional team is essential and advantageous.

Also during this time, the family needs to make preparations for home training. The preparations include child care for other siblings, transportation arrangements, parking passes, time off from work for parents, notifications to the child's school, and financial arrangements. As many of these situations as possible should be dealt with prior to training. Training has already been identified as a stress, and with each additional stress the ability of the learner to participate in the learning activities is decreased. Because of the necessity for creating a maximum learning environment, home training for CAPD should not be considered an emergency treatment.

The average number of days for pediatric CAPD home training is 8 to 10 and can be prolonged or shortened as required. Three critical elements must be satisfied during the period of CAPD home training:

1. Child or parent can safely and accurately perform CAPD exchanges.

2. Child or parent can accurately measure and record weights and blood pressures.

3. Child or parent can identify when they must seek consultation or medical attention and then do so readily.

The nurse who designs the teaching plan and provides the training has the responsibility for determining when the child or parent has successfully completed the training program.

Talabere defines teaching as "a special kind of communication that produces learning.[10] It involves various activities, both verbal and nonverbal, that change a person's knowledge, skills, or attitudes." Learning is defined as "the development of new behavior patterns that result from acquiring new knowledge, skills, or attitudes."

When designing a plan for teaching CAPD, it is valuable to recognize that the teaching-learning process is a vehicle utilized to achieve the originally stated goal. Both the teacher and the learner, whether child or parent, have responsibilities. The teacher's responsibilities include making the teaching relevant, effective, and consistent, and providing evaluation, while allowing the learner adequate time to learn. The learner's responsibilities include participating actively, giving feedback, and complying.[1, 10]

## Growth and Development Concepts

Concepts of growth and development need to be included in developing a plan for educating children and families about peritoneal dialysis. It is important to understand how children and their families think about illness, in order to make information relevant for the child or parents learning. Blas stated: "To assist children in the cognitive-affective process of learning about their bodies, health, illness and vulnerabilities, and treatment procedures, it is valuable to know how children think about these issues, how best to elicit information about such thinking, and how best to correct any wrong conclusions."[11]

A child's cognitive developmental level can be assessed chronologically as defined by Piaget[12] and psychosocially as defined by Erikson,[13] but assessing the level of a chronically ill child's development is more difficult. The latter is based on society's attitudes toward the ill child, and how that society, including parents and siblings, has allowed the child to learn about the world. Distortions of developmental tasks can be found throughout the growing years, e.g., by under or overprotective families, ranging from an aberration in basic trust to the adolescent's failed achievement of independence. A basic understanding of some factors involved in a child's development will contribute to the teaching plan.

The infant's development task is establishment of trust. This is achieved by having basic needs met through consistent mothering patterns. The major stress of illness for the infant is interruption of these mothering patterns. Teaching plans for the parents of an infant undergoing CAPD must include allowance for those patterns to be continued with as few interruptions as possible. This may also mean including plans for teaching a mother how to establish consistent patterns with her infant.

The toddler (1–3 yrs) is learning autonomy and how to separate from parents for brief periods. The major stress of illness at this age is separation anxiety. Teaching plans for the toddler include short teaching sessions for parents with frequent, brief reunions with the child during the training day.

The preschool child (3–6 yrs) is learning initiative and may tolerate longer separations from parents. However, the preschool child thinks magically and fears mutilation. The teaching plan for the preschool child includes techniques to help parents assist the child to accept the peritoneal catheter and incorporate it into the body image. This is successfully achieved in most instances. Having a favorite doll or stuffed animal accompany the child to the hospital is helpful. The doll too can have a catheter inserted and a bag attached for performing CAPD. (See Appendix B.) This concept can be continued in teaching parents to assist their child with the trauma of blood-drawing. The preschool child can learn precautionary measures, especially those related to being careful with the catheter. He learns through dramatic play about his world, and if his parent practices "bag changes" and catheter care with the doll, the child will more readily accept the procedure when it is performed on himself.

During the school years (6–12), explanations, drawings, and differentiating fact from fantasy are useful in gaining the child's cooperation. This child is achieving a sense of industry, and likes to complete tasks and receive the reward for doing so. The relationship between cause and effect is a concept which can be fully utilized, particularly since noncompliance with the dialysis regimen can result in discomfort to the child. The major stress of illness in this age group is immobilization, and provisions must be made for activities requiring the exercise of large muscles.

In conjunction with the developmental task of achieving independence, the adolescent is expected to function as the primary learner, unless physically or mentally incapacitated. A back-up person is taught, but only after the adolescent has mastered the procedures independently. The major stress of illness, however, is peer separation. In addition, being different from peers is not well tolerated. Helping the child accept a peritoneal dialysis catheter with its accompanying tubing and bag is a challenge to every team member. Successful teenage CAPD patients are the single best resource.

The developmental tasks and stresses just identified are for children progressing normally in development. Stress and chronic illness may create regressions or delays in development which require teaching plans based on the observed level of development rather than the age-expected level of development. For example, both preschoolers and teenagers have responded well to the doll or toy animal with a catheter and bag.

As a rule, children 12 years and older have the manual dexterity, judgment, and cognitive ability to perform the CAPD procedure. Younger children rarely have the judgment required. These behaviors must be assessed and identified in planning for who will assume the primary responsibility for the regimen. If the child is expected to perform CAPD independently, it is usually advantageous for him to learn independently. After he has mastered some of the essential CAPD skills, he can assist the nurse to teach his family member(s) or be the primary teacher himself, with supervision.

When planning for training of the parents of small children, the need for child care must be considered. The child will be needed for CAPD exchanges, but the parents also need undistracted learning time. This is a small problem if training occurs on an inpatient basis, but can be a major one for outpatient training. Child development staff, volunteers and other family members are possible resources.

When assessment is complete, the teaching plan is written. It includes the objectives, learning activities, and expected behaviors for each session, and all team members may contribute to its design, implementation, and evaluation. All the data gathered during the assessment is used to determine what objectives are reasonable, what learning activities will most likely help the learner, and what the pace of learning will most likely be. Then daily evaluation with the learner and the other team members will allow the training to be designed to each learner's needs and abilities.

The training environment is important. The location, which ideally is quiet and away from hospital confusion, should include the following:
— enough chairs for all involved to feel comfortable;
— desks for both the nurse and learner to take notes;
— a sink to facilitate aseptic procedures;
— adequate space to practice the dialysis techniques;
— a writing board for impromptu diagrams;
— available books and illustrations;
— audiovisual aids;
— practice equipment.

The actual content of CAPD training programs is well outlined in many other sources.[8, 9, 14] One is reproduced here (Fig. 14–1). Translating this outline into achieving the objectives outlined in the teaching plan is a four-step process: planning, implementation, testing, and review of outcome indicating additional planning.[15]

## Teaching Techniques

Repetition and dividing content into small modules are two common teaching techniques. Lectures can be used, but it is well to remember that the amount of learning achieved through hearing alone is very small and attention to a lecturer at best lasts about twenty minutes. The degree of learning increases with each sense to which the material is presented. Whenever possible the learner should see it, hear it, read it, *practice* it and take it home in writing, both his own and in the prepared materials from the program.

TEACHING OUTLINE

1. Normal kidney function
2. General pathophysiology
3. Complications of uncontrolled uremia
4. Structure of the peritoneal cavity
5. Kinetics of peritoneal dialysis
6. Description of CAPD
   a. demonstration of bag, tubing, catheter, supplies, and techniques for wearing bag and tubing
   b. exchange cycle
   c. exchange schedule
   d. glucose concentrations (1.5%, 2.5%, 4.25%)
7. Aseptic and antiseptic technique
8. Bag change procedure
9. Emergency procedures for:
   a. spike contamination or deterioration
   b. accidental disconnection
   c. tear in bag, catheter, tubing
10. Catheter care
11. Fluid balance
12. Complications: cause, symptoms, and corrective action for:
   a. fluid overload
   b. dehydration
   c. peritonitis
   d. fibrin production
   e. exit site infection
   f. tunnel infection
   g. bloody effluent
   h. difficulty establishing drainage or inflow
   i. dialysator leakage
   j. dialysis-related pain
   k. constipation
13. Addition of medication to dialysate
14. Monitoring vital signs, blood pressure, and weight
15. Maintenance of home dialysis records
16. Medications
   a. purpose
   b. appearance
   c. dosage
   d. schedule
   e. precautions or special instructions
   f. side effects
   g. relationship to blood chemistries
17. Diet
   a. meal plan
   b. caloric intake
   c. protein requirement
   d. sodium and potassium intake
   e. fluid intake
   f. diet records
18. Explanation of routine blood work
19. Description of diagnostic procedures
20. Adaptation to home environment
21. Adaptation to school schedule/environment
22. Activities and exercise regimen
23. Social, sexual function
24. Patient responsibilities
25. Ordering and inventory of supplies
26. Unit and staff directory
27. Emergency call system

**Figure 14–1.** Teaching outline for CAPD training program. (Adapted from Fruto, Prowant, and Sorrels: Nursing Management and Patient Education in Continuous Ambulatory Peritoneal Dialysis—An Introduction to Continuous Ambulatory Peritoneal Dialysis, Travenol Laboratories, Inc., 1980, p. 49.)

Talabere identifies behavior modification techniques—chaining, modeling, shaping, fading—which are widely used in successful CAPD training. "Chaining is the technique of putting together more and more complex ideas into a chain of learning."[10] For example, a client learns that glucose in dialysate removes water; more glucose removes more water; increased weight and increased blood pressure can mean excess water in the body. Ultimately, these links are connected to mean that weight gain and hypertension require dialysate with high glucose concentration.

Modeling and shaping take simple activities and move on to more complex behavior, with the teacher demonstrating and the learner imitating. Modeling and shaping are illustrated by demonstration of the exchange procedure with a doll and practice bags. The nurse demonstrates the procedure and the learner returns the demonstration. The nurse performs an exchange for the child and ultimately the learner performs the child's bag exchange. The fading occurs with the nurse's gradual withdrawal from the procedure until the learner achieves independence.[10] The bag exchange is then chained to vital signs, weights, keeping accurate records, and so on. Mastery of the simplest technique gives the learner competence and motivation to move into more complicated activities.

It is the rare child or parent who is not overwhelmed at some point with the volume and complexity of content of a CAPD training program. Parents are usually additionally overwhelmed with the burden of such major responsibility. For the child, it is often helpful to stop and ask for a step-by-step description of a familiar procedure such as how to get dressed. For the parent, you might ask for a description of how to drive a car and the responsibilities concomitant to operation of a vehicle with passengers in freeway traffic. These analogies are usually sufficient to allow the learner to gain perspective and can often provide comic relief after an intense session.

Comparisons to simple "knowns" is a technique for explaining more complex unknowns. For example, semipermeability of the peritoneal membrane can be compared to a coffee filter, a sand sieve, a colander, or items which allow small particles to pass through a membrane while withholding large particles. Keeping some of these articles on hand will allow actual experimentation during training sessions. It is helpful to look into grade school science books to get ideas on how to describe osmosis and diffusion. These books usually describe experiments easily performed with simple directions and available supplies. Colorful and stimulating presentations to both child and adult increase retention of the associated concepts.

A child or family may verbally or nonverbally communicate that this is very easy, they know what to do, and thus the teacher is wasting their time. In such a situation a good response is to give them an opportunity to teach someone else the concepts or procedures being presented in the session. Visiting doctors and nurses or other home patients are good "students" for such presentations, and the learner or the teacher may be surprised. The same technique works well for the learner who really has learned but lacks confidence.[4]

Positive reinforcement is necessary to provide the learner with a sense of mastery. However, it can be overused. An overconfident learner may make mistakes and lose all confidence. It is important to keep other team members informed of the client's progress, so that they can contribute to the overall success of the training. Also, the doctors, the dietitian, and the social worker can help to boost a patient's confidence, reinforce a protocol, and evaluate progress from their conferences with the child and family.

Evaluation can be used as a teaching technique as well as for ascertaining progress with the training program. It is a continuous process. During the period of home training, each session is followed by a time allowed for the learner to ask questions. If the learner either has no questions or is hesitant to ask them, the nurse should question the learner about the topic covered. This is a way for the child or family member to demonstrate comprehension. Written and verbal quizzes are given during the course of home training to assess the abilities of the learner and his level of comprehension.

The evaluation of procedural technique can be done through return demonstration. Supervised demonstration of each procedure must be 100% accurate. On the training nurse's evaluation, the learner will be declared competent to perform unsupervised procedures. With his freedom comes the learner's responsibility to apply the skills taught, to recognize when he may need help, and to know when to ask for this help. There comes a point in all teaching when the teacher must leave the responsibility to the learner. Only with the continued application of the concepts and skills will the learner become adept and confident with CAPD.

## Complications of Training

Complications of training may be divided into two components: behavioral and physical. Many of the problems may be anticipated and solution plans implemented before the problem actually occurs.

### Behavior Problems

Children of preschool and school age are known for having temper tantrums, which may manifest themselves as outbursts of violent behavior, directed at those involved in the child's care. This aggression can result in interruption of the training schedule and possible harm to the child or nurse or parent. One reason for uncontrolled temper tantrums can be a pattern established at home when no limits are set for the child's behavior. The nurse may take control in the training area by setting the limits and explaining to the child or parent what is acceptable behavior in the training room. Consistency is achieved with others involved in the child's care by adhering to written care plans. When appropriate expectations are not met, or the child becomes disruptive, the most immediate solution is to simply terminate the session. This is a direct way of helping the parent to identify that there is a problem, that the problem is in the child's behavior, and that the parents need to assume responsibility for their child's behavior.

Often the parents' expectations for their child's behavior are not consistent with his age and level of development. The expectations and actual behavior come in many combinations that may not be identified prior to training. Parents' expectations can be too high or too low. The child may want to follow an "ill" role, and his parents can be compliant with or try to prevent this behavior. The child may want to follow a "well" role, and his parents can be compliant with or try to prevent this behavior. These problems are best discussed with the social worker and the consulting psychiatrist or psychologist when they are identified. Changes should be made in the planned teaching program to promote appropriate changes in behavior. It is critical at this time for the team, including the parents, to make a plan which allows these situations to be dealt with over time while still allowing the training program to go safely forward.

Anger and hostility are defense mechanisms which may be incorporated into the behavior patterns of the child or family members. The causes of the anger may be multifaceted, including fear of the unknown future for the child, a sense of loss of control, a lack of understanding of the nature of the disease and resultant complications, and confusion over the various modalities of therapy. Although such anger is appropriate, hostility toward the care-giver can be expected to lead to a delay in home training. With hostility comes distrust, and if a nurse is to be an effective teacher, she or he must have the trust of the learner. Again, open acknowledgement of the action is necessary, and it will allow for communication among the adults involved in the child's care.

Finally, problems and training delays will occur when the learner is unprepared to learn. Examples include lack of sleep, missed meals leading to a nutritional state of inattentiveness or headache, illness, other scheduled appointments, lateness, learning materials left at home, or the bringing of the entire family, including young siblings, to the training area. Once problems are identified, the approach to resolve such problems must be individualized and may include termination and rescheduling of sessions.

### Physical Problems

Since home training often begins shortly after starting dialysis, multiple complications which may be the result of reversible or irreversible causes can occur during the training sessions. Changes in blood pressure and weight often are involved. Specific consideration must be given to adjustments in antihypertensive medications and volume regulation. Careful monitoring of weight, blood pressure, and medications will reduce the incidence of these problems. Also, carefully titrating dialysate concentrations of glucose to weight and blood pressure will help prevent these problems.

Any complication which occurs should be used as an opportunity to educate the child and his family. For example, peritonitis during training is a complication which can be used as a positive learning experience. The severity of the symptoms will depend on the child's level of pain tolerance and the susceptibility of the invading organism to intraperitoneal antibiotics. If the child is not already hospitalized for training, he or she may need to be hospitalized for treatment.

Constipation is a major cause of problems with dialysate inflow and outflow. The anxiety which is produced by the temporary cessation of dialysis may hinder training, and preoccupation with the symptoms of constipation may interrupt the learning process. After acute treatment with suppositories and enemas, the use of stool softeners may be necessary. The experience can be used positively to teach the child or family what can happen if regular bowel habits are not maintained.

Auditory and visual handicaps are physical complications which are not often reversible. The learner may be limited by an inability to hear in taking blood pressure and heart rates, or may be deaf. The learner may be limited by a decrease in visual acuity, or be completely blind. Blood pressures may be viewed through a lighted or digital sphygmomanometer, or amplified by a built-in device. Systolic blood pressure may be palpated. Heart rates can be taken by counting at a pulse area. There are magnifying devices which can be purchased to allow correct reading of temperature or blood pressure. Finally, CAPD vendors are becoming more sophisticated in providing equipment with emphasis on ease of visibility. There are devices on the market for blind people to perform their own exchanges. Help provided by a third party should not be ruled out. A supportive family and the proper motivation are all that is needed for a child or family member to successfully perform peritoneal dialysis at home.

The family who enters the training program may not speak the same language as the professional staff. This complication also can be solved. Interpreters can often be provided by the institution or the family. This includes sign language for the deaf. Training materials can be translated into the appropriate language. This can be done in writing or by audio tapes made by translators.

Final evaluation of the family's ability to perform home dialysis can be achieved only after the family does go home on a management regimen.

## THE MANAGEMENT PROGRAM

### Assessment

Management of the child on CAPD is the most demanding skill that families will learn. The objectives of successful CAPD management are as follows:

1. To maintain each child in a well-dialyzed and biochemically stable state;
2. To maintain each child on CAPD in an infection-free state;
3. To adjust the home peritoneal dialysis regimen so that each child attends school, as age-appropriate, on a regular basis, or otherwise achieves developmentally appropriate tasks;
4. To have each child's dialysis regimen require minimal changes in his or her family's lifestyle, and
5. To minimize hospitalizations.

Success in achieving these objectives is assessed through home visits, clinic visits, routine and impromptu telephone calls, and the use of outside professional sources.

### Home Visit

A home visit, which should be arranged as early as possible after discharge, offers the nurse a unique opportunity to observe families in their own territory.[9, 16] The major purpose of the home visit is not to see if the procedures are performed correctly—that is evaluated before discharge. It is a vehicle for offering the family an initial support system as they assume the responsibility of managing treatment for the child, and of evaluating adaptation to the home environment.

Certain concrete observations can be made by the nurse during the home visit. Suggestions may be offered regarding utilization of space and adequacy of home setup. The area of predominate usage should be scrutinized. The lighting should be adequate. Any table that is large enough to accommodate CAPD supplies can be utilized. One drawer in the bedroom dresser will be adequate for immediate supplies (i.e., syringes, medication, stethoscope, sphygmomanometer, thermometer). A closet, if available, can be used to store cases of dialysate. A sink, in the bathroom or kitchen, can be used for proper handwashing prior to performing procedures. A clock or watch with a second hand for timing a betadine soak or obtaining a heart rate helps give more organization to the peritoneal dialysis area. It is important to see how CAPD bags are heated at home, since this will probably differ from the hospital's accommodations. The family is taught to use dry heat for warming the solution, e.g., a microwave oven, heating pad, sunshine, or placement of bags near a heater.

The home visit is also a relaxed and informal time to review with the family all pertinent instructions, procedures, and information from the previous few weeks. A visit to the child's school may be included.[3, 16] When the adolescent or school-age child is regularly attending school, at least one CAPD exchange is done there. The school nurse can often assist in making the necessary arrangements, and will benefit by receiving direct or written information on CAPD. Certification of the school nurse in performing CAPD exchanges may be necessary for the young child; such training can be coordinated by the dialysis nurse.

### Clinic Visits

The vehicle by which families maintain consistent involvement with the hospital-based training staff is the monthly outpatient visit. Purposes include maintaining periodic contact among the ESRD multidisciplinary team and families and children receiving CAPD, assessing the child's status and making appropriate changes in the dialysis regimen, obtaining necessary laboratory tests and other evaluations, e.g., x-ray, EKG, etc., providing the child with ongoing educational information, and evaluating treatments, care plans, home status, and ongoing progress of the child and family.

Both parents, at least initially, should be requested to attend visits with the child.

Although the details of clinic appointments may vary, each visit has certain common goals. The nurse meets with the family to get blood samples for routine and nonroutine laboratory analysis, then reviews the day's plan. Information obtained at this time includes vital signs, a general monthly history of complaints and problems, and any questions that may arise. By performing this interview, possible complications can be detected or prevented, but it is also a time to help the family interpret symptoms.[17]

The dialysis treatment review follows. The dialysis records of the past month and the dialysis prescription are reviewed (Fig. 14–2). Questions to evaluate average weight gain or loss, and what solutions were used to achieve the gain or loss should be asked. Whether the child consistently achieves his dry weight goal is evaluated. The pattern of dialysis is established and recorded. Problems of noncompliance should be revealed.

Other items reviewed monthly include medications, blood tests, and medical evaluations. Because dialysis in children is generally viewed as preparatory to transplantation, transplantation status is reviewed monthly. As many evaluations as are needed prior to a live-related or cadaveric transplant are scheduled.

School attendance should be assessed, as well as how dialysis is affecting adaptation at school. Since a goal of home dialysis is to have the child resume normal activities, any aberration in school attendance indicates the child is not achieving that goal. The nurse can assist the family to work out any current difficulties.

Each visit is an opportunity for the nurse to provide ongoing education for the child and family. Specific educational goals can be part of a long-term care plan. The education can be a review of an organ system involved in chronic renal disease, e.g., renal osteodystrophy, or it can be a review of procedures with the aim of reassuring the family or reminding them of reasons to adhere to various procedures. The nurse and the family have a shared responsibility toward setting the agenda.

The interview is concluded with an assessment of the peritoneal dialysis catheter exit site and catheter care demonstration. The catheter is the lifeline of periotoneal dialysis, and therefore its importance should be emphasized.

The child and family are subsequently seen by a physician, dietitian, and social worker, who can collaborate on identified problems as well as perform the physical examination, dietary evaluation, anthropometric measurements, and psychosocial assessment. Meanwhile, laboratory results will begin to become available, and appropriate changes in the medications, dialysis prescriptions, and diet can be made.

### Telephone Calls

Periodically during the month, telephone calls are used as a means of updating the nurse on the child's dialysis status. After discussion among the team members regarding the child's clinic visit, a telephone call will inform the child or family of any changes in prescription. Additional calls should be made to the family if changes in dialysis prescrip-

| Date | Wt | BP | HR | T | Dialysis Solutions | | | Drainage | Exit Site | Comments |
|------|----|----|----|----|-----|-----|------|----------|-----------|----------|
| | | | | | 1.5% | 2.5% | 4.25% | | | |
| | | | | | | | | | | |
| | | | | | | | | | | |

**Figure 14–2.** Standard form for dialysis treatment review.

tions are expected to have immediate effects, i.e., to discover whether the child's dry weight goal is achieved after an increase in the number of exchanges.

If families have problems, they are instructed to call the dialysis unit or the staff member on call. Possible problems include cloudy dialysis effluent with or without accompanying complaints of abdominal pain, alterations in blood pressure status, any gastrointestinal complaints, and signs of catheter exit site infection. Telephone calls, when used judiciously, are a means of providing continued support to the families.[3, 18] However, when used too frequently, they may imply to the family a lack of their own independence and responsibility for care.

### Outside Professional Sources

Community physicians, when presented with a child who has chronic renal failure, will generally refer the child to the pediatric dialysis center closest to their practice. Pediatric dialysis centers are usually affiliated with hospitals which offer transplantation and an ongoing dialysis service. However, when the families choose CAPD, these children may continue to need the services of their referring pediatrician. For this purpose, continuous contact between the ESRD program, referring pediatrician, or local nephrologist will enhance the optimal care of the child.

The multidisciplinary team approach should be explained to these physicians. The goals of the training program also need to be explained, so that the referring physician is fully aware of the family's capabilities in recognizing symptoms of problems, and the need to report them appropriately. A report of each clinic visit should be sent to the outside physician as documentation of the child's status.

There may be times when it is necessary for the child to have blood tests or peritoneal fluid analysis performed during the month. Each family should establish a relationship with appropriate laboratories outside the primary dialysis center. A letter of introduction to the laboratory will expedite this process, particularly if the need arises to perform studies to diagnose peritonitis.

Outside pharmacies, when aware of the particular medication needs for the child on maintenance peritoneal dialysis, can serve as a resource for obtaining medications not usually found in a local pharmacy. This is par-

ticularly true for pediatric vials of intravenous antibiotics used in treatment of peritonitis. Families should have prescriptions for the antibiotics which they will use to initiate treatment for peritonitis.

### Evaluation

The ongoing evaluation of the management program reflects the program's objectives. The child's biochemical status is ascertained by analyzing the monthly blood tests. If abnormalities exist, appropriate changes can be made. Peritonitis and exit site infections are reported and treated; the treatment may serve as an impetus for future prevention. School attendance and normalization of the family's lifestyle, with minimal or no hospitalizations, will reflect a "successful" management program.

Complications invariably develop and can be subdivided into problems related to physical complaints, noncompliance, and psychosocial aberrations.

### Physical Complaints

Discomfort which continues into the home can be caused by physical or psychosocial reasons. Physical problems are more easily treated. Exchange volumes can be set at a level at which discomfort is not present. Two volumes at differing times of the day may be useful for the child on CAPD. Larger volumes can be used for the overnight dwell when the child is least active and a lesser volume used during more active times.

Hernias and dialysate leaks can be surgically repaired. Pleural effusions, a somewhat rare complication, which often does not disappear despite manipulation of dialysis volumes, may be a reason for discontinuing peritoneal dialysis.

The specific dialytic needs of children may include the use of dialysate volumes not commercially available. It is possible to partially infuse bags safely and leave small amounts in the bag outside the peritoneum. At the time of this writing, however, it appears that a greater variation in volume of commercially prepared dialysate will soon be available.

### Noncompliance

Noncompliance with the dialysis regimens and techniques will be reflected in the physical status and well-being of the child. The most serious manifestation is lapses in technique which cause peritonitis. Identification of the exact cause will alleviate the need for further investigation, and retraining is a partial solution. Unless the problem is recurrent, informal presentations during the clinic visit usually suffice. In the event of more persistent problems, scheduling of a formal retraining session should be considered.

Alterations in fluid status include the child's unexpected response to the treatment regimen. Skipping exchanges will lead to inadequate dialysis, fluid overload, and hypertension. Overdialyzing can lead to dehydration, hypotension, and symptoms of shock. The home prescription for ultrafiltration can be changed to a fixed or sliding scale routine, whatever is effective. More frequent clinic visits or telephone consultations provide more opportunities for the nurse to assess the family's understanding of changes in dialysis prescription.

Noncompliance with medications causes problems that are recognized by the results of blood tests or physical examinations. Utilization of outside support systems, such as public health nurses, school nurses, and referring physicians, can help to identify causes. It may be that prescriptions are not filled for financial reasons, in which case consultation with a LCSW may be required. Side effects of some medications may be a deterrent to compliance. This lack of compliance may be improved with continued education. Often, the form of administration can be changed to a more suitable route for compliance. For example, if a child does not like the taste of the liquid phosphate binder, and therefore does not take it, he or she may more readily accept it in a capsule or pill form.

Failure to maintain home records means a break in the communication necessary for adequate care of the child. Families must learn that written documentation provides more useful information than their memory. Any means of encouraging the use of home records is acceptable. This includes threatening, embarrassing, and cajoling the family.

### Psychosocial Aberrations

The establishment of good rapport among professional staff members and families facilitates the early recognition of psychosocial management complications and increases the chances for effective solutions.

A major complication of CAPD is what has been described as "burn-out" or treatment fatigue. Actions which indicate the presence of "burn-out" include chronic lateness or missed appointments, a decrease in previously accurate home records, the family's repeatedly forgetting to bring in daily records, frequent bouts of peritonitis, and withdrawn affect during the clinic interviews. There are several approaches to this problem. Training an additional family member is a possibility. The primary learner can train the third party, under the guidance of the Home Training Nurse; then the training center can evaluate the effectiveness. The third party can be a babysitter, but a requirement is that the person perform at least one exchange weekly so that skills are maintained.

Altered body image is a common reason for management complications. The large amount of peritoneal fluid and the attached bag and tubing may make the child feel "abnormal." This may be solved by changing the peritoneal dialysis modality, usually from CAPD to continuous cycling peritoneal dialysis (CCPD) or intermittent peritoneal dialysis (IPD). Communication with other children or parents who have dealt with the problem may offer support.

When the dialysis regimen is used as a means of rebellion, it is possibly due to the child's or family's feeling of losing control over the disease. Finding acceptable areas of control may contribute to the solution. An example is to allow the family to set their own time schedule of exchanges, provided that the dwell times conform to a written prescription. Written behavior contracts may be a tool for younger children. The rebellion, viewed as a sign of independent thought processes, can be guided toward problem-solving and goal-setting.

Responsibility shifts are common; i.e., the teenager shifts responsibility to the parent, or the parent shifts responsibility to the 10- or 11-year-old child. Recognizing and confronting this in a nonthreatening manner will identify this often subconscious behavior.

Matriculation into the school system is a means of evaluating the success of the program. How this is done varies. Appropriate steps should include educating school staff concerning CAPD and assisting the school in providing an appropriate environment for performing exchanges. Medical documentation of the child's abilities and disabilities is not only a legal necessity, but serves as a method of presenting to the child a "united front." School information packets, including introduction to peritoneal dialysis, explanation of procedures, and rationale for goals, is a means to achieve this goal.

## CONCLUSION

CAPD for the child is a treatment modality which incorporates all aspects of the child's and family's life. The role of the nurse is to support, educate, care for, and thus help the family to achieve its goal of adjusting to ESRD and fitting CAPD into their lives.

Specific procedures are individualized according to the experience of the nephrology department. Within an institution, these procedures may change according to individual family needs. Experience has shown that there are no absolute procedures. Improvements in care are developed over a period of time. What some may describe as failures in the delivery of care may instead be viewed as positive experiences designed to teach the caregivers what does not work. The most creative approaches to care come from the people who are not afraid to try new techniques. Collaboration with nursing colleagues in other centers provides the most practical source of information, but the support of peers is equally important.

# Appendix A
# Record Systems Maintained for Pediatric CAPD Programs

1. Patient Long-Term Program (Life Plan) Network Co-ordinating Council (renewed annually)
2. Patient Short-Term program
Nursing Care Plan including teaching plan—part of permanent medical record.
3. Chronic Renal Disease Medical Evidence Report HCFA #2728.
4. Prescriptions to Vendors (CAPD supplies)
   a. Prescription
   b. Insurance assignment of benefits
   c. ESRD Beneficiary Selection HCFA #382-U3
5. Consents:
   a. Peritoneal dialysis
   b. Home training
   c. All research protocols
6. Certification—Completion of Home Training
7. National Institutes of Health CAPD Patient Registry
   a. Consent to participate in CAPD Registry
   b. Patient Registration Form
   c. CAPD Patient Status Update (quarterly)
8. CAPD Program Statistics (partially maintained via 7c above) including but not limited to:
   a. Infectious complications
   b. Noninfectious complications
   c. Number of training/re-training days
   d. Peritoneal catheter data
   e. Number of hospital admissions, reasons for admissions and length of stay
   f. Transfusion records
9. Nursing Kardex
10. Patient's Daily Home CAPD Records
11. Active Outpatient Chart
    a. Standing orders for the CAPD regimen
    b. Items *1* to *10* above may be maintained in each patient's chart
    c. Other contents of the chart are dictated by the individual institution
12. Active Program List
13. Program Discharge List (including disposition)
14. Data for Research Protocols
15. Current Transplant Information
    a. Tissue typing
    b. Number of transfusions
    c. Recent measurement of cytotoxic antibodies

# Appendix B
# Procedure for Preparing a Toy for CAPD

Supplies Needed:

1. 2 bags normal saline 250 cc
2. 2 plastic adaptors (Beta adaptors I or II for peritoneum to catheter connection. Beta II or III adaptors can be used in place of a titanium connector.)
3. 1 3–4″ section of Silastic catheter or IV tubing.
4. 1 CAPD transfer set
5. 1 Prep Kit
6. Penknife or scissors and needle and thread
7. Doll or stuffed animal—provided by the child

Procedure:

1. For vinyl doll, make a midline abdominal incision with penknife and small lateral hole for "exit site."
2. For stuffed doll or animal, cut incision and exit site with scissors and remove a small amount of the stuffing.
3. Following either 1 or 2 above, make a hole into the outlet port of one bag of 250 cc saline with scissors or transfer set spike.
4. Drain solution from this bag and discard.
5. Firmly place a Beta I or II adaptor in the outlet port and attach section of IV or Silastic tubing to the other end of the adaptor. (This bag becomes the doll's peritoneum with catheter.)
6. Place empty bag in the abdominal space of the doll or toy and pull the catheter through the exit site. When "operating" on vinyl dolls, it may be necessary to hold the incision open with hemostats to insert the bag and then push a hemostat through the exit site from the outside, to grasp the catheter and pull it through the exit site.
7. Place Beta II or III adaptor in external end of catheter and attach CAPD transfer set and the full bag of saline.

8. With stuffed dolls or animals the incision is then sewn shut with needle and thread.
9. With vinyl dolls, butterfly tapes may be placed across the incision or sutures may be drawn on with marking pens.

Points to Remember:

1. Whatever is attached to the doll the child may want to imitate on himself, so any dressings placed on the doll should conform to the program requirements.
2. The child will learn about CAPD as he plays with the doll. He may repeatedly inflow and drain the fluid until he internalizes the procedure.
3. Warn parents to make a small amount of dialysis supplies available to the child for his own use or they will be likely to find an entire box of masks, gloves, and 4 × 4's strewn around the child's play area.

## REFERENCES

1. Maughton M: The patient: a partner in the health care process. Nurs Clin North Am, 17:467, 1982.
2. Renal disease: implementation of coverage of suppliers of end stage services. Department of Health, Education and Welfare, Social Security Administration, Federal Register, June 3, 1976.
3. Fielden N, Johnson S: Home training peritoneal dialysis in pediatric patients. J Am Assoc Neph Nurses Tech 8:41, 1981.
4. Hanson P: Teaching CAPD. Nephrol Nurse, 2:41, 1980.
5. Burns P: Establishing a CAPD program. Part I: The nurse's role. Nephrol Nurse, 3:43, 1981.
6. Moncrief JW, Sorrels PAJ, Kruger VJ, et al: Development of training programs for continuous ambulatory peritoneal dialysis—historical review. In: Continuous Ambulatory Peritoneal Dialysis, Legrain M (Ed). Amsterdam, Exerpta Medica, 1980, p 149.
7. Teehan BP, Schleifer CP, Cupit M, et al: Organizational aspects of a continuous ambulatory peritoneal dialysis program. In: Continuous Ambula-

tory Peritoneal Dialysis, Legrain M (ed). Amsterdam, Exerpta Medica, 1980, p 149.

8. Ray R: Establishing a CAPD program. Part II: The CAPD patient teaching program. Nephrol Nurse, 3:44, 1981.

9. Richard CJ: Peritoneal dialysis—a nursing update: technical aspects and nursing implications. Nephrol Nurse, 2:46, 1980.

10. Talabere LR: The challenge of patient and family teaching. *In:* Patient and Family Education, McCormick RM, Gilson-Parkevich T (Eds). New York, John Wiley & Sons, 1979, p 16.

11. Blas P: Children think about illness: their concepts and beliefs. *In:* Gellert E: Psychological Aspects of Pediatric Care. New York, Grune and Stratton, 1978.

12. Ginsburg H, Opper S: Piaget's theory of intellectual development. Englewood Cliffs, New Jersey, Prentice-Hall, 1979.

13. Erikson E: Childhood and Society. New York, W W Norton and Company, 1963.

14. Fruto L, Prowant B, Sorrels AJ: Nursing management and patient education in continuous ambulatory peritoneal dialysis. *In:* An Introduction to Continuous Ambulatory Peritoneal Dialysis, Travenol Laboratories, Inc., 1980.

15. Campbell C: Nursing Diagnosis and Intervention in Nursing Practice. New York, John Wiley and Sons, 1978.

16. Gross S, Algrim C: Teaching young patients—and their families—about home peritoneal dialysis. Nursing '80, 10:72, 1980.

17. Richard CJ: Peritoneal dialysis—a nursing update: physiological aspects and nursing responsibilities. Nephrol Nurse, 2:38, 1980.

18. McFarland S: Establishing a CAPD program. Part III: Nursing Management. Nephrol Nurse, 3:48, 1981.

# II

# Clinical
# Manifestations

# 15

# Nutritional Assessment and Management of Children with Renal Insufficiency

*Cyril Chantler, M.A., M.D., F.R.C.P.*

Most nutrients, other than energy in the form of fat or carbohydrate, are normally eaten in considerable excess of the body's requirement. This excess is excreted in the urine so that intake and output balance. It is important to understand that this is largely true not only in health but also in chronic renal insufficiency (CRI). Thus an individual on a normal diet and with a liberal fluid allowance will produce the same volume of urine with the same composition when renal function is normal and when moderate CRI is present. CRI is distinguished from health by the changes in body composition that have occurred in order to enable input and output to balance. As renal function declines, the alterations in body composition, and the secondary changes that occur to ameliorate

**Table 15–1.** NUTRITIONAL AND METABOLIC CONSEQUENCES OF CHRONIC RENAL INSUFFICIENCY[3, 4]

| |
|---|
| Anorexia affecting particularly energy, vitamin, and trace element intake. |
| Abnormal protein and energy metabolism. |
| Retention of nitrogenous compounds. |
| Abnormal hormone metabolism. |
| Phosphate retention, hyperparathyroidism, osteomalacia. |
| Sodium retention or depletion. |
| Metabolic acidosis. |
| Hypertension. |
| Anemia. |
| Frequent catabolic illness due to diminished immune competence. |
| Increased nutrient loss on dialysis. |

them,[1] become progressively greater until the metabolic environment becomes so poisoned by the products of nutritional intake that death is inevitable. It can be inferred from this analysis that the anorexia so common in uremia will, at least in part, serve to reduce the severity of the uremic state, thus prolonging life.[2] Anorexia, however, also causes malnutrition, which is itself harmful and a factor in the growth retardation of children with CRI.[3]

Some of the nutritional and metabolic changes in or consequences of CRI are shown in Table 15–1. It is perhaps not surprising that poor growth (see Chapter 19) is a common feature in uremic children. The purpose of this chapter is to discuss those aspects of nutritional management which can reduce these consequences.

## METABOLIC EFFECTS OF CHRONIC RENAL INSUFFICIENCY

Various nitrogenous compounds other than urea accumulate in children with CRI, and a decrease in the symptoms and signs of CRI follows the introduction of a low-protein diet. Many of these compounds are the product of bacteria in the gastrointestinal tract (phenols, aliphatic and aromatic amines, polyamines, and indoles). However, Bergstrom and Furst concluded that only urea intoxication would fulfill the criteria for a uremic toxin,[4] although the toxicity of several com-

**Table 15–2.** MALNUTRITION IN CHRONIC RENAL INSUFFICIENCY[3, 5]

| | |
|---|---|
| Body height and weight[7, 31] | decreased |
| Skeletal and sexual development[8, 9] | retarded |
| Cell mass and weight-to-height ratio[10–13] | decreased |
| Plama protein,[14] plasma albumin,[14] transferrin,[12, 15, 16] CIq,[17] C$_3$,[14, 16, 17] cholinesterase[16] | decreased |
| Plasma branch chain amino acids,[18] branch chain keto acids,[30] essential/nonessential ratio,[15, 19] tyrosine,[18, 19] tryptophan[19] | decreased |
| Muscle alkali soluble protein,[20] total albumin mass, synthesis and catabolism,[21–23] muscle mass,[14] potassium[24, 25] | decreased |
| Total protein turnover,[26] muscle protein synthesis[27, 28] | reduced |
| Muscle protein catabolism[29] | increased |

pounds which accumulate in CRI, such as choline, polyamines, cyclic AMP, guanido-succinic acid, polyols, and middle molecules, has been established.

Abnormalities of amino acid and protein metabolism in CRI are the result of biochemical alterations caused by the metabolic and hormonal changes of CRI or secondary to the protein energy malnutrition which is often present (Table 15–2).[5, 6] Most of these changes are the result of malnutrition rather than a specific effect of uremia on protein metabolism.[6] However, the alterations in energy metabolism in uremia necessarily affect protein metabolism[3] so that protein malnutrition can and does occur in spite of an adequate dietary intake of protein; in fact, protein intake in uremia is usually normal or even well above the minimum recommended daily allowances (RDA). Moreover, an adequate intake of energy will not necessarily restore protein nutrition, because of the reduced consumption of glucose as an energy source. Glucose intolerance and insulin resistance are associated with increased catabolism of protein for gluconeogenesis.[3, 30, 32, 33] Effects of uremia on protein metabolism include increased plasma concentrations of citrulline, cystine, hydroxyproline, and methyl histidine[5, 53] as well as direct effects on protein synthesis.[27]

There are similarities between CRI, protein energy malnutrition (PEM), and other catabolic states.[3, 7] The effects of these conditions on protein turnover are summarized in Table 15–3. A dialyzable constituent of uremic plasma has a direct effect on protein synthesis in vitro.[27] In addition, muscle pro-

tein synthesis can be stimulated in uremic rats by feeding carbohydrate,[28] and the tendency to increased protein degradation is enhanced by fasting.[29] Decreased growth and muscle nitrogen accretion were noted in uremic rats when compared with control pair-fed rats.[41a] The defect in normal energy metabolism is therefore of particular importance in determining the rate of net protein synthesis.

Glucose intolerance in uremia is due to reduced peripheral consumption of glucose,[37, 38] with secondary hyperinsulinemia. It has recently been demonstrated that secondary hyperparathyroidism inhibits the insulin secretion necessary to overcome the hyperglycemia and restore glucose consumption to normal.[39] The control of secondary hyperparathyroidism, either by parathyroidectomy[39] or by dietary means,[40] is associated with increased insulin secretion, and normal peripheral glucose consumption but without concomitant improvement in tissue sensitivity to insulin. Children with CRI ingesting a high carbohydrate diet tend to become obese despite having low cell masses,[41] presumably as a result of the hyperglycemia and hyperinsulinemia. The latter may be especially relevent for growth in children on continuous ambulatory peritoneal dialysis (CAPD).

Metcoff found abnormalities in glycolysis in leukocytes from uremic patients and noted improvements in the activity of pyruvate kinase, phosphofructokinase, glucose-6-phosphate dehydrogenase, and protein synthesis after dialysis.[42] Cellular glucose metabolism is reduced in the presence of uremic serum.[43] The cause of the reduction in glycolysis in uremia is not known, but uncoupling of oxidative phosphorylation by ultrafiltrates of uremic serum has been reported,[44] and low ATP levels have been found in muscle of uremic patients.[45] If glucose metabolism for energy is reduced, other sources of energy will presumably be utilized. The mobilization

**Table 15–3.** PROTEIN METABOLISM IN VARIOUS CONDITIONS

| | Protein Turnover | Protein Synthesis | Protein Degradation |
|---|---|---|---|
| Chronic Renal Insufficiency | ↓ (Ref. 26) | ↓ (Ref. 28) | ↑ or → (Ref. 29) |
| Protein Energy Malnutrition[39] | ↓ | ↓ | ↓ |
| Surgery[35] | → | ↓ | → |
| Sepsis[36] | ↑ | ↑ | ↑ ↑ |

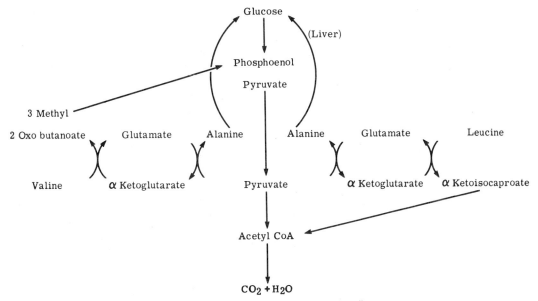

**Figure 15–1.** Oxidation of leucine and valine.

of fat may be limited in CRI by the antilipolytic action of insulin. The plasma concentrations of free fatty acids and glycerol tend to be low in children on regular hemodialysis,[32] and the low plasma fatty acid concentrations rise with adequate dialysis.[56]

A considerable amount of energy metabolism in muscle is derived from the oxidation of branch chain amino acids after transamination to their respective ketoacids[46] (Fig. 15–1). The oxidation of leucine provides acetyl CoA and serves to preserve glucose and pyruvate by the indirect transamination of pyruvate to alanine, which provides the substrate for gluconeogenesis in the liver.[47] Oxidation of valine provides citric acid cycle intermediates as well as stimulating the formation of alanine from pyruvate and aids gluconeogenesis by generating phosphoenol pyruvate (Fig. 15–1). The formation of alanine in muscle is dependent upon the availability of pyruvate and the transamination of amino acids. Whether and under what conditions alanine production in uremia is increased is controversial;[48] however, there is evidence for increased oxidation of branch chain ketoacids (BCKA). Reduced plasma concentrations of BCKA have been found in uremia,[49, 33] with a negative correlation between renal function and plasma keto isocaproic acid (KICA: ketoleucine).[49] The ratio of BCKAs to their respective amino acids is reduced.[30, 33] This reduction may be caused by increased oxidation of BCKAs, reduced pyruvate availability, or reduced protein degradation (Fig. 15–2). Metabolism of valine is reduced in CRI,[50] but increased oxidation was noted after intravenous infusion.[51] This ratio is possibly affected by pyruvate availability because it is reduced in diabetic ketoacidosis, but raised after exercise when pyruvate availability is increased.[30] Thus, in CRI, the reduction in glycolysis may, under conditions of stress such as fasting, cause an increase in protein degradation with increased oxidation of amino acids for energy. It is possible that the reduced pyruvate availability resulting from decreased glycolysis may limit this increased protein breakdown by preventing the transamination of branch chain amino acids released from muscle protein to their respective keto acids. Under these circumstances, the reduced protein synthesis might be regarded as a necessary adaptation to conserve energy. However, as yet evidence to confirm or refute this hypothesis is not available.

The low extra- and intracellular branch chain amino acid (BCAA) concentrations in uremia and the imbalance between them may affect protein synthesis.[54] Low protein diets supplemented with essential amino acids (EAA) or keto essential amino acids (KEAA) were associated with improvements in nitrogen balance[33, 52, 86] and normalization of muscle intracellular amino acid concentration in one study.[53] The low plasma concentrations of leucine, which stimulates in vitro protein synthesis,[54] may be implicated in the reduced protein synthesis in uremia. Oral administra-

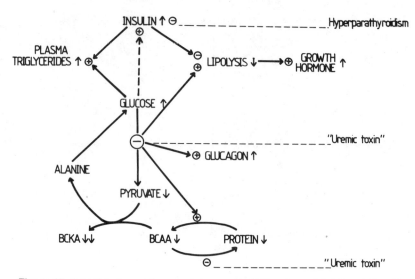

**Figure 15–2.** Metabolic and hormonal changes in CRI and possible interrelationships.

tion of KICA in normal individuals produced a marked reduction in plasma essential amino acids, either because of increased protein synthesis, or reduced protein degradation compared to the administration of other BCKA.[55]

Hypertriglyceridemia and occasionally hypercholesterolemia are found in CRI in children.[57, 58] These metabolic changes may be important in the genesis of early coronary artery disease.[58] The raised triglyceride levels have been thought to be due to both increased hepatic production and decreased clearance associated with decreased activity of plasma lipoprotein lipase. The hypertriglyceridemia is not directly related to dietary fat or total energy intake, but rather to both the proportion and total amount of carbohydrate in the diet.[57, 59] Substitution of fat, either saturated or polyunsaturated, for carbohydrate was associated with a reduction in plasma lipid levels.[59] Plasma triglyceride concentrations correlated with the plasma insulin concentration, and the continued inappropriate production of triglycerides by the liver in the face of a reduced plasma clearance are probably related to the glucose intolerance. Reducing the carbohydrate content of the diet improves glucose tolerance.[60] Plasma cholesterol concentrations are usually normal in uremic adults but variably raised in children, perhaps related to the saturated fat and cholesterol content of the diet.[57, 61] A reduction in cholesterol intake with substitution of polyunsaturated fat is associated with a fall in plasma cholesterol in children (El-Bishti, M: unpublished observations).

Plasma growth hormone concentrations are high in children on dialysis. The levels are positively correlated with the plasma fatty acid concentration,[32] but inversely correlated with the basal glucose levels.[62] Growth hormone is a lipolytic agent, and the high levels may be an adaptive response to poor glucose utilization in an attempt to mobilize endogenous fat as a noncarbohydrate source of energy in the presence of hyperinsulinemia.[63] Plasma glucagon concentrations are also high in CRI[32, 64] and increased in conjunction with a rise in insulin levels when boys on regular hemodialysis were treated with anabolic steroids.[62]

In summary (Fig. 15–2), CRI is associated with complex metabolic and hormonal changes, including a reduction in protein turnover, a reduction in protein synthesis, and a tendency to protein degradation, particularly in response to stress. Glucose intolerance is related to a reduction in glycolysis and is associated with hyperinsulinemia. Hyperparathyroidism may prevent adequate insulin secretion by the pancreas to overcome the peripheral resistance to insulin and restore peripheral glucose uptake to normal. A reduction in glycolysis implies the consumption of protein and fat as an alternative energy source. The hyperinsulinemia will reduce lipolysis, and the rise in plasma growth hormone may be a response to the antilipolytic action of insulin, while plasma glucagon may also rise as a secondary response to raised insulin levels. The glucose intolerance may also be partly responsible for the raised plasma triglycerides.

The presence of a direct inhibitor of protein synthesis in uremia has been shown, but the cause of the reduction in glucose metabolism is not known. It is, however, apparent that dialysis is associated with an improvement in glucose tolerance and the presence of a circulating inhibitor to glucose metabolism has not been excluded. Control of hyperparathyroidism does not improve tissue sensitivity to insulin,[39, 40] but reduction of nitrogen retention with a low protein diet[65] might, although this is not yet certain.[66]

## NUTRITIONAL CONSEQUENCES OF CHRONIC RENAL INSUFFICIENCY

### Energy

Resting metabolic rate and daily energy requirements per kg of body weight are about 2.5 times higher in the first year of life than in the adult.[67] The increased energy requirement is determined by the greater proportion of body mass of an infant made up by metabolically active visceral organs such as the brain.[68] Studies in malnourished children suggest that energy is only available for growth when the requirements for resting metabolism and essential physical acitivity have been fulfilled. Growth retardation occurs when energy intake falls below 70 to 80% of RDA, both in malnourished[69] and uremic children.[70] Probably only 10 to 15% of energy intake is devoted to growth except during recovery from malnutrition, and the energy cost of growth is about 5 kcal/gm of weight gain.[69] Thus, the greater the excess of energy intake over maintenance requirement, the greater the proportion available for growth. It is important to recognize that RDA values represent the average intake of normal children plus an extra allowance; intakes of normal children of the same age and height may differ by up to 50%.[71] Fat, with a higher calorie density than carbohydrate, is important in the diet if high energy intakes are to be achieved.[69]

Uremic children may have increased maintenance energy requirements. This concept is supported by the observations that uremic rats have reduced weight gain per kcal of ingested food.[72, 73] The rate of amino acid incorporation into muscle in carbohydrate gavaged uremic rats is increased;[28] the energy requirements for protein anabolism are increased in acute renal failure in children,[74]

and children on hemodialysis have a higher basal oxygen consumption per unit cell mass.[41]

The higher energy requirements of children imply a greater consumption of other nutrients such as protein, sodium, and phosphate in relation to body weight.[67, 68] All nutrients other than energy sources are usually consumed in excess and this excess is excreted by the kidney. It follows that the excess of intake compared with the requirement is greater in children than in adults; therefore, the amount requiring excretion is proportionately increased. Glomerular filtration rate (GFR) per kg body weight is higher in the child compared to the adult, but this advantage is no longer present in CRI. Thus, the normal consumption of food to satisfy the energy requirements of a child and the higher metabolic rate of a child per kg body weight mean that body composition changes more rapidly and more severely in the child with ESRD compared to an adult.[67, 68] It is not surprising, therefore, that the metabolic and hormonal consequences of CRI are more severe in children. After the first 12 months of life, the metabolic rate and energy requirements correlate with body surface area,[67, 68] and therefore the requirement for dialysis is related better to surface area than to the body mass of a child with ESRD. This necessarily implies larger dialyzers in relation to body weight or longer hours on dialysis for a child.[75, 76] A complementary strategy is to ensure an adequate energy intake by feeding energy supplements while reducing the intake of other nutrients in order to reduce the changes in body composition between dialysis sessions.

Children with CRI eat less than normal children, and there is a correlation between energy intake and growth.[77, 70] Energy supplements improve intake and growth in some but not all children.[77–79] When energy intake exceeds 80% of RDA, growth often remains inadequate and the growth rate no longer correlates with energy intake.[80–82] The foundation of the nutritional management of CRI is to ensure an adequate energy intake while reducing the intake of other nutrients in order to reduce the alterations in body composition. Energy supplements may be helpful in assuring an adequate energy intake and, by blunting appetite, may also help to reduce the intake of other nutrients.[80] There is, however, little point in pressing their use if there is no evidence of malnutrition, if energy intake is already adequate, or if their use is associated with anxiety and tension in the child and family. A supranormal energy intake may make the child obese without improving linear growth.[41]

## Protein

Protein malnutrition is frequently present in a child with CRI. It may occur despite an adequate energy intake, although it is more common in infants in whom energy intake is often low.[11, 12] Protein intake in uremic children is usually in excess of RDA[12, 62, 66, 83] (Table 15–4), although low intakes do occur in some uremic children with severe anorexia.[70] The recommended protein intake is increased for diets with low quality protein.[84] When the amino acid score of the average dietary protein is 70, then the recommended minimum protein intake is 53 gm per day for adult males with a dietary protein-energy ratio of 1.9 gm/100 kcal. The amino acid score is derived by comparing the amino acid composition of the diet with proteins having an ideal amino acid composition. The minimum protein requirement with high quality protein is 37 gm for males and 29 gm for females with a protein-energy ratio of 1.6 gm/100 kcal.[84] Uremic patients on a diet of high quality protein[85] or low quality protein supplemented with essential amino acids (EAA)[86] with a ratio of 1.5 gm protein/100 kcal will support body mass without loss of body protein as long as energy intake is adequate. A higher protein-energy ratio may be required if there is evidence of protein malnutrition.

Some of the symptoms and findings in uremia correlate with nitrogen retention, measured as the blood urea concentration, in the body. With severe uremia (GFR < 10% of normal) a low protein diet is associated with a reduction in these signs.[87, 88] A 35 to 40 gm protein diet[85, 89] or a 20 gm diet supplemented with EAA[86] will reduce the symptoms and signs of uremic toxicity and stimulate a positive nitrogen balance. Unfortunately, there are few comparable studies in children with CRI, probably because of the difficulty in performing nitrogen balance studies in children. Also, if growth is to be evaluated, the observations have to continue for a long enough period (usually 12 months) for significant changes to be detected. In addition, it is extremely difficult to get young children to consume very low protein diets while maintaining an adequate energy intake.[83] A diet calculated to provide minimum protein intake according to height[90] with a protein-energy ratio of 1.25 gm/100 kcal using nonselected protein supplemented with EAA administered to seven children over a period of six months was associated with a marked reduction in blood urea concentrations and a positive nitrogen balance.[83] Unfortunately, the strict protein limitation could not be maintained, blood urea levels rose,

**Table 15–4.** RECOMMENDED DAILY ALLOWANCES FOR CHILDREN WITH CHRONIC RENAL INSUFFICIENCY*

| Age | | Height (cm) | Energy (kcals) | Minimal Protein (gm) | Calcium (gm) | Phosphorus (gm) |
|---|---|---|---|---|---|---|
| 0–2 | months | 55 | 120/kg | 2.2/kg | 0.4 | 0.2 |
| 2–6 | months | 63 | 110/kg | 2.0/kg | 0.5 | 0.4 |
| 6–12 | months | 72 | 100/kg | 1.8/kg | 0.6 | 0.5 |
| 1–2 | years | 81 | 1100 | 18 | 0.7 | 0.7 |
| 2–4 | years | 96 | 1300 | 22 | 0.8 | 0.8 |
| 4–6 | years | 110 | 1600 | 29 | 0.9 | 0.9 |
| 6–8 | years | 121 | 2000 | 29 | 0.9 | 0.9 |
| 8–10 | years | 131 | 2200 | 31 | 1.0 | 1.0 |
| 10–12 | years | 141 | 2450 | 36 | 1.2 | 1.2 |
| 12–14 | years M | 151 | 2700 | 40 | 1.4 | 1.4 |
| 12–14 | years F | 154 | 2300 | 34 | 1.3 | 1.3 |
| 14–18 | years M | 170 | 3000 | 45 | 1.4 | 1.4 |
| 14–18 | years F | 159 | 2350 | 35 | 1.3 | 1.3 |
| 18–22 | years M | 175 | 2800 | 42 | 0.8 | 0.8 |
| 18–22 | years F | 163 | 2200 | 33 | 0.8 | 0.8 |

*Modified from Chantler, 1979;[67] sources of data: DHSS, 1969,[90] National Academy of Sciences, 1968.[128]

At least 25% of total energy should be provided by carbohydrate (normal children take about 50% total energy as carbohydrate), and at least 3% of total energy should be in the form of essential polyunsaturated fatty acids. An adequate vitamin and trace element intake must be given.[127] Sodium and potassium intake will depend on renal function but for normal children an intake of 1.5–2.5 mmol (2–3 mg)/kg body weight per day is recommended.

and the acutal diet consumed at the conclusion of the study had a mean protein-energy ratio of 1.9 gm/100 kcal. Protein nutrition, judged from plasma transferrin levels, weight-for-height ratios, and measurement of intracellular water, was reasonably well maintained. It was interesting that the one child who showed improvement in height maintained a protein-energy ratio of 1.4 gm/ 100 kcal. In a further study using a low protein diet supplemented with an EAA/ KEAA mixture[66] where growth velocity increased in the seven children studied, the protein-energy ratio averaged 1.7 gm/100 kcal.

The influence of nitrogen toxicity on nitrogen balance or growth is difficult to examine. The blood urea concentration is dependent on the GFR, on the excess, over requirement, of protein in the diet and on the proportion of dietary nitrogen which is utilized in the restoration of cell mass or in growth. The latter is, of course, influenced by many factors, including the energy content of the diet. It cannot, however, be disregarded, for a highly significant negative correlation was found between the utilization of dietary nitrogen and the blood urea concentration, with a threefold difference in blood urea concentrations according to the proportion of dietary nitrogen utilized for the maintenance of nitrogen balance.[91] Walser[92] has estimated that with a neutral nitrogen balance blood urea concentration should not exceed 30 mmol/L (180 mg/dl) in severe renal failure unless protein intake is far above requirement, or there is excessive catabolism

with a negative nitrogen balance. In fact, with a urea clearance of 4 ml/min in an adult on a minimum protein intake the blood urea would be about 20 mmol/L (120 mg/dl). A relation between nitrogen balance and blood urea concentration can be found in the data from a study of low protein diet supplemented with EAA reported by Bergstrom et al.[93] (Fig. 15–3). Unfortunately, the scatter of the data is wide; the subject with a blood urea concentration of 80 mg/dl (13 mmol/ dL) had a barely positive balance and another with a blood urea of 150 mg/dl (25 mmol/L) was in strongly positive balance. Mean blood urea concentrations in children on a low protein diet supplemented with EAA who grew poorly were 46 mmol/L (278 mg/dl),[90] while in a similar study employing KAA supplements where the children grew well the mean blood urea was 16 mmol/L (96 mg/ dl).[66] A high blood urea does not preclude adequate growth. Normal growth over a period of five years was observed in a child with a blood urea concentration consistently above 30 mmol/L (180 mg/dl) (personal observation).

## Calcium and Phosphate

Renal osteodystrophy and calcium and phosphate metabolism are discussed elsewhere in this text (Chap. 17). The anorexia of CRI and the provision of high energy diets with energy supplements may reduce calcium intake below RDA[80] (Table 15–4). Low phosphate and protein diets will also reduce cal-

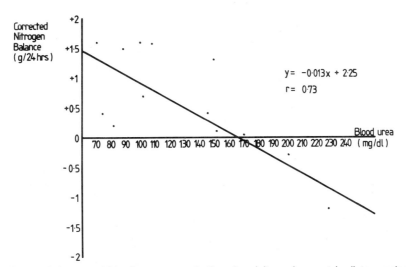

**Figure 15–3.** Nitrogen balance and blood urea concentrations in adults on low protein diets supplemented by EAA, calculated from data given by Bergstrom et al.[93]

cium intake. It is important to ensure an adequate calcium intake by feeding calcium supplements if necessary. Some calcium preparations, such as effervescent preparations of calcium glyconate, contain sodium, and if sodium retention with hypertension is a problem, then sodium-free preparations (calcium gluconate syrup) should be used.

Phosphate retention leading to secondary hyperparathyroidism is a major cause of morbidity in patients with CRI.[94, 95] The hyperparathyroidism can be substantially reversed even in established CRI by feeding a low phosphate diet with phosphate binders to prevent intestinal absorption of phosphate in both children[39, 96] and adults[97] with CRI. The diet has to be maintained over a period of months. A study conducted over a four-week period showed no effect.[98] The adequacy of the diet can be assessed by regular measurement of the fractional reabsorption of phosphate[100] calculated from the phosphate and creatinine clearances or from the Tm $PO_4$/GFR,[99] using the nomograms of Walton and Bijvoet.[101] The fractional reabsorption rises toward normal and the PTH level is suppressed as phosphate intake and absorption is reduced.[96] This is associated with the reduction in the metabolic consequence of secondary hyperparathyroidism,[39] although preliminary histologic observations on bone biopsy material suggest that the reversal of the osteitis fibrosa cystica may be less satisfactory (Mak RHK, personal communication).

The difficulty of reducing established secondary hyperparathyroidism in established CRI, even with successful transplantation,[102] suggests that prevention by controlling phosphate intake early in the renal disease is important. Fractional phosphate reabsorption and, if possible, plasma PTH concentrations should be measured in all children with CRI when GFR is below 40 ml/min/1.73 $m^2$ body surface area.[103] Because the measurement of plasma PTH is imprecise, early changes may be missed. Plasma phosphate concentrations cannot be used to determine the need for dietary phosphate control; in mild degrees of renal insufficiency values are often low, and by the time they rise outside the normal range, secondary hyperparathyroidism is established.

A substantial reduction in phosphate intake can be achieved by reducing the intake of dairy products and by a reduction in protein intake. Phosphate binders are required, in addition, in severe CRI if the di-

etary limitations are not to be too arduous. Aluminum hydroxide raises serum aluminum concentrations in renal failure[96] and has been implicated in the development of dementia;[104] calcium carbonate either alone or in combination with aluminum hydroxide is an effective binding agent.[96] The average requirement in children with moderately severe CRI is 4 to 6 gm of aluminum hydroxide or calcium carbonate daily; in addition to the usual proprietary preparations, the latter is available in custard cream biscuits containing 360 mg calcium carbonate, and these are acceptable to children.* The plasma calcium concentration should be monitored at regular intervals; hypercalcemia may require a reduction in vitamin D intake or a reduction in dietary calcium. It frequently occurs some months after treatment commences and may be due to increased vitamin D activity when the secondary hyperparathyroidism is controlled.

## Vitamins

The requirement for vitamin D or its analogs in CRI is discussed in Chapters 16 and 18. An adequate intake according to RDA should be ensured, but the difficult decision is when to use large doses of cholecalciferol or when to prescribe its active metabolites. Radiologic evidence of osteomalacia is an indication, but growth may be affected before such changes become apparent.[105, 106] It is likely that management will be easier when measurements of serum 1,25-dihydroxycholecalciferol and other vitamin D metabolites are available for clinical practice, but in the meantime it is important to check plasma calcium levels at regular intervals if vitamin D or its active metabolites are prescribed.

Vitamin $D_6$ (pyridoxine) deficiency occurs in CRI, particularly in patients on dialysis, possibly because of accelerated turnover.[5] Pyridoxine deficiency contributes to decreased immunologic competence and affects amino acid and fatty acid metabolism and neurologic function. Pyridoxine hydrochloride supplements of 10 mg each day should be given to all patients with CRI.[5]

Folic acid deficiency may occur in CRI,

---

*Obtainable from Welfare Foods Ltd., London Road South, Poynton, Stockport, Cheshire SK12 1LA, United Kingdom.

even in the presence of normal serum folic acid concentrations, owing to alterations in folate metabolism.[107]

## Trace Elements

Iron, zinc, copper, manganese, chromium, cobalt, selenium, iodine, and fluorine are essential or beneficial to man.[108] The accumulation and toxicity of aluminum and iron in dialysis patients is well recognized; copper accumulation can also occur[109] and may be associated with anemia. Tissue zinc levels, especially in the liver, brain, and heart, were increased in one study,[108] but low levels of plasma zinc have also been observed.[109] A number of abnormalities in patients with CRI, such as anorexia, impaired taste acuity, hair loss, ataxia, impotence, and poor growth, have been attributed to zinc deficiency. Zinc supplementation has been associated with increased taste acuity and appetite although changes in growth velocity were not observed.[110] It is important to ensure an adequate intake of trace elements and vitamins, if necessary by feeding supplements, in all children on special diets.

## NUTRITIONAL ASSESSMENT

Adequate nutritional management of a child with CRI either on conservative treatment, undergoing dialysis, or after renal transplantation requires careful and regular clinical assessments. It is time-consuming and each clinic visit will occupy at least one-half to one hour of the physician's time as well as involving consultation with the dietitian (nutritionist), social worker, etc. This is emphasized because to provide less inevitably will lead to less than optimal care. Certain techniques, though valuable for research, are either impractical or unnecessary for good clinical practice, and therefore will not be discussed in this section.

## Anthropometry

This is discussed in detail elsewhere.[111] Height, weight, skinfold thickness at the biceps and subscapular sites, and upper arm circumference should be measured regularly.[112–114] Weight-for-height index is a measure of muscle and adipose tissue which, al-though affected by the accumulation of extracellular fluid in uremia, provides a useful indication of the adequacy of nutritional status. Measurements of cell mass and weight-for-height index correlated ($r = 0.71$) in 21 children with CRI.[12] Skinfold and arm circumference measurements enable estimates of muscle mass and body fat to be made.[112, 113]

## Radiologic Assessment

Radiographs of the hand-wrist and knee should be obtained at tri-monthly intervals for detection and supervision of renal osteodystrophy, and assessment of skeletal age at yearly intervals.[111]

## Clinical Evaluation

A brief clinical history and examination, including the measurement of blood pressure and urine examination, should be performed at monthly to tri-monthly intervals, depending on the clinical condition. Pubertal status should be assessed at yearly intervals. Full attention should be paid to the adequacy of nutrition, the presence of edema, or evidence of dehydration. Full attention, if necessary, with skilled social or psychological assistance, should be paid to the impact of the disease and its treatment (including dietary management) on the child, his family, and the social, emotional, and intellectual growth at home and at school. Nutritional management cannot be separated from the general clinical management, and it is the responsibility of the physician to integrate the total care of the child.

## Biochemical Investigations

Full blood picture, serum ferritin level, and red cell folate level should be estimated at the initial consultation and intermittently thereafter to determine the adequacy of iron and folic acid intake. Blood electrolytes, plasma bicarbonate, calcium, phosphate, alkaline phosphatase, blood urea, serum proteins, and uric acid levels should be checked at each visit. A 24-hour urine collection should be analyzed for urea, creatinine, sodium, calcium, and phosphate content. Urea appearance rate is the urea excretion plus (or minus) the change in the body urea pool over the period of study.[92] If dietary nitrogen intake is known and it is assumed that non-urea nitrogen losses are constant, then sequential analysis of urea appearance enables an assessment of the adequacy of the nitrogen balance. Formal nitrogen balance studies are too arduous for use in clinical practice, and even the simplified balance is of little usefulness because the dietary analysis is often too variable, urine collection errors occur, and unless carefully performed the results can be misleading.

In effect, if renal function is not changing, the blood urea concentration will reflect protein intake and the nitrogen balance, because it may be assumed that any nitrogen consumed in excess of requirement is excreted. No definite statement can be made concerning levels of blood urea which reflect nitrogen toxicity, but it is our practice from the evidence discussed in the previous section to attempt to maintain the blood urea concentration below 30 mmol/L (180 mg/dl) and preferably below 20 mmol/L (120 mg/dl), or a urea:creatinine ratio of less than 10:1 (mg:mg).[116] A rising blood urea suggests a fall in renal function, an increase in protein intake, a fall in energy intake, or the presence of a catabolic state caused by infection, etc.

Urea kinetic modeling,[115] which involves the calculation of urea appearance rate, may be useful in patients on dialysis by enabling the dialysis requirement to be varied according to the individual patient's requirement, thus optimizing dietary intake and the time spent on dialysis with minimum change in body composition.

The 24-hour urine specimen obtained at each clinic visit should also be used to calculate the fractional reabsorption of phosphate so that secondary hyperparathyroidism can be adequately controlled with phosphate restriction. The urine sodium excretion provides a useful check on the adequacy of the diet assessment (see below). Serum transferrin (and plasma albumin) measurements at intervals provide a useful additional assessment on the adequacy of protein nutrition.[12]

## Dietary Assessment

The dietary intake of energy, fats, carbohydrate, protein—both quality and quantity—calcium, phosphate, sodium, and so on should be monitored at monthly to tri-

monthly intervals. Dietary intake is best estimated by a prospective recording of all items consumed over a three-day period. Parent cooperation, without causing obsessional anxiety, can usually be obtained if the estimates are not too frequent. Intakes of specific nutrients can be calculated from standard tables of food composition,[117] a task considerably simplified by having food composition tables on computer tapes[119] for comparison with RDA[84, 90, 118] (Table 15–4). This three-day prospective dietary assessment method compared well with a double-bag analysis of all food consumed, with a correlation coefficient for energy of $r = 0.92$, and for protein of $r = 0.92$; the mean discrepancy was 11%.[120]

## MANAGEMENT OF NUTRITION IN CHRONIC RENAL INSUFFICIENCY

### Conservative Management

The purpose of nutritional management in children with CRI is to promote well-being and activity and to improve growth. It is all too easy to make the treatment more arduous than the disease. While general principles can be outlined, it is important to remember that each child and family must be approached individually according to their personalities, intelligence, social integration, and culture. Simple prescriptions of diet are rarely successful; general anxiety and often a sense of failure create tension, and these often contribute to anorexia.

Recently, the possibility that nutritional therapy and, in particular, control of protein, sodium, and phosphate intake may protect the diseased kidney from further damage has been discussed.[121] A low nitrogen, low phosphate diet has been shown to slow the decline in renal function in patients with CRI.[122, 130] The importance of this concept is not yet clear, but it is of interest that no decline in renal function was observed in children with CRI maintained for one year on a low protein, low phosphate diet supplemented with KEAA.[66] If the importance of protein and phosphate intake on the progression of renal disease is confirmed, nutritional management will need to be introduced progressively from the time when GFR declines below normal and possibly in anyone with a reduced mass of normally functioning renal tissue.

At present we would undertake a nutritional assessment when the GFR is less than

40 ml/min/1.73 m$^2$ body surface area. Control of blood pressure, prevention of excess sodium intake, reduction of phosphate and protein intake to maintain a normal fractional reabsorption of phosphate, and a blood urea concentration less than 20 mmol/L (120 mg/dl) can usually be obtained with a minimum interference in the family's nutritional habits. More severe CRI requires more attention, with the progressive introduction of the nutritional assessment techniques discussed above. The requirement for each child will vary according to the severity of the uremic symptoms, growth impairment, and the disturbance in body composition.

An adequate sodium intake must be assured.[123] Children, especially infants, with obstructive uropathy or renal dysplasia often fail to conserve sodium and can become salt-depleted with a reduction in GFR or severe extracellular fluid depletion, particularly if diarrhea or vomiting supervene. Our usual practice is to increase dietary sodium or provide salt supplements to prevent hyponatremia without producing edema, a rise in blood pressure, or the development of hypernatremia. Conversely, sodium overload must be prevented by lowering dietary sodium or administering loop diuretics such as furosemide. Metabolic acidosis is corrected with alkali, usually in the form of sodium bicarbonate supplements.

Protein intake is progressively reduced according to the evidence of nitrogen toxicity, down to minimal level (Table 15–4). An adequate energy intake must be assured, and energy supplements in the form of glucose polymer or fat given as dairy cream or polyunsaturated fat emulsions are useful in increasing total energy intake while reducing an excessive intake of other nutrients.[12] In a careful study of nutrient intakes of nine children on regular hemodialysis, the total energy intake averaged 112% RDA, with supplements providing 33% of RDA, whereas energy intake without supplements was 70% of RDA (p = 0.01).[120] Protein supplements in the form of EAA also increased protein intake from 89% RDA to 103% RDA. The presence of hypertriglyceridemia will require a reduction in the carbohydrate content of the diet with subsitution of fat, while hypercholesterolemia will indicate the need to reduce cholesterol and saturated fat intake.

There is no need to prescribe energy supplements if dietary intake is satisfactory and there is no evidence of energy malnutrition. The prescription of a low protein diet to an anorectic child is often followed by food refusal. Our approach is to assess nutrient intake individually, increase energy intake if necessary, using energy supplements, and then to gently introduce protein restriction. It is not necessary to use special low protein foods, which are usually unpalatable. Every attempt should be made to accommodate the child's dietary requirements within the normal dietary pattern of the family. Above all, the generation of anxiety and tension between the child and parent must be avoided.

Very low protein diets supplemented with EAA or KEAA[66, 83] are useful for children with severe CRI who are unwell or growing poorly. These diets are difficult to apply and expensive, although they may be worthwhile in selected patients. It is often necessary to admit the child and mother to the hospital to establish dietary control, particularly if the child is anorectic with major alterations in body composition. The vicious circle of inadequate energy intake, with accelerated catabolism, from nitrogen and phosphate retention sustaining the anorexia, can sometimes only be broken by tube feeding into the stomach or jejunum, using synthetic food substitutes. If this is undertaken, then the osmolality of the feed must not be too high, and the feed should be introduced slowly to prevent vomiting, which can be a severe problem in the uremic infant.

## Dialysis

The general principles of nutritional management for children with CRI are applicable to children on dialysis. The major problem is to overcome the anorexia and ensure an adequate energy and protein intake. The vicious circle of inadequate intake leading to catabolism and anorexia may need to be broken by intensive nutritional management in the hospital, with tube feeding and the use of energy supplements. However, confrontation and tension over food intake must be avoided. Our general approach is to encourage a free diet with the avoidance of high sodium and potassium foods, no added salt at meal times, and some reduction in the salt used in cooking. No specific reductions in protein intake are advised, at least initially. Fluid intake will depend upon residual renal function. Excessive weight gain between dialysis sessions is usually primarily due to excessive sodium intake.

Diet assessments are carried out monthly, and further advice is offered with the knowledge of what the child is actually eating and the family's dietary habits. The technical quality of the dialysis[75, 76, 124] is important to prevent circulatory disturbances on dialysis, which will exacerbate the anorexia. Adequate dialysis should be provided to maintain reasonable body composition rather than adjusting dietary management to cope with inadequate dialysis. Urea kinetic modeling (Chapter 6) or some other approach to determine the need for dialysis[115, 124] is required. As long as protein intake is adequate, no advantage is gained by feeding EAA supplements.[129] Considerable protein losses may occur on CAPD, and it is important that they are replaced with extra dietary protein.

## Transplantation

The nutritional problems following transplantation are mainly caused by the necessity to use glucocorticoid steroids to prevent rejection. Sodium retention with hypertension will require reduction in sodium intake. The avoidance of high sodium foods, no added salt, and the omission of salt in cooking will reduce sodium intake to about 50 to 60 mmol (3 to 4 gm) per day. Corticosteroids are gluconeogenic, reducing net protein anabolism and increasing blood glucose levels, serum triglyceride levels, and adipose tissue. A high protein, low carbohydrate diet should be commenced early after transplantation. The diet should contain not less than 2 gm/kg body weight of protein and not more than 100 to 120 gm of carbohydrate. Dietary intake and body weight should be checked at regular intervals. Adequate calcium and phosphate intake is essential, and phosphate supplements may be required to combat hypophosphatemia.

## Parenteral Nutrition

Intercurrent illnesses are common in children with CRI and provide a serious catabolic stress in addition to the tendency to protein catabolism inherent in the uremic state in a child who is often already malnourished. If adequate oral nutrition is not possible, than parenteral nutrition should be commenced early and maintained until an adequate oral intake has been established. Anuric children, compared to adults, require more calories

and more protein, and fluid tolerance is restricted. Even with strict control of fluid intake, frequent dialysis is often required to remove water and should be undertaken rather than reducing nutritional intake. Intravenous fat emulsions in amounts greater than 1 g/kg/day are frequently inadequately metabolized owing to the reduced plasma lipoprotein lipase activity which is common in uremia, so that much of the energy requirement has to be satisfied with carbohydrate. In six anuric children, mean age 6.0 years, urea production was minimized with an energy intake of 70 kcal/kg/day.[125] Nitrogen was provided as an EAA mixture. At a mean intake of 81 mg/kg/day, nitrogen balance averaged +58 mg/kg/day. Severe catabolic states associated with major trauma or with burns may increase energy requirements by 50 to 100%, and for every degree centigrade rise in temperature there is a 13% increase in energy expenditure. The increase in protein requirements may be even greater. Glucose intolerance is common and insulin may need to be infused at 2 to 20 units/hour to maintain normoglycemia. The use of insulin in severe catabolism has been shown to reduce protein degradation.[126]

## CONCLUSION

Nutritional management is fundamental to the care of the child with CRI at all stages in the treatment of his condition and rehabilitation. Good management not only will prevent complications that arise from malnutrition but will improve growth, help to prevent or control osteodystrophy, and at times of severe catabolic stress may well prove to be the vital difference between death and survival. It is not surprising that children on regular hemodialysis in Europe managed in children's centers have a lower death rate than children in nonspecialized children's centers, nor that a common cause for death was recorded as cachexia.[75]

## REFERENCES

1. Bricker NS, Fine LG: The trade-off hypothesis: Current status. Kidney Int 13:5, 1978.
2. Betts PR, Mann WD, Wolfsdorf J: Growth and nutrition of uraemic piglets. Pediatr Res 10:937, 1976.
3. Holliday MA, Chantler C: Metabolic and nutritional factors in children with renal insufficiency. Kidney Int 14:306, 1978.

4. Bergstrom J, Furst P: Uraemic toxins. Kidney Int 13:9, 1978.
5. Kopple JD: Abnormal amino acid and protein metabolism in uraemia. Kidney Int 14:340, 1978.
6. Richards P: Protein metabolism in uraemia. Nephron 14:134, 1975.
7. Chantler C, Holliday WA: Growth in children with renal disease with special reference to the effects of calorie malnutrition: A review. Clin Nephrol 1:230, 1973.
8. Betts PR, White RHR: Growth potential and skeletal maturity in children with chronic renal insufficiency. Nephron 16:325, 1976.
9. Donckerwolcke RA, Chantler C, Brunner FP, et al: Combined report on regular dialysis and transplantation of children in Europe 1977. Proc Eur Dial Transplant Assoc 15:77, 1978.
10. Coles GA: Body composition in chronic renal failure. Quart J Med 41:25, 1972.
11. El-Bishti M, Burke J, Gill P, et al: Body composition in children on regular hemodialysis. Clin Nephrol 15:53, 1981.
12. Jones RWA, Rigdon SP, Barratt TM, Chantler C: The effects of chronic renal failure in infancy on growth, nutritional status and body composition. Pediatr Res 16:784, 1982.
13. Stickler GB, Bergen BJ: A review: short stature in renal disease. Pediatr Res 7:978, 1973.
14. Blumenkrantz MJ, Kopple JD: VA co-operative dialysis study participants: Incidence of nutritional abnormalities in uraemic patients entering dialysis therapy (Abstr). Kidney Int 10:514, 1976.
15. Kopple JD, Swendseid ME: Protein and amino acid metabolism in uraemic patients undergoing maintainance haemodialysis. Kidney Int 2 (Suppl):64, 1975.
16. Young G, Oli HA, Davison AM, Parsons FM: The effects of calorie and essential amino acid supplementation on plasma proteins in patients with chronic renal failure. Am J Clin Nutr 31:1802, 1978.
17. Heidland A, Kult J: Long term effects of essential amino acid supplementation in patients on regular haemodialysis treatment. Clin Nephrol 3:235, 1975.
18. Counahan R, Cox BD, Ogg CS, Chantler C: Plasma amino acids in children on haemodialysis. Kidney Int 10:471, 1976.
19. Kopple JD: Nitrogen metabolism. *In*: Clinical Aspects of Uraemia and Dialysis, Massry SG, Sellers AL (eds). Springfield, Illinois, CC Thomas, 1976, p 241.
20. Delaporte C, Bergstrom J, Broyer M: Variations in muscle cell protein of severely uraemic children. Kidney Int 10:239, 1976.
21. Blumenkrantz MJ, Kopple JD, Gutman RA, et al: Methods for assessing nutritional status of patients with renal failure. Am J Clin Nutr 33:1567, 1980.
22. Coles GA, Peters DK, Jones JH: Albumin metabolism in chronic renal failure. Clin Sci 39:423, 1970.
23. Bianchi R, Mariani G, Toni MG, Carmassi F: The metabolism of human serum albumin in renal failure on conservative and dialysis therapy. Am J Clin Nutr 31:1615, 1978.
24. Letteri JM, Ellis KJ, Asad SN, Cohn SH: Serial measurement of total body potassium in chronic renal disease. Am J Clin Nutr 31:1937, 1978.
25. Weber HP, Michalk D, Rauh N, et al: Total body potassium in children with chronic renal failure. Int J Pediatr Nephrol 1:42, 1980.
26. Conley SB, Rose GM, Robson AM, Bier DM: Effects of dietary intake and haemodialysis on protein turnover in uraemic children. Kidney Int 17:837, 1980.
27. Delaporte C, Gros F, Anagnostopoulos T: Inhibitory effects of plasma dialysis on protein synthesis in vitro, influence of dialysis and transplantation. Am J Clin Nutr 33:1407, 1980.
28. Holliday MA, Chantler C, McDonnell R, Keitges J: Effect of uraemia on nutritionally induced variations on protein metabolism. Kidney Int 11:236, 1977.
29. Li JB, Wassner SJ: Muscle degradation in uraemia: 3 methyl histidine release in fed and fast rats. Kidney Int 20:321, 1981.
30. Dalton N, Chantler C: The relationship between branch chain amino acids and keto acids in blood in uraemia. Kidney Int (in press).
31. Potter DE, Greifer I: Statural growth of children with renal disease. Kidney Int 14:334, 1978.
32. El-Bishti M, Counahan R, Bloom SR, Chantler C: Hormonal and metabolic responses to intravenous glucose in children on regular haemodialysis. Am J Clin Nutr 31:1865, 1978.
33. Chantler C, Jones RWA, Dalton N: Amino acid and protein metabolism in chronic renal failure. *In*: Developments in Nephrology. 3, Paediatric Nephrology. Proceedings 5th International Nephrology Symposium 1980, AB Gruskin, ME Norman (eds). Boston, Martinus Nijhoff, 1981, p 310.
34. Golden M, Waterlow JC, Picou D: The relationship between dietary intake, weight change, nitrogen balance and protein turnover in man. Am J Clin Nutr 30:1345, 1977.
35. Waterlow JC, Golden M, Picou D: The measurement of rates of protein turnover synthesis and breakdown in man and the effects of nutritional status and surgical injury. Am J Clin Nutr 30:1333, 1977.
36. Garlick PJ, McNurlan MA, Fern EM, et al: Stimulation of protein synthesis and breakdown by vaccination Br Med J 2:263, 1980.
37. De Fronzo RA: Pathogenesis of glucose intolerance in uraemia. Metabolism 27 (Suppl 2):1866, 1978.
38. Mak RHK, Haycock G, Chantler C: Glucose intolerance in children with chronic renal failure. Kidney Int (in press).
39. Mak RHK, Turner C, Haycock G, Chantler C: Glucose intolerance and secondary hyperparathyroidism in children with uraemia. Kidney Int (in press).
40. Mak RHK: Glucose intolerance in uraemia: role of secondary hyperparathyroidism (submitted for publication).
41. Chantler C, El-Bishti M, Counahan R: Nutritional therapy in children with chronic renal failure. Am J Clin Nutr 33:1682, 1980.
41a. Mehls O, Ritz E, Gilli G, et al: Nitrogen metabolism and growth in experimental uraemia. Int J Paediatr Nephrol 1:34, 1980.
42. Metcoff J, Lindemann R, Baxter D, Pederson J: Cell metabolism in uraemia. Am J Clin Nutr 30:1627, 1978.
43. Renner D, Heintz R: The inhibition of certain steps of glucose degradation in uraemia. *In*: Uraemia, Kluthe R, Berlyne G, Burton B (eds). Stuttgart, Springer Verlag 1972, p 195.
44. Glaze RP, Morgan JM, Morgan RE: Uncoupling

of oxidative phosphorylation by ultrafiltrates of uremic serum. Proc Soc Exp Biol Med 12:172, 1967.

45. Brautbar N: Muscle energy metabolism in uraemia. Kidney Int (in press).

46. Goldberg AK, Chang TW: Regulation and significance of amino acid metabolism in skeletal muscle. Fed Proc 37:2301, 1978.

47. Snell K: Muscle alanine synthesis and hepatic gluconeogenesis. Biochem Soc Trans 8:205, 1980.

48. De Fronzo RA, Felig P: Amino acid metabolism in uremia: Insights gained from normal and diabetic man. Am J Clin Nutr 33:1378, 1980.

49. Schauder P, Matthei D, Scheler F, et al: Blood levels of branched chain keto acids in uraemia: therapeutic implications. Klin Wochenschr 57:825, 1979.

50. Jones MR, Kopple JD: Valine metabolism in normal and chronically uraemic man. Am J Clin Nutr 31:1660, 1978.

51. Jones MR, Kopple JD: Valine metabolism during saline and amino acid infusion in normal and uraemic man. Abstracts of Second International Congress of Nutrition and Renal Disease, Bologna, 1979, p 76.

52. Bergstrom J, Ahlberg M, Alvestrand A, Furst P: Metabolic studies with keto acids in uraemia. Am J Clin Nutr 31:1761, 1978.

53. First P, Alvestrand A, Bergstrom J: The effects of nutrition and catabolic stress on intracellular muscle amino acid pools in uraemia. Am J Clin Nutr 33:1387, 1980.

54. Adibi SA: Roles of branch chain amino acids in metabolic regulation. J Lab Clin Med 95:475, 1980.

55. Dalton RN, Chantler C: The metabolism of orally administered branch chain keto acids. Kidney Int (in press).

56. Roth DA, Meade RC, Barboriak JJ: Glucose, insulin and free fatty acids in uraemia. Diabetes 22:111, 1973.

57. El-Bishti M, Counahan RJ, Stimmler L, et al: Abnormalities in plasma lipids in children on regular haemodialysis. Arch Dis Child 52:932, 1977.

58. Pennisi AJ, Heuser ET, Mickey MR: Hyperlipidemia in paediatric haemodialysis and renal transplant patients. Am J Dis Child 130:957, 1976.

59. Sanfelippo ML, Swenson AS, Reaven GM: Reduction of plasma triglycerides by diet in subjects with chronic renal failure. Kidney Int 11:54, 1977.

60. Sorge F, Castro LA, Nagel A, Kessel M: Serum glucose, insulin, growth hormone, free fatty acids and lipid responses to high carbohydrate and a high fat isocaloric diet in patients with chronic non-nephrotic renal failure. Horm Metab Res 7:118, 1975.

61. Broyer M, Tete MJ, Laudat MH, Dartois AM: Plasma lipid abnormalities on chronic haemodialysis: relationship to dietary intake. Proc Eur Dial Transplant Assoc 13:385, 1976.

62. Jones RWA, El-Bishti M, Bloom SR, et al: The effects of anabolic steroids on growth, body composition and metabolism in boys with chronic renal failure on regular haemodialysis. J Paediatr 97:559, 1980.

63. Glick SM, Roth J, Yalow RS, et al: The regulation of growth hormone secretion. Rec Progr Horm Res 21:242, 1965.

64. Sherwin RS, Bastl C, Finkelstein SO, et al: Influence of uraemia and haemodialysis on the turnover and metabolic effects of glucagon. J Clin Invest 57:722, 1976.

65. Snyder D, Pulido LB, Kagan A: Dietary reversal of the carbohydrate intolerance in uraemia. Proc Eur Dial Transplant Assoc 5:205, 1969.

66. Jones RWA, Dalton RW, Turner C, et al: Oral essential amino acid and keto acid supplements in children with advance chronic renal failure (submitted for publication).

67. Chantler C: Renal failure in childhood. In: Renal Disease, 4th ed, D Black, NF Jones (eds). London, Blackwell Scientific Publications, 1979, p 825.

68. Holliday MA: Calorie deficiency in children with uraemia: Effect upon growth. Pediatrics 50:590, 1972.

69. Ashworth A: Energy balance and growth: Experience in treating children with malnutrition Kidney Int 14:301, 1978.

70. Betts PR, MacGrath G: Growth pattern and dietary intake of children with chronic renal insufficiency. Br Med J 2:189, 1974.

71. Widdowson EM: A study of individual children's diets. MRC Special Report Series No 257. London, HM Stationery Office, 1947.

72. Chantler C, Lieberman E, Holliday MA: A rat model for the study of growth failure in uraemia. Pediatr Res 8:109, 1974.

73. Mehls O, Ritz E, Gilli G, et al: Effects of vitamin D on growth in experimental uraemia. Am J Clin Nutr 31:1927, 1978.

74. Abitol CL, Holliday MA: Total parenteral nutrition in uraemic children. Clin Nephrol 5:153, 1976.

75. Donckerwolcke RA, Chantler C, Broyer M, et al: Combined report on regular dialysis and transplantation in Europe 1979. Eur Dial Transplant Assoc 17:94, 1980.

76. Gardiner AOP, Sawyer AN, Donckerwolcke RA, et al: The assessment of dialysis requirement for children on regular haemodialysis. Dial Transplant 11:754, 1982.

77. Simmons JM, Wilso CJ, Potter DE, et al: Relation of calorie deficiency to growth failure in children on haemodialysis and the growth response to calorie supplementation. N Engl J Med 285:653, 1971.

78. Chantler C, El-Bishti M, Counahan R, et al: Growth in children with renal failure. Melsunger Med Mitteilungen 50 (Suppl 2):557, 1976.

79. Arnold W, Danford D, Holliday M: Effect of caloric supplementation on growth in children with uremia. Kidney Int 24:205, 1983.

80. Betts PR, MacGrath G, White RHR: Role of dietary energy supplementation in growth of children with chronic renal failure. Br Med J 1:416, 1977.

81. Chantler C, Counahan R, Wass VJ, et al: Growth in renal failure. Br Med J 1:773, 1977.

82. Broyer M: Nutritional disorders in paediatric patients with kidney failure. Kidney Int (in press).

83. Jones RWA, Dalton RW, Start K, et al: Oral essential amino acid supplements in children with advanced chronic renal failure. Am J Clin Nutr 33:1696, 1980.

84. FAO/WHO Expert Committee: Protein and energy requirements. In: WHO Technical Bulletin 522, Geneva, 1973 (WHO Sales and Services, 1211, Geneva 17, Switzerland).

85. Kopple JD, Coburn JW: Metabolic studies of low

protein diets in uraemia. 1. Nitrogen and potassium. Medicine (Baltimore) 52:583, 1973.

86. Noree LO, Bergstrom J: Treatment of chronic uraemic patients with protein poor diet and an oral supply of essential amino acids. II. Clinical results of long term management. Clin Nephrol 3:195, 1975.

87. Giordano C: Treatment of uraemia using essential amino acids and a low protein diet. *In:* Proceedings of Second International Congress of Nephrology, Basel and Karger, 1964, p 732.

88. Giovennetti S, Maggiore Q: Low nitrogen diet with proteins of high biological value for severe chronic uraemia. Lancet 1:1000, 1964.

89. Ford J, Phillips ME, Toye FE, et al: Nitrogen balance in patients with chronic renal failure on diets containing varying quantities of protein. Br Med J 1:735, 1969.

90. Department of Health and Social Security: Recommended intakes of nutrients for the United Kingdom. Reports of public health and medical subjects, No 120, London, HM Stationery Office, 1969.

91. Taylor YSM, Scimshaw NS, Young VR: The relationship between serum urea levels and dietary nitrogen utilization in young men. Br J Nutr 32:407, 1974.

92. Walser M: Determinants of urea genesis, with particular reference to renal failure. Kidney Int 17:709, 1980.

93. Bergstrom J, Furst P, Noree LO: Treatment of chronic uraemic patients with protein poor diets and an oral supply of essential amino acids. Clin Nephrol 3:187, 1975.

94. Slatopolsky E, Caglar S, Pennell JP, et al: On the pathogenesis of hyperparathyroidism in chronic experimental renal insufficiency in the dog. J Clin Invest 50:492, 1971.

95. Massry SG, Goldstein DA: Role of parathyroid hormone in uraemic toxicity. Kidney Int 13:539, 1978.

96. Mak RHK, Turner C, Powell H, et al: Treatment of secondary hyperparathyroidism in uraemic children with dietary phosphate restriction of phosphate binders (submitted for publication).

97. Barsotti G, Morelli E, Guiducci A, et al: Reversal of hyperparathyroidism in severe uraemics following very low protein and low phosphorus diet. Nephron 30:310, 1982.

98. Biswas CK, Arze RS, Ramos JM, et al: Effects of aluminium hydroxide on serum ionised calcium, immunoreactive parathyroid hormone, and aluminium in chronic renal failure. Br Med J 284:776, 1982.

99. Kruse K, Kracht U, Gopfert G: Renal threshold phosphate concentration ($TmPO_4$/GFR). Arch Dis Child 57:217, 1982.

100. Thalassinos NC, Leese B, Latham SC, et al: Urinary excretion of phosphate in normal children. Arch Dis Child 45:269, 1970.

101. Walton RJ, Bijvoet OLM: A simple slide rule method for the assessment of renal tubular reabsorption of phosphate in man. Clin Chim Acta 81:273, 1977.

102. Graf H, Kobarisk J, Stunnvoll HK, et al: Renal phosphate wasting after successful kidney transplantation (Iα Vitamin D therapy in patients with normal parathyroid gland activity). Nephron 28:285, 1981.

103. Norman ME, Mazur AT, Borden S, et al: Early diagnosis of juvenile renal osteodystrophy. J Pediatr 97:226, 1980.

104. Boukari M, Rottenbourg J, Jaudon MC, et al: Influence de la prise prolongee de gels d'alumine sur les taux seriques d'alluminium chez les patients attents d'insuffisance renale chronique. Nouv Presse Med 7:85, 1978.

105. Dent CE, Harper C, Philpot OR: The treatment of renal glomerular osteodystrophy. Quart J Med 30:1, 1961.

106. Chesney RW, Moorthy AV, Eisman JA, et al: Increased growth after long term oral 1:25 vitamin $D_3$ in childhood renal osteodystrophy. N Engl J Med 298:238, 1978.

107. Kopple JD, Swendseid ME: Vitamin nutrition in patients undergoing maintainance haemodialysis. Kidney Int 7:S-79, 1975.

108. Sandstead HH: Race elements in uraemia and haemodialysis. Am J Clin Nutr 33:1501, 1980.

109. Tsukamoto Y, Iwanami S, Marumuno F: Disturbances of trace element concentrations in plasma of patients with chronic renal failure. Nephron 26:174, 1980.

110. Eggert JV, Siegler RL, Edamkesmalee E: Zinc supplementation in chronic renal failure. Int J Paediatr Nephrol (in press).

111. Potter DE, Broyer M, Chantler C, et al: Measurement of growth in children with renal insufficiency. Kidney Int 14:378, 1978.

112. Gurney JM, Jellife DB: Arm anthropometry in nutritional assessment: nomogram for rapid calculation of muscle circumference and cross sectional muscle and fat areas. Am J Clin Nutr 26:912, 1973.

113. Frisancho AR: Triceps skin fold and upper arm muscle size norms for assessment of nutritional status. Am J Clin Nutr 27:1052, 1974.

114. Tanner JM, Whitehouse RH: Revised standards for triceps and subscapular skinfolds in British children. Arch Dis Child 50:142, 1975.

115. Sargent J, Gotch F, Borah M, et al: Urea kinetics: a guide to nutritional management of renal failure. Am J Clin Nutr 31:1696, 1978.

116. David DS, Hochgelerent E, Rubin AL, et al: Dietary management in renal failure. Lancet 2:34, 1972.

117. McCance RA, Widdowson EM: The composition of foods. Special Report Series No 297. London, HM Stationery Office, 1969.

118. Department of Health and Social Security: Recommended daily amounts of food energy and nutrients for groups of people in the U.K. London, HM Stationery Office, 1979.

119. Pennington JAT: Dietary Nutrient Guide. Westport, Connecticut, AVI Publishing Co, 1976.

120. Brown HE: The evaluation of a new diet for children on haemodialysis programmes. M Sc Thesis, Queen Elizabeth College, London, 1976.

121. Brenner BM, Meyer TW, Hostetter TH: Dietary protein intake and the progressive nature of kidney disease. N Engl J Med 307:652, 1982.

122. Barsotti G, Guiducci A, Ciardella F, Giovannetti S: Effects on normal function of a low nitrogen diet supplemented with essential amino acids and ketoanalogues and of haemodialysis and free protein supply in patients with chronic renal failure. Nephron 27:113, 1981.

123. Berlyne GM, Mallick MP, Gaan D: Dietary treatment of chronic renal failure. *In:* Nutrition in Renal Disease, Berlyne GM (ed), proceedings of a conference held at the University of Man-

chester June 29–30, 1967. Edinburgh, E&S Livingstone, 1968, p 99.

124. Donckerwolke RA, Chantler C, Broyer M: Paediatric dialysis. *In*: Replacement of Renal Function by Dialysis, Parsons M, Drukker W, Maher JF (eds). London, Martinus Nijhoff, 1978, p 444.

125. Abitol CL, Holliday MA: Total parenteral nutrition in uraemic children. Clin Nephrol 5:153, 1976.

126. Woolfson AMJ, Heatley RV, Allison SP: Insulin to inhibit protein catabolism after injury. N Engl J Med 300:14, 1979.

127. Crim MH, Calloway DH: A method for nutritional support of patients with severe renal failure. Nutr Metab 12:111, 1970.

128. National Academy of Sciences National Research Council Food and Nutrition Board: Recommended Daily Allowances, 7th edition, 1964.

129. Counahan R, El-Bishti M, Chantler C: Oral essential amino acids in children on regular haemodialysis. Clin Nephrol 9:11, 1978.

130. Walser M: Ketoacids in the treatment of uremia. Clin Nephrol 3:180, 1975.

# 16

# Principles of Nutritional Assessment and Management of the Child with ESRD

*Pauline Nelson, R.D.*
*Jean Stover, R.D.*

The growth rate of healthy children is significantly influenced by their nutritional status. Renal insufficiency in a child is associated with metabolic imbalances which lead to inadequate nutrition. The role of the nutritionist in the management of the child with chronic renal disease is to provide a comprehensive therapeutic regimen which minimizes the biochemical consequences of uremia and improves the nutritional status in an effort to maximize growth. This goal, deceptively simple, frequently becomes an inordinate challenge. In this chapter we will discuss the methods of nutritional assessment and management of infants, children, and adolescents with varying degrees of renal insufficiency and following renal transplantation.

## ASSESSMENT OF NUTRITIONAL STATUS

A comprehensive nutritional assessment of the factors affecting growth and development of the pediatric patient with chronic renal disease requires the use of a combination of tools and parameters. Anthropometric measurements, dietary histories, biochemical parameters, evaluation of water balance, and review of prescribed medications are integral parts of assessing the nutritional status and formulating the dietary prescription.

### Anthropometric Measurements

Weight, length or height, and head circumference (for children less than two years of age) measurements usually constitute the initial parameters of this assessment. These anthropometric measurements are interpreted by comparison with standardized percentiles for chronologic age and weight for height on growth charts of normal children developed by the National Center for Health Statistics (NCHS).[1] A relative body weight can be calculated for the child with renal failure by dividing the patient's body weight by the 50th percentile of weight for height of a normal child of the same sex.

Additional anthropometric measurements include mid-arm circumference (MAC) and triceps skinfold (TSF). These are obtained with the use of a metal or plastic tape and a skinfold caliper. The mid-arm muscle circumference (MAMC) can be calculated from these measurements. The combination of the MAC, MAMC, and TSF measurements reflect body protein and fat stores, which can be evaluated by comparison with published normal values.[2, 3] With serial determinations, the child serves as his own standard of comparison. Measurements are taken on the left arm, except when a vascular access is present.[4]

To increase the accuracy of these measurements, they should be performed according to a standard protocol, utilizing one individual for consistency if possible (especially for the height, MAC, and TSF measurements). Monthly repetition of height and weight measurements and at least quarterly MAC and TSF measurements are suggested for evaluation of growth in an outpatient population. The presence of edema may spuriously elevate the MAC and TSF measurements and must be noted.[4] Children on continuous peritoneal dialysis should be routinely weighed with their abdomens full for ease of evaluating repetitive measurements.

Use of the child's correct chronologic age is imperative for appropriately interpreting body weight and height measurements. Weight for height percentiles are assumed to be age-independent.[5] Height or bone age is used to evaluate the MAC, MAMC, and TSF measurements. Height age is based upon the determination of chronologic age, using standard tables where the height of the child corresponds to the 50th percentile. For example, a seven-year-old girl who measures 108 centimeters would have a height in the 50th percentile for a five-year-old girl, and thus a height age of five. Bone age is determined by roentgenographic studies of the hands and wrists. While the bone age usually lags behind the chronologic age in children with chronic renal failure, it usually surpasses the height age after puberty.[6] Body composition changes during puberty and so do the standards of comparison. Thus, for the growth-retarded adolescent, the bone age is a more reliable index for evaluation of protein and fat stores.

## Dietary Histories

When used in conjunction with physical measurements, dietary histories, including interviews and food records, are a valuable tool of nutritional assessment in the development of a nutrition care plan. Information from the patients and/or their parents or caretakers provides data about a child's current nutritional status and may identify possible future nutritional complications. Areas of importance include current appetite, any noted appetite change, recent changes in weight and activity level, previous dialytic therapies, transplantation history, prior surgery, and regularity of bowel habits. The timing of meals and participation in school lunch programs are also noteworthy. Specific food preferences may be indicative of future nutritional problems relative to a planned treatment modality (e.g., dislike of high-quality protein foods vs. protein losses associated with peritoneal dialysis). All the above data are recorded by the nutritionist and updated as necessary.

Establishing good rapport with the child and family is crucial for obtaining complete and accurate dietary information.[4] Nutritional care plans require consideration of the family's social, ethnic, economic, psychosocial, and educational status because they all impact on the child's nutrient intake.

Food intake records kept periodically by the child or caretaker for a three-day interval are an integral part of the dietary history. A three-day record has an advantage over a 24-hour recall record because a pattern of eating habits may be seen and better compliance is obtained than with a seven-day record. This written information augments the verbal information obtained in an interview.[4] The recordkeeper must be educated in the technique of weighing and measuring all foods and beverages consumed; such records may be kept during hospitalizations (by nursing staff) as well as at home.

## Laboratory Values

Biochemical assessment is another tool used in the overall nutritional assessment of children with chronic renal disease. Serum levels of electrolytes, calcium, phosphorus, blood urea nitrogen (BUN), creatinine, glucose, cholesterol (fasting), triglycerides (fasting), and specific proteins (total protein, albumin, transferrin) are measured periodically during the course of treatment. These levels are compared to normal values for evaluation of adequacy of pharmacologic, dialytic, and dietary therapy.

The determination of the urea nitrogen appearance (UNA) rate for children on peritoneal dialysis[4, 7] and protein catabolic rate (PCR) for children on hemodialysis[8] are useful estimates of dietary protein intake and can be used to validate the food records. The UNA and PCR require laboratory evaluation and are calculated from formulas to be discussed subsequently.

## Water Balance

Evaluation of water balance is a significant part of the nutritional assessment. Many children with chronic renal failure cannot excrete excess sodium and water. Following renal transplantation, excessive fluid retention may occur as a result of steroid therapy. The nutritionist must be able to differentiate between edema and dry weight gain when developing nutrient recommendations during any phase of treatment of the child with chronic renal failure.

## Medications

The mineral content of medications, their interactions with food, and effects on appetite and bowel habits are important when evaluating potential nutritional complications and dietary needs of the child with renal disease. If an ion exchange resin (Kayexelate) is required on a regular basis to maintain a normal serum potassium level, the nutritionist should realize that there are approximately 100 milligrams of sodium per gram of this medication.[9] When sodium restriction is required, dietary intake is adjusted to avoid the adverse effects of increased sodium ingestion. Sodium bicarbonate is another commonly prescribed medication which may contribute to excessive sodium intake. The Physicians' Desk Reference (PDR) can be consulted for information regarding the chemical content of specific medications.

Phosphate binders may cause constipation, and the diet may need to be altered or a stool softener prescribed prophylactically for patients taking these medications. At each visit with the nutritionist, the currently prescribed medications should be reviewed to assess compliance. Noncompliance with phosphate binders is frequent. Prescribing an alternative form (capsule, tablets, or liquid) or brand of binder may increase compliance.

## Formulating the Dietary Prescription

The dietary prescription is determined following examination of all parameters of nutritional assessment. Modifications are made in accordance with a change in the child's nutritional status, further diminution of kidney function following a change in dialytic or pharmacologic therapy, and after renal transplantation. The nutritionist must be aware of management principles at each phase of the treatment process.

A nutritional care plan is developed for each child and contains the diet prescription as well as the goals and objectives for expected patient skills and behavior. In the child with chronic renal failure, the plan is of both short and long-term duration.

## NUTRITIONAL MANAGEMENT

### Infants

Many studies relate the growth failure of children with chronic renal disease to malnutrition. (See Chapters 14 and 18.) Consequently, the additional high energy and protein needs of the infant necessitate thorough and continual assessment and management of patients in this age group. As the infant grows and develops, the nutrient needs and types of recommended foods will require adjustment.

The nutritional management of infants with chronic renal failure often requires modification of common infant nutritional practices. (Table 16–1.) In the predialysis phase, the type of formula prescribed most frequently contains a relatively low renal solute load closely resembling the mineral content of human milk. Two such formulas, SMA (Wyeth Laboratories) and PM 60/40 (Ross Laboratories) are ideal because they contain electrodialyzed whey as approximately 60% of their protein content.[10] S-29 (Wyeth Laboratories), a formula with an exceptionally low renal solute load, is also used in some situations. (Table 16–2.)

These formulas are preferred over breast milk because caloric fortification is often necessary. Many infants with chronic renal failure are poor feeders, resulting in slow weight gain and growth retardation. It has been shown that children malnourished during early infancy are less able to recover intellectual deficits suffered from poor brain growth than those malnourished later in life.[6] Malnutrition results not only from caloric deprivation but also from inadequate protein, vitamin, and mineral intake. If the total volume of formula is severely limited by voluntary intake, then nasogastric feedings may be indicated.[11]

**Table 16–1. DAILY NUTRIENT AND FLUID RECOMMENDATIONS FOR THE CHILD WITH ESRD**

| | Energy | Protein | Sodium | Potassium | Calcium | Phosphorus | Vitamins | Trace Minerals | Fluid |
|---|---|---|---|---|---|---|---|---|---|
| **Prediialysis (>15% GFR)** | | | | | | | | | |
| Infants | Minimum of RDA for statural age | RDA for statural age | 1–3 mEq/kg if necessary | 1–3 mEq/kg if necessary | Supplement as necessary | Restrict high content foods, use low content formula if necessary | 1 cc multivitamin drops if necessary + vitamin D metabolite if needed | Supplemental zinc, iron, or copper if necessary | Minimum of maintenance levels |
| Children/Adolescents | Minimum of RDA for height age | Minimum of RDA for height age | 1–3 mEq/100 kcal expended if necessary | Unrestricted until K elevated | Supplement as necessary | 500–1000 mg/day when ≤50% GFR | Multivitamin preparation if necessary + vitamin D metabolite if needed | Supplemental zinc, iron, or copper if necessary | When edema develops, give insensible + urinary output |
| **Prediialysis (<15% GFR)** | | | | | | | | | |
| Infants | Minimum of RDA for statural age | 1.5–1.6 gm/kg | 1–3 mEq/kg if necessary | 1–3 mEq/kg | Supplement as necessary | Restrict high content foods, use low content formula | Same as when GFR >15% normal | Same as when GFR >15% normal | When edema develops, give insensible + urinary output |
| Children/Adolescents | Minimum of RDA for height age | Maximum of RDA for height age | 1–3 mEq/100 kcal expended if necessary | Unrestricted until K elevated <10% GFR use 25–50 mEq/day | Supplement as necessary | 500–1000 mg/day | Same as when GFR >15% normal | Same as when GFR >15% normal | Same as when GFR >15% normal |
| **Hemodialysis** | | | | | | | | | |
| Infants | Minimum of RDA for height age | RDA for statural age | 1–3 mEq/kg if necessary | 1–3 mEq/kg | Supplement as necessary | Restrict high content foods, use low content formula | 1 cc multivitamin drops, 1 mg folic acid + vitamin D metabolite if needed | Same as during pre-dialysis period | Insensible + ultra-filtration + urinary output (if any) |
| Children/Adolescents | Minimum of RDA for height age | RDA for height age | 1–3 mEq/100 kcal expended if necessary | 25–50 mEq/day when necessary | Supplement as necessary | 500–1000 mg/day | 1 mg folic acid, 50–100 mg vitamin C, B-complex + vitamin D metabolite as needed | Same as during pre-dialysis period | Insensible + urinary output |
| **Peritoneal Dialysis (IPD)** | | | | | | | | | |
| Infants | Minimum of RDA for statural age | 2.5–3 gm/kg | 1–3 mEq/kg if necessary | 1–3 mEq/kg | Supplement as necessary | Same as for hemodialysis | Same as for hemodialysis | Same as during pre-dialysis period | Same as for hemodialysis |
| Children/Adolescents | Minimum of RDA | Usually midway between hemodialysis and CAPD recommendations | 1–3 mEq/100 kcal expended if necessary | 25–50 mEq/day when necessary | Supplement as necessary | Same as for hemodialysis | Same as for hemodialysis | Same as during pre-dialysis period | Same as for hemodialysis |
| **Peritoneal Dialysis (CAPD)** | | | | | | | | | |
| Infants | Minimum of RDA for statural age | 3–4 gm/kg | 3 mEq/kg based upon edema, BP | 3 mEq/kg and possibly not necessary | Supplement as necessary | May be liberalized based upon serum levels | Same as for hemodialysis | Same as during pre-dialysis period | Same as for hemodialysis |
| Children/Adolescents | Minimum of RDA for height age | 3.0 gm/kg–ht age 2–5 yr; 2.5 gm/kg–ht age 5–10 yr; 2.0 gm/kg–ht age 10–12 yr; 1.5 gm/kg–ht age >12 yr | Usually unlimited, 85–174 mEq/day if necessary | Usually unlimited, 25–50 mEq/day if necessary | Supplement as necessary | Generally 240 cc milk/day or equivalent in milk products | Same as for hemodialysis | Same as during pre-dialysis period | Usually not necessary |
| **Transplant** | | | | | | | | | |
| Infants | RDA for statural age after ideal weight/length is achieved | 3 gm/kg | 1–3 mEq/kg | Unlimited | Ad libitum | May need very high intakes—supplement as necessary | Usually not necessary unless severe malnutrition prior to transplant—vitamin D if needed | Should not be necessary | Usually not necessary |
| Children/Adolescents | RDA for height age—no concentrated sweets for 6 weeks post transplant | 2–3 gm/kg | 130–174 mEq/day and less if edema and BP are present | Unlimited | Ad libitum | May need very high intakes—supplement as necessary | Usually not necessary unless severe malnutrition prior to transplant—vitamin D if needed | Should not be necessary | Usually not necessary |

**Energy.** When greater caloric density of a formula is required for infants prior to initiation of dialysis, it is *not* advisable to concentrate the product (adding smaller volumes of water to the powder base or concentrate to increase calories per volume) because the renal solute load will be increased when formula is prepared this way. Once dialysis has started, it is possible to increase the protein intake and maximize the volume of formula because of the increased potential for solute removal. Modular components of carbohydrate and fat are generally added for caloric fortification, however, during all phases of treatment. A glucose polymer such as Polycose (Ross Laboratories) is tolerated by most young infants (owing to low osmolality) and is utilized for carbohydrate supplementation. The older infant (8–12 months) may tolerate corn syrup which is commercially available and is less costly. (Table 16–2.)

Medium Chain Triglyceride Oil (MCT oil) (Mead Johnson) or an unsaturated vegetable oil, such as corn or safflower oil, are acceptable sources of fat supplementation (Table 16–2). In view of the good tolerance by infants of formulas containing the latter oils reported by Fomon et al.[12] MCT oil is not usually necessary except possibly for the very young infant[11] or in instances where gastrointestinal disturbances coexist. The comparative low cost and accessibility of the other oils are the primary considerations for their use.

The modular components of carbohydrate and fat are gradually added to formula, raising the caloric content of commercial formulas from 20 kilocalories (kcal) per ounce up to 24 to 30 kcal per ounce. Caloric concentrations of 40 to 45 kcal per ounce can be achieved for infants 8 to 12 months of age without adverse effects. To promote digestibility, efforts are made to eventually keep the same proportion of total fat to carbohydrate calories which is contained in the base formula. The infant should be given a period of adjustment (24 to 72 hours) with each caloric increment. Diarrhea and/or vomiting may indicate poor tolerance due to the increased osmolality of formula. If these symptoms persist, further modification of the feeding regimen is indicated. As a precaution, a sample of the fortified formula may be tested to determine if the desired osmolality of 300 to 400 mOsm/kg water is present.[11]

When nasogastric feedings of fortified formulas are given, the rate of delivery can be decreased if vomiting or diarrhea persists.

The rate and degree of caloric fortification should not be increased simultaneously.

In a clinically malnourished infant, it is advisable to administer a fortified formula as the major source of nutrition up to one year of age. When infants begin taking small amounts of strained foods (at approximately six months of age), we often suggest adding modular components of carbohydrate and fat to these products to compensate for the decreased dietary caloric content associated with the ingestion of decreased volumes of formula.

The degree of caloric fortification of food and formula depends largely upon the infant's individual feeding habits and growth rate. Caloric needs are based upon the Recommended Dietary Allowances (RDA)[13] and the degree of growth retardation. A range of 105[13] to 200 kcal per kilogram of actual body weight is recommended.

Caloric fortification of formula and food for infants undergoing peritoneal dialysis may be altered to compensate for glucose absorption from the dialysate and the potential for hypertriglyceridemia. The latter is a controversial issue in the uremic child because of the possible development of atherosclerotic cardiovascular disease.[14] However, when the fasting serum triglyceride level is markedly elevated, the source of caloric fortification is altered to achieve a proportionally higher unsaturated fat-to-carbohydrate ratio, which may lessen the severity of this lipid abnormality.[14]

Glucose absorption from the dialysate has been reported by Balfe et al to be $2.74 \pm 1.05$ gm/kg/day in children less than six years of age undergoing Continuous Ambulatory Peritoneal Dialysis (CAPD).[15] Thus, dialysate dextrose may be considered as a caloric source when calculating the energy requirements for the infant undergoing CAPD or Continuous Cycling Peritoneal Dialysis (CCPD).

**Protein.** The RDA for protein for healthy infants is 2.2 gm/kg for statural age 0–0.5 years and 2.0 gm/kg/day for a statural age 0.5–1.0 years.[13] These recommendations are encouraged during the predialysis period when the glomerular filtration rate (GFR) is greater than 15% of normal.[16] Most infants with this degree of renal insufficiency will voluntarily consume at least this amount of protein in the first few months of life and are encouraged to do so to maximize physical growth and development. Few infants with renal disease will take significantly greater

**Table 16–2.** INFANT FORMULAS AND NUTRITIONAL SUPPLEMENTS[42–44]

| | Kcal/cc | Osmolality mOsm/kg $H_2O$ | Protein gm/L | Fat gm/L | CHO gm/l | Na/K mEq/L |
|---|---|---|---|---|---|---|
| **Infant Formulas** | | | | | | |
| PM 60/40 (Ross) | 0.68 | 260 | 16 | 38 | 69 | 7/15 |
| SMA (Wyeth) | 0.68 | 300 | 15 | 36 | 72 | 6/14 |
| S 29 (Wyeth) | 0.68 | * | 17 | 23 | 101 | <1/8 |
| Milk, cow | 0.65 | 288 | 35 | 35 | 48 | 22/37 |
| Milk, human | 0.73 | 300 | 11 | 45 | 71 | 8/14 |
| **Carbohydrate Modules** | | | | | | |
| Corn syrup | 3.9 | * | 0 | 0 | 1008 | 40/1** |
| Polycose (Ross) | 2 (4/gm) | 850 | 0 | 0 | 500 | 25/5 |
| Controlyte (Doyle) | 2 (5/gm) | 598 | 0 | 96 | 286 | 0.8/0.4 |
| Sumacal (Organon) | (4/gm) | * | 0 | 0 | 95/100 gm | 4/≤1/100gm |
| **Protein Modules** | | | | | | |
| Casec (Mead-Johnson) | (4/gm) | * | 88/100 gm | 2/100 gm | 0 | 7/ 3/100 gm |
| Pro-Mix (Nubro, Inc.) | (4/gm) | * | 85/100 gm | 0 | 9/100 gm | 7/41/100 gm |
| Propac (Organon) | (4/gm) | * | 78/100 gm | 8/100 gm | 5/100 gm | 10/13/100 gm |
| Electrodialyzed Whey (Wyeth) | (4/gm) | * | 35/100 gm | 3/100 gm | 56/100 gm | 1/ 1/100 gm |
| **Fat Modules** | | | | | | |
| MCT Oil (Mead-Johnson) | 7.7 | * | 0 | 858 | 0 | * |
| Vegetable oil, corn | 8.0 | * | 0 | 898 | 0 | * |
| **Essential Amino Acid Supplements** | | | | | | |
| Aminaid (McGaw) | 1.9 | 1095 | 19 | 46 | 366 | 14/5 |
| Travasorb Renal (Travenol) | 1.35 | 590 | 23 | 18 | 271 | 0/0 |
| **Calories/Protein Supplements** | | | | | | |
| Ensure (Ross) | 1.0 | 450 | 37 | 37 | 145 | 37/40 |
| Sustacal (Mead-Johnson) | 1.0 | 625 | 61 | 23 | 140 | 40/53 |

amounts of protein than the RDA for statural age (when infant formulas are given), and as they gain body weight, the amount of formula ingested remains the same or declines. Thus, the amount of protein ingested per kilogram of body weight will decline.

Infants with greater degrees of renal insufficiency will require less than the RDA for protein (approximately 1.5 to 1.6 gm/kg/day) to prevent azotemia.[16] Newer technical developments now permit the use of peritoneal dialysis in very young infants and enable the protein intake to be liberalized.

Protein supplementation is required for infants with renal insufficiency during the predialysis period when massive proteinuria (a minimum of 50 to 100 mg/kg body weight total protein loss daily)[17] without azotemia is present. A protein supplement, such as Casec powder (Mead-Johnson) can be added to both the formula and strained foods.

Protein needs for the infant undergoing CAPD or CCPD are always higher than those required in the predialytic period. Measured dialysate protein losses of 0.3 ± 0.06 gm/kg/ day for children less than six years of age undergoing CAPD reported by Balfe et al[15] indicate the need for supplementation of this nutrient. As mentioned previously, Casec powder may be added to infant formula and strained foods. Also, Electrodialyzed Whey (Wyeth),[11] Propac (Organon, Inc.), and Pro-mix (Nubro, Inc.) have been used successfully in this situation (Table 16–2). The addition of an amino acid preparation to the dialysate has been reported to prevent amino acid losses and provide protein supplementation with improved body weight gain.[15] Protein needs will vary depending upon individual dialysate protein losses as well as upon the serum levels of total protein, albumin, BUN, and the nutritional status based upon arm anthropometry. The needs of most infants range from 3 to 4 gm/kg/day with the daily caloric intake derived from protein being as high as 20%.

**Sodium.** Sodium needs for the infant with chronic renal insufficiency are generally in the maintenance range of 1 to 3 mEq/kg/ day[18] during all phases of renal disease. This is easily achieved by using the formulas PM 60/40 and SMA. For infants with "salt-wast-

**Table 16–2.** INFANT FORMULAS AND NUTRITIONAL SUPPLEMENTS[42-44] *(Continued)*

| Ca/PO$_4$ mg/L | Vitamin A I.U./L | Vitamin D I.U./L | Vitamin E I.U./L | Vitamin C mg/L | Folic Acid mg/L | Vitamin B$_1$/B$_2$ mg/L | Iron mg/L | Zn/Mg mg/L |
|---|---|---|---|---|---|---|---|---|
| 400/200 | 2500 | 400 | 15 | 55 | 0.05 | 0.65/1.0 | 2.6 | 4/42 |
| 440/330 | 2640 | 420 | 9.5 | 58 | 0.05 | 0.71/1.1 | 12.7 | 3.7/53 |
| 138/169 | * | * | * | * | * | * | * | * |
| 1170/920 | 1435 | 417 | 1.8 | 8.0 | 52.0 | 0.28/1.6 | 0.5 | 3.7/120 |
| 330/150 | 2500 | 22 | 1.8 | 52 | 52.0 | 0.1/0.4 | 0.21 | 1.6/40 |
| 205/12 | 0 | 0 | 0 | 0 | 0 | 0 | tr | * |
| ≤300/≤60 | * | * | * | * | * | * | * | * |
| 4/8/100 gm | * | * | * | * | * | * | * | * |
| tr/tr | * | * | * | * | * | * | * | * |
| 1600/800/100 gm | * | * | * | * | * | * | * | * |
| 225/112/100 gm | * | * | * | * | * | * | * | * |
| 600/308/100 gm | * | * | * | * | * | * | * | * |
| 700/419/100 gm | * | * | * | * | 0.025/100 gm | 0.5/2.0/100 gm | * | 0.5/61/100 gm. |
| 0 | 0 | 0 | 0 | 0 | 0 | 0 | 0 | 0 |
| 0 | 0 | 0 | 0 | 0 | 0 | 0 | 0 | 0 |
| <80/<60 | 0 | * | * | * | * | * | * | * |
| 0/0 | 0 | 0 | 0 | 45 | 0.05 | 0.75/0.85 | 0 | 0 |
| 520/520 | 2640 | 211 | 320 | 160 | 0.02 | 0.16/0.18 | 0.95 | 1.6/21 |
| 1000/917 | 4640 | 370 | 28 | 56 | 0.37 | 0.14/0.17 | 17.0 | 14/380 |

*Information not available
**Applies to product with added salt

ing" syndromes requiring phosphate and possibly potassium restrictions, a supplemental solution of sodium chloride may be necessary to compensate for the low sodium content of the above products (6 to 7 mEq/L). An estimate of the "salt-wasting" infant's sodium needs is based upon the sodium content of a 12-to-24-hour urine collection.[11, 19]

Most manufacturers in the United States do not add sodium chloride to commercial baby foods so that the introduction of solids will not be a problem when dietary sodium content must be limited. Nevertheless, the natural sodium content of foods must be considered.

For infants undergoing CAPD or a variant thereof, a liberal sodium allowance is generally tolerated. Individual needs are based upon residual renal function, etiology of the renal disease, and the presence of edema and/or hypertension.

**Potassium.** Potassium allowances for infants with renal insufficiency are dependent upon the level of GFR. When restrictions are warranted, they are usually within the maintenance range of 1 to 3 mEq/kg/day[11, 18] during both the predialysis period and during dialysis. When serum potassium levels are persistently greater than 5.5 to 6.0 mEq/L (after correction of acidosis and when potassium intakes are restricted), an ion exchange resin (Kayexelate) may be prescribed in order not to jeopardize the palatability and quantity of formula and food intake. The upper range of potassium allowance is usually feasible for infants undergoing CAPD or CCPD, and a restriction may not be necessary.

**Calcium and Phosphorus.** Calcium supplements and active vitamin D metabolites are administered based upon roentgenographic studies of the bones and serum levels of calcium, phosphorus, parathyroid hormone, and alkaline phosphatase. Aluminum-containing gels have been prescribed to maintain normal serum phosphorus levels. However, because of the potential for aluminum toxicity, calcium carbonate may be given to infants both as the phosphate binder of choice and as a calcium supplement. Phosphate levels are normally higher in neonates because of the need for rapid mineralization of growing cartilage and bone in this age group.[20]

Low phosphate formulas such as PM 60/40 and SMA are usually required for infants during the predialysis period in combination with phosphate binders to achieve the desired serum calcium and phosphate levels. However, formulas with higher phosphate concentrations as well as cow milk may be permissible for infants undergoing CAPD or CCPD.

**Vitamins and Other Minerals.** Vitamin and iron supplementation may be indicated during the predialysis period if the volume of formula intake is limited. The formulas mentioned previously, as well as all commercial infant formulas, are fortified with vitamins. Supplements are prescribed as a multivitamin preparation such as Poly-vi-sol drops (Mead-Johnson) if the estimated intake is considerably less than the RDA. The infant undergoing dialysis requires multivitamins (1 ml/day)[13] and additional folacin (1 mg/day)[21] regardless of the estimated intake because water-soluble vitamins are lost in the dialysate.[21]

Iron supplements are prescribed when indicated, based upon calculated intake and estimates of iron stores (serum iron and ferritin levels). While SMA (except new "low iron" preparation) and PM 60/40, as well as infant cereals, are fortified with iron, further supplementation may be necessary to meet the RDA. Supplementation should be prescribed cautiously because of the potential for iron overload resulting from blood transfusions. Fluoride supplementation is needed only if the water supply contains 0.3 ppm or less.[22]

**Water.** Fluid limitations are usually not required for infants prior to a decline in GFR to approximately 8 to 10% of normal.[16] Fluid needs may differ greatly, depending upon the etiology of the renal disease.[16] When nasogastric feedings are indicated, fluid intake is given according to maintenance fluid requirements (insensible water needs plus measured urine output).

When the infant is undergoing intermittent dialysis, fluids may need to be restricted, depending upon residual renal function and the amount of ultrafiltration. If strained or junior baby foods are prescribed, it must be noted that the water content of such foods ranges from 75 to 92%,[23] and this water should be considered part of the total daily fluid intake.

**Other Considerations.** The nutritional management of infants who are hemodialyzed or receive Intermittent Peritoneal Dialysis (IPD) usually requires the institution of more stringent dietary restrictions of protein, minerals, and fluid than for those receiving CAPD or CCPD. More frequent dialysis treatments, especially for ultrafiltration, may be necessary to allow the infant optimal nutritional intakes by increasing the volume of formula ingested.

As infants grow and develop, new foods are introduced in order to promote adequate nutrition. The early changeover from formula to cow milk is not recommended for infants with chronic renal insufficiency during the predialysis phase owing to its very high solute load. As the infant is weaned off formula, limited quantities of cow milk may be given, along with juices and fruit-flavored drinks if sufficient quality and quantity of solid foods are taken. Cow milk may be feasible for some infants undergoing CAPD or CCPD if solute removal of the high mineral load, including phosphorus, is adequate. In most instances, however, owing to physical and developmental delay, calorically fortified formula is encouraged into the second year of life. Solid foods should be introduced as for a normal infant.

Infants with a history of vomiting due to uremia or to the "fullness" associated with dialysate in the abdominal cavity may tolerate small frequent feedings and even the refeeding of formula and food in small amounts. In some cases, nasogastric feedings are instituted to facilitate consistent nutritional intake.[11]

When infants are successfully transplanted, a normal infant dietary regimen is maintained with emphasis on reducing excess sodium and nonessential caloric intake. Details concerning the rationale for this regimen will be discussed in the subsequent section on the nutritional management of children and adolescents following renal transplantation.

## Children and Adolescents

During all phases of chronic renal disease, the nutritional management of children and adolescents is based upon the same principles as for infants. However, integrating appropriate dietary modifications with established eating patterns as well as offering the variety of foods eaten by these age groups present significant difficulties to the nutritionist. Education about dietary limitations and nutrient needs must be directed toward the patients themselves (according to developmental level) as well as to their parents or caretakers.

In the following discussion, nutrient recommendations will be made during each treatment phase of chronic renal failure. Similar recommendations may coexist during various treatment processes; however, these, and also their rationale, will be reviewed under each section (Table 16–1).

### Predialysis

**Energy.** Caloric needs for children and adolescents with chronic renal disease should be at least equivalent to the RDA for normal children of the same height age (38 to 100 kcal/kg/day).[13, 16] However, because of the poor nutritional status often prevalent in this population, energy needs may be greater in order to promote body weight gain and linear growth.

The provision of optimal energy requirements for the child or adolescent with uremia who may be anorectic while requiring protein, mineral, and fluid restrictions is often a challenge. High calorie carbohydrate supplements are often expensive and not well accepted by children beyond infancy; therefore, it is often easier to encourage common foods of high energy but low protein and mineral content. Beverages such as soft drinks, powdered fruit drinks, and frozen fruit-flavored desserts are suggested as most of the daily fluid allowance. Some children may be responsive to encouragement of a daily intake of simple sugar-containing foods such as candy, jelly, and honey. However, the altered taste acuity associated with uremia may prevent acceptance of some of these suggestions.[24] When "sweets" are encouraged for the child with chronic renal disease, good dental care must be stressed.

In view of the tendency for altered taste acuity and the prevalence of hypertriglyceridemia in individuals with chronic renal disease, the use of unsaturated fats may be preferable to concentrated carbohydrates for increasing the caloric intake of older children and adolescents. Margarine, especially the

unsalted variety (when sodium intake must be limited), is often well accepted when added to popcorn, bread, toast, vegetables, rice, and noodles and should be encouraged. It must be noted, however, that when significant azotemia is present, the protein-sparing effect of added fat calories may not be as good as with concentrated carbohydrate calories.

Low protein wheat-starch products, if available and affordable, will provide additional low protein, low mineral calorie sources to which jelly and margarine may be added for further caloric fortification. Individualized meal plans are of paramount importance to promote adequate caloric intake and may be modified for variety on a periodic basis.

**Protein.** Since there are not extensive data suggesting evidence that protein needs are increased in children with uremia, it seems reasonable during the predialytic phase to prescribe at least the minimal amounts (RDA) recommended for normal, healthy children.[16] Recent experimental data suggest that the ingestion of protein may play a major role in further reducing the GFR in diseased kidneys.[25] Thus, it has been suggested that protein intake should be decreased even earlier in the course of treatment of chronic renal failure than warranted by the degree of azotemia. Considering the food habits in most western societies where protein ingestion is often 250% of the RDA, a restriction may be necessary when the GFR reaches 50% of normal.[16] When the GFR reaches 15 to 20% of normal, the RDA is prescribed as the maximum intake.

The practicality of enforcing a dietary protein restriction for children becomes a challenge, in view of palatability. At least 75 to 80% of this allowance should ideally be protein of high biological value (of animal origin).[16] This need places a limitation on many products made with regular wheat or corn flour, which contain lower quality proteins, such as cereals, breads, pasta, and snack foods. Although there are products manufactured with wheat-starch to reduce protein content, they are quite expensive, not easily obtained, and unpalatable to many children. Thus, diets should be planned with a dispersion of high and lower quality protein-containing foods in limited quantities throughout the day. Lists of common foods emphasizing the protein content (of each quality) may be provided to children and/or their caretakers. The percentage of protein of high biological value can be reduced to approximately 70% if it is felt the child will eat better, especially when planned dialysis therapy is imminent. Under many circumstances it is advisable to encourage increased amounts of nonprotein calories in the diet rather than decreased amounts of protein in order to decrease excessive protein catabolism with subsequent increased azotemia.

The feasibility and effectiveness of essential amino acid (EAA) supplementation for children during the predialysis interval is currently under investigation. The data available suggest that the disadvantages of the rigidity of such supplementation (half of total protein supplied by EAA) appear to outweigh the minimal advantages relative to nutritional status and growth.[26]

**Sodium.** Sodium restriction can be a difficult aspect of nutritional management during the predialytic period because of the wide availability and usage of snack and "fast" foods. The recommended maintenance allowance of 1.0 to 3.0 mEq/100 kcal expended per day[18] is modified, based upon the presence of edema, hypertension, administration of sodium-containing medications, and the etiology of the renal disease.[19, 21] If a "saltwasting" syndrome is present, increased amounts of sodium estimated by measurements of urine sodium are required.

The effective limitation of sodium intake is achieved by putting limits on preferred high sodium foods, so that irrational intake of these foods may be curtailed. For example, luncheon meats may be included in the diet in specific quantities if other high sodium foods such as table salt, canned soups, pickles, and salty snacks are eliminated totally from the diet. The judicious use of diuretics in combination with mild sodium restriction may enable the diet to be more palatable and acceptable. Individualized management is imperative to achieve compliance with sodium restriction.

**Potassium.** A potassium-restricted diet is not always necessary during the predialytic period. As renal function decreases, the renal potassium excretion capacity of each nephron increases until the GFR reaches 10% of normal,[21] and the quantity of potassium secreted into the bowel increases as well. Some diuretics, such as furosemide, which are prescribed prior to the need for dialysis increase urinary potassium excretion to the degree that potassium-rich foods may be required. Therefore, potassium restrictions may not be required until the GFR falls to less than 10% of normal or dialysis is initiated.

When elevated serum potassium levels require restriction of dietary potassium intake, a 1000 mg (25 mEq) to 2000 mg (50 mEq) limitation usually suffices. The first step is to eliminate very concentrated sources of potassium such as citrus fruits and juices, dark green leafy vegetables, and dried fruits. Methods of preparation for some vegetables, such as potatoes, may be altered to control intake (by soaking prior to cooking). Other foods, such as those containing chocolate, can be limited, but often should not be entirely eliminated owing to their wide acceptability and status as an excellent source of calories. If restricted potassium intake seriously jeopardizes overall food intake, or noncompliance with such a regimen exists, Kayexalate may be prescribed.

**Calcium and Phosphorus.** The maintenance of normal serum calcium and phosphorus levels in children with renal disease is extremely important in order to avoid bone disease and promote growth. The prevention of renal osteodystrophy is accomplished by ensuring an adequate daily calcium intake, prescribing vitamin D metabolites and preventing hyperphosphatemia. Such therapy is instituted when the GFR falls to less than 50% of normal.[27]

In order to provide adequate calcium intake for children and adolescents, oral supplements of calcium carbonate may be needed. Foods rich in calcium are also high in phosphorus content and thus must be limited to achieve control of hyperphosphatemia.

Hyperphosphatemia is treated primarily with phosphate-binding medications of aluminum hydroxide or calcium carbonate and a low phosphorus diet. The effectiveness of the binders depends upon ingestion with meals and snacks, and the child and/or caretaker is taught to distribute the binders depending upon their individual schedule of food intake. A controlled phosphorus intake is important in light of the hazards of too much aluminum hydroxide, which may lead to aluminum toxicity in patients with chronic renal failure.[28]

Phosphorus restriction is concomitantly achieved when protein intake is restricted, as dairy products, eggs, and meats are the richest sources of this mineral. If significant protein restriction is not yet warranted, limitation of milk intake to 60 to 240 cc is generally advised as the initial daily restriction. The limitations of other dairy products, such as cheese, will help maintain the total daily phosphorus intake at 500 to 600 mg daily for small children (less than 20 kg) and 600 to 1000 mg daily for larger children and adolescents. As the GFR decreases, phosphorus intake should ideally be reduced in a parallel fashion.

**Iron.** Iron supplementation is usually required only for children and adolescents in the predialysis period when depletion of iron stores is documented by laboratory studies.

**Other Vitamins and Minerals.** The need for vitamin supplementation during the predialytic period arises when the child's food and fluid intake are limited either voluntarily or by prescription. Periodic food records kept by the child or caretaker are helpful for evaluation of such needs. Vitamin D metabolites are often started early in the treatment of renal failure to prevent or treat renal osteodystrophy, as mentioned previously. Most children are given a daily multivitamin preparation.

Zinc supplementation is not routinely administered to children during the predialysis phase, but may be indicated under some circumstances. Low plasma zinc levels have been reported in nondialyzed uremic children; however, it has not been determined whether low plasma zinc levels in uremia reflect actual zinc deficiency, a redistribution of zinc in body pools, or an alteration in the binding of zinc to plasma protein.[21] Since foods rich in zinc content are often limited in protein-restricted diets or are not palatable to children (rich sources include oysters, crabs, organ meats, and other meats), supplementation by pharmacologic means based upon RDA standards for statural age is recommended when necessary.[21]

Copper depletion, as evidenced by low serum, skin, and kidney levels of copper, has been reported in uremic children prior to initiation of dialysis.[21] The encouragement of foods rich in copper (nuts, shellfish, raisins, organ meats, and legumes) when other diet restrictions permit, or supplementation of copper itself has been recommended to prevent deficiency of this trace mineral.[21]

**Water.** During the predialysis period, fluid requirements depend upon the etiology of the renal disease and the level of GFR. Increased sodium needs, such as in a "salt-wasting" syndrome, dictate increased fluid intake.

When limitations of fluid intake become necessary owing to edema and hypertension, the quantity to prescribe is based upon providing insensible water needs plus measured urine output. One method of estimating these needs is based upon the caloric expenditure of the hospitalized child.[29] Children weighing 2 to 10 kg expend approximately 100 kcal/kg/day; for each kilogram between 10 and 20 kg body weight, an additional 50 kcal/kg/day is expended; and for each kilogram greater than 20 kg body weight, an additional 10 kcal/kg is expended. The oliguric child requires 30 to 35 ml/100 kcal/day expended to meet insensible fluid losses minus the input of the water of oxidation.[29] When determining daily fluid needs, this figure would be added to the 24-hour urine output volume to arrive at the total amount of fluid which is to be prescribed.

When the child with renal failure is hospitalized during the predialysis period, foods of high fluid content such as fruits and vegetables should be included as part of the daily fluid allowance. In the outpatient population, insensible water losses may be increased, with physical activity dictating increased fluid requirements. Practically speaking, only foods which are definitely fluid at body temperature, such as gelatin, ice cream, and ice are considered in total fluid intake for outpatients.

Since diuretics are often used in the predialytic period in combination with fluid limitation to control water balance, it is important that daily (or twice daily) body weight be obtained to evaluate the appropriateness of such therapy. The child or caretaker is instructed to notify the physician if dehydration, excessive edema, or hypertension becomes apparent.

**Other Considerations.** Regular follow-up is essential to maintain effective nutritional management of children and adolescents with chronic renal disease prior to initiation of dialysis. The degree of renal insufficiency and the dietary prescription will change over time; therefore, ongoing intervention by the nutritionist will be required.

Following initial meetings with the child and/or caretaker during hospitalization, routine follow-up visits are advised. Diet restrictions are taught by priority, so as not to confuse the child and family. Nutritional status must be evaluated periodically, and the initiation of dialysis should be recommended if anorexia due to uremia or excessive dietary limitations contributes to an overall decline in the child's clinical status.

### Hemodialysis

**Energy.** Caloric needs for the child and adolescent undergoing hemodialysis are similar to those recommended during the predialysis period. Children undergoing hemodialysis who consume less than 67% of the RDA for calories have been reported to show reduced linear growth.[30]

Hemodialysis is usually prescribed for an average of 12 to 15 hours per week. This schedule is associated with limited amounts of water and solute removal; consequently, interdialytic dietary limitations are required. Encouragement of good caloric sources with low protein, mineral, and fluid content continues following initiation of hemodialysis. Flexibility in dietary composition based upon a monthly review of the child's biochemical status may promote better caloric intake. The development of nutrition/cooking programs in which children can participate during the dialysis procedure can serve to promote an increased interest in food.[31] Encouraging the use of common foods instead of caloric supplements is recommended for better acceptance and economic feasibility.

**Protein.** Protein requirements for children and adolescents undergoing hemodialysis are usually at least those of the RDA for children of the same statural age,[21] provided enough calories are ingested to avoid excessive protein catabolism. These allowances constitute a definite restriction of the normal intake commonly consumed in most western societies.

The small child (less than 20 kg) undergoing hemodialysis presents significant problems relative to a balance of actual protein and nonprotein caloric intake. It is helpful to have the small child's caretakers purchase a simple weighing scale to ensure that adequate portions of meats, fish, and poultry are consumed. Protein-containing fluids such as milk, ice cream, and pudding should also be accurately measured, as should vegetables, rice, and pasta. The importance of encouraging nonprotein caloric sources must be emphasized when protein restriction is initiated.

Predialysis elevated BUN levels greater than 100 mg/dl result from a variety of reasons. First, the technical aspects of hemodialysis, including the type of dialyzer and blood flow rates, need to be reviewed to ensure that adequate dialysis is occurring. Next, dietary aspects, including the ratio of nonprotein to protein caloric ingestion and percentage of high biological value protein to total protein content, need to be considered. Food diaries are helpful in evaluating dietary intake.

In some centers, kinetic modeling which involves the estimation of protein catabolic rate (PCR) by calculation of the urea generation rate is utilized. (See Chapter 6.) In stable patients, the PCR equals the dietary protein intake (DPI).[8] In the unstable patient, measurement of the PCR is determined so that dietary strategies can be planned and their effects monitored.[8] For the pediatric patient, this technique offers a greater degree of nutritional control. Calculations are time-consuming, however, and the efficient use of kinetic modeling for the child on hemodialysis involves access to computer systems.

Persistently low predialysis BUN levels (less than 50 mg/dl in the child with minimal residual GFR) may indicate inadequate overall protein and caloric intake rather than good nonprotein caloric intake. Food records are valuable to assess this situation. Periodic arm anthropometric measurements can document prolonged inadequate protein and caloric intake as manifested by decreasing protein stores. Serum levels of total protein and albumin are usually not decreased in hemodialysis patients unless adequate food ingestion is curtailed for prolonged periods of time.

**Sodium.** Sodium intake for children and adolescents undergoing hemodialysis is similar to that prescribed during the predialysis interval. Special emphasis is given to decreasing the sodium intake in the child with a "salt-wasting" syndrome when the urinary output decreases. A gradual decline in sodium allowance is beneficial in most cases to prevent the development of uncontrolled interdialytic weight gain and resultant hypertension, as well as to help the child adapt to altered dietary needs.

A slightly higher sodium intake may be permitted for children and adolescents undergoing hemodialysis prior to their scheduled treatments in an effort to promote an interest in food, provided that the clinical manifestations of sodium and fluid overload are not present. Ideally, if such increased allowances are made 7 to 9 hours before a dialysis treatment (which is estimated to be the time necessary for digestion and absorption of most minerals from solid food after ingestion),[32] the child on an afternoon schedule will be permitted a higher sodium breakfast. For those patients on a morning schedule, a higher intake of sodium at the dinner meal the night before scheduled morning dialysis treatments may be permitted, except at the end of the two-day interdialytic interval.

**Potassium.** Daily potassium allowances are based upon assessment of the serum levels. When the potassium level reaches 5.5 mEq/L in a nonacidotic patient, the daily dietary intake is generally limited to 1000 to 2000 mg (25 to 50 mEq). For the child weighing less than 20 kg with very minimal or *no* residual GFR, the lower range of limitation is appropriate. For the adolescent who weighs more than 40 kg, the upper end of the range is satisfactory.

When teaching potassium restrictions to all groups, it is important to emphasize that the dietary potassium intake be distributed throughout the day. Children can develop high serum concentrations of potassium when a large quantity of potassium is ingested at one time, regardless of the total dietary content for the day. High potassium foods such as chocolate and small servings of melon may be permitted on a limited basis; however, they should be avoided during the longest interdialytic interval. Dietary restrictions regarding this mineral may be taught using a "point system"[33] or by placing a limit on all fruits, vegetables, and other high potassium sources.

When serum potassium levels are repeatedly elevated prior to dialysis and the overall dietary intake is jeopardized, the use of Kayexelate is advised. This ion-exchange resin is usually given with Sorbitol to prevent constipation and promote elimination to rid the body of excess potassium.[9] If Sorbitol is not tolerated, the Kayexelate may be mixed with Kool-Aid or low potassium juices. If only one dose is prescribed, Kayexelate should be administered in the evening, after all meals and snacks are ingested, for most effective results.

**Calcium and Phosphorus.** The guidelines for calcium and phosphorus intake with regard to specific foods, supplements, and medications are the same for children undergoing hemodialysis as outlined previously. Phosphorus intake should be distributed throughout the day, with avoidance of large amounts taken at one time. The proper distribution of phosphate binders throughout the day is equally important.

**Iron.** Once children and adolescents are undergoing regular hemodialysis, blood transfusions are generally given periodically, and supplemental iron therapy is not required unless the serum ferritin level is low.

**Other Vitamins and Minerals.** Supplements of folacin and all water-soluble vitamins are indicated for children and adolescents undergoing hemodialysis. Not only do the dietary restrictions prevent adequate ingestion of all vitamins, but these substances are dialyzable. The recommendations are as follows: 1 mg folacin per day, 50 to 100 mg ascorbic acid (vitamin C) per day, 1.2 to 2.0 mg pyridoxine per day (5 mg to safely avoid deficiency), and a multivitamin preparation containing the remaining B-complex vitamins.[21]

For young children, a multivitamin preparation which also contains fat-soluble vitamins may be prescribed owing to the decreased intake of these vitamins. At this age, it is unlikely that toxic levels of vitamin A are present. A chewable vitamin preparation is often popular with this age group.

Supplemental vitamin D and trace metal therapy is similar to that prescribed in the predialysis period.

**Water.** Principles of fluid management for children and adolescents undergoing hemodialysis are the same as outlined for the predialysis period. Practically, interdialytic weight gain is generally acceptable when it does not exceed 5% of estimated dry weight. In some situations, children will respond to a "reward system" to achieve this goal. An example of reward includes choice of a favorite sticker or seal to be placed on a wall chart kept in the dialysis unit,[33] or worn personally to exhibit accomplishment.

### Peritoneal Dialysis

**Energy.** Total caloric intake is usually less than the RDA in children undergoing all forms of peritoneal dialysis (PD). Patients undergoing CAPD and CCPD may have a decreased intake due to a feeling of fullness as the indwelling dialysate exerts pressure on the stomach. The reduced intake is also attributable to the glucose level of the dialysate solution, which may affect the brain's appetite control center, thereby decreasing the desire for food.

Salusky et al reported that, in 15 patients on CAPD, the total caloric intake was 68 Kcal/kg/day, corresponding to 82% of the RDA.[34] Of the 68 Kcal/kg/day, glucose absorbed from the dialysate accounted for approximately 7.8 Kcal/kg/day.[34] Obesity, which is described in adult CAPD patients, has not been seen in preadolescent children.

The RDA for the patient's height age is used as the basis for caloric recommendations; however, the actual requirements for energy intake may be higher, as mentioned previously. The very malnourished or very active child will require additional energy above the RDA. Small frequent meals, at least five to six per day, are recommended, since the child often cannot eat a large quantity at one time.

When necessary, energy supplementation may be accomplished by using carbohydrate and/or fat modules singly or in combination with protein. Commercial products such as Ensure (Ross Laboratories) or Sustacal (Mead Johnson) are readily available (Table 16–2). However, the cost and lack of reimbursement by third-party payers may be deterrents to use of these products. When necessary, special formulas may be prepared at home using readily available foodstuffs. The need for initiating, continuing, or discontinuing energy supplements should be evaluated frequently.

Elevated serum levels of cholesterol and triglycerides are seen in patients undergoing PD,[35] as a result in part of increased protein losses via the dialysate as well as the constant infusion of glucose during CAPD. In individuals without renal disease, two dietary approaches to the treatment of hyperlipidemia are undertaken: (1) reduce carbohydrate content of the diet, and (2) reduce intake of cholesterol and saturated fats. The child undergoing PD is encouraged to increase his intake of complex carbohydrates in lieu of simple sugars and concentrated sweets and to use unsaturated fats such as oils and margarines from corn, safflower, and soy in order to control hyperlipidemia.

**Protein.** Protein requirements in children undergoing PD are higher owing to protein and amino acid losses in the dialysate. However, actual requirements for children on PD have not been established. Salusky et al reported protein losses of total protein and albumin in the dialysate in children undergoing CAPD to be 4.0 and 2.7 gm/day, respectively.[36] Higher losses were found in younger children because of their proportionally greater peritoneal surface area.[36] The use of amino acids as an osmotic agent in the dialysate of patients undergoing CAPD may help to compensate for protein and amino acid losses and improve nitrogen balance.

Current protein recommendations are adapted from those recommended for adults undergoing PD and are based on the RDA for the patient's height age plus additional quantities to replace peritoneal losses. For children with height ages of three to five years, 3.0 gm/kg/day is recommended; 2.5 gm/kg/day for height ages five to ten years (prepubertal); 2.0 gm/kg/day for height ages ten to 12 years (pubertal); and 1.5 gm/kg/day for height ages over 12 years. Protein requirements for patients undergoing intermittent PD (IPD) may be slightly lower because of the decreased dialysis time.

In CAPD patients, the urea nitrogen appearance (UNA) may be useful for estimating dietary protein intake in stable patients. There is good correlation between protein intake and UNA,[4, 7] and the accuracy of food records can be verified in this manner. A 24-hour collection of dialysate and urine output (if present) is required. The following formula is used[4]:

$$\text{UNA (gm/day)} = \text{urinary urea nitrogen (gm/day)} + \text{dialysate urea nitrogen (gm/day)}$$

In CAPD patients the body urea nitrogen is assumed to be stable.

Approximately 60 to 70% of the recommended protein intake should be of high biological value. Protein of low biological value is allowed in the diet (in controlled amounts) to increase palatability. High-protein foods with a lower saturated fat content, such as poultry and fish, are encouraged because of the propensity for elevated serum cholesterol and triglyceride levels to occur in patients undergoing PD. Eggs are limited to one per day, and milk (because of its high phosphorus content) is limited to 240 cc/day.

In our experience, some children undergoing PD have a dislike for meats, which curtails adequate protein ingestion. The reason for this aversion is not apparent. At times, increased quantities of milk, milk products, eggs, and red meats must be given to meet the protein requirements of the child. Modular protein products added to juices, cereals, or other foods may be required when protein intake is persistently very poor.

**Sodium.** The level of sodium tolerated by children undergoing CAPD or CCPD is usually greater than that tolerated by the child undergoing hemodialysis or IPD. Tolerance for sodium depends in part on the (1) size of the child, (2) original kidney disease and (3) residual renal function. Restriction of sodium intake is instituted if edema or hypertension is present, or if the child persistently requires hypertonic dialysate to increase ultrafiltration.

When sodium restriction is required in the child undergoing CAPD or CCPD, it is often minimal, approximately 3 to 4 grams (130 to 174 mEq) per day. A palatable diet containing less than 2 grams of sodium per day is difficult to achieve in the child over 12 years of age. In short, when sodium restriction is required, the mildest limitation which is effective should be instituted. Many children will not require a sodium restriction while undergoing CAPD or CCPD, while patients undergoing IPD frequently require such restriction.

**Potassium.** Many patients on PD, especially those undergoing CAPD or CCPD, do not require potassium restriction. Instead, if significant residual GFR is present, increased intake is prescribed. Most children may have unlimited potassium intake, especially if quantities are spread throughout the day rather than consumed at one time.

Restrictions of dietary potassium are indicated when the serum level persistently exceeds 5.5 mEq/L, assuming other electrolytes are within normal limits. For many patients, decreasing the intake of high potassium foods on a regular basis is sufficient to lower serum levels to within normal limits. Further limitation of dietary potassium may be necessary, however, ranging from 1 to 2 grams per day (25 to 50 mEq). It is difficult to meet the protein needs of the older child on diets containing less than one gram of potassium per day. Potassium elevation due to catabolism can be alleviated with improved protein and calorie intake.

Fecal excretion of potassium plays an important role in maintaining normal serum levels. Therefore, routine questioning about bowel habits should be a part of nutritional assessment and follow-up. Recommendations should include as high a fiber content in the diet as possible and adequate fluid intake.

Stool softeners are needed only if the above measures are inadequate to prevent constipation.

**Calcium and Phosphorus.** The calcium content of the diet is low because of the need to limit phosphorus intake. Since calcium and phosphorus commonly occur together in foods, supplements of vitamin D metabolites and calcium are used to treat the hypocalcemia. Calcium carbonate acts as both a calcium supplement (if required) and a phosphate binder.

The need for strict serum phosphorus control continues in children undergoing PD, but dietary intake must be higher to permit ingestion of higher protein levels. When other protein foods of high biological value are taken in adequate quantities, milk should be limited to 240 cc/day, or an equivalent quantity of phosphorus taken in the form of milk products. In our experience, the need for phosphate binders has continued in children undergoing CAPD and CCPD, and in many cases, increased amounts are required to accommodate the additional need for protein.

**Iron.** Routine iron supplementation is not needed unless serum ferritin levels are low.

**Other Vitamins and Minerals.** To date, there have been no published vitamin and mineral recommendations for children undergoing PD. Further investigation is necessary to quantitate nutrient losses in the dialysate. Currently, recommendations for the adult PD patients are used: 1 mg per day of folacin, 100 mg of ascorbic acid (vitamin C), and 10 mg of pyridoxine.[35] In addition to these levels, the RDA for other nutrients is given as a vitamin and mineral supplement. Commercial preparations without vitamin A are readily available, and some are available with zinc for those patients with hypogeusia possibly related to zinc deficiency. As mentioned previously, young children may be given a commercial chewable vitamin and mineral preparation because of its increased patient acceptability. Supplementation of vitamin D metabolites is individualized, depending on the serum levels of calcium, phosphorus, parathyroid hormone, and alkaline phosphatase.

**Water.** In CAPD and CCPD patients, there should be little need for fluid limitation when there is adequate ultrafiltration capacity. Patients undergoing IPD are more likely to require restrictions, because the dialysis is not continuous. If hypertension or edema is persistent, a higher glucose concentration can be used to increase ultrafiltration, and the sodium content of the diet can be decreased. Calorie-containing beverages, such as juices, can be given in place of water to the child with suboptimal energy intake.

### Transplantation

There is a paucity of information available in the literature on the nutritional management of children following renal transplantation. Long-term nutritional studies in children post-transplant have not been published, and there are few recommendations even for the adult population. With a well-functioning kidney, however, it is clear that the diet of a recently transplanted child will change. Metabolic effects of immunosuppressive therapy make it necessary to pay special attention to the child's food intake.

The metabolic effects of corticosteroids relating to nutritional status can be divided as follows: effects on (1) protein metabolism, (2), carbohydrate metabolism, (3), sodium intake, (4) bones, and (5) serum lipids. Protein metabolism is altered by increased protein catabolism, including RNA and DNA, decreased protein anabolism through decreased uptake of amino acids in muscle tissue and increased liver uptake of amino acids, resulting in increased urea production and gluconeogenesis.[37] There is also protein wasting of tissues, including muscle and bone. The effects of corticosteroids on carbohydrate metabolism include increased insulin secretion, causing elevated glucose uptake by the fat cells, impaired glucose tolerance, glycosuria, and relative resistance to insulin.[38] Glucocorticoids enhance sodium retention and potassium excretion by stimulating cation exchange in the renal tubule,[37] which may lead to hypertension and/or edema. Bones are affected by protein wasting, potentially resulting in aseptic necrosis, reduced osteoblast activity, increased calcium resorption, and lowered calcium absorption from the intestine.[37] Finally, hyperlipidemia, both hypertriglyceridemia and hypercholesterolemia, have been described following transplantation.[39] These effects improve as steroid dosage is tapered.

Azathioprine (Imuran) has been shown to inhibit DNA and RNA synthesis.[40] Nutrition-related effects of antithymocyte globulin have not been described at this time.

The effects of these medications have led us to make the following recommendations for the period following transplantation when patients are on the highest doses of glucocorticoids (greater than 1 mg/kg):

1. Protein intake is recommended to be at least 2 to 3 grams/kg/day to help alleviate protein degradation.

2. Simple sugars and concentrated sweets are eliminated from the diet for six weeks post-transplant. Liddle recommends 1 gm/kg/day of carbohydrate for adults,[41] but this is too restrictive to meet the caloric needs of pediatric patients because of their smaller body size. Complex carbohydrates, fruits, and juices are permitted ad libitum, with a goal of 40% of calorie intake from carbohydrates.

3. Energy intake, taking into consideration the above recommendations, is permitted ad libitum until ideal body weight for height age is attained. Thereafter, the patient is counseled on a calorie intake for weight maintenance.

4. In the absence of hypertension or edema, a sodium intake of 3 to 4 grams (130 to 174 mEq) per day is allowed. This is an exception to the usual practice of not restricting sodium intake prophylactically. During the period of daily high steroid dosage, hypertension and edema tend to become problems without at least a mild restriction. It is sometimes difficult to distinguish between dietary indiscretion and a rejection episode when sudden weight gain and hypertension occur.

5. Calcium is allowed ad libitum in the diet, and vitamin D supplementation is given to raise serum calcium levels if necessary. Phosphate supplementation is frequently required to replace urinary losses when the serum phosphate level approaches 2.0 mg/dl.

Essentially, this is a high protein, controlled sodium and carbohydrate diet that is generally acceptable to patients and their families. Placing a time limit such as six weeks on the concentrated sweet restriction is crucial for patients to comply with this limitation. As doses of corticosteroids are tapered, the need for dietary restrictions decreases in the patient with a well-functioning kidney. Control of sodium and energy intake, however, may need to be continued for quite some time. Ongoing follow-up should center on adequate nutrient intake ("balanced" diet) and weight control. Exercise is encouraged for its beneficial effects on carbohydrate metabolism and muscle anabolism.

Patients experiencing acute tubular necrosis immediately after transplantation require individual evaluation for nutrient recommendations. The degree of urine output and mode of dialysis (if performed) are two key factors to be considered.

The child experiencing chronic graft rejection also requires special attention. As the serum creatinine level rises, nutrient recommendations are similar to those for the predialysis period.

## CONCLUSION

It is one thing to know and understand nutritional management principles, and quite another to implement them. Patient acceptance and compliance has to be the ultimate goal. Pediatric patients with chronic renal failure offer a unique challenge to the nutritionist and other health care team members. The wide range of ages of these patients necessitates the ability to deal with many levels of intellectual, social, and emotional development. Kidney function may be only one part of a complex medical picture, and nutrients are affected in different ways, depending on the type of kidney disease.

The establishment of rapport with the patient and family members is the foundation for patient education. The framework is built by explaining to the patient and family what is expected of them and why, without overwhelming them with information. Only the information needed for that point in time should be given, and it should be kept as simple as possible, and reviewed frequently. Complicated exchange lists often are ignored, so that creative means of teaching, such as games, pictures, and puzzles are necessary in addition to written materials. It is important to have reasonable expectations for the patients and to be as flexible as possible to accommodate their desires for food. Many parents need to be taught how to set appropriate, consistent guidelines for their child's eating behavior at home. The time invested in these patients is great, but there are many rewards as well.

## REFERENCES

1. National Center for Health Statistics: NCHS growth curves for children 0–18 years, United States, Vital and Health Statistics, Series 11, No. 165, Washington, DC, Health Resources Administration, US Government Printing Office, 1977.
2. Frisancho RA: Triceps skin fold and upper arm muscle size norms for assessment of nutritional status. Am J Clin Nutr, 27:1052, 1974.
3. Frisancho RA: New norms of upper limb fat and muscle areas for assessment of nutritional status. Am J Clin Nutr 34:2540, 1981.
4. Blumenkrantz MJ, Kopple JD, Gutman RA, et al: Methods for assessing nutritional status of patients with renal failure. Am J Clin Nutr, 33:1567, 1980.
5. Ross Laboratories: Physical Growth in Children is Different, Edition 2, 1978, p 2.
6. Pipes PL: Nutrition: Growth and Development in Nutrition in Infancy and Childhood. St Louis, CV Mosby Company, 1977, p 13.
7. Blumenkrantz MJ, Kopple JD, Moran JK, et al: Nitrogen and urea metabolism during continuous ambulatory peritoneal dialysis. Kidney Int 20:78, 1981.
8. Sargent J, Gotch R, Borah M, et al: Urea kinetics: a guide to nutritional management. Am J Clin Nutr, 31:1696,1978.
9. Physician's Desk Reference, Oradell, New Jersey, Litton Industries, Inc, Edition 35:690, 1981.
10. Fomon SJ: Milks and formulas. In: Infant Nutrition. Philadelphia, WB Saunders Company, 1974, p 383.
11. Hetrick AR, Shah RV: Dietary Management of Infants on CAPD. AANNT J 9:46, 1982.
12. Fomon SJ: Fats. In: Infant Nutrition. Philadelphia, WB Saunders Company, 1974, p 162.
13. Recommended Dietary Allowances, revised 1980. Food and Nutrition Board, National Academy of Sciences, National Research Council.
14. Chantler C: Nutrition therapy in children with chronic renal failure. Am J Clin Nutr 33:1682, 1980.
15. Balfe JW, Vigneux A, Williamson J, et al: The use of CAPD in the treatment of children with end stage renal disease. Perit Dial Bull 1:35, 1981.
16. Broyer M: Conservative treatment of chronic renal insufficiency in children. Pediatrician, 8:297, 1979.
17. Grupe WE: Childhood and nephrotic syndrome. Postgrad Med 65:229, 1979.
18. Driscol JM Jr, Heird WC: Maintenance fluid and electrolyte requirements. In: Winters W, The Body Fluids in Pediatrics. Boston, Little, Brown and Company, 1973, p 272.
19. Winters RW: Maintenance fluid therapy. In: The Body Fluids in Pediatrics. Boston, Little, Brown and Company, 1973, p 130.
20. Harrison HE, Helen C: Calcium and phosphate hemostasis. In: Disorders of Calcium and Phosphate Metabolism in Childhood and Adolescents. Philadelphia, WB Saunders Company, 1979, p 38.
21. Holliday MA, McHenry-Richardson K, Portale A, et al: Nutritional management of chronic renal disease. Med Clin North Am 63:945, 1979.
22. Fomon SJ, Filer LJ, Anderson TA, et al: Recommendations for feeding normal infants. Pediatrics, 63:52, 1979.
23. Adams C: Nutritive Values of American Foods in Common Units. Agricultural Handbook No. 456, Washington, DC, 1975.
24. Grupe WE: Nutritional considerations in the prognosis and treatment of children with renal disease. In: Suskind RM (ed): Textbook of Pediatric Nutrition, New York, Raven Press, 1981, p 534.
25. Brenner B, Meyer T, Hostetter T: Dietary protein intake and the progressive nature of kidney disease: The role of hemodynamically mediated glomerular injury in the pathogenesis of progressive glomerular sclerosis in aging, renal ablation, and

intrinsic renal disease. N Engl J Med 307:652, 1982.

26. Jones R: Oral essential amino acid supplements in children with advanced chronic renal failure. Am J Clin Nutr, 33:1696, 1980.

27. Wassner SJ: The role of nutrition in the care of children with renal insufficiency. Pediatr Clin North Am 29:985, 1982.

28. Schoenman M: Dietary and pharmacologic treatment of chronic renal failure. *In*: Edelmann CM Jr, Pediatric Kidney Disease. Boston, Little, Brown and Company, 1978, p 481.

29. Gruskin AB: Fluid therapy in children. Urol Clin North Am 3:277, 1976.

30. Simmons JM, Wilson CJ, Potter DE, et al: Relation of high calorie deficiency to growth failure in children on hemodialysis and the growth response to calorie supplementation. N Engl J Med 285:653, 1971.

31. Stover J, Patton E: A cooking/nutrition program for a pediatric hemodialysis unit. AANNT J 8:9, 1981.

32. Gardner J: The GI lag and its significance to the dialysis patient. Dial Transplant 8:132, 1979.

33. Spinozzi NS: Teaching nutritional management to children on chronic hemodialysis. JADA, 75:158, 1979.

34. Salusky IB, Lucullo L, Nelson P, et al: Continuous ambulatory peritoneal dialysis in children. Pediat Clin North Am 29:1005, 1982.

35. Blumenkrantz MJ, Schmidt WR: Managing the nutritional concerns of the patient undergoing peritoneal dialysis. *In*: Nolph KD, Peritoneal Dialysis. The Hague, Martinus Nijhoff Publishers, 1981, p 295.

36. Salusky IB, Fine R, Nelson P, et al: Nutritional status of pediatric patients undergoing CAPD. Kidney Int 21:177, 1982.

37. Liddle VR, Walker PJ, Johnson HK, et al: Diet in transplantation. Dial Transplant 5:9, 1977.

38. Hill CM, Douglas JF, Rajkumar KV, et al: Glycosuria and hyperlipidemia after kidney transplantation. Lancet 2:490, 1974.

39. Casaretto A, Marcharo TL, Goldsmith R, et al: Hyperlipidemia after successful renal transplantation. Lancet 1:481, 1974.

40. Gradus D, Ettenger R: Renal transplantation in children. Pediat Clin North Am 29:1005, 1982.

41. Liddle V, Johnson HK: Dietary therapy in renal transplantation. Proc Dial Transplant Forum, 9:219, 1979.

42. Weinsier R, Butterworth C: The Handbook of Clinical Nutrition. CV Mosby Company, 1981, p 84.

43. Product information supplied by Mead Johnson and Company, Ross Laboratories, Nubro, Inc., Oraganon, Inc., Travenol Laboratories, Wyeth Laboratories, and McGaw Laboratories.

44. Selected Infant Formulas and Nutritional Supplements, Department of Dietetics, Children's Hospital, Columbus, Ohio, 1982.

# 17

# Renal Osteodystrophy in Children: Etiology and Clinical Aspects

*Otto Mehls, M.D.*

The occurrence of metabolic bone disease in uremic children has been known since the last century.[1-4] With the availability of chronic dialysis and renal transplantation for the treatment of children with ESRD, this problem has gained considerable importance. It has been noted that children with advanced renal failure may develop severe clinical and orthopedic problems within a short period of time[5] and that chronic dialysis fails to correct these skeletal abnormalities.[6]

Several recent reviews have dealt with the problem of calcium metabolism and bone disease in uremic children.[7-11] This chapter will be limited to a summary of our current understanding of the pathogenesis of renal osteodystrophy, and the clinical problems associated with this disorder.

## GENESIS OF DISTURBED CALCIUM METABOLISM IN CHRONIC RENAL FAILURE

Renal osteodystrophy is caused by a combination of disturbed *vitamin D metabolism* and *secondary hyperparathyroidism*. *Vitamin D₃* is either absorbed from the gut or synthesized by ultraviolet light in the skin. The first step in vitamin D metabolism takes place in the liver, where $25(OH)D_3$ is formed under the influence of the enzyme 25-hydroxylase. Circulating $25(OH)D_3$ is the principal form for storage of vitamin D.[12] At the same time it is a precursor for the active hormonal form of vitamin D, $1,25(OH)_2D_3$, which is produced under the influence of the enzyme 1-alpha-hydroxylase in the proximal tubules of the kidney.[13, 14] The activity of the 1-alpha-hydroxylase is regulated by a strong feedback mechanism (Fig. 17–1). Other stimuli for 1-alpha-hydroxylase include low serum calcium levels;[15] low serum phosphorus (Pi) levels,[16] high serum parathyroid hormone (PTH) levels,[14] and low vitamin D levels,[16] whereas its activity is suppressed by hypercalcemia, hyperphosphatemia, low PTH levels, and high vitamin D levels.[17]

As a rule, *$25(OH)D_3$ serum levels* are normal in patients with chronic renal failure.[18] When they are found to be low it indicates superimposed exogenous vitamin D deficiency, which is often overlooked in uremia. The causes for vitamin D deficiency are reduced dietary intake,[18] reduced sun exposure, impaired dermal generation of vitamin D,[19] heavy proteinuria,[20] and administration of phenobarbital or other drugs.[21, 22]

With progressive loss of actual or functional renal tissue *serum levels of $1,25(OH)_2D_3$* decrease,[23] leading to impaired intestinal absorption of calcium, osteomalacia, or rachitic lesions. In uremia *$24,25(OH)_2D_3$ serum levels* are usually subnormal.[24] At present there is no convincing evidence in man that $24,25(OH)_2D_3$ is not solely a biodegradation product without specific biological actions.[17]

Hyperplasia of the parathyroid glands and increased serum levels of immunoreactive parathyroid hormone (iPTH) are common in patients with reduced renal function[25] (Fig. 17–2). Several pathogenetic mechanisms are believed to contribute to *secondary hyperparathyroidism* in renal failure. One mechanism is

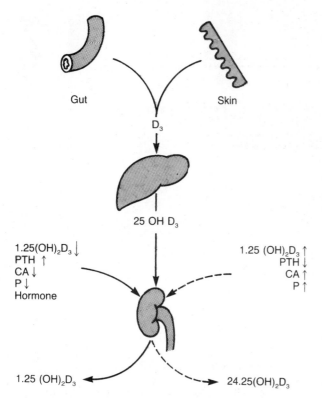

**Figure 17–1.** Scheme of vitamin D metabolism. ↓ = activation of 1-alpha-hydroxylase; ↓ = deactivation of 1-alpha-hydroxylase, concurrent with activation of 24-hydroxylase.

the above-mentioned *impaired intestinal absorption of calcium.* The resulting hypocalcemia is a strong stimulus for PTH secretion.[25] A second mechanism is the *retention of Pi* during progressive renal insufficiency (Fig. 17–3). Slatopolsky and Bricker showed that in experimental renal failure the development of secondary hyperparathyroidism is dependent upon the magnitude of the dietary Pi in-take.[26] An increase in plasma Pi produces a reciprocal fall in ionized plasma calcium by a mechanism which is poorly understood.[27] Decreased ionized calcium levels then stimulate the secretion of PTH. Serum iPTH levels increase with the decrease of renal function (Fig. 17–2). It has been claimed that this increase simply represents the accumulation of biodegradation products; however, the in-

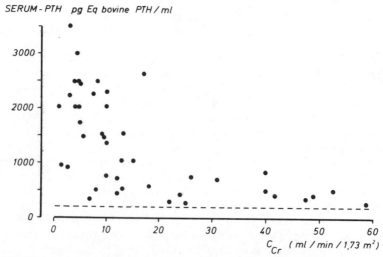

**Figure 17–2.** Relationship of serum PTH levels to GFR in children with congenital renal diseases.

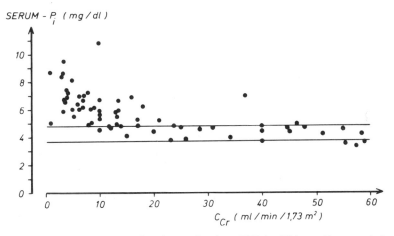

**Figure 17–3.** Relationship of fasting serum phosphatase levels to GFR in children with congenital renal diseases.

crease of urinary cAMP and histologic bone changes point to overactivity of the parathyroid glands.[28, 29]

As functional renal mass is reduced, serum iPTH levels rise if the dietary intake of Pi is maintained constant, but levels remain normal if the dietary intake of Pi is reduced in proportion to the fall of GFR.[26] In patients with advanced renal failure, hyperphosphatemia has been demonstrated to be an important stimulus for PTH secretion. However, there is no convincing evidence that such hyperphosphatemia does occur in incipient renal failure.[30] The mechanism that provokes PTH oversecretion with early impairment of renal function is not known.

In order to account for the changes seen in incipient renal failure, Bricker et al advanced the *"trade-off hypothesis."*[27] This implies that transient and possibly undetectable increases in postprandial plasma Pi occur early in renal failure. However, no difference between patients with incipient renal failure and normal subjects was found with regard to the increment of plasma Pi after a standard oral Pi load.[31] Furthermore, several investigators have found that in the fasting state both *hypophosphatemia* and *hypocalcemia* occur in patients with early renal failure.[32, 33] Such a combination cannot be completely reconciled with the theory that retention of Pi is the primary cause of secondary hyperparathyroidism in patients with incipient renal failure.

It has been suggested that the role of Pi in eliciting PTH secretion is not a direct one which is mediated by a reciprocal fall in ionized Ca, but is an indirect one[23] mediated by diminished circulating levels of $1,25(OH)_2D_3$. Indeed, in incipient renal failure $1,25(OH)_2D_3$ levels are within the normal range,[34] but they may be *inappropriately low* because one would expect elevated $1,25(OH)_2D_3$ levels in the presence of hypocalcemia, elevated iPTH levels, and hypophosphatemia, all of which are powerful stimuli known to raise plasma levels of $1,25(OH)_2D_3$.[17] Further studies are necessary to evaluate the regulatory defect of the renal 1-alpha-hydroxylase system in early renal failure.

With mild, moderate, and advanced renal failure there is *impaired responsiveness of bone* to the action of PTH in mobilizing calcium.[35] PTH resistance is not reversed by hemodialysis but disappears after transplantation. It has been argued that *resistance* to the calcemic actions of PTH is the consequence of increased amounts of skeletal osteoid that trap the calcium released for mineralized bone by the action of PTH.[36] However, PTH resistance cannot be explained exclusively as a consequence of excessive osteoid, since PTH resistance also occurs in early renal failure,[37] a condition not characterized by excessively increased amounts of osteoid.[30] Moreover, PTH resistance is also encountered acutely after bilateral nephrectomy when the amount of osteoid in the skeleton is unchanged.[38] Further studies are required to clarify the exact mechanism(s) underlying PTH resistance. It is important for clinicians to know that PTH *resistance can be corrected* at least partially by the administration of

$1,25(OH)_2D_3$. This has been demonstrated in uremic patients[39] as well as in dogs with acute bilateral nephrectomy.[40]

## CLINICAL AND MORPHOLOGICAL ASPECTS

### Clinical Manifestations (Table 17–1)

Renal bone disease is commonly associated with features of *myopathy*.[5, 11, 41] The myopathy is often overlooked or its manifestations may be interpreted as general weakness or malaise. Uremic children rarely complain of *skeletal pain;* they tend to restrict their physical activity and avoid exercising of the painful extremities. Therefore, it is advantageous to inquire about pain during heavy exercise or during long walks. When patients complain continuously of skeletal pain, it is usually a sign of serious orthopedic complications, such as a fracture or epiphyseal slippage.

*Skeletal deformities* are the hallmark of prolonged renal bone disease in children. The pattern varies with age. In *very young children* the deformities resemble those of late vitamin D deficiency rickets, and include rachitic rosary, Harrison grooves, and enlargement of wrists and ankles. Deformities of tubular bones usually occur at metaphyseal sites, and bowing of the diaphysis is only rare seen. Craniotabes and frontal bossing of the skull occur less frequently because renal osteodystrophy usually has its onset after the first year of life. The type of bone deformities that develop depends upon whether the child is crawling or walking. Characteristic deformities following metaphyseal fractures in a crawling child are shown in Fig. 17–4. Knock-

**Table 17–1.** CLINICAL SIGNS (%) OF UREMIC BONE DISEASE

|  | Before 1972 | 1978–1982 |
|---|---|---|
|  | (n = 56) $S_{CR}$ 5.9 ± 2.9 mg% | (n = 48) $S_{CR}$ 6.4 ± 3.1 mg% |
| Stunted growth | 36 | 33 |
| Skeletal deformity | 32 | 6 |
| Gait abnormality | 21 | 6 |
| Myopathy | 32 | 6 |
| Bone pain | 14 | 4 |
| Slipped epiphyses | 18 | 2 |
| Pseudogout | 2 | 0 |
| Soft tissue calcification | 0 | 0 |
| Conjunctival calcification | 7 | 4 |

knees are the most common deformity and can be seen in any age group.

The majority of children who present to the nephrologist with chronic renal failure are *above 10 years of age*. These children may have additional deformities: ulnar deviation of hands, pes varus, and "swelling" of wrists, ankles, or medial ends of clavicles. Pseudo-drumstick fingers (pseudo-clubbing) are frequently seen in nontreated patients. Epiphyseal slipping of the femoral head is commonly overlooked on physical examination unless one carefully watches for subtle abnormalities of gait which precede the more typical waddling gait. A waddling gait not only may be the result of bone disease but also may be due to myopathy, as indicated above.

*Retardation of growth* is multifactorial in origin. At the time of ESRD the height of about one third of all children is below the third percentile,[42] but the actual growth rate is subnormal in about 50% of patients.[43]

*Dental abnormalities* (enamel defects) and dental deformities (enamel defects in the form of white or brown discoloration or hypoplasia of enamel) are typical for children with congenital renal diseases because of the early disturbances of calcium metabolism and the long duration of the disease[44, 45] (Fig. 17–5).

Other signs of secondary hyperparathyroidism seen in adult patients with chronic renal failure are rare in children: *cutaneous and subcutaneous calcification, vascular calcifications, calciphylaxis, crystal-negative arthritis, pseudogout, polyarticular arthritis, spontaneous tendon ruptures,* and *olecranon bursitis.* The reason for these differences between pediatric and adult patients is not clear since the serum levels of various substances, including the product of serum calcium times phosphorus, is not different.[46]

*Itching* is a common symptom of uremic children which may improve or disappear with initiation of dialysis. It occurs especially in patients with clinical evidence of secondary hyperparathyroidism. In such children, the pruritus often improves or disappears within a few days after parathyroidectomy. However, it is important to note that pruritus is often multifactorial in origin; ultraviolet light[47] and lidocaine[48] have been reported to ameliorate the symptoms. Parathyroidectomy should not be performed unless the presence of severe hyperparathyroidism is documented by very high levels of iPTH, subperiosteal resorption by radiographic evaluation, and severe osteitis fibrosa on bone biopsy.

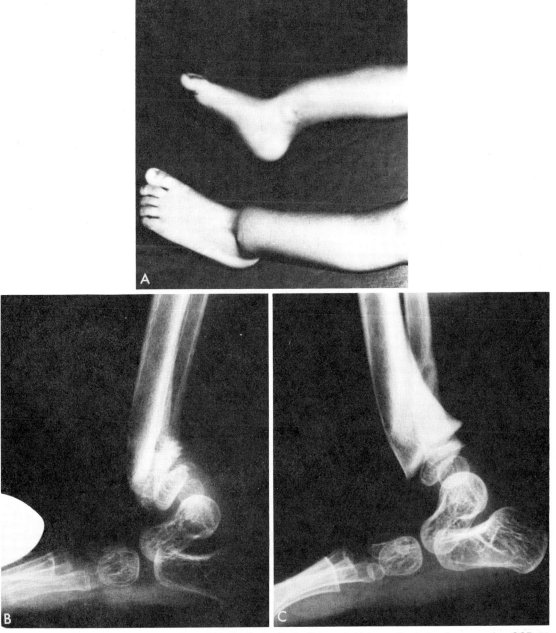

**Figure 17–4.** Metaphyseal fracture in renal osteodystrophy in 2½-year-old boy with obstructive uropathy; CCR 25 ml/min 1.73m². *A*, skeletal deformity of the lower leg. *B*, X-ray before vitamin D treatment. Metaphyseal fractures of the distal tibia with dorsal dislocation of the distal epiphysis. *C*, X-ray one year after initiating of vitamin D therapy and osteotomy. Healing of the metaphyseal fracture.

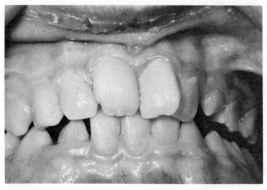

**Figure 17-5.** Hypoplasia of the upper medial incisor teeth in a 13-year-old boy with congenital renal hypoplasia undergoing dialysis treatment for two years.

## Bone Histology

In the study of renal bone disease the evaluation of bone histology is both a valuable diagnostic procedure and an important investigative tool. No single histologic lesion is specific for uremic bone disease. Renal osteodystrophy is the result of changes in the relative proportions of processes that are encountered in the normal skeleton: bone resorption and bone formation. Quantitative histologic investigation is mandatory for the proper study of renal osteodystrophy. The standard procedure is an iliac crest biopsy. This is performed either perpendicular to the iliac crest or as a through-and-through biopsy 2 cm below the iliac crest. In our experience the sampling error can be minimized when the latter technique is used.[49]

Only a few investigators have reported quantitative results by this technique in uremic children.[6, 50-56]

### Osteitis Fibrosa

All children with uremia exhibit skeletal changes of osteitis fibrosa due to secondary hyperparathyroidism. Histologic features include increased numbers of *osteoclasts, osteoblasts,* and *Howship's lacunae,* as well as increased amounts of *woven osteoid* and the appearance of *endosteal fibrosis* (Fig. 17-6). Since fibrous osteoclastic activity is essentially a nonspecific reaction of bone to local (e.g., fracture) or systemic (e.g., thyroxin, PTH) stimuli, one has to recognize the various pathogenetic mechanisms behind a rather limited number of patterns of reactions. PTH stimulates bone tissue and bone mineral turnover by activating both cells at the trabecular

surface (endosteal cells) and the cells within bone (osteocytes).[49]

One characteristic of bone showing fibroosteoclasia in the presence of increased quantities of *woven osteoid,* which differs from the usual *lamellar osteoid* is that the former exhibits a haphazard arrangement of collagen fibers. *Woven osteoid* can be mineralized in the absence of vitamin D;[57] however, the calcium may be deposited as amorphous calcium phosphate rather than as hydroxylapatite. Mineralized woven osteoid is called *woven bone.* Its appearance accounts for the loss of the normal trajectorial pattern of trabeculae in cancellous bone in uremic children (Fig. 17-7). Woven bone has an inferior mechanical stability compared to lamellar bone. To maintain the mechanical stability, more woven bone must be deposited for any given amount of lamellar bone, thus giving rise to *osteosclerosis.*

*Endosteal fibrosis,* by displacing blood-producing cells in the bone marrow, is thought to contribute to anemia.[58] We have been unable to detect a strong correlation between the degree of *endosteal fibrosis* and the degree of anemia and therefore do not believe that osteitis fibrosa is a major contributing factor to the genesis of uremic anemia.[59]

### Mineralization Defect (Osteomalacia)

Osteomalacia has been defined as an increase of unmineralized osteoid. Obviously, this assumption is incorrect, since osteoid will appear in the skeleton in increased quantities whenever the rate of bone turnover is high, as in hyperparathyroidism. At any given moment the number of osteoid lamellae (Fig. 17-8) (and osteoid volume density) is the net result of the rate of appearance of new osteoid seams and the lifespan of the individual osteoid seam. This implies that even in the presence of increased osteoid, osteomalacia cannot be diagnosed unless *delayed or defective primary mineralization* is demonstrated. Therefore, the amount of osteoid in the skeleton does not reflect the severity of the mineralization defect, as it is often implied in the literature, since the osteoid mass depends not only on the rate of mineralization but also on bone turnover and duration of the disease.

Because the definition of osteomalacia as a delay in mineralization is a *dynamic* one, direct evidence of its presence can be obtained only by markers for primary mineralization. After

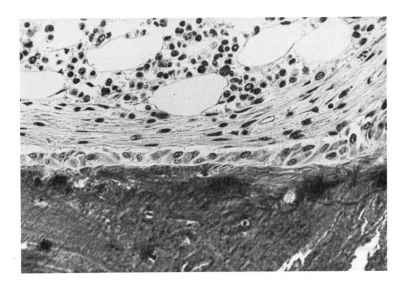

**Figure 17–6.** Endosteal fibrosis. Iliac crest biopsy in a 14-year-old boy with ESRD from renal hypoplasia. Note dense fibrous tissue with collagen fibers running parallel to the trabecular surface (on top). The trabecular surface is covered by a pseudoepithelial layer of active osteoblasts. (×230.)

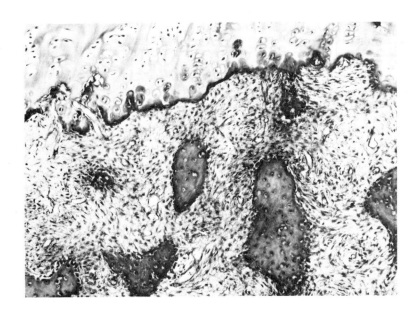

**Figure 17–7.** Growth zone of distal femoral epiphysis in a nine-year-old girl with ESRD (renal hypoplasia). Decalcified section, H and E stain (× 34). Epiphyseal cartilage on top. Degenerative cartilage is removed by chondroclasts. Cellular rich fibrous tissue with evidence of metablastic formation of trabeculae consisting entirely of woven bone is shown at the bottom.

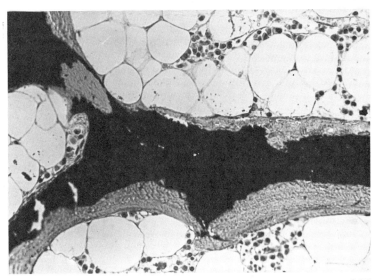

**Figure 17–8.** Iliac crest biopsy from a 16-year-old boy with nephronophthisis treated by hemodialysis. Undecalcified section, Krutsay stain (×130). Bizarre contour of remnants of the well-mineralized premorbid skeleton after osteoclastic surface resorption. Mineralized bone (black area) buried underneath broad resting osteoid seams with recognizable lamellar structure.

administration of *tetracycline* in vivo, impaired mineralization can be demonstrated by either a diminished rate of mineralization or a diminished fraction of osteoid that takes up the tetracycline label. The presence of *woven osteoid* instead of lamellar osteoid makes it impossible to identify a mineralization defect.

## Micromorphometric Studies

It is generally agreed that there are no qualitative differences in bone histology between children and adults or between patients with mild and terminal renal failure.[6, 49] The differences are only quantitative. One usually finds a mixture of both fibroosteoclastic lesions and defective mineralization, although in extreme cases either lesion may predominate. The *fibroosteoclastic pattern* corresponds to a *high turnover state* and the *osteomalacic pattern* to a *low turnover state*. Therapy can be very difficult in extremely low turnover states.

Bone abnormalities can be recognized even in *incipient renal failure*. Endosteal fibrosis[51] and woven osteoid[49] are noted at a GFR between 50 and 80 ml/min/1.73 m². Since this has not been reported uniformly,[54] it has to be kept in mind that the normal range of micromorphometric parameters is rather wide.

The *cancellous bone mass* increases with *decreasing renal function*.[51] This increase is accounted for by the increase in the amount of *osteoid*, both when calculated as a fraction of spongiosal volume (VO) and when given as a fraction of trabecular surface (OS), and by the increase in the amount of *woven bone*. Children with slipped capital femoral epiphyses because of hyperparathyroidism show extensive signs of osteitis fibrosa in their iliac bone biopsy. They have the highest degree of *osteoclastic surface resorption*, the highest volumetric density (osteosclerosis), the highest volume and surface densities of osteoid (predominantly woven), and the highest degree of *endosteal fibrosis* (Table 17–2). In these children serum iPTH levels correlate with osteoclastic resorption, with endosteal fibrosis, and with the amount of osteoid.[5] The serum calcium levels show a negative correlation with the amount of osteoid.[55]

The micromorphometric parameters in *dialyzed children* do not differ substantially from those of children with a serum creatinine level above 5 mg/dl,[6, 51] indicating that adequate dialysis treatment can prevent further deterioration of bone disease. Vitamin D,[50, 55] 25(OH)D,[52] or 1,25(OH)D[56] treatment of children with chronic renal failure may improve bone histology but fails to normalize it. It has not been determined whether early reduction of phosphorus intake[60] or early administration of 1,25(OH)$_2$D$_3$ or other vitamin D metabolites can prevent renal osteodystrophy.[30]

## Indications for Bone Biopsy

Bone biopsy is not required for the routine management of children with chronic renal failure. In certain situations (e.g., indications

Table 17–2. MICROMORPHOMETRIC PARAMETERS IN DIALYZED CHILDREN*

| | I Control group (n = 9) | II Chronic renal failure without epiphysiolysis (n = 19) | III Chronic renal failure with epiphysiolysis (n = 8) | Significance (P) of difference between† I & II | I & III | II & III |
|---|---|---|---|---|---|---|
| V$_V$ (%) | 17·7 ± 4·9 | 26·5 ± 9·0 | 33·7 ± 7·1 | 0·01 | 0·01 | 0·1 |
| V$_O$ (%) | 0·4 ± 0·2 | 2·3 ± 1·9 | 5·3 ± 4·8 | 0·01 | 0·01 | 0·05 |
| S/V (mm²/mm³) | 17·1 ± 3·1 | 12·7 ± 2·6 | 11·8 ± 3·2 | 0·01 | 0·01 | 0·1 |
| SD (mm²/cm³) | 2752 ± 813 | 3175 ± 770 | 3855 ± 908 | NS | 0·05 | 0·05 |
| HO (%) | 0·3 ± 0·7 | 3·89 ± 7·7 | 12·3 ± 7·7 | 0·01 | 0·01 | 0·01 |
| HO (mm²/cm³) | 4·1 ± 7·7 | 126 ± 17·7 | 444 ± 279 | 0·01 | 0·01 | 0·01 |
| OS (%) | 7·2 ± 4·0 | 43·6 ± 19·0 | 52·0 ± 24·9 | 0·01 | 0·01 | NS |
| OS (mm²/cm³) | 160 ± 90 | 1430 ± 739 | 2000 ± 1125 | 0·01 | 0·01 | 0·01 |
| S (μm) | 11·6 ± 2·8 | 17·1 ± 6·7 | 21·4 ± 11·7 | 0·01 | 0·01 | 0·01 |
| EOF (%) | 0 | 45·3 ± 35·2 | 88·8 ± 13·3 | 0·01 | 0·01 | 0·02 |

V$_V$, fraction of bone volume contained in unit volume of spongiosa; V$_O$, fraction of osteoid volume contained in unit volume of spongiosa; S/V, trabecular surface/unit volume of bone; SD, interface between trabecular bone and marrow cavity; HO, active Howship's lacunae (given as % trabecular surface and given as surface/unit spongiosa volume); OS, osteoid seams on trabecular surface (given as % trabecular surface and as surface/unit spongiosa volume); S, seam thickness of osteoid; EOF, fraction of trabecular surface covered by endosteal fibrosis.

*From Mehls, O, et al.[5]

†Wilcoxon test.

for parathyroidectomy, verification of aluminum osteomalacia) bone biopsy is helpful in indicating appropriate therapy. The primary indication for performing bone biopsies is clinical investigation.

## Radiographic Abnormalities

The macroscopic changes of the osseous architecture can best be visualized by appropriate radiographs.[61–63] The changes do not always reflect the changes found at the cellular level (histology). Radiographic abnormalities occur and are reversed only after the changes at the cellular level have taken place for a substantial period of time. Therefore, it is not surprising that the results of radiographic examination do not correlate with the results of quantitative bone micromorphometry as our own results in children (unpublished) as well as those of Debnam et al[64] and those of Ritz et al[65] in adults have shown.

The *incidence of radiographic abnormalities* in children with chronic renal failure varies greatly from country to country and from one center to another. This variability is partly related to the use of different radiographic techniques, including the type of film used and the interest of the involved radiologist. Because the quality of standard x-ray films developed by automated developing machines is poor, we advise the following technique: Industrial film should be exposed by a normal x-ray tube, 0.6 mm focus, 50 cm distance, 38 kV, 38 mA s. This film can be developed in an automated machine with subsequent study with a magnifying glass (magnification about 8 times). If magnification techniques are used, the physician must be familiar with the normal variations because one may easily overinterpret such films.

### Cortical Bone Lesions

In renal disease the outer *circumferential lamellae* are eroded and replaced by fibrous tissue and woven bone. This occurs primarily at points of tendon or ligament attachments, where in the normal skeleton some woven bone is found. Osteoclastic drill holes on the bone surface are directed perpendicularly to the circumferential lamellae,[66] giving a characteristic "spicular" appearance (acroosteolysis and subperiosteal resorption zones).

Whereas *subperiosteal resorption* of the inner side of the middle phalanges II and III is the most sensitive radiographic sign of secondary hyperparathyroidism in adults, a different pattern is found in children. The sites of subperiosteal resorption change with age. In infancy and in preschool age children the typical subperiosteal resorption of the phalanges is missing. Instead, only a fluffy delineation of the cortex with weak outlines is noted. In these children one should look for subperiosteal resorption zones mainly at the lateral aspect of the distal radius and ulna and at the inner side of the upper tibia. The metaphyseal shaft junction of long bones is a common site for erosions to occur. This is because there is usually an active collar of osteoclasts which acts to reduce the diameter of the epiphyseal growth plate to that of the diaphysis of the bone. The tufts of the terminal phalanges often display resorption (*acroosteolysis*). Because of severe tuft erosion, there may be a collapse of the terminal phalanges leading to the clinical sign of pseudoclubbing.

The absence of the *laminae durae* is believed to be a sensitive sign of primary and secondary hyperparathyroidism.[67] Dental films should be used to detect the *laminae durae,* and one should be familiar with the normal variations. In our experience only complete absence of the *laminae durae* is indicative of hyperparathyroidism, whereas incomplete absence can also be seen in other renal disorders such as the nephrotic syndrome without renal failure.[45]

The *histologic evidence* of resorptive defects of the outer contour of bone is not necessarily loss of bone tissue but substitution of poorly mineralized fibrous bone for well-mineralized mature lamellar bone.[65] This explains why the original shape of bone is rapidly restored after appropriate therapy. When erosions of cortical bone are treated with vitamin D therapy, bone mineral is first deposited at the inner side of the periosteal tube. At this time one notices a shell of bone separated from the cortex by a small radiolucent zone, which represents the zone of unmineralized fibrous tissue. This phenomenon is called *periosteal neo-osteosis*[68, 69] (Fig. 17–9). With further healing the radiolucent zone will become dense and the cortex appears thicker, although only the original cortical thickness is usually re-established.

In uremia increased osteoclastic activity is observed in the *core of cortical bone,* which is composed of longitudinally arranged Haversian systems. Normal remodeling is not visible roentgenologically, since resorption

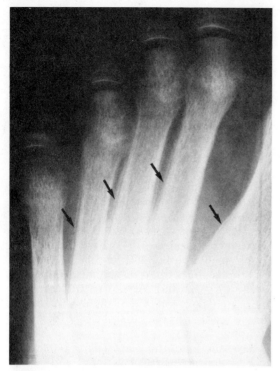

**Figure 17–9.** Periosteal neo-osteosis. X-ray of foot of a 16-year-old girl with obstructive uropathy undergoing hemodialysis treatment for more than four years. At the lateral side of the metacarpals a small shell of subperiosteal bone is seen, which is separated from the mass of cortical bone by interposition of fibrous tissue between cortical bone and periosteum.

relation between the degree of radiographic hyperparathyroidism, bone biopsy findings, serum PTH levels, and the cortical thickness (Garn Index or Nordin Index), which differs from the findings observed in adult patients (Fig. 17–10).

### Cancellous Bone Lesions

As indicated previously, the amount of cancellous bone is increased in uremia. Both the number and the diameter of trabeculae in metaphyseal bone are increased. Therefore, it is logical to look for roentgenologic evidence of *osteosclerosis* at those sites where cancellous rather than cortical bone predominates: skull, vertebrae, pelvis, and metaphyses of tubular bones. The typical signs of local osteosclerosis are the *pepper-pot skull*, the *rugger-jersey spine* (Fig. 17–11), and the *increased density of ossa iliaca and of the metaphyses* of long bones. The latter may become more apparent when remineralization occurs with vitamin D therapy.

The underlying abnormalities are well illustrated by the roentgenologic appearance of the spongiosal trabeculae. The *fuzzy contours* of the trabeculae show evidence of the osteoid coating and the *bizarre trabecular shape*

cavities are rapidly filled with mature mineralized lamellar bone. Only when resorption cavities are filled with poorly mineralized lamellar bone, woven bone, or even fibrous tissue will *longitudinal cortical striation* be observed roentgenologically.[61] Enlargement of the Haversian channels of the metacarpals is not specific for secondary hyperparathyroidism, since this appears in all situations of increased bone turnover, e.g., during the adolescent growth spurt. These findings can only be interpreted in the context of other cortical signs of secondary hyperparathyroidism.

Remodeling activity at the *endosteal surfaces* leads to bone loss even in the normal skeleton. Therefore, an increased rate of remodeling secondary to PTH overactivity must necessarily induce bone loss at the endosteal surface. This will lead to cortical thinning. The degree of thinning of cortical bone is not an indicator of the actual degree of hyperparathyroidism, but probably reflects the duration of hyperparathyroidism. This explains why we were unable to find a cor-

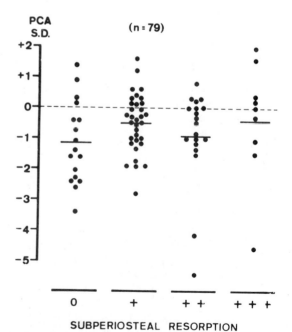

**Figure 17–10.** Percentage of cortical area (PCA) (Garn Index) of the second metacarpal associated with varying stages of renal osteodystrophy. There is no correlation between the degree of renal osteodystrophy on x-rays and the cortical thickness. (Courtesy of Dr. Gilli.)

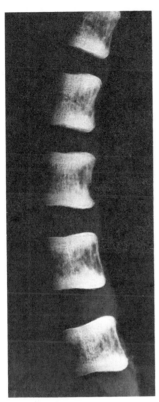

**Figure 17–11.** Rugger-Jersey spine.[75] Post-mortem x-ray of a nine-year-old girl with ESRD secondary to renal hypoplasia. Note wide band of endplate sclerosis without sharply defined margins.

points to a disorderly increased rate of remodeling.

Occasionally, *cyst formation (brown tumors)* (Fig. 17–12) may be seen. The genesis of brown tumors is poorly understood. These tumors are much more common in children than in adults.[70] The localizations we have observed are in the metacarpals, distal femur, proximal tibia, and distal radius.

The radiographic features of *osteomalacia* are far less distinctive than those of secondary hyperparathyroidism. The problem of predicting the degree of mineralization defects from radiolucent zones at the distal end of long bones will be discussed subsequently. Looser's zones, or pseudo-fractures, may be the only characteristic finding of osteomalacia.

## Mineral Content of the Uremic Skeleton

Children with chronic renal failure are at *risk of being in negative calcium balance* for several reasons. With spontaneous or pre-scribed reduction of food intake, the calcium intake is reduced concomitantly. Vitamin D deficiency as well as the reduced production of $1,25(OH)_2D_3$ leads to a decreased absorption of calcium from the gut. Metabolic acidosis may account for calcium loss by the kidney. Furthermore, dialysis may contribute to a negative calcium balance.

Measurement of the skeletal mineral content is of interest because its mineral content reflects calcium balance. Several *methodological problems* must be overcome in such studies. One problem is the appropriate base of reference, i.e., whether uremic children should be compared to control children of the same age, the same height, or the same bone age. Another issue involves skeletal heterogeneity, i.e., the divergent behavior of diaphysis versus metaphysis, and appendicular skeleton versus axial skeleton. Finally, there are technical problems in measuring the mineral content. In order for demineralization to be apparent radiographically, 30 to 50% of the skeletal bone mineral must be lost.[71] In children the methods of whole body neutron activation analysis and x-ray spectrophotometry have not been used, presumably for ethical reasons. Most studies of bone

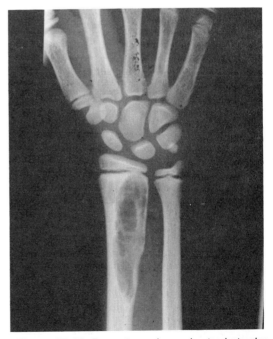

**Figure 17–12.** Brown tumor in renal osteodystrophy. X-ray of the forearm of a ten-year-old girl with renal hypoplasia with a serum creatinine level of 840 mM/L (10.0 mg/dl). The brown tumor is located at the distal radius.

density in children have been performed with photondensitometry.

Chesney et al., using the Cameron *densitometer,* found a diminished mineral density of radius and ulna when uremic children were compared to nonuremic control children of the same age or height.[72] More detailed results were reported by Mehls et al, who studied children with congenital renal diseases and growth retardation but without a history of steroid administration.[73] The mineral density was low for chronologic age but appropriate for height age when measured in the metaphysis (representing mainly spongiosa), but low for both chronologic and height age when measured in the diaphysis (mainly representing cortical) of radius and ulna. Our longitudinal studies of up to five years did not show major changes in bone mineral content following initiation of dialysis or after successful transplantation when the data were corrected for the growth increment of the patients.

These results suggest that the intestinal absorption of calcium, although diminished in absolute terms, may be appropriate to the mineral demand of the slowly growing uremic skeleton. These findings are in agreement with the observation that total body calcium in adult uremic patients, measured by whole body neutron activation analysis, is not decreased.[74] The divergent behavior of metaphysis and diaphysis is an example of heterogeneity. This finding is presumably explained by dense osteosclerosis of spongy bone in the metaphysis resulting from increased bone matrix, while in cortical bone, the diaphysis mineral resorption, which is not balanced by mineral apposition, predominates.

## Growth Zone

The histology of the growth zone is reviewed only to the extent necessary for discriminating between rickets and osteitis fibrosa and for understanding the clinical and roentgenologic signs of uremic bone disease at this particular site of tubular bone.

In the growth zone of *healthy children* (Fig. 17–13, left), growth cartilage consists of the zone of resting cartilage, the zone of degenerative cartilage, and finally the zone of provisional calcification, in which the longitudinal septa, which are juxtaposed to apparently dead chondrocytes, mineralize. Subse-

quently, at the zone of transition between cartilage and bone, necrotic chondrocytes and transverse chondroid septa are removed by vascular mesenchyma which invade from the underlying metaphysis. In the zone of primary spongiosa new bone is added to preexisting mineralized longitudinal chondroid septa by the action of the osteoblasts. Primary spongiosa is transformed into secondary spongiosa by osteoclastic resorption of the majority of the densely packed primary trabeculae, leaving only a reduced number (4:1) of trajectorially oriented secondary trabeculae.[76]

The histologic hallmark of *rickets* (Fig. 17–13, center) is an increase in the cartilaginous growth zone caused by accumulation of persisting cartilage cells in the zone of degenerative cartilage.[77] In such rachitic cartilage, the longitudinal columnar arrangement of cartilage cells is lost, and mineralization of the zone of provisional calcification is defective. As a consequence, vascular invasion from the adjacent metaphysis is disturbed. Chondroid and osteoid mingle, giving rise to a broad zone of chondroosteoid.

In *osteitis fibrosa* (Fig. 17–13, right), associated with advanced renal failure, the zone of growth cartilage is *not* increased in width but is normal or even decreased.[78] Provisional calcification of cartilage ground substance is not defective. However, the zone of transition between growth cartilage and metaphyseal zone is highly abnormal. Vascular invasion is virtually absent. Sometimes growth cartilage is occluded by a bar of dense bone. Growth cartilage is physically separated from metaphyseal bone by a zone of fibrous tissue in advanced stages. In the metaphysis, trabeculae arise de novo by metaplastic bone formation from primitive fibrous tissue. Such trabeculae differ from normal. They are not in physical contact with cartilage, are devoid of a chondroid core, and consist entirely of poorly mineralized woven bone lacking the normal trajectorial longitudinal orientation.

The *transition between the two patterns* was described in children with vitamin D deficiency rickets by Pommer in 1885.[79] Our current understanding is that the pattern of osteitis fibrosa supervenes when more advanced hyperparathyroidism is present, leading to the disappearance of accumulated chondroosteoid owing to the intensity of chondroclastic and osteoclastic resorption. In addition, mineralization of chondroosteoid may be improved by progressive hyperphos-

CONTROL                    RICKETS                    OSTEITIS  FIBROSA

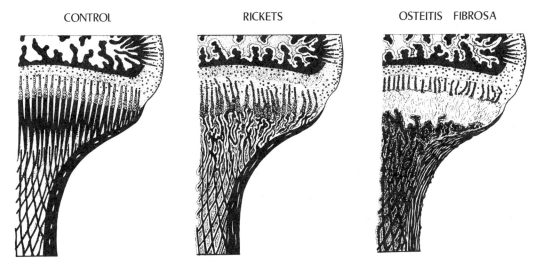

**Figure 17–13.** Diagram of the growth zone in a normal child (left), a child with rickets due to vitamin D deficiency (center), and a child with osteitis fibrosis (right). Whereas the zone of degenerative cartilage is enlarged in rickets, the zone of degenerative cartilage is resorbed by extensive chondroclasia in osteitis fibrosa. The zone of primary and secondary spongiosa is replaced by dense fibrous tissue and metaplastic woven bone. (From Mehls et al: Clin Endocrinol Metab, 9:151, 1980.)

phatemia. In support of this concept we were able to show in animal models that the rachitic pattern is transformed into the pattern of osteitis fibrosa when the degree of hyperparathyroidism is increased by decreasing the calcium content of the diet.[80]

*Radiographically*, rachitic changes and osteitis fibrosa of the growth zone are indistinguishable. Both conditions lead to radiolucent zones at the metaphyses. It is of note that identical radiographic findings are seen in primary hyperparathyroidism.[81–84] Consequently, radiolucent metaphyseal zones are not indicative of the presence or severity of the underlying mineralization defect.

## Epiphyseal Slipping and Bone Fractures

*Epiphyseal slipping* is one of the most severe clinical manifestations of renal osteodystrophy. This complication, known for decades, was considered a rare event.[84–89] However, in our experience it was a frequent complication in the natural course of uremic bone disease prior to the routine use of early prophylactic vitamin D treatment. It develops quite rapidly and can occur at an early stage of renal insufficiency.[5]

Slipping of the epiphysis in patients with renal disease is caused by mechanisms different from those operating in idiopathic slipping of the femoral epiphysis during adolescence. In the latter case, defects are initially found throughout the layer of hypertrophic cartilage adjacent to the zone of calcification. These defects are thought to be a consequence of disturbed vascular supply.

In children with renal failure, slipped epiphysis is not the result of a local process but the consequence of generalized metabolic bone disease. Our *studies* (Fig. 17–14) have shown that slipped epiphyses in uremic children are the ultimate consequence of osteitis fibrosa.[7] It should be noted that slipped epiphysis is also found in primary hyperparathyroidism.[63] In uremic children the normal transformation of cartilage into primary spongiosa is in abeyance, and the metaplastic bone from beneath the physeal plate lacks the normal connection with cartilage. Consequently, the dense fibrous tissue interposed between growth cartilage and the adjacent metaphysis provides a plane of cleavage for slipping of the epiphysis under the influence of normal shearing forces.

In contrast to the previous explanation of Kirkwood et al,[84] a history of trauma was uniformly lacking in our children with epiphyseal slipping, and our histologic findings showed no evidence of metaphyseal fractures.[78] Therefore, epiphyseal slipping represents a *nontraumatic separation of epiphyseal cartilage from metaphyseal bone* produced by intensive modeling processes.

The *sites* of epiphyseal slipping are *age-related*.[5] In preschool children slipping is ob-

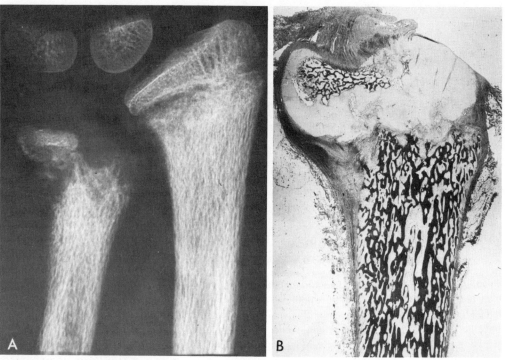

**Figure 17–14.** Epiphyseal slipping. *A,* Post-mortem X-ray of a nine-year-old girl with ESRD (oligomeganephronia). Note typical displacement of radial and ulnar epiphyses toward the ulnar side and rachitic-like lesions underneath the growth plate. *B,* Autopsy specimen of the same bone (ulna). Undecalcified section, Masson-Goldner stain (×5). Note huge erosive defect at the ulnar side of metaphyseal cortex of the ulna. Erosion has filled in with fibrous tissue and poorly mineralized woven bone. In addition, there is severe fibro-osteoclasia with destruction of primary spongiosa and dissecting cancellous cortical bone with incipient displacement of the epiphyses.

served in both upper and lower femoral epiphyses and in the distal tibial epiphyses, but not in the distal radial or distal ulnar epiphyses. In contrast, in older children the upper femoral and distal epiphyses of the forearm are primarily involved. During and after puberty slipping may occur exclusively at the forearm epiphysis. In patients with extremely severe ostcitis fibrosa epiphyseal slipping can occur, irrespective of age, in nearly all epiphyses. Severe slipping leads to *gross deformities* of the skeleton, with resultant ulnar deviation of the hand (slipping of distal radius and ulnar epiphysis) and to impairment of gait, especially *waddling gait* (slipping of upper femoral epiphyses).

When epiphyseal slipping is suspected, radiologic examination should be performed with at least two views. *Slipping of the upper femoral epiphysis* can occur in a medial or dorsolateral direction. Medial slipping can be diagnosed with anteroposterior views, whereas dorsolateral displacements are best seen with an oblique view (frog-leg position). Distal radial and ulnar epiphyses slip to the dorsolateral side.

There is no doubt that in addition to true epiphyseal slipping, *metaphyseal fractures* occur. Because the trajectorially oriented metaphyseal trabeculae are remodeled into bizarre coarse trabeculae, the mechanical stability of the metaphysis is lost, with resultant complete fractures or separations. A similar mechanism produces knock-knees or gross deformities in the metaphyseal regions of long bones. Sometimes one observes both epiphyseal slipping and metaphyseal fractures simultaneously when superimposed eccentric metaphyseal fractures, as a consequence of slipping, promote further slipping.

*Traumatic fractures* that are not metaphyseal fractures are rare in uremia. In contrast, *stress or fatigue fractures* occur more frequently, especially in the metatarsals and ribs (Fig. 17–15).

Epiphyseal slipping may provoke the temptation for early *surgical correction.* Although early operative procedure is recommended by some orthopedic surgeons,[86, 87, 89] it can lead to disastrous results when it is performed before the metabolic bone disease has been cured. Therefore, appropriate

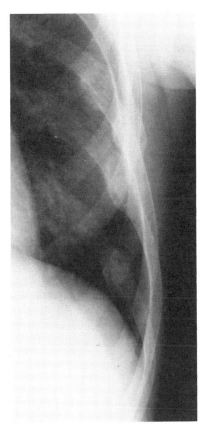

**Figure 17–15.** Spontaneous rib fractures. X-ray of the left chest skeleton in a 16-year-old girl with obstructive uropathy dialyzed for more than four years. Note the thinning of cortical bone and the blurred outlines of spongiosal bone.

treatment of the metabolic bone disease must precede orthopedic correction. Immobilization for more than three weeks to prevent slipping is unnecessary in most patients.[90] Osteotomies for correcting gross deformities or for preventing late arthrosis can be done safely thereafter.

## Dialysis-Related Bone Disease

Children undergoing chronic dialysis are at *risk for development of a negative calcium balance.* Calcium balance during dialysis depends upon the diffusive and convective transfer of calcium across the dialysis membrane. Diffusive transfer of calcium is dependent on the concentration gradient of ionized calcium between plasma and dialysate. The plasma concentration of complexed calcium is influenced by both blood flow and dialysate flow. Convective transfer of calcium

depends upon the rate of ultrafiltration. The magnitude of convective loss is often not appreciated. Negative calcium balance is inevitable when a dialysate calcium concentration of 1.5 mmol/L (6.0 mg/dl) or less is used. In contrast, a positive net gain of calcium is observed in normocalcemic patients at a dialysate calcium concentration of 1.75 mmol/L (7.0 mg/dl) or more.[91]

The prevalence of *symptomatic bone disease* and other clinical manifestations of disturbed calcium metabolism in children on maintenance hemodialysis has markedly decreased in the past decade (Table 17–1). This is due to the earlier institution of drug therapy and to improvement of the dialysis techniques. Despite these advances, osseous disorders continue to be a major unsolved problem in the management of dialyzed children. According to the 1978 report of the European Dialysis and Transplantation Association,[92] more than 14% of dialyzed children develop disabling bone disease after two to five years of treatment. Epiphyseal slipping, however, which is frequently seen prior to dialysis, is rarely observed during dialysis,[5, 93] although hyperparathyroidism and abnormal bone histology continue to be common.[6]

### Dialysis Osteopenia

One specific but not completely understood feature of renal osteodystrophy occurring during dialysis is dialysis osteopenia.[63] The incidence varies widely between different centers. There are distinctive clinical and radiologic features which together allow differentiation from renal osteodystrophy occurring in the majority of nondialyzed patients. The major differential features include a substantial reduction in the amount of bone and an increased incidence of *bone pain* and *fractures.* Both are disproportionate to the radiographic and histologic evidence of osteomalacia and osteitis fibrosa.

The variability of changes of *bone mass* in dialyzed children may be related to differences in calcium balance, catabolism, therapeutic protocols, and previously administered corticosteroids. Furthermore, the relationship of dialysis osteopenia to aluminum intoxication remains to be clarified. Many of the instances of symptomatic fracturing bone disease and osteopenia may be due to aluminum intoxication. On the other hand, we have followed two patients who were dialyzed for more than four years with the typical clinical and radiologic findings of dialysis osteopenia without finding evidence of increased aluminum levels in either their serum or dialysate (Fig. 17–15). There was widespread loss of cortical bone leading to spontaneous fractures of the ribs and metatarsals. Phalangeal subperiosteal resorption was either completely absent or present only to a mild degree. The patients did not respond to the usual treatment, including vitamin D sterols, but impressive thickening of cortical bone was noted following successful transplantation.

### Osteomalacia

In attempting to explain the occurrence of osteomalacia in children undergoing maintenance hemodialysis, one is confronted with a striking paradox. Anephric patients who are presumably deficient in $1,25(OH)_2D_3$ fail to display osteomalacic features.[94] One explanation for this observation is the high degree of secondary hyperparathyroidism which can overshadow the mineralization defect. This assumption is supported by the clinical observation that true osteomalacia may supervene after parathyroidectomy in patients in whom osteitis fibrosa was present prior to surgery.[95] In such patients the appearance of nonmineralized lamellar osteoid is evidence of de novo osteomalacia which was not demonstrable prior to parathyroidectomy.

The occurrence of osteomalacia is a *multifactorial* event. Both disturbed vitamin D metabolism and vitamin D deficiency may occur in dialyzed children. Hypocalcemia may play an important role.[96] We[97] and Duursma et al[98] have found a negative correlation between the serum calcium level and the amount of osteoid in the skeleton. Finally, many controversial findings concerning the incidence of osteomalacia in dialyzed patients and the response to treatment with vitamin D sterols[99] may be due to the role of aluminum.

### Aluminum Intoxication

Although there are no systematic data concerning aluminum (Al) osteomalacia in dialyzed children, it is appropriate to discuss this problem since there is no reason why it should not exist in children as it does in adults. High Al concentrations in

bone of dialyzed patients were reported in 1971.[100] However, it was not until Alfrey reported high Al levels in patients with encephalopathy[101-103] and fracturing osteomalacia[104] that the pathogenetic role of Al was appreciated. *High tissue Al levels* in dialyzed patients may originate from several sources, including addition of Al to dialysate water as a consequence of the electrochemical destruction of electrodes,[103] aluminum in the water supply,[104-106] chemicals from which dialysate water is produced,[105] and, finally, from ingestion of Al-containing phosphate binders.[107-110]

Clarification of the mechanism by which Al causes osteomalacia has been obtained from clinical,[111] histologic,[112] and experimental studies.[113] The so-called *Al osteomalacia* is characterized by progressive skeletal pain, proximal muscular weakness, bone pain, and unresponsiveness to vitamin D therapy.[114] Rarely, a beneficial effect of vitamin D metabolites on muscular weakness and on bone pain has been observed despite the absence of a demonstrable effect on iliac crest bone histology. The beneficial effects of vitamin D may be related to healing of Looser's zones, which consist of woven osteoid. However, in most patients vitamin D or its active sterol will induce hypercalcemia without producing healing of the osteomalacia.[115]

The *pattern of Al deposition* into bone is dependent upon the prior existence of osteitis fibrosa or osteomalacia.[116] Diffused apposition and localized uptake in cement lines have been observed in osteitis fibrosa, with preferential deposition at the mineralization front in osteomalacia. Recent studies have revealed a correlation between Al content and osteoid volume density.[112] It has been proposed that high concentrations of Al are toxic to osteoblasts and to their microtubular system; indeed, the toxic effect on osteoblasts may explain the low alkaline phosphatase levels,[117] loss of bone mass,[118] and the presence of low turnover bone disease. An important factor which can explain the low rate of bone turnover in this disease is the uniform observation of *low basal iPTH* levels which are unresponsive to stimulation by hypocalcemia.[119] This may be explained by the progressive damage of the microtubular system of the parathyroid cells by Al.[120] The interrelationship between Al and parathyroid function is complex; however, hyperparathyroidism favors intestinal absorption of Al, while Al suppresses parathyroid function.

## Bone Disease with Continuous Ambulatory Peritoneal Dialysis (CAPD) and Hemofiltration (HF)

CAPD may affect the metabolic bone disease of uremia by several mechanisms: the effect on calcium and phosphorus balance,[121] the loss of PTH into the dialysate,[122] the loss of 25OHD$_3$,[123] and the removal of putative inhibitors of bone mineralization.[123] Negative peritoneal calcium balance has been reported when dialysate calcium concentrations of 1.5 mmol/L (6.0 mg/dl) have been used. This was accompanied by unchanged total serum calcium levels.[124]

At dialysate calcium concentrations of 1.75 mmol/L (7.0 mg/dl), ionized serum calcium concentrations remain in the low normal range.[125] Because of the effect of *convective transport on calcium loss,* a greater negative calcium balance is observed when concentrated dextrose solutions are used despite identical dialysate calcium concentrations.[126] Therefore, a high dialysate concentration of calcium should be used if maintenance of fluid balance necessitates the use of large quantities of high glucose concentrations in the dialysate. *Serum Pi levels* are more easily controlled with CAPD as compared to hemodialysis.[127] However, in our experience normophosphatemia cannot be maintained in most children without the use of oral phosphate binders. In some patients on CAPD *Al plasma levels* were found to be high.[125] Al clearance with CAPD was reported to average 3.2 to 6.3 ml/min/1.73 m$^2$.[128] *Protein loss,* which influences vitamin D metabolism, varied in our children undergoing CAPD between 0.6 gm/kg/day and 1.5 gm/kg/day. During episodes of peritonitis the protein loss increased to 2.8 to 11.8 gm/kg/day. Most of the protein lost is albumin (80%). This accounts for the *loss of protein-bound 25(OH)D$_3$* into the dialysate, with a subsequent decrease of circulating 25(OH)D$_3$.[123] In our own experience, serum 25(OH)D$_3$ levels did not decrease in children treated for at least one year with CAPD and 5000 to 10,000 I.U. vitamin D/day (unpublished observations). It is controversial as to whether or not CAPD decreases *iPTH serum levels.*[121, 122, 126] CAPD removes primarily PTH fragments with a clearance of about 1.5 ml/min/1.73 m$^2$, and the decrease of serum iPTH levels can be achieved only when the iPTH secretion is controlled by an increase of the serum calcium level.[125, 126, 129]

In children undergoing regular *hemofiltration* (HF) the risk of negative calcium balance is especially high. Since the filtrate volume per kg body weight is much greater in children than in adults,[130] an adequate calcium concentration in the substitution fluid of at least 1.75–2.0 mmol/L (7.0–8.0 mg/dl) is required. It is appropriate to calculate the *calcium balance* for a hemofiltration session in an individual patient by the formula of Fournier:[131]

$$S_{CA} = \frac{UF_{Ca} \times Q_{UF}}{Q_{UF} - (Delta\ W + I)}$$

where $S_{Ca}$ = Ca concentration in substitution fluid, $UF_{Ca}$ = calcium concentration in ultrafiltrate, $Q_{UF}$ = quantity of ultrafiltrate, Delta W = weight change during HF session, and I = net fluid intake during HF session.

It has been demonstrated that *immunoreactive PTH fragments* can be removed from serum by HF.[132] However, it seems unlikely that, in the feedback controlled system, removal of the hormone will have more than a transient effect on circulating levels of the hormone. Our clinical experience with HF has not shown convincing evidence of a decrease of serum iPTH levels or improvement of metabolic bone disease over a period of one year.

## Osseous Changes Following Transplantation

After successful renal transplantation the *resolution of preexisting renal osteodystrophy* generally occurs. Roentgenologic osseous changes of secondary hyperparathyroidism may resolve within two months,[133] or may continue to improve for more than two years.[134–136] The rapidity of healing is correlated with the degree of preexisting secondary hyperparathyroidism and the degree of hyperplasia of the parathyroid glands. In our experience children treated previously with hemodialysis for more than three years show a slow resolution of secondary hyperparathyroidism compared with children treated for a shorter period of time. We have observed slightly increased iPTH and lowered Pi serum levels for up to two years after transplantation. Partial parathyroidectomy became necessary ten months after transplantation in one patient.

The administration of high doses of corticosteroids may have a deleterious effect on bone. Radiologic signs of *osteoporosis* are more frequently noted in patients who receive large amounts of corticosteroids prior to the development of ESRD. It should be emphasized that this type of osteoporosis is difficult to separate from dialysis osteopenia. Therefore, it is not surprising that the effect of renal transplantation on the radiographic evidence of dialysis osteopenia is variable. With few exceptions dialysis osteopenia is not favorably affected.

In a limited number of children in whom persistent secondary hyperparathyroidism can be excluded, persistent *hypophosphatemia* will develop after transplantation. It results from tubular damage due to graft ischemia at the time of harvesting.[137, 138] As in other forms of impaired renal tubular reabsorption of phosphate, osteomalacia may develop, but severe clinical problems have not yet been reported.

The most serious osseous complication after renal transplantation is *aseptic necrosis* (Fig. 17–16).[141–149] The incidence is high, varying from 3% to 45%.[135] The overall frequency is about 8%. Osteonecrosis usually appears within the first year after transplantation. One of our patients was found to have femoral head necrosis a few weeks after transplantation (Fig. 17–16). Late occurrence has been reported up to five years after transplantation.[122] The exact *mechanism by which osteonecrosis occurs* after transplantation is unknown. Bailey et al have suggested that *secondary hyperparathyroidism* may play a role in the genesis.[146] Hall et al found radiologic evidence of osteonecrosis prior to transplantation in three out of 140 adult patients.[147] Mehls et al reported three uremic children with femoral head necrosis prior to dialysis and transplantation, although they had never received corticosteroids.[148] Nevertheless, hyperparathyroidism appears to be a rare cause of osteonecrosis, whereas *corticosteroid* treatment appears to be *the* critical factor. However, most investigators have failed to find a correlation between the *frequency of osteonecrosis* and the daily steroid dosage. There are recent reports suggesting that low-dose steroids following transplantation will decrease the percentage of aseptic necrosis.[149]

The *femoral head* is the most common site affected in children, but in contrast to adult patients the *femoral condyles* are affected at nearly the same frequency.[141–146] Other sites in children include *os naviculare carpi, os naviculare tarsi, talus, and calcaneus.*[141, 147] *Pain* is the predominant symptom, usually preceding roentgenologic evidence of osteonecrosis by several months. On the other hand, the

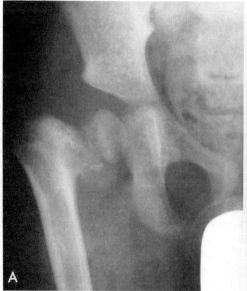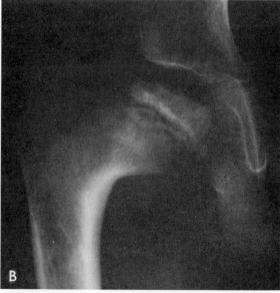

**Figure 17–16.** Femoral head aseptic necrosis after transplantation. *A,* Severe renal osteodystrophy in a four-year-old child with a serum creatinine level of 2.5 mg/dl. Note severe coxa vara. *B,* The same child at 11 years of age. The femoral head necrosis was first diagnosed a few weeks after renal transplantation. It seems possible that the preexisting coxa vara secondary to renal osteodystrophy predisposed to osteonecrosis.[148]

lesions may remain silent for longer periods. We have followed a 14-year-old boy with radiologic evidence of femoral head necrosis for one and a half years before he complained of pain.[144] The diagnosis of osteonecrosis is usually made radiologically. An early radiologic sign is a radiolucent line paralleling the joint surface of the femoral head, which represents fractures through the cancellous bone. As the lesion progresses, the osteochondrous fragment collapses at the fracture site, resulting in a "step" as noted radiographically. Subsequently bone trabeculae become more compact, leading to an increased radiographic density.

*Scintiscan* of bone performed either by [18]fluoride or [99]technetium usually reveals changes before the roentgenogram becomes abnormal. It should be remembered, however, that scintiscan diagnosis may be delayed.

We have observed spontaneous *joint effusions* (usually of the knees) in children receiving transplants, without osteonecrosis, in agreement with reports of adult patients.[11] However, *septic arthritis* seems to be rare in children.[11]

## Renal Osteodystrophy and Growth

Renal osteodystrophy is thought to be an important cause of growth failure in uremia; however, it has not been established at what stage of renal insufficiency and to what extent renal osteodystrophy contributes to stunting. In experimental uremia (creatinine clearance 20% of normal), both vitamin $D_3$[150] and $1,25(OH)_2D_3$[151] have a positive effect on bone histology and growth. We have reported a 3½-year-old child who had severe renal osteodystrophy and growth arrest at a creatinine clearance of 25 ml/min/1.73 $m^2$ and who responded to vitamin $D_3$ treatment with healing of bone disease and demonstrated true catch-up growth.[43] However, superimposed vitamin D deficiency could have been present in this child. In contrast we and others[55] have not observed convincing improvement of growth following vitamin $D_3$ treatment in patients with ESRD before or during dialysis. These results were independent of vitamin D treatment given prophylactically or to treat the roentgenologic signs of renal osteodystrophy.

Chesney et al reported increased growth velocity with administration of $1,25(OH)_2D_3$ in uremic children who had previously not responded to vitamin $D_3$ treatment;[152] however, the growth-promoting effects were only transitory.[153] Follow-up data showed that the growth curves of these patients, who were mostly not dialyzed, only paralleled the third percentile.[153] But, this in particular is a general finding in uremic children above the age of three years before institution of dialysis.[151, 154, 155] Malekzadeh,[156] Bulla,[157] and the author could not demonstrate improvement in the growth rate of dialyzed children by administration of $1,25(OH)_2D_3$.

It has not been established whether hyperparathyroidism contributes to growth failure. Children with hypoparathyroidism are stunted. There are no conclusive data concerning the growth of patients with primary hyperparathyroidism, but patients with pseudohyperparathyroidism and osteitis fibrosa are usually tall.[63] Since PTH induces mitoses in osteoprogenitor cells,[158] thymocytes, and growth cartilage cells,[159] it is likely that parathyroid hormone normally has some growth-promoting function. In uremia cAMP response of growth cartilage cells to PTH is blunted.[160] Extreme hyperparathyroidism of uremia contributes to growth failure by destroying the normal architecture of growth zones.[78] In agreement with this concept is the anecdotal report of Broyer et al, who showed that children with severe hyperparathyroidism and severe renal osteodystrophy had the poorest growth.[161] In these children parathyroidectomy led to an improvement of growth,[161] but in Broyer's (personal communication) and our experience,[90] the growth-promoting effect of parathyroidectomy was only transient.

## REFERENCES

1. Förster R: Über Schrumpfnieren im Kindesalter. Z Kinderheilk 26:38, 1887.
2. Lucas RC: On a form of late rickets associated with albuminuria, rickets of adolescents. Lancet 1:993, 1883.
3. Cameron HC: Case of osteomalacia and infantilism with renal deficiency. Proc R Soc Med 2:22,.1918.
4. Barber H: Renal dwarfism. Quart J Med 14:205, 1921.
5. Mehls O, Ritz E, Krempien B, et al: Slipped epiphyses in renal osteodystrophy. Arch Dis Child 50:545, 1975.
6. Mehls, O, Krempien B, Ritz E, et al: Renal osteodystrophy in children on maintenance hemodialysis. Proc Eur Dial Transplant Assoc 10:197, 1973.
7. Coburn JW, Slatopolsky E: Vitamin D, parathyroid

hormone and renal osteodystrophy. *In*: Brenner BM, Rector F (eds): The Kidney. Philadelphia, WB Saunders, 1981, p 2213.

8. Balsan S: Renal osteodystrophy. *In*: Liebermann E (ed): Clinical Nephrology. Philadelphia, Lippincott, 1976, p 424.

9. Beale MG, Salcedo JR, Ellis D, et al: Renal osteodystrophy. Pediatr Clin North Am 23:873, 1976.

10. Mehls O, Ritz E, Kreusser W, et al: Renal osteodystrophy in uremic children. Clin Endocrinol Metab 9:151, 1980.

11. Wright RS, Mehls O, Ritz E, et al: Musculoskeletal manifestations of chronic renal failure. *In*: Bacon PA, Hadler NM (eds): The Kidney and Rheumatic Disease. London, Butterworth Scientific, 1982, p 342.

12. Bouillon R, Van Assche FA, Van Baelen H, et al: Influence of the vitamin D-binding protein on the serum concentration of 1,25-dihydroxyvitamin $D_3$. J Clin Invest 67:589, 1981.

13. Holick MF, Schnoes HK, De Luca HF: Identification of 1,25-dihydroxycholecalciferol, a form of vitamin $D_3$ metabolically active in the intestine. Proc Natl Acad Sci 68:803, 1971.

14. Fraser DR, Kodicek E: Unique biosynthesis by kidney of a biologically active vitamin D metabolite. Nature 228:764, 1970.

15. Boyle IT, Miravet L, Gray RW, et al: The response of intestinal calcium transport to 25-hydroxy and 1,25-dihydroxy vitamin D in nephrectomized rats. Endocrinology 90:605, 1972.

16. Tanaka Y, De Luca HF: The control of 25-hydroxy-vitamin D metabolism by inorganic phosphorus. Arch Biochem Biophys 154:566, 1973.

17. De Luca HF: Vitamin D Metabolism and Function. Berlin, Heidelberg, New York, Springer, 1979.

18. Offermann G, von Herrath D, Schäfer K: Serum 25-hydroxycholecalciferol in uremia. Nephron 13:269, 1974.

19. Sallman AL, Jacob AI, Hollis B, et al: Impaired photoproduction of vitamin D in uremia. *In*: 14th Annual Meeting American Society of Nephrology, Washington DC, 1981.

20. Schmidt-Gayk H, Schmitt W, Grawunder C, et al: 25-hydroxy-vitamin D in nephrotic syndrome. Lancet 2:105, 1977.

21. Bouillon R, Reynaert J, Claes JH, et al: The effect of anticonvulsant therapy on serum levels of 25-hydroxy-vitamin $D_3$, calcium and parathyroid hormone. J Clin Endocrinol Metab 41:1130, 1975.

22. Pierides AM, Kerr DNS, Ellis HA, et al: 1-alpha-hydroxycholecalciferol in hemodialysis and renal osteodystrophy. Adverse effect of anticonvulsant therapy. Clin Nephrol 5:189, 1976.

23. Van Stone J, Frank DT, Brandsford WR: The effect of decreased renal function with and without renal mass on 1,25$(OH)_2$ cholecalciferol production in rats. J Lab Clin Med 89:1168, 1977.

24. Mawer EB, Taylor CM: Vitamin D metabolism in man, the role of the kidney. *In* Proceedings of Seventh International Congress of Nephrology, Montreal. S Karger, 1978, p 469.

25. Reiss E, Canterbury JM, Kanter A: Circulating parathyroid hormone concentration in chronic renal insufficiency. Arch Intern Med 124:417, 1969.

26. Slatopolsky E, Bricker NS: The role of phosphorus restriction in the prevention of secondary hyper-

parathyroidism in chronic renal disease. Kidney Int 4:141, 1973.

27. Bricker NS, Slatopolsky E, Rein E, et al: Calcium, phosphorus and bone in renal disease and transplantation. Arch Intern Med 123:543, 1969.

28. Kleerekoper M, Cruz C, Bernstein RS, et al: The phosphaturic action of PTH in the steady state in patients. Adv Exp Med Biol 128:145, 1980.

29. Malluche HH, Ritz E, Lange HP, et al: Bone histology in incipient and advanced renal failure. Kidney Int 9:335, 1976.

30. Ritz E, Bommer J, Kreusser W, et al: Management of disturbed calcium metabolism in renal failure. *In*: Monoclonal Antibodies and Development in Immunoassay, Albertini A, Etkins R (eds). Amsterdam, 1981, p 291.

31. Massry SG, Ritz E, Verberckmoes R: Role of phosphate in the genesis of secondary hyperparathyroidism of renal failure. Nephron 18:77, 1977.

32. Better OS, Kleeman CR, Gonick HC, et al: Renal handling of calcium, magnesium and inorganic phosphate in chronic renal failure. Isr J Med Sci 3:60, 1967.

33. Friis T, Hahnemann S, Weeke E: Serum calcium and serum phosphorus in uremia during administration of sodium phosphate and aluminum hydroxide. Acta Med Scand 183:497, 1968.

34. Slatopolsky E, Gray R, Adams ND, et al: Low serum levels of 1,25$(OH)_2D_3$ are not responsible for the development of secondary hyperparathyroidism in early renal failure. Kidney Int 14:177, 1978.

35. Coburn JW, Hartenbower DL, Massry SG: Intestinal absorption of calcium and the effect of renal insufficiency. Kidney Int 4:96, 1973.

36. Massry SG, Dua S, Garty J, et al: Role of uremia in the skeletal resistance to the calcemic action of parathyroid hormone (PTH). Kidney Int 10:A490, 1976.

37. Llach F, Massry SG, Singer FR, et al: Skeletal resistance to endogenous parathyroid hormone in patients with early renal failure. A possible cause for secondary hyperparathyroidism. J Clin Endocrinol Metab 41:339, 1975.

38. Sommerville PJ, Kaye M: Resistance to parathyroid hormone in renal failure: Role of vitamin D metabolites. Kidney Int 14:245, 1978.

39. Brickman AS, Jowsey J, Sherrand DJ, et al: Therapy with 1,25-dihydroxy vitamin $D_3$ in the management of renal osteodystrophy. *In*: Norman AW, Schaefer K, Grigoleit HG, von Herrath D, Ritz E (eds): Vitamin D and Problems Related to Uremic Bone Disease. Berlin, De Gruyter, 1975, p 241.

40. Massry SG, Stein R, Garty J, et al: Skeletal resistance to the calcemic action of parathyroid hormone. Role of 1,25$(OH)_2D_3$. Kidney Int 9:467, 1976.

41. Smith R, Stern G: Myopathy, osteomalacia and hyperparathyroidism. Brain 90:593, 1967.

42. Schärer K, Chantler C, Brunner FP, et al: Combined report on regular dialysis and transplantation of children in Europe, 1975. Proc Eur Dial Transplant Assoc 13:59, 1976.

43. Mehls O, Ritz E, Gilli G, et al: Growth in renal failure. Nephron 21:237, 1978.

44. Cadenat H, Combelles R, Fabert G, et al: Calcification du systeme dentaire sous dialyse. Rev Stomatol Chir Maxillofac 78:491, 1977.

45. Bublitz A, Machat E, Shärer K, et al: Changes in dental development in pediatric patients with chronic kidney disease. Proc Eur Dial Transplant Assoc 18:517, 1981.

46. Ritz E, Mehls O, Bommer J, et al: Vascular calcifications under maintenance hemodialysis. Klin Wochenschr 55:375, 1977.

47. Gilchrest BA, Rowe JW, Brown RS, et al: Relief of uremic pruritus with ultraviolet phototherapy. N Engl J Med 297:136, 1977.

48. Tapia L, Cheigh JS, David DS, et al: Parenteral lidocaine in treatment of pruritus in dialysis patients. N Engl J Med 279:697, 1968.

49. Ritz E, Malluche H, Krempien B, et al: Calcium metabolism in renal failure. In: Bronner F, Coburn JW (eds.): Disorders of Mineral Metabolism, Vol 3, New York, Academic Press, 1981, p 152.

50. Luciani JC, Ferran JL, Dumas ML, et al: Ostéodystrophie chez l'enfant hémodialyse. Nouv Presse Med 19:3615, 1977.

51. Mehls O, Ritz E, Krempien B, et al: Slipped epiphyses in renal osteodystrophy. In: Norman AW (ed): Vitamin D and Problems Related to Uremic Bone Disease. Berlin, De Gruyter, 1975.

52. Wittmer J, Margolis A, Fantaine O, et al: Effects of 25-hydroxycholecalciferol on bone lesions of children with terminal renal failure. Kidney Int 10:395, 1976.

53. Norman ME, Mazur AT, Borden S, et al: Early diagnosis of juvenile renal osteodystrophy. J Pediatr 97:226, 1980.

54. Hodson EM, Dunstan CR, Hillis EE, et al: Pediatric renal osteodystrophy. Pediatr Res 14:990, 1980.

55. Bulla M, Delling G, Offermann G, et al: Renal bone disorders in children. Therapy with vitamin $D_3$ or 1,25-dihydroxycholecalciferol. Proc Eur Dial Transplant Assoc 16:644, 1979.

56. Bulla M, Delling G, Offermann G, et al: Renal bone disorder in children: Therapy with vitamin $D_3$ or 1,25-dihydroxycholecalciferol. In: Norman AW, Schäfer K, von Herrath D, et al (eds): Vitamin D, Basic Research and Its Clinical Application. Berlin, De Gruyter, 1979, p 853.

57. Garner A, Ball J: Quantitative observations on mineralized and unmineralized bone in chronic renal azotemia and intestinal malabsorption syndrome. J Pathol Bacteriol 91:545, 1966.

58. Schlackman H, Green A, Naiman JL: Myelofibrosis in children with chronic renal insufficiency. J Pediatr 87:720, 1975.

59. Müller-Wiefel DE, Swoboda R, Mehls O, et al: Knochenmarkszellularität bei Kindern mit chronischer Niereninsuffizienz. In: Aktuelle Probleme der Dialyseverfahren und der Niereninsuffizienz, P van Dittrich (ed). Friedberg/Hessen, C. Bindernagel, 1981, p 208.

60. Llach F, Massry SG, Koffler A, et al: Secondary hyperparathyroidism in early renal failure: Role of phosphate retention. Kidney Int 12:459, 1977.

61. Mehls O, Ritz E, Krempien B, et al: Roentgenological signs in the skeleton of uremic children. An analysis of the anatomical principles underlying the roentgenological changes. Pediatr Radiol 1:183, 1973.

62. Meema HE, Rabinovich S, Meema S, et al: Improved radiological diagnosis of azotemic osteodystrophy. Radiology 102:1, 1972.

63. Parfitt AM: Clinical and radiographic manifestations of renal osteodystrophy. In: David DS (ed):

Calcium and Metabolism in Renal Failure and Nephrolithiasis. New York, John Wiley & Sons, 1977, p 145.

64. Debnam JW, Bates ML, Kopelman RC, et al: Radiological/pathological correlations in uremic bone disease. Radiology 125:653, 1977.

65. Ritz E, Prager P, Krempien B, et al: Skeletal X-ray findings and bone histology in patients on hemodialysis. Kidney Int 13:316, 1978.

66. Ritz E, Krempien B, Mehls O, et al: Skeletal abnormalities in chronic renal insufficiency and under maintenance hemodialysis (anatomical analysis). Kidney Int 4:116, 1973.

67. Feist HJ: The biological basis of radiologic findings in bone disease. Recognition and interpretation of abnormal bone architecture. Radiol Clin North Am 8:183, 1970.

68. Heath DA, Martin DJ: Periosteal new bone formation in hyperparathyroidism associated with renal failure. Br J Radiol 43:515, 1970.

69. Meema HE, Oreopoulos DG, Rabinovich S, et al: Periosteal new bone formation (periosteal neostosis) in renal osteodystrophy. Radiology 110:513, 1974.

70. Ritz E, Malluche HH, Krempien B, et al: Calcium metabolism in renal failure. In: Disorders of Mineral Metabolism, Vol 3. Bronner F, Coburn JW (eds). New York, Academic Press, 1981.

71. Heuck F, von Babo H: Röntgenbefunde bei primärem Hyperparathyreoidismus. Radiologe 14:206, 1974.

72. Chesney RW, Mazess RB, Rose PG, et al: Bone mineral status measured by direct photon absorptiometry in childhood renal disease. Pediatrics 60:864, 1977.

73. Mehls O, Ritz E, Broyer M: The spectrum of skeletal manifestations in renal osteodystrophy. In Pediatric Nephrology. Gruskin AB, Norman ME (eds). The Hague, M Nijhoff, 1981, p 218.

74. Letteri JM, Cohn SH: Total body neutron activation analysis in the study of mineral homeostasis in chronic renal disease. In: David DS (ed): Calcium Metabolism in Renal Failure and Nephrolithiasis. New York, John Wiley & Sons, 1977.

75. Dent CE, Hodson CJ: General softening of bone due to metabolic causes. II. Radiological changes associated with certain metabolic bone disease. Br J Radiol 27:605, 1954.

76. Rubin P: Dynamic Classification of Bone Dysplasia. Chicago, Year Book Medical Publishers, 1969, p 24.

77. Park EA: Observations on the pathology of rickets with particular reference to the changes at the cartilage shaft junctions of the growing bones. Bull NY Acad Med 15:495, 1939.

78. Krempien B, Mehls O, Ritz E: Morphological studies on pathogenesis of epiphyseal slipping in uremic children. Virchows Arch (Pathol Anat) 362:129, 1974.

79. Pommer G: Untersuchungen über Osteomalazie und Rachitis nebst Beiträgen über Kenntnis der Knochenresorption und Apposition in verschiedenen Altersgruppen. Leipzig, Vogel, 1885.

80. Mehls O, Ritz E, Gilli G, et al: Growth and bone lesions in experimental uremia. In: Vitamin D: Biochemical, Chemical and Clinical Aspects Related to Calcium Metabolism. Norman AW (ed). Berlin, De Gruyter, 1977, p 685.

81. Wood BSB, George WH, Robinson AW: Parathy-

roid adenoma in a child presenting as rickets. Arch Dis Child 33:46, 1958.

82. Rayasuria K, Peiris OA, Ratnaike UT, et al: Parathyroid adenomas in childhood. Am J Dis Child 107:442, 1964.

83. Lomnitz E, Sepulveda L, Stevenson C, et al: Primary hyperparathyroidism stimulating rickets. J Clin Endocrinol Metab 26:309, 1966.

84. Kirkwood JR, Ozonoff MB, Steinbach HL: Epiphyseal displacement after metaphyseal fracture in renal osteodystrophy. Am J Roentgenol 115:547, 1972.

85. Brailsford JF: Slipping of epiphysis of the head of the femur. Its relation to renal rickets. Lancet 1:16, 1933.

86. Shea D, Mankin HJ: Slipped capital femoral epiphyses in renal rickets. J Bone Joint Surg 48:349, 1966.

87. Catell HS, Levin S, Kopitz S, et al: Reconstructive surgery in children with azotemic osteodystrophy. J Bone Joint Surg 53:217, 1971.

88. Floman Y, Yosipovitch Z, Licht A, et al: Bilateral slipped upper femoral epiphysis. A rare manifestation of renal osteodystrophy—case report with discussion of its pathogenesis. Isr J Med Sci 11:15, 1975.

89. Goldman AB, Lane JM, Salvati E: Slipped capital femoral epiphyses complicating renal osteodystrophy: a report of three cases. Radiology 126:233, 1978.

90. Mehls O, Ritz E, Parsch K, et al: Therapeutische Erfahrungen bei urämischer Epiphysenlösung. Klin Wochenschr 54:405, 1976.

91. Johnson WJ: Optimum dialysate calcium concentration during maintenance hemodialysis. Nephron 17:241, 1976.

92. Chantler C, Donckerwolcke RA, Brunner FP, et al: Combined report on regular dialysis and transplantation of children in Europe, 1978. Proc Eur Dial Transplant Assoc 16:74, 1979.

93. Mehls O, Ritz E, Krempien B, et al: Slipped epiphyses in renal osteodystrophy. In: Norman AW, Schäfer K, Grigoleit HG, et al (eds): Vitamin D and Problems Related to Uremic Bone Disease. Berlin, De Gruyter, 1975, p 551.

94. Bordier PJ, Tunchot S, Eastwood JB, et al: Lack of histological evidence of vitamin D abnormality in bones of anephric patients. Clin Sci Mol Med 44:33, 1973.

95. Ritz E, Malluche HH, Krempien B, et al: Bone histology in renal insufficiency. In: Calcium Metabolism in Renal Failure and Nephrolithiasis, David DS (ed). New York, John Wiley & Sons, 1977, p 197.

96. Nielsen HE, Melsen F, Christensen MS: Bone histomorphometry in non-dialysed and dialysed patients with chronic renal failure. Min Electrol Metab 4:113, 1980.

97. Ritz E, Krempien B, Riedasch G, et al: Dialysis bone disease. Proc Eur Dial Transplant Assoc 8:131, 1971.

98. Duursma SA, Visser WJ, Nij EL: A quantitative histological study of bone in 30 patients with renal insufficiency. Calcif Tiss Res 9:216, 1972.

99. Massry SG, Goldstein DA, Malluche HH: Current status of the use of $1,25(OH)_2D_3$ in the management of renal osteodystrophy. Kidney Int 48:408, 1980.

100. Parsons V, Davies C, Goode GL, et al: Aluminium in bone from patients with renal failure. Br Med J 4:273, 1971.

101. Alfrey AC, Legendre GR, Kaehny WD: Dialysis encephalopathy syndrome: Possible aluminium intoxication. N Engl J Med 294:184, 1976.

102. Alfrey AC, Hegg A, Miller H, et al: Interrelationship between calcium and aluminium metabolism in dialysed uremic patients. Min Electrol Metab 2:81, 1979.

103. Flendring JA, Kruis H, Das HA: Aluminium intoxication: The cause of dialysis dementia. Proc Eur Dial Transplant Assoc 13:355, 1976.

104. Parkinson IS, Ward MK, Feest TG, et al: Fracturing dialysis osteodystrophy and dialysis encephalopathy. Lancet 1:406, 1979.

105. Elliott HL, Dryburgh F, Fell GS, et al: Aluminium toxicity during regular hemodialysis. Br Med J:1101, 1978.

106. Platts MM, Goode GL, Hislop JS: Composition of the domestic water supply and the incidence of fractures and encephalopathy in patients on home dialysis. Br Med J 2:657, 1977.

107. Pogglitsch H: Therapie mit Aluminium-haltigen Substanzen in der Nephrologie. Nieren- und Hochdruckkrankh 10:201, 1981.

108. Berlyne GM, Ben-Ari J, Pest D, et al: Hyperaluminemia from aluminium resin in renal failure. Lancet 2:494, 1970.

109. Clarkson EM, Luck VA, Hynson WY, et al: The effect of aluminium hydroxyde on calcium, phosphorus and aluminium balances, the serum parathyroid hormone concentration and the aluminium content of bone in patients with chronic renal failure. Clin Sci 93:519, 1972.

110. Kaehny WD, Hegg AP, Alfrey AC: Gastrointestinal absorption of aluminium from aluminium-containing antacids. N Engl J Med 296:1389, 1977.

111. Hodsman AB, Sherrard DJ, Wong EGC, et al: Vitamin D resistant osteomalacia in hemodialysis patients lacking secondary hyperparathyroidism. Ann Intern Med 94:629, 1981.

112. Cournot-Witmer G, Zingraff J, Plachot JJ, et al: Aluminium localisation in bone from hemodialysed patients: Relationship to matrix mineralisation. Kidney Int 20:375, 1979.

113. Ellis HA, McCarthy JH, Herrington J: Bone aluminium in hemodialysed patients and in rats injected with aluminium chloride: Relationship to impaired bone mineralisation. J Clin Pathol 32:832, 1981.

114. Henderson RG, Russel RGG, Ledingham JGG, et al: Effects of 1,25-dihydroxycholecalciferol on calcium absorption, muscle weakness and bone disease in chronic renal failure. Lancet 1:379, 1974.

115. Coburn JW, Brickman AS, Sherrard DJ, et al: Renal osteodystrophy and its relation to vitamin D: Identification of a mineralizing defect in uremia unrelated to vitamin D. In: Copp DH, Talmage RV (eds): Endocrinology of Calcium Metabolism. Amsterdam, Excerpta Medica, 1978, p 27.

116. Cournot-Witmer G, Zingraff J, Bourdon R, et al: Aluminium and dialysis bone disease. Lancet 2:795, 1979.

117. Pierides AM, Skillen AW, Ellis HA: Serum alkaline phosphatase in azotemic hemodialysis osteodys-

trophy: a study of isoenzyme patterns, their correlation with bone histology, and their changes in response to treatment with 1-alpha-(OH)D$_3$ and 1,25(OH)$_2$D$_3$. J Lab Clin Med 93:899, 1979.

118. Alvarez-Ude F, Feest TG, Ward MK, et al: Hemodialysis bone disease: Correlations between clinical, histological and other findings. Kidney Int 14:68, 1978.

119. Kraut JA, Shinaberger JH, Singer FR, et al: Reduced parathyroid response to acute hypocalcemia in dialysis osteomalacia (abstr). Min Electrol Metab 6:248, 1981.

120. Cann CE, Prussin SG, Gordan CS: Aluminium uptake by the parathyroid glands. J Clin Endocrinol Metab 49:543, 1979.

121. Gokal R, Fryer R, McHugh M, et al: Calcium and phosphate control in patients on continuous ambulatory peritoneal dialysis. In: CAPD: Proceedings of an International Symposium, Legrain M (ed). Amsterdam, Excerpta Medica, 1980, p 283.

122. Delmez J, Martin K, Harter H, et al: The effects of continuous ambulatory peritoneal dialysis on the removal of iPTH in renal failure (abstr). Am Soc Artif Organs 9:44, 1980.

123. Velentzas C, Oreopoulos DG, Brandes L, et al: Abnormal vitamin D levels. Ann Intern Med 86:198, 1977.

124. Calderaro V, Oreopoulos DG, Meema HE, et al: Renal osteodystrophy in patients on continuous ambulatory peritoneal dialysis. Proc Eur Dial Transplant Assoc 17:243, 1980.

125. Gokal R: Pathology of bone disease in CAPD. In: Atkins RC, Thomson NM, Farrell PC: Peritoneal Dialysis. New York, Churchill Livingstone, 1981, p 25.

126. Delmez J, Slatopolsky E, Martin K, et al: The effects of continuous ambulatory peritoneal dialysis (CAPD) on parathyroid hormone (PTH) and mineral metabolism. Am Soc Nephrol 1981, 38 A.

127. Oreopoulos DG: The coming age of continuous ambulatory peritoneal dialysis. Dial Transplant 8:460, 1979.

128. Chan MK, Baillod RA, Chuah P, et al: Three years' experience of continuous ambulatory peritoneal dialysis. Lancet 1:1409, 1981.

129. Khanna R, Oreopoulos DG, Dombros N, et al: Continuous ambulatory peritoneal dialysis (CAPD) after three years: "Still a promising treatment". Perit Dial Bull 1:14, 1981.

130. Müller-Wiefel DE, Rauh W, Wingen AM, et al: Hemofiltration in children. Contr Nephrol 32:128, 1982.

131. De Fremont JR, Morniere P, Pruna A, et al: Long-term evaluation of hemofiltration at home. (in press).

132. Schaefer K, Offermann G, von Herrath D, et al: Parathyroid hormone, 25-OH-vitamin D, and digoxin levels in patients treated by chronic hemofiltration. J Dial 1:619, 1977.

133. Hehrmann R, Tidow G, Offner G, et al: Plasma-Parathormon nach Nierentransplantation. Ein empfindlicher Parameter zur Beurteilung der postoperativen Transplantatfunktion. Klin Wochenschr 58:249, 1980.

134. Bricker NS, Slatopolsky E, Reiss E: Calcium, phos-

phorus and bone in renal disease and transplantation. Arch Intern Med 123:543, 1969.

135. Fine RN, Isaacson AS, Payne V, et al: Renal homotransplantation. J Pediatr 80:243, 1972.

136. Pierides AM, Ellis HA, Peart KM, et al: Assessment of renal osteodystrophy following renal transplantation. Proc Eur Dial Transplant Assoc 11:481, 1975.

137. Moorehead JF, Wills MR, Ahmed K, et al: Hypophosphatemic osteomalacia after cadaver renal transplantation. Lancet 1:694, 1974.

138. Better OS: Tubular dysfunction following kidney transplantation. Nephron 25:209, 1980.

139. Hulme B, Kenyon JR, Owen K, et al: Renal transplantation in children. Arch Dis Child 47:486, 1972.

140. Lilly JR, Giles G, Hurwitz R, et al: Renal homotransplantation in pediatric patients. Pediatrics 47:548, 1971.

141. Potter DE, Genant HD, Salvatierra O: Avascular necrosis of bone after renal transplantation. Am J Dis Child 132:1125, 1978.

142. Stern PJ, Watts HG: Osteonecrosis after renal transplantation. J Bone Joint Surg 61A:851, 1979.

143. Uittenbogaart CH, Isaacson AS, Stanley PH, et al: Aseptic necrosis after renal transplantation in children. Am J Dis Child 132:765, 1978.

144. Oppermann HC, Mehls O, Willich F, et al: Osteonekrosen bei Kindern mit chronischen Nierenerkrankungen vor und nach Nierentransplantation. Radiologe 21:175, 1981.

145. Broyer M, Gagnadoux MF, Beurton D, et al: Transplantation in children: technical aspects, drug therapy and problems related to primary renal disease. Proc Eur Dial Transplant Assoc 18:313, 1981.

146. Bailey GL, Griffiths HJL, Mocelin AJ, et al: Avascular necrosis of the femoral head in patients on chronic hemodialysis. Trans Am Soc Artif Intern Organs 18:401, 1972.

147. Hall MC, Elmore SM, Bright RW, et al: Skeletal complications in a series of human renal allografts. JAMA 208:1825, 1969.

148. Mehls O, Ritz E, Oppermann HC, et al: Femoral head necrosis in uremic children without steroid treatment or transplantation. J Pediatr 6:926, 1981.

149. McGeown MG, Douglas JF, Brown WA, et al: Low dose steroid from the following transplantation. Proc Eur Dial Transplant Assoc 16:395, 1979.

150. Mehls O, Ritz E, Gilli G, et al: Effect of vitamin D on growth in experimental uremia. Am J Clin Nutr 31:1927, 1978.

151. Gilli G, Ritz E, Mehls O, et al: Effect of vitamin D$_3$ and 1,25(OH)$_2$D$_3$ on growth in experimental uremia. Pediatr Res 14:990, 1980.

152. Chesney RW, Moorthy AV, Eisman JA, et al: Increased growth after long-term oral 1-alpha-25-vitamin D$_3$ in childhood renal osteodystrophy. N Engl J Med 298:238, 1978.

153. Chesney RW: 1,25-dihydroxy vitamin D$_3$ in the treatment of juvenile renal osteodystrophy. In: Pediatric Nephrology, Gruskin AB, Norman ME (eds). The Hague, Martinus Nijhoff Publishers, 1981, p 209.

154. Kleinknecht C, Broyer M, Huot D, et al: Growth

and development of non-dialysed children with chronic renal failure. Kidney Int 24, S-40, 1983.

155. Rizzoni G, Basso T: Growth in children with chronic renal failure. Pediatr Res 14:1016, 1980 (Abstr).

156. Malekzadeh MH, Ettenger RB, Pennisi AJ, et al: Treatment of renal osteodystrophy in children with 1-alpha-(OH)D$_3$. Fourth Workshop on Vitamin D, Berlin, 1979 (Abstr).

157. Bulla M, Stock GJ, Delling G, et al: Einfluss der Vitamin D$_3$-Therapie auf die renale Osteodystrophie im Kindesalter. Klin Wochenschr 58:237, 1980.

158. Bingham PJ, Barzell JA, Owen M: The effect of parathyroid extract on cellular activity and plasma calcium levels in vitro. J Endocrinol 45:387, 1969.

159. Shelling DH: The parathyroids in health and disease. St. Louis, CV Mosby, 1936.

160. Kreusser W, Weinkauf R, Mehls O, et. al: Effect of parathyroid hormone, calcitonin and growth hormone on cAMP content of growth cartilage in experimental uremia. Eur J Clin Invest 12:337, 1982.

161. Broyer M, Kleinknecht C, Loirat C, et al: Growth in children treated with long-term hemodialysis. J Pediatr 84:642, 1974.

# 18

# Treatment of Renal Osteodystrophy During Childhood

*Shermine Dabbagh, M.D.*
*Russell W. Chesney, M.D.*

## CLINICAL FEATURES WHICH REQUIRE CAREFUL MANAGEMENT

The association of renal failure with skeletal deformities and growth retardation in children with hyperplasia of the parathyroid glands has been known for many decades.[1, 2] Lucas, in 1883, reported four male adolescents who had albuminuria and rachitic skeletal deformities and who responded to "phosphate of iron and cod liver oil."[2] Since dialysis and transplantation allow children with chronic renal failure to have a prolonged survival and to reach adulthood, renal osteodystrophy and its sequelae have become of prime concern to physicians involved in the management of such children. The clinical manifestations of renal osteodystrophy are multifaceted and have not been completely elucidated,[3] indicating the difficulty with, but importance of, aggressive management in children (Table 18–1).

The pathologic changes in the skeleton of uremic children include osteitis fibrosa cystica, which reflects the resorptive effects of increased osteoclastic activity owing to secondary hyperparathyroidism, and osteomalacia, which is a defect in bone mineralization secondary to alterations in vitamin D metabolism. The latter is characterized by widened osteoid seams and an abnormal mineralization front. Less commonly, osteosclerosis and osteoporosis are also seen in children with chronic renal failure. These entities can exist singly or in combination.

This chapter will focus on the treatment of childhood renal osteodystrophy, detailing the newer available treatment modalities and highlighting pertinent controversial issues.

### Specific Features of Childhood Renal Osteodystrophy

Growth retardation is common in uremic children both before and during dialysis. The development of impaired renal function in infancy has a more deleterious effect on linear growth than does the onset in older children. Growth retardation can occur in the absence of overt skeletal deformities. A decrease in growth velocity may occur once the glomerular filtration rate (GFR) is <50 ml/min/1.73 $M^2$. Several factors contribute to the retarded growth, including malnutrition (secondary to anorexia and chronic protein and calorie deficiency),[4] chronic acidosis,[5] reduced intestinal absorption of calcium,[6] and low levels of somatomedin[7] as well as bone disease. Thirty to 50% of children with "preterminal" renal failure have stunted growth[8] and manifest abnormal growth velocity. He-

## ABBREVIATIONS

PTH = parathyroid hormone
iPTH = immunoreactive parathyroid hormone
cAMP = 3'-5'-cyclic adenosine monophosphate
vitamin $D_2$ = ergocalciferol
vitamin $D_3$ = cholecalciferol
25(OH)D = 25-hydroxyvitamin D or calcidiol
24,25(OH)$_2$D = 24,25-dihydroxyvitamin D
1α-(OH)D = 1-alpha-hydroxyvitamin D
1,25(OH)$_2$D = 1,25-dihydroxyvitamin D or calcitriol
DHT = Dihydrotachysterol

Supported in part by funds from Upjohn Laboratories, Hoffman-LaRoche, and Ross Laboratories. Dr. Chesney is the recipient of a U.S. Public Health Service Research Career Development Award K04–AM00421. Dr. Dabbagh is supported by the Stetler Scholarship Fund for Women Physicians.

**Table 18–1.** SPECIFIC FEATURES OF
CHILDHOOD OSTEODYSTROPHY

| | |
|---|---|
| Growth retardation | Bone pain |
| Epiphyseal slipping | Skeletal deformities |
| Pathologic fractures | Myopathy |
| Osteomalacia in transplantation | |

modialysis does not improve the growth velocity.[9]

Epiphyseal slipping is the most severe clinical manifestation of renal osteodystrophy in a growing child.[10] It has been noted in 10 of 33 untreated nondialyzed children and in one of 82 dialyzed patients. It tends to occur late in the course of uremia and to be more frequent in children with congenital renal disease who have a longer duration of renal failure. Generally, these children have more severe hyperparathyroidism and more profound hypocalcemia.[11] In adolescents, epiphyseal slipping is coincident with the onset of puberty.[12] The pattern of slipping of the epiphyses is age-related. Young children present with upper and lower femoral epiphyseal slipping. In contrast, upper femoral and/or radial and ulnar epiphyses are involved in school-age children, while adolescent patients have involvement of the forearm epiphyses. Consequently, this abnormality is associated with gross skeletal deformities and impairment of locomotion. Pathologic fractures tend to occur more frequently when osteomalacia predominates over osteitis fibrosa cystica. Fractures are less frequent in children than in adults[10] and may occur after seizures. Such fractures need to be distinguished from Looser zones (pseudofractures). Pathologic fractures tend to heal slowly. With mechanical stress and in the presence of vitamin D deficiency, Looser zones may extend across the full width of the bone and form a true fracture.

Bone pain can develop insidiously and progress slowly until a patient is bedridden. It may not be related to an underlying bony abnormality and is independent of whether the skeletal disorder is osteitis fibrosa cystica, osteomalacia, or mixed. The pain is generally vague and may be localized to the lower back, hips, legs, or knees; it is aggravated by movement and weight-bearing. Frequently, it may mimic acute arthritis. Dialysis patients with a predominance of osteomalacia exhibit symptoms restricted to the axial skeleton or stress fractures of the ribs, when tenderness becomes a physical sign.

Although skeletal findings resembling late rickets—i.e., rosary, Harrison's groove, and enlargement of the wrists and ankles—are seen in small children, typical bowing of the diaphysis of long bones is usually not seen, because the skeletal deformities of the extremities involve the metaphysis. Unless renal failure is well established during the first year of life, craniotabes and bossing are infrequent.

Renal osteodystrophy is commonly associated with a myopathy which primarily affects the proximal musculature.[11] Initially, patients experience difficulties in climbing stairs or rising from a sitting position. As the myopathy progresses, patients develop a "waddling gait." Such a myopathy is indistinguishable from that seen secondary to vitamin D deficiency due to other causes[13] and can be ameliorated by treatment with 1,25-dihydroxyvitamin $D_3$.

Although renal transplantation leads to a gradual and steady improvement in renal bone disease, osteomalacia may emerge after successful transplantation as a complication of hypophosphatemia.[14] Body phosphate stores may be depleted because of the use of antacids, increased renal excretion of phosphate due to residual hyperparathyroidism or steroids, or because of an acquired tubular phosphate leak independent of PTH.

## ROLE OF PHOSPHATE RETENTION

Hyperphosphatemia plays a central role in the development and maintenance of secondary hyperparathyroidism in uremia by affecting the levels of ionized calcium. Phosphate retention usually occurs when the GFR falls to 20 to 30% of normal.[15] Slatopolsky et al postulate that there may be transient but undetectable increases in serum phosphate levels early in renal failure that may be responsible for a decreased ionized calcium level and enhanced secretion of PTH.[16] There is considerable evidence to indicate that even with a moderate reduction in renal function there seems to be an intolerance to an oral phosphate load, which usually produces a prolonged hyperphosphatemia with subsequent elevation of iPTH levels.[15] Furthermore, hyperphosphatemia decreases the rate of conversion of 25–hydroxyvitamin $D_3$ to 1,25–dihydroxyvitamin $D_3$.[17] The low $1,25(OH)_2D_3$ may lead to skeletal resistance to the action of PTH.

Experimental evidence indicates that the

restriction of dietary phosphorus in uremic dogs in proportion to the reduction in GFR prevents the occurrence of secondary hyperparathyroidism.[16] Clinically, Maschio et al[18] and Llach et al[19] have shown that early dietary phosphate restriction was associated with a decrease in PTH levels and amelioration of the bone disease.

The dietary intake of phosphorus depends upon the ingestion of meat and dairy products. In mild renal insufficiency, the dietary phosphorus intake can be reduced by about 50 to 60% by strict adherence to low-protein diets.[20] However, with progressive renal failure, further reductions in phosphate intake may become difficult, and the use of phosphate-binding gels becomes mandatory to maintain a serum phosphate level between 4.0 and 5.0 mg/dl. The aluminum-containing compounds employed to bind phosphorus in the gastrointestinal tract include aluminum hydroxide and aluminum carbonate and are available in liquid, capsule, or tablet form. Generally, magnesium-containing antacids are not recommended because the hypermagnesemia often seen in renal insufficiency may be potentiated with the use of these compounds.

Aluminum hydroxide is not without side effects. Most patients have constipation, and many experience nausea and vomiting following ingestion, which makes compliance difficult. Furthermore, there is mounting evidence that aluminum can be absorbed from the gut.[21] Increased tissue concentrations of aluminum have been described in patients with encephalopathy and renal osteodystrophy.[22] Guillot and coworkers[23] suggest the use of magnesium-containing phosphate binders in uremic patients on hemodialysis in addition to aluminum-containing gels to control hyperphosphatemia, as long as the serum magnesium concentration is maintained below 4.5 mEq/L. It is also important to avoid reducing the serum phosphate to subnormal levels in order to prevent depletion. The resulting hypophosphatemia may be associated with anorexia, weakness, bone pain, and osteomalacia.[24]

Special attention should be paid to the effect of the administration of vitamin D analogs in renal insufficiency. These compounds increase the intestinal absorption of calcium and phosphorus,[25] thus raising the serum phosphate level. Their use in hyperphosphatemia is contraindicated because of the danger of producing metastatic calcification, unless the phosphorus level is controlled. However, $1,25(OH)_2D_3$ may suppress secondary hyperparathyroidism, thus reducing bone resorption and causing calcium and phosphorus deposition into bone and healing of osteomalacia (see further on). Thus, one may see a fall in the serum phosphorus level and a decreased need for phosphate binders during the first months of treatment.

## VITAMIN D ANALOGS

As recognized for a century,[2] abnormalities of bone and mineral homeostasis are frequent overt complications of renal insufficiency in childhood. Central to the development of renal osteodystrophy is the failure of vitamin D in usual doses to prevent hypocalcemia, osteomalacia, and secondary hyperparathyroidism.[26, 27] This apparent resistance to vitamin D is shown by intestinal malabsorption of calcium,[28] by reduced total body calcium,[29] and by a reduction in bone mineral content of the long bones.[30] Intestinal calcium absorption in uremic patients can be improved by the administration of vitamin $D_2$ (of plant origin,)[31] vitamin $D_3$ (of mammalian origin),[27] or the synthetic vitamin D analog dihydrotachysterol (DHT)[32-34] at doses that would rapidly cause hypercalcemia and hypercalciuria in normal individuals. The explanation for this vitamin D deficiency—as evidenced by negative calcium balance—despite normal serum antirachitic activity,[26-27] comes from the discovery that the kidney is the site for the synthesis of the most active metabolite of vitamin D in terms of intestinal calcium absorption—1,25-dihydroxyvitamin D $(1,25(OH)_2D)$[35-38] (Fig. 18–1).

This vitamin D metabolite cannot be detected in sera of anephric patients,[39] and the administration of μgm quantities of $1,25(OH)_2D$ will increase the serum calcium levels and intestinal calcium absorption and decrease fecal calcium,[40] thereby suggesting that "defective renal production of $1,25(OH)_2D$ in uremia" accounts for this "vitamin D resistance."[41] Using more precise assay techniques, it is clearly possible to demonstrate that $1,25(OH)_2D$ values are markedly reduced in both adults[42-48] and children[49, 50] with ESRD. A significant inverse relationship is found between creatinine or inulin clearance and serum $1,25(OH)_2D$ concentrations at clearance values less than 50 ml/min corrected for surface area[47, 49, 50] (Fig. 18–2, A). A significant reduction in serum

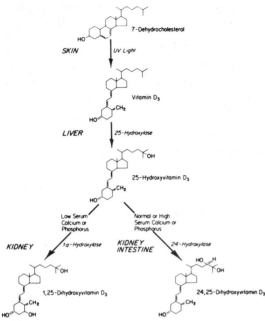

**Figure 18–1.** Vitamin D metabolism in man. (From Kumar R, Riggs, BL: Vitamin D in the therapy of disorders of calcium and phosphorus metabolism. Mayo Clin Proc 56:327, 1981.)

$1,25(OH)_2D$ can be found in patients with clearance values between 20 and 50 ml/min/1.73 $M^2$ [49,50] (Fig. 18–2, B). Further, the normal age-related variations in serum $1,25(OH)_2D$ concentrations—higher in infancy and adolescence—are not seen in uremic children.[49-51]

The kidney is also the site of production of another major circulating metabolite of vitamin D, termed 24,25-dihydroxyvitamin D or $24,25(OH)_2D$.[38,43] The possible therapeutic role of this metabolite will be discussed, but the circulating concentrations of this metabolite are reduced in uremic or anephric man.[44,47,49,52,53] Children have a circulating value of $24,25(OH)_2D$ of 1 to 4 ng/ml and a value of $1,25(OH)_2D$ of 20 to 80 pg/ml—the latter is roughly 10 times lower than normal.[49,51] The values of these metabolites in severely uremic children are 0.6 ng/ml and 10 pg/ml, respectively.[49,50] The major circulating metabolite of vitamin D in man is 25-hydroxyvitamin D or 25(OH)D,[38,43] and its concentration is usually 20 to 60 ng/ml in North American children and somewhat lower in European and British children.[54] The values of this metabolite, produced by a hepatic 25-hydroxylation, are usually normal

in uremic children,[49,55] thereby indicating that 25(OH)D deficiency is not a usual component of renal osteodystrophy and that the changes in bone and mineral homeostasis occur despite normal $25(OH)_2D$ values in the serum.

The aim of therapy in childhood renal osteodystrophy is to provide sufficient doses of whatever vitamin D analog is chosen to overcome the resistance to the action(s) of vitamin D that typify uremia and, yet, still be safe. Clearly, hypercalcemia, hypercalciuria, and the reduction in renal function that occurs with hypervitaminosis D must be avoided.[56] No analog of vitamin D is safe if the potential for hypercalcemia is forgotten and if serum calcium levels are not frequently evaluated.[57,58]

In this chapter, we will review some of the studies that have evaluated the therapeutic administration of seven vitamin D metabolites to uremic children. These agents include the natural vitamin D analogs: vitamin $D_2$ or ergocalciferol; vitamin $D_3$ or cholecalciferol; 25(OH)D or calcidiol; $1,25(OH)_2D$ or calcitriol, and $24,25(OH)_2D$. The synthetic analogs DHT and $1\alpha$-hydroxyvitamin D, or "1-alpha," have also been used to treat renal osteodystrophy.[56,59]

Several glaring problems should be noted at the outset. Firstly, most therapeutic trials in children are uncontrolled, and the vitamin D status of children prior to treatment is uncertain. Secondly, essentially no studies comparing the various vitamin D analogs against one another have been reported. Thirdly, no reports on the therapeutic use of $24,25(OH)_2D$ in children have been described. Fourthly, most studies are short-term and, therefore, long-term effects of these agents are difficult to evaluate. It is not possible to determine clearly that any single vitamin D analog is superior in terms of its therapeutic effect, particularly when appropriate doses of the D analogs are given. Nonetheless, because the kidney produces the most active vitamin D metabolite—$1,25(OH)_2D$—and because the circulating levels of this compound are extremely low in children with uremia despite concomitant hypocalcemia and elevated PTH values, there is a rational basis for the use of $1,25(OH)_2D$ and the other 1-alpha-like agents, $1\alpha$-(OH)D and DHT, in the management of the derangements of divalent mineral metabolism and of bone disease in uremia.[60]

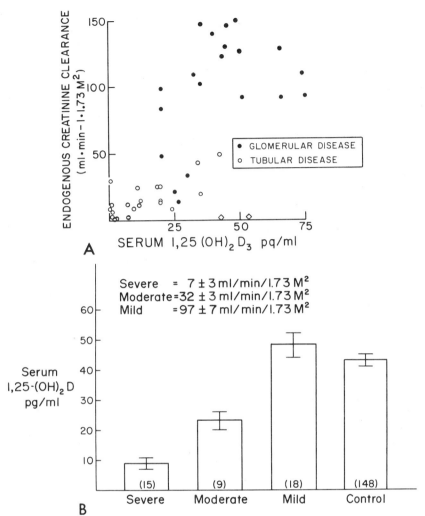

**Figure 18–2.** *A,* Serum 1,25(OH)$_2$D vs. endogenous creatinine clearance. Note prevalence of tubulo-interstitial disease in children with a clearance of less than 50 ml/min/1.73 M$^2$. *B,* Serum 1,25(OH)$_2$D values at several levels of renal function.

## Vitamin D

Vitamins D$_2$ and D$_3$ must be given in massive doses in order to overcome the uremic resistance to vitamin D.[27-31] Potter et al treated six children with vitamin D$_2$ at doses ranging from 32,000 to 57,000 IU (800 to 1425 μg) daily and demonstrated healing radiologically in three patients.[31] Hypercalcemia persisted one to five weeks post-cessation of vitamin D in three patients and conjunctival calcification was noted in three patients. Skin calcification was not increased. Bulla et al, in a multicenter, carefully controlled study of children on hemodialysis, using both vitamin D$_3$ and 1,25(OH)$_2$D, demonstrated an improvement in the serum cal-

cium level, a reduction in PTH level, and healing of osteitis fibrosa after vitamin D$_3$ at 10,000 to 50,000 units daily (250 to 1250 μg).[61] Vitamin D$_3$ appeared to act more slowly than 1,25(OH)$_2$D, and hypercalcemia, when it occurred, persisted longer after stopping vitamin D$_3$ than the 1α-hydroxylated analog. In these patients, serum 25(OH)D values increased from 15 ± 6 ng/ml to a level of 100 to 300 ng/ml after the initiation of vitamin D$_3$ therapy. The studies of Bouillon et al also demonstrated an increase in serum calcium concentration and a fall in PTH levels after vitamin D$_3$ treatment at 20,000 to 240,000 units/day.[62]

In conclusion, the main advantage of these precursor metabolites is their low cost relative to the newer metabolites. However, the disadvantages of their use are the uncertainty of dose, the slow onset of action, the very long biological half-life, and the fact that hypercalcemia may persist for weeks to months following discontinuation since these analogs are stored in fat and only slowly released.[38] Bulla et al could not demonstrate healing of the endosteal osteomalacia found in some bone biopsies,[61] whereas some patients did respond to $1,25(OH)_2D$. Finally, vitamin $D_3$ is not an approved drug in the United States even though many dairies use this metabolite to supplement their milk at 400 IU (10 μg) per quart. We do not recommend the use of these analogs in treating uremic osteodystrophy, although they are clearly useful in disorders of vitamin D in which renal function is normal.

## 25-Hydroxyvitamin D

25-Hydroxyvitamin D, which is ordinarily produced in the liver,[38] has been used orally in two trials in children.[55, 63] A standard dose of 1 to 2 μg/kg/day was found to be effective in reversing hypocalcemia, lowering PTH values, increasing linear growth, and promoting bone healing, as demonstrated by histologic evidence of improvement in both endosteal osteomalacia and osteitis fibrosa and by radiographs of bone.[55, 64] Serum $25(OH)D$ concentrations of at least 250 ng/ml were achieved, using a mean dose of 1.6 μg/kg,[55] and it was clear that $25(OH)D$ was not converted to $1,25(OH)_2D$ in these patients.[65]

This metabolite is not stored in fat to any great extent and, hence, its half-life is quite short—on the order of 14 to 16 days.[66] The finding that $25(OH)D$ itself is active, without conversion to $1,25(OH)_2D$, indicates that this analog in pharmacologic doses can stimulate intestinal calcium absorption, even in anephric man.[63, 66] Although far more studies have been reported in adults, including studies comparing $25(OH)D$ with $1,25(OH)_2D$,[67] the available studies in children indicate improvement in osteomalacia as well as in osteitis fibrosa.[55, 63, 64] Unfortunately, neither osteomalacia nor osteitis fibrosa are completely improved in every patient.

Several studies from France have reported a high incidence of osteomalacia in patients with renal osteodystrophy,[63, 66, 67] which may reflect the relatively low circulating $25(OH)D$ values found in individuals from Western Europe. The use of $25(OH)D$ in patients from Europe would seem logical if such patients have evidence of $25(OH)D$ deficiency.

One benefit of $25(OH)D$ therapy is its relatively long half-life as compared to $1,25(OH)_2D$. Thus, if a patient is poorly compliant, plasma $25(OH)D$ values will be minimally affected by skipping an occasional dose. When using $1,25(OH)_2D$ with its short half-life of four to six hours, it is imperative to take all doses to avoid vitamin D deficiency. On the other hand, since $25(OH)D$ has a half-life of 14 to 16 days, the resolution of hypercalcemia may require as long as four weeks.[68]

Patients with the nephrotic syndrome may lose $25(OH)D$ in their urine and have very low circulating levels of this metabolite.[69-71] The $25(OH)D$ is lost because vitamin D–binding protein, which has a molecular weight identical to that of albumin, is excreted in large quantities.[70] Further, the levels of both $1,25(OH)_2D$ and $24,25(OH)_2D$ are reduced.[69, 71] Since $25(OH)D$ administration can raise serum $25(OH)D$ values in nephrotic patients, it appears that there may be a role for this metabolite in treating such patients.

## Dihydrotachysterol

Despite the paucity of studies on the use of dihydrotachysterol (DHT) in children, this

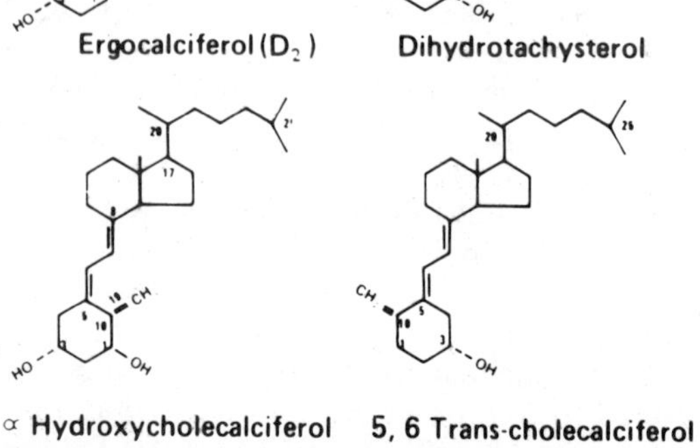

VITAMIN D$_2$ and ANALOGUES

Ergocalciferol (D$_2$)          Dihydrotachysterol

1 α Hydroxycholecalciferol    5, 6 Trans-cholecalciferol

**Figure 18–3.** The structure of several vitamin D analogs including DHT. The 3β-OH group on the A-ring can rotate to form a 1α-hydroxyl group. (From Root AW, Harrison HE: Recent advances in calcium metabolism. J Pediatr 88:1, 1982.)

synthetic agent has been used extensively in the treatment and prevention of renal osteodystrophy in children. DHT lacks the 10–19–diene on the A-ring of the vitamin D seco-steroid molecule; thus the A-ring is free to rotate. In DHT, the hydroxyl group responsible for its biological activity is a 3β-OH which can rotate to form a pseudo-1α-hydroxyl group[38, 68, 72] (Fig. 18–3). DHT then undergoes a hepatic 25-hydroxylation to form 25(OH)-DHT.[73] This compound then acts at the level of the intestine to increase active gut calcium transport without the necessity for further renal metabolic conversion.

The initial studies of Liu and Chu performed in Peking, China, in 1943 showed that the malabsorption of calcium resulting in high fecal calcium levels could be overcome by AT-10, a mixture of several vitamin D metabolites of which DHT is the active component.[32] Using crystalline DHT, Malekzadeh et al showed that renal osteodystrophy could be treated at doses of 0.125 to 1.5 mg each day.[74] The variation in the dosage required is much less than that for vitamin $D_2$ or $D_3$, and the onset of action is shorter than that observed using either vitamin $D_2$ or 25(OH)D.[75] Cordy, in an uncontrolled study, demonstrated improved bone histology following the use of DHT.[76, 77]

## 1α-Hydroxyvitamin D and 1,25-Dihydroxyvitamin D

Since the renal tubule is the site of the 1α-hydroxylation of 25(OH)D, the use of 1α-hydroxyvitamin D metabolites to reverse the calcium malabsorption in bone disorders is relevant, and "physiologic" doses of these metabolites can be employed. Brickman et al in 1972 demonstrated improved intestinal calcium absorption and correction of hypocalcemia with 1,25(OH)$_2$D[40] shortly after the discovery of the role of the kidney in the metabolism of vitamin D. A number of studies have examined the short-term and long-term use of either 1α-(OH)D or 1,25(OH)$_2$D in the treatment of childhood renal osteodystrophy.[61, 78-91] These studies are uncontrolled and compare therapy with the 1α-hydroxy metabolite to prior treatment with other analogs—usually vitamin $D_2$ or $D_3$ or DHT—except for the careful controlled study of Bulla et al.[61] In most reports, bone histomorphometry is not included, but it is available in six studies[61, 80-82, 91] (Chesney, personal communication). The clinical and laboratory findings in all these studies are quite similar; hence, they can be reported as a group.

Following treatment with 1α-(OH)D at 1 to 2 μg/day and 1,25(OH)$_2$D at 10 to 50 ng/kg/day, the hypocalcemia is corrected within one to two weeks. The first clinical improvement is usually a dramatic reversal of the myopathy of uremia and of gait disturbances, with subsequent amelioration of bone pain.

Another serum chemical change consequent to therapy is an increase in serum phosphate level, since these analogs increase intestinal phosphate absorption. The hyperphosphatemia usually responds to higher doses of phosphate binders. Serum immunoreactive PTH values fall, but usually not to the normal range.[79, 81, 84-91] Alkaline phosphatase values usually fall into the normal range within six months at a time when an improvement in the radiologic appearance of the bones is apparent. It is interesting that the reversal of bone pain, gait disturbance, and muscle weakness precedes these radiologic improvements by a substantial period of time. Following normalization of the alkaline phosphatase level and bone radiologic appearance, hypercalcemia occurs in approximately 30 to 40% of cases. Owing to the short half-life of these agents (4 hours for 1,25(OH)$_2$D), hypercalcemia can be rapidly reversed in a few days following discontinuation of therapy.[78, 81, 82, 85, 88, 91] In general, hypercalcemia is mild (<11.5 mg/dl), but the serum calcium level should be measured frequently when using these metabolites.

The potential for renal damage with use of these analogs has been emphasized,[92] but careful studies examining reciprocal serum creatinine concentrations, both before and after therapy, have failed to show any change in the slope of the lines[88, 91, 93] (Fig. 18–4). These data suggest no acceleration in the rate of deterioration of GFR in treated patients. Indeed, a few patients in these studies may have even demonstrated improved renal function for reasons that are unclear. Hypercalciuria is not a problem[87, 88, 93] (Fig. 18–5), and the careful avoidance of hypercalcemia usually precludes the rise in the serum creatinine level found with high urinary calcium concentrations.

As in adult studies, children with renal osteodystrophy have osteomalacia, osteitis fibrosa, or a mixed lesion[61, 63, 64, 80-82, 91] (Chesney, personal communication). The 1α-hydroxy analogs usually improve or heal the

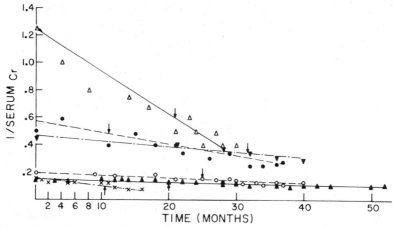

**Figure 18–4.** The reciprocal of serum creatinine (1/S$_{Cr}$) vs. time in six children with chronic renal failure. The arrow denotes the onset of 1,25(OH)$_2$D therapy. (From the data of Chesney et al, Ref. 89.)

osteitis fibrosa type of disease, as chemically evidenced by the reduction in iPTH and alkaline phosphatase values. The effect on osteomalacia is variable,[61, 91] but, in general, the osteomalacia is not completely healed.

Several investigators have reported a dramatic improvement in growth over the first 12 to 18 months of therapy[79, 83, 85, 87, 88, 91] (Fig. 18–6, *A*). However, other studies have not shown this growth acceleration.[61, 94] Patients

who are young and are not requiring dialysis appear to show this accelerated growth rate. This acceleration of growth rate is not found in all patients,[85, 88, 91] and sustained catch-up growth probably does not occur (Fig. 18–6, *B*).

The major problems with using the 1α-hydroxy compounds are: (1) their potency in terms of calcium absorption, and (2) their short half-life. The smallest currently avail-

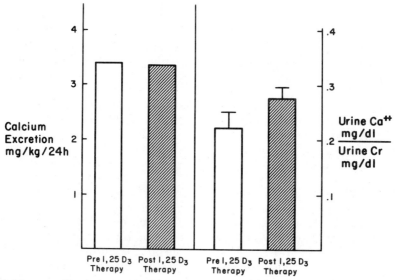

**Figure 18–5.** Calcium excretion before and after therapy with 1,25(OH)$_2$D showing no difference (from the data of Chesney et al, Ref. 87).

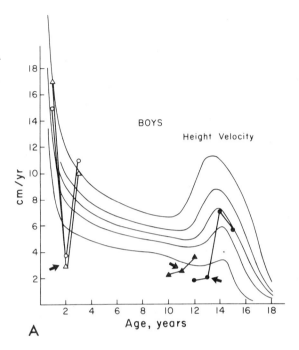

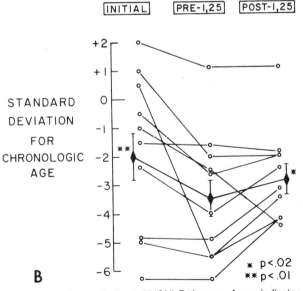

**Figure 18–6.** *A,* Growth velocity before and after 1,25(OH)$_2$D therapy. Arrow indicates the onset of therapy. Note the increase in growth velocity. (From Chesney et al in N Engl J Med 298:238, 1978.) *B,* Long-term therapy (more than 30 months) of juvenile renal osteodystrophy indicating a significant increase in growth velocity but no evidence of prolonged catch-up growth. (From the data of Chesney et al, Ref. 89.)

able form of $1,25(OH)_2D$ is a $0.25$-$\mu$g capsule which is difficult to use in infants and small children. In children who weigh up to 12 kg, this dose may be associated with hypercalcemia. In addition, the capsule is difficult to administer, to infants particularly since they cannot swallow capsules. Although these capsules can be opened or dissolved in milk, the exact dose provided cannot be known with certainty. Until a liquid form is available, it will be difficult to treat young children with oral $1,25(OH)_2D$. The second problem is that, with the short half-lives of these compounds, poorly compliant patients may have long periods of relative vitamin D deficiency.

The basic therapeutic strategy is to start $1,25(OH)_2D$ at $0.25$ $\mu$g each day and to increase the dose at intervals every two weeks until normocalcemia is achieved. A twice-daily dosage schedule is logical, since the half-life of the compound is 4 to 6 hours; however, no studies showing greater efficacy using this increased dosage schedule have been published.

### 24,25-Dihydroxyvitamin D

Recent studies in animals have suggested that $24,25(OH)_2D$ may act as a mineralizing hormone,[95–107] The evidence is summarized in Table 18–2 and indicates that $24,25(OH)_2D$ decreases PTH secretion and may be important in the healing of osteomalacia. More recent direct information indicates that $24,25(OH)_2D$ may not be of clear benefit in terms of bone mineralization or reversal of hyperparathyroidism.[108-110] The difluoro compound of vitamin D (24,24-difluoro-25(OH)D) has the same biologic activity as either $25(OH)D$ or vitamin $D_3$.[108, 111] It appears that vitamin D compounds which cannot be 24-hydroxylated evoke no disorder in bone mineralization and do not have a clear benefit in renal osteodystrophy.[109]

Clinical trials of $24,25(OH)_2D$ have been undertaken primarily in adults.[110, 112, 113] In general, patients have been treated with $24,25(OH)_2D$ in conjunction with $1,25(OH)_2D$, because patients fail to respond to $24,25(OH)_2D$ alone. Sherrard et al treated 44 patients,[109] 43 of whom had been on dialysis and had "refractory osteomalacia" and hypercalcemia, a condition which may be related to high bone aluminum levels.[114, 115] The addition of $24,25(OH)_2D$ facilitated the use of lower $1,25(OH)_2D$ doses,

**Table 18–2.** ROLE OF $24,25(OH)_2D$ IN RENAL OSTEODYSTROPHY*

1. Made predominantly in kidney, thus reduced levels in uremia (0.7 vs. 3–4 ng/ml) (Shepard et al)
2. Produced in cartilage and calvaria of *rats* (Garabedian)
3. Promotes normal ossification of bone when calcium and phosphate are supersaturated in bone ECF in *chicks* (Edelstein)
4. Reduces iPTH secretion in *dogs* when given IV or PO (Canterbury)
5. Blunts PTH resorption of bone in vitro in *rats* (Liebenherr)
6. In uremic *man* (Kanis):
    a. Increases $Ca^{++}$ absorption
    b. No rise in serum $Ca^{++}$
    c. Suggests deposition in bone
7. Reversal of "skeletal resistance to PTH" in uremic *man* by $1,25(OH)_2D$ and $24,25(OH)_2D$ (Massry)
8. Combination of $25(OH)D$ and $1,25(OH)_2D$ or $24,25(OH)_2D$ and $1,25(OH)_2D$ best heals osteomalacia in *man* (Rasmussen)
9. PTH is not always suppressed using $24,25(OH)_2D$ (Slatopolsky)
10. Difluoro-$24,25(OH)_2D$ acts the same as $25(OH)D$, casting doubts on role of $24,25(OH)_2D$ (DeLuca)

*Conclusion:* Unique biological role unclear, but may be useful in combination with $1,25(OH)_2D$. Normal man has $25(OH)D$ to $24,25(OH)_2D$ to $1,25(OH)_2D$ in 1000/100/1 ratio, and uremia changes this relationship. See text for large body of negative results.

*Adapted from Reference #93.

which resulted in the amelioration of hypercalcemia. Symptomatic improvement occurred in 21 of 36 patients, 8 patients were unchanged and 7 had further deterioration. Those patients with secondary hyperparathyroidism seemed to deteriorate, and, of patients with paired biopsies, half showed improvement and 30% showed deterioration.[110] In the other two studies reported, $24,25(OH)_2D$ alone produced no effect, and in combination with $1,25(OH)_2D$ it failed to heal osteomalacia or osteitis fibrosa any better than with $1,25(OH)_2D$ alone.[112, 113] No studies in children have been reported.

The failure of $1,25(OH)_2D$ or $25(OH)D$ alone to fully heal the osteomalacia of uremia has been disappointing and has led investigators to make great claims for the role of $24,25(OH)_2D$ in the treatment of this osteomalacia. The results of the reported clinical trials are discouraging.[110, 112, 113] Other factors such as parathyroid ablation[116] and bone aluminum[114, 115, 117] may be more relevant in the failure of matrix mineralization. Further, the metabolic clearance of $24,25(OH)_2D$ in man is very slow,[118] so that it is very hard to compare the effects of $1,25(OH)_2D$ and

24,25$(OH)_2$D on bone, particularly in vitro. Finally, the use of 24,24-difluoro-25(OH)D in vitamin D–deficient rats suggests no differences in bone histologic parameters from those found using 25(OH)D,[119] and further suggests that this metabolite may not play an important role in bone modeling and mineralization.

## ROLE OF PARATHYROIDECTOMY

Medical management usually controls the manifestations of secondary hyperparathyroidism in uremia, especially with the advent of the newer analogs of vitamin D. However, when conservative intervention fails, parathyroidectomy becomes a therapeutic option (Table 18–3). It should be considered when there is ample proof of secondary hyperparathyroidism as manifested by elevated levels of iPTH, bony erosions, or osteitis fibrosa cystica on bone biopsy, in association with one or more of the following:[120, 121] (1) Hypercalcemia, particularly if it is symptomatic. Patients develop vomiting, nausea, or ulcer disease as a result of elevated calcium levels. One should note that there are a few uremic patients who develop hypercalcemia in the absence of secondary hyperparathyroidism, in whom parathyroidectomy is not an option. (2) Progressive extraskeletal calcifications which occur in conjunction with a Ca × P product that is consistently greater than 70 to 80, despite phosphate restriction and the use of phosphate-binding gels. (3) Intractable pruritus which does not respond to aggressive dialysis. However, before considering surgical intervention, intravenous lidocaine and/or ultraviolet light is recommended. (4) Severe and progressive skeletal pain, fractures through known tumors, or epiphyseal

slipping in children.[122] Sometimes the bone disease may progress so rapidly that parathyroidectomy becomes the only option to halt and, it is hoped, reverse the debilitating disease. (5) The appearance of calciphylaxis.[123] Although rare in childhood uremia, the latter is a syndrome characterized by progressive necrosis of the fingertips and toes which tends to occur in dialysis patients or in renal transplant recipients, even with normal renal function. The disease is rapidly progressive, and many victims die because of gangrene and infection. Parathyroidectomy appears to arrest its progression and ameliorate the disease.

Frequently, we are faced with a noncompliant patient who has severe bone disease and secondary hyperparathyroidism. Parathyroidectomy will improve the bone disease, but the complications of PTH excess tend to recur if postoperative medical treatment and dietary restriction are ignored.

For many years a subtotal parathyroidectomy was recommended. The surgeon identifies the presence of four parathyroid glands and excises 3¾ glands. The remnant gland is marked by a metal clip or a long black silk suture to identify it should repeat neck exploratory surgery be required. If only three glands are identified, they are all removed, assuming that, although not seen, the fourth one is present.

Because the remnant tissue may undergo hyperplasia with recurrence of secondary hyperparathyroidism, and since a second surgical procedure is often risky and tedious, it is currently advised that these patients undergo a total parathyroidectomy.[124, 125] The excised parathyroid glands are cryopreserved and can be later autotransplanted in the brachioradialis muscle under local anesthesia without any sequelae. The main advantage of this procedure is the accessibility of parathyroid tissue, if and when hyperplasia recurs. The "take rate" of the autotransplants is greater than 90%.[126] In one study, only one patient of 16 had to have a second transplantation of cryopreserved autologous parathyroid tissue, and it was successful. It should be noted that parathyroid hormone is important in bone remodeling and mineral accretion,[127] indicating the significance of avoiding hypoparathyroidism secondary to these surgical maneuvers.

Postoperatively, it is vital to control the serum calcium level. Hypocalcemia and subsequent seizures tend to occur in the presence

**Table 18–3.** POSSIBLE INDICATIONS FOR PARATHYROIDECTOMY

1. Marked secondary hyperparathyroidism (not responsive to medical management):
   a. Increased iPTH
   b. Bony erosions
   c. Osteitis fibrosa cystica on bone biopsy
2. In association with:
   a. Hypercalcemia
   b. Progressive extraskeletal calcifications
   c. Intractable pruritus
   d. Severe bone pain, fractures through known tumors for epiphyseal slipping in children
   e. Calciphylaxis

of severe bone erosions. These are usually averted by prior treatment with $1,25(OH)_2D_3$ and oral or intravenous calcium supplements. After remineralization of "hungry" bones, the serum calcium level will increase while the serum alkaline phosphatase level will decrease, necessitating the reduction or discontinuation of vitamin D analogs and calcium supplements. Further, with the postoperative decrease in the serum phosphate level, the dose of aluminum-containing gels should be decreased or discontinued to maintain a serum phosphate level of 3.0 to 3.5 mg/dl. Both hypophosphatemia and hyperphosphatemia must be avoided.

The results of parathyroidectomy, whether subtotal or total with subsequent autotransplantation, are encouraging. In one study, 75 percent of the patients had symptomatic relief of bone pain, pruritus, and muscle cramps.[128] There was a decrease in the level of iPTH and improvement in the radiologic manifestations of renal osteodystrophy. However, Weinstein reports the occurrence of osteomalacia despite the reduction of osteitis fibrosa cystica.[129] Hypophosphatemia may have played a role in its evolution.

In general, the benefits of this surgical procedure depend on the patient's compliance with medical treatment and diet.

## EFFECT OF DIALYSIS

Dialysis can improve renal osteodystrophy; however, the response is not uniform, and there are instances of worsening of the bone disease on hemodialysis. Controlling the manifestations of secondary hyperparathyroidism prior to commencing hemodialysis is of particular importance in children. Most patients presenting for dialysis have hypocalcemia, hyperphosphatemia, and elevated iPTH levels.

There is evidence to suggest that the concentration of calcium in the dialysate seems to play a central role in the evolution of renal osteodystrophy. The dialysate calcium should be such that the ionized calcium level remains normal and that postdialysis hypercalcemia is avoided. Various concentrations have been evaluated (5.0 to 9.0 mg/dl).[130] If the patient is normocalcemic or slightly hypocalcemic, the total plasma calcium concentration increases during dialysis, regardless of whether the dialysate calcium concentration is 5.0 mg/dl or 9.0 mg/dl. With a dialysate calcium concentration of 8.0 mg/dl or more, hypercalcemia invariably occurs with resulting headache, pruritus, nausea, vomiting, and metastatic calcification when hyperphosphatemia is present. With dialysate calcium levels of 5.0 mg/dl or less, the plasma calcium level usually remains unchanged; however, with this dialysate calcium concentration patients maintain a negative calcium balance because of fecal losses. Jejunal absorption of calcium tends to be linear when intraluminal calcium is greater than 5.0 mg/dl. With the ingestion of larger quantities of calcium (either by oral supplementation or increased dialysate calcium), fecal losses do not increase proportionately, leading to a positive calcium balance.[6, 131]

Thus, it is currently recommended that a dialysate calcium concentration of 7.0 mg/dl be used. Many studies report a decrease in iPTH levels and improvement in the osteitis fibrosa cystica with this concentration.[132] However, it appears that parathyroid hyperplasia rarely involutes using a high calcium-containing dialysate, especially in children.[133] Vitamin D analogs result in a more dramatic response.

Phosphorus is poorly dialyzable and is sequestered in body tissues with a small volume of distribution. Hemodialysis and peritoneal dialysis have little effect on the serum phosphorus level. Despite dietary restrictions, most children are hyperphosphatemic, requiring aggressive use of aluminum-containing gels to maintain the scrum phosphorus level between 4.0 and 5.0 mg/dl. It should be noted that hypophosphatemia is as detrimental as hyperphosphatemia, and overzealous treatment with aluminum hydroxide should be avoided. Moreover, one should be aware of the rare patient who develops hypophosphatemia without aluminum hydroxide therapy and who needs phosphate supplementation.[134] These patients complain of weakness and often develop osteomalacia.

A significant number of the dialysis patients are magnesium overloaded.[135] The most common underlying cause appears to be related to ingestion of magnesium-containing antacids. The significance of this overload on renal osteodystrophy is unknown. However, it is known that both hypomagnesemia[136] and hypermagnesemia[137] tend to suppress PTH secretion. Consequently, most dialysate solutions contain 1.5 to 2.0 mg/dl of magnesium, which is slightly higher than normal serum levels.

The incidence of hyperparathyroid bone disease increases with the duration of renal failure,[31, 138] as well as with the duration of dialysis, if the calcium concentration in the dialysate is less than 5.6 mg/dl.[139] Potter et al reported an incidence of 47 percent in children on hemodialysis after a maximum of 17 months.[31] These findings confirmed previous reports that the incidence of bone disease is greater in children than in adults.[122] However, the frequency of epiphyseal slipping in dialyzed children is markedly decreased, which is quite puzzling in view of the fact that the secondary hyperparathyroidism persists.[11] This can be related to positive calcium balance and improved mineralization of woven bone in the metaphysis or to less severe elevated iPTH levels or to both. Moreover, some degree of secondary hyperparathyroidism is present in almost all children with ESRD with or without bone disease; it is considered by some to be a "tradeoff" for external phosphate balance in uremia.[140]

Despite the reported improvement of osteitis fibrosa cystica, including a decrease in iPTH levels on hemodialysis, with treatment with vitamin D analogs, some patients develop osteomalacia. The latter is characterized by multiple fractures, severe myopathy, and spontaneous hypercalcemia. It seems to be seen more in England. Ward et al reported an incidence of 15 percent when deionized water was used for hemodialysis and 70 percent when softened water was used.[141] There is a close association between the osteomalacia and dialysis encephalopathy. Aluminum has been implicated in the pathogenesis of the latter syndrome. It does not respond to high calcium dialysis,[142] to increasing the concentration of phosphate in the dialysate,[143] or to 1,25-dihydroxyvitamin D, which results in only symptomatic relief but causes severe hypercalcemia.[144]

Soft tissue calcification is another complication occurring with increased frequency in dialyzed patients. Multiple organs can be affected, and patients can manifest myocardial infarctions, arthritic pain, calciphylaxis, or conjunctival or vascular calcifications.[138, 145] The incidence is related to the elevated Ca × P product, which must be maintained below 70, to avert these complications.

Most of the previous discussion has been limited to hemodialysis. With the advent of continuous ambulatory peritoneal dialysis (CAPD), more and more children with ESRD are being placed on this type of treatment.

Nonetheless, only a small number of children have been treated for more than two years with CAPD. Thus, information about its effect on childhood renal osteodystrophy is limited. In one study done in adults,[146] it was found that despite a negative peritoneal calcium balance, the serum calcium level remained unchanged. This may reflect the effectiveness of compensatory mechanisms which increase intestinal absorption of calcium or increase bone resorption. Many of the patients studied had progression of bone resorption and osteitis fibrosa cystica. However, the osteomalacia seemed to respond to CAPD better than to prior treatment with vitamin D. Fractures healed rapidly and hypercalcemia was avoided. It has been postulated that CAPD may contribute to the maturation of collagen, thus facilitating its calcification by removing unidentified middle molecular weight substances that are not removed by hemodialysis.

## DOES EARLY THERAPY HAVE A ROLE?

Early therapy can include phosphate restriction and vitamin D analogs at relatively moderate degrees of renal insufficiency, or treatment at an early age in children with chronic renal insufficiency. It is clear that secondary hyperparathyroidism appears at creatinine clearance values as high as 50 to 60 ml/min/1.73 $M^2$,[147] and that $1,25(OH)_2D$ values are reduced at clearance values between 20 and 50 ml/min/1.73 $M^2$.[49, 50, 106] Thus, early treatment on a theoretical basis is indicated.

The arguments against such early treatment include: (1) that the renal disease may not be progressive (at least during childhood); (2) that phosphate restriction may cause further osteomalacia and impair bone mineralization and growth; (3) that the doses of vitamin D analogs ($25(OH)D$ and $1,25(OH)_2D$) which are used will cause hypercalcemia; (4) that hypercalcemia will further reduce renal function; and (5) that until the other factors producing renal osteodystrophy—such as nutritional elements, the osteomalacic lesion, and the defects in protein synthesis—can be adequately corrected, the role of early therapy is questionable. At present only DHT can be used in very young children, since liquid preparations of $25(OH)D$ and $1,25(OH)_2D$ are not available.

The role of early treatment remains to be elucidated.

## ASSESSMENT OF A THERAPEUTIC RESPONSE

The response to treatment of the child who has severe renal osteodystrophy, slipped epiphyses, gait disturbance, and myopathy is easy to evaluate.[85, 88, 110] Children with less severe forms of renal osteodystrophy require tools that can detect more subtle changes (Table 18–4). The clinical appearance of the patient following treatment is valuable, particularly if the patient's capacity to walk unaided, his muscle strength, and ability to participate in daily activities are evaluated.[79, 85, 88, 93] Serial determinations of serum calcium, phosphate, alkaline phosphatase activity, iPTH level, and serum magnesium concentrations can be useful. Unfortunately, iPTH may be an unrewarding indicator of the status of renal osteodystrophy, particularly if the antibody used detects the C-terminal portion of the PTH molecule. As discussed elsewhere,[93] the kidney is a major site of C-terminal PTH biodegradation and, hence, the values of this molecule are elevated in the sera of uremic subjects even though this peptide has little or no biologic activity.[89] Since antibodies directed toward the N-terminal, or active portion of the molecule, are more difficult to obtain, the accurate measurement of bioactive PTH in uremia is difficult at present.

The major problem with a serial examination of the serum $Ca \times PO_4$ solubility product is that no pathologic values are established for children, where there is such variability in the serum phosphate with age. For example, the normal neonate with a serum calcium level of 10 mg/dl and serum phosphate level of 7.0 mg/dl has a product of 70. No one knows at what value for this product the patient is endangered in terms of soft tissue calcifications. However, calcium deposits at the limbus of the eye are not infrequently seen following treatment with vitamin D analogs.[61]

The radiologic evaluation of renal osteodystrophy following treatment can show gross changes in bone appearance, but for evaluation of subtle changes, the technique of photon absorptiometry is useful.[30] This technique is used to show an improvement or decline in bone mineral content over

**Table 18–4. ASSESSMENT OF RESPONSE TO GIVEN THERAPY IN CHILDHOOD RENAL OSTEODYSTROPHY**

1. Clinical status:
   a. Gait
   b. Muscle strength
   c. Appetite
   d. Bone pain
   e. Ability to run or ride a bicycle
2. Serum chemical values:
   a. Calcium
   b. Phosphate
   c. Alkaline phosphatase
   d. iPTH (N-terminal preferable)
   e. Magnesium
   f. Creatinine
   g. $Ca \times PO_4$ solubility product
3. Radiologic evaluation:
   a. Hand films using non-grid cassette or industrial-grade film which allows one to readily see subperiosteal erosions
   b. Knee and wrist films to estimate epiphyseal slippage and metaphyseal lesions
   c. Long bone films to assess bowing
4. Photon absorptiometry:
   Used to measure bone mineral content and bone density
5. Bone histomorphometry:
   a. Define the type of lesion—osteomalacia vs. osteitis fibrosa vs. mixed
   b. Define the rate of mineralization with double time-spaced tetracycline labeling
   c. Define the change in osteoid volume, mineral opposition rate and cellular turnover after therapy
6. Vitamin D metabolite values:
   a. Assess the degree of deficiency of 25(OH)D, 24,25(OH)$_2$D and 1,25(OH)$_2$D before therapy
   b. Measure changes after therapy and determine if the patient is taking the medication or needs a higher dose
   c. Obtain 1,25(OH)$_2$D values four to six hours post-dosing to measure peak values
7. Growth:
   a. Assess with a fixed-wall stadiometer—mean of three measurements
   b. Assess using NCHS growth charts, Tanner height velocity charts, midparental height charts, or the method of standard deviation from control mean values
   c. Compare height for chronologic age vs. bone age

time[148] and detects changes as small as 2 to 3% with accuracy. The use of bone histomorphometry, particularly after employment of a time-spaced tetracycline labeling process, is the most direct means of evaluating changes in bone after treatment.[61, 91, 110, 112, 113] One difficulty encountered in using this technique is its inherent invasiveness and the need for serial biopsies. Nevertheless, this method is particularly useful in evaluating bone aluminum status and the effect of combination therapy—1,25(OH)$_2$D plus 24,25(OH)$_2$D.

Several groups have used the measurement of vitamin D metabolite concentrations[48-50, 55, 149] to better define the level of renal function at which values of $1,25(OH)_2D$ and $24,25(OH)_2D$ decline. Some of these studies have also shown the effect of therapy on vitamin D metabolite values and have indicated that 25(OH)D values should be at least seven to 10 times normal.[55] As these assays become more readily available, their use will be increased and their full utility appreciated. Certainly, they can be used to assess patient compliance.

## AN OVERALL THERAPEUTIC APPROACH TO CHILDHOOD RENAL OSTEODYSTROPHY

The caveat of most descriptions of therapy that "therapy must be individualized" is certainly relevant in childhood renal osteodystrophy. The aims of therapy are to provide adequate calcium intake, to improve intestinal calcium absorption, to improve bone mineralization, to reduce phosphate intake, to correct acidosis, and to reduce PTH secretion. Calcium supplementation is usually necessary (Table 18–5), but with the use of the $l\alpha$-hydroxyvitamin D metabolites, the supplementation should be decreased.[85, 88, 93] Calcium lactate and carbonate are particularly useful, because one can also treat the acidosis of uremia with these compounds.

The choice of a phosphate binding agent is important, because children do not readily ingest these chalky compounds.[17] Aluminum hydroxide–containing capsules can be successfully used in older children but are too large for younger children. We have not encountered great success using aluminum hydroxide–containing cookies.[56, 93] We do recommend that our younger patients continue to use low-phosphate formulas or formulas with a high calcium/phosphate ratio.

The vitamin D analog chosen is also an individual decision and, as pointed out above, the poorly compliant patient should receive a compound with a relatively long half-life, such as vitamin $D_2$, 25(OH)D, or DHT. As pointed out earlier, the main advantage of the $l\alpha$-hydroxylated vitamin D metabolites is their relatively short half-life so that hypercalcemia or an elevated Ca × $PO_4$ solubility product is managed relatively easily.

The role of parathyroidectomy has changed with our better understanding of

**Table 18–5.** ELEMENTAL CALCIUM IN AVAILABLE CALCIUM PREPARATIONS

| Preparation | Elemental Calcium |
| --- | --- |
| Calcium carbonate (supplied as tablets, suspension, and bulk powder) | 40% |
| Calcium chloride (contraindicated in acidosis) | 36% |
| Calcium citrate | 24% |
| Calcium lactate (supplied as tablet and liquid) | 18.4% |
| Calcium gluconate (supplied as tablets and IV solution) | 9.3% |
| Calcium gluconogalactogluconate syrup (supplied as syrup) | 92 mg/4 ml |

vitamin D metabolites and their role in the suppression of PTH secretion[38] and because of the availability of these metabolites for therapeutic administration. Moreover, newer methods of PTH suppression—such as β-adrenergic blocking agents and antihistaminic agents[150]—have been recognized. The role of agents such as propranolol and cimetidine in the long-term treatment of secondary hyperparathyroidism is unclear, since not all investigators have found effective suppression following the use of these drugs.[151]

The early recognition of renal osteodystrophy is a problem for all pediatric nephrologists. The use of one or a variety of techniques can often demonstrate "early" osteodystrophy. The measurement of iPTH levels indicates changes in calcium homeostasis at clearance values of 50 ml/min/1.73 $M^2$.[147] In addition, an elevation of the nephrogenous cAMP has been shown to indicate early renal osteodystrophy.[152] Bone biopsy will often reveal changes indicative of renal osteodystrophy at clearance values of 30 to 50 ml/min/1.73 $M^2$.[153] Photon absorptiometry is a useful diagnostic tool,[30, 154] but bone scans do not appear to provide therapeutically useful information.[155] Serum chemical determinations of calcium, phosphate, and alkaline phosphatase are far less useful in detecting early osteodystrophy.[50, 147, 156] Because children with congenital renal disease[32, 147] or obstructive uropathy[30, 157] are at risk for developing ESRD, this population should be assessed, probably on a semi-annual basis. After the detection of changes in the measured parameters, therapy should be instituted as outlined above in order to prevent the progression of renal osteodystrophy.

# REFERENCES

1. Albright F, Drake TG, Sulkowtich HW: Renal osteitis fibrosa cystica: report of a case with discussion of metabolic aspects. J Hopkins Med J 60:377, 1937.
2. Lucas RC: On a form of late rickets associated with albuminuria, rickets of adolescents. Lancet 1:993, 1883.
3. Lewy JE, New MI: Growth in children with renal failure. Am J Med 58:65, 1975.
4. Chantler C, Holliday MA: Growth in children with renal failure, with special reference to the effects of caloric malnutrition. Clin Nephrol 1:230, 1973.
5. McSherry E, Morris RC: Attainment and maintenance of normal status with alkali therapy in infants and children with classic renal tubular acidosis (RTA). J Clin Invest 61:509, 1978.
6. Coburn JW, Koppel MH, Brickman AS, Massry SG: Study of intestinal absorption of calcium in patients with renal failure. Kidney Int 3:264, 1973.
7. Saenger P, Wiedmann E, Schwartz E, et al: Somatomedin and growth after renal transplantation. Pediatr Res 8:163, 1974.
8. Mehls O, Ritz E, Gilli G, Kreusser W: Growth in renal failure. Nephron 21:237, 1978.
9. Kleinknect C, Broyer M, Gagnadoux MF, et al: Growth in children treated with long-term dialysis: A study of 76 patients. Adv Nephrol 9:133, 1980.
10. Mehls O, Eberhard R, Kreusser W, Krempien B: Renal osteodystrophy in uremic children. Clin Endocrinol Metab 9:151, 1980.
11. Mehls O, Ritz E, Krempien B, et al: Slipped epiphyses in renal osteodystrophy. Arch Dis Child 50:545, 1975.
12. Goldman AB, Lane JM, Salvati E: Slipped capital femoral epiphyses complicating renal osteodystrophy: A report of three cases. Radiology 126:333, 1978.
13. Schott GD, Wills MR: Muscle weakness in osteomalacia. Lancet 1:626, 1976.
14. Moorhead JF, Wills MR, Ahmed KY, et al: Hypophosphatemic osteomalacia after cadaveric renal transplantation. Lancet 1:694, 1974.
15. Kaplan MA, Canterbury J, Jaffe D, et al: Effect of dietary phosphorus in the phosphaturic and calcemic response to parathyroid hormone in the uremic dog. Kidney Int 12:457, 1977.
16. Slatopolsky E, Caglar S, Gradowska L, et al: On the prevention of secondary hyperparathyroidism in experimental chronic renal disease using "proportional reduction" of dietary phosphorus intake. Kidney Int 2:147, 1972.
17. Tanaka Y, DeLuca HF: The control of 24-hydroxyvitamin D metabolism by inorganic phosphorus. Arch Biochem Biophys 159:566, 1973.
18. Maschio G, Tessitore N, D'Angelo A, et al: Early dietary phosphorus restriction and calcium supplementation in the prevention of renal osteodystrophy. Am J Clin Nutr 33:1546, 1980.
19. Llach F, Massry SG, Koffler A, et al: Secondary hyperparathyroidism in early renal failure: Role of phosphate retention. Kidney Int 12:459, 1977.
20. Kopple JD, Coburn JW: Metabolic studies of low protein diets in uremia. II. Calcium, phosphorus and magnesium. Medicine 52:597, 1973.
21. Alfrey AC, Le Gendre GR, Kaehny WD: The dialysis encephalopathy syndrome: Possible aluminum intoxication. N Engl J Med 294:184, 1976.
22. Baluarte HF, Gruskin AB, Hiner LB, et al: Encephalopathy in children with chronic renal failure. Proc Clin Dial Transplant Forum 7:95, 1977.
23. Guillot AP, Hood VL, Runge CF, Gennari FJ: The use of magnesium-containing phosphate binders in patients with end-stage renal disease on maintenance hemodialysis. Nephron 30:114, 1982.
24. Lotz M, Zisman E, Bartter FC: Evidence for a phosphorus-depletion syndrome in man. N Engl J Med 278:409, 1968.
25. Walling MW, Kimberg DV: Effects of l-alpha, 25-dihydroxyvitamin $D_3$ and *Solanum glaucophyllum* on intestinal calcium and phosphate transport and on plasma Ca, Mg and P levels in the rat. Endocrinology 97:1567, 1975.
26. Avioli LV: Renal osteodystrophy and vitamin D. Dial Transplant 7:244, 1978.
27. Lumb GA, Mawer EB, Stanbury SW: The apparent vitamin D resistance of chronic renal failure: A study of the physiology of vitamin D in man. Am J Med 50:421, 1971.
28. Coburn JW, Sherrard DJ, Ott SM, et al: Bone disease in uremia: A reappraisal. *In*: Vitamin D: Chemical, Biochemical and Clinical Endocrinology of Calcium Metabolism. Berlin, Walter de Gruyter & Co, 1982, p 827.
29. Denney JD, Sherrard DJ, Nelp WB, et al: Total body calcium and long-term calcium balance in chronic renal disease. J Lab Clin Med 82:226, 1973.
30. Chesney RW, Mazess RB, Rose P, Jax DK: Bone mineral status measured by direct photon absorptiometry in childhood renal disease. Pediatrics 60:864, 1977.
31. Potter DE, Wilson CJ, Ozonoff MB: Hyperparathyroid bone disease in children undergoing long-term hemodialysis: Treatment with vitamin D. J Pediatr 85:60, 1974.
32. Liu SH, Chu HI: Studies of calcium and phosphorus metabolism with special reference to pathogenesis and effect of dihydrotachysterol (A.T.10) and iron. Medicine (Balt) 22:103, 1943.
33. Dent CE, Harper C, Philpott GR: The treatment of renal glomerular osteodystrophy. Q J Med 30:1, 1961.
34. Cordy PE: Treatment of bone disease with dihydrotachysterol in patients undergoing long-term hemodialysis. Can Med Assoc J 117:766, 1977.
35. Fraser DR, Kodicek E: Unique biosynthesis by kidney of a biologically active vitamin D metabolite. Nature 228:764, 1970.
36. Norman AW, Midgett RJ, Myrtle JF, et al: Studies on calciferol metabolism. I. Production of vitamin D metabolite 4B from 25-OH-cholecalciferol by kidney homogenates. Biochem Biophys Res Commun 42:1082, 1971.
37. Gray R, Boyle I, DeLuca HF: Vitamin D metabolism: The role of kidney tissue. Science 172:1232, 1971.
38. DeLuca HF: The vitamin D system in the regulation of calcium and phosphorus metabolism. WO Atwater Memorial Lecture. Nutr Rev 37:161, 1979.
39. Mawer EB, Backhouse J, Taylor CM, et al: Failure of formation of 1,25-dihydroxycholecalciferol in chronic renal insufficiency. Lancet 1:626, 1973.
40. Brickman AS, Coburn JW, Norman AW: Action

of 1,25-dihydroxycholecalciferol, a potent, kidney-produced metabolite of vitamin $D_3$, in uremic man. N Engl J Med 287:891, 1972.

41. Brickman AS, Coburn JW, Massry SG, Norman AW: 1,25-Dihydroxyvitamin $D_3$ in normal man and patients with renal failure. Ann Intern Med 80:161, 1974.

42. Eisman JA, Hamstra AJ, Kream BE, DeLuca HF: 1,25-Dihydroxyvitamin D in biological fluids: A simplified and sensitive assay. Science 193:1021, 1976.

43. Haussler MR, Brickman AS: Vitamin D: Metabolism, actions and disease states. In: Disorders of Mineral Metabolism, Vol II. New York, Academic Press, 1982, p 359.

44. Shepard RM, Horst RL, Hamstra AJ, DeLuca HF: Determination of vitamin D and its metabolites in plasma from normal and anephric man. Biochem J 182:55, 1979.

45. Slatopolsky E, Gray R, Adams ND, Lemann J: Low serum levels of $1,25(OH)_2D_3$ are not responsible for the development of secondary hyperparathyroidism in early renal failure. Kidney Int 14:733, 1978.

46. Ogura Y, Kawaguchi Y, Sakai S, et al: Plasma levels of vitamin D metabolites in renal diseases. Contrib Nephrol 22:18, 1980.

47. Christiansen C, Christensen MS, Melsen F, et al: Mineral metabolism in chronic renal failure with special reference to serum concentrations of $1,25(OH)_2D$ and $24,25(OH)_2D$. Clin Nephrol 15:18, 1981.

48. Mason RS, Lissner D, Wilkinson M, Posen S: Vitamin D metabolites and their relationship to azotaemic osteodystrophy. Clin Endocrinol 13:375, 1980.

49. Chesney RW, Hamstra AJ, Mazess RB, et al: Circulating vitamin D metabolite concentrations in childhood renal diseases. Kidney Int 21:65, 1982.

50. Portale AA, Booth BE, Tsai HC, Morris RC Jr: Reduced plasma concentration of 1,25-dihydroxyvitamin D in children with moderate renal insufficiency. Kidney Int 21:627, 1982.

51. Chesney RW, Rosen JF, Hamstra AJ, DeLuca HF: Serum 1,25-dihydroxyvitamin D levels in normal children and in vitamin D disorders. Am J Dis Child 134:135, 1980.

52. Taylor CM, Mawer EB, Wallace JE, et al: The absence of 24,25-dihydroxycholecalciferol in anephric patients. Clin Sci Mol Med 55:541, 1978.

53. Lambert PW, Stern PH, Avioli RC, et al: Evidence for extrarenal production of 1α,25-dihydroxyvitamin D in man. J Clin Invest 69:722, 1982.

54. Chesney RW: Current clinical applications of vitamin D metabolite research. In: Clinical Orthopaedics and Related Research. JB Lippincott Co, 1981, p 285.

55. Langman CG, Mazur AT, Baron R, Norman ME: 25-Hydroxyvitamin $D_3$ (calcifediol) therapy of juvenile renal osteodystrophy: Beneficial effect on linear growth velocity. J Pediatr 100:815, 1982.

56. Chesney RW: Treatment of calcium and phosphorus abnormalities in childhood renal osteodystrophy. Dial Transplant, 12:270, 1983.

57. Nordin BEC: Vitamin D analogs and renal function. Lancet 2:1259, 1978.

58. Massry SG, Goldstein DA: Is calcitriol

$(1,25(OH)_2D_3)$ harmful to renal function? JAMA 242:1875, 1979.

59. Chesney RW: Renal osteodystrophy in children. In: (Chronic Renal Disease Conference proceedings). New York, Plenum Press, in press.

60. Massry SG: Requirements of vitamin D metabolites in patients with renal disease. Am J Clin Nutr 33:1530, 1980.

61. Bulla M, Delling G, Offermann G, et al: Renal bone disorder in children: Therapy with vitamin $D_3$ or 1,25-dihydroxycholecalciferol (1,25-DHCC). In: Vitamin D: Basic Research and Its Clinical Application. Berlin, Walter de Gruyter & Co, 1979, p 853.

62. Bouillon R, Verberckmoes R, de Moor P: Influence of dialysate calcium concentration and vitamin D on serum parathyroid hormone during repetitive dialysis. Kidney Int 7:422, 1975.

63. Witmer G, Margolis A, Fontaine O, et al: Effects of 25-hydroxycholecalciferol on bone lesions of children with terminal renal failure. Kidney Int 10:395, 1976.

64. Baron R, Norman M, Mazur A, et al: Bone histomorphometry in children with early chronic renal failure treated with $25(OH)D_3$. In: Vitamin D: Basic Research and Its Clinical Application. Berlin, Walter de Gruyter & Co, 1979, p 847.

65. Norman ME, Taylor A: Interrelationship of serum $25(OH)D_3$ and $1,25(OH)_2D_3$ levels in juvenile renal osteodystrophy during therapy with $25(OH)D_3$. Calc Tissue Int 33:340A, 1981.

66. Upjohn Company Bulletin: The role of calderol capsules (calcifediol) in the management of renal osteodystrophy: Report of a clinical conference, 1981.

67. Fournier A, Bordier P, Gueris J, et al: Comparison of 1α-hydroxycholecalciferol and 25-hydroxycholecalciferol in the treatment of renal osteodystrophy: Greater effect of 25-hydroxycholecalciferol on bone mineralization. Kidney Int 15:196, 1979.

68. Haussler MR, Cordy PE: Metabolites and analogues of vitamin D: Which for what? JAMA 247:841, 1982.

69. Goldstein DA, Haldimann B, Sherman D, et al: Vitamin D metabolites and calcium metabolism in patients with nephrotic syndrome and normal renal function. J Clin Endocrinol Metab 52:116, 1981.

70. Sato KA, Gray RW, Lemann J Jr: Urinary excretion of 25-hydroxyvitamin D in health and the nephrotic syndrome. J Lab Clin Med 99:325, 1982.

71. Chesney RW, Mazess RB, Hamstra AJ, et al: Subnormal serum 1,25-dihydroxyvitamin D levels in children with glomerular disease treated with corticosteroids. In: Vitamin D: Basic Research and Its Clinical Application. Berlin, Walter de Gruyter & Co, 1979, p 935.

72. Wing RM, Okamura WH, Pirio MR, et al: Vitamin D in solution: Conformations of vitamins $D_3$, 1α,25-dihydroxyvitamin $D_3$ and dihydrotachysterol. Science 186:939, 1974.

73. Hollick RB, DeLuca HF: 25-Hydroxydihydrotachysterol: Biosynthesis in vivo and in vitro. J Biol Chem 246:5733, 1971.

74. Malekzadeh M, Stanley P, Ettenger R, et al: Treatment of renal osteodystrophy in children on haemodialysis with dihydrotachysterol. In: Vitamin D: Biochemical, Chemical and Clinical As-

pects Related to Calcium Metabolism. Berlin, Walter de Gruyter & Co, 1977, p 681.

75. Parfitt AM, Frame B: Treatment of rickets and osteomalacia. Semin Drug Treat 2:83, 1972.

76. Cordy PE: Treatment of bone disease in patients on chronic haemodialysis with dihydrotachysterol. Trans Am Soc Artif Intern Organs 22:60, 1976.

77. Cordy PE: The early detection and treatment of renal osteodystrophy. In: Vitamin D: Basic Research and Its Clinical Application. Berlin, Walter de Gruyter & Co, 1979, p 775.

78. Nielsen SP, Binderup E, Godtfredsen WO, et al: 1α-Hydroxycholecalciferol: Long-term treatment of patients with uraemic osteodystrophy. Nephron 16:359, 1976.

79. Henderson RG, Russell RGG, Ledingham JGG, et al: Effects of 1,25-dihyroxycholecalciferol on calcium absorption, muscle weakness and bone disease in chronic renal failure. Lancet 1:379, 1974.

80. Pierides AM, Ellis HA, Dellagrammatikas H, et al: 1,25-Dihydroxycholecalciferol in renal osteodystrophy: Epiphysiolysis—anticonvulsant therapy. Arch Dis Child 52:464, 1977.

81. Kanis JA, Henderson RG, Heynen G, et al: Renal osteodystrophy in nondialysed adolescents: Long-term treatment with 1α-hydroxycholecalciferol. Arch Dis Child 52:473, 1977.

82. Nielsen HE, Melsen F, Christensen MS, et al: 1α-Hydroxycholecalciferol treatment of long-term hemodialyzed patients: Effects on mineral metabolism, bone mineral content and bone morphometry. Clin Nephrol 8:429, 1977.

83. Chan JCM, DeLuca HF: Growth velocity in a child on prolonged hemodialysis: Beneficial effect of 1α-hydroxyvitamin D₃. JAMA 238:2053, 1977.

84. Balsan S, Gueris J, Levy D, et al: Suppressive effect of 1α-hydroxyvitamin D₃ on the hyperparathyroidism of children on maintenance hemodialysis. Metab Bone Dis Relat Res 1:15, 1978.

85. Chesney RW, Moorthy AV, Eisman JA, et al: Increased growth after long-term oral 1α,25-vitamin D₃ in childhood renal osteodystrophy. N Engl J Med 298:238, 1978.

86. Chan JCM, DeLuca HF: Calcium and parathyroid disorders in children: Chronic renal failure and treatment with calcitriol. JAMA 241:1242, 1979.

87. Chesney RW, Hamstra A, Jax DK, et al: Influence of long-term oral 1,25-dihydroxyvitamin D in childhood renal osteodystrophy. Contrib Nephrol 18:55, 1980.

88. Chan JCM, Kodroff MB, Landwehr DM: Effects of 1,25-dihydroxyvitamin D₃ on renal function, mineral balance and growth in children with severe chronic renal failure. Pediatrics 68:559, 1981.

89. Chesney RW, Rosen JF, Hamstra AJ, et al: The use of serum 1,25-dihydroxyvitamin D (calcitriol) concentrations in the clinical assessment of demineralizing disorders in children. In: Hormonal Control of Calcium Metabolism. Rotterdam, The Netherlands, Excerpta Medica, 1981, p 252.

90. Chan JCM, Young RB, Mamunes P: Hypercalcemia in children with disorders of calcium and phosphorus metabolism during long-term treatment with 1,25-dihydroxyvitamin D₃. Pediatrics, in press.

91. Robitaille P, Marie PJ, Delvin EE, et al: Renal osteodystrophy in children treated with 1,25-dihydroxycholecalciferol (1,25(OH)₂D₃): Histologic bone studies. Pediatrics, in press.

92. Christiansen C, Rodbro P, Christensen MS, et al: Deterioration of renal function during treatment of chronic renal failure with 1,25-dihydroxycholecalciferol. Lancet 2:700, 1978.

93. Chesney RW: 1,25-Dihydroxyvitamin D₃ in the treatment of juvenile renal osteodystrophy. In: Pediatric Nephrology. The Hague, The Netherlands, Martin Nijhoff Publishers, 1980, p 209.

94. Malekzadeh MH, Ettenger RB, Pennisi AJ, et al: Treatment of renal osteodystrophy in children with 1,25(OH)₂D₃. In: Fourth Workshop on Vitamin D. Berlin, Kongresshalle, 1979, p 200.

95. Chesney RW: Modified vitamin D compounds in the treatment of certain bone diseases. In: Nutritional Pharmacology. New York, Alan R Liss Inc, 1981, p 147.

96. Garabedian M, Liebenherr M, Corvol MT, et al: Cellular location and regulation of the 24,25-dihydroxyvitamin D₃ formation in cultured cells from bone and cartilage. In: Vitamin D: Basic Research and Its Clinical Application. Berlin, Walter de Gruyter & Co, 1979, p 391.

97. Ornoy A, Goodwin D, Noff D, Edelstein S: 24,25-Dihydroxyvitamin D is a metabolite of vitamin D essential for bone formation. Nature 276:517, 1978.

98. Canterbury JM, Lerman S, Claflin AJ, et al: Inhibition of parathyroid hormone secretion by 25-hydroxycholecalciferol and 24,25-dihydroxycholecalciferol in the dog. J Clin Invest 61:1375, 1978.

99. Canterbury JM, Bourgoignie JJ, Gavellas G, Reiss E: Metabolic consequences of oral administration of 24,25(OH)₂D₃ to uremic dogs. J Clin Invest 65:571, 1980.

100. Liebenherr M, Garabedian M, Guillozo H, et al: Interaction of 24,25-dihydroxyvitamin D₃ and parathyroid hormone on bone enzymes in vitro. Calcif Tissue Int 27:47, 1979.

101. Kanis JA, Cundy T, Bartlett M, et al: Is 24,25-dihydroxycholecalciferol a calcium-regulating hormone in man? Br Med J 1:1382, 1978.

102. Llach F, Brickman AS, Singer FR, Coburn JW: 24,25-Dihydroxycholecalciferol, a vitamin D sterol with qualitatively unique effects in uremic man. Metab Bone Dis Relat Res 2:11, 1979.

103. Massry SG, Turna S, Dua S, Goldstein DA: Reversal of skeletal resistance to parathyroid hormone in uremia by vitamin D metabolites: Evidence for the requirement of 1,25(OH)₂D₃ and 24,25(OH)₂D₃. J Lab Clin Med 94:152, 1979.

104. Bordier P, Zingraff J, Gueris J, et al: The effect of 1α-(OH)D₃ and 1,25(OH)₂D₃ on the bone in patients with renal osteodystrophy. Am J Med 64:101, 1978.

105. Rasmussen H, Bordier P: Evidence that different vitamin D sterols have qualitatively different effects in man. Contrib Nephrol 18:184, 1980.

106. Kanis JA, Cundy T, Smith R, et al: Possible function of different renal metabolites of vitamin D in man. Contrib Nephrol 18:192, 1980.

107. Chesney RW, Mazess RB, Hamstra AJ, DeLuca HF: Demineralization in hypophosphatemic rickets with normal 24,25-dihydroxyvitamin D and subnormal 1,25-dihydroxyvitamin D levels. Clin Res 27:653A, 1979.

108. Schnoes HK, DeLuca HF: Recent progress in vitamin D metabolism and the chemistry of vitamin D metabolites. Fed Proc 39:2723, 1980.

109. Olgaard K, Rothstein M, Arbelaez M, et al: Does 24,25(OH)₂D₃ have a beneficial effect in uremia?

*In:* Vitamin D: Chemical, Biochemical and Clinical Endocrinology of Calcium Metabolism. Berlin, Walter de Gruyter & Co, 1982, p 139.

110. Sherrard DJ, Ott SM, Maloney NA, et al: The use of 24,25(OH)₂-vitamin D in the refractory osteomalacia form of renal osteodystrophy. *In:* Vitamin D: Chemical, Biochemical and Clinical Endocrinology of Calcium Metabolism. Berlin, Walter de Gruyter & Co, 1982, p 169.

111. Okamoto S, Tanaka Y, DeLuca HF, et al: 24,24-Difluoro-25-hydroxyvitamin D₃–enhanced bone mineralization in rats: Comparison with 25-hydroxyvitamin D₃ and Vitamin D₃. Arch Biochem Biophys 206:8, 1981.

112. Muirhead N, Adami S, Sandler LM, et al: Long-term 24,25(OH)₂D₃ in the treatment of renal osteodystrophy. *In:* Vitamin D: Chemical, Biochemical and Clinical Endocrinology of Calcium Metabolism. Berlin, Walter de Gruyter & Co, 1982, p 187.

113. Evans RA, Hills E, Wong SYP, et al: The use of 24,25-dihydroxycholecalciferol alone and in combination with 1,25-dihydroxycholecalciferol in chronic renal failure. *In:* Vitamin D: Chemical, Biochemical and Clinical Endocrinology of Calcium Metabolism. Berlin, Walter de Gruyter & Co, 1982, p 835.

114. Hodsman AB, Sherrard DJ, Alfrey AC, et al: Bone aluminum and histomorphometric features of renal osteodystrophy. J Clin Endocrinol Metab 54:539, 1982.

115. Walker GS, Aaron JE, Peacock M, et al: Dialysate aluminum concentration and renal bone disease. Kidney Int 21:411, 1982.

116. Felsenfeld AJ, Harrelson JM, Gutman RA, et al: Osteomalacia after parathyroidectomy in patients with uremia. Ann Intern Med 96:34, 1982.

117. Cournot-Witmer G, Zingraff J, Plachot JJ, et al: Aluminum localization in bone from hemodialyzed patients: Relationship to matrix mineralization. Kidney Int 20:375, 1981.

118. Kanis JA, Taylor CM, Douglas DL, et al: Effects of 24,25-dihydroxyvitamin D₃ on its plasma level in man. Metab Bone Dis Relat Res 3:155, 1981.

119. Miller SC, Halloran BP, DeLuca HF, et al: Studies on the role of 24-hydroxylation of vitamin D in the mincralization of cartilage and bone of vitamin D-deficient rats. Calcif Tissue Int 33:489, 1981.

120. Finch T, Jacobs JK: Indications for parathyroidectomy in patients with chronic renal failure. Am Surg 40:40, 1974.

121. Popowniak KL, Esselstyn CB Jr, Nakamoto S: Parathyroidectomy for the treatment of renal osteodystrophy and tertiary hyperparathyroidism: Progress report. Surg Clin North Am 54:325, 1974.

122. Firor HV, Moore ES, Levitsky LL, Galvez M: Parathyroidectomy in children with chronic renal failure. J Pediatr Surg 7:565, 1972.

123. Gipstein RH, Coburn JW, Adams DA, et al: Calciphylaxis in man: A syndrome of tissue necrosis and vascular calcification in 11 patients with chronic renal disease. Arch Intern Med 136:1273, 1976.

124. Talwalkar YB, Puri HC, Hawker CC, et al: Parathyroid autotransplantation in renal osteodystrophy. Am J Dis Child 133:901, 1979.

125. Wells SA Jr, Gunnells JC, Shelburn JD: Transplan-

126. Mozes MF, Soper WD, Jonasson O, Lang GR: Total parathyroidectomy and autotransplantation in secondary hyperparathyroidism. Arch Surg 115:378, 1980.

127. Parfitt MA: The actions of parathyroid hormone on bone: Relation to bone remodelling and turnover calcium homeostasis and metabolic bone disease. Metabolism 25:909, 1976.

128. Swanson MR, Biggers JA, Remmers AR Jr, et al: Results of parathyroidectomy for autonomous hyperparathyroidism. Arch Intern Med 139:989, 1979.

129. Weinstein RS: Decreased mineralization in hemodialysis patients after subtotal parathyroidectomy. Calcif Tissue Int 34:16, 1982.

130. Johnson WJ: Optimum dialysate calcium concentration during maintenance hemodialysis. Nephron 17:241, 1976.

131. Juttmann JR, Hagenouw-Taal JCW, Lameyer LDF, et al: A longitudinal study of bone mineral content and intestinal calcium absorption in patients with chronic renal failure. Metabolism 28:1114, 1979.

132. Johnson JW, Hattner RS, Hampers CL, et al: Effects of hemodialysis on secondary hyperparathyroidism in patients with chronic renal failure. Metabolism 21:18, 1972.

133. Mehls O, Krampien B, Ritz E, et al: Renal osteodystrophy in children on maintenance hemodialysis. Proc Eur Dial Transplant Assoc 10:197, 1973.

134. Ahmed KY, Varghese Z, Wills MR, et al: Persistent hypophosphatemia and osteomalacia in dialysis patients not on oral phosphate binders: Response to dihydrotachysterol therapy. Lancet 2:439, 1976.

135. Cotiguglia SR, Alfrey AC, Miller N, Butkus D: Total-body magnesium excess in chronic renal failure. Lancet 1:1300, 1972.

136. Mennes P, Rosenbaum R, Martin K, Slatopolsky E: Hypomagnesemia and impaired parathyroid hormone secretion in chronic renal failure. Ann Intern Med 88:206, 1978.

137. Pletka P, Bernstein DS, Hampers CL, et al: Relationship between magnesium and secondary hyperparathyroidism during long-term hemodialysis. Metabolism 23:619, 1974.

138. Potter DE, Griefer I: Statural growth of children with renal disease. Kidney Int 14:334, 1978.

139. Fournier AE, Johnson WJ, Taves DR, et al: Etiology of hyperparathyroidism and bone disease during chronic hemodialysis. I. Association of bone disease with potentially etiologic factors. J Clin Invest 50:592, 1971.

140. Griffiths HJ, Zimmerman RE, Lazarus M, et al: The long-term follow-up of 195 patients with renal failure; a preliminary report. Radiology 122:643, 1977.

141. Ward MK, Feest TG, Ellis HA, et al: Osteomalacic dialysis osteodystrophy: Evidence for a water-borne etiological agent, probably aluminum. Lancet 1:841, 1978.

142. Evans RA, Somerville PJ: The use of high calcium dialysate in the treatment of renal osteomalacia. Aust N Z J Med 6:10, 1976.

143. Feest TG, Ward MK, Ellis HA, et al: Osteomalacic dialysis osteodystrophy: A trial of phosphate-enriched dialysis fluid. Br Med J 1:18, 1978.

144. Hodsman AB, Sherrard DJ, Wong EG, et al: Vitamin D-resistant osteomalacia in hemodialysis patients lacking secondary hyperparathyroidism. Ann Intern Med 94:629, 1981.

145. Velentzas C, Meindok H, Ozeoporilos DG, et al: Detection and pathogenesis of visceral calcification in dialysis patients and patients with malignant disease. Can Med Assoc J 118:45, 1978.

146. Calderaro V, Oreoporilos DG, Meema HE, et al: The evolution of renal osteodystrophy in patients undergoing continuous ambulatory peritoneal dialysis (CAPD). Proc Eur Dial Transplant Assoc 17:533, 1980.

147. Norman ME, Mazur AT, Borden S IV, et al: Early diagnosis of juvenile renal osteodystrophy. J Pediatr 97:226, 1980.

148. Chesney RW, Shore RM: The noninvasive determination of bone mineral content by photon absorptiometry. Am J Dis Child 136:578, 1982.

149. Loirat C, Danan JL, Nguyen Dai D, et al: l$\alpha$(OH)D$_3$ and 1,25(OH)$_2$D$_3$ plus (1,25) therapy in hemodialyzed children with reference to plasma concentration of 1,25. *In:* Vitamin D: Chemical, Biochemical and Clinical Endocrinology of Calcium Metabolism. Berlin, Walter de Gruyter & Co, 1982, p 893.

150. Jacob AI, Lanier D Jr, Canterbury J, Bourgoignie JJ: Reduction by cimetidine of serum parathyroid hormone levels in uremic patients. N Engl J Med 302:671, 1980.

151. Fuchs E, von Herrath D, Kraft D, et al: The influence of 24,25(OH)$_2$-vitamin D$_3$, beta-blockers and cimetidine on the course of experimental renal osteodystrophy in rats. *In:* Vitamin D: Chemical, Biochemical and Clinical Endocrinology of Calcium Metabolism. Berlin, Walter de Gruyter & Co, 1982, p 183.

152. Krensky AM, Harmon WE, Ingelfinger JR, et al: Elevated nephrogenous cyclic adenosine monophosphate to monitor early renal osteodystrophy. Clin Nephrol 16:245, 1981.

153. Chesney RW: Does uremic bone disease warrant early treatment with calcitriol? Arch Intern Med 140:1016, 1980.

154. Griffiths HJ, Zimmerman R, Bailey G, Snider R: The use of photon absorptiometry in the diagnosis of renal osteodystrophy. Radiology 109:277, 1973.

155. Hodson EM, Howman-Giles RB, Evans RA, et al: The diagnosis of renal osteodystrophy: A comparison of Technetium-99m-pyrophosphate bone scintigraphy with other techniques. Clin Nephrol 16:24, 1981.

156. Chesney RW, Hamstra AJ, Phelps M, DeLuca HF: Vitamin D metabolites in renal insufficiency and other vitamin D disorders of children. Kidney Int, in press.

157. Warshaw BL, Edelbrock HH, Ettenger RB, et al: Progression to end-stage renal disease in children with obstructive uropathy. J Pediatr 100:183, 1982.

# 19

# Growth in Children with Chronic Renal Insufficiency

*Karl Schärer, M.D.*
*Giulio Gilli, M.D.*

Body growth is one of the most sensitive indicators of organ dysfunction in children. Retardation of growth is a frequent sign of renal functional impairment in children and adolescents, especially in the presence of chronic renal insufficiency (CRI). Growth retardation may occur prior to a significant reduction in glomerular function. In the past growth retardation in patients with CRI was of minimal concern because early death was expected. Since dialysis and transplantation have prolonged the lives of pediatric patients with CRI, it is apparent that "renal dwarfism" has become one of the most common causes of growth failure in children and adolescents.

Short stature has a significant impact on the daily life of young patients with CRI by diminishing self-esteem and hampering rehabilitation. Final body height is often reduced; therefore, the future professional and family life of such patients may become permanently disturbed, despite restoration of renal function following successful renal transplantation.

Numerous reviews have recently appeared detailing growth retardation in children with CRI and emphasizing that the pathogenetic mechanisms involved are complex and treatment limited.[1-7] A recent conference emphasized the close relationship between growth retardation and the metabolic abnormalities of uremia.[8] In this chapter we will summarize the present knowledge on growth in children at different stages of CRI and present the current status of the pathogenetic factors which have been proposed to interfere with the normal growth process in patients with CRI.

## EVALUATION OF BODY GROWTH

Precise and uniform assessment, analysis, and expression of growth data are imperative for the appropriate interpretation of growth dynamics in children with CRI. It is advantageous to obtain measurements of body height in children with CRI together with other nutritional and developmental data, including weight, skinfold thickness, upper arm circumference, skeletal maturation, and pubertal status.

Knowledge of the normal growth process is essential for evaluating growth in disease states. *Normal postnatal growth* can be divided into three periods: (1) a period with a high but rapidly declining growth rate from birth to the age of 3–4 years; (2) a period with more or less stable growth of 6 to 7 cm/yr which occurs until the initial signs of puberty are present, i.e., at a mean age of 11 years in girls and 13 years in boys; and (3) the pubertal period, in which a growth spurt reaching a peak height velocity of about 7 cm/year in girls and 9 cm/year in boys occurs, at a mean age of 12 and 14 years, respectively. Peak height velocity is lower the later it occurs, but normally wide variations are noted.

### Assessment of Growth

Since growth in patients with CRI may be minimal over a long period of time, it is of paramount importance that rigorous procedures be applied to obtaining measurements. Inaccurate measurements may lead to erroneous conclusions about the actual growth rate. Recommendations on the precise measurements of growth in children with CRI have been detailed elsewhere.[9] Adherence to the following points is essential in order to obtain consistent and reliable data:

1. All measurements should be performed by *skilled observers* after proper training. Whenever possible, the measurements should be performed by the same observer in order to minimize variability. If more than one observer is obtaining the data, it is imperative that results be compared regularly. The assessment of skeletal maturity from radiographs is best done by an independent observer to reduce inherent biases and interpretation errors.

2. Measurements should be performed according to internationally recognized and well *standardized techniques* and procedures.[10–12] This is necessary to ensure that data from different centers around the world can be compared.

3. Measurements should be performed with *accurate instruments.* The Harpenden range of anthropometric instruments are accepted internationally because of their accuracy, consistency, and simplicity.

The following *anthropometric measurements* should be obtained in children with CRI at least every six months as well as at any major change in the mode of treatment, e.g., at the introduction of a new dietary regime or drug, at initiation of dialysis, and at transplantation. In addition, it is advantageous to have the results of prior measurements available before CRI was diagnosed.

*Stature* is measured as standing height (from 2 years of age onward) or as recumbent length (at any age). At transitional ages, *both* measurements should be performed to avoid misleading interpretations of height velocity. The use of a *stadiometer* is strongly recommended. When measuring the child, a gentle but firm pressure upward is applied by the observer under the mastoid process to help the child stretch. This procedure avoids diurnal and interobserver variations. The height should be recorded to the last completed millimeter. Whenever possible, height measurements of the parents and growth curves of siblings should be obtained.

*Weight* is preferably measured in the morning or, in dialyzed children, at the *end* of the dialysis session. Instruments accurate to at least 0.1 kg are recommended. Weighing is preferably done in the nude, but very light clothing is acceptable. The presence of edema should be recorded.

*Skinfold thickness* should be measured at the triceps site (at the midpoint between the acromion and the olecranon) and at the subscapular site (below the angle of the scapula). The use of a skinfold caliper with a constant pressure is required. These measurements should be taken on the left side. Although it has recently been recommended to obtain the measurements bilaterally in children with an arteriovenous shunt,[12] a study of 85 dialyzed children and height-matched controls failed to disclose any side difference related to the presence of an arteriovenous shunt (G. Gilli, unpublished results).

*Upper arm circumference* is measured on the left side at the same level as the measurement of the triceps skinfold thickness. A metallic tape is recommended, and linen tapes should be avoided. Skinfold thickness at the triceps site and upper arm circumference can be used to estimate body fat and muscle mass.[13, 14]

The *stage of puberty* can be determined according to the Tanner maturity ratings.[15] In males testicular size should be measured.[16] It is important to recognize the *first* clinical signs of puberty in order to determine the initiation of the adolescent growth spurt. The time of menarche should be recorded.

*Radiographs of the left hand and wrist and the left knee* should be obtained at 6-month intervals for the assessment of skeletal maturity. For the hand and wrist the scoring method developed by Tanner et al[17] and the method of Greulich-Pyle[18] are recommended. It should be stressed that if the latter method is used, the skeletal age must be assessed as the median among bone-specific skeletal ages.[19] For the knee the Roche-Wainer-Thissen (RWT) method has been developed.[20] Comparability and reliability of this method are about the same as that of the Tanner method, but positioning of the subject is somewhat more difficult and a computer is needed for calculation of skeletal age.

## Expression of Growth Data

Growth data obtained in children with CRI should be compared to *reference data* drawn from the same population. Comprehensive anthropometric reference data are limited. In the United States the Harvard growth charts have recently been superseded by the standards provided by the National Center for Health Statistics.[21] In Europe, the British height standards developed by Tanner et al[22, 23] are widely used, although they are not adequate for the majority of children in European countries. Suitable standards for mid-European children have recently been published by Prader et al.[24]

Reference data for growth are not necessarily normal or ideal. Such data simply provide a *frame of reference* for selecting the person who falls outside a predetermined level of growth performance.[25] A differentiation between normal and abnormal growth is a matter of convention. A level must be set below which an individual is considered to be at risk of growth retardation.

*Growth retardation* is usually defined as a body height corresponding to two standard deviations or more below the normal mean for chronologic age, or below the third percentile (i.e., $-1.88$ SD). Some authors prefer to relate body height to skeletal age rather than to chronologic age. Although this approach may be biologically relevant, it should be noted that normal ranges of height related to bone age are not available, and that bone age assessments by inexperienced observers will further increase the risk of misinterpretation. This is evident if an increment in growth is related to an increase in bone age rather than to the chronologic age. Therefore, we advise the *routine* use of the chronologic age for plotting growth data.

Because children with CRI are at risk of developing *malnutrition,* it is important to compare weight with height. Generally, this is done by relating the patient's weight to the expected weight for the patient's height. Charts of weight for given height can also be used.[21] Both methods assume that the expected weight for a given height is not dependent upon age; however, this assumption is not true. A more precise method of expressing the relationship of weight to height would be to compare the standard deviation scores (SDS) for weight to those for height, or to express both weight and height as a fraction of the 50th percentile for age.

*Longitudinal (serial) measurements* allow calculation of the *rate (velocity) of growth.* This can simply be done by comparing the SDS of height or weight at the beginning and at the end of a given observation period. Such a procedure perhaps allows the best mathematical description of relative loss or gain (in SDS/year); however, it should be emphasized that the physiological fluctuations in SDS of growth parameters are unknown. Alternatively, growth velocity during a given period can be calculated (cm/year) and plotted on

reference velocity charts. Whole-year velocity curves developed for British children[22, 23] may be used with sufficient accuracy for other populations. It should be noted that these curves are whole-year velocity standards and do not strictly apply if observation periods shorter than one year are considered.

It should also be kept in mind that the growth pattern of healthy children appears different when it is plotted on velocity charts rather than on longitudinal growth charts. In the latter, the individual child tends to follow the same channel throughout, a deviation of more than one channel being exceptional before puberty. On velocity charts, however, it is usual to observe that the velocity plots of the same child are scattered both above and below the 50th percentile line, with a tendency to compensate from one year to the next by crossing over the 50th percentile line. Such changes in growth velocity are physiological and do not necessarily reflect the effects of the disease or of therapeutic intervention.

It should also be remembered that at adolescence a child's growth can deviate temporarily by one or two percentile lines from the prepubertal level. This is explained by the fact that the normal adolescent growth spurt of an individual is usually more marked than the mean increment at adolescence indicated in most reference curves, because many curves are drawn from cross-sectional data and usually are not centered on peak height velocity. Therefore, an increase in growth velocity at the time of puberty should not be misinterpreted as an improvement in growth rate.

In recent years the term *"catch-up growth"* has been misused by pediatric nephrologists. Catch-up growth is a phenomenon observed when a child with a retarded pattern of growth has a restoration of the growth deficit as soon as the growth-disturbing conditions are removed. The original description implies that "at the end of a period of growth retardation consequent to illness or starvation the child grows more rapidly than usual so that he catches up toward or into his original growth curve."[26] This process, which is characterized by a sharp increase in the growth velocity above normal, is followed by a progressive deceleration until the original growth channel is reached and is called *"true catch-up growth."* Another type of catch-up growth[27] is described as a delayed maturation with a *prolonged* period of growth *without* an abnormal increase in growth velocity (Fig.

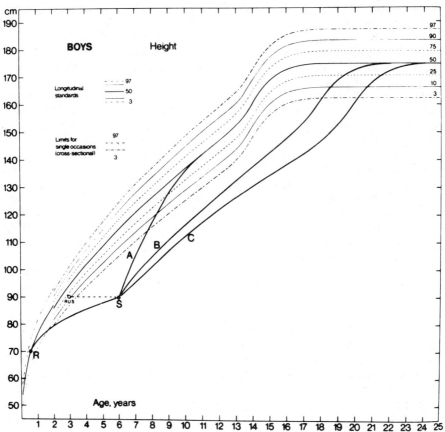

**Figure 19–1.** Two types of *complete catch-up growth*. Growth retardation occurs from R to S with rehabilitation commencing at S. *A*, Complete catch-up growth (classic). *B* and *C*, Complete catch-up by prolonged growth (delayed bone maturation). In *C*, growth is resumed at an average velocity for chronologic age, in *B* at an average velocity for bone age. (From Tanner JM: Foetus into Man: Physical Growth from Conception to Maturity. London, Open Books, 1978.)

**Table 19–1.** HEIGHT PERCENTILES AT INITIATION OF HEMODIALYSIS OR
AT FIRST TRANSPLANT (WITHOUT PRIOR DIALYSIS)*

| Primary Kidney Disorder | Height Category | | | |
| --- | --- | --- | --- | --- |
| | <3rd percentile | 3rd to 50th percentile | >50th percentile | Total number of patients |
| Glomerulonephritis | 27% | 34% | 39% | 241 |
| Pyelonephritis | 48% | 41% | 11% | 123 |
| Cystic kidney disease including nephronophthisis | 71% | 26% | 3% | 34 |
| Hereditary chronic nephropathy | 54% | 39% | 7% | 61 |
| Renal hypoplasia | 54% | 41% | 5% | 85 |
| Traumatic loss of kidney ⎫ Renal vascular disease ⎬ Cortical tubular necrosis ⎭ | 14% | 58% | 28% | 36 |
| Others and not recorded | 36% | 43% | 21% | 107 |
| Total (100%) | 271 (39%) | 267 (39%) | 149 (22%) | 687 (100%) |

*The figures indicate the percentage of children with each kidney disorder in the height category indicated in relation to all children up to age 15 years. Normal reference data by Tanner et al.[22, 23] From the Pediatric Registry of the European Dialysis and Transplantation Association.[32]

19–1). The catch-up growth can be *complete* or *partial*, depending upon whether or not the original growth percentile is regained. If a growth-depressing factor is removed only in *later* childhood, the catch-up growth is rarely complete. In most reports dealing with children with CRI the pattern of growth described does not fulfill any definition of catch-up growth.

Different methods are available for *predicting adult height* from actual height, skeletal maturity, and possibly other variables at a given age. We have found that the method proposed by Tanner et al[17] provides a reliable prognosis of future growth in most children with CRI.[28]

## GROWTH AT DIFFERENT STAGES OF CHRONIC RENAL INSUFFICIENCY

### Growth During Preterminal Stage of CRI

About one third of children with CRI receiving conservative treatment are below the third percentile for height of normal children.[29] Body growth may be inhibited early in the course of CRI when the reduction in glomerular function is minimal. At times a significant loss of height velocity is observed in children with progressive kidney disease prior to the stage of CRI. This is especially true in children with nephropathies associated with congenital metabolic disorders (e.g., cystinosis) or with severe protein malnutrition (e.g., steroid-resistant nephrotic syndrome).[30] On the other hand, normal growth may continue until the development of ESRD. We have observed a girl with oligomeganephronia who grew along the 97th percentile for normal children from birth to the initiation of dialysis at the age of 11 years.

In general terms depression of growth begins earlier and is more severe in children with congenital and hereditary nephropathies than in children with acquired kidney disorders when data are compared at the onset of dialysis[31, 32] (Table 19–1). Patients with cystinosis and renal hypoplasia are especially prone to develop severe growth failure.[33] However, retardation of growth appears to be related more to the duration of renal disease than to the primary kidney disease per se or to the degree of glomerular function. This agrees with the observation that patients with a very early onset and long course of CRI are especially prone to develop growth retardation.[5, 34] Kleinknecht et al have found that in children with congenital nephropathies growth velocity is usually retarded in the first year of life, but subsequently resumes at a normal or even an increased rate.[35] Apparently, growth velocity during the first year of life is critical for maintaining a normal height at a later age.

### Growth on Hemodialysis

Relatively few data have been published on growth in children with CRI on conservative treatment, and more information is available on growth following the onset of ESRD. Most studies of growth in dialyzed children have been reported from pediatric centers in Europe, where long-term dialysis is a common mode of treatment.[29, 36–40] A large volume of material on growth in dialyzed as well as in transplanted children has been collected for more than 10 years by the Registry of the European Dialysis and Transplant Association (EDTA)[31–33, 41–46] (Tables 19–1 and 19–2). According to the initial reports from this Registry 39% of all patients below 15 years of age had a body height below the third percentile for chronologic age when dialysis was started (Table 19–1); height was also reduced in patients starting dialysis between 15 and 20 years of age.[32] When growth velocity was compared immediately before and during the first year on regular hemodialysis, it was more or less constant in most children, although in some it diminished and in a few

**Table 19–2.** YEARLY GROWTH RATE OF PREPUBERTAL CHILDREN IN 1976 AND IN 1981*

| Year | CAPD | | Hemodialysis | | Transplantation | |
|---|---|---|---|---|---|---|
| | No. of Patients | Growth (cm/year) | No. of Patients | Growth (cm/year) | No. of Patients | Growth (cm/year) |
| 1976 | | | 40 | 2.8 ± 1.7 | 29 | 3.4[46] ± 1.7 |
| 1981 | 10 | 2.4 ± 1.3 | 79 | 3.0[46] ± 2.3 | 87 | 4.7[46] ± 2.5 |

*Data from the Registry of the European Dialysis and Transplantation Association.

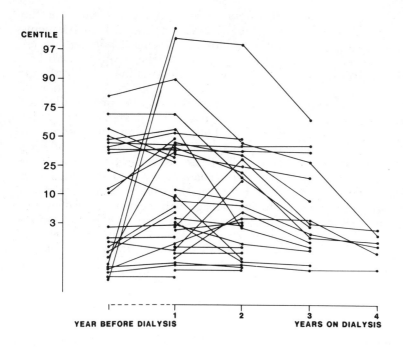

**Figure 19–2.** Growth velocity in 36 children for the year prior to and for four years after starting hemodialysis, expressed in centiles of normal growth velocity. In the year prior to dialysis, growth velocity was below the third centile in 12 of 24 children. After starting dialysis it increased above the 97th centile in two children. After the second year on dialysis growth rate decreased in almost all patients. In the third year it was below the 50th centile in 15 of 16 patients, and in the fourth year it was below the third centile in all six patients followed. (Normal standards for growth velocity from Tanner et al. Arch Dis Child 51:170, 1976.)

cases an increase was noted (Fig. 19–2). Real catch-up growth after initiating dialysis is rarely observed.[29]

Overall growth velocity on regular dialysis was found to be below the third percentile for the corresponding chronologic age in 69% of all children prior to as well as during puberty.[32] When plotted against bone age, the growth rate was similarly depressed.[42, 45] In absolute terms the mean growth rate ($\pm$ SD) of prepubertal children followed for at least 3 years on dialysis was 2.8 cm/year. In an analysis of the EDTA data in *prepubertal patients* on dialysis for more than 4 years the mean annual loss of height for chronologic age was 0.43 SD.[43] In a recent study from Paris of 51 prepubertal children treated by dialysis for more than one year, the mean loss of body height was similar (0.38 SD/year); one third of the patients had a change in height that was within normal limits (maximal loss <0.2 SD/year), whereas one third presented severe growth retardation (loss of more than 0.5 SD/year).[47]

After *several years of dialysis* growth velocity appears to remain reduced at a more or less constant rate in most European children, resulting in a progressive fall in the height percentile.[32, 44] After 5 years or more of dialysis prepubertal children had lost an average of 2.4 SD in height, compared to only 0.4 SD following transplantation.[44] Data obtained some years ago in our center suggest that some children exhibit a progressive fall

in growth velocity after 2 to 3 years of hemodialysis[29] (Fig. 19–2). In other series this phenomenon was less obvious.[32, 47]

During *puberty* growth in dialyzed children appears to be less retarded than before when the changes in the SDS for height are compared with normal children of the same chronologic age or bone age.[43, 45] In contrast to prepubertal children, some sex difference was observed during adolescence with a decrease in SDS for height of about twice as much in dialyzed boys compared to girls.[32, 43] Kleinknecht et al found a height gain during puberty of only 3 cm/year.[47] The pubertal growth spurt of children treated by regular dialysis appears to be delayed and of lesser magnitude than in normal children. When children with CRI begin their growth spurt, that of healthy children is already declining.[32] It has been shown that appreciable late growth continues in many adolescents up to 20 years or more, i.e., at an age when normal individuals already have attained their final height[43] (Fig. 19–3). This *late growth* will usually not compensate sufficiently for the height lost and therefore the original deviation from the normal mean will be regained only in rare instances.

In order to investigate the significance of late growth it is important to observe *skeletal maturation* closely. According to the EDTA Registry this is delayed an average of 0.6 years advance in bone age per one chronologic year, both on regular dialysis and after

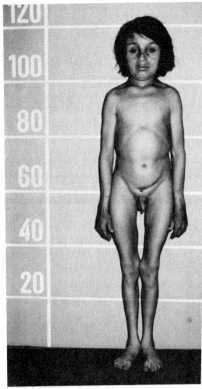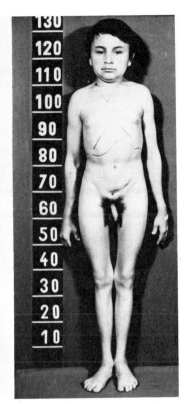

**Figure 19–3.** Late growth in a boy (S.O.) with chronic renal failure due to bilateral renal hypoplasia. Age at initiation of dialysis—18 8/12 years.

|  | Left | Right |
|---|---|---|
| Chronologic age | 18.1 yr | 21.2 yr |
| Height (height age) | 120.1 cm (6.5 yr) | 131.9 cm (8.5 yr) |
| Bone age | 9.8 yr | 14.7 yr |
| Pubertal stage | $P_2G_2$ | $P_3G_4$ |
|  |  | Testicular size 3 ml |

transplantation.[45] However, mean growth per year advance in bone age was lower in dialyzed children than in those receiving transplants (4.6 vs. 6.2 cm/year). In the study of Kleinknecht et al a similar delay in skeletal maturation was found, with a mean loss in score for age of 0.54/year in dialyzed children.[47] In the presence of a bone age of less than 12 years, skeletal maturation and statural growth were retarded to the same degree, resulting in an unchanged growth potential.

In general, variations in the *treatment modalities* of hemodialysis appear to have little influence on the growth rate in dialyzed children. Although growth rate was significantly better in prepubertal boys with three compared to two dialysis sessions per week,[32, 44] no significant difference was observed with different hours on dialysis per week, different types of dialyzer, or variable efficiency of

dialysis expressed as dialyzer surface area per body surface area.[44] Dialysis strategies have failed to influence growth, according to reports from individual centers.[37, 47] Similarly, the degree of residual renal function appears to have no effect on growth in dialyzed children.[47] On the other hand concomitant hypertension is associated with a lower growth rate.[44]

## Growth on Peritoneal Dialysis

Few data are available on the growth of children on intermittent peritoneal dialysis. These show a similar rate compared to children on hemodialysis. On CAPD growth was reported to be normal in 7 of 8 children treated for more than 6 months.[7] Balfe found significantly better growth in 17 pediatric patients treated by CAPD compared to those treated with hemodialysis.[48] On the other hand, growth data for small groups of children undergoing CAPD were less encouraging[46, 49, 50, 51] (Table 19–2).

## Growth after Renal Transplantation

Early reports of transplantation in pediatric patients have stressed that growth continues to be reduced in a large proportion of children.[2, 52–55] In the pioneer paper on the subject, Grushkin and Fine found that only 42% of pediatric patients followed for 1 to 3 years had normal post-transplant growth.[52] In a later study from the same center only 3 of 24 recipients with a functioning graft treated with daily prednisone for longer than 3 years and with a bone age of less than 12 years had a growth rate of more than 80% of that expected for height age.[56, 57] Earlier studies had given the impression that growth was normal in the majority of children receiving transplants.[58, 59] Many centers have subsequently reported on growth of children receiving transplants, providing variable results that are difficult to compare because of differences in methodology and in patient selection.[60–69]

A general impression of the effects of transplantation on growth performance can be obtained from the pediatric reports from the EDTA. Early data from this Registry had shown that only 5 of 23 children followed for more than 3 years after grafting improved their height percentile.[32] This study also demonstrated that growth in children receiving transplants is much less uniform between individuals when compared to that in children on long-term dialysis. Subsequently it became clear that in *prepubertal* children growth following transplantation is significantly superior to that observed during hemodialysis[42, 44] (Table 19–2). When calculated per one year of advance in bone age, a slight gain in SDS of height was noted at 2 to 3 years after transplantation, compared to a slight loss in dialyzed children.[45]

The general *better growth after transplantation* compared to dialysis has also been documented from individual centers.[63, 64, 68] Our experience with 10 boys receiving transplants is depicted in Fig. 19–4; all had previously been followed for various periods of time on conservative treatment and, with one exception, were prepubertal when they entered ESRD. In 8 boys growth was definitively accelerated after grafting compared to that during dialysis, but in only 5 patients was the total post-transplant growth above the expected rate of normal children, and in one boy catch-up growth was noted when the last measurement was compared to the first avail-

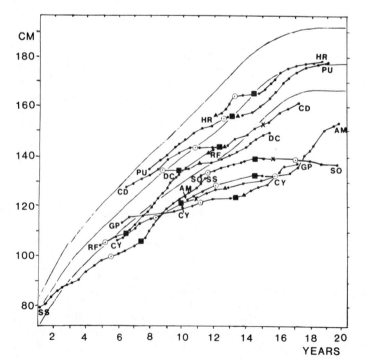

**Figure 19–4.** Changes in height of 10 male patients with chronic renal insufficiency during conservative treatment, on regular hemodialysis, and after transplantation. All patients were prepubertal at time of initiation of dialysis except HR.
⊙ start of hemodialysis
■ cadaver kidney transplantation
▲ first clinical signs of puberty (unknown in AM, missing in SO and SS).
✗ serum creatinine level after transplantation greater than 1.5 mg/dl.
In most patients growth gradually declined on conservative treatment and during dialysis therapy. The curves for third, 50th and 97th centiles of normal children are indicated. Normal standards from Prader et al.[24]

able measurement prior to ESRD. The graph shows that, in general, the starting position for catching up was more favorable if the duration of CRI without or with dialysis had been short, because during this time all children exhibited some loss of SDS in height. This applies especially to children who had received steroid treatment for the nephrotic syndrome, e.g., patients SS, CY, and SO (see Fig. 19–4). The height of SS was slightly above the 50th percentile when the disease started at the age of 1.2 years and decreased below the 3rd percentile before the serum creatinine level had risen above 1.5 mg/dl (at 3.0 years). Further loss of height occurred until the age of 7½ years when the boy received a graft. Some authors would have considered this post-transplant (prepubertal) growth as catch-up growth; however, we believe that this will only be proved if in the future the height exceeds the 50th percentile, as it was recorded at the first measurement.

Several *factors* have been proposed that affect post-transplant growth: chronologic age, skeletal maturation, sex, steroid therapy, allograft function, and growth rate prior to transplantation. It is well known that post-transplant growth rate is relatively better in *prepubertal* than in pubertal children.[45, 52] Within the prepubertal group *very young children* seem to grow better. Ingelfinger et al observed that the growth rate after transplantation was accelerated above the 50th percentile and that a normal range of height for age was reached in 7 of 11 children who were below 7 years of age at transplantation, whereas this was the case in only 1 of 16 patients receiving transplants between the ages of 7 and 11 years.[65] Apparently this difference could not be attributed to factors other than age. A similarly good growth rate in young patients was observed by other groups.[59, 65, 67, 69]

After *puberty* has begun it is frequently difficult to assess the increased growth rate in children receiving transplants (Fig. 19–4). It is usually difficult to decide if this change is due to the removal of the uremic environment, to an alteration of steroid application, or merely to the physiological pubertal growth spurt. It seems possible that removing uremic toxins improves gonadal endocrine function in these children, resulting in a steeper growth spurt.

The degree of *skeletal maturation* is critical for the gain in height after transplantation.[56] From the EDTA data cited above[45] and from more recent results,[69] it is reasonable to conclude that in children receiving transplants, at least before puberty, skeletal maturation is usually not greater than the growth rate and that, therefore, as a rule, growth potential does not decrease.

Fine et al observed that in 10 children who had already attained a *bone age of 12 years or more* (without fusion of epiphyses) total post-transplant growth was minimal, i.e., up to 3 cm.[57] Other observers found that in spite of advanced skeletal maturation the growth rate was higher in a number of adolescents receiving transplants.[43, 64] Recently Bosque et al demonstrated that boys with a bone age of less than 12 years receiving transplants had a better growth rate but at the same time exhibited a more severe degree of growth retardation when compared to patients with more advanced bone age.[69] It is possible that the described differences are due to an increased sensitivity of the growth process to corticosteroids during puberty. From our experience with children with the nephrotic syndrome, growth appears to be more depressed by similar doses of steroids in pubertal than in prepubertal children.

It has been stressed that the degree of growth retardation in children receiving transplants depends to a large extent on the amount of *glucocorticoids* given for immunosuppression. Glucocorticoids have a number of biological actions which interfere with the normal growth process: they inhibit growth hormone secretion, reduce circulating somatomedin activity, and depress growth activity of cartilage and bone cells. Furthermore, they depress calcium absorption from the gut. Individual differences in intestinal absorption, metabolism, and renal clearance of exogenous steroids may explain the great variability of growth in children receiving transplants in response to similar doses of corticosteroids.

Although a significant correlation was reported in the EDTA Registry between daily and alternate-day steroid therapy and growth rate,[44] this has not been confirmed.[45, 56, 62] However, when the daily dose exceeds 0.5 mg/kg/day the growth rate is decreased and when the dose is lower than 0.2 to 0.3 mg/kg/day it remains normal in most children receiving transplants.[45, 53, 54] Various centers have reported that the change from daily to *alternate-day therapy* is followed by an improved growth rate.[44, 52–55, 57, 61, 69] However, few studies have examined the data systematically. In 8 prepubertal children in whom a daily prednisone dose of 0.25 mg/kg/day was replaced at 2 years after grafting by an alternate-day schedule (0.625 mg/kg/48 hr), the mean SDS of height increased from −0.15 to +0.20 during a one-year period.[64] The EDTA data did not demonstrate an advantage of alternate-day therapy on post-transplant growth.[45] At present the indications and appropriate time for the change from daily to alternate-day steroid therapy in children receiving transplants remains a matter of controversy.

*Impaired allograft function* appears to diminish the growth rate in children receiving transplants.[56, 61, 68] Three examples are demonstrated in Fig. 19–4. According to Pennisi et al,[56] the critical level of GFR leading to reduction of growth is around 60 ml/min/1.73 m², although it seems that this limit may be lower in some patients.[69] It has been speculated that decreased activity of somatomedin is responsible for the retardation of growth.[70]

It was suggested that the longer the *preterminal period of CRI* the poorer growth will be after transplantation, and that growth retardation in early infancy will limit growth potential.[65] Although clinical experience (Fig. 19–4) seems to support this hypothesis, further studies are needed to resolve this question. The same is true regarding the source of kidney. It seems that, in general, growth is not different in patients who receive a kidney from a living related donor or from a cadaver donor.[69] However, the relatively good results reported in younger children[59, 61, 65, 67] may be due less to age than to the preferential use of living donors. Second transplants apparently are not associated with a more reduced growth rate than occurs after the first transplantation.[59, 60]

## Adult Height of Pediatric Patients with Chronic Renal Insufficiency

Few data exist detailing the final height attained by pediatric patients with CRI. It is a common experience that a number of patients treated by long-term hemodialysis or transplantation will continue to grow at an age when normal children have reached adult stature.[32] This observation suggests that the height retardation of children with CRI

is compensated for, at least partially, by growth at a later age.

In a study of 34 patients with CRI who had reached their final height either during conservative treatment, during dialysis, or after transplantation, we found that the distribution of final heights was markedly skewed toward the lower percentiles and that 8 patients (23%) had a final height below the third percentile[71] (Fig. 19–5); 7 of these 8 patients had a congenital or hereditary nephropathy. Final height was attained at an average of 18 years in males and 16.9 years in females. In a subsequent study from the EDTA[72] it was reported that only 9 of 30 patients who all were pubertal when treatment by dialysis or transplantation was started and were observed for more than 8 years attained a mature height within normal limits (> 154 cm in females, > 164 cm in males). The other patients were definitively stunted, with a deviation of up to −9 SD below the normal mean. According to this study, 70% of children with CRI end up with pathological height values. This study can be criticized because the adult height of the Dutch population (which is one of the tallest in Europe) was taken as the reference standard for patients from all European and Mediterranean countries.

The ability to accurately predict adult height has important implications for the management of children with CRI. In the presence of severe stunting it would be helpful in determining the choice for therapy for ESRD. In a recent study serial predictions of adult height were made in 22 pediatric patients with CRI of variable duration and severity who were followed until they were fully grown.[28] The Tanner method[17] was used for the predictions. This study showed that the prediction was accurate (± 2 cm of the actual final height) in 13 patients (59%) (Fig. 19–6). The mean prediction error at the first prediction was 2.7 cm. It was larger in patients with bone ages up to 11 years (mean 4.9 cm in 7 patients) as compared to 15 patients with more advanced bone ages (mean 1.7 cm). It was also larger in boys than in girls. Patients whose SDS for height decreased with time were overestimated by the initial assessment.

In conclusion, an accurate prediction of adult height is possible in older children with CRI. No study to date has elucidated which method of prediction is the most accurate.

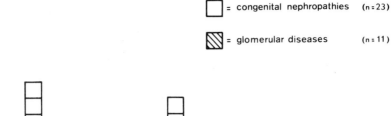

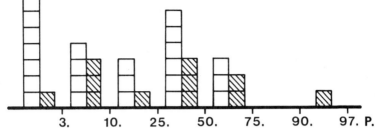

**Figure 19–5.** Adult height of 34 pediatric patients with CRI, expressed in centiles of normal population reached at the time of epiphyseal closure or minimal growth (< 1 cm/year for at least 1 year before). (From Gilli et al: Pediatr Res 14:1015, 1980.)

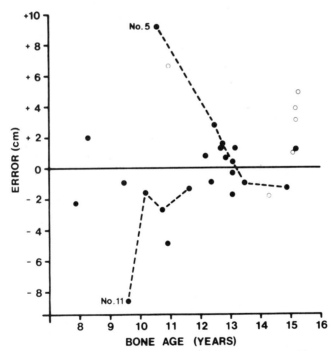

**Figure 19–6.** Errors in prediction of adult height obtained from the first assessment of bone age in 15 female (●) and 7 male (○) patients with CRI compared to actual adult height attained.

Patients above the zero line were overestimated, those below this line were underestimated. For patients no. 5 and no. 11 with the highest initial prediction errors the results of subsequent predictions from repetitive bone age assessments are shown. No. 5 had severe osteodystrophy, no. 11 was severely retarded in both height age and bone age. (From Gilli et al: Kidney Int, 24, Suppl 15:548, 1983.)

# MECHANISMS OF GROWTH RETARDATION IN RENAL INSUFFICIENCY

## Experimental Studies

Although some factors interfering with growth in children with progressive renal disease have been recognized, the pathogenesis of growth retardation in CRI is poorly understood. Recently a number of sophisticated animal studies have contributed to our understanding of growth failure in CRI.[73-78] Recent reviews have appeared on this subject.[7, 79]

In earlier studies it was difficult to produce a sufficient degree of chronic uremia experimentally which was comparable to the human situation. More recently, however, sustained CRI with a GFR below 20% of normal has been produced by combined resection and irradiation of the renal parenchyma in the rat.[77, 78]

It should be emphasized that the most widely used animal model, the *young rat* made chronically uremic by *subtotal nephrectomy*, only partially reflects the situation of the growing child suffering from CRI. This is primarily due to the different biological properties of young rats compared to children: relative immaturity, absent epiphyseal closure, absence of Haversian systems in bone, failure to require vitamin D in presence of an optimal intake of calcium and phosphorus, and incomplete catch-up growth following correction of malnutrition in the first 3 months of life. In addition, the multiple morphologic and functional derangements observed in congenital and acquired nephropathies of man are not mimicked by acute reduction in renal mass. In spite of these disadvantages, experimental uremia is an important research tool for investigating the pathophysiology of growth failure in children with CRI.[79]

## Disturbances of Water and Electrolyte Metabolism

Disturbances of water and mineral metabolism are factors proposed as being responsible for growth retardation in CRI.[80] They appear to be important primarily in slowly progressive congenital and hereditary nephropathies characterized by the tubular loss of water, electrolytes, and bicarbonate with resultant alterations of the *milieu intérieur*. In more advanced stages of CRI these losses become less important.

*Hyposthenuria* with resulting hyperosmolality of blood is said to be responsible for growth retardation in young patients with nephrogenic diabetes insipidus. Diminished capacity to concentrate the urine may also contribute to growth failure in some disorders associated with CRI, especially in those affecting the distal tubules such as juvenile nephronophthisis. The correction of hyperosmolality by fluid administration in young children with diabetes insipidus leads to dramatic improvement in growth.[81]

*Depletion of electrolytes* which are important for homeostasis is another mechanism responsible for growth retardation in CRI. Renal *potassium loss* is a frequent finding in congenital tubular disorders, notably in Bartter's syndrome.[82] It is possible that potassium loss in patients with CRI, especially with primary tubular involvement, is contributing to growth retardation. In a study by Weber et al mean total body potassium in uremic children was found to be 17% below that of healthy children with the same body size.[83] The results of this study could not determine if the reduced total body potassium was primarily due to increased potassium loss or a secondary phenomenon, simply reflecting a decrease in lean body mass.

*Salt wasting* in some renal disorders may contribute to growth failure. The mechanism of this effect is not clear but may be related to the physiologic need for sodium chloride retention during growth of connective tissue and cartilage, a process which is inhibited by extracellular volume contraction.

The role of *phosphate* in skeletal growth is evident from the accelerated growth seen in patients with familial vitamin D–resistant rickets following phosphate supplementation. Phosphorus depletion occurs in other primary tubular disorders (e.g., in cystinosis). It is sometimes observed in patients treated with excessive amounts of antacids during dialysis and is seen consequent to a phosphate leak post-transplantation.

*Calcium deficiency* is possibly responsible for growth retardation in children with idiopathic hypercalciuria and may also contribute to the development of renal osteodystrophy in children with CRI who have a reduced intestinal absorption of calcium. Mehls and Ritz have demonstrated that in uremic rats—

but not in control animals—dietary calcium is a rate-limiting growth factor.[79]

*Metabolic acidosis* was considered to be an important factor for growth failure in azotemic children by West and Smith.[80] The role of acidosis is exemplified by children with primary renal tubular acidosis, in whom catch-up growth occurs after adequate treatment with bicarbonate.[84] It was suggested that hypophosphatemia in these patients may be a causative factor for growth retardation.[85] The role of acidosis in children with CRI and growth failure is difficult to evaluate. Experimental studies indicate that the main mechanisms for this effect are the accompanying depletion of cations[5] and the inhibition of $1,25(OH)_2D_3$ production by low pH.[86] Uremic rats made acidotic by supplementation with HCl showed a diminished growth rate when compared with nonacidotic animals.[5] It should be emphasized that in some children with CRI growth is completely normal in the presence of chronic acidosis.[3] The same applies to some children without a primary kidney disorder, in whom chronic acidosis is produced by exogenous dietary hydrogen ion overload, e.g., in phenylketonuria.[87]

## Osteodystrophy (See Chapter 17)

Uremic bone disease has been suggested as an important cause for stunting in children with CRI in the absence of adequate treatment by vitamin D, calcium supplements, and phosphate binders. At present, osteodystrophy is usually preventable and, therefore, bone disease should play only a minor role in growth failure.

Two *mechanisms* are possible to explain the growth retardation in children with renal osteodystrophy: abnormal vitamin D metabolism and secondary hyperparathyroidism. *Vitamin D* levels may be deficient or active vitamin D metabolites may be lost in the urine. The administration of a vitamin D analogue may have a favorable effect on growth rate in some children with moderate degrees of CRI and severe bone disease.[88, 89] This effect may be related either to improvement in bone deformities or to a real increase in bone mass and length. It is controversial if growth is promoted by vitamin D or analogues in children with advanced CRI. Chesney et al have suggested that growth is improved by administration of $1,25(OH)_2D_3$ in uremic children unresponsive to vitamin D.[90]

Similar results were reported by Chan et al,[91] but several other groups were unable to confirm these observations.[47, 88, 89, 92] Growth of uremic rats was equally improved but not normalized by both vitamin D and $1,25(OH)_2D_3$.[89]

It is probable that *hyperparathyroidism* contributes to growth retardation by destroying the architecture of the growth zone. After parathyroidectomy some children with CRI demonstrate accelerated growth, which, however, does not persist.[47] Experimental data indicate that parathormone stimulates cell proliferation in growth cartilage.[88] This could explain the frequent association of growth retardation in children with primary hypoparathyroidism.

*Skeletal maturation* is retarded in children with CRI either receiving conservative treatment or undergoing dialysis.[3, 32, 93] The mean bone age was similar to the height age in most reported series of children with CRI.[32, 35, 45, 47] Controversy exists as to the degree of further bone maturation which occurs both before and after initiating dialysis. Some authors have observed that the bone age increases at a rate similar to that of the height age,[32, 35, 45, 47] and others have reported a relatively higher rate of skeletal maturation, thereby leading to a decrease of the future growth potential.[36, 94]

The degree to which osteodystrophy contributes to retardation of skeletal maturation is unclear. Studies suggested that during vitamin D therapy growth potential may improve by normalization of the relationship between statural height and bone maturation.[7, 47] Long-term studies are required before this concept can be validated.

## Hormonal Disturbances

A number of hormonal alterations present in uremia have been implicated as the cause of growth retardation in children with CRI; however, a precise role has not been established. Immunoreactive plasma *growth hormone* levels have been repeatedly found to be increased in uremic subjects.[95] In contrast plasma *somatomedin* activity has been reported to be decreased in some pediatric patients with CRI when measured by bioassay[53, 56] and protein-binding assay, but not when measured by radioreceptor assay.[96] During hemodialysis somatomedin activity has been shown to increase, possibly as a result of the removal of low molecular weight inhibitors.[96] Following transplantation, somatomedin activity increases to normal levels and has been correlated with an improved growth rate.[70] At present no conclusive role of somatomedin activity for growth in children with CRI has been delineated.[97] Experimental data have shown that uremic rats grow better after injections of superphysiological doses of porcine growth hormone.[79] These data indicate that end-organ responsiveness should be considered in interpreting the above clinical studies on somatomedin activity in children with CRI.

Abnormalities of *thyroid* function, which could contribute to growth retardation in children, have been reported in patients with CRI.[95] However, definite thyroid insufficiency is rare, occurring primarily in children with cystinosis. No data are available to indicate that administration of thyroid hormone stimulates growth in uremic children.

The rapid increase in *testosterone* production contributes substantially to the sharp increase in growth velocity during puberty. In boys with CRI plasma testosterone levels before and after stimulation with human chorionic gonadotropin (HCG) were found to be low prior to and during puberty.[98, 99] It must be assumed that insufficient androgen production is at least partially responsible for the flat and delayed pubertal growth spurt observed in most of these children. It remains speculative if similar changes in production of estrogens interfere with growth in girls with CRI.

## Uremic Toxins

Many metabolic and hormonal changes observed in CRI are related to the accumulation of waste products. It is possible that these waste products directly influence body growth. Early investigators indicated that the degree of azotemia did not correlate with the growth rate.[80, 100] Betts and Magrath[94] reported that growth is usually reduced when the GFR declines to values below 25 ml/min/1.73 m². The exact relationship between GFR and growth retardation is, however, not well established. In the recent study by Kleinknecht et al of nondialyzed children, height loss was less in children when the GFR was greater than 25 ml/min/1.73 m² than in those with a GFR < 12 ml/min/1.73 m², although the difference was not significant.[35] The au-

thors concluded that reduction of GFR per se is not a primary cause for subnormal growth velocity as long as the GFR is > 5 ml/min/1.73 m².

In children treated by regular dialysis an inverse correlation was reported between growth velocity and the levels of various *uremic waste products*, e.g., predialysis serum levels of creatinine, uric acid, and phosphorus.[38, 47] Other studies have failed to observe such a relationship.[37, 46] None of the substances measured have been shown to cause growth retardation directly; however, high plasma levels could indicate the presence of unknown substances accumulating in uremia which would have a direct toxic effect on growth.

*Experimental data* indicate that the degree of renal dysfunction is critical in the pathogenesis of growth retardation in uremic rats compared to pair-fed control rats.[74, 75, 79] Recent experiments have revealed that spermine, a substance that accumulates in uremic serum, possibly has a specific toxic effect. High concentrations of spermine were shown to inhibit incorporation of ³H-thymidine into growth cartilage of uremic rats.[79] Since spermine accumulates in uremic man, it could have a role in the production of growth retardation in children with CRI.

## Energy and Protein Malnutrition

It has been generally accepted that nutritional factors are important in the pathogenesis of the growth failure in uremic children.[1, 4, 5, 34] Lack of appetite is frequent and can be attributed to a number of factors: altered taste perception, polydipsia, hypertension, and psychological stress. Deficient energy and protein intake is frequently observed in children with CRI, whether in the preterminal stage or with ESRD.[4, 100, 101–104] Children with advanced CRI are in negative nitrogen balance if calorie and protein intake is reduced minimally below the rates recommended for normal children.[105]

A number of authors have emphasized the similarity between the clinical and biochemical changes seen in *calorie malnutrition* and those seen in CRI. Both clinical states are accompanied by growth retardation. Among the common features of the two conditions are the diminished weight-to-height ratio in patients with significantly stunted growth,[4, 43, 80, 102, 104] the reduction in body cell mass,[83, 104, 106] and evidence of protein depletion, as indicated by a decreased ratio of essential-to-nonessential amino acids. It should be stressed that in uremia no study has demonstrated that these findings are the direct result of reduced calorie or protein intake.[79]

In order to study this problem further a number of *experiments* have been undertaken in growing uremic animals. Rats with advanced (but not with moderate) degrees of uremia grow less than pair-fed controls.[75, 77, 78, 107] In addition, a correlation has been found between growth retardation and reduced overall intake.[73] Despite these detailed studies, the importance of dietary intake in producing the growth retardation in children with CRI remains unanswered. This question would only be answered in experimental animals by providing uremic animals with an energy intake above that spontaneously consumed; however, this poses methodological problems.[79]

It has been suggested that with uremia the requirements of *energy and protein for growth are increased*.[73] At a given protein intake conversion to body protein is less efficient in uremic than in pair-fed control animals.[77, 79] Both decreased synthesis and increased catabolism of protein appear to contribute to this reduced gain in body protein in uremic animals.[108] The efficiency by which dietary protein is converted into body protein declines as the protein intake increases, and at the same time more protein is used as a source of energy.[79] In the normal rat protein intake should not exceed 17% of total calorie intake in order to guarantee an optimal degree of anabolism; however, it is not known if this relationship is maintained in uremic animals. Obviously, the answer to this question would have an impact on the dietary recommendations required for growth-retarded children with CRI.

Studies in humans have been forced to evaluate the relationship between energy and protein intake and growth by methods that are unsatisfactory because of the practical difficulties of performing long-term balance studies in chronic diseases. In 1972 Simmons et al reported an increase of growth velocity in a few children undergoing regular dialysis after receiving daily *energy supplements*.[109] This study, which has been criticized because of the short periods of dietary assessments, resulted in the widespread use of additional oral supply of energy in uremic children. Although some authors have shown some improvement of growth velocity with calorie supplements in dialyzed children,[37] others were less optimistic. Betts et al pointed out the difficulties of maintaining a high energy intake in children with CRF and did not observe a definite increase of growth rate when supplementation was possible.[110] Kleinknecht et al reported that overall calorie and protein intake were similar in dialyzed children during periods of good and poor growth. However, in a select group of 8 children the only nutritional or biochemical parameter found to be significantly different during these different growth periods was calorie intake (13% higher during periods of good growth). In our own experience with dialyzed and nondialyzed children, some of whom were treated with energy supplements, we found no correlation between calorie intake and growth rate (Fig. 19–7.)[103] Even if nasogastric hyperalimentation was given to young children, growth did not improve, but was followed by an increase in the weight/height ratio, indicating that the energy was utilized for adipose tissue formation rather than for an increase in height.[111] Therefore, we believe that the current clinical studies do not allow the conclusion that energy intake is a prominent factor contributing to the growth failure of children with CRI unless obvious signs of malnutrition are present.

It is less clear to what extent *protein intake* contributes to growth in children with CRI. Protein requirements for normal children are in dispute.[4] Clear-cut signs of protein malnutrition are rare in children with CRI except when persistent protein losses occur. Kleinknecht et al found that a moderate restriction of protein intake to 75% of the RDA was associated with better growth than in children with a higher intake.[47] In our patients with CRI we weighed all foods given during a 5- to-7-day period and found the mean protein intake to be around 100% of RDA both in children in the preterminal stage and in those on dialysis. A correlation between protein intake and growth rate was not observed.[103] In the multicentric study reported by EDTA the one-year growth rate was significantly less in prepubertal children with unrestricted protein intake compared to children receiving 100% of RDA (2.6 vs. 4.3 cm/yr), while that of patients with protein restriction was 3.2 cm/yr.[46] It should be emphasized that this study was not based on exact dietary proto-

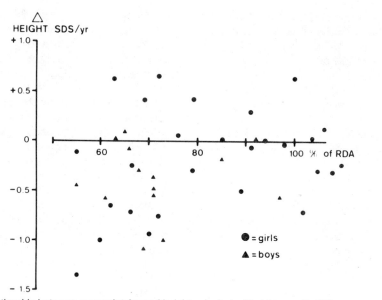

**Figure 19–7.** Relationship between energy intake and height velocity in 43 children with CRI on conservative treatment and on regular hemodialysis. The assessment of dietary intake was based on dietary protocols over 5 to 7 days. The minimal period for calculating corresponding growth rates was 12 months. (From Mehls et al: Third International Congress on Nutrition and Metabolism in Renal Disease, Marseille, 1982.)

cols and, therefore, the results may be invalid.

At present precise recommendations cannot be given regarding protein and amino acid requirements in uremic children necessary for promoting growth. It is important to consider not only the degree of anabolism but also the effect on kidney function when altering the protein intake in children with CRI. Animal experiments have shown that protein restriction has a beneficial effect on the degree of deterioration of renal function and is associated with improved growth rates.[75] Similar trials in children are not available. Optimal growth in children with CRI probably requires the provision of protein intake in the range allowed for normal children (100% RDA) with a preference for high quality proteins containing a high proportion (about 50%) of essential amino acids. A lower intake will produce malnutrition and an excess will provoke uremic toxicity. Both clinical experience[4] and experimental data[112] suggest that protein intake should be carefully monitored and adjusted so that the total calorie intake will be similar to that proposed for healthy children (2 gm protein per 100 kcal of total diet).

## Other Disturbances

Besides the accumulation of uremic toxins and protein-energy malnutrition, further metabolic alterations have been considered as possible growth-depressing factors in uremia. Most of these are related to the profound changes in carbohydrate, lipid, protein, and trace element metabolism present in uremia. *Disturbed utilization of nutrients* by enzymatic inhibition or by hormonal changes may also impact on skeletal growth. Hypertension and hypoxia secondary to chronic anemia may be other growth-depressing factors, the latter either by causing loss of appetite or by reducing aerobic metabolism. Finally, the association between severe growth failure and progressive encephalopathy must be mentioned.[113]

## THERAPEUTIC IMPLICATIONS

Since the etiologic factors leading to growth retardation in children with CRI are hard to define, it is difficult to propose a successful treatment. No specific therapeutic intervention assures normal growth in CRI.[114] From the initial stage of CRI one should aim at eliminating all the known causes of growth failure. *Factors capable of responding to therapy* include metabolic acidosis, electrolyte depletion, hyposthenuria, osteodystrophy, chronic infection, and protein-calorie malnutrition. Correction of acidosis, electrolyte loss, and hyperosmolality in congenital nephropathies are probably essential for promoting normal growth in the critical period of the *first two years of life*. In the presence of poor calorie intake, transient parenteral nutrition, especially in infants, may possibly improve growth, but for practical reasons such therapy is difficult to continue over longer periods of time. Because forced feeding by tube may lead to poor appetite responses in later life, this technique should be used in young anorectic children only when other approaches fail.

Other means should be sought to *combat anorexia*. In many children appetite can be improved by removing unacccptable (e.g., salt-free) diets and by adapting the nutritional demands to the child's taste. In advanced CRI appetite is often compromised by the administration of calcium salts and phosphate binders. For patients with CRI due to inherited renal tubular disorders therapeutic guidelines have been given elsewhere.[115] In any case, the help of a capable dietitian is advantageous.

In the terminal stage of CRI, *adequate dialysis therapy* should not be delayed. It seems, however, that the choice of dialysis strategy does not affect future growth. Increasing dialysis time does not appear to improve the growth rate. The preservation of an optimal nutritional state, reduction in the accumulation of waste products, absence of osteodystrophy, and limitation of severe cardiovascular impairment are the most important factors facilitating optimal growth. *Caloric supplements* are indicated only when a deficiency of energy is present. Oral amino acid supplements may be indicated in the presence of obvious protein losses not replaced by oral intake. *Anabolic steroids* have rarely been used in children with CRI because of their well-known risks. A recent study demonstrated improvement in growth velocity in boys on regular dialysis therapy without accelerating bone maturation with anabolic steroid therapy.[116] The long-term effect in pediatric patients remains to be defined.

The importance of specialized *pediatric care* for promoting growth in dialyzed children is emphasized by the results collected by the EDTA. Prepubertal children treated in specialized pediatric centers had a significantly higher growth rate than those treated in nonspecialized (adult) centers.[43]

The desire for optimal growth is one of the most important reasons for promoting *early transplantation* in children with ESRD. In order to prevent further growth retardation in transplant patients it seems important to *reduce the dosage of glucocorticoids* rapidly after grafting and to change from a daily to an alternate-day schedule as early as possible. Data from the EDTA Registry have shown that from 1976 to 1981 the mean one-year growth rate in prepubertal children has significantly increased after transplantation (from 3.5 to 4.7 cm/yr). This improvement is probably related to a reduction in steroid dosage as well as improved graft function.[46] At the same time, mean growth in a similar group of children treated by dialysis remains unchanged (3.0 cm/yr in 1981). Future studies are required to determine if replacement of steroids by other immunosuppressive agents, e.g., cyclosporin A, leads to improved growth performance in children receiving transplants.

It should be stressed that the results of a given treatment in a child with CRI can be evaluated only on the basis of *frequent and precise recordings* of body height and skeletal maturity, followed by a careful assessment of data. Final evaluation of any therapeutic strategy requires the serial evaluation of a representative group of children until adult height is reached.

In the management of children with growth retardation, *psychosocial factors* should not be neglected. The importance attributed to the attainment of normal body height varies among patients and depends on the severity of and stress by other manifestations of kidney disease and on the presence of achievements in school, profession, and family life. In addition, the social and racial background should be considered. It must be questioned if reaching "normal height" should invariably be regarded as a primary goal in such patients.

## REFERENCES

1. Chantler C, Holliday MA: Growth in children with renal disease with particular reference to the effects of calorie malnutrition: A review. Clin Nephrol 1:230, 1973.
2. Lewy JE, New MI: Growth in children with renal failure. Am J Med 58:65, 1975.
3. Stickler GB: Growth failure in renal disease. Pediatr Clin North Am 23:885, 1976.
4. Holliday MA: Growth retardation in children with renal disease. *In*: Edelmann CM Jr (ed), Pediatric Kidney Disease, Vol 1. Boston, Little, Brown Co, 1978, p 331.
5. Mehls O, Ritz E, Gilli G, Kreusser W: Growth in renal failure. Nephron 21:237, 1978.
6. Schärer K: Growth in children with chronic renal failure. Kidney Int 13 (Suppl 8):68, 1978.

7. Broyer M: Growth in children with renal insufficiency. Pediatr Clin North Am 29:991, 1982.

8. Holliday MA, Chantler C, Potter DE (eds): Symposium on metabolism and growth in children with kidney disease. Kidney Int 14:299, 1978.

9. Potter DE, Broyer M, Chantler C, et al: Measurement of growth in children with renal insufficiency. Kidney Int 14:378, 1978.

10. Cameron N: The methods of auxological anthropometry. In: Falkner F, Tanner JM (eds), Human Growth, Vol. 2. London, Bailliere Tindall, 1978, p 35.

11. Weiner JS, Lourie JA: Practical Human Biology. London, Academic Press, 1981.

12. Roche AF: Growth assessment in abnormal children. Kidney Int 14:369, 1978.

13. Gurney JM, Jelliffe DB: Arm anthropometry in nutritional assessment: Nomogram for rapid calculation of muscle circumference and cross-sectional muscle and fat areas. Am J Clin Nutr 26:912, 1973.

14. Frisancho AR: Triceps skinfold and upper arm muscle size norms for assessment of nutritional status. Am J Clin Nutr 27:1058, 1974.

15. Tanner JM: Growth at Adolescence. Oxford, Blackwell, 1962.

16. Zachmann M, Prader A, Kind HP, et al: Testicular volume during adolescence: cross-sectional and longitudinal studies. Helv Paediatr Acta 29:61, 1974.

17. Tanner JM, Whitehouse RH, Marshall WA, et al: Assessment of Skeletal Maturity and Prediction of Adult Height (TW 2 Method). London, Academic Press, 1975.

18. Greulich WW, Pyle SI: Radiographic Atlas of Skeletal Development of the Hand and Wrist, 2nd edition. Stanford CA, Stanford University Press, 1959.

19. Roche AF: Predicting Adult Stature for Individuals. Basle, Karger, 1975.

20. Roche AF, Wainer H, Thissen D: Skeletal Maturity: the Knee Joint as a Biological Indicator. New York, Plenum Medical Books Co, 1975, p 91.

21. Hamill PVV: NCHS growth curves for children, birth–18 years, United States DHEW Publication No (PHS) 78–1960. Hyattsville, US Department of Health, Education, and Welfare, 1977.

22. Tanner JM, Whitehouse RH, Takaishi M: Standards from birth to puberty for height, weight, height velocity and weight velocity. Arch Dis Child 41:454, 631, 1966.

23. Tanner JM, Whitehouse RH: Clinical longitudinal standards for height, weight, height velocity, weight velocity and stages of puberty. Arch Dis Child 51:170, 1976.

24. Prader, A, Issler C, Molinari L, et al: Physical growth in Swiss children from birth to 20 years of age. Helv Paediatr Acta (in press).

25. Neumann CG: Reference data. In: Jelliffe DB, Jelliffe EFP (eds): Nutrition and Growth. New York/London, Plenum Press, 1979, p 299.

26. Prader A, Tanner JM, von Harnack GA: Catch-up growth following illness or starvation—An example of developmental canalization in man. J Pediatr 62:646, 1963.

27. Tanner JM: Catch-up growth in man. Br Med Bull 37:233, 1981.

28. Gilli G, Mehls O, Wallstein B, et al: Prediction of adult height in children with chronic renal insufficiency. Kidney Int 24(Suppl 15):48, 1983.

29. Gilli G: Therapie der Wachstumsstörung bei chronischer Niereninsuffizienz. Mschr Kinderheilk 123:772, 1975.

30. Schärer K, Jura E, Mehls O: Long-term growth of children with idiopathic nephrotic syndrome. Pediatr Res 14:1001, 1980 (Abstract).

31. Schärer K, Chantler C, Brunner FP, et al: Combined report on regular dialysis and transplantation of children in Europe, 1974. Proc Eur Dial Transplant Assoc 12:65, 1975.

32. Schärer K, Chantler C, Brunner FP, et al: Combined report on regular dialysis and transplantation of children in Europe, 1975. Proc Eur Dial Transplant Assoc 13:59, 1976.

33. Broyer M, Donckerwolcke RA, Brunner FP, et al: Combined report on regular dialysis and transplantation of children in Europe, 1980. Proc Eur Dial Transplant Assoc 18:60, 1981.

34. Betts PR, Magrath G: Growth pattern and dietary intake of children with chronic renal insufficiency. Br Med J 2:189, 1974.

35. Kleinknecht C, Broyer M, Huot D, et al: Growth and development of non-dialysed children with chronic renal failure. Kidney Int 24(Suppl 15):40, 1983.

36. Broyer M, Kleinknecht C, Loirat C, et al: Growth in children treated with long-term hemodialysis. J Pediatr 84:642, 1974.

37. Chantler C, El-Bishti M, Cox BD, et al: Growth in children with chronic renal failure. Melsungen Med Mitt 50 (Suppl 2):57, 1976.

38. Degoulet P, Lauwers E, Aime F, et al: Programme dialyse-informatique. Hémodialyse chez l'enfant. J Urol Néphrol 84:895, 1978.

39. Gusmano R, Gilli G, Perfumo F: Valutazione critica dei risultati del trattamento emodialitico in età pediatrica. Minerva Nefrol 19:60, 1972.

40. Bulla M: Stoffwechsel- und Wachstumsstörung bei chronischer Niereninsuffizienz des Kindes. Habilitationsschrift, Köln, 1982.

41. Chantler, C, Schärer K, Gilli, G, et al: Dialysis and renal transplantation of children in Europe, 1975. Acta Paediatr Scand 67:5, 1978.

42. Chantler C, Donckerwolcke RA, Brunner FP, et al: Combined report on regular dialysis and transplantation of children in Europe, 1976. Proc Eur Dial Transplant Assoc 14:70, 1977.

43. Donckerwolcke RA, Chantler C, Brunner FP, et al: Combined report on regular dialysis and transplantation of children in Europe, 1977. Proc Eur Dial Transplant Assoc 15:77, 1978.

44. Chantler C, Donckerwolcke RA, Brunner FP, et al: Combined report on regular dialysis and transplantation of children in Europe, 1978. Proc Eur Dial Transplant Assoc 16:74, 1979.

45. Donckerwolcke RA, Chantler C, Broyer M, et al: Combined report on regular dialysis and transplantation of children in Europe, 1979. Proc Eur Dial Transplant Assoc 17:87, 1980.

46. Donckerwolcke RA, Broyer M, Brunner FP, et al: Combined report on regular dialysis and transplantation of children in Europe, XI, 1981. Proc Eur Dial Transplant Assoc 19:61, 1982.

47. Kleinknecht C, Broyer M, Gagnadoux MF, et al: Growth in children treated with long-term dialysis. A study of 76 patients. Adv Nephrol 9:133, 1980.

48. Balfe JW: Metabolic effects of CAPD in the child. Perit Dial Bull 3(Suppl):21, 1983.

49. Kohout EC: Growth in children with end-stage

renal disease treated with continuous ambulatory peritoneal dialysis for at least one year. Perit Dial Bull 2:159, 1982.

50. Salusky IB, Kopple JD, Fine RN: Continuous ambulatory peritoneal dialysis (CAPD) in pediatric patients—20 month experience. Kidney Int 24(Suppl 15):101, 1983.

51. De Santo NG, Capodicasa G, Gilli G, et al: Metabolic aspects of continuous ambulatory peritoneal dialysis with reference to energy-protein input and growth. Int J Pediatr Nephrol 3:279, 1982.

52. Grushkin CM, Fine RN: Growth in children and adolescents following renal transplantation. Am J Dis Child 121:514, 1973.

53. Saenger P, Wiedemann E, Schwartz E, et al: Somatomedin and growth after renal transplantation. Pediatr Res 8:163, 1974.

54. Potter DE, Holliday MA, Wilson CJ, et al: Alternate day steroids in children after renal transplantation. Transplant Proc 7:79, 1975.

55. Hoda Q, Hasinoff DJ, Arbus GS: Growth following renal transplantation in children and adolescents. Clin Nephrol 3:6, 1975.

56. Pennisi AJ, Costin C, Phillips LS, et al: Linear growth in long-term renal allograft recipients. Clin Nephrol 8:415, 1977.

57. Fine RN, Malekzadeh MH, Pennisi AJ, et al: Long-term results of renal transplantation in children. Pediatrics 61:641, 1978.

58. Lilly JR, Giles G, Hurwitz R: Renal homotransplantation in children. Pediatrics 47:548, 1971.

59. De Shazo CV, Simmons PL, Bernstein DM, et al: Results of renal transplantation in 100 children. Surgery 76:461, 1974.

60. Lawson RK, Murphy JB, Talwalkar YB: Special problems in pediatric renal transplantation. Urol Clin North Am 3:667, 1976.

61. Martin LW, McEnery PT, Rosenkrantz JG, et al: Renal homotransplantation in children. J Pediatr Surg 14:571, 1979.

62. Offner G, Brandis M, Brodehl J, et al: Nierentransplantation bei Kindern in Hannover, 1970–1977. Dtsch Med Wochenschr 104:393, 1979.

63. Chantler C, Carter JE, Bewick M, et al: 10 years' experience with regular haemodialysis and renal transplantation. Arch Dis Child 55:435, 1980.

64. Broyer M, Gagnadoux MF, Beurton D, Pascal B: La transplantation rénale chez l'enfant. 26 ème Congrès des pédiatres de langue francaise, Toulouse, 1981, Vol 2, p 567.

65. Ingelfinger JR, Grupe WE, Harmon WE, et al: Growth acceleration following renal transplantation in children less than 7 years of age. Pediatrics 68:255, 1981.

66. Rizzoni G, Malekzadeh MH, Pennisi AJ, et al: Renal transplantation in children less than 5 years of age. Arch Dis Child 55:523, 1980.

67. Miller LC, Bock GH, Lum CT, et al: Transplantation of the adult kidney into the very small child: long-term outcome. J Pediatr 100:675, 1982.

68. Schärer K, Mehls O, Dreikorn K, et al: Nierentransplantation bei Kindern und Jungendlichen. Nieren- und Hochdruckrankh 12:1, 1983.

69. Bosque M, Munian A, Bewick M, et al: Growth after renal transplants. Arch Dis Child 58:110, 1983.

70. Pennisi AJ, Costin C, Phillips LS, et al: Somatomedin and growth hormone studies in pediatric renal allograft recipients who receive daily prednisone. Am J Dis Child 133:950, 1979.

71. Gilli G, Mehls O, Fischer W, Schärer K: Final height of children with chronic renal failure. Pediatr Res 14:1015, 1980 (Abstract).

72. Chantler C, Broyer M, Donckerwolcke RA, et al: Growth and rehabilitation of long-term survivors of treatment for end-stage renal failure in childhood. Proc Eur Dial Transplant Assoc 18:329, 1981.

73. Chantler C, Lieberman E, Holliday MA: A rat model for the study of growth failure in uremia. Pediatr Res 8:109, 1974.

74. Diaz M, Kleinknecht, Broyer M: Growth in experimental renal failure: Role of calorie and amino acid intake. Kidney Int 8:349, 1975.

75. Kleinknecht C, Salusky I, Broyer, M, Gubler MC: Effect of various protein diets on growth, renal function and survival of uremic rats. Kidney Int 15:534, 1979.

76. Mehls O, Ritz E, Gilli G, et al: Skeletal changes and growth in experimental uremia. Nephron 18:288, 1977.

77. Mehls O, Ritz E, Gilli G, et al: Nitrogen metabolism and growth in experimental uremia. Int J Pediatr Nephrol 1:34, 1980.

78. Schalch DS, Burstein PJ, Tewel SJ, et al: The effect of renal impairment on growth in the rat: relationship to malnutrition and serum somatomedin levels. Endocrinology 108:1653, 1981.

79. Mehls O, Ritz E: Skeletal growth in experimental uremia. Kidney Int 24(Suppl 15):53, 1983.

80. West CD, Smith WC: An attempt to elucidate the cause of growth retardation in renal disease. Am J Dis Child 91:460, 1956.

81. Vest M, Talbot NB, Crawford JD: Hypocaloric dwarfism and hydronephrosis in diabetes insipidus. Am J Dis Child 105:175, 1963.

82. Simopoulos AP: Growth characteristics in patients with Bartter's syndrome. Nephron 23:130, 1979.

83. Weber HP, Michalk D, Rauh W, et al: Total body potassium in children with chronic renal failure. Int J Pediatr Nephrol 1:42, 1980.

84. McSherry E, Morris RC Jr: Attainment and maintenance of normal stature with alkali therapy in infants and children with classic renal tubular acidosis. J Clin Invest 61:509, 1978.

85. Harrison HE, Harrison HC: Disorders of Calcium and Phosphate Metabolism in Childhood and Adolescence. Philadelphia, WB Saunders Company, 1979.

86. Cunningham J, Avioli LV: Systemic acidosis and the bioactivation of vitamin D. In: Norman AW, Schaefer K, von Herrath D, Grigoleit HG (eds): Vitamin D, Chemical, Biochemical and Clinical Endocrinology of Calcium Metabolism. Berlin, New York, Walter de Gruyter, 1982, p 443.

87. Manz F, Schmidt H, Schärer K, Bickel H: Acid-base status in dietary treatment of phenylketonuria. Pediatr Res 11:1084, 1977.

88. Mehls O, Ritz E, Kreusser W, Krempien B: Renal osteodystrophy in children. Clin Endocrinol Metab 9:151, 1980.

89. Gilli G, Mehls O, Ritz E: Wirkung von Vitamin $D_3$ und 1.25(OH)$_2$D$_3$ auf das Wachstum bei Niereninsuffizienz. Nieren- und Hochdruckkrankh 10:259, 1981.

90. Chesney RW, Moorthy AV, Eismann JA: Increased

growth after long-term oral 1-α-25-vitamin $D_3$ in childhood renal osteodystrophy. N Engl J Med 298:238, 1978.

91. Chan JCM, Kodroff MB, Landwehr DM: Effects of 1,25-dihydroxy vitamin $D_3$ on renal function and growth in children with severe chronic renal failure. Pediatrics 68:559, 1981.

92. Bulla M, Delling G, Offermann G, et al: Renal bone disorders in children: Therapy with vitamin $D_3$ or 1.25-dihydroxycholecalciferol. Proc Eur Dial Transplant Assoc 16:644, 1979.

93. Johannsen A, Nielsen HE, Hansen HE: Bone maturation in children with chronic renal failure—Effect of 1-α-hydroxy vitamin D and renal transplantation. Acta Radiol (Diagn) 20:193, 1979.

94. Betts PR, White RHR: Growth potential and skeletal maturity in children with chronic renal insufficiency. Nephron 16:325, 1976.

95. Rauh W, Oertel PJ: Endocrine function in children with end-stage renal disease. *In*: Fine RN, Gruskin A (eds): End-stage Renal Disease in Children. Philadelphia, WB Saunders, 1984, Chap 21.

96. Spencer EM, Uthne K, Arnold W: Elevated somatomedin A by radioreceptor assay in children with growth retardation and chronic renal insufficiency. *In*: Giordano C, van Wyck JJ, Minuto F (eds): Somatomedin and Growth. New York, London, Academic Press, 1979, p 34.

97. Philips LS, Kopple JD: Circulating somatomedin activity and sulfate level in adults with normal and impaired renal function. Metabolism 30:1091, 1981.

98. Schärer K, Broyer M, Vecsei P, et al: Damage to testicular function in chronic renal failure of children. Proc Eur Dial Transplant Assoc 17:725, 1980.

99. Oertel PJ, Lichtwald K, Häfner S, et al: Hypothalamo-pituitary-gonadal axis in children with chronic renal failure. Kidney Int 24(Suppl 15):34, 1983.

100. Bergström WH, De Leon AS, van Gemund JJ: Growth aberrations in renal disease. Pediatr Clin North Am 11:563, 1964.

101. Schärer K: Spezielle Aspekte der Diättherapie der Niereninsuffizienz im Kindesalter. *In*: Canzler H (ed): Aktuelle Fragen der Ernährungstherapie in Nephrologie und Gastroenterologie. Stuttgart, G. Thieme, 1978, p 23.

102. Broyer M, Kleinknecht C, Gagnadoux MF, Dartois AM: Growth in uremic children. *In*: Strauss J (ed): Pediatric Nephrology, Vol 4. New York, Garland STPM Press, 1978, p 185.

103. Mehls O, Gilli G, Schärer K: Analysis of growth and food intake in uremic children. Third International Congress on Nutrition and Metabolism in Renal Disease, Marseille, 1982 (Abstract).

104. Jones RWA, Rigden SP, Barratt TM, Chantler C: The effects of chronic renal failure in infancy on growth, nutritional status and body composition. Pediatr Res 16:784, 1982.

105. Alatas H, Schärer K: Wirkungen von L-Histidin auf die Stickstoffbilanz bei Kindern mit chronischer Niereninsuffizienz. Nieren- und Hochdruckkrankh 2:67, 1975.

106. El-Bishti M, Murke J, Gill D: Body composition in children on regular hemodialysis. Clin Nephrol 15:53, 1981.

107. Wang M, Vyhmeister I, Kopple JD, Swendseid ME: Effect of protein intake on weight gain and plasma amino acid levels in experimental uremia. Am J Physiol 230:122, 1976.

108. Harter HR, Birge SJ, Martin KJ, et al: The effects of vitamin D metabolites on protein catabolism of muscle from uremic rats. Kidney Int 23:465, 1983.

109. Simmons JM, Wilson CJ, Potter DE, Holliday MA: Relation of calorie deficiency to growth failure in children on hemodialysis and the growth response to calorie supplementation. N Engl J Med 285:653, 1971.

110. Betts PR, Magrath G, White RHR: Role of dietary energy supplementation in growth of children with chronic renal insufficiency. Br Med J 1:416, 1977.

111. Guillot M, Broyer M, Cathelineau L: Nutrition entérale a débit constant en néphrologie pédiatrique. Arch. Franc Péd 37:497, 1980.

112. Abitbol C, Jean G, Broyer M: Urea synthesis in moderate experimental uremia. Kidney Int 19:648, 1981.

113. Rotundo A, Nevins TE, Lipton H, et al: Progressive encephalopathy in children with chronic renal insufficiency. Kidney Int 21:486, 1982.

114. Fine RN: Can growth retardation in renal failure be influenced? Controversies in Nephrology 1:346, 1980.

115. Manz F, Schärer K: Long-term management of inherited renal tubular disorders. Klin Wochenschr 60:1115, 1982.

116. Jones RWA, El-Bishti M, Bloom SR, et al: The effects of anabolic steroids on growth, body composition and metabolism in boys with chronic renal failure on regular hemodialysis. J Pediatr 97:559, 1980.

# 20

# Sexual Maturation in Children with Renal Insufficiency: Response to Dialysis and Transplantation*

*Frank G. Boineau, M.D.*
*John E. Lewy, M.D.*

## CHARACTERIZATION OF SEXUAL MATURATION IN CHILDREN WITH RENAL INSUFFICIENCY

Delayed sexual maturation is a common complication in children with chronic renal disease and renal insufficiency. As renal insufficiency advances and end stage renal disease (ESRD) develops, the problem becomes more severe. Both hemodialysis and peritoneal dialysis do not alter the events which retard sexual maturation.[1,2,3] Renal transplantation usually restores normal sexual maturation, provided the maintenance dose of glucocorticoids is low and renal graft function is good.[2,4]

### Normal Pubertal Development

Puberty is characterized by an increase in linear growth rate and the appearance of secondary sexual characteristics. The increase in linear growth rate and somatic changes actually antedate the appearance of secondary sex characteristics by a few years. Thus, sexual maturation is a considerably longer process than the period of visible changes induced by marked increments in gonadal hormones.

The changes in growth during puberty are, of course, most impressively reflected by increments in height and weight. The age of initiation of the adolescent growth spurt precedes the onset of secondary sex characteristics by approximately one year in boys and girls. The first sign of pubertal development in boys (enlargement of testicular size) occurs only about six months later than the first change in girls, which is usually breast development (Table 20–1). Thus, the timing of the onset of the pubertal process may be similar for boys and girls, in contrast to the progressive development of secondary sexual characterization. Pubic hair, for instance, appears about 1.5 years later in boys than in

Table 20–1. PATTERNS OF PUBERTAL DEVELOPMENT IN BOYS AND GIRLS

| Pubertal Event | Mean Age of Onset* | |
|---|---|---|
| | *Boys* | *Girls* |
| Breast development | — | 11.2 |
| Testicular enlargement | 11.6 | — |
| Pubic hair development | 13.4 | 11.7 |
| Peak height velocity | 14.1 | 12.1 |
| Menarche | — | 13.5 |
| Adult pubic hair configuration | 15.2 | 14.4 |
| Adult-type breast | — | 15.3 |

*SD for each event is approximately 1 year. Data based on British children. Standards for American children are 6 to 12 months earlier for girls and 2 to 6 months earlier for boys. (From Marshall and Tanner: Arch Dis Child 44:291, 1969; 45:13, 1970; adapted from Reference 5.)

*The authors wish to thank Ms. Kate de Vaux for assistance in preparing this manuscript.

girls, and peak height velocity is reached almost two years later in boys than in girls.

Although the secretory products of the hypothalamic-pituitary-gonadal axis are the primary modulators of the somatic changes that appear during puberty, other hormones also play a role. Both growth hormone and thyroxine must be present in normal amounts for sexual maturation to occur. Adrenal androgen production also increases before pubertal activation of gonadal hormone secretion. Although adrenal androgens are not required for the pubertal growth spurt, they have an effect on the development of pubic and axillary hair.

Serum levels of gonadal hormones and pituitary gonadotropins show a progressive rise throughout pubertal development. However, the degree of somatic development and the serum level of the responsible sex hormone do not always correspond.[5]

## Somatic Changes in Children with ESRD

A recent study of growth of children on long-term dialysis discusses the delayed somatic changes of pubertal age children with ESRD. Thirty-five patients who had reached pubertal age, which for girls was over 11 years and for boys over 13 years, were closely followed for more than one year after initiation of dialysis. Of these 35 early adolescents, 7 boys and 5 girls had signs of pubertal development. Bone maturation was documented in 15 boys and 12 girls. In 8 boys and 8 girls bone maturation remained below 13 years for boys and 11 years for girls during the period of observation.[1]

Pubertal growth was analyzed in 7 boys and 4 girls, whose bone maturation was greater than 13 years for boys and 11 years for girls. Ten exhibited an accelerated growth rate, sometimes following a period of growth arrest. The accelerated growth rate began in boys whose bone age was 13.5 to 14.8 years and in girls whose bone age was around 12 years. This level of bone maturity was reached later, at chronologic age 15–18 years for boys and 14–16 years for girls. During pubertal development, height increment remained limited, with a mean value of 2.7 cm/year in boys and 2.0 cm/year in girls.[1]

Thus, pubertal growth in dialyzed patients was variable but never equal to that of normal children. Most often growth was severely reduced and abnormally prolonged, but

eventually led to some catch-up of height for age. The catch-up growth rate was insufficient, however, to achieve normal adult stature.[1, 6]

## HORMONAL CHANGES IN ADULTS WITH CHRONIC RENAL FAILURE

Changes in gonadal function in adult males on chronic dialysis are well recognized.[7–12] Elevated levels of luteinizing hormone (LH), follicle stimulating hormone (FSH), and prolactin (PRL) and reduced levels of testosterone (T) have been reported in males who are on maintenance hemodialysis or peritoneal dialysis.[7–12] Also, elevated cortisol levels have been found in these same groups.[12]

Severe spermatogenic changes have also been reported in males on chronic dialysis.[9, 11] Holdsworth and colleagues reported reduced or absent spermatogenesis in 19 males on chronic hemodialysis. These 19 males all had open testicular biopsy performed at the time of renal transplantation. Quantitative analysis of the testicular histology was possible in 15 of 19 patients. In all 15 males studied, there was a significant reduction in spermatogenesis at all stages, ranging from spermatogonia to late spermatids. Sertoli cell number was normal in all 15 patients studied.[9]

The origin of the elevated LH levels has been studied by Holdsworth and colleagues. The metabolic clearance rate of LH was determined in 9 males on chronic hemodialysis and was only 30% that of the normal males (p < 0.01). Production of LH was also abnormal, being significantly higher (p < 0.05) in males with chronic renal failure than in normal individuals. This finding is attributed to significant impairment of Leydig cell function.[9] Luteinizing-hormone–releasing hormone (LHRH) was given to these same subjects and caused a rise in serum LH. Luteinizing hormone levels remained higher than normal following LHRH, suggesting reduced clearance of either LH or LHRH by the uremic male.[9]

Alterations of the hypothalamic-pituitary-ovarian axis have not been studied in females as thoroughly as in males.[13, 14] With decreasing renal function, alterations in menstrual function appear, and when ESRD supervenes, secondary amenorrhea invariably occurs. The progression of these abnormalities is closely correlated with the severity of renal insufficiency. Although menstruation may return after a variable length of hemodialysis treatment, it may still be irregular in cycle length or flow.[15, 16]

Swamy and colleagues studied 13 adult females on chronic hemodialysis. Six were premenopausal and seven postmenopausal. Menstrual problems were present in all premenopausal women. Luteinizing hormone values were elevated in premenopausal women, but not in postmenopausal women. Follicle stimulating hormone values in the women on hemodialysis were in the normal range, as were total plasma estrogen levels. Luteinizing hormone response to LHRH was tested in three women and was normal.[13]

## PUBERTAL DEVELOPMENT IN CHILDREN WITH RENAL INSUFFICIENCY

Delayed pubertal development is a well-described complication in children with ESRD.[1, 2] Hormonal changes in adolescents with renal insufficiency have been studied in males[2] but not, to our knowledge, in females.

Ferraris and colleagues[2] evaluated 31 male adolescents ranging in age from 11.7 to 20 years and at all pubertal stages. Three groups were studied. Group I patients had chronic renal insufficiency but were not on dialysis; Group II patients were on chronic hemodialysis, and Group III patients had undergone renal transplantation. Group III patients were receiving prednisone (0.2 mg/kg/day) and azathioprine 2 mg/kg/day.

Bone age and secondary sexual characteristic development were delayed in the majority of children when compared with chronologic age (Fig. 20–1, A). Bone age showed a closer correlation with genital development (Fig. 20–1, B). Eight of 11 children with Tanner Stage IV development had delayed genital maturation relative to bone age.

Serum testosterone and dihydrotestosterone were normal in all but one patient when correlated with pubertal stage. Luteinizing hormone was normal in all groups. In contrast FSH was increased in all patients in Groups I and II.

The adrenal androgens were slightly reduced in many Group I and Group II patients. The serum concentration of $\Delta$ 4-androstenedione was normal in Group I and Group II patients. Dehydroepiandrosterone and dehydroepiandrosterone sulfate were at the lower end of normal for Group I and Group II patients.

Several important facts emerge from this study. The severity and duration of renal failure correlates well with bone age delay. Thus, adolescents who have not required dialysis or transplanation (Group I) show less of a delay in bone age and sexual maturation than do patients on hemodialysis (Group II). Bone age correlates better than chronologic age with attained degree of sexual maturation. Serum testosterone and dihydrotestosterone were normal relative to pubertal stage in all but one patient.[2] Previously reported[7-12] serum testosterone levels in male adults on hemodialysis have been low. The normal testosterone-to-dihydrotestosterone ratio in

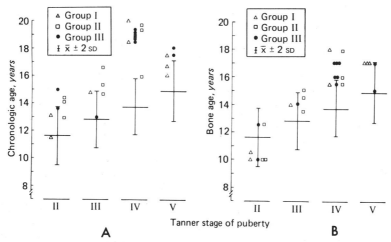

**Figure 20–1.** *A,* Bone age (± 2 SD) versus chronologic age in three groups of males with renal disease. (See text for group description.) *B,* Chronologic age and bone age versus degree of sexual maturation (Tanner stage of puberty). The mean ± 2 SD refers to the ages at which normal boys pass through the successive Tanner stages of puberty. (From Ferraris et al: Delayed puberty in males with chronic renal failure. Kidney Int 18:344, 1980.)

these patients suggests that 5α-reductase activity was nomal. Thus, Leydig cell function appears intact in adolescent males with chronic renal failure.

Elevated FSH levels in all Group I and II patients appear to reflect damage to the seminiferous epithelium. The fact that FSH was elevated regardless of the pubertal stage suggests that germinal epithelium damage can occur early in puberty. Hemodialysis does not improve this abnormality. In fact, the highest FSH levels were found after several years of chronic dialysis.[2] This is similar to the reported elevation in FSH in adult males on hemodialysis.[9, 10, 11]

## EFFECT OF RENAL TRANSPLANTATION ON SEXUAL MATURATION

Successful renal transplantation for chronic renal failure has been shown to improve the growth rate of children.[16, 17] Prepubertal children show a greater rate of growth than do children who have entered puberty.[6] Sexual maturation and bone age maturation correlated after transplantation, as reported in the study by Ferraris et al.[2]

The hormonal aberrations reported in adult males are improved or corrected by renal transplantation. Serum testosterone returns to normal after transplantation[7, 10, 11] but FSH and LH remain elevated.[10, 11] The FSH and LH levels after transplantation do return to values closer to normal. Sperm count and fertility also improve after renal transplantation in males.[11] Pubescent males also show a fall in FSH toward normal after renal transplantation. Ferraris et al reported that 67% of pubertal males had a normal FSH after renal transplantation if the serum creatinine was below 2 mg/dl. Those with a serum creatinine above 2 mg/dl all had elevated FSH levels after transplantation.[2]

The slightly suppressed serum adrenal androgen levels in Group I and Group II patients in the study by Ferraris et al did not improve after renal transplantation. Indeed, a large percentage of Group III patients had values in the lower range of normal than Group I and II patients.[2] In post-transplant patients, the lowering of adrenal androgen levels with prednisone may contribute to blunting the desirable post-transplant growth response.[2, 18]

## SUMMARY

Sexual maturation is delayed in children with ESRD. The degree of delay is greater with increasing impairment of renal function. In pubertal males, Leydig cell function appears to be normal, whereas in adult males serum LH is elevated and testosterone reduced. Follicle stimulating hormone concentration is elevated, a fact which may signify injury to germinal epithelium. Following successful renal transplantation, pubertal progression occurs and the elevated serum FSH levels usually return to normal. Presumably there has been repair of germinal epithelium and a consequent fall in serum FSH levels.

## REFERENCES

1. Kleinknecht C, Broyer M, Gagnadoux M, et al: Growth in children treated with long-term dialysis: a study of 76 patients. *In*: Hamburger J, Crosnier J, Grunfeld J, Maxwell MH (eds), Advances in Nephrology, Vol 9. Chicago, Year Book Medical Publishers, 1980, p 133.
2. Ferraris J, Saenger P, Levine L, et al: Delayed puberty in males with chronic renal failure. Kidney Int 18:344, 1980.
3. Lewy JE, New MI: Growth in children with renal failure. Am J Med 58:65, 1975.
4. Najarian JS, Simmons RL, Tallent MB, et al: Renal transplantation in infants and children. Ann Surg 174:583, 1971.
5. Kulin HE: Normal pubertal development. *In*: Rudolph AM, Hoffman JIE (eds), Pediatrics, 17th ed. Norwalk, Appleton-Century-Crofts, 1982, p 1558.
6. Donckerwolcke RA, Chantler C, Broyer M, Brunner FP, et al: Combined report on regular dialysis and transplantation of children in Europe, 1979. Proc Eur Dial Transplant Assoc 17:87, 1980.
7. Zadeh JA, Koutsaimanis KG, Roberts AP, et al: The effect of maintenance hemodialysis and renal transplantation on the plasma testosterone levels of male patients in chronic renal failure. Acta Endocrinol 80:577, 1975.
8. Hagen C, Olgaard K, McNeilly AS, Fisher R: Prolactin and the pituitary-gonadal axis in male uremic patients on regular dialysis. Acta Endocrinol 82:29, 1976.
9. Holdsworth S, Atkins RC, deKretser DM: The pituitary-testicular axis in men with chronic renal failure. N Engl J Med 296:1245, 1977.
10. Chopp RT, Mendez R: Sexual function and hormonal abnormalities in uremic men on chronic dialysis and after renal transplantation. Fertil Steril 29:661, 1978.
11. Holdsworth SR, de Kretser DM, Atkins RC: A comparison of hemodialysis and transplantation in reversing the uremic disturbances of male reproduction function. Clin Nephrol 10:146, 1978.
12. Zumoff B, Walter L, Rosenfeld RS, et al: Subnormal

plasma adrenal androgen levels in men with uremia. J Clin Endocrinol Metab 51:801, 1980.

13. Swamy AP, Woolf PD, Cestero RVM: Hypothalmic-pituitary-ovarian axis in uremic women. J Lab Clin Med 93:1066, 1979.

14. Olgaard K, Hagen C, McNeilly AS: Pituitary hormones in women with chronic renal failure: the effect of intermittent hemo and peritoneal dialysis. Acta Endocrinol 80:237, 1975.

15. Rice GG: Hypermenorrhea in the young hemodialysis patient. Am J Obset Gynecol 116:539, 1973.

16. Larsen NA: Sexual problems of patients on RDT and after renal transplantation. Proc Eur Dial Transplant Assoc 9:271, 1972.

17. Saenger P, Wiedemann E, Schwartz E, et al: Somatomedin and growth after renal transplantation. Pediatr Res 8:163, 1974.

18. Keough B, Chu TM, Murphy GP: The effects of long-term alternate day steroids on parameters of adrenal function in renal transplant patients. J Urol 115:487, 1976.

# 21

# Endocrine Function in Children with ESRD

Wolfgang Rauh, M.D.
Peter-Joachim Oertel, M.D.

The endocrine system is of paramount importance in regulating and integrating various body functions. Hormonal changes in chronic renal failure (CRF) may be responsible for disturbances of several body functions in uremic patients. CRF may affect the endocrine system by altering synthesis, release, protein binding, degradation, elimination, receptor binding, and postreceptor activity of hormones. Treatment of renal insufficiency by regular hemodialysis often improves endocrine abnormalities induced by uremia. Conversely, additional endocrine changes may be caused by hormone elimination and disruption of physiological feedback mechanisms during dialysis. Endocrine function in uremia has been studied extensively in adults and a comprehensive review of the literature has recently been published.[1]

Despite the important role of endocrine function in a developing organism, pediatric data about hormonal changes in uremia are remarkably scarce. The following analysis of hormone systems in ESRD will concentrate on pediatric aspects. Findings will be included where applicable from studies in uremic adults or from animal experiments. Because of the broad spectrum of endocrine changes in uremia, our review has to remain incomplete. This chapter will focus on thyroid and adrenal hormonal alterations and selected clinical aspects of sexual maturation, growth, carbohydrate metabolism, and blood pressure regulation. The hormonal regulation of calcium metabolism and of erythropoiesis is described in Chapters 17, 18, and 25.

## SEX HORMONES

Disturbances of sexual function are common in chronic renal disease. Menstrual abnormalities, infertility, and diminished libido have been reported in uremic women.[2–4] Gynecomastia, impotence, and decreased sexual activity are frequently observed in uremic men prior to and after initiation of dialysis treatment.[5–7] Delayed sexual maturation is characteristic of children with CRF.[8, 9] These disturbances have been attributed to hormonal alterations at both the hypothalamo-pituitary and gonadal level.

In *adult males* with CRF, low plasma testosterone concentrations with an inadequate rise after administration of human chorionic gonadotropin (HCG) suggest decreased testicular function.[6, 10, 11] Oligospermia and hypomotility of the sperm population are also common findings.[10] Testicular biopsies reveal tissue atrophy, especially of the Leydig cells.[11] A reduced conversion of testosterone to the active metabolite dihydrotestosterone due to a decreased 5α-reductase activity[12] and increased plasma binding of androgens[13] may also contribute to disturbed sexual function in uremic men.

In *prepubertal and pubertal boys* with CRF, low or low normal plasma testosterone levels have been reported.[9, 14] We found that total plasma testosterone and dihydrotestosterone concentrations were decreased while the ratio of testosterone to dihydrotestosterone and the percentage of free testosterone in plasma were normal in prepubertal boys with CRF (Figs. 21–1 and 21–2). This indicates that

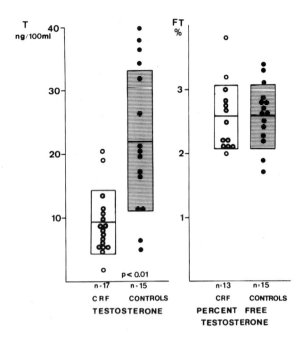

**Figure 21–1.** Total plasma testosterone and percentage of free testosterone in prepubertal boys (age 5–12 yrs) with chronic renal failure ($S_{CR}$> 2 mg/dl, open circles) and normal age-matched controls (closed circles). The shaded columns represent mean ± SD.

Leydig cell function is impaired, whereas 5α-reductase activity and plasma protein binding of testosterone are not disturbed in prepubertal boys with CRF. Testosterone response to HCG stimulation is decreased in prepubertal and pubertal uremic boys.[15] Thus, in CRF, damage to testicular tissue may be present before and during puberty.

In *adult women* with ESRD, plasma estrogen and progesterone levels tend to be decreased and secondary amenorrhea or anovulatory cycles are frequently seen.[2, 3] *Ovarian function* in *prepubertal or pubertal girls* with CRF has not been studied systematically. Gonadal function is not ameliorated by hemodialysis treatment but is often normalized after successful renal transplantation.[10, 16, 17]

In addition to a gonadal defect, a disturbance at the hypothalamo-pituitary level may be involved in the delay of puberty and in sexual dysfunction in uremia. In *adults* with CRF, increased basal levels of *luteinizing hor-*

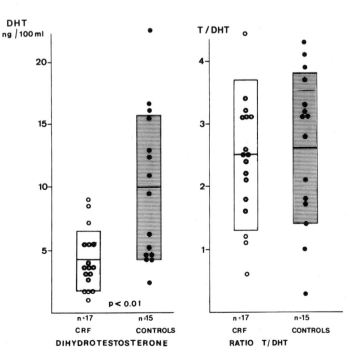

**Figure 21–2.** Dihydrotestosterone and ratio of testosterone/dihydrotestosterone in the plasma of prepubertal boys (age 5–12 yrs) with chronic renal failure ($S_{CR}$>2 mg/dl, open circles) and age-matched controls (closed circles). The shaded columns represent mean ± SD.

mone *(LH)* and less frequently of *follicle stimulating hormone (FSH)* have been found.[2, 10, 11, 17, 18] Data on gonadotropin levels in uremic *children* are controversial. In one study, normal LH and elevated FSH concentrations were reported in boys with CRF before and during different stages of puberty.[9] More recent investigations have indicated that LH levels tend to be increased in uremic boys of all age groups,[14, 19, 20] while FSH levels are raised only in boys above the age of 13 years.[14] In prepubertal girls with CRF, elevated LH and normal FSH concentrations have been found.[19, 20] The pattern of gonadotropins in uremic girls after the onset of puberty is at present not known.

Decreased gonadal hormones and increased gonadotropins in CRF are compatible with the presence of hypergonadotropic hypogonadism. It has, however, been suggested that the elevation of gonadotropins in CRF is inadequate in relation to the decrease in gonadal hormones, thus indicating a disturbance at the hypothalamo-pituitary level.[16] This concept is supported by the recent finding of a blunted response of LH and FSH to LH-releasing hormone in prepubertal children with CRF.[19, 20]

High circulating *prolactin* levels and an abnormal prolactin response to thyrotropin releasing hormone (TRH) have been reported in a large number of uremic children and adults.[7, 21–23] The hyperprolactinemia of renal failure may be attributed in part to altered renal metabolism.[21] There is, however, evidence for a deranged hypothalamo-pituitary control, probably due to a decrease in hypothalamic prolactin inhibiting factor.[21, 24] Elevated prolactin levels may affect central and gonadal function,[25] and long-term administration of the dopaminergic agonist bromocriptine may result in a decrease of prolactin levels and in improved sexual activity in uremic men.[26] Hyperprolactinemia may also play a role in the pathogenesis of *gynecomastia* in CRF; but no correlation between increased prolactin levels and occurrence of gynecomastia has been demonstrated.[7] Considerable differences in the incidence of gynecomastia have been reported and its pathogenesis remains poorly understood.[6, 7, 24]

Altered *vitamin D metabolism* and *hyperparathyroidism* have recently been implicated in central and gonadal disturbances in CRF.[27] Other factors such as *zinc deficiency* may also contribute to sexual dysfunction in uremia.[28]

The role of a delayed *adrenarche* in the disturbance of pubertal development in children with CRF requires further elucidation. In uremic boys, the levels of adrenal androgens (dehydroepiandrosterone and androstenedione) are normal or decreased, depending on whether they are related to chronologic age, height age, or bone age.[9, 14] In post-transplant patients the lowering of adrenal androgens with glucocorticoid therapy may blunt the post-transplant growth response.[9]

Thus, the disturbances of pubertal development and of sexual function in CRF involve a multitude of hormonal abnormalities. The precise pathophysiological mechanisms leading to these abnormalities are poorly understood. Most of the endocrine changes in uremia appear to be transient in nature, as they are often reversed after successful renal transplantation.

## GROWTH HORMONE AND SOMATOMEDINS

**Growth Hormone.** Growth retardation is a well known but poorly understood concomitant of CRF in children.[29–31] The concentration of circulating immunoreactive growth hormone is normal or elevated in uremia and the degree of elevation tends to parallel the rise in serum creatinine.[32–34] An exaggerated rise of plasma growth hormone after administration of TRH has been reported.[22, 35] The response of growth hormone secretion to known stimuli such as hypoglycemia or arginine infusion is increased in most uremic children.[36] After glucose loading, a lack of suppression or a stimulation of plasma growth hormone has been observed.[37, 38] Growth hormone has an antagonistic effect on insulin-induced cellular glucose uptake, but the degree of insulin resistance in uremia does not appear to correlate with the increased level of growth hormone.[32, 34, 37] After renal transplantation, a normalization of growth hormone levels has been reported.[39] Decreased metabolic clearances of growth hormone may contribute to the elevation of growth hormone in CRF,[40, 41] but the pathogenetic mechanisms of the increase and of the altered release pattern of growth hormone in uremia remain poorly understood.

**Somatomedins.** The somatomedins are a family of growth-hormone–dependent, insulin-like peptides which have been postulated to mediate the actions of pituitary growth hormone on skeletal tissue. The role of somatomedins in the pathogenesis of growth retardation in uremia is controversial and the interpretation of the available data is hampered by differences in assay techniques.[42] Somatomedins have been measured by bioassay (as "sulfation factor"), radioreceptor assay, competitive protein binding assay, and radioimmunoassay.

Serum levels of somatomedin as measured by *bioassay* are either normal or decreased in children with ESRD,[39, 43] even when corrected for elevated sulfate concentration in uremia. Following hemodialysis, an increase of somatomedin levels into the normal range has been reported.[43] It has been suggested that dialysis may remove somatomedin inhibitors.[43] Heparinization during hemodialysis may also contribute to the observed rise in bioassayable somatomedin following hemodialysis.[44] After renal transplantation somatomedin levels are not different from healthy controls and correlate with growth velocity.[39]

In *radioreceptor* studies increased somatomedin levels have been found in patients on chronic hemodialysis.[45–48] A correlation between somatomedin levels and calorie intake in uremic children has been observed.[45] Following renal transplantation somatomedin levels decrease to the normal range.[48]

Somatomedin levels measured by *protein binding assay* or *radioimmunoassay* are increased and do not decrease after hemodialysis in uremic patients.[45, 49]

Thus, somatomedin levels in uremic patients have been found to be low, normal, or high in various assay systems. Bioassays, even when corrected for sulfate content, have tended to give normal or low values in children with CRF, whereas radioreceptor and radioimmunoassays have tended to give high values. All bioassays are sensitive to both stimulatory and inhibitory factors, and the presence of inhibitory factors could explain the discrepancy between levels found by radioligand techniques and those determined by bioassay. A dialyzable substance may inhibit somatomedin activity in vitro and perhaps also in vivo. The role of an end-organ resistance to the action of somatomedins remains to be elucidated.

## ENDOCRINE ASPECTS OF CARBOHYDRATE METABOLISM

It is well known that carbohydrate metabolism is abnormal in CRF. In uremic children and adults on regular hemodialysis, increased blood glucose levels are associated with elevated *insulin* levels in the fasting state.[38, 50]

After glucose loading, hyperinsulinemia and glucose intolerance have been demonstrated.[38] Plasma *glucagon* levels are also high and fail to decrease normally after intravenous glucose administration.[38] The pattern of immunoreactive fragments of insulin[51] and glucagon[52] may be altered in CRF.

The pathogenesis of glucose intolerance in uremia is controversial, and several pathophysiological concepts have been developed in recent years. In uremic rats binding of glucagon to liver cellular membranes is increased, whereas, in contrast, that of insulin is diminished when compared with normal rats.[53] Thus the tissue resistance to insulin and the hyperglycemic action of glucagon have been attributed to alterations of receptor binding in uremia. Decreased insulin binding has, however, not been observed in monocytes of patients on regular hemodialysis.[54] This finding, in combination with the results of hyperglycemic and euglycemic glucose clamp technique studies in uremic patients, has led to the hypothesis of a disturbance at a step beyond the insulin receptor. There is increasing evidence that insulin resistance in uremia is mediated by post-binding defects.[55]

In addition, a relative insensitivity of the pancreatic beta cells to glucose,[54, 56] altered insulin metabolism,[57] and increased gluconeogenesis from alanine[58, 59] may contribute to the disturbance of carbohydrate metabolism in uremia. An increase in gluconeogenesis which is partially normalized by regular hemodialysis treatment has been observed in uremic patients.[58, 59]

Increased growth hormone, cortisol, and catecholamines may antagonize the action of insulin in terminal renal failure.[38, 60] Hyperparathyroidism, a frequent concomitant of CRF, has also been suggested to play a role in glucose intolerance. Hyperparathyroidism may stimulate gluconeogenesis.[61] An improvement of glucose intolerance following parathyroidectomy was recently reported in children on regular hemodialysis.[62]

On the basis of the pathophysiological concepts mentioned above, insulin resistance evolves as the major cause of glucose intolerance of uremia. The relative importance of the various factors contributing to insulin resistance and the exact nature of the postulated post-binding defect in insulin action await clarification.

## THYROID FUNCTION

Some clinical manifestations of CRF such as dry skin, yellowish complexion, lethargy, fatigue, and cold intolerance resemble the features of hypothyroidism. The reported increased incidence of goiter in uremic patients[63, 64] has not been confirmed by other authors.[65] Despite extensive studies, thyroid function in uremia remains inconclusive because of the complexity of the system. Disturbances of thyroid function in uremia have been attributed to changes at the hypothalamo-pituitary level, intrathyroidal abnormalities, abnormal peripheral conversion, and metabolism of thyroid hormones.[63]

In most studies normal basal levels of *thyroid stimulating hormone (TSH)* have been found in uremic children[22, 66] and adults.[63, 67] After administration of thyrotropin releasing hormone (TRH) a subnormal or a delayed and prolonged rise of TSH has been reported in patients undergoing regular hemodialysis.[22, 63, 66] The prolonged elevation of TSH after TRH stimulation may be due to an increased half-life of TSH in renal failure.[68] The TSH response to TRH may vary considerably during the course of the disease.[69] TSH responsiveness and thyroid function are probably influenced by the clinical status of uremic patients. In a recent investigation, patients on regular hemodialysis who were in a stable clinical condition showed a normal pituitary responsiveness to TRH and a normal thyroidal response to endogenous TSH secretion.[67]

*Plasma iodine* and *iodine uptake* by the thyroid gland have been reported to be increased in CRF before the onset of dialysis treatment.[70] In patients undergoing intermittent peritoneal dialysis or hemodialysis, iodine uptake is normal or decreased.[64, 65, 71]

Total plasma *thyroxine ($T_4$)* and *triiodothyronine ($T_3$)* have been found to be low or low normal in uremic patients before and after the onset of hemodialysis treatment.[22, 63-66] Most authors agree that $T_3$ is more markedly depressed than $T_4$ in uremia. Increased weekly dialysis time tends to normalize the levels of circulating thyroid hormones.[72] The concentration of circulating *thyroxine binding globulin* appears to be normal in CRF.[64] Plasma levels of *free $T_4$* may be decreased,[63, 65] but normal levels have been reported in recent studies.[72, 73] In uremic patients, plasma concentrations of *free $T_3$* are reduced both prior to and during dialysis therapy.[73, 74]

There is evidence for a disturbed peripheral metabolism of thyroid hormones in uremia.[75] Conversion of $T_4$ to $T_3$ is significantly decreased.[63] *Reverse $T_3$* has been found to be either normal or slightly elevated.[74, 76] After successful transplantation thyroid parameters usually return to normal.[63, 66]

In view of the conflicting reports in the literature, it is difficult to draw any definite conclusions about thyroid function in uremia. Differences in nutritional and metabolic status of the patients in various studies may explain some of the discrepant findings. There is no agreement whether the observed hormonal alterations in uremia actually represent a hypothyroid state. Therapeutic trials with thyroid hormones have produced inconclusive results.[64, 65] In most of the recent studies, uremic patients have been considered to be euthyroid.[67, 73, 75] It has been suggested that the reported changes of thyroid hormones are not distinctive for CRF, but reflect the "euthyroid sick" state found in serious systemic illnesses.[73, 74]

It is possible that the decreased $T_3$ levels provide a protective mechanism against the catabolic effects of chronic uremia. This mechanism has been suggested to play a role in patients with other nonthyroidal illnesses as well as during fasting.[77] Future studies of cellular effects of thyroid hormones may contribute to a better understanding of thyroid status in uremia.

In certain diseases producing CRF such as cystinosis[78] or congenital nephrotic syndrome,[79] hypothyroidism requiring thyroid hormone replacement has been documented. At this point no general recommendation regarding thyroid hormone therapy in uremic children can be given. Repeated clinical and laboratory evaluations appear mandatory in order to assess the necessity of thyroid hormone administration in individual patients.

## THE ADRENOCORTICOTROPIN (ACTH)-CORTISOL AXIS

The literature concerning the pituitary-adrenal axis in CRF is confusing. Most of the studies in uremic children and adults have found normal basal plasma concentrations of *cortisol*.[34, 80-83] Elevated cortisol levels have, however, also been reported[84, 85] and mean total 24-hour cortisol concentrations may be increased.[85] Circadian rhythmicity, as evidenced by times of peak secretory activity and number of peaks, appears to be normal in patients on chronic hemodialysis.[83, 85] A rise of plasma cortisol has been observed in children and adults during hemodialysis or hemofiltration.[83, 86, 87] Stimulation with ACTH results in a normal rise of plasma cortisol in most uremic patients.[82, 84, 86] After administration of dexamethasone, both a normal[81] and an incomplete suppression of cortisol[84, 88] have been reported.

There is also no agreement about plasma *ACTH* levels in CRF. Basal plasma ACTH has been found in low,[89] normal,[34] and high normal[84] levels in uremic adults. In children with CRF, increased basal ACTH levels and an impaired response to insulin-induced hypoglycemia have been reported.[83] In a recent study in uremic adults, neither cortisol nor ACTH was suppressed by dexamethasone administration.[84] In addition, metyrapone, given orally or intravenously, failed to produce the expected rise in ACTH or 11-deoxycortisol.[84] These results suggest a disturbance in the normal feedback control of the hypothalamo-pituitary-adrenocortical axis. The apparent autonomy of ACTH secretion is compatible with a Cushing's syndrome–like state in patients on maintenance hemodialysis. It has been speculated that some complications of uremia such as osteopathy, negative nitrogen balance, and glucose intolerance may be attributable in part to this state of hormonal dysfunction.[84] It is, however, currently not clear whether the *hormonal* abnormalities of the hypothalamo-pituitary-adrenal axis are actually associated with a *clinical* state of hypercorticism in CRF.

## THE RENIN-ANGIOTENSIN-ALDOSTERONE SYSTEM

Under normal conditions, body sodium and volume status and the functional activity of the renin-angiotensin-aldosterone system are linked by a complex feedback mechanism which maintains a state of equilibrium. In CRF, this equilibrium is often disturbed.[90–92] High levels of *plasma renin activity (PRA)* may be due to some degree of autonomy of the renin secretory process, responding only partially to the controlling mechanisms. In most adults with ESRD, PRA is normal or low when compared with that in healthy subjects. Excessively elevated PRA levels are found in some patients with severe hypertension which is not corrected by hemodialysis. Normal or low PRA levels in CRF may, however, be inappropriately high in relation to increased body sodium and blood volume.[90, 91] The importance of the renin-angiotensin system in maintaining arterial hypertension in uremic children and adults has recently been underlined by the antihypertensive effect of the angiotensin-converting enzyme inhibitor captopril.[93, 94]

Pediatric data about PRA in CRF are scarce. In children with CRF before the onset of dialysis treatment, we found PRA levels ranging from low to extensively high (Fig. 21–3). PRA is markedly elevated in *hypertensive* children with reflux nephropathy as well as in some *normotensive* children, e.g., in patients with nephronophthisis. In the preterminal stage of nephronophthisis and other renal disorders PRA is often increased as a result of sodium loss. This state of hyperreninism may persist in the terminal stage of the disease when renal sodium loss is no longer present.[95]

Following hemodialysis or hemofiltration a rise of PRA has been reported by several authors.[90, 95–97] Renin release may be stimulated by the fall in blood pressure during hemodialysis, either directly via a renal baroreceptor mechanism or indirectly via β-adrenergic stimulation.[97] Recurrent stimulation of the renin-angiotensin system during dialysis may play a role in hypertension of uremic patients since angiotensin levels are slow to fall while the patient is reaccumulating volume.[97] After renal transplantation high levels of renin originating from the patient's remaining kidneys or from the graft, e.g., due to stenosis of the renal artery, may cause serious hypertension.

Uremic children and adults show a wide range of basal plasma *aldosterone* concentrations.[91, 95] There is a significant correlation between PRA and plasma aldosterone levels in children with terminal renal failure and in normal controls (Fig. 21–4). This indicates that the renin-angiotensin system is a major determinant of aldosterone secretion both under normal conditions and in ESRD. Raised serum potassium levels may be responsible for the elevation of plasma aldosterone in CRF.[91, 98] The response of aldosterone to hemodialysis is variable because of the interaction of several factors stimulating or suppressing aldosterone release.[95, 98] During dialysis aldosterone secretion is enhanced by stimulation of the renin-angiotensin sys-

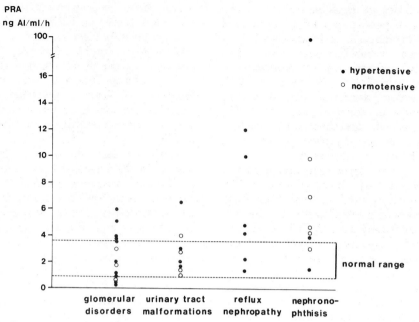

**Figure 21–3.** Plasma renin activity (PRA) in normotensive (open circles) and hypertensive (closed circles) children (age 6–15 yrs) with chronic renal failure ($S_{CR} >$ 2 mg/dl) due to different primary renal disorders.

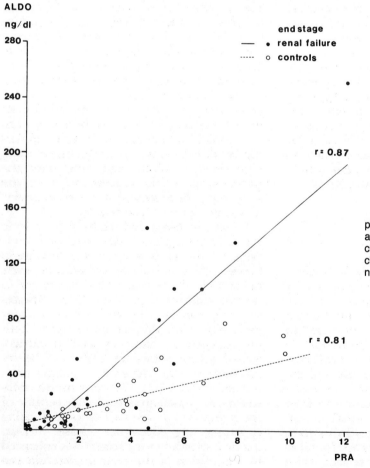

**Figure 21–4.** Relationship between plasma renin activity (PRA) and plasma aldosterone concentration (ALDO) in children (age 8–18 yrs) with ESRD on chronic hemodialysis (closed circles) and normal controls (open circles).

tem and possibly by a stress-induced rise of ACTH, while the fall in serum potassium level inhibits aldosterone release. In the preterminal stage of renal disease, aldosterone contributes to the development of hypertension. Since the hypertensinogenic action of aldosterone is predominantly related to the effect of the hormone on tubular reabsorption of sodium, it is unlikely that aldosterone plays a role in the hypertensive process once the kidney has ceased to have excretory function.

## VASOPRESSIN (ANTIDIURETIC HORMONE)

Basal plasma vasopressin concentrations are elevated in uremic children[95] and adults.[99] Increased serum osmolality may be responsible for the rise of vasopressin in CRF, but osmotic and nonosmotic regulation of vasopressin in uremia is poorly understood. Vasopressin has been implicated in the pathogenesis of various forms of hypertension.[100] It is, however, at present unknown whether elevated vasopressin levels contribute to hypertension in CRF.

## CATECHOLAMINES

The investigation of the sympathetic nervous system has been considerably facilitated by the introduction of sensitive and specific methods for the determination of plasma catecholamine levels.[101] Plasma *epinephrine* largely reflects the hormone released from the adrenal medulla. Plasma *norepinephrine* is generally acknowledged to be a suitable index for the activity of the sympathetic nervous system,[97, 102, 103] although plasma levels may not always directly reflect conditions at the receptor sites. In uremic adults, increased plasma norepinephrine levels have been reported by most authors,[102, 104, 105] while there is no agreement on plasma epinephrine concentrations.[102–104] Raised plasma catecholamines in uremia could theoretically be explained by increased synthesis, diminished reuptake at the nerve terminals,[106] deficient enzymatic degradation, or decreased renal excretion.[107]

Autonomic dysfunction, abnormal baroreceptor reflexes and an inadequate response to dialysis hypotension have been suggested as evidence for an abnormality of the sympathetic nervous system in uremic adults.[108–110]

Disturbances in adrenergic blood pressure control could contribute to arterial hypertension as well as to orthostatic and dialysis-associated hypotension.[109, 111]

In our studies, basal plasma epinephrine and norepinephrine levels were normal or slightly elevated in uremic children when compared to normal age-matched controls.[95] In addition, a marked rise of plasma catecholamines was found in children during hemodialysis or hemofiltration, indicating an adequate response of the adrenergic system to the observed fall in blood pressure. It has been suggested that the dysfunction of the autonomic nervous system in CRF is a part of a more generalized uremic polyneuropathy. There may be a considerable difference in incidence and severity of uremic polyneuropathy between children and adults.[112]

## FUTURE DEVELOPMENTS

The information on hormonal disturbances in CRF has been accumulating in recent years. Many studies have remained purely descriptive, but in some instances a better understanding of the pathogenetic mechanisms underlying the hormonal disturbances has emerged from clinical and experimental investigations. Further studies dedicated to the cellular effects of various hormones may provide new insights into endocrine dysfunction in uremia. The development of new methods for the treatment of children with ESRD, such as hemofiltration and chronic peritoneal dialysis, poses a challenge to the pediatrician. Because the long-term clinical usefulness of a new form of treatment of CRF can be expected in part to be determined by its effect on the endocrine system, an adequate evaluation of endocrine function will be required before the precise role of the new therapeutic modality for ESRD in children can be established.

## REFERENCES

1. Drüeke T: Endocrine disorders in chronic hemodialysis patients (with the exclusion of hyperparathyroidism). *In:* Hamburger J, Crosnier J, Grünfeld JP, Maxwell MH (eds), Advances in Nephrology, Vol 10. Chicago, Year Book Medical Publishers, 1981, p 351.
2. Swamy AP, Woolf PD, Cestero RVM: Hypothalamic-pituitary-ovarian axis in uremic women. J Lab Clin Med 93:1066, 1979.
3. Wass VJ, Wass JAH, Rees L, et al: Sex hormone changes underlying menstrual disturbances on

haemodialysis. Proc Eur Dial Transplant Assoc 15:178, 1978.

4. Morley JE, Distiller LA, Epstein S, et al: Menstrual disturbances in chronic renal failure. Horm Metab Res 11:68, 1979.

5. Levy NB: Coping with maintenance hemodialysis. Psychological considerations in the care of patients. *In:* Massry SG, Sellers AL (eds), Clinical Aspects of Uremia and Dialysis. Springfield, Illinois, Charles C Thomas, Publisher, 1976, p 53.

6. Fichman MP: Pituitary, gonadal and thyroid function. *In:* Massry SG, Sellers AL (eds), Clinical Aspects of Uremia and Dialysis. Springfield, Illinois, Charles C Thomas, Publisher, 1976, p 273.

7. Nagel TC, Freinkel N, Bell RH, et al: Gynecomastia, prolactin and other peptide hormones in patients undergoing chronic hemodialysis. J Clin Endocrinol Metab 36:428, 1973.

8. Broyer M, Kleinknecht C, Loirat C, et al: Maturation osseuse et development pubertaire chez l'enfant et l'adolescent en dialyse chronique. Proc Eur Dial Transplant Assoc 9:81, 1972.

9. Ferraris J, Saenger P, Levine L, et al: Delayed puberty in males with chronic renal failure. Kidney Int 18:344, 1980.

10. Lim VS, Fang VS: Gonadal dysfunction in uremic men. A study of the hypothalamo-pituitary-testicular axis before and after renal transplantation. Am J Med 58:655, 1975.

11. Stewart-Bently M, Gans D, Horton R: Regulation of gonadal function in uremia. Metabolism 23:1065, 1974.

12. Gupta D, Bundschu HD: Testosterone and its binding in the plasma of male subjects with chronic renal failure. Clin Chim Acta 36:479, 1972.

13. Rager K, Bundschu HD, Gupta D: The effect of HCG on testicular androgen production in adult men with chronic renal failure. J Reprod Fertil 42:113, 1975.

14. Roger M, Broyer M, Schärer K, et al: Gonadotropines et androgènes plasmatique chez les garcons traités pour insufficance rénale chronique. Pathol Biol 29:378, 1981.

15. Schärer K, Broyer M, Vecsei P, et al: Damage to testicular function in chronic renal failure of children. Proc Eur Dial Transplant Assoc 17:725, 1980.

16. Lim VS, Auletta F, Kathpalia S: Gonadal dysfunction in chronic renal failure. Dial Transplant 7:896, 1978.

17. Mies R, von Baeyer H, Figge H, et al: Investigation on pituitary and Leydig cell function in chronic hemodialysis and after renal transplantation. Klin Wochenschr 53:611, 1975.

18. Geisthövel W, von zur Mühlen A, Bahlmann J: Studies on the pituitary-testicular axis in male patients with chronic renal failure with different glomerular filtration. Klin Wochenschr 54:1027, 1976.

19. Oertel PJ, Schärer K, Lichtwald K, Schönberg D: The hypothalamo-pituitary-gonadal axis in children with chronic renal failure (CRF). Abstracts of the International Workshop on Recent Advances in Diagnosis and Treatment of Children with Chronic Renal Failure, Heidelberg, May 21–22, 1982.

20. Oertel PJ, Lichtwald K, Rauh W, et al: The hypothalamo-pituitary-gonadal axis in prepubertal children with chronic renal failure (CRF). Kidney Int (submitted for publication).

21. Cowden EA, Ratcliffe WA, Ratcliffe JG, et al: Hyperprolactinemia in renal disease. Clin Endocrinol 9:241, 1978.

22. Czernichow H, Dauzet MC, Broyer M, Rappaport R: Abnormal TSH, PRL, and GRH response to TSH releasing factor in chronic renal failure. J Clin Endocrinol Metab 43:630, 1976.

23. Ijaiya K, Roth B, Schwenk A: Serum prolactin levels in renal insufficiency in children. Acta Paediatr Scand 69:299, 1980.

24. Sawin CT, Longcope GW, Ryan RJ: Blood levels of gonadotropins and gonadal hormones in gynecomastia associated with chronic hemodialysis. J Clin Endocrinol Metab 36:988, 1973.

25. Fonzo D, Sivieri R, Gallone G, et al: Effect of a prolactin inhibitor on libido, sexual potency and sex hormones in men with hyperprolactinemia, oligospermia and/or impotence. Acta Endocrinol 85(Suppl 212):142, 1977.

26. Bommer J, Ritz E, Del Pozo E, Bommer G: Improved sexual function in male haemodialysis patients on bromocriptine. Lancet 2:496, 1979.

27. Massry SG, Goldstein DA, Procci WR, Kletzky OA: Impotence in patients with uremia: a possible role for parathyroid hormone. Nephron 19:305, 1977.

28. Antoniou LG, Shalhoub RJ, Sudhakar T, Smith JC Jr: Reversal of uremic impotence by zinc. Lancet 2:895, 1977.

29. Chantler C, Holliday MA: Growth in children with renal disease with particular reference to the effects of calorie malnutrition: Review. Clin Nephrol 1:230, 1973.

30. Lewy JE, New MI: Growth in children with renal failure. Am J Med 58:65, 1975.

31. Stickler GB: Growth failure in renal disease. Pediatr Clin North Am 23:885, 1976.

32. Wright AD, Lowy D, Fraser TR: Serum growth hormone and glucose intolerance in renal failure. Lancet 2:798, 1968.

33. Samaan NA, Freeman RM: Growth hormone levels in severe renal failure. Metabolism 19:102, 1970.

34. Bonomini V, Orgoni G, Stefoni S, Vangelista A: Hormonal changes in uremia. Clin Nephrol 11:275, 1979.

35. Gonzales-Barcena D, Kastin AJ, Schalch DS, et al: Responses to thyrotropin releasing hormone in patients with renal failure and after infusion in normal men. J Clin Endocrinol Metab 36:117, 1973.

36. Ijaiya K: Pattern of growth hormone response to insulin, arginine and hemodialysis in uremic children. Eur J Pediatr 131:185, 1979.

37. Swenson RS, Weisinger JR, Reaven GM: Effect of chronic uremia and hemodialysis on carbohydrate metabolism. Clin Res 22:209A, 1974.

38. El-Bishti MM, Counahan R, Bloom SR, Chantler C: Hormonal and metabolic responses to intravenous glucose in children on regular hemodialysis. Am J Clin Nutr 31:1865, 1978.

39. Saenger P, Wiedemann E, Schwartz E, et al: Somatomedin and growth after renal transplantation. Pediatr Res 8:163, 1974.

40. Cameron DP, Burger HG, Catt KJ, et al: Metabolic clearance rate of human growth hormone in patients with hepatic and renal failure, and in the isolated perfused pig liver. Metabolism 21:895, 1972.

41. Johnson V, Maack T: Renal extraction, filtration, absorption, and catabolism of growth hormone. Am J Physiol 233:F185, 1977.

42. Lewy JE, Van Wyk JJ: Somatomedin and growth retardation in children with chronic renal insufficiency. Kidney Int 14:361, 1978.

43. Phillips LS, Pennisi AJ, Belosky DC, et al: Somatomedin activity and inorganic sulfate in children undergoing hemodialysis. Clin Endocrinol Metab 46:165, 1978.

44. Wiedemann E, Ackad AS, Lewy JE, Schwartz E: Bioassayable serum somatomedin activity (SMA) in chronic renal failure: Age dependence and role of dialysis and heparin. Clin Res 25:402A, 1977.

45. Arnold WC, Spencer EM, Uthne KO, et al: Radioreceptor assay for somatomedin-A in uremic children. Pediatr Res 11:546A, 1977.

46. Spencer EM, Uthne K, Arnold W: Elevated somatomedin A by radioreceptor assay in children with growth retardation and chronic renal insufficiency. In: Giordano C, Van Wyk JJ, Minuto F (eds), Somatomedins and Growth. New York, Academic Press, 1979, p 341.

47. Schiffrin A, Guyde H, Robitaille P, Posner B: Increased plasma somatomedin in reactivity in chronic renal failure as determined by acid gel filtration and radioreceptor assay. J Clin Endocrinol Metab 46:511, 1978.

48. Takano K, Hall K, Kastrup KW, et al: Serum somatomedin A in chronic renal failure. J Clin Endocrinol Metab 48:371, 1979.

49. Frye D, Lum G, Schalch DS, Diehl M: Serum somatomedins and their carrier proteins during hemodialysis in uremic children with growth retardation. Clin Res 30:101A, 1982.

50. De Fronzo RA, Andres R, Edgar P, Walker WG: Carbohydrate metabolism in uremia: A review. Medicine 52:469, 1973.

51. Jaspan JB, Mako ME, Kuzuya H, et al: Abnormalities in circulating beta cell peptide in chronic renal failure: Comparison of C-peptide, proinsulin and insulin. J Clin Endocrinol Metab 45:441, 1977.

52. Kuku SF, Jaspan JB, Emmanouel DS, et al: Heterogeneity of plasma glucagon. Circulating components in normal subjects and patients with chronic renal failure. J Clin Invest 58:742, 1976.

53. Soman V, Felig P: Glucagon and insulin binding to liver membranes in a partially nephrectomized rat model. J Clin Invest 60:224, 1977.

54. De Fronzo RA: Pathogenesis of glucose intolerance in uremia. Metabolism 27:1866, 1978.

55. Smith D, De Fronzo RA: Insulin resistance in uremia mediated by postbinding defects. Kidney Int 22:54, 1982.

56. De Fronzo RA, Tobin JD, Rowe JW, Reubin A: Glucose intolerance in uremia. Quantification of pancreatic beta cell sensitivity to glucose and tissue sensitivity to insulin. J Clin Invest 62:425, 1978.

57. Ferrannini E, Pilo A, Navalesi R, Citti L: Insulin kinetics and glucose-induced insulin delivery in chronically dialyzed subjects: Acute effects of dialysis. J Clin Endocrinol Metab 49:15, 1979.

58. Rubenfeld S, Garber AJ: Abnormal carbohydrate in chronic renal failure. The potential role of accelerated production, increased gluconeogenesis, and impaired glucose disposal. J Clin Invest 62:20, 1978.

59. Rubenfeld S, Garber AJ: Impact of hemodialysis on the abnormal glucose and alanine kinetics of chronic azotemia. Metabolism 28:934, 1979.

60. Holliday MA, Chantler C: Metabolic and nutritional factors in children with renal insufficiency. Kidney Int 14:306, 1978.

61. Hruska KA, Blondin J, Bass R, et al: Effect of intact parathyroid hormone on hepatic glucose release in the dog. J Clin Invest 64:1016, 1979.

62. Mak RHK, Turner C, Bosque M, et al: Metabolic and hormonal responses to constant hyperglycemia in children with chronic renal failure (CRF). Abstracts of the International Workshop on Recent Advances in Diagnosis and Treatment of Children with Chronic Renal Failure, Heidelberg, May 21–22, 1982.

63. Lim VS, Fang VS, Katz AI, Refetoff S: Thyroid dysfunction in chronic renal failure. A study of pituitary-thyroid axis and peripheral turnover kinetics of thyroxine and triiodothyronine. J Clin Invest 60:522, 1977.

64. Ramirez G, Jubiz W, Gutch CF, et al: Thyroid abnormalities in renal failure. A study of 53 patients on chronic hemodialysis. Ann Intern Med 79:500, 1973.

65. Silverberg DS, Ulan RA, Fawcett DM, et al: Effects of chronic hemodialysis on thyroid function in chronic renal failure. Can Med Assoc J 109:282, 1973.

66. Ijaiya K: TSH and PRL response to thyrotropin-releasing hormone in children with chronic renal failure undergoing hemodialysis. Arch Dis Child 54:937, 1979.

67. Davis FB, Spector DA, Davis PJ, et al: Comparison of pituitary-thyroid function in patients with end-stage renal disease and in age- and sex-matched controls. Kidney Int 37:362, 1982.

68. Fang VS, Lim VS, Refetoff S: Sustained thyrotropin elevation in patients with renal failure. Studies of mechanism in azotemic rats. American Thyroid Association, abstract T6, 1973.

69. Marti-Henneberg C, Domenech JM, Montoya E: Thyrotropin-releasing hormone responsiveness and degradation in children with chronic renal failure: effect of time of evolution. Acta Endocrinol 99:508, 1982.

70. Becker C, van Ypserle de Strihou C, Coche E, et al: Iodine metabolism in severe renal insufficiency. J Clin Endocrinol Metab 29:293, 1969.

71. Oddie TH, Flanigan WJ, Fisher DA: Iodine and thyroxine metabolism in anephric patients receiving chronic peritoneal dialysis. J Clin Endocrinol Metab 31:277, 1970.

72. Savdie E, Stewart JH, Mahony JF, et al: Circulating thyroid hormone levels and adequacy of dialysis. Clin Nephrol 9:68, 1978.

73. Spector DA, Davis PJ, Helderman JH, et al: Thyroid function and metabolic state in chronic renal failure. Ann Intern Med 85:724, 1976.

74. Chopra IJ, Chopra U, Smith SR, et al: Reciprocal changes in serum concentrations of 3,3′,5′-triiodothyronine (reverse T3) and 3,3′,5-triiodothyronine (T3) in systemic illness. J Clin Endocrinol Metab 41:1043, 1975.

75. Kaptein EM, Feinstein EI, Massry SG: Thyroid hormone metabolism in renal disease. Contrib Nephrol 33:122, 1982.

76. Kosowicz J, Malczewska B, Czekalski C: Serum reverse triiodothyronine (3,3′,5′-L-triiodothyronine) in chronic renal failure. Nephron 26:85, 1980.

77. Utiger RD: Decreased extrathyroidal triiodothyronine production in nonthyroid illnesses: Benefit or harm? Am J Med 69:807, 1980.

78. Burke JR, El-Bishti MM, Maisey MN, Chantler C:

Hypothyroidism in children with cystinosis. Arch Dis Child 53:947, 1978.

79. McLean RH, Kennedy TL, Rosoulpour M, et al: Hypothyroidism in the congenital nephrotic syndrome. J Pediatr 101:72, 1982.

80. Feldman HA, Singer I: Endocrinology and metabolism in uremia and dialysis. A clinical review. Medicine 54:345, 1976.

81. Barbour GL, Sevier BR: Adrenal responsiveness in chronic hemodialysis. N Engl J Med 290:1258, 1974.

82. Klett M, Gilli G, Schärer K, Schönberg D, Vecsei P: Plasma-HGH,-TSH and cortisol in children with chronic renal failure (CRF). Pediatr Res 10:897, 1976.

83. Stahnke N, Willig RP, Kollenrott H, et al: Effect of chronic renal failure on insulin, GH, thyroid hormone, gluco- and mineralocorticoid, ACTH and gonadotropin levels. Pediatr Res 15:1551, 1981.

84. McDonald WJ, Golper TA, Mass RD, et al: Adrenocorticotropin-cortisol axis abnormalities in hemodialysis patients. J Clin Endocrinol Metab 48:92, 1979.

85. Wallace EZ, Rosman P, Toshav N, et al: Pituitary-adrenocortical function in chronic renal failure. Studies of episodic secretion of cortisol and dexamethasone suppressibility. J Clin Endocrinol Metab 50:46, 1980.

86. Akmad M, Manzier AD: Simplified assessment of pituitary-adrenal axis in a stable group of chronic hemodialysis patients. Trans Am Soc Artif Intern Organs 23:703, 1977.

87. Rauh W, Steels P, Klare B, et al: Plasma catecholamines, renin and aldosterone during hemodialysis and hemofiltration in children. In: Bulla M (ed), Renal Insufficiency in Children, 3rd International Symposium, Cologne, May 2–3, 1981. Berlin, Heidelberg, New York, Springer Verlag, 1982, p 110.

88. Rosman PM, Faray A, Peckham R, et al: Pituitary-adrenocortical function in chronic renal failure: blunted suppression and early escape of plasma cortisol levels after intravenous dexamethasone. J Clin Endocrinol Metab 54:528, 1982.

89. Bertagna X, Donnadieu M, Idatte JM, Girard F: Dynamics and characterization of plasma immunoreactive β-melanocyte stimulating hormone in hemodialysis patients: Its relationship to ACTH. J Clin Endocrinol Metab 45:1179, 1977.

90. Schalekamp MADH, Schalekamp-Kuyken MPA, De Moor-Fruytier M et al: Interrelationship between blood pressure, renin, renin substrate and blood volume in terminal renal failure. Clin Sci Mol Med 45:417, 1973.

91. Maxwell MH, Weidman P: The renin-angiotensin system in parenchymal renal disease. In: Hamburger J, Crosnier J, Maxwell MH (eds), Advances in Nephrology, Vol 5. Chicago, Year Book Medical Publishers Inc, 1975, p 301.

92. Weidman P, Beretta-Piccoli C, Steffen F, et al: Hypertension in terminal renal failure. Kidney Int 9:294, 1976.

93. Brunner HR, Waeber B, Wauters JP, et al: Inappropriate renin secretion unmasked by captopril (SQ 14225) in hypertension of chronic renal failure. Lancet 2:704, 1978.

94. Friedman A, Chesney RW, Ball D, Goodfriend T: Effective use of captopril (angiotensin I–converting enzyme inhibitor) in severe childhood hypertension. J Pediatr 97:664, 1980.

95. Rauh W, Hund E, Sohl G, et al: Vasoactive hormones and sympathetic nervous system in children with terminal renal failure. Kidney Int, in press.

96. Quellhorst E, Schuenemann B, Hildebrand U, Falda Z: Response of the vascular system to different modifications of hemofiltration and hemodialysis. Proc Eur Dial Transplant Assoc 17:197, 1980.

97. Textor SC, Gavras H, Tifft CP, et al: Norepinephrine and renin activity in chronic renal failure. Evidence for interacting roles in hemodialysis hypertension. Hypertension 3:3, 1981.

98. Ghione S, Fommei E, Clerico A, et al: Major determinants of plasma aldosterone levels in chronic uremia on dialytic treatment. Nephron 30:110, 1982.

99. Horky K, Sramkova J, Lachmanova J, et al: Plasma concentration of antidiuretic hormone in patients with chronic renal insufficiency on maintenance dialysis. Horm Metab Res 11:241, 1979.

100. Möhring J, Kintz J, Schaun J, et al: The antidiuretic hormone and arterial hypertension: recent observations in rats. In: Hamburger J, Crosnier J, Grünfeld JP, Maxwell MH (eds): Advances in Nephrology, Vol 10. Chicago, Year Book Medical Publishers Inc, 1981, p 75.

101. Da Prada M, Zürcher G: Simultaneous radioenzymatic determination of plasma and tissue adrenaline, noradrenaline and dopamine within the femtomole range. Life Sci 19:1161, 1976.

102. Ksiazek A: Beta dopamine hydroxylase activity and catecholamine levels in the plasma of patients with renal failure. Nephron 24:170, 1979.

103. McGrath BP, Ledingham JGG, Benedict CR: Catecholamines in peripheral venous plasma in patients on chronic hemodialysis. Clin Sci Mol Med 55:89, 1978.

104. Henrich WL, Katz FH, Molinoff PB, Schier RW: Competitive effects of hyperkalemia and volume depletion on plasma renin activity, aldosterone and catecholamine concentrations in hemodialysed patients. Kidney Int 12:297, 1977.

105. Brecht HM, Ernst W, Koch KM: Plasma noradrenaline levels in regular hemodialysis patients. Proc Eur Dial Transplant Assoc 12:218, 1976.

106. Hennemann H, Hevendehl G, Reble B, Heidland A: Untersuchungen zur urämischen Sympathikopathie in vitro und in vivo. Dtsch Med Wochenschr 98:1630, 1973.

107. Atuk NO, Bailey CJ, Turner S, et al: Red blood cell catechol-O-methyl transferase, plasma catecholamines and renin in renal failure. Trans Am Soc Artif Intern Organs 22:195, 1976.

108. Kersh FS, Kronfield SJ, Unger A, et al: Autonomic insufficiency in uremia as a cause of hemodialysis-induced hypotension. N Engl J Med 290:650, 1974.

109. Lilley JJ, Golden J, Stone RA: Adrenergic regulation of blood pressure in chronic renal failure. J Clin Invest 57:1190, 1976.

110. Nies AS, Robertson D, Stone WJ: Hemodialysis hypotension is not the result of uremic peripheral autonomic neuropathy. J Lab Clin Med 94:395, 1979.

111. Tomiyama O, Shigai T, Ideura T, et al: Baroreflex sensitivity in renal failure. Clin Sci 58:21, 1980.

112. Reitter B, Müller-Wiefel DE, Schärer K: Motor nerve conduction in children with chronic renal failure. In: Bulla M (ed), Dialysis and Kidney Transplantation in Children. Bibliomed Melsungen, 1979, p 98.

# 22

# Neurologic Complications of ESRD, Dialysis, and Transplantation

*Martin S. Polinsky, M.D.*

## ABBREVIATIONS USED

| | |
|---|---|
| ESRD | – end stage renal disease |
| GFR | – glomerular filtration rate |
| CRT | – Choice Reaction Time Test |
| CPT | – Continuous Performance Test |
| CMT | – Continuous Memory Test |
| WISC-R | – revised Wechsler Intelligence Scales for Children |
| EEG | – electroencephalogram |
| PTH | – parathyroid hormone |
| HPTH | – hyperparathyroidism |
| Hz | – Hertz (cycles/sec) |
| CNS | – central nervous system |
| IV | – intravenous |
| NCV | – nerve conduction velocity |
| VPT | – vibratory perception threshold |
| TKA | – transketolase activity |
| VER | – visual evoked response |
| DDS | – dialysis disequilibrium syndrome |
| RHD | – rapid hemodialysis |
| SHD | – slow hemodialysis |
| CSF | – cerebrospinal fluid |
| PML | – progressive multifocal leukoencephalopathy |
| CPM | – central pontine myelinolysis |
| CVA | – cerebrovascular accident |

Disturbances in central and peripheral nervous system function account for an appreciable proportion of the morbidity associated with severe chronic renal insufficiency in children and adults.[1-3] As the glomerular filtration rate (GFR) approaches levels consistent with ESRD, i.e., < 5 ml/min/1.73 m², an increasing number of patients will develop evidence of neurologic dysfunction. Adequate dialysis or successful transplantation may stabilize or reverse these disturbances; however, both therapeutic modalities have themselves been associated with the development of unique neurologic syndromes, which may, in turn, cause death or permanent disability. Patient age and the premorbid state of the nervous system appear to determine, in part, susceptibility to certain uremia-related forms of neurologic injury. Peripheral neuropathy, for example, occurs more commonly in adults,[4, 5] while disturbances such as those which follow the initiation of dialysis, e.g., the dialysis dysequilibrium syndrome, are seen more frequently in children.[1, 6, 7] Still other forms of neurologic dysfunction may be unique to the very young child with renal disease.[8-13] Nonetheless, because similar patterns of neurologic disease may be seen in renal patients of widely disparate ages, this chapter will review the spectrum of neurologic complications of ESRD, dialysis, and transplantation in all age groups, with major emphasis on those relevant to pediatrics.

Several syndromes of neurologic dysfunction are identifiable in children on the basis of clinical, psychometric, and electrophysiologic studies. These include uremic, hypertensive, and drug-induced encephalopathies, an as yet unexplained form of progressive neurologic deterioration resembling that of adult dialysis dementia, and peripheral and cranial neuropathies.

## ESRD AND NEUROLOGIC FUNCTION

### Uremic Encephalopathy

**Cognitive Disturbances.** The earliest signs of uremic encephalopathy usually appear in association with marked azotemia (e.g., BUN concentrations ≥ 300 mg/dl), and a reduction of the GFR to 4 to 10 ml/min,[14] although subtler disturbances in mentation may appear with renal decompensation of lesser degrees of severity. The *rate* of deterioration, more than the absolute level of the GFR, appears to determine the specific pattern of symptoms seen and the time of their appearance.[2, 15] The premorbid personality also influences the nature of the psychiatric manifestations of uremic encephalopathy found in individual patients.[16, 17]

As renal insufficiency progresses, the earliest and most sensitive indicator of developing encephalopathy is the appearance of sensorial clouding,[15] i.e., a decrease in the level of interaction between patient and environment, which often manifests as indifference, preoccupation, and fatigue. Subtle disturbances in cognitive function appear, in the form of a decreased ability to concentrate and diminished attention span.[2, 3, 15, 18] Teschan et al[19] have defined two forms of attention deficits, "sustained" and "selective." The former relates to an "[in]ability to focus . . . on a given task for a period of time," and the latter to an "[in]ability to respond only to relevant stimuli among other extraneous and irrelevant [ones]. . . ." These early cognitive disturbances also include a diminished capacity for performing the repetitive mental manipulation of symbols, and reduced speed of decision making.[19] The Choice Reaction Time (CRT), Continuous Performance Test (CPT), Continuous Memory Test (CMT), and the ability to perform mental arithmetic have proved particularly useful in identifying these disturbances of higher cortical function in adults.[19, 20] Progressively poorer performances have been associated with increasingly higher serum creatinine concentrations, beginning at levels corresponding to only moderately diminished GFRs.[19] Recently, the CPT was used to evaluate attention span in a group of children with ESRD 7 to 14 days prior to the initiation of maintenance dialysis.[21] Interestingly, no significant difference was observed between the mean test score in these patients and that of a group of normal children matched for age, intelligence, and years of parental education.

Little information is available regarding the evolution of cognitive disturbances in the uremic infant and very young child, but the delayed acquisition of developmental milestones, or the actual regression of those previously achieved, is to be expected.[8] The Denver Developmental Screening Test[22] has been used to detect the presence of developmental delay in children with congenital nephropathies.[8] The revised Wechsler Intelligence Scales for Children (WISC-R), Peabody Individual Achievement Test, Halstead-Reitan Category Test, and a Free Recall Memory Task have been used to evaluate intelligence, problem-solving ability, and memory in children with ESRD.[21] Concomitant drug therapy (e.g., with anticonvulsants),[23] the presence of chronic anemia, uremia-associated nutritional deficiency,[8, 24–28] and trace metal intoxication (see below) may also interfere with cognitive function and psychomotor development in very young children with ESRD due to congenital nephropathies.

The early diagnosis of uremic encephalopathy may be difficult. Initially, periods of normal mentation and reactivity may be interspersed with those in which symptoms are manifest. Moreover, the electroencephalogram (EEG) may or may not be abnormal at this time (see below).[2] Finally, if the rate of deterioration is sufficiently rapid, a delirium (toxic psychosis) may develop, characterized by the acute onset of agitation, delusions, and hallucinations.[2, 15, 16, 29] These findings are not specific for uremia and may be seen in patients with other disorders, including drug

---

**Table 22–1.** DIFFERENTIAL DIAGNOSIS OF UREMIC ENCEPHALOPATHY*

1. Hypertensive encephalopathy
2. Drug-induced encephalopathy
3. Electrolyte imbalance
   (a) Water intoxication (dilutional hyponatremia)
   (b) Hypocalcemia
   (c) Severe acidemia
4. Unexplained, progressive encephalopathy (Dialysis dementia–like syndrome of childhood)
5. CNS infection
6. Pre-existing neuropsychiatric conditions
   (a) Functional psychiatric disorders
   (b) CNS vasculitis associated with multisystem disease (e.g., SLE)
   (c) Idiopathic seizure disorder

*All conditions may be associated with seizures.

intoxication and metabolic encephalopathies of nonrenal etiology (Table 22–1).

As renal insufficiency progresses, additional cognitive disturbances appear. Recent memory deteriorates, followed much later by remote memory. Personality deterioration becomes more apparent as patients manifest increasing irritability and lack of cooperation. More profound alterations in the content of consciousness develop as confusion and disorientation appear. Finally, the level of consciousness declines, with lethargy progressing to stupor and then coma. Normal ventilation is replaced by Kussmaul breathing, followed by Cheyne-Stokes respirations and, ultimately, respiratory arrest.[16]

**Motor Disturbances.** Motor disturbances almost always accompany cognitive dysfunction in developing uremic encephalopathy, and include muscle cramps, manifestations of neuromuscular hyperirritability, myopathy, weakness due to peripheral neuropathy, and seizures[2, 3, 14, 15, 29] (Table 22–2). The earliest signs are those of muscle cramps, tremor, and asterixis. Cramps are exacerbated by movement. They are usually nocturnal at first, but later begin to occur during, or to persist into, the waking hours as well. Their occurrence has been noted more commonly in patients with water intoxication[2] and in association with worsening acidosis and an increase in the serum Na:K concen-

tration ratio.[18] Asterixis, which is usually present by the time sensorial clouding develops,[15] is not specific for uremia and may be seen in other forms of metabolic encephalopathy. Muscle tremor is more readily apparent with motion and during attempts to elicit asterixis.

Myoclonus and muscle fasciculations are generally seen with advanced encephalopathy, and often in the presence of stupor or coma.[15, 30] "Diffuse neuronal dysfunction," alterations in the cerebrospinal fluid (CSF) K:Ca ratio, and an increase in the CSF phosphate concentration have all been implicated in the pathogenesis of these changes.[2] Other manifestations of the neuromuscular hyperirritability which may be seen in advanced uremia include hypertonia with marked stretch reflex asymmetry,[29, 31] calcium unresponsive tetany,[2] meningismus, opisthotonus, and decorticate posturing.[15]

Myopathy occurs in patients with ESRD, and may be proximal or distal in distribution. Distal myopathy usually develops in association with severe peripheral neuropathy (see below). A primary polymyopathy also occurs, as characterized by proximal muscle weakness, wasting, and tenderness,[2, 32] and must be differentiated from polymyositis[2] and the ischemic myopathy associated with secondary hyperparathyroidism (HPTH).[33, 34] A severe proximal myopathy has also been described

**Table 22–2. MOTOR DISTURBANCES IN ESRD**

| Disturbance | Clinical Setting in Which Seen | Etiology |
|---|---|---|
| 1. Muscle cramps | "Early" uremic encephalopathy | Decreased muscle intracellular pH.[2] Fluid shift into muscle cells.[102] Effects of uremic "toxins."[102] |
| 2. Muscle tremor | "Early" uremic encephalopathy | "Increased CNS irritability."[102] |
| 3. Asterixis | "Early" uremic encephalopathy | "Diffuse CNS dysfunction of a metabolic nature."[102] |
| 4. Myoclonus | "Advanced" uremic encephalopathy | "Diffuse neuronal dysfunction."[2] Elevated blood, neuronal urea concentrations.[3] |
| 5. Fasciculations | "Advanced" uremic encephalopathy | Elevated CSF $K^+$:$Ca^{++}$ ratio.[2] Elevated CSF $PO_4^{-3}$ concentration.[2] |
| 6. Distal muscle weakness, wasting | Advanced peripheral neuropathy (GFR $\leq$ 5–13 ml/min/1.73 m²) | Multiple uremic "toxins" implicated.[100] |
| 7. Proximal muscle weakness, wasting | (a) Severe secondary hyperparathyroidism | Skeletal muscle ischemia due to circumferential medial arteriolar calcinosis and intimal fibrosis.[33, 34] |
| | (b) Primary polymyopathy (i) Mild (weakness only) | Nonspecific, minor changes on muscle biopsy.[2] |
| | (ii) Severe | Skeletal muscle ischemia due to luminal arteriolar phospholipid deposition. |
| | (c) Hemodialysis patients with osteomalacia and multiple bone fractures | Aluminum accumulation in bone.[36, 80] |

in adult dialysis patients with osteomalacia and multiple bone fractures, absence of osteitis fibrosa, and normal or low serum parathyroid hormone (PTH) levels.[35, 36] Bone aluminum levels were markedly elevated in these patients.

Seizures may be focal or generalized and are not an uncommon manifestation of uremic encephalopathy, occurring in 33 to 46% of patients in various series.[17, 29, 31] A significantly higher incidence of seizures was seen in patients with BUN concentrations above 250 mg/dl than in those with levels of 50 to 199 mg/dl.[17] Seizures occurring during early uremic encephalopathy are often attributable to the presence of superimposed severe hypertension or drug toxicity.[15] Rapid serum pH or electrolyte shifts may provoke seizures, and an increase in the serum K:Ca concentration ratio has been noted to be a good indicator of seizure risk.[2]

Analysis of CSF obtained from uremic patients has shown the presence of elevated opening pressures and protein concentrations.[2, 15, 18, 29] However, earlier reports documenting the finding of CSF pleocytosis in uremic patients[31, 37] have not been confirmed in more recent studies.[2] The presence of a CSF pleocytosis should be considered a sign of infection until proven otherwise.[18]

**EEG Changes in Uremic Encephalopathy.** Alterations in the resting EEG are seen in most adults when BUN concentrations exceed 60 mg/dl.[2] Recordings in mild uremic encephalopathy may be normal or of the "low voltage" pattern and may occur in association with a less clearly defined alpha component to the fundamental (background) rhythm than that expected for age.[2] Psychometric testing has demonstrated cognitive dysfunction in adults with ESRD when slow, i.e., < 7 Hz (cycles/sec) waves are present in 40% of the EEG recording.[38] With worsening of uremia, progressive slowing and disorganization (poor regulation) of the fundamental rhythm occurs. Ultimately, diffuse slowing for age appears, associated with paroxysmal bursts of bilaterally synchronous, high amplitude slow waves; the largest amplitudes generally arise from the anterior (fronto-parietal) parasagittal scalp regions.[2, 39] A paradoxical response to eye opening and abnormal arousal responses are also seen.[39] In an early study,[38] the presence of slow wave (< 7 Hz) activity in >15 to 25% of the EEG record was taken as an indication for initiation of dialysis. In children, however, age-related variations in

the fundamental frequency make such judgments difficult when based solely on visual inspection of brain electrical activity.[40] Moreover, hypertension and anemia may also alter the EEG.[38]

***Quantitative Analysis of Brain Electrical Activity in Children with Chronic Renal Failure and ESRD.*** Visual inspection of the EEG in patients with chronic renal insufficiency does not provide data which can be quantitatively related to attendant clinical and biochemical disturbances. To solve this problem, manual and automated methods have been applied to the quantitative evaluation of brain electrical activity in patients with chronic renal insufficiency and ESRD.[41–47] Quantitative measures, which have been found particularly useful in evaluating the degree of slowing of the fundamental rhythm which occurs as uremia worsens, include: (1) the percentage of EEG power (area) < 5 Hz;[42, 43, 46] (2) the percentage of EEG frequencies < 7 Hz;[42, 46] and (3) the percentage of slow wave–associated EEG power.[19] Analogous to (1) above, the last measure depicts slow frequency–associated electrical energy by the ratio: % EEG Power $[(3–7)Hz/(3–13)Hz] \times 100$. A statistically significant, positive linear correlation has been shown to exist between the percentage of slow wave–associated EEG power and serum creatinine concentrations between 2 and 29 mg/dl $(r = 0.63, p < 0.001)$, suggesting that as GFR falls below 50 ml/min/1.73 m$^2$ progressive slowing of the fundamental EEG rhythm occurs.[19]

Normal values for the above indices are age-dependent.[19, 40] Thus, they have not yet been applied to the evaluation of the EEG in children, since a major problem in this regard has been the development of a normative electrophysiologic data base for comparison. A major step in this direction was taken with the development of neurometrics.[48] This technique utilizes computer analysis of the EEG to quantitatively assessed brain electrical activity at rest and in response to somatosensory stimuli. To date, a pool of 648 normal children has been studied in an attempt to obtain normative data regarding the distribution of EEG frequencies at all ages from 5 to 21 years.[40] Recently, neurometrics was applied to the evaluation of resting EEG data from 26 children with chronic renal insufficiency of varying degrees of severity.[49] Quantitative electrophysiologic data were obtained from each of 20 scalp electrode positions.

These were then referenced to age-related norms by Z-transformation, and a multivariate statistic, the EEG Severity Index (SI), was calculated by "summing" the corresponding univariate probabilities from individual electrodes. As such, the SI represents the probability of obtaining the observed *overall* pattern of brain electrical activity in a normal child *of the same age*. As calculated, an SI = 1,2,3 ... n corresponds to a 10%, 1%, 0.1% ... $(10^{-n} \times 100)\%$ probability of normal, respectively. Statistically significant linear correlations were observed between: (a) SI and duration of chronic renal insufficiency (r = 0.77, p < 0.05, Fig. 22–1, A), and (b) SI and the calculated creatinine clearance $(C_{Cr})^{50}$ (r = 0.77, p < 0.05, Fig. 22–1, B). Interestingly, these relationships resemble those derived by Teschan et al[19] for percentage of EEG power [(3–7) Hz/(3–13)Hz] × 100 versus serum creatinine concentration in adults, except that, with neurometrics, elec-

trophysiologic data are obtained from all scalp electrode positions and the data are adjusted by referencing to age-matched norms.

Thus, when corrected for age-related variations in brain electrical activity, quantitative electrophysiologic data can be related to severity of disease in both adults and children with chronic renal insufficiency. Through the application of these or similar techniques to the evaluation of EEG data in the future, it may ultimately be possible to quantitate adequacy of dialysis as a function of the extent to which patterns of brain electrical activity are normalized.

**Pathologic Changes.** An extensive study of CNS pathology in patients dying with chronic renal insufficiency was conducted by Olsen.[51] These data have been reviewed recently.[3]

Using computed tomography, it has been shown that diffuse cerebral cortical atrophy occurs in patients with long-standing ESRD.[52]

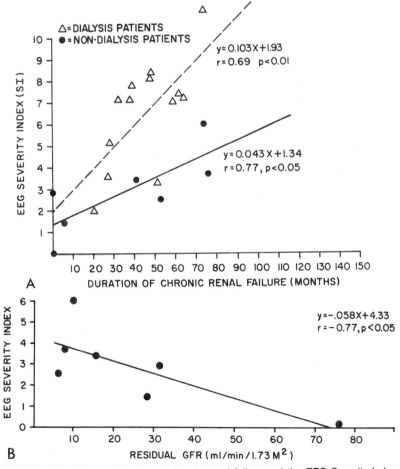

**Figure 22–1.** *A,* Relationship between duration of chronic renal failure and the EEG Severity Index for dialysis (△) and non-dialysis (●) patients. (From Polinsky M et al: Proc Dial Transplant Forum 10:299, 1980, with permission.) *B,* Relationship between residual GFR and the EEG Severity Index for non-dialysis patients.

Although significant differences in ventricular size were seen in patients versus controls in all age groups under 70, the most marked differences were found in two children, aged four and ten years. Cortical atrophy was recently identified in eight of 16 children with ESRD, and isolated ventricular enlargement in another two.[53] Additional reports of cerebral atrophy in children with ESRD and unexplained progressive encephalopathy have also appeared.[9-11]

**Etiology of Uremic Encephalopathy.** The etiology of uremic encephalopathy is not known. Studies using animal models of acute and chronic renal failure have provided some insight into the nature of the biochemical, metabolic, and physiologic disturbances which may be present in uremic patients. Increases in brain, CSF, and plasma urea concentrations and osmolalities occur in uremic animals versus controls,[54] but to comparable extents in all compartments, so that no change in brain water content is observed. Thus, uremia per se does not cause cerebral edema. Cerebral cortical energy metabolism is, however, disordered in uremic rat brain.[15, 55, 56] The disturbances are characterized by diminished cerebral glucose and, perhaps, oxygen consumption in the resting state, and by impaired utilization of high energy phosphate (ATP and creatinine phosphate). The permeability of the blood-brain barrier to ionic and nonionic substances is altered over a wide range of molecular weights. Rates of uptake of $^{35}SO_4$ and $^{42}K$ are increased, and those of $^{24}Na$ and $^{14}C$ penicillin decreased in the uremic brain,[57-59] whereas permeability to $^{14}C$ inulin and $^{14}C$ sucrose are both increased.[57, 58] The activity of brain Na-K–activated ATPase has been found to be normal in recent studies.[55, 57] The significance of these observations remains unclear.

*Role of PTH and Brain Calcium.* A significant increase in brain calcium content has been demonstrated in adults dying with secondary HPTH,[46] and in acutely uremic animals.[42, 46, 54, 60] This increase has been produced in animals with normal renal function by administration of parathyroid extract, but is prevented by parathyroidectomy when performed prior to induction of uremia.[42, 60] Giving Vitamin $D_3$ in quantities sufficient to produce persistent hypercalcemia or infusing sufficient phosphate into Vitamin $D_3$-treated animals to markedly elevate the calcium-phosphorus product also failed to significantly increase cortical gray matter calcium levels in the absence of HPTH.[60] EEG abnormalities and impaired performance on cognitive function studies have been demonstrated in adults with primary and secondary HPTH, the latter due to acute and chronic renal insufficiency.[43, 46] The electrophysiologic disturbances observed in patients with HPTH were similar to those described in adults with renal failure. Following either subtotal parathyroidectomy or recovery from acute renal failure, the percentage of EEG power < 5 Hz and percentage of EEG frequencies < 7 Hz and >9 Hz achieved or approached normal values.[43, 46] Moreover, improved performance on cognitive function studies was seen post-parathyroidectomy in patients with secondary HPTH.[46]

The above data suggest that PTH may be a neurotoxic substance when present in elevated concentrations, and may exert its detrimental effects either directly, or indirectly by promoting the accumulation of other toxic substances in the brains of patients with chronic renal insufficiency. Of interest are the reports that PTH enhances the accumulation of aluminum in cortical gray matter.[61, 62] However, the potential role of PTH in the pathogenesis of uremia-related neurologic dysfunction remains controversial.[63]

## Hypertensive Encephalopathy

Disturbances in neurologic function commonly occur in children with hypertension and chronic renal disease.[64] In such patients, hypertension severe enough to precipitate encephalopathy may result from one or more of the following: an acute exacerbation of the underlying renal disease; volume overload associated with dietary non-compliance or the sudden loss of residual renal function; non-compliance with antihypertensive medications; or complications of drug therapy per se, such as rebound hypertension following abrupt clonidine withdrawal[257] or clonidine-beta blocker interactions.[258] Hypertensive encephalopathy is a reversible disorder characterized by the subacute onset of generalized, rather than focal, disturbances in cerebral function.[65-68] If not recognized and treated promptly, permanent brain damage or death may result. Symptoms usually begin with severe generalized headache, which has been present for several hours to 1 to 2 days, and is followed by the appearance of alterations in cognition and in the level of consciousness. The latter manifest initially as somnolence and confusion, progressing to stupor and then coma if therapeutic intervention has not occurred. Restlessness is also a prominent early symptom.[65]

Other prominent clinical manifestations include: vomiting; visual disturbances (blurring, amaurosis); VIth and VIIth cranial nerve palsies manifesting as diplopia, facial weakness, and dysarthria; transient, migratory focal neurologic deficits; and seizures.[64-66] Retinal arteriolar vasospasm is nearly always present. Retinal hemorrhages and exudates, the "clinical hallmark of the disease,"[69] and papilledema, are present in most, but not all, patients.[29, 65]

CSF examination shows normal or elevated opening pressure and protein concentration; pleocytosis is not seen unless subarachnoid hemorrhage has occurred. The EEG may show transient focal changes and/or the bilateral slowing characteristic of uremia per se, with superimposed sharp waves.[65] Radiographic, sonographic, and scintigraphic studies are normal.

Uremic and hypertensive encephalopathies may coexist. Both can cause altered cognition, a decreased level of consciousness, and seizures. Moreover, the onset of uremic encephalopathy may be acute. However, visual disturbances are not as common in uremic encephalopathy and headache is not as prominent a complaint. The above-noted funduscopic findings, combined with a positive response to antihypertensive therapy, should differentiate these two conditions. The rapid resolution of symptoms and signs which occurs following control of the hypertension is, perhaps, the most important observation for confirming the diagnosis of hypertensive encephalopathy.[65, 66, 70]

Other causes of encephalopathy which may be associated with systemic and intracranial hypertension in patients with ESRD, with or without focal neurologic signs, include intracranial hemorrhage, brain tumor, brain abscess (see below), cerebral infarction, and thromboembolism. The persistence of a focal neurologic sign, e.g., cranial nerve palsy or hemiparesis, following control of hypertension, should raise the suspicion of an intracranial mass lesion and is an indication for further diagnostic work-up, including computed tomography.

The presence of hypertensive encephalopathy is an indication for the immediate reduction of systemic arterial pressure. The most effective agents in this regard are diazoxide and nitroprusside. Neither drug interferes with the clinical evaluation of central nervous system function.[71] It is recommended that diazoxide be given by rapid (bolus) IV infusion in a dose of 2 to 10 mg/kg (maximum 300 mg) with constant blood pressure monitoring.[72, 73] Lower doses are often as effective as higher ones initially, and may prevent the development of sequelae associated with too rapid or excessive lowering of the blood pressure (see below). Excessive dosing also may be "associated with overshoot of the return blood pressure to levels exceeding pretreatment readings."[71] The onset of effect is usually within one minute, while maximum hypotension is seen at two to five minutes.[73] The duration of effect has been variably reported as 3 to 15[73] and 4 to 24 hours.[72]

Nitroprusside is the drug of choice when cerebral hemorrhage is suspected, and in the presence of congestive heart failure. It is administered in 5% dextrose in water as a continuous infusion, commonly at rates of 0.5 to 8 $\mu$g/kg/min[72] but doses as high as 400 $\mu$g/kg/min have been administered for short periods of time,[74] and in situations where other drug therapy has failed to halt a progressively rising blood pressure. A stepwise increase in the dose of nitroprusside above 8 $\mu$g/kg/min is indicated until the desired degree of hypotensive effect is obtained. The antihypertensive effect ceases within 5 to 10 minutes of its discontinuation.[71, 74] Nitroprusside does not increase cardiac work and is therefore well suited for use in patients with congestive heart failure, with or without pulmonary edema. Serum thiocyanate concentrations should be monitored in children with renal insufficiency and therapy modified when levels exceed 10 mg/dl.

The development of permanent blindness has been reported recently in association with the use of potent antihypertensives to control malignant hypertension in children and adults with renal disease.[64, 75-79] These reports are worrisome because dramatic reductions in systemic arterial pressure may, in fact, further compromise cerebral perfusion.[80] In some of these cases, partial or complete loss of vision either preceded initiation of therapy[64, 78] or occurred in association with a *gradual* lowering of blood pressure over 24 hours,[79] suggesting that the loss of vision may have developed as a consequence of the hypertension itself. Prompt reduction of blood pressure in patients with hypertensive encephalopathy is still indicated to prevent permanent neurologic sequelae or death due to cerebral edema.[64, 66] Adherence to guidelines regarding dosage and mode of administration may help avoid complications related to inordinately rapid blood pressure reduction, with resulting further compromise of cerebral perfusion.

## Drug-Induced Encephalopathy in the Pediatric ESRD Patient

Drug-related disturbances in cognitive function occur commonly in patients with ESRD.[81, 82] Of 178 episodes of neurologic dysfunction occurring in adults with chronic renal failure, 61 (34.3%) were attributed by process of exclusion to "definite" or "probable" drug toxicity.[82] In most cases of drug-induced encephalopathy the clinical presentation is that of delirium (toxic psychosis), decreased consciousness, or seizures. Delirium, as previously described, has been observed following the administration of therapeutic doses of chlorpromazine, promethazine, diphenhydramine, tripolidine, and cyproheptadine, alone[83] or in combination,[84, 85] and is similar to that produced by atropine.[82] The clinical manifestations are indistinguishable from those of the central anticholinergic syndrome,[84] and may be accompanied by signs of peripheral cholinergic blockade such as mydriasis, warm, flushed, dry skin, xerostomia, and fever. The penicillins, including some of the newer, semisynthetic ones, are known cortical irritants;[81, 86] in addition to delirium, ESRD patients have developed myoclonus, asterixis, and seizures following their administration.[87] The benzodiazepines (diazepam, flurazepam) have produced an encephalopathy characterized by confusion, asterixis, and diffuse slowing of the fundamental EEG rhythm.[88] A reversible encephalopathy characterized by confusion, dysarthria, and diffuse EEG slowing has followed the administration of amitriptyline to an adult hemodialysis patient.[88] Reversible psychic disturbances also have occurred in patients with ESRD to whom aminoglycosides, colistin, barbiturates, and haloperidol were administered.[82]

The pathogenesis of drug-induced neurotoxicity appears, to some extent, to involve an increase in the amount of free drug or

active metabolite available for entry into the CSF.[81] The factors involved may vary with the particular class of compound in question, but, in general, toxic levels of drug may accumulate in the CNS owing to decreased plasma protein binding, the absence of appreciable renal excretion, and diminished outward transport across the blood-brain barrier via the choroid plexus. All three mechanisms may be operative in the pathogenesis of penicillin neurotoxicity.[89, 90] Similarly, the delirium accompanying the use of atropine, phenothiazines, antihistamines, and tricyclic antidepressants has been attributed to a combination of diminished renal clearance and an increase in the unbound plasma drug fraction.[84]

The differential diagnosis of a neuropsychiatric disorder which occurs suddenly and unexpectedly in a child with ESRD should always include drug toxicity. The resolution of symptoms following withdrawal of the suspected agent confirms the diagnosis and may be the only form of therapy required, unless respiratory depression or seizures have occurred. The time required for resolution of symptoms varies greatly between drugs. The neurologic symptoms and EEG disturbances associated with phenothiazine toxicity have required up to 7 to 29 days to resolve,[83] while those attributed to the benzodiazepines were gone in 4 to 5 days.[88] Penicillin-related neurotoxicity usually resolves in 24 to 72 hours, although that specifically associated with ticarcillin therapy disappeared only after 7 to 14 days, in a single patient.[87] The delirium associated with parasympathetic blockade has been successfully treated, in otherwise normal patients, with physostigmine salicylate. Since the use of this drug is contraindicated in the presence of renovascular hypertension,[84] physostigmine should be reserved for those children with ESRD in whom respiratory depression due to parasympathetic blockade is present.

## Unexplained (Dialysis Dementia-Like) Progressive Encephalopathy in Children with ESRD

A relatively new and, as yet, unexplained neurologic syndrome has been described in an increasing number of young children with chronic renal insufficiency during the past 5 years. In 1977, Baluarte et al first reported the development of a syndrome of progres-

**Table 22–3.** STAGING OF NEUROLOGIC DETERIORATION IN CHILDREN WITH ESRD AND UNEXPLAINED ENCEPHALOPATHY*

| Stage | Neurologic Manifestations |
|---|---|
| I | Tremor<br>Dysmetria (infants; very young children)<br>Ataxia (ambulatory patients)<br>Arrested acquisition of new motor skills<br>Hyperreflexia<br>Positive Babinski sign |
| II | Marked ataxia<br>Myoclonus (face and extremities)<br>Seizures<br>Regression of previously acquired developmental milestones<br>Hypotonia |
| III<br>(Chronic Vegetative State) | Unresponsiveness to visual/auditory stimuli<br>Absence of voluntary movement<br>Generalized myoclonus<br>Marked hypotonia<br>Absent swallowing function with retention of gag reflex |

*Modified from Foley CM et al, Arch Neurol 38:656, 1981, with permission.

sive neurologic deterioration, clinically indistinguishable from that of adult dialysis dementia (see below), in five children with congenital nephropathy and severe renal insufficiency.[9] All had bilateral renal hypoplasia/dysplasia, initially diagnosed at 3 weeks to 14 months of age in 4 children and at 6½ years in the fifth patient. Neurologic dysfunction appeared at 2 to 9½ years of age, at which time all patients had elevated BUN and creatinine concentrations (ranges: 60–105 and 4.27–7.2 mg/dl, respectively) and GFRs of 5–10 ml/min/1.73 m².

The major clinical abnormalities seen included speech disorder (lingual apraxia, dysarthria), tremor, myoclonus, seizures, and dementia; in the younger children, dementia was characterized by regression of previously achieved developmental milestones. In all patients a stereotyped pattern of progressive deterioration occurred in three stages, the clinical characteristics of which are summarized in Table 22–3.[12]

In the three patients in whom it was performed, computed tomography was abnormal and demonstrated ventricular dilation with cortical atrophy. EEGs were abnormal in all patients; sequential studies demonstrated progressive slowing of the fundamental rhythm with superimposed bursts of sharp waves and 2–4 Hz polyspike-wave discharges (Fig. 22–2), abnormalities similar to those

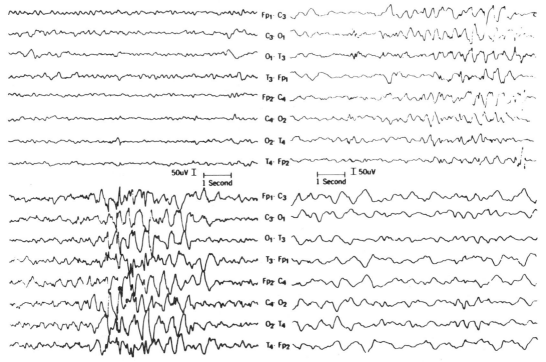

**Figure 22–2.** Serial tracings from EEG recordings obtained at six-month intervals beginning at 3½ years of age, in a boy with unexplained, progressive encephalopathy. See text for interpretation. (Earliest tracing is in upper left; latest, lower right.)

described in adults with dialysis dementia.[91, 92] Clinical and electrophysiologic deterioration occurred in parallel.

Renal osteodystrophy was present in all patients within 18 to 30 months of the time renal disease was diagnosed, as documented by the presence of hyperphosphatasia, characteristic radiographic changes, and markedly elevated serum PTH concentrations.[9] All children received massive doses of phosphate binding gels (240–800 mg/kg/day) for 9 to 62 months, resulting in considerable exposure to aluminum, and all experienced the onset of neurologic deterioration within 6 months of the time when maximal dose phosphate binder therapy was initiated. Of note is the development of symptoms in all children *prior to* the onset of dialysis, a phenomenon only recently described in adults,[93, 94] in whom the onset of neurologic deterioration usually occurs after months to years of maintenance dialysis (see below).

In a survey of 96 United States and foreign pediatric ESRD centers,[95] 24 of 728 patients, from 14 of 61 responding centers, were reported to have developed a syndrome of progressive mental deterioration (personality changes, dementia, regression of developmental milestones), speech disturbances, and seizures (Fig. 22–3). Abnormal EEGs similar to those described above were recorded in patients from 77% of reporting institutions. In 69% of the centers reporting cases, the appearance of neurologic deterioration had *followed* the initiation of maintenance dialysis, whereas in 31% it had not. All centers reported that patients had received or were receiving aluminum-containing phosphate binders prior to or at the time of appearance of symptoms, and all but one patient had secondary HPTH.

Additional cases of progressive and unexplained encephalopathy have occurred in children with ESRD (Table 22–4).[8, 10, 11, 13, 96] These patients also had congenital nephropathies, and developed a progressive encephalopathy characterized by dementia, regression of developmental milestones, speech disorder, ataxia, myoclonus, and seizures. Characteristic EEGs were recorded in association with these clinical findings, and CT scans showed cortical atrophy in all of them. All had severe secondary HPTH. The patient of Nathan et al[13] had received aluminum-containing phosphate binding gels for 5½ years and was found to have a markedly elevated aluminum level in brain gray matter of 80 μg/gm dry weight (normal 2.2–2.4 μg/gm[97, 98]). However, this child did not receive a trial of dialysis, so that a component of uremic encephalopathy cannot be excluded from having contributed to the pathogenesis of his neurologic disease. Another child[96] received large quantities of phosphate binders and had a serum aluminum concentration of 651 μg/L at the time of appearance of encephalopathy (M. Polinsky, unpublished data); discontinuation of phosphate binder therapy led to clinical improvement. One of Geary et al's[11] patients had a markedly elevated serum aluminum concentration of 601 μg/L, and the other, a brain gray matter

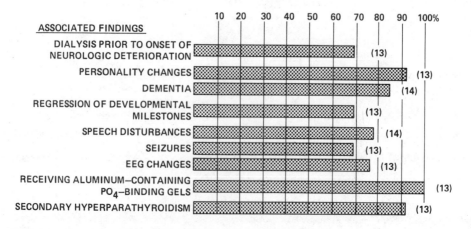

% OF CENTERS REPORTING CASES WITH FINDING NOTED*

*Numbers in parentheses indicate total number of centers responding to each item.

**Figure 22–3.** Results of a multicenter survey of unexplained, progressive encephalopathy occurring in childhood end stage renal disease: distribution of associated findings by centers reporting cases.

**Table 22–4.** CLINICAL FEATURES OF UNEXPLAINED ENCEPHALOPATHY OF CHILDHOOD CHRONIC RENAL FAILURE (CRF)*

| Reference # | (9,12)** | (11) | (10) | (13) | (8) | Totals | (%) |
|---|---|---|---|---|---|---|---|
| # Cases | 5 | 2 | 3 | 1 | 20 | 31 | (35.5) |
| Male:female | 4:1 | 2:0 | 3:0 | 1:0 | 17:3 | 27:4 | |
| *Etiology of CRF:* | | | | | | | |
| Hypodysplasia | 5/5 | 2/2 | 1/3 | 1/1 | 4/20 | 11/31 | (35.5) |
| Obstruction | — | — | 2/3 | — | 14/20 | 18/31 | (58.1) |
| Polycystic kidneys | — | — | — | — | 1/20 | 1/31 | (3.2) |
| Medullary cystic disease | — | — | — | — | 1/20 | 1/31 | (3.2) |
| *Age at onset of:* | | | | | | | |
| CRF | 1–78 mo | 2–6 mo | 0–2 mo | 6 mo | 0–13 mo | — | |
| CNS Disease | 24–114 mo | 6–12 mo | 17–66 mo | 72 mo | 0.5–83 mo | — | |
| Microcephaly | N**** | N | 2/3 | N | 15/20 | 17/23 | (73.9) |
| Hypotonia | 5/5 | N | 3/3 | N | 13/20 | 21/28 | (75) |
| Hyperreflexia | 5/5 | N | 0/3 | N | N | 5/8 | (62.5) |
| Tremor | 5/5 | N | N | N | 3/20 | 8/26 | (30.8) |
| Dysmetria/ataxia | 4/5 | 1/2 | 3/3 | 1/1 | 4/20 | 13/31 | (41.9) |
| Myoclonus | 5/5 | 2/2 | N | 1/1 | 3/20 | 11/28 | (39.3) |
| Seizures | 5/5 | 2/2 | 3/3 | 1/1 | 13/20 | 24/31 | (77.4) |
| *Abnormal:* | | | | | | | |
| CT scan | 2/2 | 2/2 | 1/3 | Not Done | 7/12 | 12/19 | (63.2) |
| EEG | 5/5 | 2/2 | 3/3 | 1/1 | 17/18 | 28/29 | (96.6) |
| Hyperparathyroidism | 5/5 | 2/2 | N | 1/1 | 4/8 | 12/16 | (75) |
| Aluminum intake*** | 5/5 | 2/2 | N | 1/1 | 16/20 | 24/28 | (85.7) |
| Dialysis*** | 0/5 | 0/2 | 0/3 | 0/1 | 0/20 | 0/31 | 0 |
| *Results of therapy:†* | | | | | | | |
| Anticonvulsants | TI: 5/5 | I: 1/1 | I: 2/3 | NI: 1/1 | N | | — |
| Dialysis | NI: 3/3 | Not Done | Not Done | Not Done | N | | — |
| Transplantation | NI: 2/3 | Not Done | Not Done | Not Done | I: 1/4 | | — |
| | S: 1/3 | | | | NI: 3/4 | | |
| Parathyroidectomy | NI: 1/1 | TS: 2/2 | Not Done | Not Done | Not Done | | — |
| Mortality | 4/5 | 1/2 | 2/3 | 1/1 | 10/20 | 18/31 | (58.1) |

*Also see Fig. 22–3.
**Included in Fig. 22–3 data.
***Prior to onset of CNS disease.
****Not noted.
†KEY:
  I = Improvement
  TI = Transient improvement
  NI = No improvement
  S = Stabilization
  TS = Transient stabilization

aluminum concentration of 13.6 μg/gm dry weight (normal 3.3, 3.4, and 8.7 μg/gm).

The above data appear to support an association between secondary HPTH, aluminum intake, and the unexplained progressive encephalopathy of childhood ESRD. Both HPTH and aluminum ingestion have been identified as potential risk factors for the development of dialysis dementia, a syndrome attributable, in its acute form, to aluminum intoxication[99, 100] (see below). However, as noted by Geary et al,[11] their patient's brain aluminum level was not appreciably different from that of a child who died of chronic renal failure without encephalopathy (12.1 μg/gm), suggesting that aluminum alone may have not been responsible for the observed symptoms. Similar observations made by Arieff et al[101] suggest that cortical gray matter aluminum levels may be elevated in a number of pathologic states associated with alterations in the permeability characteristics of the blood-brain barrier. Finally, a patient of Bale et al[10] with progressive encephalopathy was reported to have a "normal" CSF aluminum concentration, although no value was cited.

Rotundo et al[8] recently reported 20 children with congenital nephropathy and progressive, unexplained encephalopathy. Nearly all had microcephaly and exhibited developmental delay, hypotonia, and seizures. Motor disturbances similar to those described above—tremor, ataxia, myoclonus, and dyskinesias—were seen in a variable number of patients (Table 22–4). Seventeen of 18 patients had abnormal EEGs. In 7 of 12 patients, evidence of cortical atrophy or ventricular enlargement was noted by computed tomography, thus confirming similar observations made in other children with ESRD.[52, 53] None of these patients had received dialysis prior to developing symptoms. However, unlike most of the previously reported cases, only 4 of 8 patients tested had HPTH, and 4 of 20 had not received aluminum-containing phosphate binding gels prior to the appearance of neurologic symptoms. As in most of the cases already cited (Table 22–4), no aluminum determinations were performed on serum or bone, or on postmortem specimens of cerebral cortex from those patients who died.

Perhaps the most important feature of the report by Rotundo et al[8] is the striking association between the occurrence of progressive encephalopathy and the presence of marked developmental delay, cortical atrophy, and microcephaly in children, all of whom had congenital nephropathy and impaired renal function from an early age. In keeping with this is the observation that, of the centers reporting children with ESRD and unexplained encephalopathy in the above-noted survey,[95] nearly 75% noted its occurrence in patients with congenital renal disease. These findings are consistent with the suggestion that the metabolic and biochemical derangements associated with severe chronic renal insufficiency may be particularly detrimental to the still-developing CNS of the child with congenital or acquired nephropathy in whom renal function deteriorates to end-stage levels within the first year of life, the most critical period of postnatal brain growth.[24] Damage to the immature CNS also may result from the toxic side effects of drugs given to treat the complication of renal failure, or from calorie malnutrition.[25, 26] The latter commonly occurs in these children[25, 26] and is known to be associated with impaired brain growth and cognitive dysfunction.[24, 27, 28] Finally, the resemblance of the unexplained encephalopathy to adult dialysis dementia may or may not reflect the detrimental effects of hormonal or metabolic disturbances (e.g., HPTH), or trace metal intoxication, on the developing nervous systems of these children. Alternatively, the similarity may simply reflect a limited range of responsiveness of the CNS, at any age, to diverse insults.

The management of suspected aluminum intoxication is discussed in the section on dialysis dementia.

## Peripheral Neuropathy

Uremic peripheral neuropathy is a mixed, symmetric, sensorimotor polyneuropathy, which tends to involve the distal more than the proximal portions of the extremities.[2, 102] The lower extremities are usually the first to be affected and tend to be the most severely involved areas. Clinically apparent peripheral neuropathy is a major cause of morbidity in adults with ESRD, occurring in 11 to 75% of patients,[103] but has been reported in only a few children, all over 10 years of age.[103–107] Conversely, electrophysiologic evidence of peripheral nerve involvement occurs more frequently in children.[108, 109] Although clinically apparent peripheral neuropathy usually occurs in patients with severe chronic renal failure or ESRD, and is thus an indication for initiating maintenance dialysis, it may be overlooked in children because of the relative infrequency with which it occurs.

**Clinical Manifestations.** Clinical peripheral neuropathy appears when the GFR has diminished to 5–13 ml/min/1.73 m$^2$.[108–110] Early symptoms include both sensory and motor disturbances: paresthesias, and muscle cramps and restless legs, respectively.[103, 104, 108] Paresthesias are usually experienced distally, in fingers, toes, and the soles of the feet. Severe and painful paresthesias involving the soles of the feet were the primary clinical manifestations of peripheral neuropathy in 2 of 18 (11%) patients aged 12 to 16 years reported by Fine et al.[104] Muscle cramps tend to be nocturnal and painful, and involve muscle groups in the legs. The "restless legs" syndrome, another motor symptom, is characterized by "peculiar creeping, crawling, prickling, and itchy sensations"[107] experienced deep within the muscles of the legs, most often between the knees and ankles. Present more commonly during periods of muscular inactivity, the sensations are more intense at night and are relieved by movement. Restless legs tend to appear somewhat later than muscle cramps, the latter usually disappearing as the BUN rises above 100 ml/dl with progression of renal failure.[2] Muscle weakness, dysesthesias, pain, and "burning feet" generally appear much later, i.e., after the aforementioned symptoms have been present for months to years.[103] Muscle weakness is usually first detectable in the extensor digitorum brevis,[103] resulting in a diminished ability to dorsiflex the big toe. The "burning foot" syndrome is a relatively uncommon symptom of advanced sensory neuropathy in which "unpleasant tingling, band-like constrictions, swelling sensations, and tenderness"[102] are experienced in the distal extremities. Of the symptoms noted, however, only paresthesias have been shown to correlate well with the presence of objective signs of neuropathy.[111]

The earliest objective signs of peripheral neuropathy are hyporeflexia (decreased ankle jerk) and loss of vibratory sensation over the pulp of the big toe and medial malleolus. The latter may be shown to develop more or less abruptly over a period of weeks when quantitative testing (vibrometry) is carried out to detect an elevation of the so-called vibratory perception threshold (VPT).[108, 111–113] Testing for both hyporeflexia

and VPT will correctly identify 91% of patients with clinical peripheral neuropathy.[111]

As neuropathy worsens, muscle weakness progresses to involve the distal lower extremities more generally, and atrophy develops. Stocking-glove anesthesia may appear as another sign of advanced polyneuropathy.

Age, sex, and the severity and duration of chronic renal insufficiency have been shown to influence the risk of development of peripheral neuropathy. The male:female ratio in adults with clinical neuropathy ranges from 1.5 to 3.8:1 in unselected series.[4, 114, 115] Moreover, if linear regression analysis is carried out, with residual GFR (measured as creatinine clearance or log serum creatinine) as a function of patient age, it is possible to correctly discriminate between male patients with objective signs of moderate to severe neuropathy and those with none or only mild involvement, with a 12% rate of misclassification (Fig. 22–4).[4] The younger the patient is, therefore, the more severe renal insufficiency must be before clinical neuropathy develops. For example, a male patient 20 years of age would theoretically need a GFR corresponding to a serum creatinine concentration of at least 20 mg/dl; for a 10-year-old the corresponding serum creatinine level would have to be nearly 30 mg/dl (Fig. 22–

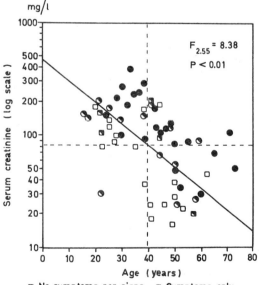

**Figure 22–4.** Relationship between age, serum creatinine concentration, and the presence or absence of clinical peripheral neuropathy in male patients with chronic renal failure. (From Nielsen VK et al: Acta Med Scand 190:119, 1971, with permission.)

4). In fact, of 25 patients aged 16 to 61 years and with serum creatinine concentrations above 5 mg/dl, only those 38 years or older developed clinical neuropathy.[116] These data provide a possible explanation for the relative infrequency with which clinically manifest peripheral neuropathy occurs in children and adolescents with ESRD, that is, since nearly all receive dialysis before the serum creatinine concentration reaches the above-noted levels. It is also known that progressive anatomic and functional deterioration of peripheral nerves occurs as part of the normal aging process,[5, 117, 118] so that the lower incidence of clinical neuropathy in younger patients also may reflect the healthier premorbid condition of their peripheral nervous systems.

**Electrophysiologic Studies.** The electrophysiologic studies of peripheral nerve function most commonly used in evaluating patients for the presence of uremic neuropathy are the testing of sensory and motor nerve conduction velocities (NCVs). Abnormally low values for one or both of these parameters are demonstrable in most adults and children with ESRD just prior to the time of initiation of maintenance dialysis.[105–110, 114, 118–120] NCVs are usually diminished from an earlier stage of renal functional deterioration than that at which clinical manifestations of neuropathy appear. Diminished NCVs have been detected at or below GFRs of 10 to 40 ml/min, and with serum creatinine concentrations as low as 2.1 mg/dl in adults[108–110] and 1.5 mg/dl in children.[120]

Significant correlations have been demonstrated between NCV and creatinine clearance ($r = 0.68$, $p < 0.001$), NCV and the log serum creatinine concentration ($r = -0.51$, $p < 0.001$), and the percentage change in NCV and serum creatinine concentration.[109, 110, 121] In one study of 21 children with ESRD, NCVs were significantly lower than normal just prior to beginning maintenance dialysis, but no attempt was made to correlate these changes with the level of renal function.[119] Arbus et al also failed to show significant correlations between mean serum creatinine concentration and motor NCVs in 31 children evaluated prior to beginning dialysis,[120] nor was significant deterioration demonstrable by serial testing of patients using the paired t test. However, in this study, comparisons were made between *mean* NCVs in *groups* of children, ordered by increasing serum creatinine concentrations which were

not adjusted for body size. Moreover, since day-to-day intrapatient variation in NCV may be as great as $25\%$[50] and since interpatient determinations are likely to be even more variable, group comparisons of NCVs may exhibit variation for reasons other than those being studied. The use of linear regression analysis to compare serum creatinine concentrations and NCVs in individual patients might have yielded different results.[109, 110] Therefore, the extent to which a relationship may exist between the severity of renal failure and the degree of slowing of NCVs in children remains unclear.

**Etiology and Pathogenesis of Peripheral Neuropathy.** Histologic studies of peripheral nerve biopsy specimens from adults with chronic renal insufficiency have shown the presence of paranodal segmental demyelination and axonal degeneration in varying proportions.[122–124] Axonal degeneration may occur in the absence of significant demyelination, and is most severe in the distal segments of sensory nerves, where clinical neuropathy tends to begin, but affects all fibers to some extent.[123] It is felt by some experts to be the primary pathologic process underlying the development of uremic peripheral neuropathy.[102] However, neither segmental demyelination nor axonal degeneration occurs exclusively in uremia, and pathologic changes may be present in peripheral nerves in the absence of clinical neuropathy. Thus, whether one or both of the above-noted processes is of primary importance in the development of uremic neuropathy remains uncertain.

A variety of abnormal circulating uremic "toxins" have been held responsible, at one time or another, for the pathogenesis of peripheral neuropathy.[100] Most of these substances were presumed to interfere with nerve conduction in proportion to their plasma concentrations, although the precise mechanism whereby interference occurred varied with each one. It has been suggested by Nielsen that for a substance to be considered a uremic "toxin," its correlation with NCV must be better than that between GFR and NCV ($r = 0.68$, $p < 0.001$),[109] a criterion not fulfilled by most of them.[100] For example, the percentage of inhibition, by uremic serum, of the activity of transketolase (% TKA inhibition), an enzyme essential for the maintenance of the myelin sheath,[125] was shown to correlate only weakly with NCVs in adults with ESRD ($r = 0.468$, $p < 0.05$).[126]

Table 22–5. DRUGS ASSOCIATED WITH PERIPHERAL NEUROPATHY*

| Clinical Presentation | Antimicrobial Drugs | Antineoplastic Drugs | Cardiovascular Drugs | Hypnotics and Psychotropics | Antirheumatic Drugs | Other Drugs |
|---|---|---|---|---|---|---|
| *Sensory neuropathy* | Ethionamide Chloramphenicol Thiamphenicol Diamines | Procarbazine Nitrofurazone | | | | Calcium carbimide Sulfoxone Ergotamine Propylthiouracil |
| *Paresthesiae only* | Colistin Streptomycin Nalidixic acid | Cytarabine | Propranolol | Phenelzine | | Sulthiame Chlorpropamide Methysergide |
| *Sensorimotor neuropathy* | Isoniazid** Ethambutol Streptomycin Nitrofurantoin Clioquinol Metronidazole | Vincristine Podophyllum Chlorambucil | Perhexiline Hydralazine** Amiodarone Disopyramide Clofibrate | Thalidomide Methaqualone Glutethimide Amitriptyline | Gold Indomethacin Colchicine Chloroquine Phenylbutazone | Phenytoin Disulfiram Carbutamide Tolbutamide Chlorpropamide Methimazole |
| *Predominantly motor* | Sulfonamides Amphotericin | | | Imipramine | | Dapsone |
| *Localized neuropathies* | Amphotericin Penicillin | Mustine Ethoglucid | | | | Anticoagulants |

*From: Argov Z, et al, Br Med J 1:663, 1979, with permission.
**Pyridoxine-responsive.

Moreover, changes in % TKA inhibition were monitored in the serum of an 11½-year-old female with clinical peripheral neuropathy, and were found to decline progressively with dialysis, while NCVs improved little or not at all.[106] PTH has also been shown to exhibit a weak but significant inverse linear correlation with peroneal NCVs (r = −0.45, p < 0.01),[127] a relationship which could not be duplicated by another investigator.[128] In neither of these cases is Nielsen's criterion for the identification of a uremic "toxin" fulfilled.[109]

**Differential Diagnosis and Management.** Nutritional and drug-related causes of peripheral nerve damage must be excluded. Thiamine and pyridoxine deficiencies can cause peripheral neuropathy; the clinical features of both are nonspecific, involve sensory and motor nerve dysfunction, and are likely to occur in children receiving maintenance dialysis only if multivitamin supplements have not been prescribed. A number of drugs may also cause peripheral neuropathy (Table 22–5), and should be avoided in children with ESRD when possible.

Clinically significant peripheral neuropathy generally responds to the initiation of maintenance dialysis. The "restless legs" syndrome has been successfully treated with clonazepam in adults,[129] the recommended dose being 0.5 mg given two times daily (at 6 P.M. and bedtime). Symptomatic relief has also been achieved in a single adolescent treated with this regimen (M. Polinsky, unpublished observation).

## Cranial Neuropathy

Cranial nerve involvement may occur in patients with ESRD. A small number of patients have developed "uremic amaurosis," characterized by the onset of blindness occurring over several hours, associated with a normal funduscopic examination and pupillary light reflexes.[2] Recovery generally occurs spontaneously. Reversible amaurosis also has occurred in patients with ESRD following general anesthesia, and as a complication of hypertensive encephalopathy.[130]

High frequency (> 2000 Hz) sensorineural hearing loss has been reported in 61 to 70% of adults with ESRD prior to beginning maintenance dialysis, with hearing loss attributed to presbyacusis, "noise exposure," and "multiple factors."[131, 132] Dialysis per se does not appear to have any effect on hearing; in one study, 75% of the patients followed showed no hearing loss during the period of evaluation.[132] Deafness has also occurred with the use of ototoxic drugs, particularly furosemide and the aminoglycosides,[2] and has been irreversible in several patients.[133]

Decreased taste acuity, as characterized by elevated detection (concentration at which the taste was first perceived) and recognition (concentration at which the taste was distinguished from distilled water) thresholds, occurs in most patients with ESRD.[134, 135] Diminished taste acuity may be primarily due to cranial neuropathy, i.e., to a malfunction of taste receptors or the special sensory components of the seventh cranial nerve. Zinc deficiency may also contribute to the development of hypogeusia in some patients.[134, 135] Maintenance dialysis does not appear to improve taste acuity.[136]

## EFFECTS OF DIALYSIS ON NEUROLOGIC FUNCTION

### Beneficial Effects of Dialysis

**Cognitive and EEG Disturbances.** The institution of therapy with hemodialysis or peritoneal dialysis in patients with ESRD generally results in progressive improvement in cognitive function. This has been demonstrated in adults by improved performances on the Choice Reaction Time Test, Continuous Memory Test, and Continuous Performance Test.[19] Improvement has also been demonstrated with repeat testing performed as little as two weeks following the initiation of maintenance hemodialysis.[20] Suggestive improvement in cognitive function and affect was noted in 5 of 18 children reported by Grushkin et al[7] within weeks to several months after the initiation of maintenance hemodialysis. No differences between the results of neurobehavioral testing have been demonstrated between groups of patients receiving maintenance hemodialysis versus peritoneal dialysis.[137]

Recently, quantitative analysis of EEGs in adults by computer-assisted methods has demonstrated progressive normalization of brain electrical activity following initiation of maintenance dialysis, as demonstrated by a decrease in the % EEG Power [(3–7) Hz/(3–13) Hz] × 100,[19] a shortened visual evoked response (VER) latency,[19] and a reduction in the % EEG Power <7 Hz.[44] Improvement was noted to be most dramatic within two months of beginning dialysis. Although comparable data are not available for children, neurometrics analysis of brain electrical activity (see below) in 8 children studied both pre- and postdialysis in a single week, failed to demonstrate any significant short-term changes in the overall pattern of brain electrical activity by paired t test[49] (Fig. 22–5). Conversely, significant positive linear correlations were observed between the Severity Index and duration of chronic renal failure (r = 0.69, p < 0.01) for 13 children who had been receiving maintenance dialysis for 20 to 74 months, suggesting that progressive deterioration in the overall pattern of brain electrical activity occurred in these children with increasing time on otherwise adequate dialysis (Fig. 22–1, A upper regression line).[49] These findings have yet to be confirmed by subsequent studies, and there remains the need to obtain additional longitudinal, quantitative electrophysiologic data to further characterize the long-term effects of dialysis on brain electrical activity in children with ESRD.

**Peripheral Neuropathy.** The clinical manifestations of peripheral neuropathy either improve or do not progress in most adult patients receiving adequate maintenance hemodialysis for periods of 1 to 7 years.[108, 116, 121, 138] Significant improvement in objective indices of clinical neuropathy, such as the vibratory perception threshold (VPT), was noted by Nielson within 12 months of initiation of maintenance dialysis.[113] The acute deterioration reported in a few patients shortly after beginning therapy was apparently due to underdialysis, in that it generally responded to an increase in treatment time and/or dialyzer surface area.[116, 121] Improvement followed three months of dialysis in one of two adolescents with clinical peripheral neuropathy reported by Fine et al;[104] the second failed to improve after one month of dialysis, no further follow-up having been reported.

The effect of adequate dialysis on NCVs is more variable. Several early reports indicated that NCVs remained unchanged in most adults during the first year of dialysis despite clinical improvement.[113, 116, 121] An increase (improvement) in NCVs then seemed to occur after the first year of dialysis in those reports, although, in a more recent study, continued deterioration was noted during a 7-year follow-up period.[138]

No significant improvement or deterioration in NCVs has been noted in children receiving maintenance hemodialysis for periods of up to 60 months,[119, 120, 139] although the overall proportion of patients with abnormal studies varied considerably between reports. Chan et al noted that median, peroneal, and posterior tibial NCVs remained normal in 82% (9 of 11) of children receiving dialysis for up to 24 months, and in 75% (3 of 4) of those treated for up to 60 months.[139] Arbus et al reported abnormally low peroneal NCVs in 57% (16 of 28) of examinations in 20 children, with no significant improvement

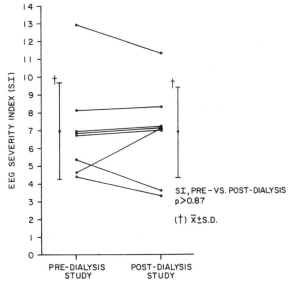

**Figure 22–5.** Changes in the EEG Severity Index with acute dialysis in eight children.

SI, PRE- VS. POST-DIALYSIS
p>0.87

(†) x̄±S.D.

noted after 12 months of dialysis.[120] Mentser et al likewise reported persistently lower mean peroneal NCVs versus controls in a group of 58 children followed for more than 24 months.[119] Decreased NCVs have been noted to occur more commonly in lower than upper extremities in children,[120] similar to the situation in adults, in whom motor conduction in the common peroneal nerve was shown to be more severely affected than that in the median nerve.[118] However, the *ratio* of conduction velocities in lower versus upper extremity motor nerves should remain constant, since deterioration appears to occur in parallel everywhere.[118, 140, 150]

NCVs may also deteriorate in adults and children receiving maintenance dialysis. Identifiable factors which may adversely affect NCVs in such patients include underdialysis, too vigorous ultrafiltration,[248] the use of high magnesium-containing dialysate[247] or of disproportionately large surface area dialyzers,[249, 252] intercurrent infection with hepatitis B virus,[250] and severe, renin-dependent hypertension with resultant ischemia of the vasa nervorum.[105, 251]

**Value of Electrophysiologic Studies in the Management of Pediatric ESRD.** Studies in both adults and children have failed to demonstrate the existence of significant correlations between clinical and electrophysiologic evidence of peripheral nerve disease. Decreased NCVs were seen in 97% (28 of 29) of adults with, but also in 70% (19 of 27) of those without, clinical neuropathy.[109] None of the patients of Mentser et al had clinical neuropathy, yet most had abnormally low NCVs.[119] These data, along with the above-noted day-to-day intrapatient variation in NCV,[150] and the observed failure of NCVs to consistently improve with increasing time on dialysis, suggest that serial measurements of these parameters in children would be of little value in determining the need to alter the dialysis prescriptions of individual patients, as originally suggested by Babb et al.[141] However, such testing may still be indicated in children and adolescents in whom clinical evidence of neuropathy appears, without reason, during the course of dialysis.

## Neurologic Complications Associated With Dialysis

### Dialysis Disequilibrium Syndrome (DDS)

The DDS is a common and potentially serious cause of acute illness in children receiving maintenance hemodialysis. It occurs in a third of pediatric patients so treated,[7] an incidence four times that reported in adults.[1] DDS is less common at all ages in patients undergoing peritoneal dialysis.[102] The syndrome tends to develop toward the end of a hemodialysis treatment or within 8 to 24 hours thereafter,[1, 102] and is more likely to occur in new patients, particularly those who are markedly azotemic and are treated at blood flow rates associated with disproportionately high urea clearances.

The classic clinical picture begins with restlessness, irritability, muscle cramps, headache, drowsiness, nausea, and, occasionally, vomiting.[1, 102, 142, 143] If ignored or not recognized, progression to confusion, disorientation, and somnolence occurs, accompanied by hypertension, visual disturbances (blurring), muscle twitching, myoclonus, and asterixis. With further deterioration, life-threatening complications may develop: convulsions, coma, and cardiac arrhythmias, including ventricular tachycardia.[142] Deaths have occurred in children and adolescents.[142, 144] Transient amaurosis, with normal optic fundi, has been described in a 5-year-old boy with acute renal failure following 2½ hours of his third hemodialysis treatment, in association with a decrease in the BUN concentration from 195 to 100 mg/dl.[145] Characteristically, the EEG shows an acute deterioration in the pattern of brain electrical activity, with further generalized slowing and episodic bursts of high voltage, rhythmic or dysrhythmic delta waves.[146]

In recent years, a milder form of DDS has become increasingly prevalent. It is characterized by restlessness, headache, nausea, muscle cramps, and increased fatigue and weakness. Its relatively benign nature is probably due to avoidance of overly efficient dialysis, the tailoring of urea clearances to the body mass of the individual child, and more frequent recognition and treatment of earlier stages of the syndrome.[147]

The symptoms and signs of DDS appear to result from cerebral edema, which occurs in association with the development of osmotic disequilibrium between the intracerebral and plasma compartments. Early theories concerning the pathogenesis of the cerebral edema variably attributed it to the "reverse urea effect" (disproportionate rates of urea clearance from brain and plasma),[39, 143, 146] rapid lowering of the serum sodium concentration,[148] acute alterations in arterial pH,[143] dialysis against low glucose-containing dialysate,[149] an increase in the serum K:Ca ratio,[2] and relative cerebral hypoxia due to a shift to the left of the hemoglobin-oxygen dissociation curve, as a consequence of the acute correction of acidosis and hyperphosphatemia.[150] More recently, using an animal model of experimental dialysis disequilibrium to compare biochemical changes in brain, CSF, and plasma during rapid (RHD) versus slow (SHD) hemodialysis, Arieff et al have demonstrated the following:[54, 151–153]

1. A disproportionate fall in the urea nitrogen concentration of blood occurs relative to that of CSF and brain, resulting in the generation of modest brain:blood and CSF:blood urea concentration gradients (6–8 mg/dl and 14–18 mg/dl, respectively), which are no greater during RHD than SHD;

2. During either RHD or SHD a similar CSF:plasma osmotic gradient exists, of approximately 14–16 mOsm/kg;

3. A significantly large brain:blood osmotic gradient exists only during RHD;

4. Brain $H_2O$ content increases only with RHD;

5. Intracerebral and CSF pH and bicarbonate concentrations decline only with RHD;

6. No significant changes in brain or CSF Na, K, Cl, or lactate concentrations occur with SHD or RHD.

It was concluded that cerebral edema resulted only from RHD, and was due to an increase in intracerebral osmolality, which could not be attributed to identifiable, osmotically active solutes. The observed decreases in intracerebral and CSF pH and bicarbonate concentrations suggested that *de novo* generation of organic acids had occurred in the brain to account for the observed increase in osmolality, in the form of so-called "idiogenic osmoles"[151] (Fig 22–6), in a manner similar to that reported in hypernatremic dehydration.[154]

The differential diagnosis of DDS includes other causes of neurologic dysfunction associated with dialysis, and is summarized in Table 22–6. In the presence of the more severe manifestations of DDS, particularly seizures, or when progression of symptoms occurs in spite of the institution of corrective therapy, hypertensive encephalopathy and intracranial hemorrhage should be seriously considered. The dialysis dementia-like syndrome of childhood and vitamin $B_6$ defi-

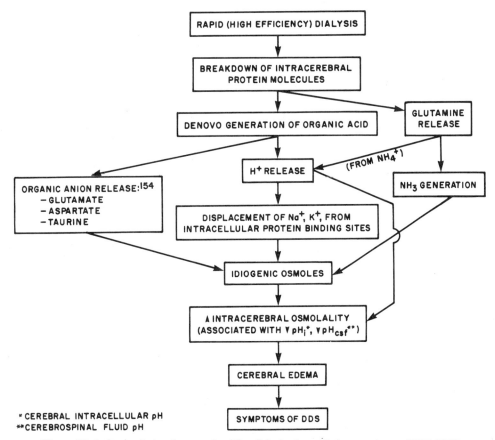

**Figure 22–6.** Suggested pathogenesis of the dialysis disequilibrium syndrome (DDS).[152, 154]

**Table 22–6.** NEUROLOGIC COMPLICATIONS
ASSOCIATED WITH DIALYSIS

1. Dialysis disequilibrium syndrome (DDS).*
2. Isolated headache.
3. Isolated muscle cramps, weakness.
4. Complications attributable to:
   a. Acute electrolyte and acid-base derangements.*
   b. Acute changes in blood glucose concentration.*
5. Symptomatic hypotension/hypertension.*
6. Neurovascular complications:
   a. Intracranial hemorrhage.*
   b. Cerebral embolization (Scribner shunt declotting).[180]
7. Dialysis dementia–like syndrome of childhood.*
8. Acute copper intoxication.
9. Vitamin deficiency.
   a. $B_1$ (Wernicke).
   b. $B_6$.*
10. CNS infection.*†
11. Drug-related.*†

---

*Can cause seizures.

†Not a complication of dialysis per se, but may be responsible for seizures or altered consciousness in a patient receiving dialysis.

ciency are uncommon causes of seizures or acute alterations in the level or content of consciousness in a child receiving hemodialysis. These are discussed below.

**Management of DDS.** In the aforementioned model of experimental DDS, rapid hemodialysis against a mannitol-containing bath prevented the observed fall in intracerebral pH and the development of cerebral edema and seizures, although it failed to maintain a normal CSF pH or to prevent deterioration of the EEG, both of which are components of the experimental DDS. The addition of glycerol to the dialysis bath prevented the development of *all* DDS-related disturbances.[153] These observations provide a rationale for the use of mannitol or glycerol in the prophylaxis and therapy of this disorder.

Mannitol should be used prophylactically in children undergoing their first few dialyses, particularly if the BUN is very high (e.g., above 100 mg/dl[147]). It is given in a dose of 1 gm/kg (maximum, 50 mg), distributed over the course of the dialysis. We have found 0.5 mg/kg given at onset, and 0.25 mg/kg given at hourly intervals for 2 total doses, to be a safe and effective regimen. Prophylactic mannitol should also be considered for the treatment of chronic dialysis patients under circumstances in which the BUN has risen acutely to well above pre-existing levels: e.g., following dietary indiscretions or the development of a hypercatabolic state associated with intercurrent illness.

For the treatment of the milder symptoms of DDS, mannitol may be administered as a 25% solution in a dose of 0.5 gm/kg, and may be repeated once. If symptoms of dysequilibrium persist, blood flow should be reduced. If more severe manifestations of DDS are present, e.g., seizures, or decreased consciousness, or if symptoms progress in spite of therapy, dialysis should be discontinued immediately, and appropriate blood studies performed (see below) to rule out other causes for the observed disturbances.

The excessive use of mannitol in a child with ESRD may produce the clinical manifestations of water intoxication with dilutional hyponatremia,[155] and may lead to the development of congestive heart failure and pulmonary edema, whether or not pre-existing myocardial disease is present.[156] The child with dilutional hyponatremia due to mannitol intoxication may be identified by the presence of the so-called "osmolality gap," i.e., a measured serum osmolality in excess of the calculated one.

### Other Neurologic Complications of Dialysis

**Isolated Headache and Neuromuscular Irritability.** Causes of isolated, dialysis-related headache, other than DDS, include hypotension associated with vigorous ultrafiltration (cerebral hypoxia),[157] hypercalcemia (usually associated with delirium),[29] and intracranial hemorrhage. It has also been suggested that the rapid correction of hyperphosphatemia and acidosis may cause cerebral hypoxia and headache by increasing hemoglobin-oxygen binding affinity in the face of chronic anemia.[158]

Isolated, painful muscle cramps have been noted to occur twice as frequently in patients dialyzed against fluid with a relatively low (132 meq/L), versus a high (145 meq/L), Na concentration.[159] It has been suggested that acutely lowering the serum Na concentration toward 132 meq/L during "low sodium" dialysis allows movement of extracellular water into cells from a vascular volume already acutely contracted as a result of ultrafiltration, and that the "extra" reduction was critical to the pathogenesis of the muscle cramps. However, volume expansion with isotonic saline (5–10 ml/kg in 1 to 2 boluses) has been used successfully to treat isolated muscle cramps, as well as those occurring as part of the DDS. Thus, the extent to which isolated cramps may represent either a mild form of the DDS or a pathogenetically distinct entity is unknown. If the infusion of isotonic saline fails to effect symptomatic improvement, muscle cramps may respond to a decrease in ultrafiltration rate.

Generalized muscle weakness may occur in patients who are receiving maintenance dialysis. The development of a myasthenia gravis–like, edrophonium (Tensilon)-responsive syndrome of limb and jaw muscle weakness followed the administration of carnitine to adults, and may have resulted from the accumulation of acetylcholine-like carnitine metabolites in the presence of anuria.[160] Muscle weakness with a predominantly proximal distribution is usually the result of secondary HPTH.[161] Dialysis per se has not been shown to have any immediately beneficial or detrimental effect on limb and respiratory muscle strength in 10 men evaluated before and 1½ hours after a single treatment.[162]

**Electrolyte and Metabolic Disturbances Associated with ESRD and Dialysis.** Sudden or profound disturbances in electrolyte or acid-base balance may cause seizures or acute alterations in consciousness. When associated with neurologic dysfunction, these disturbances should be corrected promptly, but in a controlled manner.

*Hypo- and Hypernatremia.* In children with ESRD, hyponatremia is most commonly dilutional and due to the ingestion of excessive quantities of fluid in the absence of adequate glomerular ultrafiltration. In dialysis patients, hypo- or hypernatremia may result from iatrogenic errors in dilution of dialysate concentrate, or from malfunction of the central apportioning mechanisms of peritoneal or hemodialysis machines.[100, 161] Hypernatremia may also result from the "sieving," or convective transport which occurs during hypertonic peritoneal dialysis,[163, 164] and is more likely to occur with shorter exchange times.[165] Symptoms may appear when the serum Na concentration falls below 120 meq/L[29] or rises above 160 meq/L,[166] or with even smaller deviations from normal when the *rate* of change exceeds 1 to 2 meq/L/hr. Hypernatremia manifests clinically with intense thirst, irritability, and restlessness, followed by a progressive deterioration in the level of consciousness from lethargy to stupor to coma, associated with heightened muscle tone. Seizures may occur.[166] The neurologic manifestations of hyponatremia include weakness, increased fatigue, hyporeflexia with positive

Babinski signs, bulbar or pseudobulbar palsy (dysarthria, dysphagia, emotional lability), decreased consciousness, and seizures.

ESRD patients with symptomatic hyponatremia should be severely water-restricted and sufficient 3% NaCl should be given to raise the serum Na concentration to 125 meq/L; this should alleviate neurologic disturbances in most patients until dialysis can be initiated.[167] Seizures occurring in a child receiving dialysis should prompt at least temporary discontinuation of treatment. If present, hyponatremia is corrected with 3% NaCl, as just noted. Hypernatremia is best treated with hypotonic saline solutions at a rate such that the serum Na concentration is not reduced by greater than 1 meq/L/hr. Dialysis may then be resumed in 12 to 24 hours if vital signs are stable and seizures have been adequately controlled.

*Acidosis.* Rapid changes in arterial pH are particularly epileptogenic in patients with ESRD.[143] Unless severe, e.g., serum $CO_2$ content <10 mM/L, the correction of metabolic acidosis in the child with ESRD is best accomplished following the institution of dialysis, since the administration of $NaHCO_3$ may also worsen hypertension and foster the development of congestive heart failure, pulmonary edema, or hypertensive encephalopathy. In addition, if hypocalcemia is present, acutely elevating arterial pH may lower the ionized calcium concentration and precipitate tetany and/or convulsions. This has also occurred following initiation of acute peritoneal dialysis.[168] Rapid correction of acidosis with hemodialysis has been associated with development of cerebral edema and death due to brain stem herniation in an 18-year-old male with ESRD.[144] Thus, the treatment of metabolic acidosis may still be hazardous, even when attempted with dialysis.

*Hypo- and Hypercalcemia.* Symptomatic hypocalcemia manifests with increased neuromuscular irritability (tetany) and seizures. Initially, 10% Ca gluconate, 0.5 ml/kg may be given by *slow* IV infusion over 3 to 5 minutes to control seizures, followed by a constant infusion of 4 mg of elemental Ca/kg/hr for each 1 mg/dl by which the serum Ca concentration is to be elevated. Overcorrection should be avoided, since hypocalcemia is often accompanied by hyperphosphatemia, and calcium infusion may precipitate metastatic calcification if the Ca-P product of the blood is iatrogenically elevated above 70. Hyperphosphatemia may be controlled with dialysis, dietary phosphate restriction, and aluminum-containing phosphate binding gels, the latter in a dose of 50 to 150 mg/kg/24 hr.

Hypercalcemia may develop within weeks of initiation of hemodialysis, and has been attributed to an increased sensitivity of bone to the calcemic effects of PTH and vitamin D.[169, 170, 171] It has also resulted from the addition of excessive calcium to the dialysis bath.[172] Clinical symptoms are progressive: initially, headache and delirium are seen, but progression to stupor and coma may occur; seizures are uncommon.[29] Delirium, myoclonus, dysarthria, and seizures have been described in association with the accidental *acute* elevation of the serum calcium concentration to 11.8 to 13.7 mg/dl in 8 adults receiving maintenance dialysis.[172] Thus, the clinical picture of acute hypercalcemia may resemble that of dialysis dementia, from which it must be differentiated. Treatment of hypercalcemia may require temporary discontinuation of calcium supplements and vitamin D metabolites. Subtotal parathyroidectomy may be necessary for control of severe or persistent hypercalcemia due to intractable secondary hyperparathyroidism.

*Phosphate Depletion.* When combined with the use of low phosphorus-containing dialysate and severe dietary phosphate restriction, the ingestion of large quantities of aluminum-containing phosphate binding gels by hemodialysis patients may result in severe hypophosphatemia.[173, 174] The cognitive disturbances may mimic any form of psychosis, except that hallucinations are absent,[174] and usually appear at serum phosphate concentrations well below 2 mg/dl.[173] This syndrome may be clinically indistinguishable from that of dialysis dementia.[175, 176] Treatment to bring the serum phosphate concentration above 2 mg/dl has resulted in the disappearance of symptoms.

*Hyperosmolality.* Nonketotic, hyperosmolar coma may result from the use of hypertonic glucose-containing solutions to perform peritoneal dialysis.[177, 178] The clinical features are similar to those of hypernatremia, and may appear at serum glucose concentrations above 400 mg/dl.[29] They develop more commonly when 7% glucose-containing dialysate is used during peritoneal dialysis, but may also occur with successive exchanges of 4.25%. The blood glucose concentration should be monitored at regular intervals during peritoneal dialysis when frequent exchanges of 4.25% glucose are being used, or in children simultaneously receiving cortico-

steroids. If hyperglycemia develops, it may be necessary to use alternating exchanges of 1.5% and 4.25% solutions, and to add insulin directly to the bottles of dialysate,[179] at least temporarily.

**Neurovascular Complications.** Cerebral thromboembolization from Scribner arteriovenous shunts has occurred during declotting procedures employed in an attempt to reestablish shunt patency.[180] Intracranial hemorrhage occurs in 0.6 to 9.8% of adults receiving maintenance hemodialysis,[1, 181–187] but only isolated cases have been reported in patients 16 years of age or less.[7, 187, 188] Prompt recognition of this condition is important in all age groups if survival is to occur without neurologic sequelae. In most patients more than one predisposing factor is present: hypertension, and a history of chronic or excessive oral anticoagulant therapy and/or heparin overdose during dialysis, is a common combination.[183–185, 187] Of the patients reported by Leonard et al,[183] 82% of those developing intracranial hemorrhage had received long-term therapy with oral anticoagulants to maintain shunt patency, and 68% had a prolonged prothrombin time and/or partial thromboplastin time beforehand. Moderate to severe hypertension, and/or excessive weight gain necessitating vigorous ultrafiltration, was present in 45% of these patients, while a history of minor head trauma was noted in fewer than one-third.[183] Of the three cases reported to date in patients 16 years of age or less, two have survived. The third patient died while receiving maintenance hemodialysis, 24 hours after irreversible rejection of a renal transplant. Intracranial hemorrhage developed in a 16-year-old dialysis patient in association with the use of large doses of heparin and a concomitant episode of viral hepatitis.[187] Subdural hematoma in an 11½-year-old female receiving maintenance intermittent peritoneal dialysis was associated with severe nutritional deficiency, a prolonged prothrombin time, and two recent episodes of hypertensive encephalopathy (Baluarte, H.J., personal communication). A single intramuscular dose of vitamin K, 5 mg, restored the prothrombin time to normal.

The clinical manifestations of intracranial hemorrhage include protracted headaches which acutely worsen during dialysis, fluctuating focal or multifocal neurologic signs, acute alterations in consciousness, and meningismus occurring in the absence of fever.[183, 186, 187] Occasionally, an acute drop in hematocrit[184] or evidence of gastrointestinal, mucosal, or cutaneous bleeding[186, 187] is also present. The current diagnostic procedure of choice is computed tomography, although arteriography has been diagnostic in patients so studied.[183] It should be remembered that a normal skull radiograph and EEG do not exclude the presence of subdural hematoma. The treatment is surgical evacuation of the hematoma.

**Dialysis Dementia (Dialysis Encephalopathy).** Initially described by Alfrey et al[91] in adults who had been stable on maintenance dialysis for periods of 3 to 6 years, this syndrome of progressive encephalopathy has also developed in patients with ESRD prior to the initiation of dialysis,[93, 94] and following renal transplantation.[189, 190] Mortality rates have been as high as 85% in Europe[191] and 97% in the United States.[92] A clinically indistinguishable syndrome of progressive encephalopathy with seizures, which has been described in children with ESRD, has already been discussed.

The clinical syndrome is heralded by the onset of speech disturbances: dysarthria, dyspraxia, and dysphasia.[192, 193] Mental changes have begun insidiously in some, with forgetfulness, decreased ability to concentrate, and changes in affect. In others, delirium (toxic psychosis) may occur acutely during dialysis. Ultimately, progressive dementia becomes apparent. Motor disturbances include asterixis, myoclonus, apraxia, facial grimacing, tremor, and twitching. Focal or generalized seizures are characteristic. These disturbances usually first appear during dialysis and disappear during interdialytic periods, eventually becoming persistent. Characteristic, but not pathognomonic, EEG changes, which may predate the clinical manifestations by up to 3 to 6 months, include generalized slowing of the fundamental (background) rhythm, with multifocal, paroxysmal discharges of high amplitude delta waves.[91, 92]

The etiology of this progressive encephalopathy remains unknown, although multiple factors have been considered, including slow virus infection, altered cerebrospinal fluid dynamics, and accumulation of calcium or tin in cerebral cortex.[101] Particular emphasis has been placed on the potential roles of aluminum and PTH in the pathogenesis of this syndrome.[99] Major sources of increased body aluminum burden in adults and children with ESRD are considered to be the phosphate binding gels taken for control of hyperphosphatemia, and the water used to prepare dialysate.[99, 194] PTH may also increase the risk of developing aluminum intoxication, by enhancing gastrointestinal uptake of the metal and its distribution to various tissues, including brain gray matter.[61, 62]

Until recently, therapy had been exclusively supportive, and included the use of diazepam and clonazepam to control seizures, EEG disturbances, and the movement and speech disorders;[91, 92, 195, 196] but these failed to prevent death in most patients. More recently, improvement has been documented in some patients following attempts to reduce body aluminum burden by withdrawal of aluminum-containing phosphate binding gels,[197, 198] successful renal transplantation,[199] and chelation with deferoxamine in conjunction with hemodialysis.[200–202] While these associations serve to strengthen the postulated etiologic role for aluminum in this syndrome, convincing arguments to the contrary also have been presented.[101]

Dialysis encephalopathy appears to occur in epidemic and sporadic forms. While the etiology of the latter remains unknown, the epidemic form may represent the consequences of acute aluminum intoxication,[100] and has followed exposure to dialysate heavily contaminated with this metal.[99] Aluminum is amphoteric and becomes increasingly soluble as dialysate pH rises above 7.6 or falls below 6.5.[203] Within that narrow pH range most of the metal exists in the form of a colloidal suspension and cannot cross the dialyzer membrane. Thus, increasing the pH and alkalinity of dialysate by increasing its bicarbonate concentration may enhance the risk of development of symptomatic aluminum intoxication. The mean serum aluminum concentration of patients dialyzed against bicarbonate-containing dialysate (pH 7.8) was found to be significantly higher than that of another group dialyzed against a standard acetate-containing solution (pH 6.9).[203] Moreover, the mean dialysate pH obtained from a group of centers reporting cases of dialysis encephalopathy was significantly higher than that from centers in which no cases occurred (mean pH difference, 8.1 versus 7.5, $p < 0.005$).[203] These data may explain why all patients with comparable degrees of aluminum exposure do not share the same risk of developing symptomatic intoxication.

Moreover, interpatient differences with respect to state of nutrition, degree of intercurrent stress, and drug therapy may also affect this relative risk.[189] It has recently been proposed that asymptomatic patients with chronic aluminum poisoning may acutely develop the clinical manifestations of dialysis encephalopathy in association with any intercurrent stress which favors catabolism of bone, such as immobilization, surgery, the administration of corticosteroids, and hypophosphatemia.[204] The latter has previously been associated with the development of a dialysis encephalopathy-like syndrome.[175, 176] The sudden release of bone aluminum stores into the circulation might promote deposition of considerable quantities of this metal in brain gray matter, particularly in the presence of secondary HPTH. Symptoms of dialysis dementia might then appear in a manner analogous to that in which acute encephalopathy may be precipitated in a previously asymptomatic child with chronic lead poisoning.[205] The failure of successful renal transplantation to reverse the clinical manifestations of the syndrome in some patients[92, 206] also might be explained in this way.

The relevance of the above findings to the child with ESRD lies in the apparent similarities between the adult syndrome of dialysis dementia and the unexplained, progressive encephalopathy of childhood (see above).[8-13] Most of these children had symptoms identical to those seen in adults with dialysis dementia, had secondary HPTH, and were receiving large quantities of aluminum-containing compounds. Therefore, the *potential* neurotoxicity of aluminum should be considered in the management of all children with ESRD. The following recommendations are made:

1. Dialysate should be prepared from water treated by reverse osmosis or deionization, and the aluminum levels monitored and maintained below 15 μg/L.[207] Dialysate pH should be checked periodically and maintained within the range of 6.5–7.6,[203] unless bicarbonate dialysis must be performed for other reasons.

2. Wherever possible, serum aluminum concentrations* should be monitored in pa-

tients receiving bicarbonate dialysis and/or aluminum-containing phosphate binding gels in doses exceeding 150 mg/kg/day for prolonged periods of time.

3. In patients exhibiting clinical and EEG evidence of unexplained, progressive, dialysis-unresponsive encephalopathy, the presence of elevated plasma aluminum concentrations should prompt temporary discontinuation of therapy with aluminum-containing compounds, and a search for possible sources of dialysis contamination.[208] Consideration should be given to temporarily discontinuing bicarbonate dialysis when serum aluminum concentrations are markedly elevated. These patients should be followed for a prolonged period of time, since clinical improvement may occur up to 9 months after discontinuation of phosphate binding gels.[198] Clinical improvement should then be taken as evidence that aluminum intoxication was present, and the future use of phosphate-binding gels limited. It should be noted that the use of magnesium-containing antacids to control hyperphosphatemia remains controversial.[97, 209, 210]

4. Particular emphasis should be placed on the control of secondary HPTH in patients with markedly elevated serum aluminum levels, particularly if unexplained, progressive neurologic deterioration develops. Subtotal parathyroidectomy has not been shown to be consistently beneficial to either adults or children with unexplained encephalopathy.[9, 92, 211]

5. Hemofiltration may be of benefit to children with hyperaluminemia and progressive, unexplained encephalopathy in whom increased dialysis time and elimination of all potential sources of aluminum intake have failed to effect improvement.[212] Chelation therapy, using deferoxamine in conjunction with hemodialysis, has been reported to arrest or reverse neurologic deterioration in adults[200-202] and may be tried if other methods have failed. No reports are currently available to document the efficacy or hazards associated with the use of this treatment in children. Recommendations may be followed for the use of deferoxamine in the treatment of iron poisoning in children.[213] This may be given in an initial dose of 600 mg/m² (20 mg/kg) intramuscularly or by slow IV drip, at a rate not to exceed 15 mg/kg/hr. The above dose may be given after every dialysis treatment until symptomatic improvement occurs. Side effects of deferoxamine therapy

---

*Serum aluminum concentrations have been reported in normal children (16.9 ± 2.9 μg/L;[49a] <10 μg/L;[194] mean=23 μg/L[49b]) and do not differ from those in adults.[99] In two children with ESRD and progressive, unexplained encephalopathy who had aluminum determinations performed, the levels were markedly elevated, i.e., 601[11] and 651 μg/L (Polinsky, M., unpublished data).

include acute hypersensitivity reactions, hypotension with rapid IV infusion, and local irritation at the injection site.[213]

**Vitamin Deficiency.** When taken daily, the contents of a single multivitamin tablet should prevent the development of any deficiency syndromes. However, patients who do not receive B-complex vitamin supplements may develop thiamine ($B_1$) or pyridoxine ($B_6$) deficiency. The former may cause the Wernicke encephalopathy, which is characterized by confusion and disorientation with or without memory deficit, ocular disturbances (bilateral ophthalmoplegia, nystagmus), and gait and stance ataxia.[29] Improvement of ocular disturbances occurs within hours of administration of parenteral thiamine; the other manifestations improve more gradually. Pyridoxine deficiency manifests as seizures and peripheral neuropathy. Seizures should respond to vitamin $B_6$, 100 mg given intramuscularly.

**Acute Copper Intoxication.** Copper may be leeched from copper tubing which is bathed by acidic dialysate (pH 6.5). Under such circumstances, acute intoxication may develop, as manifested by headache, abdominal pain, nausea, vomiting, and diarrhea.[214] Cutaneous flushing, hepatitis, pancreatitis, hemolytic anemia, and myoglobinemia may also occur.[214] The initial symptoms may be indistinguishable from those of the DDS, except for the diarrhea, which, along with evidence of an acute drop in the hematocrit and of hepatocellular injury, should suggest the diagnosis.

## NEUROLOGIC COMPLICATIONS OF RENAL TRANSPLANTATION

### Beneficial Effect of Transplantation

Successful renal transplantation generally reverses most of the neurologic complications of uremia. Performance on cognitive function studies such as the CRT, CMT, and CPT improves in adults,[19] as does slowing of the fundamental EEG rhythm, the latter evidenced by a decrease in the % EEG power [(3–7) Hz/(3 + 3) Hz] × 100 to normal.[19] Significantly improved performance on intelligence tests such as the WISC-R, mathematics and reading subtests of the Peabody Individual Achievement Test, and the Halstead-Reitan Category Test has been demonstrated in children at one month post-transplant, when compared with predialysis studies.[21] However, no significant improvement in attention span was demonstrable by the CPT when group mean predialysis and post-transplant performances were compared.[21] Recovery from peripheral neuropathy occurs clinically and electrophysiologically in both adults[116, 215–217] and children,[120] the degree of improvement depending, in part, upon the extent of pretransplant nerve damage and the age of the patient.[215, 216] After the prompt establishment of allograft function, clinical recovery generally proceeds in a cephalocaudad and proximal-distal direction. A biphasic pattern of recovery has been observed, with rapid resolution of paresthesias and dramatic improvement in the VPT occurring within weeks of transplantation. This is followed by a slower phase, during which improvement in motor function (deep tendon reflexes, muscle strength) and additional recovery of sensory function take place over months to years. Motor function which has not been recovered by 6 months post-transplant may be permanently lost.[215]

NCVs also tend to follow a biphasic pattern of recovery in both adults and children; the period of most rapid improvement is the first 4 to 10 weeks post-transplant in most adults.[217] Improvement appears to take longer in children, with some NCVs still abnormally slow 2 to 3 years later.[120] The most dramatic improvements in NCVs have been observed in those patients with the worst electrophysiologic studies pretransplant. Nonetheless, in some patients with severe and long-standing disease, NCVs fail to fully recover.[216, 217]

### Neurologic Complications of Transplantation

**Peripheral Neuropathy.** Some patients have experienced worsening of clinical neuropathy following successful transplantation, usually in one of several situations: following a sudden worsening of renal function as, e.g., in association with acute rejection;[215] as an iatrogenic complication of transplant surgery, due to femoral nerve compression resulting from the use of self-retaining retractors;[218, 219] and as a complication of spinal cord compression in a 15-year-old male, due to a midline accumulation of fat in the epidural space.[220] The latter followed multiple bouts of acute rejection and the repeated use of high doses of corticosteroids, and was characterized by weakness and numbness of the lower extremities in association with normal NCVs and an extradural occlusion of the spinal canal at $T_9$–$T_{12}$. All clinical manifestations resolved following surgical removal of the benign fatty tissue. Finally, the development of a Guillain-Barre–like polyradiculopathy has occurred, with muscle weakness and bulbar involvement, associated with elevated serum and CSF complement-fixing antibody titers to cytomegalovirus.[221]

### CNS Dysfunction Following Renal Transplantation

*Hypertensive Encephalopathy.* The clinical picture of hypertensive encephalopathy was discussed earlier. During the immediate post-transplant period, hypertension may result from sodium and water retention associated with acute tubular necrosis (ATN), corticosteroid therapy, and acute rejection.[222–224] Causes of persistent hypertension include chronic rejection, hypercalcemia, renal artery stenosis, segmental renal ischemia due to sacrifice of a polar artery, recurrence of the original renal disease in the allograft, and the development of pseudotumor cerebri in association with the tapering of corticosteroid dosage.[225]

*Infection.* Infection is the major cause of death in children following renal transplantation, and is an important cause of morbidity.[226, 227] Bacterial (*Listeria monocytogenes, Nocardia asteroides, Streptococcus pneumoniae*), fungal (Aspergillus, Cryptococcus, Histoplasma), protozoan (Toxoplasma), and viral (papovavirus, ?CMV) agents have been identified as causes of infection in children and adults.[102, 228, 229, 254, 255] Collectively, Listeria, Cryptococcus, and Aspergillus are responsible for more than 75% of all CNS infections.[228] The clinical syndromes caused by these organisms include:

*Acute meningitis,* most often due to *Listeria monocytogenes,*[222] and characterized by fever, headache, meningismus, and abnormal CSF (pleocytosis and elevated protein). Listeria may cause meningoencephalitis,[230] cerebritis,[231] and rhombencephalitis.[232] *S. pneumoniae* has caused acute meningitis in a 7-year-old child, three years post-renal transplantation.[233]

*Subacute to chronic meningitis,* usually due to Cryptococcus.

*Focal brain infection,* usually due to Aspergillus. Listeria, Toxoplasma, Nocardia, and Histoplasma may also be responsible. Lister-

iosis may occur at any time after the first month post-transplant.[228] Aspergillus, Toxoplasma, and Nocardia usually cause infection one to four months after transplant, while Cryptococcus occurs later. The clinical picture of CNS fungal infection includes fever, delirium, and seizures. A positive chest roentgenogram is almost always seen, since nervous system involvement usually occurs secondary to pulmonary infection, and is helpful in excluding brain tumor as a cause of the associated neurologic disturbances.

*Complications of Corticosteroid Therapy.* When given in doses usually prescribed in the immediate post-transplant period and for the treatment of acute rejection, corticosteroids may produce neurologic disturbances through a variety of mechanisms. The role of corticosteroids in the pathogenesis of post-transplant hypertension, and the opportunistic infections which immunosuppressive medication may promote have been discussed. Corticosteroids may also cause an acute psychosis, which appears to be dose-related and is reversible upon reduction of drug dose.[234] Symptoms include violent behavior, hallucinations, delusions, profound depression, or mania. In the immediate post-transplant period, corticosteroids may also induce hypophosphatemia, with its attendant neurologic problems, by increasing phosphaturia and stimulating muscle phosphate uptake.[171]

*Electrolyte Disturbances.* Hypercalcemia may occur following successful renal transplantation in adolescents and adults,[171] and has been attributed to delayed resolution of secondary HPTH and, in some patients, to concomitant phosphorus depletion. The signs, symptoms, and therapy of specific electrolyte disorders have been discussed.

*Neurovascular Complications.* Cerebrovascular accidents (CVAs) may occur in the post-transplant period owing to thromboembolic phenomena,[235] systemic fat embolization,[236] and intracranial hemorrhage.[237] CVAs due to intracranial hemorrhage are relatively uncommon in patients under 20 years of age. However, in a recent survey, subdural hematoma was noted as a cause of death exclusively in patients 8 to 18 years of age.[237] Additional fatal cases have been reported by Potter el al.[226] Presentation is usually with headache, focal neurologic signs, and seizures. Thromboembolic phenomena, an unusual cause of CVAs in young transplant recipients,[235] are most likely to occur in the first three postoperative months, a period during which the blood is unusually hypercoagulable. However, Hulme et al reported a 15-year-old male who presented 200 days post-transplant with a 7-hour history of fever and occipital headaches, which were followed by the development of stupor and seizures.[238] At postmortem examination, thrombosis of the basilar and anterior, middle, and posterior cerebral arteries was noted, with associated cerebral infarction. Systemic fat embolization has occurred in association with marked hypertriglyceridemia (1600 mg/dl) in a 25-year-old female who developed drowsiness and lethargy following high-dose corticosteroid therapy for acute rejection.[236]

*Neoplasia.* CNS neoplasia has occurred in 32 of 19,631 renal transplants reviewed in the most recent report of the Advisory Committee to the Human Renal Transplant Registry.[239] Several of these patients were under 20 years of age, and had lymphomas or reticulum cell sarcomas.[227, 240, 241] The symptoms are those associated with increasing intracranial pressure and rapidly evolving focal neurologic signs. CSF examination may show elevated opening pressure and protein concentration. The EEG shows focal slowing in the portion of the recording corresponding to the involved brain area. Computed tomograms may be normal initially, only to become abnormal within days owing to rapid tumor growth.[241] Neoplasms of multifocal origin have occurred.[240] In a child with focal neurologic signs, the absence of fever and the presence a normal chest roentgenogram is strongly suggestive of neoplasia, as opposed to fungal brain abscess. Because neoplasia and infection may coexist in the same patient, however, brain biopsy may be needed for definitive diagnosis.[240]

*Progressive Multifocal Leukoencephalopathy (PML).* This is a subacute, progressive papovavirus infection of the CNS, characterized pathologically by multiple foci of demyelination involving cerebral subcortical white matter ("U" fibers) and, to a lesser extent, the cortex and white matter of the cerebellum and brain stem.[242-244] The characteristic lesions include the presence of oligodendroglia containing amphophilic intranuclear inclusions. The latter have been shown, by electron microscopy, to contain particles having the dimensions of papovavirus.[242-244] The disease has occurred predominantly in patients with lymphoreticular malignancies, only six adult renal transplant patients having been

described. To date no pediatric cases have been reported. Brain biopsy may be necessary to establish the diagnosis and, thus, to rule out the presence of other, treatable conditions, including fungal and protozoan infections. Death due to PML has occurred in all reported patients, between two and five months after the onset of symptoms.

*Central Pontine Myelinolysis (CPM).* This is a progressive, demyelinating disease of unknown etiology, which has developed in both pediatric and adult renal transplant recipients.[245, 246] Affected patients have all been nutritionally debilitated, and often have had concomitant systemic infections and/or have been receiving immunosuppressant medication. CPM has been noted as an incidental postmortem finding in the two pediatric patients in whom it has been described. However, symptomatic patients, with flaccid quadriparesis, pseudobulbar palsy, sensorial clouding, and facial diplegia, also have been described.[102] Symptoms have progressed to death within weeks in patients with extensive lesions.

## REFERENCES

1. Tyler HR: Neurological complications of dialysis, transplantation, and other forms of treatment in chronic uremia. Neurology 15:1081, 1965.
2. Tyler HR: Neurologic disorders in renal failure. Am J Med 44:734, 1968.
3. Nissenson AR, Levin ML, Klawans HL, Nausieda PL: Neurologic sequelae of end stage renal disease. J Chron Dis 30:705, 1977.
4. Nielsen VK: The peripheral nerve function in renal failure. III. A multivariate statistical analysis of factors presumed to affect the development of clinical neuropathy. Acta Med Scand 190:119, 1971.
5. Thomas PK, Hollinrake K, Lascelles RG, et al: The polyneuropathy of chronic renal failure. Brain 94:761, 1971.
6. Bower JD, Magee JH: The use of the Seattle hemodialysis system in renal homotransplantation. Trans Am Soc Artif Intern Organs 10:251, 1964.
7. Grushkin CM, Korsch B, Fine RN: Hemodialysis in small children. JAMA 221:869, 1972.
8. Rotundo A, Nevins TE, Lipton M, et al: Progressive encephalopathy in children with chronic renal insufficiency in infancy. Kidney Int 21:489, 1982.
9. Baluarte HJ, Gruskin AB, Hiner LB, et al: Encephalopathy in children with chronic renal failure. Proc Clin Dial Transplant Forum 7:95, 1977.
10. Bale JF Jr, Siegler RL, Bray PF: Encephalopathy in young children with moderate chronic renal failure. Am J Dis Child 134:581, 1980.
11. Geary DF, Fennell RS, Andriola M, et al: Enceph-

alopathy in children with chronic renal failure. J Pediatr 96:41, 1980.

12. Foley CM, Polinsky MS, Gruskin AB, et al: Encephalopathy in infants and children with chronic renal disease. Arch Neurol 38:656, 1981.

13. Nathan E, Pedersen SE: Dialysis encephalopathy in an undialyzed uremic boy treated with aluminum hydroxide orally. Acta Paediatr Scand 69:793, 1980.

14. Dinapoli RP, Johnson WJ, Lambert EH: Experience with a combined hemodialysis renal transplantation program: Neurologic aspects. Mayo Clin Proc 41:809, 1966.

15. Raskin NH, Fishman RA: Neurologic disorders in renal failure. N Engl J Med 294:143, 1976.

16. Schreiner, GE: Mental and personality changes in the uremic syndrome. Med Ann DC 28:316, 1959.

17. Stenback A, Haapanen E: Azotemia and psychosis: Acta Psychiatr Scand 43:81, 1967.

18. Halverston D: Neurologic complications of renal failure and renal transplantation. In: The Practice of Pediatric Neurology, 2nd Ed, Swaiman KF, Wright FS (eds). St. Louis, CV Mosby Co, 1975.

19. Teschan PE, Ginn HE, Bourne JR, et al: Quantitative indices of clinical uremia. Kidney Int 15:676, 1979.

20. Ginn HE: Neurobehavioral dysfunction in uremia. Kidney Int 7:S217, 1975.

21. Rasbury WC, Fennell, RS, III, Morris MK: Cognitive functioning of children with end-stage renal disease before and after successful renal transplantation. J Pediatr 102:589, 1983.

22. The Denver Developmental Screening Test. In: VC Vaughan III, RJ McKay, WE Nelson (eds). Nelson Textbook of Pediatrics, 10th Edition, Philadelphia, WB Saunders Company, 1975, p 1809.

23. Solomon GE, Plum F: General treatment of epilepsy. In: Clinical Management of Seizures: A Guide for the Physician. Philadelphia, WB Saunders Company, 1976, p 96.

24. Winick M, Rosso P: Head circumference and cellular growth of the brain in normal and marasmic children. J Pediatr 74:774, 1969.

25. Holliday MA: Calorie deficiency in children with uremia: effect upon growth. Pediatrics 50:590, 1972.

26. MacDonnell RC Jr, Buzon MM, Holliday MA: Growth failure in uremic rats: The role of caloric deficiency. Pediatr Res 7:411, 1973.

27. Stoch MD, Smythe PM: Does undernutrition during infancy inhibit brain growth and subsequent intellectual development? Arch Dis Child 38:546, 1963.

28. Evans D, Bowie MD, Hansen JDL, et al: Intellectual development and nutrition. J Pediatr 97:358, 1980.

29. Plum F, Posner JB (eds): The Diagnosis of Stupor and Coma, 2nd Edition. Philadelphia, FA Davis Company, 1972, p 142.

30. Tyler HR: Asterixis (Editorial). J Chron Dis 18:409, 1965.

31. Locke S, Merrill JD, Tyler HR: Neurologic complications of acute uremia. Arch Intern Med 108:75, 1961.

32. Chazan JA, Ambler M, Kalderan A, et al: Vascular deposits causing ischemic myopathy in uremia:

Two brothers with hereditary nephritis. Ann Intern Med 73:73, 1970.

33. Goodhue WW, Davis JN, Porro RS: Ischemic neuropathy in uremic hyperparathyroidism. JAMA 221:911, 1972.

34. Richardson JA, Herron G, Reitz R, Layzer R: Ischemic ulcerations of skin and necrosis of muscle in azotemic hyperparathyroidism. Ann Intern Med 71:129, 1969.

35. Ott SM, Maloney NA, Coburn JW, et al: The prevalence of bone aluminum in renal osteodystophy and its relation to the response to calcitriol therapy. N Engl J Med 307:709, 1982.

36. Hodsman AB, Sherrard DJ, Wong EGC, et al: Vitamin D-resistant osteomalacia in hemodialysis patients lacking secondary hyperparathyroidism. Ann Intern Med 94:629, 1981.

37. Madonick MJ, Berke K, Schiffer I: Pleocytosis and meningeal signs in uremia. Arch Neurol Psychiatr 64:431, 1950.

38. Kiley J, Hines O: Electroencephalographic evaluation of uremia. Arch Intern Med 116:67, 1965.

39. Jacob JC, Gloor P, Elwan OH, et al: Electroencephalographic changes in chronic renal failure. Neurology 15:419, 1965.

40. John ER, Ahn H, Prichep L, et al: Developmental equations for the electroencephalogram. Science 210:1255, 1980.

41. Engel GL, Romano J, Ferris EB, et al: A simple method of determining frequency spectra in the electroencephalogram: observations on physical variations in glucose, $O_2$, protein, and acid-base balance on the normal electroencephalogram. Arch Neurol Psychiatry 51:124, 1944.

42. Guisado R, Arieff AI, Massry SG: Changes in the electroencephalogram in acute uremia. J Clin Invest 55:738, 1975.

43. Cooper JD, Lazarowitz VC, Arieff AI: Neurodiagnostic abnormalities in patients with acute renal failure. J Clin Invest 61:1448, 1978.

44. Kiley JE, Pratt KL, Gisser DG, Schaffer CA: Techniques of EEG frequency analysis for evaluation of uremic encephalopathy. Clin Nephrol 5:279, 1976.

45. Bourne JR, Ward JW, Teschan PE, et al: Quantitative assessment of the electroencephalogram in renal disease. Electroencephalogr Clin Neurophysiol 39:377, 1975.

46. Cogan MG, Covey CM, Arieff AI, et al: Central nervous system manifestations of hyperparathyroidism. Am J Med 65:963, 1978.

47. Teschan PE: Electroencephalographic and other neurophysiologic abnormalities in uremia. Kidney Int 7:S210, 1975.

48. John ER, Karmel BZ, Corning WC, et al: Neurometrics. Science 196:1393, 1977.

49. Polinsky M, Baird H, Gruskin A, et al: Evaluation of neurologic dysfunction in children with chronic renal disease by neurometrics. Proc Clin Dial Transplant Forum 10:299, 1980.

49a. Polinsky MS, Baird H, Gruskin AB, et al: Evaluation of neurologic dysfunction in children with chronic renal failure by neurometrics. Pediatr Res 15:698, 1981.

49b. Andreoli SP, Bergstein JM, Sherrard DJ: Elevated serum aluminum levels and osteomalacia in nondialyzed uremic children due to oral aluminum hydroxide. Pediatr Res 17:344A, 1983.

50. Schwartz GJ, Haycock GB, Edelmann CM Jr,

Spitzer A: A simple estimate of glomerular filtration rate in children derived from body length and plasma creatinine. Pediatrics 58:259, 1976.

51. Olsen S: The brain in uremia. Acta Psychiatr Neurol Scand 36:1, 1961.

52. Passer JA: Cerebral atrophy in end stage uremia. Proc Dial Transplant Forum 7:91, 1977.

53. Schnaper HW, Robson AM: Cerebral cortical atrophy in pediatric patients with end stage renal disease. Pediatr Res 16:327A, 1982.

54. Arieff AI, Guisado R, Massry SG: Uremic encephalopathy: Studies on biochemical alterations in the brain. Kidney Int 7:S194, 1975.

55. Van den Noort S, Eckel RE, Brine KL, Hrdlicka J: Brain metabolism in experimental uremia. Arch Intern Med 126:831, 1970.

56. Schienberg P: Effects of uremia on cerebral blood flow and metabolism. Neurology 15:101, 1954.

57. Fishman RA, Raskin NH: Experimental uremic encephalopathy, permeability, ion exchange, and brain "spaces." Trans Am Neurol Assoc 90:71, 1965.

58. Fishman RA, Raskin NH: Experimental uremic encephalopathy. Permeability and electrolyte metabolism of brain and other tissues. Arch Neurol 17:10, 1967.

59. Fishman RA: Permeability changes in experimental uremic encephalopathy. Arch Intern Med 126:835, 1970.

60. Arieff AI, Massry SG: Calcium metabolism of brain in acute renal failure: Effects of uremia, hemodialysis and parathyroid hormone. J Clin Invest 53:387, 1974.

61. Mayor GH, Keiser JA, Makdani D, Ku PK: Aluminum absorption and distribution: Effect of parathyroid hormone. Science 197:1187, 1977.

62. Mayor GH, Sprague SM, Hourani MR, Sanchez TV: Parathyroid hormone-mediated aluminum deposition and egress in the rat. Kidney Int 17:40, 1981.

63. Arieff AI, Armstrong DK: Parathyroid hormone and uremic neurotoxicity: An unproven association. Contrib Nephrol 20:56, 1980.

64. Hulse JA, Taylor DSI, Dillon MJ: Blindness and paraplegia in severe childhood hypertension. Lancet 2:553, 1979.

65. Gifford RW Jr, Westbrook E: Hypertensive encephalopathy: Mechanisms, clinical features and treatment. Prog Cardiovasc Dis 17:115, 1974.

66. Healton EB, Brust JCM: Hypertensive encephalopathy and the neurological manifestations of malignant hypertension. Trans Am Neurol Assoc 104:212, 1979.

67. Ziegler DK, Zosa A, Zileli T: Hypertensive encephalopathy. Arch Neurol 12:472, 1963.

68. Clarke E, Murphy EA: Neurologic manifestations of malignant hypertension. Br Med J 2:1319, 1956.

69. Perry HM Jr: Minoxidil and improvement of renal function in uremic malignant hypertension. Ann Intern Med 93:769, 1980.

70. Healton, EB, Brust JC, Feinfeld DA, Thomson GE: Hypertensive encephalopathy and the neurologic manifestations of malignant hypertension. Neurology 32:127, 1982.

71. Blaschke TF, Melmon KL: Antihypertensive agents and the therapy of hypertension. *In*: AG Gilman, LS Goodman, A Gilman (eds). The Pharmacologic Basis of Therapeutics, 6th Edition. New York, Macmillan Publishing Co, Inc, 1980, p 793.

72. Ingelfinger, JR: Hypertensive emergencies and acute hypertension. *In*: JR Ingelfinger (ed). Pediatric Hypertension, Philadelphia, WB Saunders Company, 1982, p 222.

73. Koch-Weser J: Diazoxide. N Engl J Med 294:1271, 1976.

74. Palmer RF, Lasseter KC: Sodium nitroprusside. N Engl J Med 292:294, 1975.

75. Editorial: Thought for autoregulation in the hypertensive patient. Lancet 2:510, 1979.

76. Deming QB: Blindness and paraplegia in severe childhood hypertension. Lancet 2:847, 1979.

77. Pryor JS, Davies PD, Hamilton DV: Blindness and malignant hypertension. Lancet 2:803, 1979.

78. Cove DH, Seddon M, Fletcher RF, Dukes DC: Blindness after treatment for malignant hypertension. Br Med J 2:245, 1979.

79. Wetherill JH: Blindness after treatment for malignant hypertension. Br Med J 2:550, 1979.

80. Ingelfinger JR: Hypertension and the central nervous system. *In* JR Ingelfinger (ed). Pediatric Hypertension. Philadelphia, WB Saunders Company, 1982, p 207.

81. Tyler HR: Neurologic aspects of uremia: An overview. Kidney Int 7(1 Suppl 2):S188, 1975.

82. Richet G, Lopez de Noveles E, Verroust P: Drug intoxication and neurologic episodes in chronic renal failure. Br Med J 1:394, 1970.

83. McAllister CJ, Scowden EB, Stone WJ: Toxic psychosis induced by phenothiazine administration in a patient with chronic renal failure. Clin Nephrol 10:191, 1978.

84. Zetin, MZ: Letter to the editor. Clin Nephrol 11:95, 1979.

85. Berger M, White J, Travis LB, et al: Toxic psychosis due to cyproheptadine in a child on hemodialysis. Clin Nephrol 7:43, 1977.

86. Mandell GL, Sande MA: Antimicrobial agents (continued): penicillins and cephalosporins. *In* AG Goodman, LS Gilman, A Gilman (eds). The Pharmacologic Basis of Therapeutics, 6th Edition. New York, Macmillan Publishing Co, Inc, 1980, p 1150.

87. Kalloy MC, Tabechian H, Riley GR, Chessin LN: Neurotoxicity due to ticarcillin in patients with renal failure. Lancet 1:608, 1979.

88. Taclob L, Needle M: Drug-induced encephalopathy in patients on maintenance hemodialysis. Lancet 1:704, 1976.

89. Spector R, Lorenzo AN: The effects of salicylate and probenecid on the cerebrospinal fluid transport of penicillin, aminosalicylic acid, and iodide. J Pharmacol Exp Ther 188:55, 1974.

90. Fishman RA: Blood-brain and CSF barriers to penicillin and related organic acids. Arch Neurol 15:113, 1966.

91. Alfrey AC, Mishell JM, Burks JM, et al: Syndrome of dyspraxia and multifocal seizures associated with chronic dialysis. Trans Am Soc Artif Intern Organs 18:257, 1972.

92. Burks JS, Alfrey AC, Huddlestone J, et al: A fatal encephalopathy in chronic hemodialysis patients. Lancet 1:764, 1976.

93. Mehta RP: Encephalopathy in chronic renal failure appearing before the start of dialysis. Can Med Assoc J 120:1112, 1979.

94. Etheridge WB, O'Neill WM Jr: The "dialysis encephalopathy syndrome" without dialysis. Clin Nephrol 10:250, 1978.

95. Polinsky MS, Prebis JW, Elzouki AY, et al: A dialysis-encephalopathy-like syndrome in children: results of a survey to determine incidence and geographic distribution of cases. Pediatr Res 14:1017, 1980.

96. Holland N: Personal communication, 1980.

97. Alfrey AC, LeGendre GR, Kaehny WD: The dialysis encephalopathy syndrome: possible aluminum intoxication. N Engl J Med 294:184, 1976.

98. McDermott JR, Smith AI, Ward MK, Kerr DNS: Brain aluminum concentration in dialysis encephalopathy. Lancet 1:901, 1978.

99. Polinsky MS, Gruskin AB, Baluarte HJ, et al: Aluminum in chronic renal failure: A pediatric perspective. *In*: J Strauss (ed). Pediatric Nephrology, Vol 6: Current Concepts in Diagnosis and Management. New York, Plenum Publishing Corp, 1981, p 315.

100. Arieff AI: Neurological complications of uremia. *In* BM Brenner, FC Rector (eds). The Kidney, 2nd Edition. Philadelphia, WB Saunders Company, 1981, p 2320.

101. Arieff AI, Cooper JD, Armstrong D, Lazarowitz VC: Dementia, renal failure and brain aluminum. Ann Intern Med 90:741, 1979.

102. Raskin NH, Fishman RA: Neurologic disorders in renal failure (Part II). N Engl J Med 294:204, 1976.

103. Nielsen VK: The peripheral nerve function in chronic renal failure: I. Clinical signs and symptoms. Acta Med Scand 190:105, 1971.

104. Fine RN, Korsch BM, Grushkin CM, Lieberman E: Hemodialysis in children. Am J Dis Child 119:498, 1970.

105. Romagnoni M: Neuropathy in uremia. N Engl J Med 282:1271, 1970.

106. McVicar M, Gauthier B, Goodman CT: Uremic neuropathy: Monitoring of transketolase activity inhibition in a child. Am J Dis Child 125:263, 1973.

107. Callaghan N: Restless legs syndrome in uremic neuropathy. Neurology (Minn) 16:359, 1961.

108. Jennekens FGI, Dorhout Mees EJ, van der Most van Spijk D: Clinical aspects of uremic polyneuropathy. Nephron 8:414, 1971.

109. Nielsen VK: The peripheral nerve function in chronic renal failure. VI: The relationship between sensory and motor conduction and kidney function, azotemia, age, sex and clinical neuropathy. Acta Med Scand 194:455, 1973.

110. Savazzi GM, Migone L, Cambi V: The influence of glomerular filtration rate on uremic polyneuropathy. Clin Nephrol 13:64, 1980.

111. Nielsen VK: The peripheral nerve function in uremia. II. Intercorrelation of clinical symptoms and signs and clinical grading of neuropathy. Acta Med Scand 190:113, 1971.

112. Daniel CR III, Bower JD, Pearson JE, Halbert RD: Vibrometry and uremic peripheral neuropathy. South Med J 70:1311, 1977.

113. Nielsen VK: The peripheral nerve function in chronic renal failure. VII. Longitudinal course during terminal renal failure and regular hemodialysis. Acta Med Scand 195:155, 1974.

114. Versaci AA, Olsen KJ, McMain PB, et al: Uremic polyneuropathy and motor nerve conduction velocities. Trans Am Soc Artif Intern Organs 10:328, 1964.

115. Nielsen VK: The Peripheral Nerve Function in Chronic Renal Failure: A Survey. Copenhagen, Christtrev and Petersens, 1974, p 9.

116. Tenckhoff HA, Boen FST, Jebsen RH, Spiegler JH: Polyneuropathy in chronic renal insufficiency. JAMA 192:91, 1965.

117. Lascelles RG, Thomas PG: Changes due to age in internodal length in the sural nerve in man. J Neurol Neurosurg Psychiatry 29:40, 1966.

118. Nielsen VK: The peripheral nerve function in chronic renal failure. V. Sensory and motor conduction velocity. Acta Med Scand 194:445, 1973.

119. Mentser MI, Clay S, Malekzadeh MH, et al: Peripheral motor nerve conduction velocities in children undergoing chronic hemodialysis. Nephron 22:337, 1978.

120. Arbus GS, Barnor NA, Hsu AC, et al: Effect of chronic renal failure dialysis, and transplantation on motor nerve conduction velocity in children. Can Med Assoc J 113:517, 1975.

121. Jebsen RH, Tenckhoff H, Honet JC: Natural history of uremic polyneuropathy and effects of dialysis. N Engl J Med 277:327, 1967.

122. Appenzeller O, Kornfeld M, MacGee J: Neuropathy in chronic renal disease: A microscopic, ultrastructural and biochemical study of sural nerve biopsies. Arch Neurol 24:499, 1971.

123. Dyck PJ, Johnson WJ, Lambert EH, O'Brien PC: Segmental demyelination secondary to axonal degeneration in uremic neuropathy. Mayo Clin Proc 46:400, 1971.

124. Dinn JJ, Crane DL: Schwann cell dysfunction in uremia. J Neurol Neurosurg Psychiatry 33:605, 1970.

125. Lonergan ET, Semar M, Sterzel RB, et al: Erythrocyte transketolase activity in dialyzed patients. N Engl J Med 284:1309, 1971.

126. Lange K, Lonergan ET, Semar M, Sterzel RB: Transketolase inhibition as a mechanism in uremic neuropathy. Trans Assoc Am Physicians 84:172, 1971.

127. Avram MM, Feinfeld DA, Huatuco AH: Search for the uremic toxin: Decreased motor nerve conduction velocity and elevated parathyroid hormone in uremia. N Engl J Med 298:1000, 1978.

128. DiGiulio S, Chkoff N, Lhoste F, et al: Parathormone as a nerve poison in uremia. N Engl J Med 299:1134, 1978.

128a. Argov Z, Mastaglia F: Drug-induced peripheral neuropathies. Br Med J 1:663, 1979.

129. Read DJ, Feest TG, Nassim MA: Clonazepam: Effective treatment for restless leg syndrome in uraemia. Br Med J 283:885, 1981.

130. Lennon PA, Adam WR, Bladin P, et al: Transient blindness associated with renal failure. Aust NZ J Med 4:346, 1971.

131. Mirahmadi MK, Vazini ND: Hearing loss in end-stage renal disease—effect of dialysis. J Dial 4:159, 1980.

132. Henich WI, Thompson P, Bergstrom L, Lum GM: Effect of dialysis on hearing activity. Nephron 18:348, 1977.

133. Quick CA, Happe W: Permanent deafness associated with furosemide administration. Ann Otol 84:94, 1975.

134. Mahajan SK, Prasad AS, Lambujon J, et al: Im-

provement of uremic hypogeusia by zinc: a double blind study. Am J Clin Nutr 33:1517, 1980.

135. Ciechanover M, Persecenschi G, Aviram A, Steiner JE: Malrecognition of taste in uremia. Nephron 26:20, 1980.

136. Mahajan SK, Gardiner WH, Abbasi AA, et al: Hypogeusia in patients on hemodialysis. Proc Dial Transplant Forum 8:20, 1978.

137. Blumenkrantz MJ, Lindsay RM: Comparisons of hemodialysis and peritoneal dialysis: A review of the literature. Contrib Nephrol 17:20, 1979.

138. Caccia MR, Mangili A, Mecca G, et al: Effects of hemodialysis treatment on uremic polyneuropathy: A clinical and electrophysiologic study. J Neurol 217:123, 1977.

139. Chan JCM, Eng G: Long-term hemodialysis and nerve conduction in children. Pediatr Res 13:591, 1979.

140. Honet JC, Jebsen RH, Tenckhoff HA: Motor nerve conduction velocity in chronic renal insufficiency. Arch Phys Med 47:647, 1966.

141. Babb A: The genesis of the square meter-hour hypothesis. Trans Am Soc Artif Intern Organs 17:81, 1971.

142. Kennedy AC: Dialysis disequilibrium syndrome. Electroenceph Clin Neurophys 29:206, 1970.

143. Wakim KG: The pathophysiology of the dialysis disequilibrium syndrome. Mayo Clin Proc 44:406, 1969.

144. Milutinovich J, Warren J, Graefe U: Death caused by brain herniation during hemodialysis. South Med J 72:418, 1979.

145. Moel DI, Kwun YA: Cortical blindness as a complication of hemodialysis. J Pediatr 93:890, 1978.

146. Kennedy AC, Linton AL, Luke RG, Renfrew S: Electroencephalographic changes during haemodialysis. Lancet 1:408, 1963.

147. Mauer, SM, Lynch RM: Hemodialysis techniques for infants and children. Pediatr Clin North Am 23:843, 1976.

148. Wakim KG, Johnson WJ, Klass DW: Role of blood urea and serum sodium concentrations in the pathogenesis of the dialysis disequilibrium syndrome. Trans Am Soc Artif Intern Organs 14:394, 1968.

149. Hampers CL, Doak PB, Callaghan MN, et al: The electroencephalogram and spinal fluid during hemodialysis. Arch Intern Med 118:340, 1966.

150. Kominami N, Taylor HR, Hampers CL, Merrill JP: Variation in motor nerve conduction velocity in normal and uremic patients. Arch Intern Med 128:235, 1971.

150a. Kerr DNS: Clinical and pathophysiologic changes in patients on chronic dialysis: The central nervous system. Adv Nephrol 9:109, 1980.

151. Arieff AI, Guisado R, Massry SA, Lazarowitz V: Central nervous system pH in uremia and the effects of hemodialysis. J Clin Invest 58:306, 1976.

152. Arieff AI, Massry SG, Barriendos A, Kleeman CR: Brain water and electrolyte metabolism in uremia: effects of slow and rapid hemodialysis. Kidney Int 4:177, 1973.

153. Arieff AI, Lazarowitz VC, Guisado RG: Experimental dialysis of disequilibrium syndrome: Prevention and glycerol. Kidney Int 14:270, 1978.

154. Finberg L: Hypernatremic dehydration. In: Water and Electrolytes in Pediatrics: Physiology, Pathophysiology, and Treatment, L Finberg, RE Kravath, AR Fleischman (Eds). Philadelphia, WB Saunders Company, 1982, p 81.

155. Borges HF, Hocks J, Kjellstrand CM: Mannitol intoxication in patients with renal failure. Arch Intern Med 142:63, 1982.

156. Mudge GH: Drugs affecting renal function and electrolyte metabolism. In: AG Gilman, LS Goodman, A Gilman (eds), The Pharmacologic Basis of Therapeutics, 6th Edition. New York, Macmillan Publishing Co, Inc, 1980, p 896.

157. Bana DS, Graham JR: Renin response during hemodialysis headache. Headache 16:168, 1976.

158. Chillar RK, Desforges JF: Muscular cramps during maintenance dialysis. Lancet 2:285, 1972.

159. Stewart WR, Fleming LW, Manual MA: Muscle cramps during maintenance dialysis. Lancet 1:1049, 1972.

160. Bazzato G, Mezzina E, Ciman M, Guarnieri G: Myasthenia-like syndrome associated with carnitine in patients on long-term hemodialysis. Lancet 1:1041, 1979.

161. Lazarus JM: Maintenance dialysis and proximal muscle weakness. JAMA 46:2629, 1981.

162. Sakai JK, Vazeri ND, Naeim F, Meshkinpour H: Dialysis-induced changes in muscle strength. J Dial 4:191, 1980.

163. Smith RJ, Block MR, Arieff AI, et al: Hypernatremic, hyperosmolar coma complicating chronic peritoneal dialysis. Proc Dial Transplant Forum 4:96, 1974.

164. Nolph KD, Twardowski ZJ, Popovich RP, Rubin J: Equilibration of peritoneal dialysis solutions during long-dwell exchanges. J Lab Clin Med 93:246, 1979.

165. Ribot S, Jacobs MG, Frankel HJ, Bernstein A: Complications of peritoneal dialysis. Am J Med Sci 35:505, 1966.

166. Hagan GR: Hypernatremia—problems in management. Pediatr Clin North Am 23:569, 1976.

167. Gruskin AB, Baluarte HJ, Prebis JW, et al: Serum sodium abnormalities in children. Pediatr Clin North Am 29:907, 1982.

168. Whang R, Draney D, Ryan M: Postdialysis convulsions: Treatment with calcium infusion. Rocky Mt Med J 68:41, 1971.

169. David DS: Calcium metabolism in renal failure. Am J Med 58:48, 1975.

170. Coburn JW, Massry SG, DePalma R, Shinaberger JH: Rapid appearance of hypercalcemia with initiation of hemodialysis. JAMA 210:2276, 1969.

171. Schwartz GH, David DS, Riggio RR, et al: Hypercalcemia after renal transplantation. Am J Med 49:42, 1970.

172. Rivera-Vazquez AB, Noriega-Sanchez A, Ramirez-Gonzales R, Martinez-Maldonado M: Acute hypercalcemia in hemodialysis patients: Distinction from dialysis dementia. Nephron 25:243, 1980.

173. Lotz M, Sisman E, Barittez FC: Evidence for a phosphorus depletion syndrome in man. N Engl J Med 278:409, 1968.

174. Kreisberg RA: Phosphorus deficiency and hypophosphatemia. Hosp Pract 12:121, 1977.

175. Pierides AM, Ward MK, Kerr DNS: Haemodialysis encephalopathy: Possible role of phosphate depletion. Lancet 1:1234, 1976.

176. Ward MK, Pierides AM, Fawcett D, et al: Dialysis encephalopathy syndrome. Proc Eur Dial Transplant Assoc 13:348, 1976.

177. Bayer J, Gill GN, Epstein FH: Hyperglycemia and hyperosmolality complicating peritoneal dialysis. Ann Intern Med 67:568, 1967.

178. Iatrogenic non-ketotic hyperglycemic coma. (Editorial.) JAMA 203:173, 1968.

179. Cohen IM, Lee S: Diabetes, intraperitoneal insulin, and CAPD. J Dial 5:269, 1981.

180. Gaan D, Mallick NP, Brewis RAL, et al: Cerebral damage from declotting Scribner shunts. Lancet 2:77, 1969.

181. Leonard CD, West E, Scribner BH: Subdural hematomas in patients undergoing hemodialysis. Lancet 2:239, 1969.

182. Leonard CD: Subdural hematoma and dialysis: Survey of reprint requesters. N Engl J Med 282:1433, 1970.

183. Leonard A, Shapiro FL: Subdural hematoma in regularly hemodialyzed patients. Ann Intern Med 82:650, 1975.

184. DelGreco FO, Kramlovsky F: Subdural hematoma in the course of haemodialysis. Lancet 2:1009, 1969.

185. Siddiqui JY, Fitz AE, Lawton RL, Kirkendall WM: Causes of death in patients receiving long-term hemodialysis. JAMA 212:1350, 1970.

186. Talalla A, Halbrook H, Barbour BH, Kurze T: Subdural hematoma associated with long-term hemodialysis for chronic renal disease. JAMA 12:1847, 1970.

187. Bechar M, Lakke JPWF, van der Hem GK, et al: Subdural hematoma during long-term dialysis. Arch Neurol 26:513, 1972.

188. Fine RN, Malekzadeh MH, Pennisi AJ, et al: Long term results of transplantation in children. Pediatrics 61:641, 1978.

189. Platts MM, Anastassiades E: Dialysis encephalopathy: Precipitating factors and improvement in prognosis. Clin Nephrol 15:223, 1981.

190. Masramon J, Ricait MJ, Caralps A, et al: Dialysis encephalopathy. Lancet 1:1370, 1978.

191. Report of the registration committee of the European Dialysis and Transplant Association. Dialysis dementia in Europe. Lancet 2:190, 1980.

192. Rosenbek JC, McNeil MR, Leme ML, et al: Speech and language findings in a chronic hemodialysis patient: a case report. J Speech Hear Dis 40:245, 1975.

193. Madison DP, Baehr ET, Bazell M, et al: Communicative and cognitive deterioration in dialysis dementia: Two case studies. J Speech Hear Dis 42:238, 1977.

194. Sedman AB, Alfrey AC, Warady BA, Lum GM: Aluminum levels in children with chronic renal failure. Pediatr Res 17:356A, 1983.

195. Trauner DA, Clayman M: Dialysis encephalopathy treated with clonazepam. Ann Neurol 6:555, 1979.

196. Pascoe MD: Clonazepam in dialysis encephalopathy. Ann Neurol 9:200, 1981.

197. Masselot JP, Adhemar JP, Jaudon MC, et al: Reversible dialysis encephalopathy: Role for aluminum-containing gels. Lancet 2:1386, 1978.

198. Buge A, Poisson M, Masson S, et al: Encephalopathie reversible des dialysees apres l'apport d'aluminum. Nouv Presse Med 8:2729, 1979.

199. Sullivan PA, Murnaghan DJ, Callaghan N: Dialysis dementia: recovery after transplantation. Br Med J 2:740, 1977.

200. Ackrill P, Ralston AJ, Day JP, Hodge KC: Successful removal of aluminum from patients with dialysis encephalopathy. Lancet 2:692, 1980.

201. Pogglitsch H, Peter W, Wawschenek O, Holzer W: Treatment of early stage of dialysis encephalopathy by aluminum depletion. Lancet 2:1344, 1981.

202. Arze RS, Parkinson IS, Cartlidge NEF, et al: Reversal of aluminum dialysis encephalopathy after deferoxamine treatment. Lancet 2:1116, 1981.

203. Gacek EM, Babb AL, Uvelli DA, et al: Dialysis dementia: the role of dialysate pH in altering the dialyzability of aluminum. Trans Soc Artif Intern Organs 25:409, 1979.

204. Platts M: Dialysis encephalopathy. Lancet 2:1035, 1980.

205. Browder A, Joselow MM, Louria DB: The problem of lead poisoning. Medicine (Baltimore) 52:121, 1973.

206. Mattern WD, Krigman MR, Blythe WB: Failure of successful renal transplantation to reverse the dialysis associated encephalopathy syndrome. Clin Nephrol 7:275, 1977.

207. Hodge KC, Day JP, O'Hara M, et al: Critical concentrations of aluminum in water used for dialysis. Lancet 2:802, 1981.

208. Flendrig JA, Kruis H, Das HA: Aluminum and dialysis dementia. Lancet 1:1235, 1976.

209. Diamant UH, Gambertoglio JG: Aluminum intoxication (letter). N Engl J Med 294:1129, 1976.

210. Alfrey AC, Kaehny WD: Aluminum intoxication (letter). N Engl J Med 294:1131, 1976.

211. Ball JH, Butkus DE, Madison DS: Effect of subtotal parathyroidectomy on dialysis dementia. Nephron 18:151, 1977.

212. Adhemar JP, Laederich J, Jaudon MC, et al: Removal of aluminum from patients with dialysis encephalopathy. Lancet 2:1311, 1980.

213. Shirkey HC: Pediatric Therapy, 5th edition. St. Louis, CV Mosby, 1975, p 1238.

214. Klein WJ, Metz EN, Price AR: Acute copper intoxication: A hazard of hemodialysis. Arch Intern Med 129:578, 1972.

215. Nielsen VK: The peripheral nerve function in chronic renal failure. VIII. Recovery after renal transplantation. Clinical aspects. Acta Med Scand 195:163, 1974.

216. Bolton CF, Baltzan MA, Baltzan RB: Effects of renal transplantation on uremic neuropathy: A clinical and electrophysiologic study. N Engl J Med 284:1170, 1971.

217. Nielsen VK: The peripheral nerve function in chronic renal failure. IX. Recovery after renal transplantation. Electrophysiologic aspects (sensory and motor nerve conduction). Acta Med Scand 195:171, 1974.

218. Vaziri ND, Barnes J, Mirahmadi K, et al: Compression neuropathy subsequent to renal transplantation. Urology 7:145, 1976.

219. Vaziri ND, Barton CH, Ravikumar GR, et al: Femoral neuropathy: a complication of renal transplantation. Nephron 28:30, 1981.

220. Lee M, Lekins J, Gubbay SS, Hurst PE: Spinal cord compression by extradural fat after renal transplantation. Med J Aust 1:201, 1975.

221. Bale JF, Rote NS, Bluomer LC, Bray PF: Guillain-Barre-like polyneuropathy after renal transplant: Possible association with cytomegalovirus infection. Arch Neurol 37:784, 1980.

222. Fine RN, Korsch BM, Stiles Q, et al: Renal homotransplantation in children. J Pediatr 76:347, 1970.

223. Malekzadeh MH, Brennan LP, Payne VC Jr, Fine

RN: Hypertension after renal transplantation in children. J Pediatr 86:370, 1975.

224. Arbus GS, DeMaria JE, Churchill BM: Transplantation and complications of chronic renal failure. Can Med Assoc J 120:659, 1980.

225. Mauer SM, Howard RJ: Renal transplantation in children. In: CM Edelmann Jr (ed). Pediatric Kidney Disease. Boston, Little, Brown, and Company, 1978, p 524.

226. Potter DE, Holliday MA, Piel CF, et al: Treatment of end-stage renal disease in children: A 15 year experience. Kidney Int 18:103, 1980.

227. Novello AJ, Fine RN: Renal transplantation in children—a review. Int J Pediatr Nephrol 3:87, 1982.

228. Rubin RH, Wolfson JS, Cosimi AB, Tolkoff-Rubin NE: Infection in the renal transplant recipient. Am J Med 70:405, 1981.

229. Schneck SA: Neuropathologic features of human organ transplantation. I. Probable cytomegalovirus infection. J Neuropathol Exp Neurol 24:415, 1965.

230. Lechtenberg R, Sierra MF, Pringle G, et al: Listeria monocytogenes: Brain abscess or meningoencephalitis? Neurology 29:86, 1979.

231. Watson GW, Fuller TJ, Elms J, Kluge RM: Listeria cerebritis: Relapse of infection in renal transplant patients. Arch Intern Med 138:83, 1978.

232. Mahoney JF, Manbyah JH, Dalton VC, Wolfenden WH: Pontomedullary listeriosis in renal allograft recipient. Br Med J 1:705, 1974.

233. Hodson EM, Najarian JS, Kjellstrand CM, et al: Renal transplantation in children ages 1–5 years. Pediatrics 61:458, 1978.

234. The Boston Collaborative Drug Surveillance Program. Acute adverse reactions to prednisone in relation to dosage. Clin Pharmacol Ther 13:694, 1972.

235. Rao KV, Smith EJ, Alexander JW, et al: Thromboembolic disease in renal allograft recipients. Arch Surg 111:1086, 1976.

236. Jones JP Jr, Engleman EP, Najarian JS: Systemic fat embolism after renal homotransplantation and treatment with corticosteroids. N Engl J Med 273:1453, 1965.

237. Harris RD, Campbell JK, Howard FM, et al: Neurovascular complications of dialysis and transplantation. Stroke 5:725, 1974.

238. Hulme B, Kenyon JR, Owen K, et al: Renal transplantation in children. Arch Dis Child 47:486, 1972.

239. Advisory Committee to the Renal Transplant Registry: The 13th Report of the Human Renal Transplant Registry. Transplant Proc 9:9, 1977.

240. Schneck SA, Penn I: Cerebral neoplasms associated with renal transplantation. Arch Neurol 22:226, 1970.

241. Mirra SS, Check IJ, Porter JD, et al: Rapid evolution of central nervous system lymphoma in a renal transplant recipient. Lancet 2:868, 1981.

242. ZuRhein GM, Varakis J: Progressive multifocal leukoencephalopathy in a renal allograft recipient. Lancet 2:798, 1974.

243. McCormick WF, Schochet SS Jr, Sarles HE, Calverley JR: Progressive multifocal leukoencephalopathy in renal transplant recipients. Arch Intern Med 136:829, 1976.

244. Garcia JH, Dismukes WE, Duvall ER: Medical Pathology Conference. Ala J Med Sci 18:61, 1981.

245. Lopez RI, Collins GN: Wernicke's encephalopathy: A complication of chronic hemodialysis. Arch Neurol 18:248, 1968.

246. Schneck SA: Neuropathologic features of human organ transplantation. II. Central pontine myelinolysis and neuroaxonal dystrophy. J Neuropathol Exp Neurol 25:18, 1966.

247. Fleming LW, Lennon JAR, Steward WK: Effect of magnesium on nerve conduction velocity during regular dialysis treatment. J Neurol Neurosurg Psychiatry 35:342, 1972.

248. Meyrier A, Fardeau M, Richet G: Acute asymmetrical neuritis associated with rapid ultrafiltration dialysis. Br Med J 2:252, 1972.

249. Teehan BP, Smith LJ, Gilgore GS, Sigler MH: Adverse effects of large surface area dialysis on motor nerve conduction velocity. Proc Dial Transplant Forum 4:166, 1974.

250. Davison AM, Williams IR, Mawdsley C, Robson JS: Neuropathy associated with hepatitis in patients maintained on haemodialysis. Br Med J 1:409, 1972.

251. Popovtzer MM, Rosenbaum BJ, Gordon A, Maxwell MH: Relief of uremic polyneuropathy after bilateral nephrectomy. N Engl J Med 281:949, 1969.

252. Bosl R, Shideman JR, Mayer RM, et al: Effects and complications of high efficiency dialysis. Nephron 15:151, 1975.

253. Holden FA, Kaczmer JE, Kinahan CC: Listerial meningitis and renal allografts: A life-threatening affinity. Postgrad Med 68:69, 1980.

254. Barmeir E, Mann JH, Marcus RH: Cerebral nocardiosis in renal transplant patients. Br J Radiol 54:1107, 1981.

255. Karalakulasingam R, Krishan KA, Adams G, et al: Meningoencephalitis caused by Histoplasma capsulatum. Arch Intern Med 136:217, 1976.

256. Dintenfass L, Ibels LS: Blood viscosity factors and occlusive arterial disease in renal transplant recipients. Nephron 15:456, 1975.

257. Pettinger WA: Clonidine, a new antihypertensive drug. N Engl J Med 293:1179, 1975.

258. Bailey RR, Neale TJ: Rapid clonidine withdrawal with blood pressure overshoot exaggerated by beta-blockade. Br Med J 1:942, 1976.

# 23

# Hypertension in Children with ESRD

*Julie R. Ingelfinger, M.D.*

Children with ESRD, whether predialysis, undergoing dialysis, or post-transplant, often have hypertension. Hypertension may be asymptomatic or may cause considerable morbidity. This chapter will review mechanisms of hypertension in children with ESRD, including clinical aspects, methods of evaluation, and pharmacologic treatment.

## MECHANISMS OF HYPERTENSION IN ESRD

In the normal child, blood pressure is the product of cardiac output and peripheral vascular resistance. All factors contributing to blood pressure must be considered to understand the mechanism of hypertension in children with chronic renal disease—cardiovascular parameters, extracellular and plasma fluid volumes, and hormonal and neurogenic factors.

### Cardiovascular Factors

Heart rate and stroke volume determine cardiac output. Effective blood volume, circulatory filling pressure, and venous return all contribute to cardiac output. Heart rate, which is determined by oxygen demand and adrenergic function as well as the condition of the heart muscle, also contributes to cardiac output. With chronic increases in cardiac output, autoregulation may lead to increased peripheral vascular resistance, returning cardiac output toward normal.

In essential hypertension with normal renal function, there is often a phase of increased cardiac output followed by a permanent phase of increase in peripheral vascular resistance.[1-4] In chronic renal failure the same findings are generally present.[5] Concomitant anemia and volume expansion in patients with chronic renal failure contribute to the observed increase in cardiac output.[6-12] Anemia is a large contributor to this finding[11, 13] because when the marked anemia is discounted, the difference in cardiac output between normotensive and hypertensive patients with uremia disappears. The rise in cardiac output is neither the initiating nor perpetuating factor in systemic hypertension in chronic renal failure.

The use of echocardiography in children with ESRD has permitted determination of systolic time intervals, particularly the pre-ejection period (PEP), as an index of myocardial performance. In a recent study by Scharer et al, hypertensive children with ESRD were found to have longer PEP than normotensive children with ESRD (Fig. 23–1).[14] The authors concluded that volume expansion and anemia in children with ESRD, when combined with arterial hypertension, led to significantly impaired left ventricular function.

### Peripheral Vascular Resistance

Numerous factors promote an increase in peripheral vascular resistance, including neural factors via stimulation of alpha-adren-

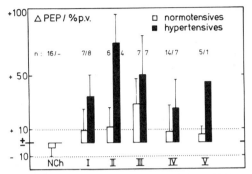

**Figure 23–1.** Pre-ejection period (PEP) in children at different stages of chronic renal failure: NCh = normal children. I: conservative treatment ($S_{cr}$ < 2 mg/dl). II: conservative treatment ($S_{cr}$ 2–5 mg/dl). III: conservative treatment ($S_{cr}$ > 5 mg/dl). IV: Regular hemodialysis. V: After transplantation. The columns indicate mean PEP values (mean ± SD) of the deviations from the predicted individual normal values (in per cent). *White bars:* normotensive patients; *black bars:* hypertensive children; n = number of children examined. The upper limit of normal values is at + 10%. (From Scharer K, Rauh W, and Ulmer HE: The management of hypertension in children with chronic renal failure. *In* Giovannelli G, New MI, and Gorini S: Hypertension in Children and Adolescents. New York, Raven Press, 1981.)

ergic receptors, catecholamines, angiotensin II, vasopressin, certain prostaglandins, and serotonin.[15] Increased peripheral vascular resistance also occurs with changes in cation concentration consequent to alkalosis, with hypothermia, and with decreased osmolality. A passive increase in peripheral vascular resistance may occur with an increase in extra luminal pressure because of edema, with thrombosis or embolism, with hemoconcentration, or with increased blood or plasma viscosity.[15] In chronic renal failure there are perturbations in the levels of various hormonal substances, particularly angiotensin II and vasoactive factors.[16-19] In addition, the vessel walls may be abnormal, owing to derangements in calcium and phosphorus homeostasis.[20]

Peripheral vascular resistance in uremic hypertensive patients may be higher than in those with normotension. Kim et al compared 52 hypertensive to 23 normotensive uremic patients.[11] Cardiac index was similar in both groups, whereas peripheral vascular resistance was increased in the hypertensive patients.[11] Frohlich et al obtained similar results,[4] whereas other investigators have found an elevated cardiac index.[7] This apparent disparity is clearly due to concomitant anemia, because correcting the anemia decreases

the cardiac output. Prospective studies evaluating the progression of hemodynamic changes in patients with renal insufficiency are needed for definitive answers.

## Neurogenic Factors

Autonomic dysfunction is common in patients with chronic renal failure.[21] This may be associated with postural hypotension and abnormalities on Valsalva maneuver.[22-23] The actual contributions of autonomic dysfunction to hypertension are unknown. Some studies have shown that on Valsalva maneuver patients with ESRD have a short Valsalva ratio, which is defined as the ratio between the longest RR interval during the release phase and the shortest RR interval during the strain phase of the Valsalva maneuver. Patients with chronic renal failure also have evidence of decreased baroreceptor activity. It has been postulated that the abnormality resides within baroreceptors because the cold pressor test is normal (tests efferent pathway), while the amyl nitrate inhalation test is abnormal (tests entire reflex arc).[24]

Since norepinephrine (NE) levels tend to be elevated in patients with chronic renal failure, it has been suggested that the autonomic nervous system (ANS) dysfunction is due to end-organ insensitivity to NE. Recently, Campese et al studied the ANS in dialysis patients, predialysis patients, and normal controls.[24] The authors confirmed both reduced end-organ response to NE, using infusion as well as baseline measurements, and low Valsalva ratios, and the blood pressure rose with handgrip efforts.[24]

No *primary* neurogenic component contributing to hypertension in patients with ESRD has been found. Nonetheless, treatment with neurogenically active drugs may augment volume changes in situations of either volume expansion or diuresis.

Exogenous drugs may lead to exaggerated hemodynamic responses in renal insufficiency. For instance, the administration of trimethaphan may lead to an exaggerated response to rapid volume expansion.[25] Since patients with chronic renal failure often have increased extracellular fluid volume,[26-27] antihypertensive agents that would normally work by marked vasodilatation, such as diazoxide or hydralazine, may have a blunted effect.[25] Volume-dependent blood pressure changes may be related to ANS dysfunction in uremia.

## Vasoactive Substances

The major pressor hormone system is the renin-angiotensin system[28-30] (Fig. 23–2). Renin substrate, an alpha-2 globulin synthesized in the liver, is acted upon by renin after its release into the circulation from the juxtaglomerular apparatus (JG).[28] Angiotensin I (AI) is thus produced, a decapeptide with little physiological activity. Following a single passage through the pulmonary bed, AI is cleaved by a converting enzyme bound in the membranes of endothelial cells, yielding angiotensin II (AII), which is a very potent vasoconstrictor.[28] Subsequently, angiotensin III (AIII), a heptapeptide, is produced. The angiotensins are eliminated from the plasma by enzymatic hydrolysis.[31] Many factors determine renin release, including renal perfusion pressure, beta-adrenergic tone, and sodium concentration.[28] Renin production generally is inversely proportional to blood flow. With decreased effective blood volume, renin production is stimulated, promoting an increase in effective blood volume which suppresses its subsequent release. In some patients with ESRD hypertension is clearly renin-mediated; nephrectomy is indicated in this form of hypertension.

In an individual with normal renal function, several mechanisms are responsible for renin release[32]: (a) receptors within the kidney—the macula densa and a renovascular receptor; (b) sympathetic nerves to the kid-

ney, and (c) interaction of electrolytes, vasopressin, and other hormones, including catecholamines, AII, and perhaps AIII. The interaction of these factors in patients with ESRD is unknown. A number of studies have investigated the relationship between sodium excretion and plasma renin activity in uremic subjects.[16-18, 33] Though not all studies agree, some have demonstrated a positive correlation between plasma renin activity and blood pressure elevation, provided that renin was profiled against blood volume and exchangeable sodium.[33]

Several hypotensive substances, such as those emanating from renal medullary cells, have been described experimentally.[34-36] It is possible that in patients with renal insufficiency there is a deficiency in an antihypertensive substance. In uremia there is evidence that renin inhibitors and/or accelerators are present.[37] The contribution of such substances remains to be elucidated.

## Aldosterone

The usual periodic variations in plasma aldosterone levels[38-41] occur in patients with chronic renal failure.[42-44] Since renin and angiotensin interact with aldosterone, and because aldosterone exerts much of its effect via the kidney,[45] important differences in the aldosterone effect on blood pressure exist in the patient with renal insufficiency. Most pa-

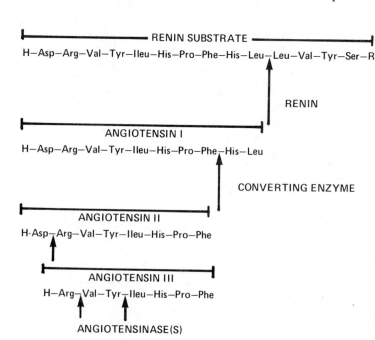

**Figure 23–2.** Schematic representation of the chemical structures and sequence involved in the generation of angiotensin from renin substrate. (From Lifschitz, M. D., and Stein, J. H.: Renal vasoactive hormones. *In* Brenner, B. M., and Rector, F. C., Jr. (Eds.): The Kidney. 2nd Ed. Vol. 1. Philadelphia, W. B. Saunders Co., 1981, p. 651.)

tients with ESRD will respond with a natruresis to the administration of spironolactone, thus demonstrating that mineralocorticoid function is preserved. Occasionally, impressive sodium wasting occurs in patients with chronic renal failure and resistance of renal tubules to mineralocorticoid action appears to be present.[46-48]

It has been suggested that aldosterone may facilitate the control of plasma potassium levels in the uremic patient.[49-52] Aldosterone enhances the fecal excretion of potassium in addition to its renal tubular secretion and may enhance potassium flux into cells once nephrectomy has occurred. In ESRD patients with adrenocortical deficiency, marked hyperkalemia may occur.[53-54]

## The Azotemic Patient's Control of Blood Pressure — Overview

Most patients with moderately severe renal failure appear to respond to changes in volume status in the same manner as do normal individuals. In many patients the renin-angiotensin system has been activated during the course of the chronic renal disease. These

individuals generally are hypertensive during the development and progression of their renal failure. The interaction of various factors resulting in hypertension in patients with chronic renal failure is summarized in Fig. 23–3. As children approach ESRD there appear to be two distinct groups of patients—those with previous hypertension who have had previous glomerular disease,[55] and those with renal dysplasia, generalized hypoplasia, or a structural defect, in whom hypertension is less common.[55] Of the children initiating dialysis at The Children's Hospital Medical Center, 98% of those with glomerular disease had predialysis hypertension, whereas only 23% of those with a structural lesion had hypertension.[55]

## Hypertension in Dialysis Patients

Once patients are anephric, cardiac output and peripheral resistance correlate directly with changes in arterial pressure.[56-57] In nephric patients, it would appear that volume depletion during hemodialysis will increase plasma renin activity.[57] Adjusting the sodium and potassium balance of dialysis patients to

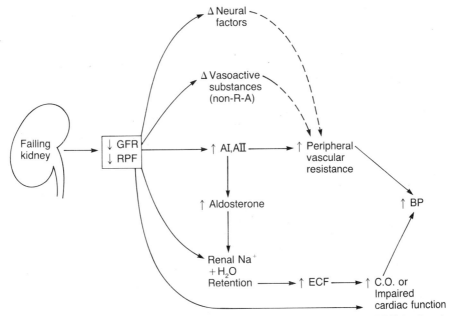

**Figure 23–3.** With failing kidneys, glomerular filtration rate (GFR) and renal plasma flow (RPF) lead to alterations (△) in neural factors, and vasoactive substances. Increases in angiotensin I (AI) and angiotensin II (AII) also occur, leading to increases in peripheral vascular resistance and rise in blood pressure. Increases in AI and AII also stimulate aldosterone production which causes salt and water retention, which is already favored with decreased GFR and RPF. Resultant increases in extracellular fluid (ECF) lead to increased cardiac output (CO) and rise in blood pressure. Furthermore, anemia and impaired cardiac function may contribute to hypertension.

that of control subjects is difficult.[13] This is necessary in order to evaluate the renin-angiotensin system response in various groups of individuals. There is evidence that volume administration will suppress plasma renin activity in dialysis patients.

Following bilateral nephrectomy, renin disappears in a two-component curve. One rapid component disappears over 13 ± 1.1 minutes and the slower component takes 280 ± 94.7 minutes.[58] Although some studies have suggested the presence of renin-like material in basal conditions in anephric patients, it is felt that hypertension in anephric patients is unrelated to the renin-angiotensin system. Plasma concentration of potassium and aldosterone levels correlate directly in anephric patients.[59-61] In addition there may be ACTH unresponsiveness, and the aldosterone response to angiotensin II is either blunted or absent.

## Mechanisms of Post-Transplant Hypertension

Post-transplant hypertension is a common problem in children.[62-63] The hypertension may be either volume-mediated or renin-mediated (Table 23–1).[55] Volume-mediated hypertension is seen with volume expansion due to administration of salt, water, and colloid in the immediate postoperative period. Glucocorticoids induce a volume-mediated hypertension, and renal artery stenosis of the graft may produce volume-mediated hypertension after the stenosis has been present for a period of time.

### Table 23–1. POST-TRANSPLANT HYPERTENSION*

*Renin-Mediated*
1. Multiple kidneys present
2. Hypoperfusion
3. Transplant artery stenosis —— multiple kidneys
   —— single-early
4. Rejection episodes
   —acute
   —chronic
5. Recurrent nephritis
6. ? Residual pressor factors
7. ? Hydronephrosis with obstruction
8. ? Hypercalcemia

*Volume-Mediated*
1. Fluid overload
2. Steroid induced
3. Single kidney stenosis (late)

*Adapted from Ingelfinger.[55]

Renin-mediated hypertension occurs with the presence of multiple kidneys, with hypoperfusion of the graft, with renal artery stenosis, with recurrent nephritis, and with rejection episodes. It has also been hypothesized that residual pressor factors in the graft may cause transient renin-mediated hypertension postoperatively. Hydronephrosis and obstruction may be associated with relative hypoperfusion and renin-mediated hypertension. With acute pyelonephritis of the graft, hydronephrosis and hypoperfusion may lead to hypertension.

## CLINICAL ASPECTS OF PRESENTATION AND EVALUATION OF HYPERTENSIVE PATIENTS

### The Azotemic Patient[64-68]

Patients presenting de novo with hypertension may have renal insufficiency. It is of utmost importance to determine whether such patients have hypertension associated with acute renal failure, with chronic renal failure, or with renal failure due to accelerated hypertension. Because renal insufficiency in some patients may be reversible, the evaluation for a newly discovered hypertensive patient with renal insufficiency should simultaneously consider the causes of hypertension and renal insufficiency. In those patients presenting with both renal failure and hypertension, it is expedient to obtain a renal ultrasonogram to assess the size of the kidneys and a radionuclide renal scan in order to look at segmental perfusion. This approach avoids the need to administer the large volumes of contrast media which would be necessary for an IVP or infusion IVP. A flow diagram for evaluation of such a patient is shown in Figure 23–4.

Control of hypertension during the predialysis period in a patient with ESRD is significant in preventing future morbidity.[67] Control of the hypertension prevents complications, as well as halting or slowing the progression of the renal failure.[68]

Hypertension is frequently seen in patients with membranoproliferative glomerulonephritis, focal segmental glomerulonephritis, systemic lupus nephritis, and immune complex nephritis, as well as rapidly progressive nephritis.[66] Discovery of chronic renal failure with hypertension demands full evaluation of the etiology of the chronic renal failure.

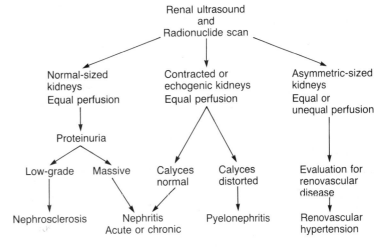

**Figure 23–4.** Suggested pathways for evaluating the hypertensive patient with renal insufficiency.

Diagnostic biopsy is helpful in assessing the underlying disease.

## Clinical Aspects of Hemodialysis Patients with Hypertension

Virtually all children on hemodialysis have periods of hypertension.[63, 69-70] Ultrafiltration to dry weight controls the blood pressure in more than 90% of patients. In children, however, ultrafiltration to dry weight often produces hypotension. Those patients whose blood pressure is not controlled by dialysis alone will require antihypertensive therapy. A minority of children undergoing dialysis will not have their blood pressure controlled with the currently available antihypertensives.

The major mechanism operative for blood pressure elevation in dialysis patients is volume expansion.[56, 71] Thus, ultrafiltration leading to a reduction of the intravascular volume will control the blood pressure. When ultrafiltration fails to control the blood pressure, patients should be evaluated for renin-dependent hypertension and other forms of hypertension.[72-74]

Peripheral plasma renin activity determinations should be evaluated in relationship to sodium intake. In adult patients with hypertension undergoing dialysis, the use of saralasin has been suggested to determine if the blood pressure elevation is renin-dependent.[73] If hypertension appears to be renin-dependent by the saralasin test, bilateral nephrectomy should control the hypertension. The use of saralasin in children is limited, and the predictability of the saralasin test in patients undergoing dialysis remains unclear.

Because vascular volume control is important in blood pressure regulation in hemodialysis patients, evaluation of the adequacy of dialysis therapy with persistent hypertension is important. Is the child really at dry weight? Additional fluid removal can be achieved by using a dialyzer with a larger surface area, by increasing the ultrafiltration pressure, or by substituting a more effective dialytic membrane. Monitoring interdialytic weight gain and assessing nutritional status is of paramount importance in managing the child with persistent hypertension despite dialysis.

Persistent hypertension despite apparent adequate dialysis mandates searching for additional factors, such as the use of drugs with pressor activity (for instance, ephedrine nose drops),[75] change in vessel calcium content,[76] or high output states due to a large vascular access.[77]

If a controllable cause of the persistent hypertension is not found, bilateral native nephrectomy or transplant nephrectomy should be considered.[77-81] Most postnephrectomy hypertension is volume-related.[80-82] The decision to undertake a nephrectomy should be weighed against the negative effects of the anephric state—loss of urine output, loss of erythropoietin, and loss of 1,25 DHCC production. After bilateral nephrectomy persistent hypertension may be due to changes in total peripheral resistance which cannot promptly reverse,[77-81] or due to vasoactive substance produced outside the kidney.[83-84]

Although virtually all children entering dialysis have some elevation in blood pressure for age and some instability of blood pressure while on hemodialysis, blood pressure control generally improves once the patient is well dialyzed (Fig. 23–5).

## Hypertension in Patients Undergoing Chronic Peritoneal Dialysis

At the initiating of continuous ambulatory peritoneal dialysis (CAPD), patients have just as much hypertension as do those initiating hemodialysis (Fig. 23–5). However, it has been reported that both children and adults on CAPD have far better blood pressure control than those on hemodialysis.[85-87] The reasons for this are unclear. Perhaps it is better fluid control, or less frequent fluid shifts.

In patients on chronic peritoneal dialysis, the blood pressure may drop or go up.[86] The content of the dialysis solutions may influence blood pressure shifts, e.g., the induction of hypernatremia may aggravate both hypertension and thirst (the latter leading to fluid intake).[86]

Hemodialysis has been stated to be superior to intermittent peritoneal dialysis for control of hypertension.[14] Recently, with the advent of CAPD, claims have been made that blood pressure control is better.[85-87] With adequate dialysis, it appears that *all* methods of dialysis can control hypertension in pediatric ESRD patients. On occasion, sequelae of ma-lignant hypertension precipitate the need to initiate dialytic care, e.g., intractable heart failure or sudden deterioration of renal function. Such patients initially require drug therapy despite dialysis.

## Hypertension after Transplantation

Sudden onset of acute hypertension may occur in various situations post-transplant: with rapid volume-loading,[55] with hypoperfusion of the graft, with release of pressor factors,[88] with acute rejection,[89] with stenosis of the renal artery, with large bolus steroid administration,[90-91] with hypercalcemia,[92] or rarely with pseudotumor cerebri.[55]

Hypertension in pediatric recipients is extremely common.[55, 93-104] Close to 100% of children are hypertensive during the initial post-transplant week. Late or sustained hypertension has been reported in 6 to 86% of pediatric recipients.[55, 93-104]

Colloid and intravenous electrolyte administration may lead to volume expansion, and hypertension, which is seen most commonly in the first few days following transplantation.[94, 95] This is generally transient, lasting 7 to 10 days and remits with diuresis. The

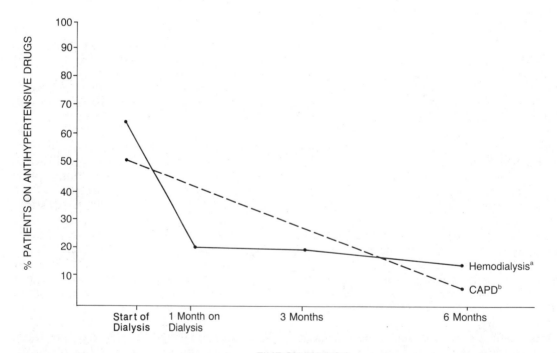

**Figure 23–5.** Percentage of dialytic patients requiring antihypertensive medications. Solid line is for hemodialysis patients; dashed, for CAPD patients. a = Patients at Children's Hospital Medical Center (N = 24); b = estimated from Salusky et al.[85] and Brem, personal communication (N = 30).

younger the patient, the more frequently this type of hypertension is seen.[65] In all ten patients under three years of age who received renal allografts from live-related donors at The Children's Hospital Medical Center, volume expansion resulted in elevations of blood pressure, which subsequently responded to diuresis.

Severe acute hypertension may be due to residual vasoactive factors in the graft. This concept has been promulgated by McDonald et al,[88] who noted that hypertension occurred following engraftment of a cadaver donor kidney from a donor with the hepatorenal syndrome. The authors postulated that high renin and renin substrate levels in the graft were present at the time of transplantation. The recipient, who was previously anephric and renin-sensitive, generated high levels of AI and AII following transplantation.[88] Since the half-life of renin is very short, this form of hypertension is transient. In a well-perfused kidney from a related donor this phenomenon is rarely, if ever, seen.

## Acute Rejection

Hypertension as a sign of acute rejection has been described since the early days of renal transplantation.[89] A direct relationship between elevated plasma renin activity and acute rejection has been noted. Following reversal of the acute rejection episode, plasma renin activity is reduced. It is frequently difficult to demonstrate this finding, since with severe acute rejection there is a decrease in renal perfusion and GFR, leading to salt and water retention, which blunts the renin response.

## Steroid-Related Hypertension

Hypertension decreases in pediatric recipients following conversion to alternate-day steroid dosage[104-107] (Fig. 23–6). Similar circumstantial evidence has been reported by Jacquot et al,[105] who found a decrease in mean arterial pressure in renal transplant recipients over time, coincident with decreases in steroid dosage. At the Children's Hospital Medical Center recipients who had neither rejection nor recurrent disease had lower blood pressure at six months than immediately post-transplant and lower at 12 months than at six months post-transplant, all coinciding with lower steroid doses compared to those with structural lesions. Children with nephritis had higher levels of blood pressure six months after transplant.[108] (Fig. 23–7).

Acute increases in blood pressure occur after high dose steroid administration for rejection, even though the blood pressure was relatively well controlled before steroid treatment was initiated. In assessing the development of hypertension the role of steroid administration and the role of rejection and vascular disease must be considered.

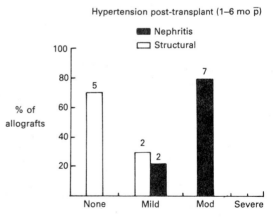

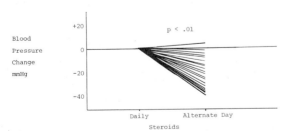

**Figure 23–6.** Drop in diastolic blood pressure in 74 patients who gradually were tapered from daily to alternate-day steroid therapy. (From Ingelfinger JR: Hypertension in children with kidney transplants. *In* Gruskin AB, and Norman ME (eds), Pediatric Nephrology. Proceedings of the Fifth International Pediatric Nephrology Symposium, Boston, Martinus Nijhoff, 1981.)

**Figure 23–7.** In patients without rejection or recurrent disease, blood pressure 1 to 6 months (mo) post (p̄) transplant is higher in those with a previous nephritis. Dark bars show nephritis patients; clear bars, those with a structural disease leading to ESRD. (From Ingelfinger J, Grupe WE, and Levey RH: Post-transplant hypertension in the absence of rejection or recurrent disease. Clin Nephrol, 15:236, 1981.)

## Hypercalcemia in Hypertension Post-Transplant

Calcium homeostasis contributes to the regulation of blood pressure via changes in peripheral vascular resistance, cardiac output, or both.[92, 109] Parathyroid hormone interacts with calcium leading to the release of renin and/or catecholamines. Following transplantation elevated serum calcium levels may occur, leading to acute hypertension. Treatment of the hypercalcemia will lower the blood pressure.

## Transplant Renal Artery Stenosis

Transplant renal artery stenosis is fairly common.[90-91, 110-121] It is caused by a variety of factors—surgical implantation problems, injury to the vessel during nephrectomy, perfusion injury and rejection.[110-121] A continuous suture line may produce a significant stenosis as the child grows, and thus, placing interrupted sutures in the transplanted artery is advantageous. Late stenosis may occur from adhesions around the anastomosis, causing extrinsic pressure. During rejection episodes there may be vascular deposition of immunoglobulin and complement with fibrin, causing an immune reaction which secondarily may lead to stenosis. The onset of renal artery stenosis may be insidious, though a rapid and sudden increase in blood pressure may result,[90-91] leading to symptomatic hypertension. The signs of renal artery stenosis may appear concomitantly, with rapid increases in creatinine mimicking acute rejection. Thus, this lesion should be considered whenever a rise in blood pressure occurs.

Renal arteriography has been advocated for the evaluation of possible graft renal artery stenosis.[55, 114] The presence of hypertension unresponsive to usual therapy with stable renal function or situations in which the distinction between rejection and renal artery stenosis is difficult are the usual indications.[114] Though the presence of a bruit often indicates renal artery stenosis, a lesion may occur without bruit, and bruit need not mean stenosis.[114, 122]

Currently, evaluation of a recipient for possible renal artery stenosis is less invasive. Doppler flow may make it possible to detect changes in arterial perfusion.[123] The development of venous digital subtraction angiography obviates the need for direct arterial injections to study the vasculature.[124-125]

Therapy of graft renal artery stenosis is focused on correction of the affected area, using either transluminal angioplasty[125-127] or surgical revascularization. Medical management should be reserved only for those patients in whom repair is not possible or has been unsuccessful.[55]

## Graft Hypoperfusion

Small children are often the recipients of an adult kidney. One obvious difference between the child and adult recipient is the increase in cardiac output which could be demanded by the graft. It has been hypothesized that a higher cardiac output and changes in peripheral vascular resistance might increase blood pressure.[128] Furthermore, large kidneys in small recipients would have a relatively lower blood flow following engraftment which would lead to high renin production and angiotensin generation, especially in the early post-transplant period.[128]

Increasing renal mass per se has been studied in dogs.[128] It has been shown that pup recipients of adult kidneys do not develop hypertension in DLA-matched beagles. Studies of cardiac output pre- and post-transplant in children at Children's Hospital Medical Center indicate that, at least initially, cardiac output changes do not account for blood pressure changes. Of ten patients studied with noninvasive echocardiography pre- and post-transplant, there was no significant increase in cardiac output, nor was there a correlation with post-transplant blood pressure fluctuations and increases in cardiac output (unpublished data).

## Chronic Rejection

The presence of chronic hypertension is directly related to the serum creatinine level in grafts which are functioning poorly.[129, 130] Small vessel lesions in the graft occur with chronic rejection and may lead to renin-mediated hypertension. Mean renal cortical blood flow in chronic rejection is decreased when studied with isotopic washout techniques (xenon-133 or chromium-85).[89, 131] Verniori et al[132] published a large study using blood samples in 75 consecutive patients in whom an inverse correlation was found between endogenous creatinine clearance and the log of the plasma renin concentration.

Others have found plasma renin activity to be elevated or normal in chronic rejection, but not all of these studies correlated the plasma renin activity with the sodium excretion.

In the first 150 transplants at The Children's Hospital Medical Center, we found a positive correlation between blood pressure level, renal function, serum creatinine level, and the number of hypotensive agents required to maintain blood pressure within the normal range for age.

## Multiple Kidneys in Post-Transplant Hypertension

In transplant recipients who have retained their native kidneys or who still have a previously failed renal allograft present, hypertension may be due to renin release from one or more of the old "nonfunctioning" kidneys.[133, 134] Linas et al demonstrated lateralization of renal vein renin to the old kidneys.[133] The authors also showed that saralasin infusion led to a fall in blood pressure in patients with multiple kidneys, whereas in those with a single kidney and hypertension the saralasin test was negative. It has been claimed that even without positive renal vein renin lateralization or a positive saralasin test the presence multiple kidneys contributes to hypertension, and many have advocated nephrectomy of those native kidneys or previously failed allografts if hypertension is a severe problem. Review of the Children's Hospital Medical Center series suggests that native kidney nephrectomy does not prevent post-transplant hypertension. Neither does it result in immediate control of hypertension. However, over time there appears to be some benefit of native nephrectomy in severe hypertension.[55, 110]

## Pyelonephritis, Hydronephritis, and Recurrent Nephropathy

When the original renal disease recurs in the graft, there is a frequent concomitant occurrence of hypertension.[55, 100, 109] Furthermore, patients with previous glomerulonephritis are often hypertensive; such individuals are likely to be hypertensive when they initiate dialysis and with recurrent disease in the graft all become hypertensive. Evaluation in this instance requires a search for recurrent disease as well as for other forms of post-transplant hypertension.

Acute pyelonephritis as well as transplant hydronephrosis are associated with post-transplant hypertension.[55]

## Demographic Features of Post-Transplant Hypertension in Children

Coinciding events often obscure the clinical presentation of post-transplant hypertension. The hypertension frequently is silent and the symptoms depend on the cause of the hypertension. It is important to remember that children with post-transplant hypertension may present with hypertensive crisis.

We have found a consistent association of post-transplant sustained hypertension with the original disease.[104, 108] Various nephritides account for close to half of our patients, and virtually all of them are hypertensive. In contrast, patients with renal dysplasia or obstructive uropathy are less likely to be hypertensive at the start of dialysis or post-transplant.[104, 108] General findings include the following:[55, 104, 108]

1. In the immediate post-transplant patient period most children develop hypertension.

2. Patients with stable function have less hypertension than those with chronic rejection. Recipients of cadaver donor kidneys (with more rejection problems) have more moderate to severe hypertension than those with live related donor grafts.

3. The most common etiology of post-transplant hypertension is rejection. Next is steroid-related hypertension. Recurrent nephropathy, renal artery stenosis, and other causes account for a minority of sustained episodes of hypertension. In our experience fewer than 10% of patients remain normotensive throughout their post-transplant course following the first postoperative week.

4. Patients with prior nephritides have more hypertension than all other groups.

5. Diurnal variation of blood pressure appears to be significantly altered in transplanted children. Whereas normal blood pressure tends to vary throughout the day, and the highest pressures are observed in the late afternoon or early evening, in children with renal transplants, blood pressure typically is most elevated in the middle of the night. This must be duly noted in treating patients for post-transplant hypertension.

## Evaluation of Patients with Post-Transplant Hypertension

During the first post-transplant days when most patients become hypertensive, it is important to carefully monitor colloid and fluid administration. Cardiovascular status, fluid intake, urinary output, and the central venous pressure must be checked. With hypertension, chest x-ray, electrocardiogram, and blood chemistries should be monitored. Based upon these parameters most hypertensive patients will be found to have volume expansion; their hypertension should respond to diuresis and fluid restriction. Occasional patients with hypovolemia may have vasoconstriction leading to hypertension, and some patients may have volume abnormalities in association with acute tubular necrosis. When the etiology of the hypertension is in doubt it is important to do a renal scan to verify the presence of adequate graft blood flow. If a major vascular problem is suspected, arteriography may be indicated.

Should a vascular abnormality be detected, surgical correction should be undertaken. In children who develop acute tubular necrosis, supportive measures (medication and dialysis) should be undertaken and hypertension managed medically.

Hypotension in the early days post-transplant may lead to acute renal failure. For this reason decreasing fluid administration and using diuretics are often more helpful than using potent antihypertensive therapy. Pain medication may also help to lower blood pressure. If the blood pressure becomes dangerously high, parenteral vasodilators, e.g., nitroprusside drip, diazoxide, or hydralazine, may be used.

The evaluation of hypertension developing after the early postoperative period is usually staged. The detection of hypertension necessitates evaluation for rejection. Whether or not screening studies are positive a renal scan should be done with marked hypertension; and, if rejection is discovered, it should be treated. Irrespective of findings with severe

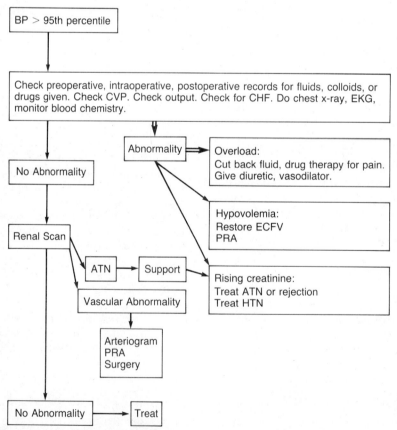

**Figure 23–8.** Evaluation of postoperative, post-transplant hypertension. CVP = central venous pressure; CHF = congestive heart failure; EKG = electrocardiogram; ATN = acute tubular necrosis; PRA = plasma renin activity; ECFV = extracellular fluid volume; HTN = hypertension.

hypertension, venous angiography or arteriography should be done along with selective renal vein renin determination if multiple kidneys are present. An approach to evaluating post-transplant hypertension is outlined in Figures 23–8 and 23–9.

## PHARMACOLOGIC TREATMENT OF HYPERTENSION IN ESRD[135–141]

Use of antihypertensive drugs in children with ESRD arises in several situations. In a hypertensive crisis, the drugs are used as in "normal" children. Several caveats must be observed: (1) metabolic half-lives of drugs may be prolonged; (2) children with precarious renal function may develop further acute reduction in renal function with rapid lowering of blood pressure, and (3) adjunctive diuretics may be largely ineffective. If control of the hypertensive crisis fails, dialysis may be utilized for blood pressure control.

Both diuretic and antihypertensive drugs may have altered effective half-lives and elimination with renal insufficiency. Diuretics in patients with renal failure are generally ineffective in inducing diuresis.[135–143] Of the diuretics most commonly used in children, furosemide is most effective. Furosemide may aid in moderating the fluid retention seen with various vasodilators. The dosage of diuretics in children with renal insufficiency is shown in Table 23–2. The changes in antihypertensive drug dosages in children with chronic renal failure are summarized in Table 23–3. Hypertension in children with chronic renal insufficiency may require multiple antihypertensive agents for control. The fewer the number of medications and the fewer the number of doses for control of hypertension, the better. In the absence of left ventricular dysfunction and/or bronchospasm, beta blockers are often very helpful. If renally excreted agents such as nadolol (Corgard) and atenolol (Tenormin) are being used, once-daily dosage or less may be acceptable.

Antihypertensive therapy of dialyzed patients present a special problem. Vasodilating agents may make dialysis technically difficult. The choice of antihypertensive agents for dialyzed children and adolescents is shown in Table 23–4. Note that vasodilators must be held on the morning of dialysis. Over time, an effort should be made to wean patients

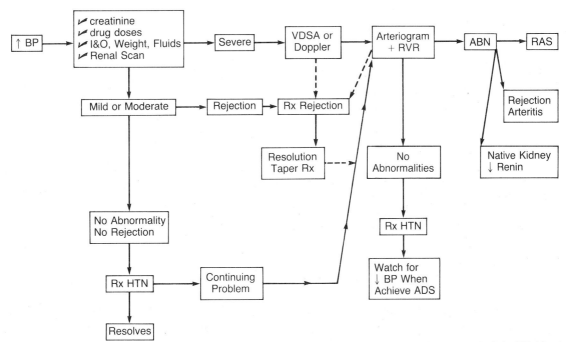

**Figure 23–9.** Management of hypertension after the immediate postoperative period. Abbreviations include: BP, blood pressure; I & O, intake and output; VDSA, venous digital subtraction angiography; RVR, renal vein renin; ABN, abnormality; RAS, renal artery stenosis; Rx, treat; HTN, hypertension; ADS, alternate-day steroids. Note that severe hypertension warrants full investigation. VDSA or Doppler flow studies may obviate the need for arteriography in severe hypertension. Modified from reference 55.

**Table 23–2. DIURETICS IN RENAL FAILURE***

| Drug | Oral Absorption | Protein Binding | Metabolism and Elimination | Half-Life (Hours) | | Dosage Change with Renal Failure |
|---|---|---|---|---|---|---|
| | | | | *Normal* | *Anephric* | |
| Acetazolamide | Well absorbed | 80% protein bound; distributed in 30% of body weight | Not metabolized; 90% excreted in urine within 24 hours | ? | ? | Not effective if GFR <30 ml/min |
| Ethacrynic acid | Well absorbed | Unknown | Some hepatic metabolism; renal excretion of unchanged drug and metabolites | ? | ? | No change required†; monitor hearing, renal function, and electrolytes |
| Furosemide | 50% absorbed | 90–95% protein-bound | 75% eliminated unchanged in urine | 1 | 2–14 | No change required†; monitor renal function and electrolytes |
| Mercurials | Poor | Unknown | Primarily renal elimination | 2–3 | 22–48 | Avoid repeated dose if GFR <25 ml/min because of nephrotoxic potential |
| Spironolactone | Well absorbed | 90% protein-bound | Extensive hepatic metabolism; renal excretion of active and inactive metabolites | 37 | ? | Not effective and may induce hyperkalemia if GFR <25 ml/min |
| Thiazides | 50–70% absorbed | 75% protein-bound | 75% excreted in urine | 12 | Increased | Not effective if GFR <25 ml/min |
| Triamterene | Well absorbed | 50% protein-bound | Extensive hepatic metabolism; renal excretion of small amount of unchanged drug and metabolites | 2 | ? | Not effective and may induce hyperkalemia if GFR <30 ml/min |

*Modified from Anderson RJ, et al: Fate of drugs in renal failure, *in* Brenner BM, Rector FC Jr, The Kidney, 2nd Edition. Philadelphia, WB Saunders, 1981, p 2694.

†The dosage changes with daggers were modified from the cited source.

**Table 23–3.** ANTIHYPERTENSIVE DRUGS IN RENAL FAILURE

| Drug | Metabolism/Elimination | Half-Life (Hours) | | Dosage Change in Renal Failure | Effect of Dialysis |
|------|------------------------|-------------------|---|-------------------------------|--------------------|
| | | *Normal* | *Anephric* | | |
| ***Vasodilators*** | | | | | |
| Diazoxide | Excretion of unchanged drug and metabolites by kidney | 20–36 | ↑ | Slight ↓ | Dialyzable |
| Hydralazine | Hepatic acetylation; renal excretion of metabolites | 3 | 16 | None ? | ? |
| Minoxidil | Mainly hepatic; renal excretion of 10% unchanged drug | 1–4 | 1–4 | None | ? Probably little |
| Nitroprusside | Renal excretion of thiocyanate | ? | ? | ↓ | Dialyzable Thiocyanate dialyzable |
| Prazosin | Mainly hepatic; <5% excreted renally | 9 | ? | Slight ↓ | ? Probably little |
| ***Central and Peripheral Inhibitors*** | | | | | |
| Reserpine | <1% in urine | 50–100 | ? | None | Not dialyzable |
| ***False Transmitter*** | | | | | |
| Methyldopa | Renal excretion of 60% of unchanged drugs plus metabolites | 2–4 | >4 | Slight ↓ | Dialyzable |
| ***B-Blockade*** | | | | | |
| Propranolol | Mainly hepatic; renal excretion of metabolites | 2–3 | 3–5 | None | Not well dialyzable |
| Metoprolol | Mainly hepatic; renal excretion of metabolites | 3–4 | ? | None | Not well dialyzable |
| Nadolol | Renal excretion | 14–24 | >24 | GFR 31–50 q 24–36h 10–30 q 24–48h <10 q 40–60h | Dialyzable |
| Atenolol | Renal excretion; largely unchanged | 6–9 | <24 | GFR 15–35 half dose <15 qod | Dialyzable |
| Timolol | Renal (~20%) | 3–4 | ↑ | Slight ↓ | Not well dialyzable |
| Pindolol | Primarily hepatic; also renal (40% unchanged) | 3–4 | slight ↑ | None | ? |
| ***Neuroeffector Blockade*** | | | | | |
| Guanethidine | Renal excretion of unchanged drug (50%) and metabolites | 120 | ? | Slight ↓ | Probably little |
| ***Central Alpha-Adrenergic Stimulation*** | | | | | |
| Clonidine | 60% renal excretion of metabolites | 10–14 | ? | None | Probably little |
| ***Converting Enzyme Inhibitor*** | | | | | |
| Captopril | Renal (40–50% unchanged) | 1–3 | ↑ | GFR 15–30 slight ↓ 5–15 half-dose <5 ¼-dose | Dialyzable |

**Table 23–4.** CHOICE OF ANTIHYPERTENSIVE AGENTS FOR CHILDREN ON DIALYSIS

| *Moderate Hypertension* | **Comments** |
|---|---|
| Beta blocker | (may give on dialysis day) |
| Hydralazine | (hold on AM of dialysis) |
| Methyldopa | (may give on dialysis day) |
| Clonidine | (beware of rebound) |
| *Severe Hypertension* | |
| Minoxidil | |
| Captopril | |
| Diazoxide | |
| Nitroprusside | |
| ? Verapamil | (not FDA approved for this indication) |
| *Limited Usefulness* | |
| Guanethidine | |
| *Useless* | |
| Diuretics | |

from the antihypertensive agents. In addition, the removal of agents during the dialysis must be considered (Table 23–3).

Beta blockade may be very helpful in the treatment of hypertension in children with ESRD[74, 136–144, 145] However, complete atrioventricular block has occurred in children.[146] Propranolol has been reported to have a normal half-life in uremia. However, recently massive retention of metabolites of propranolol have been reported in uremia,[147] and some of these are biologically active. Additional beta blockers are now available in the United States, however, their usefulness in dialysis patients remains to be evaluated. The half-lives of atenolol and nadolol are clearly prolonged,[135] and they perhaps can be given infrequently.

Methyldopa has been used in dialysis patients for some time.[140] It is dialyzable; however, the dosage may need to be adjusted in patients undergoing dialysis.[135] Post-ganglionic nerve ending blockers (e.g., guanethidine) may produce hypotension during dialysis.[141] Clonidine has been used for controlling hypertension in dialysis patients without causing hemodynamic instability.[137]

Severe hypertension in uremic children has been controlled with minoxidil.[148–149] The side effects of minoxidil are significant, making long-term therapy questionable, even if the alternative is nephrectomy.

The oral angiotensin-converting enzyme inhibitor, captopril, has been successfully used in patients with hemodialysis-resistant hypertension,[72, 150–152] even in anephric patients. Others drugs which have been helpful include oral prazosin and nitroprusside (with the help of intermittent dialysis of the toxic thiocyanate).[153–155] Calcium channel blockers such as verapamil have been used in Europe

to treat hypertensive crisis and chronic hypertension in children with ESRD.[14]

The experience in treating hypertension in ESRD patients has been largely uncontrolled; however, de Fremont et al[156] compared the effects of several antihypertensive drugs in an open cross-over trial. Using metoprolol, alpha methyldopa, and clonidine in a randomized sequential manner for six weeks each, the blood pressure was brought to normal range in the 13 subjects. The authors found that blood pressure could be controlled on all regimens. They suggest no reason for preferring one drug to another, unless there is cardiomegaly (contraindication to metoprolol) or increased susceptibility to hypotension (contraindication to alpha methyldopa). Differences were observed in metabolic risk factors (clonidine led to higher blood sugar, calcium and phosphate levels; metoprolol led to lowering of cholesterol), but these differences did not lead to long-term predictions, in view of the short-term nature of the study. Renin secretion was inhibited equally by each agent. Similar studies are needed using other drug regimens.

There is suggestive evidence that hypertension is a negative risk factor in the dialysis patient.[157–159] For example, in a recent report by Vincenti et al, 35% of patients under 30 years of age had atherosclerosis compared to zero % of non-uremic controls, and 90% of those with moderate or severe atherosclerosis were hypertensive.[158]

Treatment of post-transplant hypertension with drugs is necessary if blood pressure remains elevated.[55] With normal renal function, no special precautions concerning drug metabolism are needed. With hypertension and renal insufficiency in the graft recipient an adjustment in dosage may be necessary. Since steroid-related hypertension is to some extent volume-related, it is useful to use diuretic therapy and a vasodilator or beta blocker for treatment. With renin-mediated post-transplant hypertension, a beta blockade and/or the use of converting enzyme inhibitor are recommended. Vigilance for drug-drug interaction is important in this setting.

Because patients with ESRD are receiving multiple medications, it is important to enlist the help of the child and family in monitoring blood pressure. Such monitoring provides objective evidence for adequacy of blood pressure control. In addition to drug therapy, dietary control, exercise,[160] relaxation techniques, and biofeedback may be useful in the control of hypertension.

Hypertension in children with ESRD can be controlled in the majority of patients and undoubtedly reduces morbidity. Long-term studies in children remain to be done. Patients with hypertension tend to have concomitant problems with other organ systems. This makes the contribution of hypertension to morbidity and mortality in patients with ESRD difficult to assess. However, extrapolating information from other studies suggests that blood pressure control remains of utmost importance and will add to improved quality of life for these children.

## REFERENCES

1. Chau NP, Safar ME, Weiss YA, et al: Relationships between cardiac output, heart rate, and blood volume in essential hypertension. Clin Sci Mol Med 54:175, 1978.
2. London GM, Safer ME, Simon AC, et al: Total effective compliance, cardiac output and fluid volumes in essential hypertension. Circulation 57:995, 1978.
3. Weiss YA, Safar ME, London GM, et al: Repeat hemodynamic determinations in borderline hypertension. Am J Med 64:382, 1978.
4. Frohlich ED, Tarazi RC, Dustan HP: Re-examination of the hemodynamics of hypertension. Am J Med Sci 257:9, 1969.
5. Frohlich ED, Tarazi RC, Dustan HP: Hemodynamic and functional mechanisms in two renal hypertensions: Arterial and pyelonephritis. Am J Med Sci 261:189, 1971.
6. Cangiano JL, Ramirez-Muxo O, Ramirez-Gonzalez R, et al: Normal renin uremic hypertension. Study of cardiac hemodynamics, plasma volume, extracellular fluid volume, and the renin angiotensin system. Arch Intern Med 136:1723, 1976.
7. Brod J, Fencl V, Ulrych M: General and regional hemodynamics in hypertension in chronic renal disease. Clin Nephrol 5:1751, 1975.
8. Nitatpumin T, Yipintsoi T, Penpargkul S, et al: Increased cardiac contractility in acute uremia: Interrelationships with hypertension. Am J Physiol 229:501, 1975.
9. Onesti G: Dialysis and volume control. Postgrad Med 56:51, 1974.
10. Coleman TG, Neff MS: Hemodynamics of uremic anemia. Circulation 45:510, 1972.
11. Kim KE, Onesti G, Schwartz AB, et al: Hemodynamics of hypertension in chronic end-stage renal disease. Circulation 46:456, 1972.
12. Neff MS, Kim KE, Persoff M, et al: Hemodynamics of uremic anemia. Circulation 43:876, 1971.
13. Kim KE, Onesti G, Swartz CD: Hemodynamics of hypertension in uremia. Kidney Int 8:S155, 1975.
14. Scharer K, Rauh W, Ulmer HE: The management of hypertension in children with chronic renal failure. In: Giovanelli G, New MI, Gorini S, Hypertension in Children and Adolescents. New York, Raven Press, 1981, p 239.
15. Frohlich ED: Hemodynamics of hypertension. In: Genest J, Koiw E, Kuchel O (eds), Hypertension. New York, McGraw-Hill, 1977, p 18.
16. Kotchen TA, Rice TW, Walters DR: Renin activity in normal, hypertensive and uremic plasma. J Clin Endocrinol Metab 34:928, 1972.
17. Sambhi MP, Wiedemann CE: Renin activation in the venous plasma from the involved kidney in the patient with renal hypertension. J Clin Invest 51:22, 1972.
18. Blaufox MD, Goodman A, Weseley S, et al: The renin-angiotensin system in patients receiving hemodialysis. In Assaykeen TA (ed), Control of Renin Secretion. New York, Plenum Press, 1972, p 193.
19. Maebashi M, Miura Y, Yoshinaga K: Renin inhibitor in plasma of uraemic patients. Lancet 1:1146, 1968.
20. Lazarus JM, Lowrie EG, Hampers CL, et al: Cardiovascular disease in uremic patients on hemodialysis. Kidney Int 2(Suppl): 167, 1975.
21. Goldberger S, Thompson A, Guha A, et al: Autonomic nervous dysfunction in chronic renal failure. Clin Res 19:531, 1971.
22. Ewing DJ, Winney R: Autonomic function in patients with chronic renal failure on intermittent hemodialysis. Nephron 15:424, 1975.
23. Lilley JJ, Golden J, Stone RA: Adrenergic regulation of blood pressure in chronic renal failure. J Clin Invest 57:1190, 1976.
24. Campese VM, Romoff MS, Levitan D, et al: Mechanisms of autonomic nervous system dysfunction in uremia. Kidney Int 20:246, 1981.
25. Frye RL, Braunwald E: Studies on Starling's law of the heart. I. The circulatory response of acute hypervolemia and its modification by ganglionic blockade. J Clin Invest 39:1043, 1960.
26. Dustan HP, Tarazi RC, Bravo EL: Dependence of arterial pressure on intravascular volume in treated hypertensive patients. N Engl J Med 286:861, 1972.
27. Coleman TG, Bower JD, Langford HG, Guyton AC: Regulation of arterial pressure in the anephric state. Circulation 42:509, 1970.
28. Oparil S, Haber E: The renin-angiotensin system. N Engl J Med 291:389, 446, 1974.
29. Stein JH, Ferris TF; The physiology of renin. Arch Intern Med 131:860, 1973.
30. Davis JO: The control of renin release. Am J Med 55:333, 1973.
31. Semple PF, Boyd AS, Dawes PM, et al: Angiotensin II and its heptapeptide (2-8), hexapeptide (3-8) and pentapeptide (4-8) metabolites in arterial and venous blood of man. Circ Res 39:671, 1976.
32. Ingelfinger JR: The renin-angiotensin system and other hormonal systems in the control of blood pressure. In Ingelfinger JR, Pediatric Hypertension. Philadelphia, WB Saunders, 1982, p 45.
33. Weidmann P, Beretta-Piccoli, Steffen F, et al: Hypertension in terminal renal failure. Kidney Int 9:294, 1976.
34. Muirhead EE, Brown GB, Germain GS, et al: The renal medulla as an antihypertensive organ. J Lab Clin Med 76:641, 1970.
35. Lee JB, Gougoutas JZ, Takman BH, et al: Vasopressor and antihypertensive prostaglandins of PGE type with emphasis on the identification of medullin as PGE₂-217. J Clin Invest 45:1036, 1966.
36. Tobian L: A viewpoint concerning the enigma of hypertension. Am J Med 52:595, 1972.
37. Muirhead EE, Brooks B, Pitcock JA, et al: Renomedullary antihypertensive function in accelerated (malignant) hypertension. Observations on

renomedullary intersititial cells. J Clin Invest 51:181, 1972.

38. Liddle GW, Duncan LE, Jr, Bartter FC: Dual mechanisms regulating adrenocortical functions in man. Am J Med 21:380, 1956.

39. Laragh JH, Stoerk HC: A study of the mechanism of secretion of the sodium-retaining hormone (aldosterone). J Clin Invest 36:383, 1957.

40. Ganong WF, Biglieri EG, Mulrow PJ: Mechanisms regulating adrenocortical secretion of aldosterone and glucocorticoids. Recent Prog Horm Res 22:381, 1966.

41. Michelakis AM, Horton R: The relationship between plasma renin and aldosterone in normal man. Circ Res 26(Suppl 1):1, 1970.

42. Cope CL, Pearson J: Aldosterone secretion in renal failure. Clin Sci 25:331, 1963.

43. Gold EM, Kleeman CR, Ling S, et al: Sustained aldosterone secretion in chronic renal failure. Clin Res 13:135, 1965.

44. Wilkinson R, Luetscher JA, Dowdy AJ, et al: Studies on the mechanism of sodium excretion in uraemia. Clin Sci 42:711, 1972.

45. Fanestil DD: Mode of spironolactone action: Competitive inhibition of aldosterone binding to kidney mineralocorticoid receptors. Biochem Pharmacol 17:2240, 1968.

46. Thorn GW, Koepf GF, Clinton M Jr: Renal failure stimulating adrenocortical insufficiency. N Engl J Med 231:76, 1944.

47. Stanbury SW, Mahler RF: Salt-wasting renal disease. Metabolic observations on a patient with "salt-losing nephritis." Q J Med 28:425, 1959.

48. Walker WG, Jost LJ, Johnson JR, Kowarski A: Metabolic observations on salt wasting in a patient with renal disease. Am J Med 39:505, 1965.

49. Adler S: An extrarenal action of aldosterone on mammalian skeletal muscle. Am J Physiol 218:616, 1970.

50. Charron RC, Leme CE, Wilson DR, et al: The effect of adrenal steroids on stool composition as revealed by in vivo dialysis of faeces. Clin Sci 37:151, 1969.

51. Levitan R, Ingelfinger FJ: Effects of d-aldosterone on salt and water absorption from the intact human colon. J Clin Invest 44:801, 1965.

52. Alexander EA, Levinsky NG: An extrarenal mechanism of potassium adaptation. J Clin Invest 47:740, 1968.

53. Gerstein AR, Kleeman CR, Gold EM, et al: Aldosterone deficiency in chronic renal failure. Nephron 5:90, 1968.

54. Vagnucci AH: Selective aldosterone deficiency in chronic pyelonephritis. Nephron 7:524, 1970.

55. Ingelfinger JR: Hypertension in end-stage renal disease and renal transplantation. In: Ingelfinger JR, Pediatric Hypertension. Philadelphia, WB Saunders, 1982, p 252.

56. Onesti G, Kim E, Greco JA, et al: Blood pressure regulation in end-stage renal disease and anephric man. Circ Res 36(Suppl 1): 1, 1974.

57. Dustan HP, Page JA: Some factors in renal and renoprival hypertension. J Lab Clin Med 64:948, 1964.

58. Michelakis AM, Mizukoshi H: Distribution and disappearance rate of renin in man and dog. J Clin Endocrinol Metab 33:27, 1971.

59. Cooke CR, Ruiz-Maza F, Kowarski A, et al: Regulation of plasma aldosterone concentration in anephric man and renal transplant recipients. Kidney Int 3:160, 1973.

60. Weidmann P, Horton R, Maxwell MH, et al: Dynamic studies of aldosterone in anephric man. Kidney Int 4:289, 1973.

61. Williams GH, Bailey GL, Hampers CL, et al: Studies on the metabolism of aldosterone in chronic renal failure and anephric man. Kidney Int 4:280, 1973.

62. Ingelfinger JR, Lazarus JM, Levey RH, et al: Hypertension in pediatric renal transplant patients. Pediatr Res 9:376, 1976.

63. Loggie JMH, McEnery PJ: Hypertension in childhood and adolescence. In Rubin MI, Barratt TM, Pediatric Nephrology. Baltimore, Williams and Wilkins, 1975, p 433.

64. Perry HM, Jr.: Minoxidil and improvement of renal function in uremic malignant hypertension (editorial). Ann Intern Med 93:769, 1980.

65. Vincenti FG, Heymsfield S: Reversible malignant hypertension and azotemia due to urethral stricture. Arch Intern Med 137:370, 1977.

66. Ingelfinger JR: Renal parenchymal and structural causes of hypertension in childhood. In: Ingelfinger JR, Pediatric Hypertension. Philadelphia, WB Saunders, 1982, p 168.

67. Wing AJ: Diseases of the urinary system: Prospects for the treatment of renal diseases. Br Med J 2:881, 1977.

68. Adelman RD, Russo J: Malignant hypertension: Recovery of renal function after treatment with antihypertensive medications and hemodialysis. J Pediatr 98:766, 1981.

69. Ingelfinger JR, Harmon WE: Pediatric dialysis. In Press.

70. Schoeneman M: Dietary and pharmacologic treatment of chronic renal failure. In: Edelmann C (ed), Pediatric Kidney Disease. Vol I. Boston, Little, Brown and Co., 1978, p 475.

71. Fine RN, Korsch BM, Gruskin CM, et al: Hemodialysis in children. Am J Dis Child 119:495, 1970.

72. Vaughan ED, Carey RM, Ayers CR, et al: Hemodialysis-resistant hypertension: Control with an orally active inhibitor of angiotensin-converting enzyme. J Clin Endocrinol Metab 48:869, 1979.

73. Lifschitz MD, Kirschenbaum MA, Rosenblatt SG, et al: Effect of saralasin in hypertensive patients on chronic hemodialysis. Ann Intern Med 88:23, 1978.

74. Lindner A, Douglas SW, Adamson JW: Propranolol effects in long-term hemodialysis patients with renin-dependent hypertension. Ann Intern Med 88:457, 1978.

75. Messerli FH, Frohlich ED: High blood pressure—a side effect of drugs, poisons and foods. Arch Intern Med 139:682, 1979.

76. Ibels LS, Alfrey AC, Huffer WE, et al: Arterial calcification and pathology in uremic patients undergoing dialysis. Am J Med 66:790, 1979.

77. Haines JG, Sherrard DJ, Tremann JA: Nephrectomy for renovascular hypertension in azotemic patients. J Urol 114:828, 1975.

78. Lazarus JM, Hampers C, Merrill JP: Hypertension in chronic renal failure; treatment with hemodialysis and nephrectomy. Arch Intern Med 133:1059, 1974.

79. Schupak E, Urichek P, Merrill JP: The long-term maintenance of bilaterally nephrectomized man by periodic hemodialysis. Trans Am Soc Artif Intern Organs 9:24, 1963.

80. Onesti G, Swartz C, Ramirez O, et al: Bilateral nephrectomy for control of hypertension in ure-

mia. Trans Am Soc Artif Intern Organs 14:361, 1968.

81. Kolff WJ, Nakamoto S, Poutasse EF, et al: Effect of bilateral nephrectomy and kidney transplantation on hypertension in man. Circulation II (Suppl 2):23, 1964.

82. Wilkinson R, Scott DF, Uldall PR, et al: Plasma renin and exchangeable sodium in the hypertension of chronic renal failure. Q J Med 34:377, 1970.

83. McKenzie JK, Montgomerie JZ: Renin-like activity in the plasma of anephric men. Nature 223:1156, 1969.

84. Capelli JP, Wesson LG, Jr, Aponte GE, et al: Characterization and source of a renin-like enzyme in anephric humans. J Clin Endocrinol Metab 28:221, 1968.

85. Salusky IB, Lucullo L, Nelson P, et al: Continuous ambulatory peritoneal dialysis in children. Pediatr Clin North Am 29:1005, 1982.

86. Oreopoulos DG, Khanna R, Williams P, et al: Continuous ambulatory peritoneal dialysis— 1981. Nephron 30:293, 1982.

87. Gault MH, Ferguson EL, Sidhu JS, et al: Fluid and electrolyte complications of peritoneal dialysis. Ann Intern Med 75:253, 1971.

88. McDonald FD: Severe hypertension and elevated plasma renin activity following transplantation of "hepatorenal donor" kidneys into anephric recipients. Am J Med 54:39, 1973.

89. Bennett WM, McDonald WJ, Lawson RK: Post-transplant hypertension:, Studies of cortical blood flow and the renal pressor system. Kidney Int 6:99, 1974.

90. Schramek A, Better OS, Adler O, et al: Hypertensive crisis, erythrocytosis, and uraemia due to renal artery stenosis of kidney transplants. Lancet 1:70, 1975.

91. Simmons RL, Tallent MB, Kjellstrand CM, et al: Renal allograft rejection simulated by arterial stenosis. Surgery 68:800, 1970.

92. Weidmann P, Massry SG, Coburn JW, et al: Blood pressure effects of acute hypercalcemia: Studies in patients with chronic renal failure. Ann Intern Med 76:741, 1972.

93. Malekzadeh MH, Brennen LP, Payne VC, et al: Hypertension after renal transplantation in children. J Pediatr 86:370, 1975.

94. Gonzales LL, Martin L, West CD, et al: Renal homotransplantation in children. Arch Surg 101:232, 1970.

95. Najarian JS, Simmoni RL, Tallent MB, et al: Renal transplantation in infants and children. Ann Surg 174:583, 1971.

96. Williams GM, Lee HM, Hume DM: Renal transplants in children. Transplant Proc 1:262, 1969.

97. Fine RN, Korsch BM, Stiles Q, et al: Renal homotransplantation in children. J Pediatr 76:347, 1970.

98. LaPlante MP, Kaufman JJ, Goldman R, et al: Kidney transplantation in children. Pediatrics 46:665, 1970.

99. Belzer FO, Schweitzer RT, Holliday M, et al: Renal homotransplantation in children. Am J Surg 124:270, 1972.

100. Loggie JMH, McEnery PT: Hypertension in childhood and adolescence. In: Rubin MI, Barratt TM, Pediatric Nephrology. Baltimore, Williams and Wilkins, 1975, p 433.

101. Cerelli J, Evans WE, Sotos JF: Renal transplanta-

tion in infants and children. Transplant Proc 4:633, 1972.

102. Lilly JR, Giles G, Hurwitz R, et al: Renal homotransplantation in pediatric patients. Pediatrics 47:548, 1971.

103. Potter D, Belzer FO, Rames L, et al: The treatment of chronic uremia in childhood. I. Transplantation. Pediatrics 45:432, 1970.

104. Ingelfinger JR: Hypertension in children with kidney transplants. In: Gruskin AM, Norman ME, Pediatric Nephrology. Proceedings of the Fifth International Pediatric Nephrology Symposium, 1980. Boston, M Nijhoff, 1981, p 376.

105. Jacquot C, Idatte JM, Bedrossian J, et al: Long-term blood pressure changes in renal homotransplantation. Arch Intern Med 138:233, 1978.

106. Sampson D, Albert DJ: Alternate day therapy with methylprednisolone after renal transplantation. J Urol 109:345, 1973.

107. Sampson D, Kirdani RY, Sandberg AA: The aetiology of hypertension after renal transplantation in man. Br J Surg 61:819, 1973.

108. Ingelfinger JR, Grupe WE, Levey RH: Post-transplant hypertension in the absence of rejection or recurrent disease. Clin Nephrol 15:236, 1981.

109. Earll JM, Kurtzman NA, Moser RH: Hypercalcemia and hypertension. Ann Intern Med 64:378, 1966.

110. Pollini J, Guttmann RD, Beaudoin JG, et al: Late hypertension following renal allotransplantation. Clin Nephrol 11:202, 1979.

111. Lifschitz MD, Rios M, Radwin HM, et al: Renal failure with posttransplant renin-angiotensin mediated hypertension. Arch Intern Med 138:1409, 1978.

112. Collins GM, Johansen K, Bookstein J, et al: Transplant renal artery stenosis occurring in both recipients from a single donor. Arch Surg 113:767, 1978.

113. Potter DE, Schambelan M, Salvatierra O, et al: Treatment of high-renin hypertension with propranolol in children after renal transplantation. J Pediatr 90:307, 1977.

114. Beachly MC, Pierce JC, Boykin JV, et al: The angiographic evaluation of human renal allotransplants. Arch Surg 111:134, 1976.

115. Ernst CM, Daugherty ME, McRoberts JW, et al: Renal transplant arterial stenosis: Amelioration of hypertension and improvement of transplant function after revascularization. Am J Surg 42:319, 1976.

116. Smith RB, Cosimi AB, Lordon R, et al: Diagnosis and management of arterial stenosis causing hypertension after successful renal transplantation. J Urol 115:639, 1976.

117. Doyle TJ, McGregor WE, Fox PS, et al: Homotransplant renal artery stenosis. Surgery 77:53, 1975.

118. Lacombe M: Arterial stenosis complicating renal allotransplantation in man: A study of 38 cases. Ann Surg 181:283, 1975.

119. Lindsey ES, Garbus SB, Golladay ES, McDonald JC: Hypertension due to renal artery stenosis in transplanted kidneys. Ann Surg 181:604, 1975.

120. Margules RM, Belzer FO, Kountz SL: Surgical correction of renovascular hypertension following renal allotransplantation. Arch Surg 106:13, 1973.

121. Morris PJ, Yadav VS, Kincaid-Smith P, et al: Renal

artery stenosis in renal transplantation. Med J Aust 1:255, 1971.

122. Jachuck SM, Wilkinson R: Abdominal bruit after renal transplantation. Br Med J 3:202, 1972.

123. Greene ER, Venters MD, Avasthi PS, et al: Noninvasive characterization of renal artery blood flow. Kidney Int 20:523, 1981.

124. Mistretta CA, Kruger RA, Ergun DL, et al: Digital vascular imaging. Medicamundi 26:1, 1981.

125. Osborne RW, Goldstone J, Hillman BJ, et al: Digital video subtraction angiography: screening technique for renovascular hypertension. Surgery 90:932, 1981.

126. Barth KH, Brosilow SW, Kaufman SL: Percutaneous transluminal angioplasty of homograft renal artery stenosis in a 10-year-old girl. Pediatrics 67:675, 1981.

127. Diamond NG, Casarella WJ, Hardy MA, et al: Dilatation of critical transplant renal artery stenosis by percutaneous transluminal angioplasty. Am J Radiol 133:1167, 1979.

128. Ingelfinger JR, Caldicott WJH: Cardiovascular function in pups receiving allografts from adult dogs. Pediatr Res 15:935, 1981.

129. Rao TKS, Grupta SK, Butt KMH, et al: Relationship of renal transplantation to hypertension in end-stage renal failure. Arch Intern Med 138:1236, 1978.

130. Bachy, Van Ypersele de Strihou, Alexandre GPJ, et al: Hypertension after renal transplantation. Proc Eur Dial Transplant Assoc 12:461, 1976.

131. Grunfeld JP, Kleinknecht D, Moreau JF, et al: Permanent hypertension after renal homotransplantation in man. Clin Sci 48:391, 1975.

132. Verniory A, Potvliege P, VanGeertruyden JJ, et al: Renin and control of arterial blood pressure during terminal renal failure treated by hemodialysis and by transplantation. Clin Sci 42:685, 1972.

133. Linas SL, Miller PD, McDonald KM, et al: Role of the renin-angiotensin system in post-transplantation hypertension in patients with multiple kidneys. N Engl J Med 298:1440, 1978.

134. Zawada ET, Maxwell MH, Marks LS, et al: The diagnostic and therapeutic uses of saralasin in renal transplant hypertension. J Urol 123:148, 1980.

135. Anderson RJ, Bennett WM, Gambertoglio JG, et al: Fate of drugs in renal failure. *In* Brenner BM, Rector FC Jr, The Kidney, 2nd edition. Philadelphia, WB Saunders, 1981, p 2659ff.

136. Mirkin BL, Green TP, O'Dea RF: Disposition and pharmacodynamics of diuretics and antihypertensive agents in renal disease. Eur J Clin Pharm 18:109, 1980.

137. Mauer SM: Pediatric renal dialysis. *In*: Edelmann CM (ed.), Pediatric Kidney Disease. Boston, Little Brown, 1978, p 487.

138. Mitus JA 2nd, O'Connor DT, Stone RA: Hypertension in renal insufficiency: A major therapeutic problem. Postgrad Med 64:113, 1978.

139. Swartz CD, Kim KE: Management of hypertension in the patient with chronic renal disease. Cardiovasc Clin 9:263, 1978.

140. Onesti G: Management and treatment of hypertension secondary to acute and chronic renal disease. *In*: Genest J, Koiw E, Kuchel O, Hypertension. New York, McGraw-Hill, 1977, p 1118.

141. Curtis JR, Williams GB: Clinical management of chronic renal failure. Oxford, Blackwell Scientific Publications, 1975, pp 84–89, 151–153.

142. Mroczek WJ, Moir D, Davidov ME, et al: Sodium intake and furosemide administration in hypertensive patients with renal insufficiency. Am J Cardiol 39:808, 1977.

143. Rose HJ, O'Malley K, Pruitt AW: Depression of renal clearance of furosemide in man by azotemia. Clin Pharmacol Ther 21:141, 1977.

144. Maggiore Q, Biagini M, Zoccali C, et al: Long-term propranolol treatment of resistant arterial hypertension in haemodialysed patients. Clin Sci Mol Med 48(Suppl)2:73s, 1975.

145. Smith EC, Dhar SK, Freedman P: Propranolol in the management of hypertension in a long-term dialysis program. JAMA 229:1777, 1974.

146. Zeis PM, Thanopoulos B, Pierroutsakos IN, et al: Complete atrioventricular block associated with propranolol therapy. J Pediatr 98:326, 1981.

147. Stone WJ, Walle T: Massive propranolol metabolite retention during maintenance hemodialysis. Clin Pharmacol Ther 28:449, 1980.

148. Perry HM, Jr: Minoxidil and improvement of renal function in uremic malignant hypertension. Ann Intern Med 93:769, 1980.

149. Pettinger WA, Mitchell HC: Minoxidil—an alternative to nephrectomy for refractory hypertension. N Engl J Med 289:167, 1973.

150. Onoyama K, Hirakata H, Iseki K, et al: Blood concentration and urinary excretion of captopril (SQ14,225) in patients with chronic renal failure. HTN 3:456, 1981.

151. Warren SE, O'Connor DT: Hyperkalemia resulting from captopril administration. JAMA 244:2551, 1980.

152. Man In't, Veld AJ, Schect IM, et al: Effects of an angiotensin-converting enzyme inhibitor (captopril) on blood pressure in anephric subjects. Br Med J 1:288, 1980.

153. Harter HR, Delmez JA: Effects of prazosin in the control of blood pressure in hypertensive dialysis patients. J Cardiovasc Pharmacol 1:543, 1979.

154. Elberg AJ, Gorman HM, Baker R, et al: Prolonged nitroprusside and intermittent hemodialysis as therapy for intractable hypertension. Am J Dis Child 132:988, 1978.

155. Gordillo-Paniagua G, Velasquez-Jones L, Martini R, et al: Sodium nitroprusside treatment of severe arterial hypertension. J Pediatr 87:799, 1975.

156. de Fremont JF, Coevoet B, Andrejak M, et al: Effects of antihypertensive drugs on dialysis-resistant hypertension, plasma renin, and dopamine beta-hydroxylase activities, metabolic risk factors and calcium-phosphate homeostasis: Comparison of metoprolol, alphamethyldopa and clonidine in a cross-over trial. Clin Nephrol 12:198, 1979.

157. Ikaheimo M, Huttunen K, Kakkunen J: Cardiac effects of chronic renal failure and hemodialysis treatment. Hypertensive versus normotensive patients. Br Heart J 45:710, 1981.

158. Vincenti F, Ament WJ, Abele J, et al: The role of hypertension in hemodialysis-associated atherosclerosis. Am J Med 68:363, 1980.

159. Lindner A, Charra B, Sherrard DJ, et al: Accelerated atherosclerosis in prolonged maintenance hemodialysis. N Engl J Med 290:697, 1974.

160. Goldberg AP, Hagberg J, Delmez JA, et al: The metabolic and psychological effects of exercise training in hemodialysis patients. Am J Clin Nutr 33:1620, 1980.

# 24

# Cardiovascular Abnormalities in Pediatric Patients with ESRD

*Sean O'Regan, M.B., Bch., F.R.C.P. (C)*

Cardiovascular complications are important determinants of the long-term survival of children with chronic renal failure.[1] Renal failure is associated with severe anemia, electrolyte, acid-base, and humoral abnormalities, and alterations in intravascular volume, all of which may adversely influence cardiac performance. Chronic pressure load due to hypertension as well as possible impairment of myocardial metabolism due to chronic exposure to uremic toxins has adverse effects on myocardial function in uremia. In addition, the therapeutic necessity of arteriovenous fistula construction required for hemodialysis as well as the hemodialysis procedure itself alters cardiovascular hemodynamics. These various factors may contribute to functional derangements, which may be manifested by latent or overt cardiac failure in both children and adults. Because of the multiplicity of elements that potentially influence cardiac performance in ESRD, attempts have been made to define the cardiodepressant potential of each individual factor. In addition, the hemodynamic effects of construction of vascular access, bilateral nephrectomy, hemodialysis, hemofiltration, and renal transplantation have also been studied.

A pediatric patient with ESRD provides an opportunity for study of cardiac performance that is uninfluenced by factors that might adversely alter cardiac performance, such as arteriosclerosis, smoking, and diabetes, which are present in adult patients. However, limited studies have been undertaken on effects of chronic renal failure on cardiovascular hemodynamics in pediatric patients.

Thus an analysis of data on adults is required to adequately assess the effects of ESRD on the cardiovascular system

## MYOCARDIAL FUNCTION IN CHRONIC RENAL FAILURE AND ESRD

A limited number of studies have evaluated cardiac function in children with chronic renal failure. These studies have utilized mechanocardiography and echocardiography to study left ventricular function in pediatric patients with renal disease of varying etiology and severity. The study of systolic time intervals provides a sensitive and noninvasive approach to assessment of left ventricular dysfunction.[2] The basic systolic time intervals measured are the following:

1. The pre-ejection period (PEP), which is measured from the onset of electrical ventricular depolarization to the beginning of mechanical ventricular ejection.

2. The left ventricular ejection time (LVET), which is the phase of systole during which the left ventricle ejects into the aorta.

3. The total electromechanical systole ($QS_2$), the time interval comprising the period of systole from the onset of the $QS_2$ complex on the EKG to the closure of the aortic valve as measured by the second heart sound.

With the progressive deterioration of left ventricular function, PEP increases, left ventricular ejection time shortens, and the total electromechanical systole remains unchanged. The determination of the

PEP/LVET ratio is found to correlate very well with angiographic measurements of ejection fraction. Echocardiography provides measurements of cardiac chamber size and, in addition, allows for the noninvasive measurement of cardiac output, cardiac index, peripheral vascular resistance, and parameters of contractility, such as shortening fraction (SF) and mean velocity of circumferential fiber shortening (MVCF). Limited angiographic investigations have been performed in children with chronic renal failure.[3]

Children with chronic renal failure have elevated cardiothoracic ratios by chest x-ray, and this is attributable mainly to a physiologic adaptation to an increased stroke volume and is not a reflection of pathologic cardiac dilatation. A uniform pattern of decreased left ventricular performance, which is most marked during the period of hemodialysis,[4] occurs in children with chronic renal failure. When systolic time intervals were compared with calculated normal standards in children with chronic renal failure, the pre-ejection period was found to be significantly prolonged, the ejection time was significantly shortened, and the PEP/LVET ratio was markedly increased, suggesting the presence of latent, clinically undetectable depression of left ventricular function.[4] A study on 20 pediatric patients with chronic renal failure demonstrated that in the majority of patients the systolic time intervals, i.e., PEP, LVET, the PEP/LVET ratio, were within the 95% confidence limits established for a normal control population. Parameters of contractility such as mean velocity of circumferential fiber shortening (MVCF) as well as shortening fraction (SF) were within normal established ranges.[5] However, it was noted that those patients with more severe degrees of renal failure had increased PEP intervals and PEP/LVET ratios, suggesting diminished left ventricular performance.

The presence of depressed left ventricular function in adults with chronic renal failure has also been inferred by studies of systolic time intervals.[6-9] In contrast, others have reported that normal or near normal cardiac performance is maintained in adult patients in the predialytic period.[10, 11] The preponderance of evidence suggests that children and adults, especially those on chronic hemodialysis, have varying degrees of depression of left ventricular performance and contractility.

Various echocardiographic abnormalities have been described in adult patients with chronic renal failure. These include right and left ventricular dilatation, concentric left ventricular hypertrophy, asymmetric hypertrophy of the interventricular septum, and frank cardiomyopathic patterns. Blanchard et al retrospectively studied the echocardiograms of 52 pediatric patients and divided the observed patterns into three groups. Group 1 patients had a normal echocardiogram or evidence of right ventricular dilatation; group 2 patients had echocardiograms that demonstrated concentric left ventricular hypertrophy manifested by symmetric thickening of both the interventricular septum and the posterior wall of the left ventricle with normal or decreased left ventricular dimensions measured in diastole; group 3 patients had left ventricular dilatation with commonly decreased excursion of the interventricular septum and decreased shortening fraction of the left ventricle.[12] The authors defined a cardiomyopathic pattern as a combination of left ventricular dilatation associated with decreased shortening fraction. Group 1 patients, with normal or near normal echocardiograms had the shortest mean duration on dialysis and the lowest systolic and diastolic blood pressures and a lower incidence of glomerulonephritis. Patients in group 2 had the smallest left ventricular size and tended to have a greater incidence of diastolic hypertension than the patients in group 1. Group 3 patients had the longest time on dialysis and the highest incidence of glomerulonephritis. These patients did not appear to have left ventricular dilatation or depression of contractility secondary to beta blockade.

Schott et al described three distinct echocardiographic patterns of left ventricular function and dimension in adult patients with chronic renal failure:[13] (1) hyperkinetic heart characterized by normal left ventricular size and increased excursion of the intraventricular septum and left ventricular posterior wall; (2) left ventricular dilatation with a left ventricular internal dimension in diastole equal to or greater than 5.5 cm, but with normal or hyperkinetic motion of the interventricular septum and left ventricular posterior wall; (3) a cardiomyopathic pattern with reduced excursion of the interventricular septum and left ventricular posterior wall associated with left ventricular dilatation and decreased shortening fraction of the left ventricle. A similar pattern of depression of left ventricular contractility was observed by DeCruz et al.[14]

Asymmetric septal hypertrophy observed both in adult[11, 14-16] and pediatric patients[5] with ESRD appears to be common and associated in the majority of patients with poorly controlled hypertension.

EKG changes are rarely observed in pediatric patients with ESRD and when they occur are most commonly observed in patients with arterial hypertension. The majority of EKG abnormalities noted by Ulmer et al were observed in patients on hemodialysis.[4] The authors attributed the rarity of EKG abnormalities in the predialytic stage to the fact that hyperkalemia was treated much earlier. In addition, the authors felt that the incidence of arrhythmias was reduced by a more restrictive use of digitalis glycosides.

Arrhythmias have been observed during hemodialysis and have been attributed to hypokalemia and the presence of preexisting ischemic heart disease in adult patients.[17, 18] The reported incidence has ranged from 9% to 40%, the lower incidence being associated with a dialysate potassium concentration of 3 mEq/L.[18] Atrial and ventricular arrhythmias occurred in patients dialyzed with a dialysate potassium concentration of <2 mEq/L.[19] Other EKG abnormalities in patients with ESRD are usually due to effects of electrolyte imbalance[20] or hypertension.[19]

In uremic patients abnormal vagal function as indicated by an absence of appropriate bradycardia in response to the Valsalva maneuver has suggested the presence of an autonomic neuropathy.[21, 22] The normal response of an increased blood pressure and pulse pressure to bradycardia is absent or depressed in uremic patients, similar to that observed in patients with cardiac failure[23] and suggests dysfunction of the autonomic system in uremia.[24, 25] In addition, depression of baroreflex sensitivity as indicated by a reduced slowing of the pulse induced by a rise in arterial pressure following intravenous administration of pressor drugs has been described in hemodialysis patients.[26] Heart rate variation as measured by continuous monitoring by electrocardiography is also decreased compared to normal.[27] Therefore, substantial evidence exists that autonomic reflexes involving cardiac rate are abnormal in patients with chronic renal failure.

Ulmer et al in their studies of children with ESRD noted that one of the most striking cardiovascular findings was the presence of heart murmurs.[4] A common observation was a holosystolic diamond-shaped murmur best heard along the left sternal border or in the aortic region, which the authors attributed to a functional aortic stenosis. These murmurs were preceded by an early systolic ejection click originating from a dilated aortic root. Other murmurs attributed to functional stenosis of the aortic or mitral valves were also noted. In addition, transitory diastolic murmurs suggesting the presence of aortic valvular incompetence, which were similar to those observed in adult patients, were noted.[28-32] Both the adult and pediatric patients were severely anemic, overhydrated, and hypertensive.[4, 28] The diastolic murmurs resolved promptly with fluid removal and aggressive antihypertensive therapy. In adult patients with signs of aortic incompetence the aortic ostium has previously been found to be normal at autopsy even if previous angiographic findings have indicated overt aortic insufficiency.[28]

Although adult patients with severe uremia have been described with normal cardiac performance,[33] both adult[34-37] and pediatric patients[5, 38] with severe uremia have presented with a uremic cardiomyopathy. Four children with severe uremia had marked abnormalities of systolic time intervals, suggesting depression of left ventricular function.[5] In addition, parameters of contractility such as mean velocity of circumferential fiber shortening and shortening fraction were markedly depressed in association with severe left ventricular dilatation. Adult patients have been observed with a uremic cardiomyopathy[34-37] and depression of contractility and cardiac dilatation.[13, 14] However, despite these descriptions, controversy exists concerning the presence of a true uremic cardiomyopathy.[39, 40] Because of the multifactorial origin of heart disease in uremia, the term "uremic heart disease," as suggested by Ulmer et al,[4] is perhaps more appropriate.

Although numerous factors capable of altering cardiac function are present in uremia, the individual contribution of each potential cardiodepressant element is unknown. A significant negative correlation has been observed between cardiac index and hemoglobin level,[5] and hemoglobin level and systolic time intervals[38] in pediatric patients. These findings indicate that the anemia, which is more severe in pediatric than in adult patients,[41] is a major cause of the increased cardiac output and hyperkinetic circulation in chronic renal failure.[42-45] Ono studied the exercise capacity of children with chronic renal failure and noted that there was a significant correlation between heart rate and hemoglobin.[46] Studies in adult patients have substantiated the role of anemia in causing an augmented cardiac index in patients with ESRD.

Anemia is associated with a reduced capacity for oxygen transport, which necessitates compensatory adjustments of the cardiac output and pulmonary ventilation.[47-49] There is also a shift to the left of the hemoglobin dissociation curve and a rise in red cell 2,3-diphosphoglycerate. Duke and Abelman found that anemic patients with normal renal function have an increased cardiac index and decreased peripheral resistance, similar to that observed in anemic uremic patients.[50] However, owing to the complex metabolic abnormalities in patients with ESRD, it is difficult to determine the exact contribution of the anemia to alterations in cardiac performance. An improvement in physical working capacity after correction of the anemia was observed in 6 of 10 patients with ESRD studied by Sill et al.[51] Similarly, when patients undergoing hemodialysis were transfused to achieve a hematocrit of 30 or higher, the cardiac index decreased to normal while peripheral resistance increased.[52, 53] Kim et al suggested that the most likely explanation for the increased blood pressure in response to transfusion is related to the fact that severe anemia is associated with reduced oxygen delivery to the tissues, resulting in peripheral vasodilation.[53] Correcting the anemia abolishes hypoxic vasodilatation and increases arteriolar resistance and blood pressure. Increased myocardial oxygen consumption and cardiac work is present in chronic renal failure.[54] Increased myocardial mass and consequent myocardial oxygen demand may not be met as a result of the anemia in uremic patients. Thus anemia contributes to the depression of cardiac performance in uremic patients.

Schiffrin et al investigated the role of anemia in 10 patients with chronic renal failure who had no prior history of heart disease.[55] Systolic time intervals were studied prior to and after plasmapheresis, which consisted of the injection of packed cells and simultaneous extraction of a similar volume of blood. Systolic time intervals were abnormal in nine patients prior to transfusion. An increase in mean hematocrit from 15 to 25% was associated with a decrease in pre-ejection period without alteration in the left ventricular ejection time. This resulted in a decrease in the PEP/LVET ratio, thus suggesting that anemia is a significant contributing factor to depression of left ventricular function in ESRD. In addition, Todesco et al noted a high diastolic pressure/isometric contraction ratio in anemic uremic patients.[56]

Numerous studies in adult patients (utilizing systolic time intervals) have substantiated the possibility that progression of chronic renal failure is associated with left ventricular dysfunction, which may be correlated significantly with the plasma creatinine concentration as an indicator of severity of renal disease.[6] Depression of left ventricular performance has also been attributed to the presence of arterial hypertension.[6, 57, 58] Accelerated atherosclerosis,[59] though its presence has been disputed,[60] has been attributed to concomitant hypertension.[61]

Humoral factors have been suggested as contributive factors in depressing cardiac performance. Intracellular as well as extracellular metabolic and electrolyte abnormalities are observed with secondary hyperparathyroidism.[62] Myocardial high energy phosphate and calcium ion concentrations are major factors determining the contractile performance of the myocardial fiber.[63] Synthetic parathormone administration decreased the stimulatory effects of isoproterenol on myocardial contractility of isolated guinea pig auricles.[64] Secondary hyperparathyroidism may cause areas of cardiac necrosis in uremic animals.[65] Drüeke et al, using radionuclide angiocardiography and echocardiography, evaluated 22 patients with secondary hyperparathyroidism on chronic hemodialysis prior to and two weeks after parathyroidectomy.[66] An improvement in left ventricular function resulted in an increased shortening fraction, an increased cardiac index, and an increased mean velocity of circumferential fiber shortening. Other studies have also implicated altered calcium metabolism in cardiac complications of renal disease.[67, 68] Severe disturbances in calcium/phosphate homeostasis have resulted in cardiac calcification in uremia.[69, 70]

Raab et al considered increased circulating catecholamines to be an important cardiotoxic factor in clinical and experimental uremia.[71] Clinical and experimental evidence suggests that elevated circulating catecholamines may cause lesions in a healthy myocardium.[72, 73] Catecholamine levels are increased in chronic renal failure.[74, 75] In assessing left ventricular function in stable chronic hemodialysis patients, Miach et al were unable to attribute myocardial impairment to hypertension or ischemic heart disease; however, they noted a significant negative correlation between shortening fraction and plasma catecholamine levels. The authors suggested that chronic exposure to elevated plasma catecholamine levels might contribute to the observed decreased myocardial contractility.[76]

Other potential cardiodepressant factors in chronic renal failure are hyperkalemia and acidosis. Acidosis may depress cardiac contractility,[77] especially in the presence of beta blockers such as propranolol.[78] Similarly, hyperkalemia has a negative inotropic effect, which is more profound in the presence of pre-existing cardiac disease.[79] Beriberi-associated cardiac failure has been reported in one chronic hemodialysis patient,[80] related to the loss of vitamin $B_1$ during hemodialysis.

Trznadel et al have demonstrated an improvement in left ventricular function after digoxin administration in patients with chronic renal failure,[8] although no clinical signs of congestive cardiac failure were evident prior to digoxin therapy. Pre-ejection periods and PEP/LVET ratios were greater and left ventricular ejection times were shorter than those of normal individuals in the study. Digoxin administration resulted in a reduction in $QS_2$, PEP, and PEP/LVET ratios. This study suggested that the use of digitalis preparations in patients with renal failure despite the absence of clinical signs of heart failure was advantageous. Other investigators, however, have found the response to digitalis glycosides to be clinically satisfactory in only a few cases.[81] In addition, the difficulties in adequately controlling serum levels of digoxin preparations in chronic renal failure, and the associated increase in cardiac arrhythmias discourage its use in all but those individuals with overt cardiac failure.

A limited number of studies have been performed in animals to determine the influence of uremic toxins on left ventricular performance in uremia. Indeed, some experimental evidence suggests that hearts of acutely uremic animals may actually have augmented cardiac contractility.[82] Raab added human uremic sera to isolated frog hearts and observed a decrease in the amplitude of contraction.[83] Penpargkul and Scheuer studied hearts isolated from rats 24 hours after bilateral nephrectomy. They perfused the hearts with solutions free of nitrogenous compounds and observed normal or augmented cardiac function.[82]

In dogs, a two-week period of uremia results in the depression of parameters of left ventricular performance, which is reversible by dialysis. This suggests that uremia per se is associated with deterioration in cardiac function.[84]

Acquatella et al[85] suggested that guanidosuccinic acid was a cardiotoxin in uremia by its depressant effect on contractility in healthy dogs. However, this was not confirmed by further studies[86] or by using isolated guinea pig hearts.[87] Urea in high concentration decreased oxygen consumption in isolated guinea pig hearts.[87, 88] The effects of urea in depressing cardiac contractility by altering $O_2$ uptake and carbohydrate metabolism have also been confirmed in perfusion of isolated rat hearts.[89, 90] The modification, by a specific middle molecule fraction isolated from ultrafiltrates of uremic patients, of cardiac rhythm of chick hearts has recently been described by Bernard et al.[91]

In summary, accumulated evidence indicates that progressive deterioration in left ventricular performance occurs with progression of renal failure. Both clinical and experimental studies indicate that anemia, electrolyte and acid-base abnormalities, hypertension, humoral factors, and accumulation of uremic compounds all appear to contribute to depression of myocardial performance.

## CARDIOVASCULAR ABNORMALITIES ASSOCIATED WITH ARTERIOVENOUS COMMUNICATIONS

The construction of an arteriovenous communication with a sufficient blood flow rate to allow for a vascular access for hemodialysis may have dramatic effects on cardiovascular hemodynamics in anemic uremic patients. Great variations in blood flow rates of the vascular access have been observed in adult patients. Blood flow has been measured using manometric methods,[92] electromagnetic flow meters,[93, 94] plethysmographic methods,[95] and dye dilution and radiotracer methods.[96-98]

Blood flow through the vascular access has been assessed by measurement of cardiac output prior to and after acute occlusion of the shunt or the arteriovenous fistula.[99-103] The accuracy of determination of fistula flow by differences in cardiac output has been questioned; however, a significant correlation may be obtained between direct measurement of fistula flow and that obtained by difference in cardiac output associated with fistula occlusion.[97, 98] Wide variability is observed between actual measurement and extrapolated measurements.[104] Indeed, cardiac index alterations may provide a more accurate determination than that obtained by cardiac output studies.[97]

Dilutional and other methods of measurement have determined that flow rates are in the range of 300 to 850 ml/min. Higher flow rates have also been measured in patients using dilutional isotope flow methods and have been successfully used to select patients who might appropriately require procedures such as banding to treat or prevent cardiac decompensation due to high fistula flow.[105] Also the hemodynamic response to fistula compression can be used for this purpose.[106] Though isolated cases of congestive cardiac failure due to high flow rates have been reported in adult patients,[107-112] the high fistula flow rates appear in general to be well tolerated.[113, 114]

Arteriovenous communications with adequate flow rates for hemodialysis may be successfully constructed in a majority of children weighing less than 20 kg.[115] Fistula flow rates in pediatric patients are similar to those observed in adult patients[116]; however, cardiac failure attributable to the vascular access has been reported in only one pediatric patient.[3] The rarity of cardiac decompensation due to arteriovenous communications in children may reflect the lack of age-related ischemic heart disease commonly observed in adult patients. In studies on the direct effects of fistulae on cardiac function and hemodynamics, most authors have utilized fistula compression. Changes in cardiac hemodynamics are observed. The main features are a decrease in heart rate and cardiac output associated with an increase in peripheral resistance.[117, 118] However, in one group of children with ESRD studied by echocardiography prior to and after maturation of the Brescia-Cimino fistula, changes in indices of cardiac contractility, i.e., ejection fraction and velocity of circumferential fiber shortening, suggested that deterioration of myocardial

performance occurred following construction of the arteriovenous communication.[119] Similarly, physical working capacity in children deteriorated following arteriovenous fistula construction.[120]

Acute occlusion of an arteriovenous fistula may result in a decrease in cardiac output to a mean level lower than that observed in normal patients, suggesting that time-related cardiac decompensation may occur.[100, 101] This has been attributed to the presence of a fistula. Buckberg et al found that opening an arteriovenous fistula in dogs decreased systolic coronary arterial flow significantly below control levels.[121] In addition, there was an increased intraventricular volume associated with an increase in myocardial oxygen consumption, presumably as a result of an obligatory increase in ventricular wall stress with increased volume. Therefore, it was suggested that the presence of a vascular access increases stroke work and myocardial oxygen consumption, which in the presence of a possibly decreased diastolic coronary blood flow may be deleterious to the heart. Similar studies by Krumhaar et al in dogs demonstrated time-related cardiac decompensation.[122] Therefore, the revision of a vascular access is occasionally necessary to prevent myocardial failure, especially if the venous outflow tract is dilated, thereby decreasing the resistance to arteriovenous flow.[106] In the vast majority of patients with cardiac failure associated with an arteriovenous fistula, occlusion or banding of the fistula may result in a dramatic improvement in cardiac performance. However, caution is advised because the decrease in peripheral resistance resulting in decreased afterload may, with occlusion, accentuate cardiac failure in patients with pre-existing cardiac decompensation.[123]

## CARDIOVASCULAR CONSEQUENCES OF BILATERAL NEPHRECTOMY

Patients with chronic renal failure requiring long-term hemodialysis commonly have associated hypertension. Though the majority of patients can be successfully managed with available antihypertensive medications, occasionally patients are resistant to aggressive therapy and require a bilateral nephrectomy. The recent availability of powerful antihypertensive agents such as minoxidil[124] or angiotensin convertase inhibitor (Captopril) has reduced significantly the number of patients requiring bilateral nephrectomy for control of hypertension. However, some patients with ESRD are still subjected to bilateral nephrectomy.[124-127] Bilateral nephrectomy is occasionally required for the removal of huge polycystic kidneys to allow placement of a renal allograft.[128] Patients with chronically infected kidneys require a bilateral nephrectomy to remove a source of potential catastrophic infection when a transplant requiring immunosuppression is performed.

The effects of the acute loss of the major source of vasopressor, in addition to the removal of the main source of fluid and electrolyte excretion, on cardiovascular hemodynamics in these patients have been subjected to limited study. Studies in adults indicate that the total peripheral resistance was increased following bilateral nephrectomy.[129] More recent studies have determined that neither indices of preload (blood volume, cardiac index, pulmonary artery occlusion pressure, or central venous pressure) nor factors relating to myocardial contractility (cardiac index, left ventricular stroke work, or stroke work/filling pressure ratios) change significantly after bilateral nephrectomy in patients with nonmalignant hypertension. Mean arterial pressure and systemic vascular resistance fall when intravascular volume is stabilized. An increase in extracellular fluid and exchangeable sodium with an increase in cardiac output has been observed in patients one month after bilateral nephrectomy.[130] These alterations in body composition returned to preoperative values four months postoperatively. Decreases in mean arterial pressure and systemic vascular resistance were evident, but the cardiac output remained unchanged from initial values. Thus, bilateral nephrectomy results in decreased mean blood pressure and systemic vascular resistance, and indices of cardiac performance are unchanged.[131] However, after bilateral nephrectomy in patients with malignant hypertension, cardiac index and stroke volume increased.[53]

## PERICARDITIS IN PATIENTS WITH ESRD

Patients who develop pericarditis in association with ESRD can be divided into two groups. In the first group are those patients who develop pericarditis, usually with effusion, prior to initiation of dialysis. The incidence of pericarditis approximates 50% in untreated patients with uremia. The pericarditis observed in this group is very responsive to dialysis, and commonly all associated signs and symptoms rapidly resolve with dialysis therapy alone.

In the second group of patients are those with dialysis-associated pericarditis. Between 2 and 19% of patients who have been stabilized on chronic dialysis therapy develop pericarditis.[132-136] The variable incidence reported may be attributable to the methods of diagnosis utilized. A high incidence has been reported in series in which echocardiography was used to diagnose effusion in otherwise asymptomatic patients.[137-139] Dialysis-associated pericarditis may develop years after initiation of dialysis, but it usually develops within the first three months.[133, 136, 140, 141]

Gusmano et al reported an incidence of pericarditis in a pediatric population of 11.5% (7 of 61 patients).[142] Ulmer et al reported 12 cases of pericarditis in children on chronic hemodialysis.[143] The symptoms at presentation in both groups of children were similar to those documented in adult patient populations. The major presenting physical findings included fever, pericardial friction rub, congestive heart failure, elevated central venous pressure, and a gallop rhythm. On chest x-ray patients demonstrate cardiomegaly, often with a silhouette suggestive of pericardial effusion and associated pleural effusion. Electrocardiography is abnormal in approximately 80% of patients.[133, 134] Typical electrocardiographic findings of pericarditis, consisting of ST elevation in standard limb leads and precordial leads without reciprocal ST depression and occasional ST depression in Vl and AVR, are seen in 30% of patients.[133, 144-146] With successful therapy these electrocardiographic abnormalities return to normal. Atrial arrhythmias, including fibrillation, may occur in 20 to 25% of patients.[133, 144] These arrhythmias, if present after successful therapy of the pericarditis, may indicate underlying myocardial abnormalities.[147]

Echocardiography appears the most helpful diagnostic tool for assessment of patients with pericarditis because abnormalities of chamber size and myocardial contractility can also be measured.[13, 14] In addition, estimates can be made of the volume of fluid present, and fluid loculation with fibrin formation can be identified.[13, 14] Cardiac scanning may also be used as a diagnostic tool for the presence of effusion.

Major hemodynamic complications of pericarditis in patients with ESRD occur as a result of cardiac tamponade and constrictive pericarditis. The development of pericardial tamponade, the most serious and acute life-threatening complication of pericarditis, has been reported in up to 20% of patients with dialysis-associated pericarditis and is usually observed in those who are symptomatic.[133, 134, 141, 144, 146] The major clinical manifestations are elevated central venous pressure, a narrow pulse pressure, pulsus paradoxus, and hypotension. These hemodynamic abnormalities usually respond to rapid removal of accumulated pericardial fluid.[148-150] Dialysis may occasionally precipitate hypotension and signs of acute tamponade.[133, 150] Alfrey et al evaluated a patient with pericardial effusion who had elevated right atrial pressure and increased intrapericardial pressure.[148] During dialysis the cardiac index and stroke index fell to 50% of their initial values. Femoral arterial pressure after four hours of dialysis also dropped. The patient developed hypotension and evidence of tamponade. When pericardiocentesis was performed, the cardiac index and stroke index increased with a decrease in right atrial and intrapericardial pressure, suggesting that volume depletion associated with fluid removal during dialysis caused the hypotension.

Constrictive pericarditis may occur as early as six weeks or up to 11 months following acute pericarditis. Compty et al have suggested an incidence of 12% for this complication.[133]

The acute treatment required for pericardial tamponade is pericardiocentesis. However, this is associated with an appreciable mortality rate. In patients with dialysis-associated pericarditis, intensive dialysis alone is successful in approximately 40% of cases.[133, 136, 141, 151] However, the recurrence rate can be quite high. Other treatment modalities include peritoneal dialysis and charcoal hemoperfusion.[152, 153] Indomethacin has also been used,[154] although a control study has failed to confirm benefit from this drug.[155] In addition, systemic steroids[133] as well as intrapericardial steroids have been used.[156] It would appear that triamcinolone administration by indwelling pericardial catheter provides the highest success rate, with minimal recurrence and the lowest morbidity rate.[156-158] Construction of pericardial windows as well as pericardiostomy and pericar-

diectomy may be required for intractable effusions, with pericardiectomy providing the highest success rate.[134, 141, 159, 160]

## CARDIOVASCULAR ALTERATIONS ASSOCIATED WITH HEMODIALYSIS AND HEMOFILTRATION

The correction of electrolyte and acid-base imbalance and the removal of fluid and uremic toxins by hemodialysis or hemofiltration may result in acute alterations in cardiovascular hemodynamics. Previous studies have shown that left ventricular performance of hemodialysis patients, as assessed by systolic time interval analysis,[6, 8, 9, 161, 162] echocardiography,[76] and cardiac catheterization,[54] is depressed. Studies performed on pediatric patients undergoing chronic hemodialysis have shown both the presence[5] and progression[4] of depression of left ventricular performance by systolic time intervals.

In adults, unfavorable hemodynamic effects that occur during dialysis, such as variations in intravascular volume and blood pressure and cardiac arrhythmias, commonly cause an abnormal rise in pulmonary arterial pressure, indicating that cardiac reserve, especially that of the left ventricle, is markedly restricted.[163] Although left ventricular failure may not be detectable at rest, Aigner et al noted a progressive reduction in the cardiac index from 3.7 L/min/m$^2$ to 2.94 L/min/m$^2$ in adult patients undergoing hemodialysis.[164] The authors demonstrated a decreased left ventricular minute work index with progressive depression of left ventricular function. Work capacity in exercise testing was also reduced in these patients.

In contrast, in a selected group of stable patients who had been undergoing hemodialysis for more than five years, and on whom maximum oxygen consumption and echocardiographic assessment of left ventricular function was performed, the majority of patients had both oxygen consumption and echocardiographic indices within the range established for normal individuals.[165] Others have reported similar observations in young stable chronic hemodialysis patients.[166] In a large group of adult patients studied after a period of 30 months on chronic hemodialysis, left ventricular function did not appear to deteriorate and, in fact, systolic time intervals suggested an improvement in cardiac performance.[167]

Studies on the acute effects of hemodialysis on cardiac performance have provided conflicting results. Pertinent factors appear to be patient age, intravascular volume status, and the presence or absence of underlying heart disease. In pediatric patients assessed by systolic time intervals and echocardiography, an improvement in left ventricular function, as indicated by a decrease in the PEP/LVET ratio[38, 168] as well as an increase in mean velocity of circumferential fiber shortening, suggested that hemodialysis results in an improvement in left ventricular function. These indices were not influenced by changes in blood pressure or intravascular volume status.[168]

More recent studies by Koji et al utilizing systolic time intervals suggest that any improvement in hemodialysis was mainly observed in patients who were without cardiomegaly, and that left ventricular function tended to improve in younger patients.[169] Studies performed by Hung et al, using radionuclide ventriculography, on patients with cardiomegaly and congestive cardiac failure in whom mean velocity of circumferential fiber shortening was already depressed, showed an improvement post-dialysis.[170] These studies have been substantiated by Macdonald et al in studying a group of 22 stable patients undergoing hemodialysis.[17]

Others have also noted an improvement in left ventricular function with hemodialysis, using systolic time intervals[171, 172] and echocardiography.[173] Based on these and other studies,[169, 174, 175] it would appear that patients with cardiomegaly, depressed mean velocity of circumferential fiber shortening, and associated circulatory congestion appear to derive the greatest benefit from hemodialysis. However, other patients with cardiac failure and indices of contractility within the normal range do not show any acute improvement in contractility. Underlying left ventricular dysfunction may explain shortened ejection times in some patients post-dialysis.[176] Younger patients in particular derive the greatest benefit from hemodialysis in improving left ventricular performance.

Other studies have emphasized that the benefit produced by hemodialysis was due to decreasing circulatory congestion.[81, 129, 177-179] In contrast, several studies using systolic time interval analysis indicated a worsening or no change in left ventricular performance.[180-184]

Thayssen et al concluded that in elderly patients dialysis-induced hypotension resulted in deterioration of left ventricular performance.[180] Studies on changes of left ventricular transverse diameter and contractility after hemodialysis by Hanrath et al indicated no improvement in contractility.[181] Bornstein et al studied 15 patients who were maintained free of circulatory congestion and noted that left ventricular ejection time decreased significantly after an episode of dialysis.[182] The pre-ejection period rose significantly with an increase in PEP/LVET. These changes were consistent with a reduction in stroke volume, as reflected by decreased ejection time index, and also a reduced Starling effect with or without decreased contractility, as reflected by an increased PEP. Similarly, Oreto et al, studying the effect of hemodialysis on 28 patients, noted an increase in the pre-ejection period and an increase in the PEP/LVET ratio.[185] They and others[182] interpreted their results as not indicating a worsening of myocardial performance but attributed the findings to a lowering of preload produced by a reduction in circulating blood volume. Prakesh et al studied 10 patients without evidence of circulatory congestion and concluded that the primary circulatory effect of hemodialysis was a reduction in plasma volume, which resulted in a reduction in the left ventricular ejection index and ejection fraction index.[186] PEP was maintained at a constant length, and the authors suggested that an acute improvement of the dialyzable biochemical abnormalities did not appear to result in improved cardiac function.

Studies by Ikahimo et al on the cardiac effects of hemodialysis in hypertensive and normotensive patients concluded that the left atrial and left ventricular end-diastolic diameter decreases were in response to decreased left ventricular filling pressure because of decreased blood volume.[187] Decreases in cardiac output without decreased peripheral vascular resistance resulting from hemodialysis have also been described.[188-190]

The conflicting results may be explained in part by the intravascular volume status of the patients prior to dialysis and the relief of circulatory congestion produced by ultrafiltration.[191] In many of these studies ischemic heart disease was present in some patients. In others, while not specifically stated, the age range of the patients suggested the possibility that some age-related ischemic heart disease may have been present, though it was not detailed.

During hemodialysis patients may have an increased or decreased[19] cardiac index and normal peripheral vascular resistance. A decrease in cardiac output has been demonstrated in dialyzed patients during hypotensive episodes,[180] indicating that hemodialysis may induce peripheral dilatation in addition to fluid volume loss, resulting in hypotension and postdialysis decreases in cardiac output. Aizawa et al, utilizing systolic time intervals, studied the effects of hemodialysis with dialysate containing acetate and demonstrated an increase in the PEP/LVET ratio, thus indicating the depression of left ventricular function and decreased peripheral resistance.[192] This increased PEP/LVET ratio was higher when acetate rather than bicarbonate was used in the dialysate. The authors inferred that acetate, as had been observed in previous studies with infused sodium acetate in dogs,[193] had a cardiac depressant effect and also decreased total peripheral resistance. However, recent studies have failed to demonstrate a cardiodepressant effect with acetate in the dialysate.[168] Subsequent studies in dogs have indicated that the intravenous infusion of acetate did not have a cardiodepressant effect.[194] The acute hypotensive episodes that occur during hemodialysis[189] have been attributed to both the autonomic neuropathic effects of uremia[195] and alterations in plasma osmolality.[196]

Both hemofiltration and sequential hemodialysis with ultrafiltration are associated with decreases in mean blood pressure.[197] However, studies comparing the two modalities have demonstrated that hemodynamic variations induced by hemofiltration have a different pattern to that observed with hemodialysis.[198] There is a slight decrease in cardiac output with a moderate reduction in stroke volume and absence of acute hypotension.[198-200] The stability of cardiac output and stroke volume associated with hemofiltration suggests that venous return is maintained in the presence of blood volume contraction and fluid depletion. The data suggest that venous constriction occurs in order to initiate a redistribution of blood in the venous compartment. Such a venoconstrictive phenomenon does not appear to occur with conventional hemodialysis.[201] In addition, the decrease in plasma osmolality that is associated with hypotension[196, 202] is less with hemofiltration than that observed with hemodialysis.[200] The latter may explain the hemodynamic homeostasis observed with hemofiltration.

## CARDIOVASCULAR STATUS FOLLOWING RENAL TRANSPLANTATION

Successful renal transplantation results in the resolution of anemia, the elimination of uremic toxins, and the achievement of normal fluid and electrolyte homeostasis. In serial studies of children by Ulmer et al, systolic time interval analysis indicated persistence of depressed left ventricular function in the immediate post-transplant period.[4] Normal cardiac performance was only achieved by one year after transplantation, suggesting that the depressed left ventricular function associated with chronic renal failure resolved slowly even after the elimination of uremia and anemia. Similar observations in adults have been reported by Riley et al.[100] In the latter studies achievement of normal left ventricular function was not reached until three months after transplantation. Newmark and Kohn noted progressive improvement in left ventricular function up to five years after transplantation, as indicated by systolic time intervals.[203] Other investigators have also noted a progressive improvement in systolic time intervals.[161] Tuckman et al, utilizing an indicator dilution method for determination of cardiac output, and heart catheterization, studied recipients five to 14 months following transplantation.[204] Cardiac index was normal in six of seven patients, and the presence of a Brescia-Cimino arterial fistula did not appear to cause an increase in cardiac index.

Echocardiographic studies on children prior to construction of arteriovenous fistulae and repeated examination six months or more after transplantation revealed systolic time intervals indicative of normal left ventricular function, as well as normal indices of myocardial contractility.[205] The maintenance of a patent Brescia-Cimino fistula in the pediatric recipient did not appear to depress cardiac performance; however, post-occlusion alterations in cardiac index and systemic vascular resistance were observed.[97] The echocardiographic studies demonstrating normal indices of contractility in the children with ESRD and the achievement of normal indices of contractility following transplantation in the presence of patent Brescia-Cimino fistulas indicate that anemia may be the major pathogenetic mechanism for decreased exercise tolerance and cardiovascular impairment in children with ESRD. Similarly, Ulmer et al noted that near normal indices of physical working capacity were attained in four children after transplantation.[120]

In summary, it is not possible to determine the role of each potential factor causing cardiodepression in chronic renal failure. There appears to be an increased volume load on the left ventricle in the presence of hypervolemia. Patients may be subjected to increased pressure load from chronic arterial hypertension and, in addition, anemia and metabolic and endocrine factors may be relevant. Hemodialysis appears to acutely improve left ventricular performance of patients with pre-existing depressed contractility. However, ventricular function may deteriorate or remain stable during longterm hemodialysis. Renal transplantation, by eliminating uremia and anemia, and by achieving normal fluid and electrolyte homeostasis, allows for recovery of normal left ventricular performance.

# REFERENCES

1. Donckerwolcke RA, Chantler C, Broyer M, et al: Combined report on regular dialysis and transplantation of children in Europe, 1979. Proc Eur Dial Transplant Assoc 17:89, 1980.
2. Ulmer HE, Heupel EW, Weckasser G: Mechanocardiographic assessment of systolic time intervals in normal children. Basic Res Cardiol 77:197, 1982.
3. Potter D, Larsen D, Leumann E, et al: Treatment of chronic uremia in childhood. II. Hemodialysis. Pediatrics 46:678, 1970.
4. Ulmer HE, Heupel EW, Schärer K: Longterm evaluation of cardiac function utilizing systolic time intervals in children with chronic renal failure. Int J Pediatr Nephrol 3:79, 1982.
5. O'Regan S, Matina D, Ducharme G, Davignon A: Recent advances in diagnosis and treatment of children with chronic renal failure. International Workshop, Heidelberg, May 21–22, 1982.
6. Trznadel, K, Luciak, M: Analysis of contractile activity of the left ventricle in the initial stage of chronic renal failure. Pol Tyg Lek 32:39, 1977.
7. Juskowa J: Left ventricular function in chronic uremia treated with repeated dialysis and kidney transplantation on the basis of polycardiography. Acta Med Pol 19:4, 1978.
8. Trznadel K, Luciak M, Wyszogrodzka M: The left ventricular systolic function after digoxin administration in patients with chronic renal failure. Clin Nephrol 13:231, 1980.
9. Juskowa J, Lapinska K, Swiderska-Kulikowa B, Deka A: Wydolnosc lewej komory serca oceniana metodami nieinwazyjnymi (polikardiograficzna I

echokardiograficzna) U chorych przewiekla niewydolnoscia nerek leczonych poczonych powtarzanymi dializami. Pol Arch Med Wewn 65:17, 1981.
10. Lewis BS, Milne FJ, Goldberg B: Left ventricular function in chronic renal failure. Br Heart J 38:1229, 1976.
11. Ikäheimo M, Huttunen K, Takkunen J: Cardiac effects of chronic renal failure and haemodialysis treatment. Hypertensive versus normotensive patients. Br Heart J 45:710, 1981.
12. Blanchard WB, Fenell RS, Buciarelli RL, Victoria BE: Echocardiographic patterns in children and adolescents with chronic renal failure. Int J Pediatr Nephrol 1:222, 1980.
13. Schott CR, LeSar JF, Kotler MN, et al: The spectrum of echocardiographic findings in chronic renal failure. Cardiovasc Med 3:217, 1978.
14. D'Cruz IA, Bhatt GR, Cohen HC, Glick G: Echocardiographic detection of cardiac involvement in patients with chronic renal failure. Arch Intern Med 138:720, 1978.
15. Abbasi AS, Slaughter JC, Allen MW: Asymmetric septal hypertrophy in patients on long-term hemodialysis. Chest 74:548, 1974.
16. Kuroda M, Murakami K: Variety of cardiomegaly showing asymmetric septal hypertrophy or dilatation in long-term hemodialyzed patients: an echocardiographic study. Nephron 24:155, 1979.
17. Macdonald IL, Uldall R, Buda AJ: The effect of hemodialysis on cardiac rhythm and performance. Clin Nephrol 15:321, 1981.
18. Morrison G, Brown ST, Michelson EL, Morenroth J: Mechanism and prevention of cardiac arrhythmias during hemodialysis. Am J Cardiol 43:360, 1979.
19. Endou K, Kamijima J, Kabubari Y, Kikawada R: Hemodynamic changes during hemodialysis. Cardiology 63:175, 1978.
20. Papadmitriou M, Roy RR, Varkarakis M: Electrocardiographic changes and plasma potassium levels in patients on regular hemodialysis. Br Med J 2:268, 1970.
21. Ewing DJ, Winney R: Autonomic function in patients with chronic renal failure on intermittent hemodialysis. Nephron 19:424, 1975.
22. Soriano G, Eisinger RP: Abnormal responses to the Valsalva maneuver in patients on chronic hemodialysis. Nephron 9:251, 1972.
23. Sharpey-Schafer EP: Effects of Valsalva's maneuver on the normal and failing circulation. Br Med J 1:693, 1956.
24. Kersh ES, Kronfeld SJ, Unger A, et al: Autonomic insufficiency in uremia as a cause of hemodialysis-induced hypotension. N Engl J Med 290:650, 1975.
25. Mostert JW, Evers JL, Hobika GH, et al: The Valsalva maneuver as a clinical test for circulatory congestion in chronic uremia. J Surg Oncol 2:207, 1970.
26. Pickering TG, Gribbin B, Oliver DO: Baroflex sensitivity in patients on long-term hemodialysis. Clin Sci 43:645, 1972.
27. Burgess ED: Cardiac vagal denervation in hemodialysis patients. Nephron 30:228, 1982.
28. Storstein O, Örjavik O: Aortic insufficiency in chronic renal failure. Acta Med Scand 203:175, 1978.
29. Adam WR, Dawborn JK, Rosenbaum M: Transient

early diastolic murmurs in patients with renal failure. Med J Aust 2:1085, 1970.

30. Bowman D: Murmur of aortic insufficiency. Ann Intern Med 78:451, 1973.

31. Garvin CF: Functional aortic insufficiency. Ann Intern Med 13:1799, 1940.

32. Matalon R, Moussalli AR, Nidus BD, et al: Functional aortic insufficiency—a feature of renal failure. N Engl J Med 285:1522, 1971.

33. Acquatella H, Pérez-Rojas M, Burger B, Guinand-Baldo A: Left ventricular function in terminal uremia. A hemodynamic and echocardiographic study. Nephron 22:160, 1978.

34. Bailey GL, Hampers CL, Merrill JP: Reversible cardiomyopathy in uremia. Trans Am Soc Artif Intern Organs 13:263, 1967.

35. Drüeke T, LePailleur C, Meilhac B, et al: Congestive cardiomyopathy in uraemic patients on long term haemodialysis. Br Med J 1:350, 1977.

36. Scheer, RL, Ozdemir AI, Bernstein BA, Gensini GG: Ventriculography and hemodynamic studies in uremic cardiomyopathy. Kidney Int 8:419, 1975.

37. Ianhez LE, Lowen J, Sabbaga E: Uremic myocardiopathy. Nephron 15:17, 1975.

38. Ulmer HE, Gilli G, Schärer K: Assessment of uremic cardiomyopathy in childhood by systolic time intervals. Pediatr Res 10:897, 1976.

39. Gueron M, Berlyne GM, Nord E, Ben Ari J: The case against the existence of a specific uraemic myocardiopathy. Nephron 15:2, 1975.

40. Prosser D, Parsons V: The case for a specific uraemic myocardiopathy. Nephron 15:4, 1975.

41. Müller-Wiefel DE, Schärer K, Ulmer HE, et al: Verlauf der Anämie bei Kindern mit chronischer Niereninsuffizienz. Monatsschr Kinderheilkd 124:323, 1976.

42. Pippig L: Herz-und Kreislauffunktion bei Urämie. Archiv für Klinische Medizin 214:244, 1968.

43. Mostert JW, Evers JL, Hobika GH, et al: The haemodynamic response to chronic renal failure as studied in the azotaemic state. Br J Anaesth 42:397, 1970.

44. Mostert JW, Evers JL, Hobika GH, et al: Cardiac evaluation in renal and pulmonary insufficiency. NY State J Med 70:1196, 1970.

45. Dziuk E, Wankowicz Z: The use of 51-Cr-labelled erythrocytes for assessment of influence of arteriovenous fistula on haemodynamic conditions in patient with chronic renal failure treated with haemodialysis. Strahlentherapie 72:459, 1973.

46. Ono M: Exercise capacity of children with chronic renal failure. Jpn J Nephrol 21:1089, 1979.

47. Payne RM, Soderblom RE, Lobstein P, et al: Exercise-induced hemodynamic effects of arteriovenous fistulas used for hemodialysis. Kidney Int 2:344, 1972.

48. Sproule BJ, Mitchell JH, Miller WF: Cardiopulmonary physiologic responses to heavy exercise in patients with anemia. J Clin Invest 39:378, 1960.

49. Roy SB, Bhatia ML, Mathur VS, Virmani S: Hemodynamic effects of chronic severe anemia. Circulation 28:346, 1963.

50. Duke M, Abelmann WH: The hemodynamic response to chronic anemia. Circulation 39:503, 1969.

51. Sill V, Lanser KG, Bauditz W: Einfluss der Anämie und der arteriovenosen Fistel anf die körperliche Leistungsfähigkeit der Dauerdialysepatienten. Z Kardiol 62:164, 1973.

52. Neff MS, Kim KE, Persoff M, et al: Hemodynamics of uremic anemia. Circulation 43:876, 1971.

53. Kim KE, Onesti G, Swartz CD: Hemodynamics of hypertension in uremia. Kidney Int 7(Suppl): S155, 1975.

54. Capelli JP, Kasparian H: Cardiac work demands and left ventricular function in end-stage renal disease. Ann Intern Med 86:261, 1977.

55. Schiffrin EL, Morales JC, Agrest YA: Influencia de la anemia sobre la funcion cardiovascular en la insuficiencia renal cronica. Medicina (Buenos Aires) 37(Suppl 2):163, 1977.

56. Todesco S, Maschio G, Poli D, et al: Su alcuni aspetti della meccanica cardiaca in corso di insufficienza renale cronica iperazotemica. Loro correlazione con i disordini humorali propri dell'uremia. Folia Cardiol 26:285, 1967.

57. Brass H, Krückels ED, Müller G, Heintz R: Pathomechanismen der Herzinsuffizienz bei Hamodialyseptatienten. Dtsch Med Wochenschr 33:1319, 1971.

58. Sodi A, Rizzo M, Durval A, et al: I tempi della sistole ventricolare in pazienti uremici in trattamento emodialitico periodico. Malattie Cardiovascolari 9:441, 1968.

59. Lindner A, Charra B, Sherrard DJ, Scribner BH: Accelerated atherosclerosis in prolonged maintenance hemodialysis. N Engl J Med 290:697, 1974.

60. Rostand SG, Gretes JC, Kirk KA, et al: Ischemic heart disease in patients with uremia undergoing maintenance hemodialysis. Kidney Int 16:600, 1979.

61. Vincenti F, Amend WJ, Abele J, et al: The role of hypertension in hemodialysis-associated atherosclerosis. Am J Med 68:363, 1980.

62. Guisado R, Arieff AI, Massry SG: Muscle water and electrolytes in uremia and the effects of hemodialysis. J Lab Clin Med 80:322, 1977.

63. Katz AM: Congestive heart failure. Role of altered myocardial cellular control. N Engl J Med 293:1184, 1975.

64. Lhaste F, Drucke T, Larno S, Boissier JR: Cardiac interaction between parathyroid hormone, beta-adrenoceptor agents, and verapamil in the guinea pig in vitro. Clin Exp Pharmacol Physiol 7:119, 1980.

65. Ejerbkad S, Eriksson I, Johansson H: Uraemic arterial disease. An experimental study with special reference to the effect of parathyroidectomy. Scand J Urol Nephrol 13:161, 1979.

66. Drüeke T, Fleury J, Toure Y, et al: Effect of parathyroidectomy on left-ventricular function in haemodialysis patients. Lancet 1:112, 1980.

67. Kramer P, Schmidt-Lauber M, Langenheim N, et al: Reno-kardiale Wechselwirkungen bein Niereninsuffizienz. Klin Wochenschr 58:1043, 1980.

68. Lhoste F, Drüeke T, Man NK, et al: Anti-beta adrenoceptor blockade activity of plasma ultrafiltrate in two uraemic patients. Effect of parathyroidectomy. Biomedicine 25:181, 1976.

69. Therman DS, Alfrey AC, Hammond WS, et al: Cardiac calcification in uremia. Am J Med 50:744, 1971.

70. Arora KK, Lacy JP, Schackt RA, et al: Calcific cardiomyopathy in advanced renal failure. Arch Intern Med 135:603, 1975.

71. Raab W, Lepeschkin E, Starcheska YK, Gigee W: Cardiotoxic effects of hypercatecholemia in renal insufficiency. Circulation 14:614, 1956.

72. Garcia R, Jennings JM: Phaeochromocytoma masquerading as a cardiomyopathy. Am J Cardiol 29:568, 1972.

73. Szakacs JE, Mehlman B: Pathologic changes by l-norepinephrine: Quantitative aspects. Am J Cardiol 5:619, 1960.

74. Atuk NO, Bailey CJ, Tunr S, et al: Red blood catechol-O-methyl transferase, plasma catecholamines and renin in renal failure. Trans Am Soc Artif Intern Organs 22:195, 1976.

75. Miach PJ, Louis WJ, Dawhorn JK, Doyle AE: Plasma catecholamines in dialysed uraemic patients. Eur J Clin Invest 7:245, 1977 (Abstract).

76. Miach PJ, Dawborn JK, Louis WJ, McDonald IG: Left ventricular function in uremia: echocardiographic assessment in patients on maintenance dialysis. Clin Nephrol 15:259, 1981.

77. Wildenthal K, Mierzwiak DS, Myers RW, Mitchell JH: Effects of acute lactic acidosis on left ventricular performance. Am J Physiol 214:1352, 1968.

78. Rocamora JM, Downing SE: Preservation of ventricular function by adrenergic influences during metabolic acidosis in the cat. Circ Res 24:373, 1969.

79. Kaseno K, Sugmoto T, Hirasawa K, et al: The effects of hyperpotassemia on cardiac performance. Cardiovasc Res 9:212, 1975.

80. Gotloib L, Servadio C: A possible case of beriberi heart failure in a chronic hemodialyzed patient. Nephron 14:293, 1975.

81. DelGreco F, Simon NM, Roguska J, Walker C: Hemodynamic studies in chronic uremia. Circulation 40:87, 1969.

82. Penpargkul S, Scheuer J: Effect of uremia upon the performance of the rat heart. Cardiovasc Res 6:702, 1972.

83. Raab W: Cardiotoxic substances in the blood and heart muscle in uremia. J Lab Clin Med 29:715, 1944.

84. Uraoka T, Sugimoto T, Inasaka T, et al: Changes of cardiac performance in renal failure. Jpn Heart J 16:489, 1975.

85. Acquatella H, Perez Rojas M, Burger B, Lozano RJ: Modificaciones experimentales de la contractilidas miocardica producidas por un toxico retenido en la uremia: el acido guanido succinico. Arch Inst Cardiol Mex 44:624, 1974.

86. Giovannetti S, Balcstri PL, Barsotti G: Mcthylguanidine in uremia. Arch Int Med 131:709, 1973.

87. Kersting F, Brass H, Heintz R: Uremic cardiomyopathy: studies on cardiac function in the guinea pig. Clin Nephrol 10:109, 1978.

88. Kersting F, Brass H: The effects of uraemic compounds on oxygen consumption and mechanical activity of isolated guinea pig hearts. Proc Eur Dial Transplant Assoc 13:472, 1976.

89. Scheuer J, Stezoski W: The effects of uremic compounds on cardiac function and metabolism. J Mol Cell Cardiol 5:287, 1973.

90. Penpargkul S, Kuziak J, Scheuer J: Effects of uremia upon carbohydrate metabolism in isolated perfused rat heart. J Mol Cell Cardiol 7:499, 1975.

91. Bernard P, Crest M, Rinaudo JB, et al: A study of the cardiotoxicity of uremic middle molecules on embryonic chick hearts. Nephron 31:135, 1982.

92. Langescheid C, Kramer P, Scheler F: Anastomosis-pressure-dynamic method for determining AV fistula blood flow rate. Dial Transplant 6:54, 1977.

93. Anderson CB, Etheredge EE, Harter HR, et al: Blood flow measurements in arteriovenous dialysis fistula. Surgery 81:459, 1977.

94. Ehrenfeld WK, Grausz H, Wylie EJ: Subcutaneous arteriovenous fistulas for hemodialysis. Am J Surg 124:200, 1972.

95. Hurwich BJ: Plethysmographic forearm blood flow studies in maintenance hemodialysis with radial arteriovenous fistula. Nephron 6:673, 1969.

96. Kaye M, Lemaitre P, O'Regan S: A new technique for measuring blood flow in polytetrafluoroethylene grafts for hemodialysis. Clin Nephrol 8:533, 1977.

97. Révillon L, O'Regan S, Robitaille P, et al: The effects of Brescia-Cimino fistulas on cardiac function in transplanted pediatric patients. Clin Nephrol 12:26, 1979.

98. Dongradi G, Rocha P, Kahan JC, et al: Arteriovenous fistula blood flow in chronic dialyzed patients: comparison of values obtained by the dye-dilution method and by the variations in cardiac output during temporary occlusion of the arteriovenous fistula. Proc Eur Dial Transplant Assoc 16:690, 1979.

99. Conte J, Durand D, Ton That H, et al: Etude du retentissement hémodynamique des fistules artérioveineuses chirurgicales chez les malades en hémodialyse périodique. J Urol Néphrol 4–5:351, 1973.

100. Riley SM Jr, Blackstone EH, Sterling WA, Diethelm AG: Echocardiographic assessment of cardiac performance in patients with arteriovenous fistulas. Surg Gynecol Obstet 146:203, 1978.

101. Fee HJ, Levisman JA, Dickmeyer JP, Golding AL: Hemodynamic consequences of femoral arteriovenous bovine shunts. Ann Surg 184:103, 1975.

102. Zebe H, Ritz E, Ziegler M, et al: Hämodialyse mit der Oberarmfistel. Dtsch Med Wochenschr 98:395, 1973.

103. Johnson G, Blythe WB: Hemodynamic effects of arteriovenous shunts used for hemodialysis. Ann Surg 171:715, 1970.

104. Dongradi G, Rocha P, Baron B, et al: Hemodynamic effects of arteriovenous fistulae in chronic hemodialysis patients at rest and during exercise. Clin Nephrol 15:75, 1981.

105. O'Regan S, Lemaitre P, Kaye M: Hemodynamic studies in patients with expanded polytetrafluoroethylene (PTFE) forearm grafts. Clin Nephrol 10:96, 1978.

106. Cerra FB, Shapiro R, Anthone R, Anthone S: Physiologic response patterns to occlusion of clinically significant arteriovenous fistulas. J Dial 1:665, 1977.

107. Anderson CB, Groce MA: Banding of arteriovenous dialysis fistulas to correct high-output cardiac failure. Surgery 78:552, 1975.

108. Ahearn DJ, Maher JF: Heart failure as a complication of hemodialysis arteriovenous fistula. Ann Intern Med 77:201, 1972.

109. Draur RA: Heart failure and dialysis fistulas. Ann Intern Med 79:765, 1973.

110. George CRP, May J, Schieb M: Heart failure due to arteriovenous fistula for hemodialysis. Med J Aust 1:696, 1973.

111. Zerbino VR, Tice DA, Katz LA, Nidus BD: A 6 year clinical experience with arteriovenous fistulas and bypasses for hemodialysis. Surgery 76:1018, 1974.

112. Bergrem H, Flatmark A, Simonsen S: Dialysis

fistulas and cardiac failure. Acta Med Scand 204:191, 1978.

113. Dotremont G, Piessens J, Verberckmoes R, De Geest H: Hemodynamic studies in patients on chronic hemodialysis by venipuncture of a peripheral arteriovenous fistula. Acta Cardiol (Brux.) 25:230, 1970.

114. Izquierdo GF, Vivero RR: Venous autograft for hemodialysis. Operative technique, its systemic effects. Nephron 8:57, 1971.

115. Gagnadoux MF, Pascal B, Bronstein M, et al: Arteriovenous fistulae in small children. Dial Transplant 9:318, 1980.

116. O'Regan S, Robitaille PO, Davignon A, et al: Assessment of Brescia-Cimino fistula blood flow rates in pediatric patients. Nephron 24:138, 1979.

117. Chvatikova J, Tomasek R, Johanovska K, et al: Arteriovenozni pistel U nemocnych S chronickym selhanim ledvin V pravidelnem dialyzachim leceni. Zmeny systolickych casovych intervalu V zavislosti na pisteli. Cas Lek Cesk 117:556, 1978.

118. Klütsch VK, Ross W, Christ V, Scheitza E: Die hämodynamischen Auswirkungen der subkutanen arteriovenösen Fistel bien chronischer Urämie. Z Kreislaufforsch 61:497, 1972.

119. O'Regan S, Villemant D, Ducharme G, et al: Effects of Brescia-Cimino fistulae on myocardial function in pediatric patients. Dial Transplant 10:202, 1981.

120. Ulmer HE, Greiner H, Schüler HW, Schärer K: Cardiovascular impairment and physical working capacity in children with chronic renal failure. Acta Paediatr Scand 67:43, 1978.

121. Buckberg GD, Fixler DE, Archie JP, et al: Variable effects of heart rate on phasic and regional left ventricular muscle blood flow in anesthetized dogs. Cardiovasc Res 9:1, 1975.

122. Krumhaar D, Schmidt HD, Schulz U: Acute and chronic flow-measurements in experimental arteriovenous fistulas. Basic Res Cardiol 69:447, 1973.

123. Timmis AD, McGonigle RJS, Weston MJ, et al: The influence of hemodialysis fistulas on circulatory dynamics and left ventricular function. Int J Artif Organs 5:101, 1982.

124. Piettinger WA, Mitchell HC: Minoxidil—an alternative to nephrectomy for refractory hypertension. N Engl J Med 289:167, 1973.

125. Lazarus JM, Hampers CL, Bennett AH, et al: Urgent bilateral nephrectomy for severe hypertension. Ann Intern Med 76:733, 1972.

126. Mahony JF, Gibson GR, Sheil AGR, et al: Bilateral nephrectomy for malignant hypertension. Lancet 1:1036, 1972.

127. Konnak JW, Hyndman CW, Cerny JC: Bilateral nephrectomy prior to renal transplantation. J Urol 107:9, 1972.

128. Salvatierra O, Kountz SL, Fackert OB: Polycystic renal disease treated by renal transplantation. Surg Gynecol Obstet 137:431, 1973.

129. Hampers CL, Skillman JJ, Lyons JH, et al: A hemodynamic evaluation of bilateral nephrectomy and hemodialysis in hypertensive man. Circulation 35:272, 1967.

130. Zollinger RM, Skillman JJ, Gumpert JRW, et al: Effects of bilateral nephrectomy on hemodynamics and body composition in patients with chronic renal failure. Surg Forum 20:38, 1969.

131. Civetta JM, Lynne CM, Carrion HM, et al: Cardiovascular changes after bilateral nephrectomy. J Surg Res 18:301, 1975.

132. Compty CM, Wathen RL, Shapiro FL: Uremic pericarditis. Cardiovasc Clin 7:219, 1976.

133. Compty CM, Cohen SL, Shapiro FL: Pericarditis in chronic uremia and its sequels. Ann Intern Med 75:173, 1971.

134. Ribot S, Frankel HJ, Gielchinsky I, Gilbert L: Treatment of uremic pericarditis. Clin Nephrol 2:127, 1974.

135. Silverberg S, Oreopoulos DG, Wise DJ, et al: Pericarditis in patients undergoing long-term hemodialysis and peritoneal dialysis. Am J Med 63:874, 1977.

136. Bailey GL, Hampers CL, Hager EB, Merrill JP: Uremic pericarditis: clinical features and management. Circulation 38:582, 1968.

137. Goldstein DH, Nagar C, Srivastava N, et al: Clinically silent pericardial effusions in patients on long-term hemodialysis. Chest 72:744, 1977.

138. Horton JD, Gelfand MC, Sherber HS: Natural history of asymptomatic pericardial effusions in patients on maintenance hemodialysis. Proc Clin Dial Transplant Forum 7:76, 1977.

139. Kleiman JH, Motta J, London E, et al: Pericardial effusions in patients with end-stage renal disease. Br Heart J 40:190, 1978.

140. Fuller TF, Knochel JP, Brennan JP, et al: Reversal of intractable uremic pericarditis by triamcinolone hexacetonide. Arch Intern Med 136:979, 1976.

141. Marini P, Hull AR: Uremic pericarditis: A review of incidence and management. Kidney Int 7 (Suppl 2):163, 1975.

142. Gusmano R, Perfumo F, Formicucci L, Bertolini A: La pericarditide uremica in età pediatrica. Minerva Nefrol 24:239, 1977.

143. Ulmer HE, Gilli G, Schärer K: Urämische perikarditis im Kindesalter. Nieren-und Hochdruckkrankh 9:193, 1980.

144. Mitchell AG: Pericarditis during chronic haemodialysis therapy. Postgrad Med J 50:741, 1974.

145. Morin JE, Mulder DS, Long R: Pericardiectomy for uremic tamponade. Can J Surg 19:109, 1976.

146. Winney RJ, Wright N, Summerling MD, Lambie AT: Echocardiography in uraemic pericarditis with effusion. Nephron 18:201, 1977.

147. Spodick DH: Arrhythmias during acute pericarditis. A prospective study of 100 consecutive cases. JAMA 235:39, 1976.

148. Alfrey AC, Goss JE, Ogden DA, et al: Uremic hemopericardium. Am J Med 45:391, 1968.

149. Baldwin JJ, Edwards JE: Uremic pericarditis as a cause of cardiac tamponade. Circulation 53:896, 1976.

150. Shabetai R, Fowler NO, Guntheroith WG: The hemodynamics of cardiac tamponade and constrictive pericarditis. Am J Cardiol 26:480, 1970.

151. Wray TM, Stone WJ: Uremic pericarditis: a prospective echocardiographic and clinical study. Clin Nephrol 6:295, 1976.

152. Kramer P, Wigger W, Scheler F: Management of uraemic pericarditis. Br Med J 2:564, 1975.

153. Martin AM, Gibbins JK, Kimmitt J, Rennie F: Hemodialysis and hemoperfusion in the treatment of uremic pericarditis. A study of 13 cases. Dial Transplant 8:135, 1979.

154. Minuth ANW, Nottebohm GA, Eknoyan G, Suki WN: Indomethacin treatment of pericarditis in

chronic hemodialysis patients. Arch Intern Med 135:807, 1975.

155. Spector D, Alfred H, Siedlecki M, Briefel G: Indomethacin treatment of uremic pericarditis. Am Soc Nephrol p 30A, 1978 (Abstract).

156. Buselmeir TJ, Davin TD, Simmons RL, et al: Treatment of intractable uremic pericardial effusion. Avoidance of pericardiectomy with local steroid instillation. JAMA 240:1358, 1978.

157. Krikorian JG, Hancock EW: Pericardiocentesis. Am J Med 65:808, 1978.

158. Fuller TJ, Knochel JP, Brennan JP, et al: Reversal of intractable uremic pericarditis by triamcinolone hexacetonide. Arch Intern Med 136:979, 1976.

159. Ali-Regiaba S, Gay WA, Sullivan JF, et al: Treatment of uraemic pericarditis by anterior pericardiectomy. Lancet 2:12, 1974.

160. Jungers P, Zingraff J, Brefort G, et al: Uremic pericarditis: beneficial effect of surgical pericardiostomy. Kidney Int 14:202, 1978 (Abstract).

161. Jahn H, Schohn D, Schmitt R: Etudes hémodynamiques en cours de l'insufficience rénale chronique terminale—effets des techniques d'épuration extrarénale. Néphrologie 2:53, 1981.

162. Dongradi G, Dubois D, Bécart J, et al: Fonction myocardique de l'hémodialysé chronique. Evaluation par la mesure des intervalles de temps systoliques. Nouv Presse Méd 6:23, 1977.

163. Brass H, Brückels ED, Müller G, Heintz R: The mechanism of heart failure in patients undergoing haemodialysis. Dtsch Med Wochenschr 96:1319, 1971.

164. Aigner VA, Skrabal F, Knapp E, et al: Ruhehämodynamik und körperliche leistungsfähigkeit von chronisch hämodialysierten patienten. Wien Klin Wochenschr 88:232, 1976.

165. Lundin AP, Stein RA, Frank F, et al: Cardiovascular status in long-term hemodialysis patients: an exercise and echocardiographic study. Nephron 28:234, 1981.

166. Cohen MV, Diaz P, Scheuer J: Echocardiographic assessment of left ventricular function in patients with chronic uremia. Clin Nephrol 12:156, 1979.

167. Astorri E, Cambi V, Assanelli D, et al: Comparison of the left ventricular function after 1 year in 67 patients under periodical hemodialysis for renal insufficiency. Boll Soc Ital Cardiol 23:505, 1978.

168. O'Regan S, Villemand D, Révillon L, et al: Effects of hemodialysis on myocardial function in pediatric patients. Nephron 25:214, 1980.

169. Koji T, Sugawa M, Izumi K, et al: Left ventricular performance in chronic renal failure before and after hemodialysis assessed by systolic time intervals. Jpn Circ J 45:397, 1981.

170. Hung J, Harris PJ, Uren RF, et al: Uremic cardiomyopathy—Effect of hemodialysis on left ventricular function in end-stage renal failure. N Engl J Med 302:547, 1980.

171. Strangfeld D, Günther KH, Bohm R, et al: Cardiac function in chronic renal failure before and after hemodialysis. Cardiology 58:109, 1973.

172. Shvaro SV: Changes of the contractile function of the myocardium in patients with renal failure treated by programmed hemodialysis. Vrach Delo 9:79, 1981.

173. Chen TS, Friedman HS, Del Monte M, Smith AJ: Hemodynamic changes during dialysis: relationship to arterial pO$_2$. Proc Clin Dial Transplant Forum 9:30, 1979.

174. Fernando HA, Friedman HS, Zaman O: Echocardiographic assessment of cardiac performance in patients on maintenance hemodialysis. Cardiovasc Med 4:459, 1979.

175. Cini G, Camici M, Pentimone F, Palla R: Echocardiographic hemodynamic study during ultrafiltration sequential dialysis. Nephron 30:124, 1982.

176. Mahajan S, Kinhal V, Gardiner H, et al: Cardiac function changes during hemodialysis. Proc Clin Dial Transplant Forum 7:99, 1977.

177. Chvatikova J, Tomasek R, Kral M, et al: Systolic time interval changes in patients with chronic renal failure receiving regular dialysis treatment. Cas Lek Cesk 117:1092, 1978.

178. Tomasak R, Lisy Z, Souckova Pick P, Lachmanova J: Cardiac volume and cardiac output quotient in patients with renal failure on days 1, 2, and 3 after dialysis. Cas Lek Cesk 116:361, 1977.

179. Del Greco F, Shere J, Simon NM: Effect of hemodialysis on cardiac dynamics. Trans Am Soc Artif Intern Organs 10:353, 1964.

180. Thayssen P, Andersen KH, Pindborg T: Noninvasive monitoring of cardiac function during haemodialysis. Scand J Urol Nephrol 15:313, 1981.

181. Hanrath P, Schweizer P, Bleifeld W, et al: Changes of left ventricular transverse diameter and of contractility after haemodialysis. Dtsch Med Wochenschr 101:655, 1976.

182. Bornstein A, Sanchez Zambrano S, Morrison RS, Spodick DH: Cardiac effects of hemodialysis: noninvasive monitoring by systolic time intervals. Am J Med Sci 269:189, 1975.

183. Wiecko W, Herczka S: The effect of haemodialysis on left ventricular function in patients with chronic renal failure. Wiad Lek 30:3, 1977.

184. Astorri E, Cambi V, Manca C, et al: Left ventricular function (LVF) in 103 patients with chronic renal failure in dialytic treatment and 1 year follow up on LVL in 67 of the same patients. Minerva Nefrol 26:65, 1978.

185. Oreto G, Arrigo F, Melluso C, et al: Effetti cardiovascolari dell'emodialisi. Minerva Cardioangiol 29:195, 1981.

186. Prakash R, Wegner S: Indirect assessment of left ventricular function following hemodialysis in patients with chronic renal disease. Am J Med Sci 264:127, 1972.

187. Ikäheimo M, Huttunen K, Takkunen J: Cardiac effects of chronic renal failure and haemodialysis treatment. Br Heart J 45:710, 1981.

188. Goss JE, Alfrey AC, Vogel JHK, Holmes JH: Hemodynamic changes during hemodialysis. Trans Am Artif Intern Organs 8:68, 1967.

189. Azancot I, Degoulet P, Juillet Y, et al: Hemodynamic evaluation of hypotension during chronic hemodialysis. Clin Nephrol 8:312, 1977.

190. Handt A, Farhen MO, Szwed JJ: Intradialytic measurement of cardiac output by thermodilution and impedance cardiography. Clin Nephrol 7:61, 1977.

191. Vaziri ND, Prakash R: Echocardiographic evaluation of the effect of hemodialysis on cardiac size and function in patients with end-stage renal disease. Am J Med Sci 278:201, 1979.

192. Aizawa Y, Ohmori T, Imai K, et al: Depressant action of acetate upon the human cardiovascular system. Clin Nephrol 8:477, 1977.

193. Kirkendol PL, Devia CJ, Bower JD, Holbert RD:

A comparison of the cardiovascular effects of sodium acetate, sodium bicarbonate and other potential sources of fixed base in hemodialysate solutions. Trans Am Soc Artif Intern Organs 23:399, 1977.

194. Kirkendol PL, Robie NW, Gonzalez FM, Devia CJ: Cardiac and vascular effects of infused sodium acetate in dogs. Trans Am Soc Artif Intern Organs 24:714, 1978.

195. Imai Y, Abe K, Otsuka Y, et al: Blood pressure regulation in chronic hypotensive and hypertensive patients with chronic renal failure. Jpn Circ J 45:303, 1981.

196. Aizawa Y, Hirasawa Y, Shibata A: A fall of plasma osmolality created at dialyzer and its possible effect on circulating blood volume. Clin Nephrol 12:269, 1979.

197. Quellhorst E, Schuenemann B, Doht B: Treatment of severe hypertension in chronic renal failure by hemofiltration. Proc Eur Dial Transplant Assoc 14:129, 1977.

198. Hampl H, Paeprer H, Unger V, Kessel M: Hemodynamic studies during hemodialysis in comparison to sequential ultrafiltration and hemofiltration. J Dial 3:51, 1979.

199. Baldamus CA, Ernst W, Fassbinder W, Koch KM: Differing hemodynamic stability due to differing sympathetic response: comparison of ultrafiltration, hemodialysis and hemofiltration. Proc Eur Dial Transplant Assoc 17:205, 1980.

200. Chaignon M, Aubert P, Martin MF, et al: Hemodynamic effects of hemodialysis and hemofiltration. Int Soc Artif Organs 6:27, 1982.

201. Chaignon M, Chen WT, Tarazi RC, et al: Effect of hemodialysis on blood volume distribution and cardiac output. Hypertension 3:327, 1981.

202. Henrich WL, Woodard TD, Blachley JD, et al: Role of osmolality in blood pressure stability after dialysis and ultrafiltration. Kidney Int 18:480, 1980.

203. Newmark KJ, Kohn P: Myocardial function improvement in the post renal transplantation state assessed by systolic time intervals. Kidney Int 6:79A, 1974 (Abstract).

204. Tuckman J, Benninger JL, Reubi F: Haemodynamic and blood volume studies in long-term haemodialysis patients, and in patients with successfully transplanted kidneys. Clin Sci Mol Med 45:155s, 1973.

205. O'Regan S, Douste-Blazy MY, Ducharme G, et al: Renal transplantation and cardiac function in pediatric patients. Clin Nephrol 17:237, 1982.

# 25

# Anemia in Children with ESRD

*Frank G. Boineau, M.D.*
*James W. Fisher, Ph.D.*
*John E. Lewy, M.D.*

Anemia is a cardinal feature of chronic renal failure in children. The severity of anemia is frequently proportional to the degree of renal failure and is almost invariably present when ESRD develops. Characteristically, the reduction in hemoglobin is proportional to the reduction in hematocrit, and erythrocytes appear normochromic and normocytic. The reticulocyte response is inadequate for the degree of anemia.[1] Anemia in children is usually more severe than in adults.[2]

Our knowledge of the effects of anemia in children with ESRD is incomplete. When severe, anemia contributes to fatigue, limited exercise tolerance, and increased cardiac demand. Its severity does not, however, correlate with the growth rate of children with ESRD who are on dialysis.[2] Ulmer and colleagues[3] reported on cardiovascular impairment and physical work in children with mild to severe renal insufficiency, including a group on hemodialysis. Physical work capacity was measured using a cycle ergometer. The work capacity of all subjects was compared with that of a group of normal children by the percentile method. Children whose serum creatinine was below 2 mg/dl had normal work capacity. In those with more severe renal insufficiency the physical work capacity was inversely related to the serum creatinine level, with a high degree of correlation (r = 0.79) between the two. There

was also a significant correlation (r = 0.81) between physical work capacity and the degree of anemia, which was described by an exponential relationship. Work capacity of children on hemodialysis was slightly better than that of those not on hemodialysis with a serum creatinine level above 5 mg/dl. When work capacity was measured before and after a hemodialysis session, it was found to be worse immediately after hemodialysis than before hemodialysis.[3]

The cause of anemia in ESRD is undoubtedly multifactorial. The model proposed by Fisher and colleagues[4] may serve as a useful conceptual guide to review this problem (Fig. 25–1). Important mechanisms in the origin of the anemia include:

1. Relative deficiency in the level of erythropoietin (Ep);
2. Accumulation of toxins, which are inhibitors of erythropoiesis, in the serum of patients with ESRD;
3. Decreased erythrocyte life span;
4. Blood loss from the gastrointestinal tract, dialyzer, and prolonged bleeding;
5. Deficiency of iron and folic acid.

This chapter explores the role of these factors in the anemia of ESRD in children.

## MECHANISMS OF ANEMIA OF CHRONIC RENAL FAILURE

### Normal Maturation of Red Blood Cells

The normal maturation of red blood cells and the influence of erythropoetin are shown

The authors wish to thank Ms. Terri White for assistance in preparing this manuscript. Supported in part by a grant from the Thrasher Research Fund.

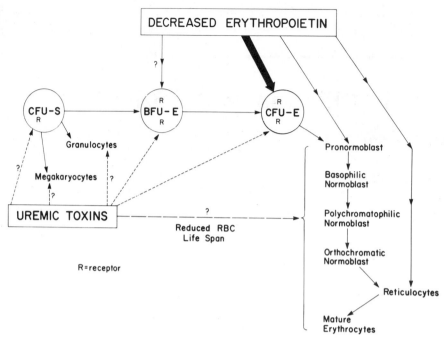

**Figure 25–1.** Model for mechanism of anemia of chronic renal failure, R = receptor. (Adapted from Reference 4 with permission.)

in Figure 25–1. Pluripotent stem cells in the bone marrow give rise to several cell lines. The stem cell is called colony-forming unit-spleen (CFU-S) because it forms granulocytic, erythrocytic, and megakaryocytic colonies in the spleens of irradiated mice. The relationship between the myeloid and lymphoid stem cells is highly conjectural. Presumably, the lymphoid lines diverge at an early stage, but they appear to share a common ancestry with the myeloid line.

The pluripotent stem cells can become differentiated into progenitor cells committed to either granulocytic/myelocytic (CFU-GM), erythrocytic (BFU-E, CFU-E), or megakaryocytic (CFU-M) progenitors. The earliest cell that can be identified as an erythroid progenitor is called burst-forming unit-erythroid (BFU-E), which differentiates into the colony-forming unit-erythroid (CFU-E). This late BFU-E may be responsive to high concentrations of erythropoietin (Fig. 25–1), but its proliferation and differentiation are controlled by a burst-promoting factor. More mature BFU-E's become increasingly responsive to Ep. They subsequently evolve into colony-forming unit-erythroid (CFU-E) cells, which are the target cells for Ep. High concentrations of Ep may also directly stimulate the recognizable nucleated erythroid cell compartment to increase its numbers and may stimulate the marrow to release reticu-

locytes into the circulation when there is an extreme demand for new red blood cells.

## Erythropoietin Deficiency

Numerous studies have established that renal hypoxia increases Ep production.[5] Hypoxia may be produced by reduced arterial blood supply to the whole kidney or segments of the kidney.[6] There exists also an extrarenal source of Ep, which is probably the liver in that the production of Ep is enhanced after partial hepatectomy.[7]

Until recently, there have been conflicting results on the level of serum Ep in chronic renal failure (CRF). However, recent bioassays[8, 9] and radioimmunoassays[10] have shown both normal and elevated levels of serum Ep in patients with CRF.

Radtke et al[8] studied patients with a creatinine clearance ranging from normal to 2 ml/min/1.73 m². The degree of anemia (hematocrit) was directly related to the creatinine clearance between 2 and 40 ml/min/1.73 m². Above a creatinine clearance of 40 ml/min/1.73 m² the hematocrit was not proportional to the creatinine clearance, and in most patients the hematocrit was normal when the creatinine clearance exceeded 40 ml/min/1.73 m². Ep was measured using the fetal mouse liver cell culture technique, and correlated with the endogenous creatinine clearance. The mean value of serum Ep was greater in those patients with reduced creatinine clearance ($<90$ ml/min/1.73 m$^2$) than in normals (p $<0.01$). However, the serum Ep concentration was not related to the degree of anemia. There was, in those patients whose creatinine clearance ranged from 2 to 40 ml/min/1.73 m$^2$, a direct relationship between creatinine clearance and serum Ep. Thus, a parallel decrease in excretory (creatinine clearance) and endocrine function (Ep production) was present in this study.

Caro et al measured Ep in anephric and nephric adult patients on stable hemodialysis.[9] Ep was measured by bioimmunoassay. In the anephric patients, the Ep concentration was similar to that in a group of normal subjects who were not anemic and had normal renal function. The group of nephric hemodialysis patients had an elevated Ep level compared to normal controls. There was no relationship between the Ep levels and the degree of anemia (hematocrit). The Ep levels in both nephric and anephric patients on hemodialysis were considerably less than Ep levels in patients with the same degree of anemia having normal renal function. Thus, when judged against appropriate controls, patients on hemodialysis with anemia have a relative deficiency of Ep. The level of Ep is inadequate for the degree of anemia.

More direct evidence for the effect of Ep on the anemia of CRF was reported by Van Stone and Max[11] and Eschbach, Mladenovic and Adamson.[12] Van Stone and Max[11] studied the response to Ep in rats made uremic by bilateral nephrectomy. After bilateral nephrectomy, peritoneal dialysis was performed daily for 6 hours using 15 peritoneal exchanges. The nephrectomized rats receiving peritoneal dialysis had a BUN of 118 mg/dl (group mean). The control group was composed of non-nephrectomized rats who were also receiving peritoneal dialysis in an identical fashion and had a BUN of 18 mg/dl (group mean). Half of the nephrectomized and non-nephrectomized rats were given subcutaneous Ep 2 U s.c. each day for 12 days. Nephrectomized rats given Ep had a significantly (p $< 0.05$) higher hematocrit, red cell mass, and erythron iron turnover than nephrectomized rats not given Ep. However, the nephrectomized, Ep-treated rats did not have as high a hematocrit and red cell mass as non-nephrectomized rats given Ep or not given Ep. Thus, other factors, including (a) insufficient Ep to restore normal red blood cell mass and production, (b) inhibitors of red blood cell production, and (c) shortened red blood cell life span, may account for incomplete correction of the anemia in this model.

Eschbach, Mladenovic, and Adamson[12] reported preliminary observations on the effect of Ep in sheep with renal insufficiency having serum creatinine values ranging from 3.3 to 10 mg/dl. Studies were performed on four sheep with varying degrees of renal insufficiency. Ep was intravenously infused for ten days at a dose of 4 to 10 units/kg/day. The reticulocyte count and plasma iron turnover increased significantly in those given Ep for 10 days. In a smaller group of sheep with renal insufficiency, Ep was infused intravenously for 15 to 40 days at the same dose. The anemia was completely corrected with normalization of hematocrit and red cell mass in this smaller group. However, serum Ep levels were not measured and compared to appropriate controls during Ep infusions and, thus, the amount of Ep needed to correct the anemia in relation to normal is unknown.

## Inhibitors of Erythropoiesis

Several investigators have reported inhibition of heme synthesis with sera from anemic CRF patients.[13-18] Wallner et al reported that sera from 22 adult males on hemodialysis inhibited erythropoiesis.[13] The assay system utilized dog bone marrow cells incubated in the presence and absence of both sera from dialysis patients and sheep Ep. Radioiron incorporation into heme of erythroid cells in culture was an index of erythropoiesis. Iron concentration in the culture media was the same in all groups. Erythropoiesis was inhibited by sera from ESRD patients when compared with normal controls (p $< 0.001$). There was a linear relation between erythropoiesis and decreasing amounts of dialysis patient's sera used in the incubation media. Erythropoiesis was not affected by urea or creatinine added to the bone marrow cultures[13]

Moriyama and Fisher[14] and Ohno and Fisher[15] have reported an inhibitor of CFU-E in the sera of uremic rabbits, using a nephrectomy ESRD model and an inhibitor of both CFU-E and BFU-E in the sera of patients with anemia and ESRD.[16] This inhibitor was partially removed by hemodialysis.[16]

Radtke and colleagues[17] found indirect evidence of an inhibitor of erythropoiesis in adult patients on chronic hemodialysis. Hematocrits and Ep levels were measured in 44 adult patients immediately before regular hemodialysis was instituted and 3 to 27 months later while the patients were still on regular hemodialysis. Hematocrits increased during chronic hemodialysis from 22% to 29%, (p < 0.01) and Ep concentrations fell during chronic hemodialysis from 509 mU/ml to 182 mU/ml (p < 0.001). Thus, the improvement in anemia was not a consequence of increased Ep production nor blood transfusion but was most likely due to the elimination of an inhibitor of erythropoiesis by hemodialysis.

Radtke and colleagues have further characterized the inhibition of erythropoiesis in patients with ESRD.[18] Their patient population consisted of eight adults with ESRD. The patients were studied immediately before regular hemodialysis was initiated. The mean BUN was 177 mg/dl; serum creatinine level, 24 mg/dl; and hematocrit, 16% for the group of patients. Sera from these patients significantly inhibited (p < 0.01) CFU-E formation in fetal mouse liver cell cultures when compared to the effect of ten pooled normal human sera. In vitro dialysis of the uremic sera for 48 hours using a dialysis membrane with an exclusion limit of 3500 daltons resulted in a significant (p < 0.01) reduction in the inhibition of CFU-E. Pooled dialysate of the uremic sera after freeze-drying and readjusting to the original volume of the uremic serum samples demonstrated an inhibitory effect on CFU-E formation similar to that in the predialysis sera. These observations have been extended to human bone marrow cultures. Sera from uremic patients were added to human bone marrow cultures and significantly inhibited human CFU-E formation.[19] Thus, uremic sera inhibit CFU-E formation in fetal mouse liver cell cultures and human bone marrow cultures, proving the validity of fetal mouse liver cell technique in testing inhibitors of erythropoiesis.

**Polyamines and Suppression of Erythropoiesis.** Radtke and colleagues have also demonstrated that uremic serum dialysates applied to biogel columns, which permitted the assessment of molecular weight fractions of uremic sera down to 100 daltons, contained an inhibitor of erythropoiesis (CFU-E) in the low molecular weight range.[18] Polyamines which are in the 200-dalton range have been found to be significantly elevated in the serum of uremic patients[20, 21] and have

been reported to suppress cell proliferation.[22] The serum level of the polyamines putrescine, spermidine, and spermine have been quantitated using high performance liquid chromatography. Serum was collected from 12 subjects with advanced renal insufficiency whose mean serum creatinine level was 9.2 mg/dl and whose hematocrit was 29%. Of all polyamines, spermine concentration was the only one significantly elevated (p < 0.01) compared with that in normal subjects. The mean spermine concentration was approximately 9 times higher than that of normal controls.[19] The major endogenous mammalian polyamines, spermine and spermidine, were tested in the fetal mouse liver cell culture and spermine was tested in human marrow cultures to determine whether they might elicit an inhibitory effect on erythroid colony formation. Both spermine and spermidine produced a dose-related inhibition of erythroid colony formation in fetal mouse liver preparations, and spermine produced such an effect in human bone marrow cultures.[18]

In an attempt to evaluate whether spermine present in sera from uremic patients was the only inhibitor of erythroid colony formation, specific spermine antiserum was added to the in vitro test system. Spermine antiserum completely neutralized the inhibitory activity of each of eight different uremic sera. Spermine antiserum added to normal human serum and normal rabbit serum did not influence CFU-E formation in the fetal mouse liver cell culture.[18]

In a long-term animal experiment the effect of spermine continuously infused into the peritoneal cavity was investigated. Spermine at a rate of 0.5 micromoles/hour was continuously infused into the peritoneal cavity by a micropump in five normal rats for three weeks. Before the infusion was started, the mean hematocrit was 50% and after three weeks had fallen to 43% (p < 0.01). The hematocrit in five sham-operated controls decreased from 50 to 46% (p = n.s.). Thus, a mild anemia was initiated in normal rats by continuous spermine administration, which was normochromic and normocytic in nature, resembling the anemia of CRF.[19] These observations provide evidence that spermine may be responsible for the inhibition of erythropoiesis in patients with the anemia of CRF.

**Effect of Parathyroid Hormone on Erythropoiesis.** Elevated levels of parathyroid hormone (PTH) are nearly always present in patients with ESRD.[23, 24] There is indirect evidence that the high levels of PTH found in these patients may contribute to the anemia of ESRD. Zingraff and colleagues reported that 18 patients who were on chronic hemodialysis had a significant ($p < 0.001$) increase in hematocrit after subtotal parathyroidectomy.[23] In a smaller subgroup of these patients, serial bone marrow biopsies showed a decrease in bone marrow fibrosis and a corresponding increase in hematocrit. Podjarny and colleagues also reported improvement in the degree of anemia after parathyroidectomy in patients with ESRD who were on hemodialysis.[24] Eighteen patients had parathyroidectomies and 44% (10 patients) had a rise in hematocrit following surgery. Since elevated levels of PTH stimulate myelofibrosis, the decrease in PTH resulting from parathyroidectomy may result in less myelofibrosis and an increase in bone marrow mass. Comparison was also made by Podjarny[24] between the degree of anemia (hematocrit) and serum PTH, calcium, phosphorus, and alkaline phosphatase levels in 96 patients on chronic hemodialysis. There was no correlation between the degree of anemia and these indices of secondary hyperparathyroidism.

More direct evidence for an effect of PTH on erythropoiesis has been reported by Meytes and colleagues.[25] Test systems to determine the effect of PTH on erythropoiesis included human peripheral blood and mouse bone marrow burst-forming unit-erythroid (BFU-E) and mouse bone marrow erythroid colony-forming cells. When 1-84 bPTH was added to the cell culture medium, it significantly ($p < 0.01$) reduced mouse BFU-E. There was also a significant ($p < 0.01$) effect of 1-84 bPTH on human peripheral blood BFU-E when PTH concentration was greater than 1 U/ml in the culture medium. The amino terminal fragment of PTH, 1-34 bPTH, did not inhibit mouse or human BFU-E. Mouse marrow CFU-E colonies were not inhibited by 1-84 bPTH 20 U/ml in the culture media. Ep when added to the culture medium was able to reverse the effects of 1-84 bPTH 7.5 U/ml, on human peripheral blood BFU-E. When the concentration of Ep was increased from 0.67 to 1.90 U/ml, the human peripheral blood BFU-E was normal even in the presence of 1-84 bPTH 7.5 U/ml. The same culture medium with 1-84 bPTH but without Ep resulted in a reduction of BFU-E to 33% of control value.

These results by Meytes[25] indicate an inhibitory effect of the intact PTH molecule or a C-terminal fragment larger than the 53 to 84 moiety on erythropoiesis at the level of the BFU-E but not CFU-E. The levels of PTH used in the culture medium are similar to blood levels found in ESRD patients. There was also a dynamic interplay between PTH levels and Ep levels in these experiments.

On the other hand, other investigators have reported that PTH actually produced dose-dependent stimulation of erythropoiesis in fetal mouse liver cell cultures at 10 to 100 times normal serum levels, and 240 times normal PTH levels were required to inhibit heme synthesis.[26] These findings cast doubt on the hypothesis that PTH is directly responsible for the anemia of uremia. This stimulatory effect of PTH at one dose and inhibitory effect at extremely high doses was confirmed by Levi et al[27] and Zevin et al.[28] Therefore, it would appear that the role of PTH as a uremic toxin in the mechanisms of anemia in CRF has yet to be elucidated.

**Shortened Red Cell Life Span.** Even though the principal cause of anemia of renal insufficiency seems to be a failure of erythropoiesis, which is due, at least in part, to inadequate production of Ep by the diseased kidney, another factor contributing to the anemia is a shortened red cell life span.[29-31] Hemolysis, which contributes to the anemia of renal disease, appears to be due to an extracorpuscular hemolytic factor and not to any abnormality in the red cell itself. Red blood cells from patients with renal disease have been transfused into healthy recipients and appear to have a normal life span. However, when normal red cells have been transfused into uremic recipients their life span has been found to be shortened. The hemolysis is usually mild or may not be present at all until the development of ESRD.

## EFFECT OF DIALYSIS ON THE ANEMIA OF ESRD

Chronic dialysis in adults has been shown to improve the degree of anemia in various studies when compared with the level of anemia before regular dialysis was initiated. Radtke[17] studied 42 adult patients with ESRD immediately before regular hemodialysis was initiated. None had been bilaterally nephrectomized. At that time the mean hematocrit was 22%. After 3 to 27 months of regular hemodialysis, which consisted of three 6- to 8-hour treatments per week, the hematocrit had increased to 29% ($p < 0.01$ compared with predialysis). During this time no blood transfusions or androgens were given. Similar studies have not been done in children.

Continuous ambulatory peritoneal dialysis (CAPD) has also been shown to improve the degree of anemia in adults and children.[32-36] Nolph et al[32] reported that CAPD led to a significant (p < 0.05) improvement in hematocrit after six months of CAPD compared to the hematocrit before CAPD was initiated. Amair et al[33] reported on CAPD in diabetics with ESRD. Twenty diabetics were studied before and after the initiation of CAPD. None had been on dialysis prior to initiation of CAPD. The hemoglobin increased from a mean of 8.7 gm/dl to 10.6 gm/dl (p < 0.005) after one year of CAPD. Baum and colleagues[36] compared the degree of anemia in 16 children receiving hemodialysis to that in 20 children receiving CAPD. Both groups had similar ages, body weights, and length of time on either mode of dialysis. The mean hematocrit was 22% in patients receiving CAPD and 20% in patients receiving hemodialysis (p < 0.05).[36] Unfortunately, in none of these studies was red blood cell mass measured. Thus, the degree of anemia may not actually have been influenced by the type of dialysis used, since both the hematocrit and hemoglobin may have increased in patients receiving CAPD because of a decrease in plasma volume.

## MANAGEMENT OF ANEMIA IN ESRD

This review has concentrated on the characteristics of the anemia of ESRD, which is hypoproliferative, normocytic, and normochromic, with inadequate Ep for the degree of anemia. Other causes of anemia must, however, be recognized. These include: (1) accelerated red blood cell destruction, (2) reduced body stores of iron, (3) deficiency states of water-soluble vitamins, and (4) deficiency of folic acid. Additionally, children experience a greater relative blood loss from hemodialysis (small amounts of blood left in hemodialyzer and tubing) than do adults when compared to body size.

At the initiation of dialysis the hematocrit, hemoglobin, red blood cell indices, serum ferritin level, and reticulocyte count should be measured and a peripheral blood smear examined. If there is evidence of accelerated red cell destruction from the red cell smear and reticulocyte count, then appropriate studies such as Coombs' test, hemoglobin electrophoresis, and haptoglobin concentration need to be obtained.

A deficiency of iron and vitamins is common in patients whose intake of these and other nutrients is impaired owing to anorexia, depression, and restricted dietary intake. Most children should be placed on a multivitamin preparation. When evidence of diminished iron stores is present, an oral iron supplement should be prescribed until the anemia is corrected.

Throughout dialysis for ESRD, the hematocrit, hemoglobin, and red blood cell indices need to be measured on a monthly basis. Unusual changes in the degree of anemia or red blood cell indices should be investigated to determine the cause. Iron deficiency may develop during dialysis therapy even in patients receiving adequate amounts of oral iron. The best indicator of this is the serum ferritin concentration. Bell and colleagues studied 55 adult patients on hemodialysis for an average of four years.[37] The average daily iron intake was 189 mg of elemental iron. Bone marrow specimens were obtained from each patient and the hemosiderin content of bone marrow was graded semiquantitatively and compared with hematocrit, red cell volume, serum iron level, transferrin saturation, and serum ferritin level. Bone marrow iron stores correlated best (0.884) with the serum ferritin level but not as strongly with the serum iron level (0.543) or hematocrit (0.312). Thus, iron deficiency may develop even in patients on an adequate iron intake, and the serum ferritin level is the best indicator of bone marrow iron stores. The serum ferritin level should be regularly measured. The frequency needed is unknown and probably every four months is reasonable. Changes in red blood cell indices suggestive of iron deficiency require investigation of this possibility, including measurement of the serum ferritin and iron levels.

Hemodialysis removes folic acid from the blood. Thus, it is rational to administer folic acid orally, 1 mg daily or after each hemodialysis episode. The exact requirement of folic acid in dialysis patients has not been determined, but this dose of folic acid has been shown to prevent deficiency.

The mainstay of treatment of the anemia of ESRD is red blood cell transfusion. The transfusion needs of children are highly variable and relative indications include (1) fatigue, (2) chest pain, (3) reduction in exercise tolerance, (4) evidence of congestive heart failure in association with severe anemia, and (5) anorexia. It is safest to give transfusions during dialysis so that excessive plasma volume can be removed to prevent or manage hypertension or congestive heart failure. Transfusion is indicated when the hematocrit approaches 20% in the absence of specific symptoms. Transfusion requirements in children undergoing CAPD are less than those of children receiving hemodialysis.[36]

## SUMMARY

The anemia of ESRD is multifactorial. The most important factor is a relative deficiency of Ep. Erythropoietin given to animals with renal insufficiency has significantly improved their anemia. Inhibitors of erythropoiesis also contribute to the development of anemia. Inhibitors have been best demonstrated using in vitro cell culture systems containing the sera of humans with CRF and ESRD. The improvement in the anemia of ESRD with hemodialysis and sometimes dramatically with CAPD suggests that inhibitors may play a secondary role as causal factors in the anemia of ESRD.

## REFERENCES

1. Erslev AJ, Shapiro SS: Hematologic aspects of renal failure. *In:* Earley LE, Gottschalk CW (eds), Strauss and Welts Diseases of the Kidney. Boston, Little, Brown and Co, 1979, p 277.
2. Combined report on regular dialysis and transplantation of children in Europe, 1979. Proc Eur Dial Transplant Assoc 17:87, 1980.
3. Ulmer HE, Greiner H, Schuler HW, Scharer K: Cardiovascular impairment and physical work capacity in children with chronic renal failure. Acta Paediatr Scand 67:43, 1978.
4. Fisher JW, Radtke HW, Rege AB: Mechanism of the anemia of chronic renal failure. *In:* Dunn CDR (ed), Current Concepts in Erythropoiesis. Sussex, England, John Wiley and Sons, Ltd, 1983 (in press).
5. Fisher JW, Busuttil R, Rodgers GM, et al: The kidney and erythropoietin production: A review. *In:* Nakao K, Fisher JW, Takaku F (eds), Erythropoiesis. Tokyo, University of Tokyo Press, 1975, p 315.
6. Eschback JW, Detter JC, Adamson JW: Physiologic studies in normal and uremic sheep: II. Changes in erythropoiesis and oxygen transport. Kidney Int 18:732, 1980.
7. Naughton BA, Kaplan SM, Roy M, et al: Hepatic regeneration and erythropoietin production in the rat. Science 196:301, 1977.
8. Radtke HW, Claussner A, Erbes PM, et al: Serum erythropoietin concentration in chronic renal fail-

9. Caro J, Brown S, Miller O, et al: Erythropoietin levels in uremic nephric and anephric patients. J Lab Clin Med 93:449, 1979.
10. Lertora J, Dargon JL, Rege AB, et al: Studies on a radioimmunoassay for human erythropoietin. J Lab Clin Med 86:140, 1975.
11. Van Stone JC, Max P: Effect of erythropoietin on anemia of peritoneally dialyzed anephric rats. Kidney Int 15:370, 1979.
12. Eschbach JW, Mladenovic J, Adamson JW: Erythropoietin action in chronic renal failure (Abst). Kidney Int 21:260, 1982.
13. Wallner SF, Kwinick JE, Ward HP, et al: The anemia of chronic renal failure and chronic diseases: in vitro studies of erythropoiesis. Blood 47:561, 1976.
14. Moriyama Y, Fisher JW: Effects of erythropoietin on erythroid colony formation in uremic rabbit bone marrow cultures. Blood 45:659, 1975.
15. Ohno Y, Fisher JW: Inhibition of bone marrow erythroid colony forming cells (CFU-E) by serum from chronic anemic uremic rabbits. Proc Soc Exp Biol Med. 156:56, 1977.
16. Ohno Y, Rege AB, Fisher JW, et al: Inhibitors of erythroid colony-forming cells (CFU-E and BFU-E) in sera of azotemic patients with anemia of renal disease. J Lab Clin Med 92:916, 1978.
17. Radtke HW, Frei U, Erbes PM, et al: Improving anemia by hemodialysis: effect on serum erythropoietin. Kidney Int 17:382, 1980.
18. Radtke HW, Rege AB, LaMarche MB, et al: Identification of spermine as an inhibitor of erythropoiesis in patients with chronic renal failure. J Clin Invest 67:1623, 1981.
19. Radtke HW, Scheuermann EH, Desser H: Polyamine induced in vivo and in vitro suppression of erythropoiesis in uremia. Haematologia 1983 (in press).
20. Bergstrom J, Furst P: Uremic toxins. Kidney Int 8:59, 1978.
21. Swendseid M, Panaque M, Kopple JD: Polyamine concentrations in red cells and urine of patients with chronic renal failure. Life Science 26:533, 1980.
22. Grahl WA, Changus JW, Pitot AC: The effect of spermine and spermidine on proliferation in vitro of fibroblasts from normal and cystic fibrosis patients. Pediatr Res 12:531, 1976.
23. Zingraff J, Druke T, Marie P, et al: Anemia and secondary hyperparathyroidism. Arch Intern Med 138:1650, 1978.
24. Podjarny E, Rathaus M, Korzets Z, et al: Is anemia of chronic renal failure related to secondary hyperparathyroidism? Arch Intern Med 141:453, 1981.
25. Meytes D, Bogin E, Ma A, et al: Effect of parathyroid hormone on erythropoiesis. J Clin Invest 67:1263, 1981.
26. Dunn CDR, Trent D: The effect of parathyroid hormone on erythropoiesis in serum free cultures of fetal mouse liver cells. Proc Soc Exp Biol Med 166:556, 1981.
27. Levi JH, Bessler H, Hirsch I, et al: Increased RNA and heme synthesis in mouse erythroid precursors by parathyroid hormone. Acta Haematol 61:125, 1979.
28. Zevin D, Levi J, Bessler H, et al: Effect of parathy-

roid hormone and 1,25-dihydroxyvitamin $D_3$ on RNA and heme synthesis by erythroid precursors. Mineral Electrolyte Metab. 6:125, 1981.

29. Loge JP, Lange RD, Moore CV: Characterization of the anemia associated with chronic renal insufficiency. Am J Med 24:4, 1958.

30. Joske RA, McAlister JM, Prankerd TAJ: Isotope investigation of red cell production and destruction in chronic renal disease (Abst). Clin Res 4:511, 1956.

31. Shaw AB: Haemolysis in chronic renal failure. Br Med J 2:213, 1967.

32. Nolph K, Sorkin M, Rubin J, et al: Continuous ambulatory peritoneal dialysis: three-year experience at one center. Ann Intern Med 92:609, 1980.

33. Amair P, Khanna R, Leibele B, et al: Continuous ambulatory peritoneal dialysis in diabetics with end-stage renal disease. N Engl J Med 306:625, 1982.

34. Lacke C, Senekjian HO, Knight TF, et al: Twelve months' experience with continuous ambulatory and intermittent peritoneal dialysis. Arch Intern Med 141:187, 1981.

35. Zappacosta AR, Caro J, Erslev A: Normalization of hematocrit in patients with end-stage renal disease on continuous ambulatory peritoneal dialysis. Am J Med 72:53, 1982.

36. Baum M, Powell D, Calvin S, et al: Continuous ambulatory peritoneal dialysis in children: comparison with hemodialysis. N Engl J Med 307:1537, 1982.

37. Bell JD, Kincaid WR, Morgan RG, et al: Serum ferritin assay and bone-marrow iron stores in patients on maintenance hemodialysis. Kidney Int 17:242, 1980.

# 26

# Pulmonary Function in ESRD

*Daniel V. Schidlow, M.D.*

Respiratory function can be deranged in end stage renal disease (ESRD) as a result of muscle weakness, congestive heart failure, calcium deposition in the lung, viral and bacterial respiratory infections, and several other conditions known to occur in patients with chronic renal failure.

After an initial description of the techniques used to evaluate pulmonary function, this chapter will briefly discuss the effects of chronic renal failure and dialysis on respiratory physiology. While this subject has been studied relatively well in adults, little information concerning children is available. Some of the data presented here regarding pediatric patients are the product of ongoing investigations and are largely preliminary. Each section of this chapter will start with a brief review of the available information in adults, followed by that concerning children.

## EVALUATION OF PULMONARY FUNCTION

Standard pulmonary function testing in most laboratories includes the measurement of lung volumes and capacities, analysis of air flows, and determination of diffusion capacity. Patient understanding and cooperation with the test is essential to obtain meaningful data; usually, children under 6 years of age are unable to satisfactorily perform the necessary maneuvers. Measurements of pulmonary function are expressed in units of volume and time (i.e., liters, liters per second) and compared with normal standards for height. The usual manner in which results are reported is in percentages of pre-

dicted normal (in order to facilitate comparisons between individuals of different size).

**Lung Volumes and Capacities.** The "physiologic size" of the lung is assessed by the measurement of volumes and combinations of volumes called "capacities" (Table 26–1).

Pulmonary disorders give rise to two functional patterns which may occur singly or in combination (Fig. 26–1):

1. *Restrictive disease,* characterized by reduced lung volumes, particularly vital capacity (VC) and total lung capacity (TLC). This condition is caused by a loss of functioning parenchyma, such as in lung fibrosis, or by

**Table 26–1. LUNG VOLUMES AND CAPACITIES**

**Volumes**
1. *Tidal Volume* (TV) is the volume of gas inspired or expired in each respiratory cycle.
2. *Inspiratory Reserve Volume* (IRV) is the maximal amount of gas that can be inspired from the end of a normal inspiration.
3. *Expiratory Reserve Volume* (ERV) is the maximal volume of gas expired from the end of a normal expiration.
4. *Residual Volume* (RV) is the volume of gas remaining in the lung at the end of a maximal expiration.

**Capacities***
1. *Total Lung Capacity* (TLC) is the amount of gas contained in the lung at the end of a maximal inspiration.
2. *Vital Capacity* (VC) is the maximal volume of gas that can be exhaled from the lungs following a maximal inspiration.
3. *Inspiratory Capacity* (IC) is the maximal volume of gas inspired from the resting expiratory level.
4. *Functional Residual Capacity* (FRC) is the volume of gas remaining in the lungs after a normal expiration.

*Each capacity comprises two or more volumes.

383

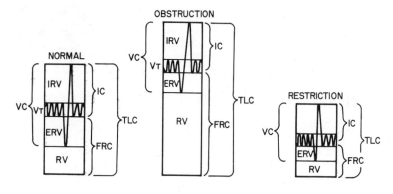

**Figure 26–1.** Lung volumes and capacities—patterns of abnormality. Obstruction results in increase in residual volume and total lung capacity. Restriction results in overall reduction in lung volumes. (Adapted after Netter).

nonpulmonary conditions that cause mechanical impediment to lung inflation, such as chest deformities, neuromuscular diseases, or severe ascites.

2. *Obstructive disease,* characterized by increased TLC and residual volume (RV). Obstruction to air flow, particularly on expiration, due to narrowing of the lumen of the airways because of edema, secretions, or bronchospasm, results in decreased expiratory reserve volume (ERV) and characteristically an increased TLC and RV.

**Analysis of Air Flows.** The presence and magnitude of airway obstruction is detected by measuring the amount of air exhaled during a forced maximal expiration following a maximal inspiration. This is called the forced vital capacity (FVC) maneuver. In normal individuals, this maneuver lasts for 3 or 4 seconds and approximately 80% of the total volume is exhaled in the first second. This measurement, which is called the forced expiratory volume in one second ($FEV_1$), is also expressed as a percentage of the total FVC ($FEV_1/FVC\%$) and represents a good

measure of patency or obstruction of the airways. By drawing a straight line between the points where 25% and 75% of the FVC have been exhaled and prolonging this line so that it encompasses one second, the forced expiratory flow 25–75%, also called maximum mid-expiratory flow rate (MMEFR), can be obtained. This value represents the flow through small airways (Fig. 26–2).

A more sensitive test to detect airway obstruction is the flow-volume curve, which represents the continuous plotting of air flow against lung volumes. In this manner, an instantaneous determination of flow at a given degree of lung inflation can be obtained. Maximal flows ($\dot{V}_{max}$) at 25 and 50% of VC represent the degree of patency of small airways (Fig. 26–3).

**Diffusion Capacity for Carbon Monoxide (DLCO).** This test measures the amount of known gas (carbon monoxide) entering the blood through the alveolar-capillary units. During the single breath technique used in our studies, the patient inhales a gas mixture containing a known concentration of CO and

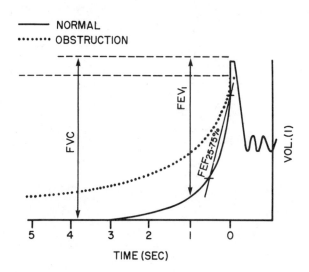

**Figure 26–2.** Forced vital capacity maneuvers and expiratory flow rates. Obstructive disease results in decreases in the volume of air exhaled per second, with the resulting prolongation of the curve. In restrictive disease the curve is reduced in size but not prolonged.

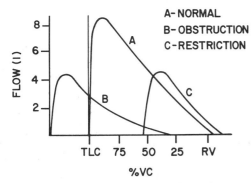

**Figure 26-3.** Maximal expiratory flow-volume curve. Obstructive disease results in breathing at higher volumes owing to lung hyperinflation and sharp reductions in flows, especially at lower lung volumes. Restrictive disease is manifested by uniformly decreased flows, resulting in a curve of normal shape but reduced size.

holds his breath. Carbon monoxide is an inert, easily measured gas with great affinity for hemoglobin; therefore, once in contact with the cell, it is taken up very quickly. Factors which determine the DLCO include the total area available for diffusion, the thickness of the diffusion path, and the amount of hemoglobin available for binding. Decreases in DLCO may be due to loss of alveolar-capillary units, fibrosis or thickening of pulmonary interstitium, and anemia.

## PULMONARY FUNCTION ABNORMALITIES IN PATIENTS UNDERGOING MAINTENANCE DIALYSIS

Spirometric determinations are normal in many patients with renal failure.[1, 2] Fluid overload, congestive heart failure, pleuropericarditis, and lung fibrosis, frequently seen in ESRD, can result in decreases in lung volumes, especially VC.[1-8] In one study VC was found to drop to as low as 40% of predicted normal in patients with congestive heart failure.[4] While restoration of fluid balance toward normal tended to correct the abnormalities in these individuals, pulmonary function measurements remained below expected normal values.

Accumulation of fluid in the lung also causes loss of elastic recoil and preferential edema in the dependent areas of the lung; the resulting physiologic defects include decreases in ventilation and perfusion of the lung bases as well as trapping of air behind closed small airways.[3, 7] Significant increases in MMEFR and ventilation to previously un-

deraerated areas following dialysis has been interpreted as an indication that air flow through small airways is impaired in ESRD patients who are in positive water balance prior to dialysis.[3]

We studied the pulmonary function of eight adolescents with ESRD, ages 12 to 16 years, undergoing maintenance hemodialysis, and found several abnormalities.[2] Five of the eight patients studied prior to dialysis had normal lung volumes. VC and TLC ranged from 55 to 82% and 62 to 84% of predicted normal, respectively, in three subjects. Evidence of small airway obstruction was also found in five children in the same group; mean flows at 25% and 50% of VC were 55% and 65% of predicted normal, respectively.

The most consistent abnormality in respiratory function found in ESRD is the impairment of diffusion capacity of carbon monoxide (DLCO).[1, 3, 5, 9] Reduction in DLCO is directly correlated with decrease in red cell mass, a constant finding in patients with ESRD. In order to determine whether the cause for the decrease in DLCO is anemia alone or whether other factors are also present, it is possible to calculate DLCO using a correction factor that takes into account the concentration of hemoglobin.[10] In many ESRD patients, the calculated DLCO, once "corrected," reaches normal levels, while in others it remains abnormally low.[10] This finding suggests that other conditions such as interstitial pulmonary fibrosis may cause impaired gas transfer across alveolar-capillary membranes and reductions in DLCO in these individuals.[2, 10] In our population, DLCO was decreased in all patients (mean 42% of predicted); "corrected" values were normal in three patients and significantly diminished in the remaining five (mean 63.5% of predicted).[2]

The magnitude of diffusion defects and restrictive pulmonary abnormalities has been directly correlated with the severity of histopathologic changes in the lung in ESRD patients. Conger et al showed that increases in calcification and interalveolar thickening (fibrosis) correlate with decreases in lung volumes and DLCO measurements.[11] The pathologic changes are severe and irreversible and help explain the inability to correct functional defects in some patients even after improvement of anemia and fluid balance has occurred. Interestingly, the radiographic appearance of the lung in patients with ESRD can be entirely normal and shows no correlation whatsoever with the degree of histopathologic damage or functional impairment.[2, 11] Even though a wide range of variability and heterogeneity in structural and functional lung damage can be seen in ESRD patients, a clear-cut correlation between the extent of renal disease and the impairment in respiratory function has not been established.

## Changes Associated with Dialysis

The nature of the lung involvement will determine whether pulmonary function will be affected by dialysis. Since patterns of restrictive disease and diffusion impairment are largely due to irreversible changes in the pulmonary interstitium, lung volumes and DLCO tend to change little with dialysis. Exceptions to this trend are patients with severe fluid overload and congestive heart failure; in these instances, removal of excess water by dialysis usually results in significant increase in vital capacity.[4]

In our experience with adolescents with ESRD, hemodialysis did not result in significant changes in either spirometric values or DLCO.[12] This fact supports the notion that irreversible lung damage can be present in younger patients with ESRD as well, even though their disease may have had a shorter course than that of many adults.

Patterns of obstructive disease clearly can be affected by dialysis. The decrease in bronchiolar wall edema and the enhancement of air flow following removal of fluid is usually reflected in improvement of tests of small airway function such as MMEFR.[3] In our group, some patients responded to dialysis by improving their small airway flows, while others did not.[12] Again, the correction of fluid overload probably accounts for these results.

The introduction of large amounts of fluid into the abdominal cavity which occurs during peritoneal dialysis (PD) can induce mechanical impairment to respiration similar to that experienced by patients with ascites. The infusion of several liters of fluid into the peritoneum results in slight decreases in RV, FRC, and TLC,[13, 14] probably as a result of decreased diaphragmatic excursion in the presence of increased intraabdominal pressure. This effect is transitory, and pulmonary function values revert to the predialysis status once the dialysate fluid is withdrawn.[13, 14] Theoretically, at least, basal atelectasis and pneumonia are more likely to develop in patients undergoing frequent or continuous PD, especially if the patients remain in the supine position, suffer from peritonitis, and are weak or hypoventilate. Prophylactic measures, such as close monitoring of breathing patterns, incentive spirometry and chest physiotherapy, should be instituted in these situations. Studies of respiratory function in children undergoing PD are conspicuously absent.

**Dialysis-Induced Changes in Arterial Blood Gases and Acid-Base Balance.** The process of acetate-buffered hemodialysis almost uniformly alters acid-base homeostasis and blood oxygenation leading to hypoxemia. The latter has been explained on the basis of two major mechanisms: (1) leukocyte sequestration in lung capillaries causing areas of ventilation-perfusion mismatch[15–17] (this hypothesis has been challenged because both leukopenia and hypoxemia have been shown to occur during dialysis independently of each other[18]), and (2) decreased alveolar ventilation. Some studies have demonstrated an increase in oxygen consumption and decrease of $CO_2$ production in the lung because of loss of $CO_2$ from the blood into the dialysate. This results in hypoventilation because of decreased $CO_2$ stimulation of the respiratory center.[19–20] These changes are of lesser magnitude or do not occur when bicarbonate rather than acetate is used as a buffer.[21, 22]

When compared to the predialysis state, postdialysis pH is higher, frequently in the alkalemic range; arterial $CO_2$ tension ($PaCO_2$) is lower, and bicarbonate concentration is elevated.[23, 24] In children undergoing hemodialysis, Kaiser et al demonstrated that as plasma acetate increases during the procedure, $PaCO_2$ falls progressively, as does bicarbonate, albeit to a lesser extent, while pH becomes increasingly alkalemic.[25] Within one hour following discontinuation of the procedure, acetate is rapidly metabolized, bicarbonate levels increase sharply, $PaCO_2$ increases nearly to predialysis levels, and pH stabilizes in the alkalemic range (Fig. 26–4).

We have found a similar trend in our studies.[26] Furthermore, we observed a trend toward increased minute ventilation ($\dot{V}_E$) after dialysis on the basis of slightly larger tidal volumes ($\dot{V}_E = T_V \times$ respiratory rate). Mean tidal volumes were 248 and 288 ml while minute volumes were 5.8 and 6.21

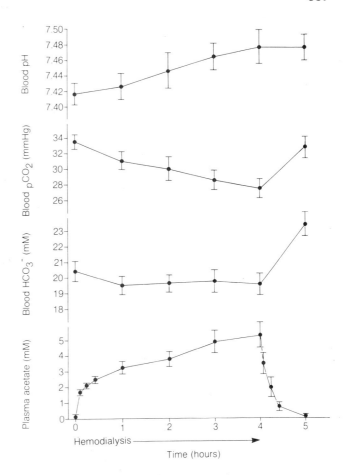

**Figure 26–4.** Acid-base and acetate changes during hemodialysis in children. (Data are means ± SEM.) (Reprinted from Kaigh et al, Kidney International 19:70–79, 1981, with permission).[25]

liters/minute before and after dialysis, respectively. A slight decrease in $PaCO_2$ from a mean of 32.4 mm Hg to 29.6 mm Hg was also observed. Others have also found that hyperventilation as well as respiratory and metabolic alkalosis may follow dialysis and suggested increased respiratory center sensitivity to $CO_2$ as a cause.[27] Similar alterations in acid base homeostasis have been recently reported to occur with acetate-buffered peritoneal dialysis.[28]

Some of the discrepancies noted between reports can be attributed to the small number of patients in each series, differences in buffer concentration in the dialysate, length and aggressiveness of the procedure, patient condition prior to dialysis, and age differences (children may metabolize acetate faster than adults[24]). Finally, an important source of differences may be the time at which measurements are obtained, since the first hour after discontinuation of dialysis is one of rapid metabolic changes.

## KIDNEY TRANSPLANTATION

Neither the short nor the long-term effects of this mode of therapy on pulmonary function have been adequately investigated in adults or children.

Increased maximum voluntary ventilation has been seen after successful renal transplantation.[5] This phenomenon may very well represent a measure of overall well-being and ability to endure a sustained effort rather than improvement in lung function. It is conceivable, however, that, as fluid and acid-base balance improves, some of the reversible defects of respiratory function will improve as well. Patients who receive renal transplants not only undergo long surgical procedures but also receive large doses of immunosuppressive drugs, may experience reactivation of latent pulmonary infections or suffer new ones, and, finally, may undergo rejection of their graft with generalized immunologic reaction; all these situations may result in added insult to the lung. Furthermore, it is to be expected that pulmonary parenchymal changes, fibrosis, and calcifications which have taken place over the years will not suffer regression even if kidney transplantation is successful. Hence, it is likely that the patient's respiratory status will improve after transplant only to the extent that its derangement is caused by fluid, electrolyte and acid-base abnormalities.

In summary, long-standing abnormalities in respiratory function characterize the course of patients with ESRD. Periodic pulmonary function testing and careful long-term assessment of the extent and rate of progression of lung damage in renal disease are needed in order to more clearly establish the clinical relevance of these findings. Greater knowledge of the effects of loss of renal function on pulmonary parenchyma and their role in the overall growth, development, and functional capabilities of children with ESRD may conceivably influence the choice of therapy or its timing. Furthermore, the effects of kidney transplantation and newer therapeutic modes such as continuous ambulatory peritoneal dialysis on respiratory function merit further evaluation by means of carefully conducted multidisciplinary investigations.

## REFERENCES

1. Lee HY, Stretton TB: The lungs in renal failure. Thorax 30:46, 1975.
2. Schidlow DV, Morgenstern BZ, Haas JM, Baluarte HJ: Pulmonary function in adolescents with chronic renal failure. Pediatr Res 17:389A, 1983 (Abstract).
3. Zidulka A, Despas PJ, Milic-Emili J, Anthoninsen NR: Pulmonary function with acute loss of excess lung water by hemodialysis in patients with chronic uremia. Am J Med 55:134, 1973.
4. Robson M, Levin S, Ravid M: Serial measurements of vital capacity in patients on chronic hemodialysis. Nephron 19:60, 1977.
5. Zarday Z, Benjamin JJ, Koerner SK, et al: Effects of hemodialysis and renal transplantation on pulmonary function. Chest 63:532, 1973.
6. Myersk BD, Rubin AE, Schey G, et al: Functional characteristics of the lung in chronic uremia treated by renal dialysis therapy. Chest 68:191, 1975.
7. Stanescu DC, Veriter C, DePlaey JF, et al: Lung function in chronic uraemia before and after removal of excess of fluid by haemodialysis. Clin Sci Mol Med 47:143, 1974.
8. Fairshter RD, Vaziri ND, Wilson AF, Fugl-Meyer AR: Respiratory physiology before and after he-

modialysis in chronic renal failure patients. Am J Med Sci 278:11, 1979.
9. Forman DW, Ayers LN, Miller WC: Pulmonary diffusing capacity in chronic renal failure. Br J Dis Chest 75:81, 1981.
10. Dinakara P, Blumenthal WS, Johnston RF, et al: The effect of anemia on pulmonary diffusing capacity with derivation of a correcting equation. Am Rev Resp Dis 102:965, 1970.
11. Conger JD, Hammond WS, Alfrey AC, et al: Pulmonary calcification in chronic dialysis patients. Clinical and pathologic studies. Ann Intern Med 83:303, 1975.
12. Schidlow DV, Morgenstern BZ, et al: Unpublished observations.
13. Ahluwalia M, Ishikawa S, Gellman M, et al: Pulmonary functions during peritoneal dialysis. Clin Nephrol 18:251, 1982.
14. Epstein SW, Inouye T, Robson M, Oreofoulos DG: Effect of peritoneal dialysis fluid on ventilatory function. Perit Dial Bull 2:120, 1982.
15. Craddock PR, Fehr J, Brigham KL, et al: Complement and leukocyte-mediated pulmonary dysfunction in hemodialysis. N Engl J Med 296:769, 1977.
16. Bischel MD, Scole BG, Mohler JG: Evidence for pulmonary microembolization during hemodialysis. Chest 67:333, 1978.
17. Torem M, Gaffret JA, Kaplow LS: Pulmonary bed sequestration of neutrophils during hemodialysis. Blood 36:337, 1970.
18. Dumler F, Levin NW: Leukopenia and hypoxemia. Unrelated effects of hemodialysis. Arch Intern Med 139:1103, 1979.
19. Aurigemma NM, Feldman NT, Gottlieb M, et al: Arterial oxygenation during hemodialysis. N Engl J Med 297:871, 1977.
20. Dolan MJ, Whipp BJ, Davidson WE, et al: Hypopnea associated with acetate hemodialysis: carbon dioxide-flow-dependent ventilation. N Engl J Med 305:72, 1981.
21. Eiser AR, Jayamanne D, Kokseng C, et al: Contrasting alterations in pulmonary gas exchange during acetate and bicarbonate hemodialysis. Am J Nephrol 2:123, 1982.
22. Ikeda T, Hirasawa Y: Effect of acetate upon arterial gases. J Dial 3:135, 1979.
23. Ernest DL, Sadler JH, Ingram RH, Macon EJ: Acid base balance in chronic hemodialysis. Trans Am Soc Artif Intern Organs 14:434, 1968.
24. Weller JM, Swan RC, Merrill JP: Changes in acid-base balance of uremic patients during hemodialysis. J Clin Invest 32:729, 1953.
25. Kaiser BA, Potter DE, Bryant RE, et al: Acid-base changes and acetate metabolism during routine and high-efficiency hemodialysis in children. Kidney Int 19:70, 1981.
26. Schidlow DV, Morgenstern BZ, Haas JM, Baluarte HJ: Ventilatory and acid-base changes following hemodialysis in adolescents. Pediatr Res 17:389(A), 1983 (Abstract).
27. Hamilton RW, Epstein PE, Henderson LW, et al: Control of breathing in uremia: ventilatory response to CO2 after hemodialysis. J Appl Physiol 41:216, 1976.
28. La Greca G, Biasiolo S, Chiaramonte S, et al: Acid-base balance in peritoneal dialysis. Clin Nephrol 16:1, 1981.

# Liver Problems Associated with ESRD in Children

*Robert S. Fennell, III, M.D.*
*Joel M. Andres, M.D.*
*Eduardo H. Garin, M.D.*
*Abdollah Iravani, M.D.*
*George A. Richard, M.D.*

The association between liver dysfunction and ESRD is well known. Hepatic fibrosis and cystic disease of the liver are associated with polycystic and dysplastic kidneys in several congenital syndromes;[1-5] chronic active liver disease occurs in patients with glomerulonephritis;[6-10] and fulminant liver failure may produce kidney failure (hepatorenal syndrome).[11-12] This chapter will consider those liver diseases which are noted in children with ESRD.

The liver in patients with ESRD has certain typical patterns of injury to noxious stimuli of toxic or immunologic origin. The etiology of liver dysfunction is often difficult to determine and may be multifactorial. A broad spectrum of response is encountered, from asymptomatic elevation of the serum transaminase levels secondary to mild hepatocyte membrane damage to overt hepatonecrosis. Acute viral hepatitis is characterized by parenchymal lymphocytic infiltration, hepatocyte vacuolization, and nonspecific cell necrosis. This is usually a self-limiting process, but may lead to massive hepatic necrosis. Acute cholestatic hepatitis and the rarer granulomatous hepatitis are also observed in patients with ESRD; the latter tissue reaction consists of mononuclear cell infiltration with random granulomata noted within the hepatic lobules (Fig. 27–1). Chronic persistent hepatitis or "triaditis" is characterized by the lymphocytic infiltration of portal tracts with minimal infiltration of the parenchyma, and preservation of the hepatocyte limiting plates (Fig. 27–2). It is usually benign but may progress to chronic active hepatitis. Chronic active hepatitis is a histologic lesion with lymphocytic and plasma cell infiltration involving portal tracts and parenchyma. Pathologic findings consist of piecemeal hepatocellular necrosis, disruption of the portal tract limiting plate, and bridging fibrosis (Fig. 27–3), which may be a precirrhotic lesion. Viruses, drugs, other toxins, and immunologic mechanisms are implicated as causes of these diseases.

The following nonspecific hepatic changes are also seen in patients with ESRD: hemosiderosis (iron deposition in hepatocytes and Kupffer cells) in patients on hemodialysis receiving frequent blood transfusions, and steatosis (fatty infiltration of liver) in dialyzed or transplanted patients after receiving certain antibacterial and immunosuppressive agents. Peliosis hepatitis is an uncommon liver abnormality consisting of endothelial-lined, blood-filled cavities, randomly distributed in the liver parenchyma, which may be associated with immunosuppression in the renal transplant recipient. Neoplastic degeneration of the liver with histologic features typical of hepatoma is reported in transplant recipients.[13-15]

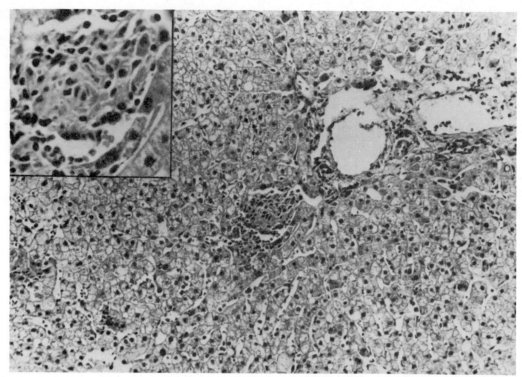

**Figure 27–1.** Mild mononuclear cell infiltrate involving hepatic lobule with granuloma adjacent to portal tract (hematoxylin-eosin, ×100); inset: detailed enlargement of noncaseating granuloma (×250). (From Fennell RS III, Andres JM, Pfaff WW, Richard GA: Liver dysfunction in children and adolescents during hemodialysis and after renal transplantation. Pediatrics 67:855, 1981.)

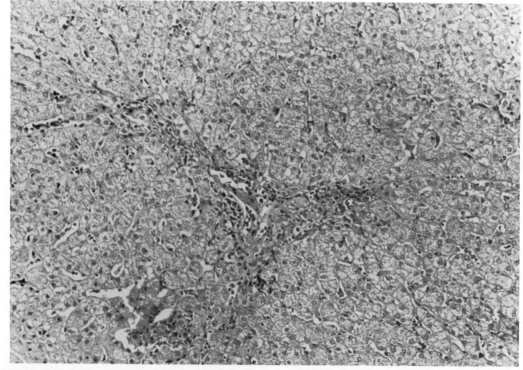

**Figure 27–2.** Liver section showing mild mononuclear cell infiltrate in portal tract ("triaditis") with minimal lobular inflammation (hematoxylin-eosin, ×100). (From Fennell RS III, Andres JM, Pfaff WW, Richard GA: Liver dysfunction in children and adolescents during hemodialysis and after renal transplantation. Pediatrics 67:855, 1981.)

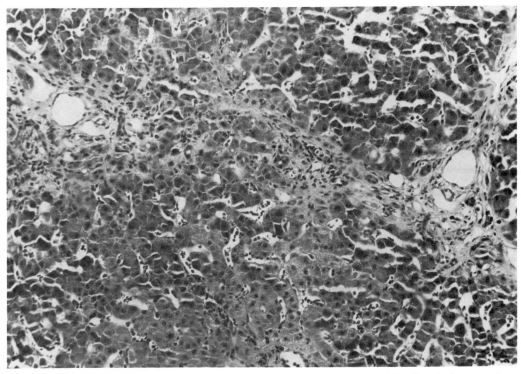

**Figure 27–3.** Mild portal tract infiltrate with patchy liver cell necrosis and early bridging fibrosis (hematoxylin-eosin, ×100). (From Fennell RS III, Andres JM, Pfaff WW, Richard GA: Liver dysfunction in children and adolescents during hemodialysis and after renal transplantation. Pediatrics 67:855, 1981.)

## VIRUSES

*Hepatotoxic viruses* are the most common cause for the hepatic dysfunction seen in the patient on hemodialysis or after kidney transplantation. Hepatitis B virus (HVB), cytomegalic inclusion disease virus (CMV), Epstein-Barr virus (EBV), non-A, non-B hepatitis virus, hepatitis A virus (HAV), herpes simplex virus type I (HSV₁), and varicella-zoster virus are most often implicated. The incidence of these viral infections is difficult to determine, since the signs and symptoms of hepatitis, especially in the hemodialysis patient, are generally mild and nonspecific.[16-20] Jaundice is usually absent. However, patients with minimal or no symptoms can have advanced lesions on liver biopsy.[20-23] Patients on hemodialysis may be chronic carriers of viruses, and thus be significant reservoirs of infection for the general population. Transmission of these viral infections to medical personnel, family members of the patient, and occasionally to other ESRD patients may lead to severe hepatitis.

Therefore, it is essential to undertake routine surveillance for persistent liver enzyme elevations and evidence of viral antigens and antibodies.[16, 24]

Occult viral hepatitis in patients undergoing hemodialysis may become clinically apparent following renal transplantation. Degos et al., in a prospective study, found that 40% of transplant recipients had histologic evidence of hepatitis at surgery, and on a rebiopsy three years later the prevalence had increased by only 15%.[25] The prevalence of liver disease reported in retrospective surveys of patients receiving transplants is 4% to 50%, depending upon the author's definition of hepatitis and whether patients with asymptomatic transaminasemia are included.[26-37] The clinical course of these patients is usually benign, but some may develop cirrhosis and hepatic failure.[30, 31, 38] In several reports, death of transplant recipients is attributed to hepatitis.[29, 31, 39] The susceptibility of these patients to infection may be related to the immunodeficiency of ESRD and to the antirejection regimens employed in the kidney allograft recipient.[40-43]

## Hepatitis B Virus

Hepatitis B virus is reported to be the most common virus producing liver dysfunction in patients with ESRD. This infection is identified by the presence of hepatitis B surface antigen (HBsAg) or antibody to the surface antigen (anti-HBs) in the serum. Patients known to be HBsAg-positive are highly infectious and may have active liver disease, whereas patients who are anti-HBs-positive are usually non-infectious and are less likely to have liver disease.[44, 45] Many children and adults who acquire HBV infection while on hemodialysis do not develop anti-HBs and remain carriers of this virus.[46, 47]

A specific antigen and antibody to the HBV core (HBcAg and anti-HBc) may be found in the absence of HBsAg.[48, 49] Significant titers of anti-HBc suggest the persistence of active viral replication and not acquired host resistance to the viral antigen.[20] The "e" antigen (HBeAg) appears to be associated with the presence of HBsAg, active infection, and liver disease.[50-53] However, positive serology for HBeAg is not as likely to indicate liver disease in the patient with ESRD as in the patient without renal disease.[21, 22, 54, 55] Development of antibody (anti-HBe) to the "e" antigen is associated with recovery from HBV infection.[50, 53]

Patients with ESRD tend to remain HBsAg, anti-HBc and HBeAg positive for longer periods than do normal individuals.[49, 56-59] This is more common in males than females, perhaps because of a similarity between HBsAg and antigens on the surface of male cells.[60] Patients who remain antigen-positive for longer than six months rarely develop antibodies, and serve as reservoirs for this viral infection.

Hepatitis B viral disease in hemodialysis centers was reported to be endemic and even epidemic by the late 1960's and early 1970's. Screening programs conducted throughout Europe and the United States discovered infected patients in as many as 82% of the renal dialysis units surveyed.[16, 22, 61, 62] When these units began HBV screening, about 10% of the patients were noted to be positive for HBsAg, with some programs reporting up to 90% of patients exhibiting a present or prior history of the infection.[16, 22, 46, 61-69] One pediatric center reported that 58% of their children developed serologic evidence of HBV since the initiation of hemodialysis.[24]

The HBV is usually introduced into a hemodialysis center by infected blood products and spread from patient to patient within the unit.[69-70] This may occur because of venipuncture with contaminated needles, while cannulating arteriovenous fistulae, or during injection of medications into venous access lines. Contamination of the environment also occurs when blood leaks from infected dialysis equipment. The virus may also cross dialyzer membranes to infect the patient.[71-74]

Hemodialysis patients who develop HBV liver disease are more likely to have milder symptoms than the general population with a similar infection.[20, 21] However, chronic liver disease may result,[23, 25, 35, 74] and even fulminant hepatitis occurs in the patient on hemodialysis.[75, 76] The mortality rate of these infected patients is higher than that observed in the general hemodialysis population.[22]

The danger of exposure to HBV by hemodialysis personnel and family members of ESRD patients is a major problem.[75, 77-80] They may develop symptomatic liver dysfunction leading to significant morbidity and mortality.[16-19, 81] In 1974, a survey of 795 centers by the European Dialysis and Transplant Association recorded 800 cases of HBV hepatitis among dialysis personnel, with 13 deaths.[61] Several dialysis and transplant centers curtailed their ESRD programs because of the high incidence of HBV seroconversion and illness in hospital personnel. This resulted in the denial of therapy to some ESRD patients.[19, 82]

The effects of HBV infections on patient and allograft survival rates following kidney transplantation are well studied.[83-102] Most investigators feel that renal transplantation should not be undertaken while the patient's liver enzymes are elevated. However, some programs report that the HBsAg-positive patients are at no risk for increased morbidity if transplantation takes place after the liver enzymes return to normal.[83-87] These authors have suggested that renal transplantation can be used to decrease the reservoir of HBsAg carriers in the hemodialysis population.[87, 88] Torisu and Starzl[34] found a high incidence of hepatic dysfunction not associated with the HBsAg carrier state in their transplant recipients. Briggs[75] reported a benign course of HBV hepatitis in his transplant patients. In a series of 36 HBsAg-positive children receiving transplants, liver biopsies revealed chronic persistent hepatitis in six patients and chronic active hepatitis in two.[89] The liver disease was not responsible for the death of any patient. On the other hand, some investigators have reported a high incidence of morbidity and mortality associated with the presence of HBV in the transplant recipient.[90-93] Fulminant hepatitis and death occurred in one patient, and severe hepatic dysfunction in 7 of 33 HBsAg-positive patients in one series of 200 transplant recipients.[91] In another study, 18 of 125 HBsAg-positive transplant recipients developed hepatitis; 8 of these patients had chronic active hepatitis, and death attributable to the liver disease occurred in 7 patients.[92] Pirson et al reported their experience with HBV surface antigenemia in 218 transplant recipients. Six to 12 months after transplantation 63% had become HBsAg-positive; 80% of the patients with hepatic dysfunction were HBsAg-positive and 7% of the transplant patients exhibited hepatic failure. Twenty percent of the deaths were the result of hepatitis.[93]

Hepatic dysfunction due to HBsAg-positive hepatitis occurs most often between six and 12 months after transplantation, although mortality from chronic liver disease may occur several years later.[93, 94] Azathioprine and other immunosuppressive drugs predispose to the development of a chronic viremia[43] and subsequent hepatic dysfunction. The viral infections may be newly acquired or develop because of reactivation of a previous infection as evidenced by the reappearance of HBsAg in patients with anti-HBs titers.[95, 96]

Some reports describe no adverse effect of chronic HBV antigenemia on graft survival.[84, 86, 89] In fact, several authors have demonstrated better kidney allograft survival or a delay in the initial allograft rejection episode in patients who were HBsAg-positive.[61, 100, 101] The presence of this antigen was purported to be an indicator of graft tolerance; however, Opelz and Terasaki attributed this apparent improvement in graft survival to a possible protective effect of multiple blood transfusions.[102] In contrast, Pirson et al reported a greater renal allograft loss in patients who were HBsAg-positive. This loss was due to the increased incidence of late deaths from liver failure occurring in this group of patients.[94]

Also of interest is the renal allograft survival rates in the anti-HBs-positive patients. London et al[100] reported a high rate of renal allograft rejection in anti-HBs-positive patients during the first year following transplantation, especially if the renal allograft

donor was a male. This phenomenon was attributed to either a better immunologic responsiveness among this subgroup of patients or the influence of y-linked histocompatability antigens on host responsiveness to HBsAg and HLA antigens.[44, 100, 103, 104]

**Prevention of HBV Infections.** The majority of evidence supports the conclusion that infection with HBV increases morbidity and mortality in both the hemodialysis and transplant patients. Therefore, prevention of the transmission of this virus is very important. Standards and policies have been established to decrease the incidence of HBsAg-positive hepatitis among patients and staff of hemodialysis units. These include provision of gowns and gloves for the staff; use of disposable equipment; routine HBV screening of patients and staff; assignment of machines and individual equipment for each patient; dialysis of HBsAg-positive patients in isolation; and the utilization of home dialysis.[45, 62, 105-112] Peritoneal dialysis, with its decreased need for venipuncture, has not been fully evaluated in the epidemiology of HBV infections. However, HBV has been transmitted in peritoneal fluid.[113, 114] The screening of blood donors for HBsAg protects hemodialysis patients from acquisition of the virus.[44, 105, 112] Washed frozen red cells also decrease the transmission of viral infections;[112, 115-117] however, cells prepared in this manner are less effective than packed red cells in promoting renal allograft tolerance in transplant recipients.[118] HBV infections may be transmitted by a HBsAg-positive kidney donor. Therefore, all prospective donors should be screened for the HBV surface antigen.

Gammaglobulin prepared from regular blood bank donors has no prophylactic effect against HBV exposure since only a small portion of the general population is infected,[81, 119] whereas hyperimmune serum prepared from patients recovering from HBsAg-positive hepatitis may provide passive immunity. Hyperimmune serum is used successfully to prevent the development of hepatitis in patients exposed to HBV by accidental puncture with a contaminated needle.[107, 120] It may also be given prophylactically to ESRD patients and hemodialysis staff to contain or prevent an epidemic of HBV hepatitis.[105, 121-127] These programs are effective in preventing the spread of the viruses to uninfected individuals. However, they are costly and require continued administration of the hyperimmune serum for indefinite periods.

A recently developed vaccine is now being used to actively immunize hemodialysis personnel and patients with ESRD against HBV infection.[128] The vaccine is made from formalin-inactivated HBsAg particles. It has few side effects with no reported cases of antigenemia or significant transaminasemia after use in healthy high-risk volunteers.[129] A series of four injections provides active immunity to most healthy individuals and to approximately 60% of patients with ESRD.[128, 130, 131] One trial of immunization in 10 pediatric hemodialysis patients produced protective antibody levels in all children.[132] Patients developing anti-HBs after vaccination appeared to be protected from the native virus. An unanswered question regarding the use of the vaccine is whether patients who develop anti-HBs will be at an increased risk for renal allograft rejection.[131] As previously noted, this phenomenon has been documented in ESRD patients who develop antibodies to the native virus. Thus, protection against HBsAg-positive hepatitis could conceivably jeopardize chances for a successful renal transplant.

With the introduction of these control methods in hemodialysis units, the incidence of HBV disease in ESRD patients has decreased dramatically. Over a four-year period, a survey from the United Kingdom reported a tenfold decline in the prevalence to 0.3%;[110] other investigators reported a 67.9% decrease in the HBV carrier rate over a three-year period.[109] Therefore, HBV infections are clearly on the decline and may be effectively eliminated from the ESRD population in the near future.

## Cytomegalovirus

Cytomegalovirus may be acquired during hemodialysis through blood transfusions but does not produce liver disease until after the patient has received a renal transplant and is immunosuppressed.[133] The virus may be transmitted by the renal allograft to the patient.[134, 135] An infectious mononucleosis-like syndrome occurs in many of these patients following transplantation.[134-137] The diagnosis is made by seroconversion or a fourfold rise in CMV titers, or the isolation of the virus from the urine or blood. In one pediatric series the virus was isolated from the blood

or urine of 38% of the recipients tested.[138] In another pediatric study the same percentage of patients exhibited a seroconversion after kidney transplantation.[139] Among adult patients 72% had a significant rise in titers for CMV following renal transplantation.[140] Usually, hepatic dysfunction associated with CMV viremia is mild and transient.[27, 136, 141] However, fulminant hepatitis and death are occasionally reported.[26] The prevalence of CMV-induced hepatic dysfunction following transplantation may be as low as 1.6% and as high as 21%.[142-145] Unfortunately, the high incidence of CMV seroconversion following renal transplantation makes a causal relationship difficult to establish, and few investigators have actually isolated CMV from the liver of these patients.

The liver pathology is similar to that of acute viral hepatitis or chronic persistent hepatitis;[134, 141, 146] however, a granulomatous response may occasionally be observed.[147] Autopsy studies were performed on renal transplant recipients with documented CMV infections and hepatic dysfunction, but not hepatic failure, at the time of death. The hepatic pathology consisted of focal necrosis, and moderate fibrosis.[29, 35] Several authors suggest that CMV is an important cause of chronic hepatic dysfunction in renal transplant recipients.[35, 36, 140, 148] Ware et al observed CMV seroconversion associated with the onset of hepatic dysfunction in 9 of 21 transplant recipients with chronic active hepatitis.[36] In 81 transplant recipients, CMV was implicated in 6 of 12 patients with chronic hepatitis.[35] We have suggested that renal transplantation be delayed in children with hepatic dysfunction, if they experience a recent change in CMV serologic status and have a prior history of allograft rejection.[145]

## Other Viruses

Other viruses are associated with hepatitis in ESRD patients. *Epstein-Barr virus* produced an epidemic of hepatitis in at least one hemodialysis center.[149] The clinical syndrome was mild with moderate transaminase elevations. Liver biopsies were not performed. Transplant recipients may shed the EBV from the oropharynx,[150] but no clinical symptomatology is related to this observation, and evidence for EBV hepatitis as a major cause of post-transplant liver dysfunction remains speculative.[144, 150]

*Hepatitis A virus* was implicated during a hepatitis epidemic in a hemodialysis unit, but this was not substantiated by appropriate serologic studies.[151] In fact, when hepatitis A disease was investigated epidemiologically in a population on hemodialysis, there was no evidence for viral dissemination by the dialysis process or for the development of associated liver dysfunction.[65, 152-154]

*Herpes simplex virus Types I and II* are known to cause disseminated disease in the immunosuppressed host.[155, 156] Herpes simplex virus is reported to occasionally cause disease in the transplant recipient but an asymptomatic rise in antiviral titers is more common. In one series, 45% of patients had titers to $HSV_1$ at the time of transplantation, but only 18.2% had a significant rise in titers in the post-transplantation period.[140] There was no association of hepatic dysfunction with these rises in $HSV_1$ titers. However, a few recipients have been reported to develop fulminant hepatitis and disseminated $HSV_1$ infections; this complication is rare and almost always results in death from hepatic failure.[27, 157-161] The results of antiviral drug therapy[162, 163] in renal transplant patients with fulminant hepatitis are disappointing.[158-160] Moreover, some of these agents may be potentially neurotoxic in patients with renal insufficiency.[164] $HSV_2$ may rarely be associated with disseminated disease and fulminant hepatitis in the immunosuppressed or immunodeficient patient.[156] We have observed a case of fulminant $HSV_2$ hepatitis in a 20-year-old transplant recipient resulting in hepatic necrosis and death. The virus was isolated from the liver at postmortem examination.

*Herpes zoster* and *varicella* infections are associated with liver enzyme elevations in renal transplant recipients. Hepatitis in these patients is usually associated with a more severe clinical course.[165-167] Withdrawal of azathioprine and reduction in steroid dosage is indicated with these acute viral infections.

Some ESRD patients demonstrate elevated liver enzymes and histologic findings of hepatitis in the absence of the previously mentioned viral entities. These episodes of hepatitis are often seen in clusters suggesting an infectious etiology.[168-171] *Non-A, non-B viral hepatitis* is responsible for most epidemics of post-transfusion hepatitis in the general population.[169, 172, 173] Since a reliable serologic test is not available, the diagnosis of this disease is made by the exclusion of other viral and toxic insults. Epidemiologic studies suggest that there may be at least two separate viruses responsible for this disease.[152, 169] The liver pathology varies from mild acute hepatitis to chronic active hepatitis.[174] Epidemics of non-A, non-B hepatitis are reported in patients on chronic hemodialysis. The disease appears likely to be transmitted by blood products. The patients usually have minimal symptoms, mild-to-moderate elevations in liver enzymes, and no evidence of cholestasis.[152, 170, 171] The serum transaminase elevations may persist for several months with eventual resolution. However, the histologic diagnosis is frequently either chronic persistent or chronic active hepatitis, with progression to cirrhosis in some patients.[152, 175] There are a number of renal transplant recipients in whom chronic active hepatitis is discovered without an apparent etiology; non-A, non-B virus disease is perhaps the putative hepatic insult in some of these patients.[30, 36, 37, 83, 145, 169, 176] Prevention of the spread of this virus remains a problem. However, screening of the blood donors for elevated liver enzymes appears to decrease non-A, non-B post-transfusion hepatitis.[177]

## HEPATOTOXIC DRUGS

The liver is a prime target for *drug injury* in patients with compromised renal function. It is the only effective site of intermediary metabolism of drugs which are converted to water-soluble metabolites normally excreted by the kidney. The pattern of toxic or "allergic" drug injury encompasses a broad spectrum of hepatic damage, from asymptomatic acute hepatitis to postnecrotic cirrhosis. The long-term effects of drug-induced hepatitis remain unknown. However, continued drug administration associated with clinically apparent hepatitis may lead to cirrhosis, and, therefore, prompt withdrawal of the offending agent is indicated. The evaluation of suspected drug-induced liver disease in patients with decreased renal function should include the search for atypical clinical features and evidence for hypersensitivity, changes in clinical disease after stopping the drug, and consideration of liver biopsy.

*Azathioprine* is the most commonly implicated drug in the allograft recipient. Hepatocellular dysfunction may occur months after initiation of this immunosuppressive drug or its metabolites.[178-181] One pediatric study attributed liver enzyme elevations to azathioprine in its transplant recipients.[142] Cholestatic hepatitis without hepatonecrosis[181] is the most frequent histologic abnormality. In addition, hepatic veno-occlusive disease[182] and peliosis hepatis are occasionally seen.[183] Exceptional cases of severe hepatocellular dysfunction and hepatic fibrosis leading to death from liver failure are reported.[176, 184-186] Liver function usually improves after reducing the dosage or discontinuing the drug. Cyclophosphamide may be substituted for azathioprine in order to maintain stable kidney function.[28, 75, 97, 187] Other investigators were unable to show an improvement in hepatic function following drug withdrawal, and found no clear evidence that azathioprine was hepatotoxic.[30, 36, 37, 188]

*Methyldopa* may cause mild symptomatic hepatitis, especially in middle-aged women. The liver dysfunction usually disappears soon after the drug is discontinued. Five percent of patients are reported to improve even with continued use of methyldopa.[23, 189] However, chronic active hepatitis may occur, and the severity seems to be correlated with the duration of treatment following the appearance of the prodromal symptoms. A hypersensitivity or "allergic" response is suggested, since some patients develop fever and rash, positive serum antinuclear antibodies, and a positive direct Coombs test. Methyldopa should be discontinued and another antihypertensive agent substituted if a severe reaction occurs.

Other drugs are associated with liver dysfunction in patients with ESRD. *Furosemide* may be converted to a reactive arylating metabolite which at toxic levels produces massive hepatic necrosis.[190] However, the usual therapeutic doses of up to 600 mg/day are not hepatotoxic. *Isoniazid*, in therapeutic doses, may cause hepatic injury in ESRD patients. The hepatic injury is mediated by reactive toxic metabolites. Although mild liver dysfunction may subside despite continuation of the drug, chronic active hepatitis has been reported, with progression to fulminant hepatic failure.[191, 192] Antibacterial agents, such as *sulfonamide* and *nitrofurantoin*, are reported in association with chronic active hepatitis and hepatocellular cholestasis.[193-195] Sulfonamides may infrequently cause a hepatonecrosis or a granulomatous reaction in the liver. *Cyclosporin A*, a new immunosuppressive agent undergoing clinical trials in transplant recipients, may cause liver enzyme elevations, and its potential for hepatotoxicity is a major concern.[196, 197]

## OTHER TOXINS

Some instances of hepatic dysfunction in ESRD patients cannot be attributed to viruses or hepatotoxic drugs. Mattenheimer et al reported minor histologic changes in the liver histology of patients on hemodialysis, which they attributed to hypoxia.[198] Others have described mild elevation of liver enzymes and nonspecific infiltration of lymphocytes in the portal tracts in the absence of a specific viral or toxic etiology.[199] Six of 12 children on hemodialysis in our program exhibited hepatic dysfunction with normal liver histology and no identifiable etiologic agent.[145]

*Hemosiderosis* is observed in many dialysis and transplant patients as a result of multiple blood transfusions.[200-203] The iron deposition may contribute to acute liver dysfunction.[152, 175] Massive iron deposits may be seen in Kuppfer cells and hepatocytes along with an increase in hepatic fibrous tissue. The serum ferritin level is the most reliable indicator of this hepatic iron deposition.[202, 204-206] The long-term effect of excessive iron stores in patients on hemodialysis has yet to be determined.[202, 207] The role of iron in the production of progressive hepatic fibrosis is unknown but it may be involved in other organ dysfunction.[201] Parenteral deferoxamine is used in hemodialysis patients exhibiting massive iron overload but the results have been inconsistent. A decrease in iron stores and the removal of iron-deferoxamine complexes during dialysis is reported in some patients, although others failed to respond to this chelating agent.[201, 206] An increased biliary loss of iron is also reported in hemodialysis patients treated with deferoxamine.[206] We were able to reduce liver iron stores with deferoxamine administered during dialysis in one adolescent patient with liver dysfunction.

*Synthetic substances* leached into the circulation from hemodialysis equipment may be hepatotoxic. Neergaard et al reported a hepatitis-like syndrome in patients hemodialyzed with tubing manufactured from *polyvinyl chloride* (PVC) *diethylphalate*.[208, 209] A nonspecific hepatitis without hepatonecrosis was the pathologic finding. *Plasticizers* from the PVC tubing were thought to exert a direct toxic effect on the liver. Symptoms resolved rapidly with the substitution of other tubing and reappeared with the reuse of the PVC equipment. *Silicone* was identified recently in the liver tissues of a number of hemodialysis patients with hepatic dysfunction.[210] Granulomatous hepatitis with giant cells containing silicone were seen in the liver biopsies of some of these patients. Silicone is a component of the roller pump segments of the hemodialysis tubing and was noted to be present in the blood pumped through these segments under ordinary dialysis conditions. The exact role of silicone in the production of liver damage is not fully established.

## SUMMARY

*Acquired liver disease* in children with ESRD remains a significant problem. Patients with liver dysfunction are often asymptomatic but still may have significant liver damage. The etiologic agent for the liver dysfunction is difficult to determine and requires careful investigation. A hepatotoxic virus is the most common cause. Children with ESRD often become chronic carriers of the virus and disseminate the infection to the general population and other ESRD patients. Hepatitis acquired during hemodialysis may adversely affect the life expectancy of adult patients with ESRD and decrease the chances for a successful renal transplantation. Recently, there have been new developments for control of HBV. The perfection of a formalin-inactivated vaccine may eliminate this important viral infection in the future. Certain drugs in the ESRD patient may produce hepatotoxicity and should be eliminated if suspected. Other substances introduced into the circulation during hemodialysis are either metabolized by or stored in the liver and may produce hepatotoxicity. A liver biopsy is often necessary to establish a diagnosis, determine prognosis, and define therapy.

## Acknowledgments

The authors wish to acknowledge the medical support of Drs. John K. Orak, William W. Pfaff, Richard J. Howard, and R. Dixon Walker, III. We also wish to acknowledge the support of the Children's Medical Services of the State of Florida Department of Health and Rehabilitative Services given to children with ESRD. Finally, we wish to acknowledge the help of Ms. Johnette Arnold and Ms. Oonagh Kater, who provided editorial assistance.

## REFERENCES

1. Blyth H, Ockenden BG: Polycystic disease of kidneys and liver presenting in childhood. J Med Genet 8:257, 1971.
2. Danks DM, Tippett P, Adams C, Campbell P: Cerebro-hepato-renal syndrome of Zellweger. J Pediatr 86:382, 1975.
3. Lieberman E, Salinas-Madrigal L, Gwinn JL, et al: Infantile polycystic disease of the kidneys and liver: Clinical, pathological and radiological correlations and comparison with congenital hepatic fibrosis. Medicine 50:277, 1971.
4. Passarge E, McAdams AJ; Cerebro-hepato-renal syndrome. J Pediatr 71:691, 1967.
5. Thaler MM, Ogata ES, Goodman JR, et al: Congenital fibrosis and polycystic disease of liver and kidneys. Am J Dis Child 126:374, 1973.
6. Dobrin RS, Hoyer JR, Nevins TE, et al: The association of familial liver disease, subepidermal immunoproteins, and membranoproliferative glomerulonephritis. J Pediatr 90:901, 1977.
7. Hirschel BJ, Benusiglio LN, Favre H, et al: Glomerulonephritis associated with hepatitis B. Report of a case and review of the literature. Clin Nephrol 8:404, 1977.
8. Nagy J, Bajtai G, Brasch H, et al: The role of hepatitis B surface antigen in the pathogenesis of glomerulopathies. Clin Nephrol 12:109, 1979.
9. Nochy D, Callard P, Bellon B, et al: Association of overt glomerulonephritis and liver disease: a study of 34 patients. Clin Nephrol 6:422, 1976.
10. Slusarczyk J, Michalak T, Nazarewicz-de Mezer T, et al: Membranous glomerulopathy associated with hepatitis B core antigen immune complexes in children. Am J Pathol 98:29, 1980.
11. Epstein M: Deranged renal function in liver disease. Contrib Nephrol 7:250, 1977.
12. Papper S: The hepatorenal syndrome. Clin Nephrol 4:41, 1975.
13. Chan MK, Fernando ON, Moorhead JF: Hepatic malignancy after renal transplantation in an HBsAg positive patient. Br J Clin Pract 34:294, 1980.
14. Arbus GS, Hung RH: Hepatocarcinoma and myocardial fibrosis in an 8¾-year-old renal transplant recipient. Can Med Assoc J 107:431, 1972.
15. Pritzker K: Neoplasia in renal transplant recipients. Can Med Assoc J 107:1059, 1972.
16. Garibaldi RA, Forrest JN, Bryan JA, et al: Hemodialysis-associated hepatitis. JAMA 225:384, 1973.
17. London WT, DeFiglia M, Sutnick AI, Blumberg BS: An epidemic of hepatitis in a chronic-hemodialysis unit. Australia antigen and differences in host response. N Engl J Med 281:571, 1969.
18. Nordenfelt E, Lindholm T, Dahlquist E: A hepatitis epidemic in a dialysis unit. Occurrence and persistence of Australia-antigen among patients and staff. Acta Pathol Microbiol Scand 78:692, 1970.
19. Ogg CS, Bewick M, Cameron JS, Ellis FG: Hepatitis at Guy's Hospital. Proc Eur Dial Transplant Assoc 9:228, 1972.

20. Soulier J-P, Jungers P, Zingraff J: Virus B hepatitis in hemodialysis centers. Adv Nephrol 6:383, 1976.

21. Nordenfelt E, Lindholn T, Henrikson H: The relationship between hepatitis B antigen, e-antigen, and liver pathology in patients treated with dialysis. Scand J Urol Nephrol 9:277, 1975.

22. Piccinino F, Giusti G: The spread of viral hepatitis in Italian dialysis units. Acta Hepato-Gastroenterol 23:392, 1976.

23. Simon P, Herry D, Brissol P, et al: Long-term follow-up of chronic hepatitis by serial liver biopsies in HBsAg-positive haemodialysis patients, role of hepatotoxic drugs. Proc Eur Dial Transplant Assoc 15:596, 1978.

24. Fine RN, Malekzadeh MH, Wright HT: Hepatitis B in a pediatric hemodialysis unit. J Pediatr 86:355, 1975.

25. Degos F, Degott C, Bedrossian J, et al: Is renal transplantation involved in post-transplantation liver disease? Transplantation 29:100, 1980.

26. Aldrete JS, Sterling WA, Hathaway BM, et al: Gastrointestinal and hepatic complications affecting patients with renal allografts. Am J Surg 129:115, 1975.

27. Anuras S, Piros J, Bonney WW, et al: Liver disease in renal transplant recipients. Arch Intern Med 137:42, 1977.

28. Berne TV, Chatterjee SN, Craig JR, et al: Hepatic dysfunction in recipients of renal allografts. Surg Gynecol Obstet 141:171, 1975.

29. Evans DB, Millard PR, Herbertson BM: Hepatic dysfunction associated with renal transplantation. Lancet 2:929, 1968.

30. Ireland P, Rashid A, von Lichtenberg F, et al: Liver disease in kidney transplant patients receiving azathioprine. Arch Intern Med 132:29, 1973.

31. Moore TC, Hume DM: The period and nature of hazard in clinical renal transplantation: I. The hazard to patient survival. Ann Surg 170:1, 1969.

32. Pierides AM, Skillen AW: Serum gamma-glutamyl transferase activity in chronic renal failure during regular haemodialysis and after successful renal transplantation. Clin Chim Acta 77:83, 1977.

33. Reeve CE, Martin DC, Gonick HC, et al: Kidney transplantation. A comparison of results using cadaver and related living donors. Am J Med 47:410, 1969.

34. Torisu M, Yokoyama T, Amemiya H, et al: Immunosuppression, liver injury, and hepatitis in renal, hepatic, and cardiac homograft recipients: With particular reference to the Australia antigen. Ann Surg 174:620, 1971.

35. Toussaint C, DuPont E, Vanherweghem JL, et al: Liver disease in patients undergoing hemodialysis and kidney transplantation. Adv Nephrol 8:269, 1979.

36. Ware AJ, Luby JP, Eigenbrodt EH, et al: Spectrum of liver disease in renal transplant recipients. Gastroenterology 68:755, 1975.

37. Ware AJ, Luby JP, Hollinger B, et al: Etiology of liver disease in renal-transplant patients. Ann Intern Med 91:364, 1979.

38. Berne TV, Butler J, Silberman H: Hepatic dysfunction in renal transplant recipients: A serious problem. Transplant Proc 11:1282, 1979.

39. Sopko J, Anuras S: Liver disease in renal transplant recipients. Am J Med 64:139, 1978.

40. De Gast GC, Houwen B, van der Hem GK, The TH: T-lymphocyte number and function and the course of hepatitis B in hemodialysis patients. Infect Immun 14:1138, 1976.

41. Huges-Law G, de Gast GC, Houwen B, et al: Phytohemagglutin-induced lymphocyte cytotoxicity in hemodialysis patients with hepatitis B virus infection. Hepato-Gastroenterol 28:93, 1981.

42. Tong MJ, Bischel MD, Scoles B, Berne TV: T and B lymphocytes in uremic patients with type B hepatitis infection. Nephron 18:162, 1977.

43. Skinhoj P, Steiness I: Radioimmunoassay of hepatitis B antigen and antibody in dialysis and transplant patients. A five-year follow-up study. Acta Pathol Microbiol Scand 83:125, 1975.

44. Blumberg BS: Australia antigen and the biology of hepatitis B. Science 197:17, 1977.

45. Blumberg BS, Sutnick AI, London WT, Millman I: Australia antigen and hepatitis. N Engl J Med 283:349, 1970.

46. London WT, Drew JS, Lustbader ED, et al: Host responses to hepatitis B infection in patients in a chronic hemodialysis unit. Kidney Int 12:51, 1977.

47. Turner GC, White GBB: S. H. antigen in haemodialysis-associated hepatitis. Lancet 2:121, 1969.

48. Wasnich RD, Puapongsakorn R, Seto DSJ: Significance of antibody to hepatitis B core antigen in a hemodialysis unit. West J Med 132:297, 1980.

49. Yameda E, Ohori H, Ishida N: Physicochemical heterogeneity of hepatitis B e antigen detected in asymptomatic carriers and carriers in a hemodialysis unit. J Med Virol 4:33, 1979.

50. Eleftheriou N, Thomas HC, Heathcote J, Sherlock S: Incidence and clinical significance of e antigen and antibody in acute and chronic liver disease. Lancet 2:1171, 1975.

51. Magnius LO, Lindholm A, Ludin P, Iwarson S: A new antigen-antibody system. Clinical significance in long-term carriers of hepatitis B surface antigen. JAMA 231:356, 1975.

52. Nielsen JO, Dietrichson O, Juhl E: Incidence and meaning of the "e" determinant among hepatitis-B-antigen positive patients with acute and chronic liver diseases. Lancet 2:913, 1974.

53. Smith JL, Murphy BL, Auslander MO, et al: Studies of the "e" antigen in acute and chronic hepatitis. Gastroenterology 71:208, 1976.

54. Coughlin GP, Van Deth AG, Disney APS, et al: Liver disease and the e antigen in HBₓAg carriers with chronic renal failure. Gut 21:118, 1980.

55. Werner BG, Blumberg BS: E antigen in hepatitis B virus infected dialysis patients: Assessment of its prognostic value. Ann Intern Med 89:310, 1978.

56. Gibson PE: E antigen and antibody in outbreaks of hepatitis B in two renal dialysis units. J Clin Pathol 30:717, 1977.

57. Howard CR, Zanetti AR, Thal S, Zuckerman AJ: Viral antigens and antibodies in hepatitis B infection. J Clin Pathol 31:681, 1978.

58. Miller DJ, Williams AE, Le Bouvier GI, et al: Hepatitis B in hemodialysis patients: Significance of HBeAg. Gastroenterology 74:1208, 1978.

59. Ohori H, Yamada E, Tateda A, Ishida N: Prevalence of Williams $e_1$ antigen in comparison with $e_2$ antigen in hepatitis B antigen carriers and patients in hemodialysis unit. J Med Virol 6:61, 1980.

60. London WT, Drew JS: Sex differences in response to hepatitis B infection among patients receiving chronic dialysis treatment. Proc Natl Acad Sci USA 74:2561, 1977.

61. Brunner FP, Giesecke B, Gurland HJ, et al: Combined report on regular dialysis and transplant in Europe, V, 1974. Proc Eur Dial Transplant Assoc 12:3, 1975.

62. Goldsmith HJ: Viral hepatitis in dialysis units. Nephron 12:355, 1974.

63. Sengar PPS, Rashid A, McLeish WA, et al: Hepatitis B surface antigen (HB$_S$Ag) infection in a hemodialysis unit. II. Factors affecting host immune response to HB$_S$Ag. Can Med Assoc J 113:945, 1975.

64. Andrassy K, Ritz E, Sanwald R: Australia antigen in chronic hemodialysis. Vox Sang 19:369, 1970.

65. Gmelin K, v. Ehrlich B, Kommerell B, et al: Viral hepatitis A and B in hemodialysed patients. Klin Wochenschr 58:365, 1980.

66. Jacobs C, Brunner FP, Chantler C, et al: Combined report on regular dialysis and transplantation in Europe, VII, 1976. Proc Eur Dial Transplant Assoc 14:3, 1977.

67. Pattison CP, Maynard JE, Berquist KR, Webster HM: Serological and epidemiological studies of hepatitis B in haemodialysis units. Lancet 2:172, 1973.

68. Polakoff S, Cossart YE, Tillett HE: Hepatitis in dialysis units in the United Kingdom. Br Med J 3:94, 1972.

69. Szmuness W, Prince AM, Grady GF, et al: Hepatitis B infection. A point-prevalence study in 15 US hemodialysis centers. JAMA 227:901, 1974.

70. Hamilton JD, Hatch MH, Gutman RA: Serological evidence of cross infection in a dialysis unit hepatitis-B epidemic. Kidney Int 6:118, 1974.

71. Almeida JD, Chisholm GD, Kulatilake AE, et al: Possible airborne spread of serum-hepatitis virus within a haemodialysis unit. Lancet 2:849, 1971.

72. Snydman DR, Bryan JA, London WT, et al: Transmission of hepatitis B associated with hemodialysis: role of malfunction (blood leaks) in dialysis machines. J Infect Dis 134:562, 1976.

73. LaForce FM, Nelson M: Air-rinsing after dialysis. A mode of transmission of hepatitis virus. JAMA 233:331, 1975.

74. Snydman DR, Bryan JA, Macon EJ, Gregg MB: Hemodialysis-associated hepatitis: Report of an epidemic with further evidence on mechanisms of transmission. Am J Epidemiol 104:563, 1976.

75. Briggs WA, Lazarus JM, Birtch AG, et al: Hepatitis affecting hemodialysis and transplant patients. Arch Intern Med 132:21, 1973.

76. Nielsen V, Clausen E, Ranek L: Liver impairment during chronic hemodialysis and after renal transplantation. Acta Med Scand 197:229, 1975.

77. Acchiardo SR: Nonpercutaneous transmission of hepatitis B to the families of hemodialysis patients. Proc Dial Transplant Forum 6:58, 1976.

78. Chan MK, Moorhead JF: Hepatitis B and the dialysis and renal transplantation unit. Nephron 27:229, 1981.

79. Finn R: Haemodialysis-associated hepatitis. Postgrad Med J 47:499, 1971.

80. Gahl GM, Vogl E, Kraft D, et al: Hepatitis B virus markers among family contacts and medical personnel of 239 hemodialysis patients. Clin Nephrol 14:7, 1980.

81. Ringertz O, Nyström B, Ström J: Clinical aspects of an outbreak of hepatitis among personnel in hemodialysis units. Scand J Infect Dis 1:51, 1969.

82. Collste LG, Blomstrand R, Magnusson G: Six-year survey of staff and patient hepatitis in a renal transplantation unit. Scand J Infect Dis 3:113, 1971.

83. Berne TV, Fitzgibbons TJ, Silbern H: The effect of hepatitis B antigenemia on long-term success and hepatic disease in renal transplant recipients. Transplantation 24:412, 1977.

84. Chatterjee SN, Payne JE, Bischel MD, et al: Successful renal transplantation in patients positive for hepatitis B antigen. N Engl J Med 291:62, 1974.

85. Reed W, Lucas ZJ, Kempson R, Cohn R: Renal transplantation in patients with Australia antigenemia. Transplant Proc 3:343, 1971.

86. Shons AR, Simmons RL, Kjellstrand CM, et al: Renal transplantation in patients with Australia antigenemia. Am J Surg 128:699, 1974.

87. Steiness I, Skinhoj P: Hepatitis associated antigen: elimination from a dialysis unit and persistence in renal transplant recipients. Acta Pathol Microbiol Scand 79:721, 1971.

88. Thomas DR, Bogie W, Blainey JD, et al: Hepatitis in a renal transplant unit. Br J Surg 59:310 1972.

89. Ettenger RB, Tong MJ, Landing BH, et al: Hepatitis B infection in pediatric dialysis and transplant patients: Significance of e antigen. J Pediatr 97:550, 1980.

90. Galbraith RM, Sheikh N El, Portmann B, et al: Immune response to HBsAg and the spectrum of liver lesions in HBsAg-positive patients with chronic renal disease. Br Med J 1:1495, 1976.

91. Disler PB, Meyers AM, Kew MC, Myburgh JA: Hepatitis B virus-associated liver disease after renal transplantation. S Afr Med J 59:97, 1981.

92. Aronoff A, Gault MH, Huang S-N, et al: Hepatitis with Australia antigenemia following renal transplantation. Can Med Assoc J 108:43, 1973.

93. Pirson Y, van Ypersele de Strihou C, Noel H, et al: Liver disease in transplanted patients. Proc Eur Dial Transplant Assoc 10:434, 1973.

94. Pirson Y, Alexandre GPJ, van Ypersele de Strihou C: Long-term effect of hbs antigenemia on patient survival after renal transplantation. N Engl J Med 296:194, 1977.

95. De Flora S, Ferroni P, Chekikian G: Hepatitis B infections in renal transplanted patients. Immunologia 55:23, 1976.

96. Nagington J: Reactivation of hepatitis B after transplantation operations. Lancet 1:558, 1977.

97. Campion EC, Wangel AG, Lawrence JR: Hepatitis B antigen, autoantibodies and liver disease in a haemodialysis and transplantation unit. Aust NZ J Med 5:314, 1975.

98. Czaja AJ, Ludwig J, Baggenstoss AH, Wolf A: Corticosteroid-treated chronic active hepatitis in remission. Uncertain prognosis of chronic persistent hepatitis. N Engl J Med 304:5, 1981.

99. Lam KC, Lai CL, Ng RP, et al: Deleterious effect of prednisolone in HBsAg-positive chronic active hepatitis. N Engl J Med 304:380, 1981.

100. London WT, Drew JS, Blumberg BS, et al: Association of graft survival with host response to hepatitis B infection in patients with kidney transplants. N Engl J Med 296:241, 1977.

101. Toussaint C, Thiry L, Kinnaert P, et al: Prognostic

significance of hepatitis B antigenemia in kidney transplantation. Nephron 17:335, 1976.

102. Opelz G, Terasaki PI: Graft survival rates and HLA antigen frequencies in renal cadaver transplant recipients with hepatitis B antigenemia. Transplantation 25:159, 1978.

103. Hillis WD, Hillis A, Bias WB, Walker WG: Associations of hepatitis B surface antigenemia with HLA locus B specificities. N Engl J Med 296:1310, 1977.

104. Sengar DPS, McLeish WA, Sutherland M, et al: Hepatitis B antigen (HBAg) infection in a hemodialysis unit. I. HL-A8 and immune response to HBAg. Can Med Assoc J 112:968, 1975.

105. Bosch E, Kolk-Vegter AJ: Control of serum hepatitis in a dialysis unit. Neth J Med 16:200, 1973.

106. Desmyter J, Fiasse R, Verberckmoes R, et al: Anti-HAA immunity in renal units with a high and low incidence of serum hepatitis. Proc Eur Dial Transplant Assoc 9:84, 1972.

107. Lucas CR, Williamson HG, Dimitrakakis M, Gust ID: Maintenance dialysis of patients infected with hepatitis B virus. Med J Aust 1:343, 1981.

108. Gold CH: Hepatitis in the haemodialysis unit, Baragwanath Hospital, 1973–1977. A cross-sectional and longitudinal survey. S Afr Med J 56:214, 1979.

109. Najem GR, Louria DB, Thind IS, et al: Control of hepatitis B infection. The role of surveillance and an isolation hemodialysis center. JAMA 245:153, 1981.

110. Polakoff S: Hepatitis B in retreat from dialysis units in United Kingdom in 1973. Br Med J 1:1579, 1976.

111. Postic B, Schreiner DP, Hanchett JE, Atchison RW: Containment of hepatitis B virus infection in a hemodialysis unit. J Infect Dis 138:884, 1978.

112. Snydman DR, Bryan JA, Dixon RE: Prevention of nosocomial viral hepatitis, Type B (Hepatitis B). Ann Intern Med 83:838, 1975.

113. Salo RJ, Salo AA, Fahlberg WJ, Ellzey JT: Hepatitis B surface antigen (HB$_s$Ag) in peritoneal fluid of HB$_s$Ag carriers undergoing peritoneal dialysis. J Med Virol 6:29, 1980.

114. Spector D: Hepatitis B miniepidemic in a peritoneal dialysis unit. Arch Intern Med 137:1030, 1977.

115. Carr JB, de Quesada AM, Shires DL: Decreased incidence of transfusion hepatitis after exclusive transfusion with reconstituted frozen erythrocytes. Studies in a dialysis unit. Ann Intern Med 78:693, 1973.

116. Huggins CE, Russell PS, Winn HJ, et al: Frozen blood in transplant patients: hepatitis and HL-A isosensitization. Transplant Proc 5:809, 1973.

117. Shires DL Jr: Transfusion of frozen-washed red cells in preventing hepatitis. Clinical uses of frozen-thawed red blood cells. Proc Clin Biol Res 11:183, 1976.

118. Opelz G, Terasaki PI: Dominant effect of transfusions on kidney graft survival. Transplantation 29:153, 1980.

119. Kaboth U, Junge U: Prophylaxis of viral hepatitis. Clin Gastroenterol 3:453, 1974.

120. Seeff LB, Wright EC, Zimmerman HJ, et al: Type B hepatitis after needle-stick exposure: Prevention with hepatitis B immune globulin. Ann Intern Med 88:285, 1978.

121. Burck HC, Berg P: Is passive immunization against hepatitis B a luxury, danger or necessity for dialysis patients and staff? Dialysis Transplantation Nephrology. Proc Eur Dial Transplant Assoc 15:130, 1978.

122. Delons S, Naret C, Ciancioni C, et al: An attempt to prevent hepatitis B in a haemodialysis unit's team utilisation of specific immunoglobulins. Proc Eur Dial Transplant Assoc 11:237, 1975.

123. Desmyter J, Bradburne AF, Vermylen C, et al: Hepatitis-B immunoglobulin in prevention of HBs antigenaemia in haemodialysis patients. Lancet 2:377, 1975.

124. Kleinknecht D, Courouce AM, Delons S, et al: Prevention of hepatitis B in hemodialysis patients using hepatitis B immunoglobulin. A controlled study. Clin Nephrol 8:373, 1977.

125. Nik-Akhtar B, Khakpour M, Panahi F, Hesabi AM: Prevention of hepatitis Type B with specific immune serum globulin. Nephron 17:402, 1976.

126. Prince AM, Szmuness W, Mann MK, et al: Hepatitis B "immune" globulin: Effectiveness in prevention of dialysis-associated hepatitis. N Engl J Med 293:1063, 1975.

127. Prince AM, Szmuness W, Mann MK, et al: Hepatitis B immune globulin: Final report of a controlled multicenter trial of efficacy in prevention of dialysis-associated hepatitis. J Infect Dis 137:131, 1978.

128. Crosnier J, Jungers P, Courouce A-M, et al: Randomised placebo-controlled trial of hepatitis B surface antigen vaccine in French haemodialysis units: I, Medical staff. Lancet 1:455, 1981.

129. Szmuness W, Stevens CE, Harley EJ, et al: Hepatitis B vaccine. Demonstration of efficacy in a controlled clinical trial in a high-risk population in the United States. N Engl J Med 303:833, 1980.

130. Maupas P, Goudeau A, Coursaget P, et al: Vaccine against hepatitis B—18 months' prevention in a high risk setting. Med Microbiol Immunol 166:109, 1978.

131. Stevens CE, Szmuness W, Goodman AI, et al: Hepatitis B vaccine: Immune responses in haemodialysis patients. Lancet 1:1211, 1980.

132. Nivet H, Drucker J, Dubois F, et al: Vaccine against hepatitis B in children: prevention of hepatitis in a pediatric hemodialysis unit. Int J Pediatr Nephrol 3:25, 1982.

133. Spencer ES: Cytomegalovirus antibody in uremic patients prior to renal transplantation. Scand J Infect Dis 6:1, 1974.

134. Fiala M, Payne JE, Berne TV, et al: Epidemiology of cytomegalovirus infection after transplantation and immunosuppression. J Infect Dis 132:421, 1975.

135. Ho M: Virus infections after transplantation in man. Brief review. Arch Virol 55:1, 1977.

136. Armstrong D, Balakrishnan SL, Steger L, et al: Cytomegalovirus infections with viremia following renal transplantation. Arch Intern Med 127:111, 1971.

137. Cappel R, Hestermans O, Toussaint C, et al: Cytomegalovirus infection and graft survival in renal graft recipients. Arch Virol 56:149, 1978.

138. Fine RN, Grushkin CM, Anand S, et al: Cytomegalovirus in children: Postrenal transplantation. Am J Dis Child 120:197, 1970.

139. Fennell RS III, Garin EH, Pfaff W, et al: Renal transplantation in children and adolescents. Clin Pediatr 19:518, 1979.

140. Luby JP, Burnett W, Hull AR, et al: Relationship

between cytomegalovirus and hepatic function abnormalities in the period after renal transplant. J Infect Dis 129:511, 1974.

141. Fine RN, Grushkin CM, Malekzadeh MH, Wright HT Jr: Cytomegalovirus syndrome following renal transplantation. Arch Surg 105:564, 1972.

142. Malekzadeh MH, Grushkin CM, Wright HT Jr, Fine RN: Hepatic dysfunction after renal transplantation in children. J Pediatr 81:279, 1972.

143. Rubin RH, Cosimi AB, Tolkoff-Rubin NE, et al: Infectious disease syndromes attributable to cytomegalovirus and their significance among renal transplant recipients. Transplantation 24:458, 1977.

144. Toussaint C, Thiry L, Vereerstraeten P, et al: Clinical aspects of infections due to herpesviruses in renal transplant recipients. Transplant Clin Immunol IX. Proceedings of NiWL Intern Course, Lyon, June, 1977. Excerpta Medica, Amsterdam-Oxford, 1978, p 5.

145. Fennell RS III, Andres JM, Pfaff WW, Richard GA: Liver dysfunction in children and adolescents during hemodialysis and after renal transplantation. Pediatrics 67:855, 1981.

146. Foster KM, Ralston M, Field PR, et al: Primary cytomegalovirus infection and hepatitis in a renal allograft recipient. Aust NZ J Med 2:148, 1972.

147. Clarke J, Craig RM, Saffro R, et al: Cytomegalovirus granulomatous hepatitis. Am J Med 66:264, 1979.

148. Dickerman RM, Niederhuber JE, Eigenbrodt E, Fry WJ: Portal hypertension following renal transplantation. Surgery 84:322, 1978.

149. Corey L, Stamm WE, Feorino PM, et al: HB$_S$Ag-negative hepatitis in a hemodialysis unit. Relation to Epstein-Barr virus. N Engl J Med 293:1273, 1975.

150. Strauch B, Andrews L-L, Siegel N, Miller G: Oropharyngeal excretion of Epstein-Barr virus by renal transplant recipients and other patients treated with immunosuppressive drugs. Lancet 1:234, 1974.

151. Eastwood JB, Curtis JR, Wing AJ, de Wardener HE: Hepatitis in a maintenance hemodialysis unit. Ann Intern Med 69:59, 1968.

152. Galbraith RM, Dienstag JI, Purcell RH, et al: Non-A Non-B hepatitis associated with chronic liver disease in a haemodialysis unit. Lancet 1:951, 1979.

153. Kelly TJ, Patterson MJ, Hourani MR, et al: Antibody to hepatitis A among Michigan hemodialysis patients. Proc Dial Transplant Forum 9:174, 1979.

154. Szmuness W, Dienstag JL, Purcell RH, et al: Hepatitis type A and hemodialysis. A seroepidemiologic study in 15 United States centers. Ann Intern Med 87:8, 1977.

155. Goyette RE, Donowho EM, Hieger LR, Plunkett GD: Fulminant herpesvirus hominis hepatitis during pregnancy. Obstet Gynecol 43:191, 1974.

156. Sutton AL, Smithwick EM, Seligman SJ, Kim D-S: Fatal disseminated herpesvirus hominis Type 2 infection in an adult with associated thymic dysplasia. Am J Med 56:545, 1974.

157. Anuras S, Summers R: Fulminant herpes simplex hepatitis in an adult: Report of a case in renal transplant recipient. Gastroenterology 70:425, 1976.

158. Elliott WC, Houghton DC, Bryant RE, et al:

159. Holdsworth SR, Atkins RC, Scott DF, Hayes K: Systemic herpes simplex infection with fulminant hepatitis post-transplantation. Aust NZ J Med 6:588, 1976.

160. Taylor RJ, Saul SH, Dowling JN, et al: Primary disseminated herpes simplex infection with fulminant hepatitis following renal transplantation. Arch Intern Med 141:1519, 1981.

161. Walker DP, Longson M, Lawler W, et al: Disseminated herpes simplex virus infection with hepatitis in an adult renal transplant recipient. J Clin Pathol 34:1044, 1981.

162. Hirsch MS, Swartz MN: Antiviral agents. N Engl J Med *Part 1,* 302:903 and *Part 2,* 302:949, 1980.

163. Whitley RJ, Ch'ien LT, Dolin R, et al: Adenine arabinoside therapy of herpes zoster in the immunosuppressed NIAID. Collaborative antiviral study. N Engl J Med 294:1193, 1976.

164. Marker SC, Howard RJ, Groth KE, et al: A trial of vidarabine for cytomegalovirus infection in renal transplant patients. Arch Intern Med 140:1441, 1980.

165. Millard PR, Herbertson BM, Nagington J, Evans DB: The morphological consequences and the significance of cytomegalovirus infection in renal transplant patients. Q J Med, New Series 42:585, 1973.

166. Feldhoff CM, Balfour HH, Simmons RL, et al: Varicella in children with renal transplants. J Pediatr 98:25, 1981.

167. Groth KE, McCullough J, Marker SC, et al: Evaluation of zoster immune plasma. Treatment of cutaneous disseminated zoster in immunocompromised patients. JAMA 239:1877, 1978.

168. Leski M, Grivaux C, Courouce-Pauty AM: Australia antigen in hemodialysis and renal transplantation units. Vox Sang 19:359, 1970.

169. Dienstag JL: Non-A, non-B hepatitis. Adv Intern Med 26:187, 1980.

170. Avram MM, Feinfeld DA, Gan AC: Non-A, non-B hepatitis: A new syndrome in uraemic patients. Proc Eur Dial Transplant Assoc 16:141, 1979.

171. Simon N, Méry JP, Trépo C, et al: A non-A non-B hepatitis epidemic in a HB antigen-free haemodialysis unit. Demonstration of serological markers of non-A non-B virus. Proc Eur Dial Transplant Assoc 17:173, 1980.

172. Feinstone SM, Kapikian AZ, Purcell RH, et al: Transfusion-associated hepatitis not due to viral hepatitis type A or B. N Engl J Med 292:767, 1975.

173. Prince AM, Brotman B, Grady GF, et al: Long-incubation post-transfusion hepatitis without serological evidence of exposure to hepatitis-B virus. Lancet 2:241, 1974.

174. Wyke RJ, Williams R: Clinical aspects of Non-A, non-B hepatitis infection. J Virol Meth 2:17, 1980.

175. Galbraith RM, Portmann B, Eddleston ALWF, Williams R: Chronic liver disease developing after outbreak of HBsAg-negative hepatitis in haemodialysis unit. Lancet 2:886, 1975.

176. Freiberger Z, Anuras S, Koff RS, Bonney WW: Chronic active hepatitis without hepatitis B antigenemia in renal transplant recipients. Gastroenterology 66:1187, 1974.

177. Aach RD, Szmuness W, Mosley JW, et al: Serum alanine aminotransferase of donors in relation

to the risk of non-A, non-B hepatitis in recipients. The transfusion-transmitted viruses study. N Engl J Med 304:989, 1981.

178. Starzl TE, Marchioro TL, Porter KA, et al: Factors determining short- and long-term survival after orthotopic liver homotransplantation in the dog. Surgery 58:131, 1965.

179. Drinkard JP, Stanley TM, Dornfeld L, et al: Azathioprine and prednisone in the treatment of adults with lupus nephritis. Medicine 49:411, 1970.

180. Shorey J, Schenker S, Suki WN, Combes B: Hepatotoxicity of mercaptopurine. Arch Intern Med 122:54, 1968.

181. Sparberg M, Simon N, del Greco F: Intrahepatic cholestasis due to azathioprine. Gastroenterology 57:439, 1969.

182. Marubbio AT, Danielson B: Hepatic veno-occlusive disease in a renal transplant patient receiving azathioprine. Gastroenterology 69:739, 1975.

183. Degott C, Rueff B, Kreis H, et al: Peliosis hepatis in recipients of renal transplants. Gut 19:748, 1978.

184. Nataf C, Feldmann G, Lebrec D, et al: Idiopathic portal hypertension (perisinusoidal fibrosis) after renal transplantation. Gut 20:531, 1979.

185. Krawitt EL, Stein JH, Kirkendall WM, Clifton JA: Mercaptopurine hepatotoxicity in a patient with chronic active hepatitis. Arch Intern Med 120:729, 1967.

186. Zarday Z, Veith FJ, Gliedman ML, Soberman R: Irreversible liver damage after azathioprine. JAMA 222:690, 1972.

187. Franksson C: Hepatitis and liver damage among patients and staff in a transplantation unit. Transplant Proc 1:209, 1969.

188. Zazgornik J, Schmidt P, Kopsa H, Deutsch E: Liver function after renal transplantation. Med Chir Dig 4:81, 1975.

189. Goldstein GB, Lam KC, Mistilis SP: Drug-induced active chronic hepatitis. Am J Dig Dis 18:177, 1973.

190. McMurtry RJ, Mitchell JR: Renal and hepatic necrosis after metabolic activation of 2-substituted furans and thiophenes, including furosemide and cephaloridine. Toxicol Appl Pharmacol 4:285, 1977.

191. Thomas NA, Mozes MF, Jonasson O: Hepatic dysfunction during isoniazid chemoprophylaxis in renal allograft recipients. Arch Surg 114:597, 1979.

192. Maddrey WC, Boitnott JK: Isoniazid hepatitis. Ann Intern Med 79:1, 1973.

193. Berger M, Potter DE: Pitfall in diagnosis of viral hepatitis on haemodialysis unit. Lancet 2:95, 1977.

194. Dujovne CA, Chan CH, Zimmerman HJ: Sulfon-

amide hepatic injury. Review of the literature and report of a case due to sulfamethoxazole. N Engl J Med 277:785, 1968.

195. Fries J, Siraganian R: Sulfonamide hepatitis. Report of a case due to sulfamethoxazole and sulfisoxazole. N Engl J Med 274:95, 1966.

196. Morris PJ: Transplantation overview: Cyclosporin A. Transplantation 32:349, 1981.

197. Starzl TE, Weil R, Iwatsuki S, et al: The use of cyclosporin A and prednisone in cadaver kidney transplantation. Surg Gynecol Obstet 151:17, 1980.

198. Mattenheimer H, Friedel R, Schwartz FD: Hepatopathy of chronic hemodialysis in the absence of hepatitis. Gastroenterology 58:310, 1970.

199. Bergman LA, Thomas W Jr, Reddy CR, et al: Nonviral hepatitis in patients maintained by long-term dialysis. Arch Intern Med 130:96, 1972.

200. Ali M, Fayemi AO, Rigolosi R, et al: Hemosiderosis in hemodialysis patients. JAMA 244:343, 1980.

201. Baker LRI, Barnett MD, Brozovic B, et al: Hemosiderosis in a patient on regular hemodialysis: treatment by desferrioxamine. Clin Nephrol 6:326, 1976.

202. Kothari T, Swamy AP, Lee JCK, et al: Hepatic hemosiderosis in maintenance hemodialysis (MHD) patients. Dig Dis Sci 25:363, 1980.

203. Hill RB, Porter KA, Massion CG: Hepatic reaction to renal transplants modified by immunosuppressive therapy. Arch Pathol 81:71, 1966.

204. Aljama P, Ward MK, Pierides AM, et al: Serum ferritin concentration: a reliable guide to iron overload in uremic and hemodialyzed patient. Clin Nephrol 10:101, 1978.

205. Ellis D: Serum ferritin compared with other indices of iron status in children and teenagers undergoing maintenance hemodialysis. Clin Chem 25:741, 1979.

206. Gokal R, Millard PR, Weatherall DJ, et al: Iron metabolism in haemodialysis patients. Q J Med, New Series 48:369, 1979.

207. Pitts TO, Barbour GL: Hemosiderosis secondary to chronic parenteral iron therapy in maintenance hemodialysis patients. Nephron 22:316, 1978.

208. Neergaard J, Nielsen B, Faurby V, et al: Plasticizers in PVC and the occurrence of hepatitis in a haemodialysis unit. Scand J Urol Nephrol 5:141, 1971.

209. Neergaard J, Nielsen B, Faurby V, et al: On the exudation of plasticizers from PVC haemodialysis tubings. Nephron 14:263, 1975.

210. Leong AS-Y, Disney APS, Gove DW: Spallation and migration of silicone from blood-pump tubing in patients on hemodialysis. N Engl J Med 306:135, 1982.

# 28

# PRINCIPLES OF DRUG THERAPY IN CHILDREN WITH ESRD

*Alan R. Sinaiko, M.D.*
*Thomas P. Green, M.D.*

Patients with ESRD receive a variety of pharmacologic agents to control the broad spectrum of pathophysiologic disorders associated with chronic renal failure. Most of these drugs are used regularly during the course of daily pediatric practice, providing the clinician with practical experience relating to dosing regimens and potential adverse reactions. However, ESRD imposes conditions that may require substantial adjustments in usual treatment regimens. Reduction in drug excretion by the kidney is only the most obvious of these. Associated changes in hepatic drug metabolism, serum drug-protein binding, and drug distribution in body tissues and fluids may have an equally important impact on drug therapy and toxicity.

Dependable analytic techniques for drug measurement have added a new dimension to drug therapy. It has been possible to determine drug disposition, construct dosing regimens, and determine the therapeutic index, i.e., the relationship between toxic and therapeutic drug concentrations, for many drugs. Because the majority of these studies have been conducted in adults, they neglect considerations of drug absorption, distribution, metabolism, and excretion that may undergo significant change during the course of biological development. Thus, recent reviews of drug disposition in patients with renal failure[1, 2] must be used with the caveat that they may be imprecise estimates of dosage requirements in children.

This chapter is devoted to a discussion of the principles controlling drug disposition in ESRD. While an extensive catalogue of individual drugs and explicit dosing recommendations will not be provided, drugs will be categorized according to characteristics that may be influenced by a reduction in renal function. The intent of this information is to provide guidelines for the rational design of dosing regimens in this age group until such time as data on disposition of specific drugs in children with renal failure are available.

## CHANGES IN DRUG DISPOSITION DURING MATURATION

The adverse influence of ESRD on drug disposition occurs in children against a background of developmental changes that are a normal component of biological maturation. The processes that determine drug absorption, distribution, metabolism, and excretion undergo considerable change between birth and adulthood. It is generally accepted that the most dramatic changes take place during the first weeks and months of life. Consequently, the majority of investigations of the effect of maturation on drug disposition have been conducted in this age group. This chapter and the accompanying table (Table 28–1) will summarize these data.[3–18] More complete reviews can be found elsewhere.[19–21]

The rate and extent of enteral drug absorption reach adult standards for most drugs after early infancy. The principal physiologic determinants of absorption, including

**Table 28–1.  MATURATION OF PHYSIOLOGICAL VARIABLES THAT DETERMINE DRUG DISPOSITION‡**

| Aspect of Drug Disposition | Physiological Variable | Representative Values* | | | | Examples |
|---|---|---|---|---|---|---|
| | | Premature | Newborn | One Year Old | Adult | |
| Absorption (oral) | Gastric acid secretion (mEq/kg/h) | | 0.015 | | 0.2 | Penicillin G—increased bioavailability in newborns[3] |
| | Gastric emptying time (minutes) | | 87 | | 65 | Phenobarbital—slower rate of absorption in newborns[4] |
| | Intestinal peristalsis | ↓† | ↓† | | | Phenobarbital—slow rate of absorption in newborns[5] |
| Absorption (intramuscular) | Regional muscular blood flow | △ | △ | | | Digoxin, gentamicin—erratic absorption in newborns[5,6] |
| Distribution | Total body water (% of total body weight) | 87 | 79 | 67 | 60 | |
| | Extracellular water (% of total body weight) | 62 | 45 | 27 | 20 | Amikacin, ticarcillin—increased distribution volumes in young subjects[7,8] |
| | Adipose tissue (% of total body weight) | 3 | 12 | 23 | 12–25 | |
| | Total serum proteins (g/dl) | 5.9 | 6.0 | 6.4 | 7.2 | |
| | Serum albumin (g/dl) | 3.7 | 4.5 | 4.9 | 4.9 | Sulfadiazine—decreased serum drug protein binding in newborns[9] |
| Metabolism | Sulfation* | | ↔ | ↔ | | Acetaminophen—predominantly sulfated in infants[10] |
| | Glucuronidation* | → | → | ↔ | | Chloramphenicol—delayed elimination in prematures and newborns[11] |
| | Mixed-function oxidase | → | → | ↔ | | Theophylline—decreased rate of metabolism in newborns[12] |
| Elimination | Glomerular filtration (ml/min/m²) | 5 | 15 | 50 | 70 | Gentamicin—delayed elimination in newborns[13] |
| | Tubular anion secretion (PAH clearance—ml/min/1.73 m²) | 50 | 50 | 245 | 380 | Furosemide—delayed elimination in newborns[14] |

*For physiological variables for which no quantitation in children is available, the values are qualitatively expressed relative to the adult (References 15 to 18).

†Peristalsis tends to be slow and irregular in premature and newborn infants.

△Muscular blood flow appears to be more labile in very young subjects.

‡Table reproduced from Reference 19 with permission from the publisher, Raven Press.

gastric pH, gastric emptying time, intestinal surface area, and intestinal motility, attain functional maturity early in the first year of life.

Drug disposition is dependent on the interaction between cardiovascular factors, body composition, and the numerous plasma components that determine drug-protein binding (i.e., albumin, other drug binding proteins, and competing small molecular weight ligands). Body composition appears to change the most dramatically of these factors during development.

In early infancy, the largest component of body mass is water, with a predominance of extracellular fluid.[22] An adult distribution pattern for body water is achieved within the first year of life. The lipid fraction of body mass is considerably greater in infants than in adults but rapidly changes to approach that found in lean adults shortly after infancy. Plasma drug protein binding changes most abruptly early in the newborn period.[23] This is primarily the result of modifications in drug albumin affinity, secondary to changes in configuration or charge on the albumin molecule and competition for binding sites by ligands such as bilirubin.

Metabolic pathways for drug biotransformation develop at independent rates. The pathway for sulfate conjugation is relatively mature in infancy, whereas glucuronidation is poorly developed and undergoes maturation during the first year of life. As is well known, compounds such as chloramphenicol and bilirubin that are virtually totally dependent on glucuronidation for excretion accumulate in newborns and young infants.[24] In other cases, drugs which are inactivated in adults by glucuronidation may be metabolized during infancy via an alternate pathway. One such drug is acetaminophen, which is primarily dependent on glucuronidation for clearance in adults but does not accumulate in infants because of efficient metabolism through the sulfation pathway.[10] During development the primary organ system involved in the clearance of drugs may also change. Lidocaine is excreted by the kidney in infancy[25]; as hepatic metabolic pathways mature, the liver becomes the major organ of clearance.

The maturational sequence of the kidney is perhaps most familiar to clinicians dealing with ESRD. Glomerular filtration rate standardized for body size approximates adult norms during the latter half of the first year of life; renal tubular function matures slightly later.[26] Therefore, drugs that rely on the kidney for excretion achieve adult clearance rates at this time. Although less well studied than the changes occurring in early infancy, renal drug clearance rates in the preadolescent child appear to be slightly higher than those in adults,[26, 27] thus conforming to the pattern established for hepatic drug clearance in the age group.[28]

## GENERAL PRINCIPLES OF DRUG CLEARANCE

Plasma half-life (T½) is the clinical term commonly used to express the rate of drug removal from the body. It is related to the elimination rate constant ($k_{el}$) for a given drug by the following equation:

$$T\frac{1}{2} = \frac{0.693}{k_{el}} \qquad (1)$$

Because drug concentration decreases in an exponential fashion (dependent on $k_{el}$) once a drug is completely distributed within the body, the T½ describes the duration of time required for drug elimination. After a period of time equal to one half-life, the original plasma concentration will be reduced to 50%, after two half-lives to 25%, after three half-lives to 12.5%, etc.

A major determinant of plasma half-life is the efficiency with which drug is removed from the body, i.e., drug clearance. Total drug clearance ($Cl_T$) represents the summated effect of drug elimination via renal ($Cl_R$), pulmonary ($Cl_P$), and intestinal ($Cl_I$) excretion, hepatic metabolism ($Cl_H$), and, in patients who are functionally anephric, via dialysis ($Cl_D$). It is the clearance of drug per unit time from the volume of drug distribution (Vd) within the body that determines the elimination rate constant as follows:

$$k_{el} = \frac{Cl_T}{Vd} \qquad (2)$$

By combining equations 1 and 2 to achieve the following equation

$$T\frac{1}{2} = \frac{0.693 \times Vd}{Cl_T} \qquad (3)$$

it can be seen that the elimination half-life of

a drug is inversely related to its total clearance and directly related to its volume of distribution.

Once steady-state conditions of drug therapy have been achieved, i.e., when amount of drug administered and amount of drug eliminated are equal over a given period of time, the plasma drug concentration is dependent primarily on drug clearance, as expressed in the following equation:

$$C_{SS} = \frac{D}{Cl_T} \qquad (4)$$

where $C_{SS}$ equals plasma concentration at steady state and D equals the drug dose per unit time. Because the clearance of most drugs is almost entirely dependent on renal excretion or hepatic degradation to inactive or active metabolites, Equations 3 and 4 can be expressed as:

$$T\tfrac{1}{2} = \frac{0.693 \times Vd}{(Cl_R + Cl_H)} \qquad (5)$$

and

$$C_{SS} = \frac{D}{(Cl_R + Cl_H)} \qquad (6)$$

## RENAL DRUG CLEARANCE

The kidney is directly involved with the excretion of most drugs from the body. It may act as the primary organ of clearance of unchanged drug, or it may be secondarily involved through the excretion of metabolic products produced by drug biotransformation in the liver.

**Table 28–2.** SOME FREQUENTLY USED DRUGS DEPENDENT ON THE KIDNEY FOR EXCRETION

| Glomerular Filtration | Tubular Excretion |
|---|---|
| | *Organic Acids* |
| Amikacin | Carbenicillin |
| Digoxin | Cephalexin |
| Flucytosine | Ethacrynic Acid |
| Gentamicin | Furosemide |
| Kanamycin | Methotrexate |
| Tetracycline | Penicillin G |
| Tobramycin | Thiazide diuretics |
| Vancomycin | *Organic Bases* |
| | Procainamide |
| | Triamterene |

The clearance of drugs that are excreted in an unchanged form by the kidney and do not have appreciable nonrenal clearance (Table 28–2) (i.e., $Cl_H = 0$), is correlated with glomerular filtration rate (GFR). Therefore, drug concentration can be expected to respond to a reduction in renal function with changes approximating the rise in the serum creatinine level. Equation 5, in which plasma half-life is inversely related to drug clearance from the body, has been used to construct a graphic representation of this relationship (Fig. 28–1).[29] Each decrement in GFR and renal drug clearance is accompanied by an equivalent increase in drug half-life and steady-state serum concentration (Equation 6). In other words, each time the creatinine clearance is reduced by one-half, the drug half-life doubles. For most drugs, at least a twofold increase in plasma concentration must be reached before adverse effects directly associated with concentration become evident.

It is apparent from Figure 28–1 that dosage modifications for drugs excreted unchanged by the kidney are rarely necessary until GFR is reduced to 50% of normal renal function. However, each additional decrement in GFR results in a corresponding prolongation of drug half-life and an increase in drug concentration, unless dosing regimens are altered accordingly. An example of this principle is applicable to diuretic therapy. The tubular response to diuretics is determined by the amount of drug reaching the luminal side of the nephron[30–32] (Fig. 28–2). As GFR decreases, the effectiveness of thiazides and furosemide, both of which are dependent on the tubular organic acid transport system for excretion, also decreases.[30] The effect of renal failure on serum hydrochlorothiazide concentrations in children is shown in Figure 28–3 (Mirkin BL, Sinaiko AR, unpublished observations). When the GFR is greater than 50 ml/min, the concentration of hydrochlorothiazide is independent over a wide dosage range (0.1–0.5 mg/kg), whereas, in children with a creatinine clearance less than 50 ml/min, hydrochlorothiazide excretion is significantly reduced and drug accumulation is directly correlated with dose.

### Renal Tubular Excretion

Renal tubular transport is the primary excretory pathway for many drugs cleared by

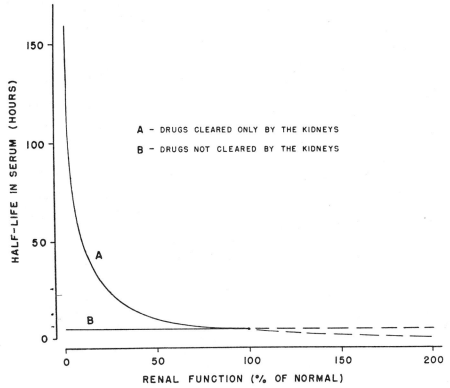

**Figure 28–1.** Representation of hypothetical relationship between half-life of drugs in serum and renal function. (From Kunin CM, Finland M: Persistence of antibiotics in blood in patients with acute renal failure. J Clin Invest 38:1509, 1959.)

the kidney (Table 28–2). Nevertheless, GFR remains a valid indicator of drug accumulation for these agents, since both GFR and renal blood flow usually decrease proportionately with renal mass in severe kidney disease. The proximal renal tubule is the site of drug extraction and secretion into the urine and contains both organic acid and organic base transport systems. Many organic acids may share the same tubular transport system; consequently, when multiple acidic drugs are administered, they compete for excretion. This principle forms the well-established basis for the prolongation of penicillin half-life by concurrent administration of probenecid.

Clearance of drugs dependent on renal tubular organic acid transport for excretion is adversely affected in renal failure by a second factor in addition to the reduction in clearance attributable to compromised renal blood flow. In vivo experiments in dogs[33] and man[34] have shown a linear relationship between extraction and clearance of acidic drugs, e.g., furosemide, and degree of uremia, expressed as the serum creatinine level or blood urea nitrogen (BUN) level. It appears that this reduction in extraction is dependent upon the presence of an interfering uremic substance. Serum from patients in renal failure depresses uptake of p-amino-hippurate (PAH) by isolated rabbit renal tu-

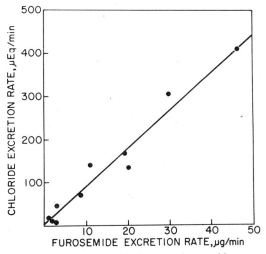

**Figure 28–2.** Relationship between furosemide excretion rate and urinary chloride excretion. (From Green TP, Mirkin BL: Determinants of the diuretic response to furosemide in infants with congestive heart failure. Pediatr Cardiol 3:47, 1982.)

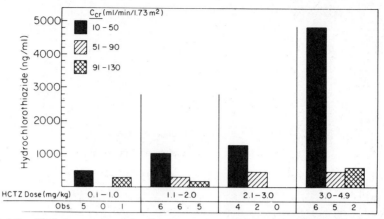

**Figure 28–3.** Relationship between glomerular filtration rate and plasma levels of hydrochlorothiazide in children.

bules, an effect that is reduced when serum is obtained from patients immediately after hemodialysis.[35] Although the humoral agents responsible for this phenomenon have not been isolated, it is generally accepted that the reduction in organic acid clearance results from competition for tubular transport sites by endogenous organic acids that accumulate in renal failure.[36] In contrast to the situation for organic acids, the extraction of organic bases is preserved,[33, 37] and the reduction in clearance of these compounds remains proportional to GFR.

## Influence of Proteinuria on Renal Drug Excretion

The inhibitory influence of proteinuria on drug-mediated diuresis is not widely recognized. Investigations of this relationship in aminonucleoside-treated rats have shown that urine protein concentration is positively correlated with percentage of bound furosemide[38] (Fig. 28–4). As would be expected, responsiveness of the nephron to furosemide was directly related to concentration of unbound drug, since water and chloride excretion were inversely related to urinary protein excretion. These findings may help to explain the unusual resistance of some nephrotic patients to aggressive furosemide therapy.

Elevated concentrations of protein in the urine also inhibit drug reabsorption by the renal tubule. Reabsorption is inversely related to degree of ionization. Reduction of urinary pH enhances reabsorption of organic acids by increasing the un-ionized fraction of drug. When the urine of normal rats was acidified by infusion of hydrochloric acid,[39]

furosemide excretion was significantly reduced because of increased drug reabsorption by the renal tubule; under similar experimental conditions in proteinuric rats, this effect was significantly blunted. While this relationship has not been studied in humans, it may be of clinical importance during treatment with drugs such as the sulfonamides or salicylate that are highly protein bound, cleared by the kidney, and undergo tubular reabsorption.

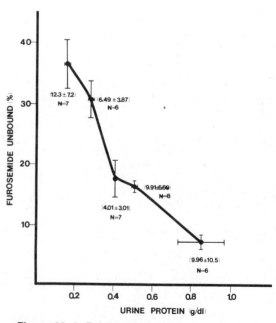

**Figure 28–4.** Relationship between amount of urine protein and urinary drug-protein binding of furosemide in nephrotic rats. Values in parentheses are mean ± SD furosemide concentration (μg/ml). (From Green TP, Mirkin BL: Resistance of proteinuric rats to furosemide: Urinary drug protein binding as a determinant of drug effect. Life Sci 26:623, 1980.)

## HEPATIC DRUG CLEARANCE

Drugs that are totally dependent on hepatic biotransformation for clearance should conform to the pattern represented by Line B in Figure 28–1. Because renal clearance is insignificant and hepatic clearance is independent of GFR, the relationships established in Equations 5 and 6 suggest that dosage adjustments for these drugs are not required to maintain patterns of drug disposition observed in normal individuals. These theoretical considerations are not borne out in all cases. For some drugs in this classification, hepatic metabolism is adversely influenced by renal failure.[40] While the degree of interference with drug clearance may not be as severe as noted for drugs that are subject to renal clearance, the impact on clinical response may be substantial.

Hepatic drug biotransformation is effected through a number of independent metabolic processes, including oxidation, reduction, glucuronide and sulfate conjugation, acetylation, and ester hydrolysis. It appears that uremia may have a selective influence on each of these processes according to a specific pattern.[40] The rate of metabolism for drugs undergoing ester hydrolysis and acetylation is generally slower than normal. Conjugation reactions proceed at a normal rate despite renal failure.

The effect on oxidation remains questionable; it appears to be unchanged for the majority of drugs studied but has been reported to be increased in the case of phenytoin and propranolol. It is not clear whether this is truly a function of increased hepatic metabolism or a consequence of reduced protein-drug binding, as discussed in detail subsequently. In favor of a direct effect of renal failure on this reaction is the evidence that antipyrine, a drug that is minimally protein bound, also appears to have an increased rate of clearance.[41]

The concentration of certain drugs in the portal circulation is reduced by highly efficient hepatic extraction and metabolism after absorption from the gut and prior to reaching the systemic circulation. This phenomenon, known as "first-pass effect," has been extensively investigated with the beta-adrenergic blocking agent, propranolol. In normal subjects, approximately 70% of an initial oral dose of propranolol is extracted in this fashion by the liver.[42]

When the disposition of propranolol was investigated in patients with chronic renal failure, it was discovered that after the initial dose, plasma drug concentrations were threefold greater than levels obtained in normal subjects.[43] Absorption, hepatic blood flow, and elimination rate were not significantly different between the two groups; therefore, it was concluded that hepatic first-pass extraction is inhibited by chronic renal failure. If propranolol represents the prototype for drugs subject to the first-pass effect, reduction in *initial* dosage may be indicated for agents that undergo extensive first-pass metabolism to prevent excessive plasma concentrations.

This observation does not appear to be relevant to the chronic administration of propranolol. More recent studies conducted under steady-state conditions (i.e., after at least 48 hours of continuous propranolol therapy) were unable to confirm differences in plasma drug concentration, drug clearance, apparent hepatic blood flow, or drug extraction ratio between individuals with normal and chronically impaired renal function.[44]

Adjustments for drugs subject to a first-pass effect are best individualized. The high therapeutic index for propranolol[45] suggests that dosage reductions are not necessary. In contrast, greater care may be indicated for initiation of therapy with calcium-entry blocking drugs where the risk of adverse reactions may be more closely related to moderate changes in serum concentrations.[46]

### Drug Clearance by Kidney and Liver

Drug clearance for some drugs may be dependent on a combination of renal excretion and hepatic metabolism (Table 28–3). One such drug is cimetidine.[47] In patients with normal renal function, the drug is cleared predominantly via the kidney. As renal function deteriorates, the proportion of total clearance attributable to hepatic clearance increases. Therefore, plasma half-life never exceeds twice the normal rate, even in patients with a GFR below 10 ml/min. In

**Table 28–3.  DRUGS CLEARED BY RENAL EXCRETION AND HEPATIC METABOLISM**

Cephalothin
Cephapirin
Cimetidine
Dicloxacillin
Penicillin G

patients with both kidney and liver failure, the half-life can be expected to reach 10 times the normal value, requiring alterations in dosage.

Determination of the route and rate of clearance for a given drug is not necessarily predictive of patterns of clearance for other congeners within that class. As an example, penicillin G follows a pattern similar to that described for cimetidine. Under usual conditions, it is cleared by renal tubular transport; however, nonrenal clearance and a wide therapeutic index permit only modest dosage adjustments with renal failure.[48] In contrast, ticarcillin,[49] carbenicillin,[50] and ampicillin[51] appear to have less efficient hepatic clearances than penicillin G in renal failure and therefore require a greater degree of dosage modification with advanced renal failure. Nafcillin is virtually totally cleared by hepatic metabolism.[52] Similar differences can be found within the cephalosporin and tetracycline classes of antibiotics.

## Metabolic Products of Hepatic Drug Clearance

When compared to their parent compounds the metabolic products of hepatic drug biotransformation are generally more polar and less lipid-soluble, characteristics that enhance their renal excretion. Because these metabolites in most cases are also less pharmacologically active than their parent compounds, the consequences of metabolite accumulation during renal failure are commonly given little consideration when drugs that are known to be cleared primarily by the liver are used. Metabolic conversion may, however, result in metabolites that exert an independent or additive pharmacologic effect[53] (Table 28–4). In patients with normal renal function, these metabolites make an insignificant contribution to the therapeutic response. When renal clearance becomes compromised with ESRD, a significant accu-

mulation may occur and result in unexpected toxicity.

Adverse reactions attributable to drug metabolites are generally difficult to assess accurately since laboratory measurements for these compounds are less frequently available. For some drugs such as methyldopa, it is not always clear which metabolite is responsible for the toxicity.[54] Design of drug regimens to compensate for production of active metabolites will be imprecise in most cases. While reduction in dosage can be recommended, final therapeutic considerations may, of necessity, be determined by clinical response.

## INFLUENCE OF RENAL FAILURE ON DRUG DISTRIBUTION; ALTERATIONS IN PLASMA BINDING

The quantity of drug bound to protein as well as the volume of distribution of many drugs are significantly altered in renal failure (Table 28–5). The volume of distribution is determined by dividing the amount of drug in the body at a given time by the concentration of drug measured in the plasma at the same point in time:

$$Vd = \frac{D}{C} \qquad (7)$$

To fully understand this relationship it is important to consider three factors: (1) drugs circulate in two fractions: (a) a free form, dissolved in plasma water; and (b) a fraction bound to plasma proteins; (2) it is only the free fraction of circulating drug that equilibrates with body tissues and fluids; (3) laboratory analytic methods measure total amount of circulating drug and do not distinguish between the bound and free fractions. Therefore, Equation 7 represents an *apparent*

**Table 28–4.** SOME DRUGS THAT FORM ACTIVE METABOLITES BY HEPATIC BIOTRANSFORMATION

| |
|---|
| Allopurinol |
| Cephalothin |
| Diazepam |
| Imipramine |
| Meperidine |
| Procainamide |

**Table 28–5.** SOME DRUGS WITH DECREASED PROTEIN BINDING IN ESRD

| |
|---|
| Cephalothin |
| Diazoxide |
| Furosemide |
| Dicloxacillin |
| Penicillin G |
| Phenobarbital |
| Phenytoin |
| Salicylate |
| Warfarin |

rather than absolute volume of drug distribution and is highly dependent on the degree of drug protein binding. The decreased binding is not compensated by an increase in free drug, since hepatic clearance maintains the total amount of free drug at previous steady-state conditions.[55]

The maintenance of free drug concentration by hepatic metabolism after changes in drug-protein binding has been confirmed in a group of patients with the nephrotic syndrome and hypoalbuminemia.[41] When phenytoin was administered under steady-state conditions, total plasma concentrations were significantly lower in the nephrotic (2.9 µg/ml) than in normal patients (6.8 µg/ml). Despite an increase in the percentage of unbound drug in the nephrotic group (19.2%) compared to the normal group (10.1%), plasma concentrations of free drug were not significantly different (0.59 and 0.69 µg/ml).

The increased volume of distribution for highly protein-bound drugs in uremic patients has been attributed to an impairment of protein binding. Reduced binding is probably unrelated to the relatively small reductions in the serum protein level that may be present, since the concentration of albumin in these patients is in great molar excess of drug concentration. It seems more likely that reduced protein binding can be attributed to displacement of drug by organic acids,[36] fatty acids,[56] or peptides[57] that are retained in high concentration in patients with renal failure. This view is supported by evidence that the protein binding of weakly acidic drugs is decreased in renal failure, whereas drug-protein binding for weak bases remains unchanged.[58]

The implications of the above for clinical practice have recently been discussed.[59] The recognition that levels of free drug under steady-state conditions do not differ significantly between patients with normal and reduced drug-protein binding suggests that modifications of dosing regimens based upon reduced protein binding need not be made to achieve usual therapeutic effects. Yet the incidence of adverse drug reactions has been reported to be increased in hypoproteinemic patients,[60] and therapeutic response may be exaggerated in uremic patients treated with drugs that are highly protein-bound.[61]

These findings may be explained by the principles of pharmacokinetics discussed above and illustrated by Levy.[62] Figure 28–5 demonstrates that under normal conditions (solid line) the concentration of free drug immediately after administration (Time 0) is lower and half-life is longer than under conditions of decreased renal function (interrupted line), in which the concentration of free drug is increased and drug half-life becomes shorter. Thus, despite equivalent concentrations at steady state (noted in the illustration by the identical concentration of free drug at midpoint of the 12-hour dosing interval), the actual drug concentration in patients with reduced protein binding will be considerably higher for a significant amount of time during the dosing schedule. These unexpectedly high concentrations may account for an increase in pharmacologic effect

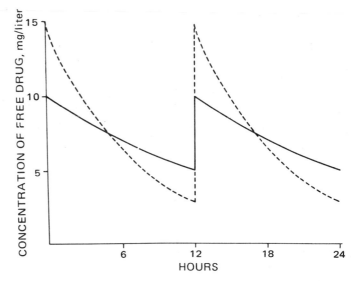

**Figure 28–5.** Effect of renal failure on drug-protein binding, expressed as concentration of free drug. Solid line represents patients with normal renal function. Interrupted line represents uremic patients. (From Levy, G.: Effect of plasma protein binding of drugs on duration and intensity of pharmacologic activity. J Pharmaceut Sci 65:1264, 1976. Reproduced with permission.)

and potential for adverse reactions. To accommodate for these wide swings in concentration, drug dosage should be reduced but administered more frequently. This maneuver will adjust peak and nadir concentrations toward the mean while the steady-state concentration remains unchanged.

Changes in body compartment volumes may accompany ESRD and produce corresponding changes in drug distribution volumes. Drugs that are highly water-soluble and have small apparent volumes of distribution, such as the aminoglycoside antibiotic, are most affected by this process. Patients with ESRD may have expanded or contracted extracellular fluid volumes, depending on the type of renal disease, the effectiveness of diuretic therapy, and the use of dialysis.

## INFLUENCE OF DIALYSIS ON DRUG CLEARANCE

Peritoneal dialysis and hemodialysis may significantly alter the rate of drug clearance and established pharmacokinetic conditions. This effect is not uniform but is dependent on physical and drug disposition characteristics for each agent.

Drugs that normally rely on glomerular filtration for clearance, such as the aminoglycoside antibiotics, have the highest dialysis clearance rates, whereas drugs that are highly protein-bound,[63] such as phenytoin and nafcillin, are cleared to a lesser extent. Limitations of the dialysis membrane may restrict filtration of high-molecular-weight drugs, independent of the above principles. Thus, the antibiotic vancomycin which is excreted via the kidney in individuals with normal renal function and is not highly bound to protein, is poorly dialyzed.

It is usually desirable to replace dialyzable drugs at the completion of dialysis. If the volume of drug distribution is known, the amount of drug removed during dialysis can be approximated by application of Equation 7 as follows:

$$D_{rep} = Vd \, (C_{pre} - C_{post}) \qquad (8)$$

where $D_{rep}$ equals the replacement dose, $C_{pre}$ equals the plasma concentration of drug immediately before, and $C_{post}$ the plasma concentration immediately after dialysis. Drug clearance during dialysis can be measured more accurately if drug concentrations are obtained during dialysis and applied to spe-

cific flow characteristics of the dialyzer being used as follows:

$$Cl_{HD} = Q \, \frac{A-V}{A} \qquad (9)$$

where Q is the dialyzer blood flow, A is the drug concentration in blood entering the dialyzer, and V is the drug concentration in blood leaving the dialyzer. (This equation assumes that drug does not accumulate in the dialyzer.)

Drug clearance is generally less efficient during peritoneal dialysis than during hemodialysis. Not only can technical problems contribute to the considerable variability observed between patients, but, in addition, clearance of drug has been known to vary significantly between dialyses in the same patient. The calculation for dialysate clearance is similar to that used to determine renal clearance:

$$Cl_{PD} = \frac{DV}{P} \qquad (10)$$

where D is the concentration of drug in dialysis fluid, V is the rate of dialysate removal from the peritoneal cavity, and P is the concentration of drug in the plasma at the midpoint of dialysis.

Direct administration of antibiotics into the peritoneal dialysate has been used to treat patients with peritonitis. Under these conditions, the potential for a drug to pass from the peritoneal cavity into the plasma will be correlated with the drug's usual dialysis clearance. When aminoglycoside antibiotics are added to each dialysate in a constant concentration, equilibrium will be reached within a few hours and stady-state plasma conditions maintained for the duration of dialysis.[64] In the case of the aminoglycosides, the potential for toxicity to develop at serum concentrations usually not associated with adverse reactions may be greater when constant levels are maintained than when usual kinetic peak-and-trough conditions prevail.[65] The use of peritoneal dialysate as a portal for drug administration should be approached with caution until additional data have been obtained.

## DESIGNING DOSAGE REGIMENS IN END STAGE RENAL DISEASE

Drug disposition in patients with ESRD is complicated by the general complex physiologic and metabolic changes affecting all patients with renal failure and the variability in response between individual patients. The availability of analytic methods for measurement of drug concentrations has greatly improved the design of dosing regimens. However, the use of these methods demands a clear understanding of the limitations of the information provided, so that blood samples for analysis are timed appropriately after dosing and pharmacokinetic data are properly interpreted for application to patient management.

Some general principles can be established:

1. When therapy is initiated, the usual loading dose can be administered for almost all drugs. Adverse reactions more commonly are associated with drug accumulation because of reduced drug clearance during ongoing therapy.

2. Drugs that are cleared entirely by hepatic metabolism can be administered without modification of dosing regimens when active metabolites are not produced.

3. The usual total daily dose can be administered for drugs that are highly protein-bound and cleared by hepatic metabolism. Displacement from binding sites on serum albumin may require modification of dosing regimens. This can be accomplished by dividing the total daily dose into smaller aliquots and administering these at more frequent intervals to provide a narrower range of concentration.

4. Drugs cleared entirely by the kidney require the most careful monitoring, even when their hepatic clearance increases in renal failure. Pharmacokinetic studies appear to be most useful for these agents. Exceptions to this rule are drugs such as penicillin, which has a broad therapeutic index. This class of drugs requires calculation of pharmacokinetic constants to ensure adequate therapeutic concentrations and to minimize the risk of adverse reactions in patients with renal failure. By obtaining blood samples immediately prior to a dose, at the peak concentration following an intravenous dose and at two or more additional points during the elimination phase, it is possible to determine drug clearance, half-life, and volume of distribution and to construct reliable dosing regimens. A variety of computer programs are now available for this purpose[66] and greatly facilitate the precision and effectiveness of therapy.

The utility of plasma concentrations to assess therapy with drugs that have reduced protein binding and, consequently, significantly lower levels in patients with renal failure remains unclear at the present time. Under ideal circumstances, the level of free or unbound drug should be measured, since this fraction is closely correlated with therapeutic effect and toxicity. Because analytic methods are not usually available to provide this measurement, pharmacokinetic data must be integrated with clinical response to construct appropriate dosing regimens.

## REFERENCES

1. Bennett WM, Porter GA, Bagby SP, McDonald WJ (Eds): Drug therapy in patients with reduced renal function. *In:* Drugs and Renal Disease. New York, Churchill Livingstone, 1978, pp 21–64.
2. Anderson RJ, and Schrier RW (Eds): Clinical Use of Drugs in Patients with Kidney and Liver Disease. WB Saunders Company, Philadelphia, 1981, pp 311–333.
3. Huang NN, High RH: Comparison of serum levels following the administration of oral and parenteral preparation of penicillin to infants and children of various age groups. J Pediatr 42:657, 1953.
4. Heimann G: Enteral absorption and bioavailability in children in relation to age. Eur J Clin Pharmacol 18:43, 1980.
5. Morselli PL: Clinical pharmacokinetics in neonates. Clin Pharmacokin 1:81, 1976.
6. Assael BM, Gianni V, Marnin A, et al: Gentamicin dosage in preterm and term neonates. Arch Dis Child 52:883, 1977.
7. Sardemann H, Colding H, Hendel J, et al: Kinetics and dose calculations of amikacin in the newborn. Clin Pharmacol Ther 20:59, 1976.
8. Nelson JD, Kusmiesz H, Shelton S, Woodman E: Clinical pharmacology and efficacy of ticarcillin in infants and children. Pediatrics 61:858, 1978.
9. Wallace S: Factors affecting drug protein binding in the plasma of newborn infants. Br J Clin Pharmacol 3:510, 1976.
10. Miller RP, Robert RJ, Fischer LJ: Acetaminophen elimination kinetics in neonates, children and adults. Clin Pharmacol Ther 19:284, 1976.
11. Friedman CA, Lovejoy FC, Smith AL: Chloramphenicol disposition in infants and children. J Pediatr 95:1071, 1979.
12. Aranda JV, Turmen T, Sasynuik BI: Pharmacokinetics of diuretics and methylxanthines in the neonate. Eur J Clin Pharmacol 18:55, 1980.
13. Haugey DB, Hilligoss DM, Grassi A, Schentag JJ: Two compartment gentamicin pharmacokinetics in premature infants: A comparison to adults with decreased glomerular filtration rates. J Pediatr 96:325, 1980.
14. Peter RG, Simmons MA, Rumak BH, et al: Pharmacology of furosemide in premature infants. J Pediatr 97:139, 1980.
15. Hilligoss DM: Neonatal pharmacokinetics. *In:* Evans WE, Schentag JJ, Jusko WJ (Eds), Applied Pharmacokinetics. San Francisco, Applied Therapeutics, Inc, 1980, pp 76–94.

16. Winters RW: Regulation of normal water and electrolyte metabolism. *In:* Winters RW (Ed), The Body Fluids in Pediatrics. Boston, Little, Brown, 1973, pp 95–112.

17. Fomon SJ: Infant Nutrition. Philadelphia, WB Saunders Company, 1974, p 575.

18. Vaughn VC, McKay JR, Nelson WE: Textbook of Pediatrics. Philadelphia, WB Saunders Company, 1975, p 1876.

19. Green TP, Mirkin BL: Clinical pharmacokinetics: Pediatric considerations. *In:* The Pharmacokinetic Basis of Drug Treatment, Benet LZ, Gambertoglio JG, Massoud N (Eds). New York, Raven Press, 1982, Chapter 14.

20. Shirkey AC (Ed): Drug administration with special emphasis on techniques and problems related to infants and children. *In:* Pediatric Therapy, Shirkey HC (Ed). St. Louis, CV Mosby, 1972, pp 14–27.

21. Morselli PL, Franco-Morselli R, Bossi L: Clinical pharmacokinetics in newborns and infants. Clin Pharmacokin 5:485, 1980.

22. Frus-Hansen B: Body water compartments in children. Pediatrics 28:169, 1961.

23. Kurz H, Mauser-Ganshorn A, Stickel HH: Differences in the binding of drugs to plasma proteins from newborn and adult man, I. Eur J Clin Pharmacol 2:463, 1977, and Kurz H, Michaels H, Stickel HH: Differences in the binding of drugs to plasma proteins from newborn and adult man, II. Eur J Clin Pharmacol 2:469, 1977.

24. Lietman PS: Chloramphenicol and the neonate—1979 view. Clin Perinatol 6:151, 1979.

25. Mihaly GW, Moore RG, Thomas J, et al: The pharmacokinetics and metabolism of the anilide local anesthetics in neonates. Eur J Clin Pharmacol 13:143, 1978.

26. Rane A, Wilson JT: Clinical pharmacokinetics in infants and children. Clin Pharmacokin 1:2, 1976.

27. Echeverria T, Siber GR, Paisley J, et al: Age-dependent dose response to gentamicin. J Pediatr 87:805, 1975.

28. Ginchansky E, Weinberger M: Relationship of theophylline clearance to oral dosage in children with chronic asthma. J Pediatr 91:655, 1977.

29. Kunin CM, Finland M: Persistence of antibiotics in blood of patients with acute renal failure. III. Penicillin, streptomycin, erythromycin and kanamycin. J Clin Invest 38:1509, 1959.

30. Odlind B, Baerman B: Renal tubular secretion and effects of furosemide. Clin Pharmacol Ther 27:784, 1980.

31. Fuller R, Hoppel C, Ingalls ST: Furosemide kinetics in patients with hepatic cirrhosis with ascites. Clin Pharmacol Ther 30:461, 1981.

32. Green TP, Mirkin BL: Determinants of the diuretic response to furosemide in infants with congestive heart failure. Pediatr Cardiol 3:47, 1982.

33. Rose HJ, Pruitt AW, McNay JL: Effect of experimental azotemia on renal clearance of furosemide in the dog. J Pharmacol Ther 196:238, 1976.

34. Rose HJ, O'Malley K, Pruitt AW: Repression of renal clearance of furosemide in man by azotemia. Clin Pharmacol Ther 21:141, 1977.

35. Preuss HG, Massry SG, Maher JF, et al: Effects of uremic sera on renal tubular p-aminohippurate transport. Nephron 3:265, 1966.

36. Kramer B, Seligson H, Baltrush H, Seligson D: The isolation of several aromatic acids from the hemodialysis fluids of uremic patients. Clin Chir Acta 11:363, 1965.

37. Bourke E, Frindt G, Preuss H, et al: Studies with uraemic serum on the renal transport of hippurates and tetraethylammonium in the rabbit and rat: Effects of oral neomycin. Clin Sci 38:41, 1970.

38. Green TP, Mirkin BL: Resistance of proteinuric rats to furosemide: Urinary drug protein binding as a determinant of drug effect. Life Sci 26:623, 1980.

39. Green TP, Mirkin BL: Furosemide disposition in normal and proteinuric rats: Urinary drug-protein binding as a determinant of drug excretion. J Pharmacol Exp Ther 218:122, 1981.

40. Reidenburg MR: The biotransformation of drugs in renal failure. Am J Med 62:484, 1977.

41. Gugler R, Shoeman DW, Huffman DH, et al: Pharmacokinetics of drugs in patients with the nephrotic syndrome. J Clin Invest 55:1182, 1189, 1975.

42. Shand DG, Rangno RG: The disposition of propranolol. I. Elimination during oral absorption in man. Pharmacology 7:159, 1972.

43. Lowenthal DT, Briggs WA, Gibson TP, et al: Pharmacokinetics of oral propranolol in chronic renal disease. Clin Pharmacol Ther 16:761, 1974.

44. Wood AJJ, Vestal RS, Spannuth CL, et al: Propranolol disposition in renal failure. Br J Pharmacol 10:562, 1980.

45. Mirkin BL, Sinaiko AR: Clinical pharmacology and therapeutic utilization of antihypertensive agents in children. *In:* Juvenile Hypertension, New MI, Levine CS (Eds), New York, Raven Press, 1977, p. 223

46. Piepho RW, Bloedow DC, Lacz JP, et al: Pharmacokinetics of diltiazem in selected animal species and human beings. Am J Cardiol 49:525, 1982.

47. Schentag JJ, Cerra FB, Calleri GM, et al: Age, disease, and cimetidine disposition in healthy subjects and chronically ill patients. Clin Pharmacol Ther 29:737, 1981.

48. Bryan CS, Stone WJ: Comparably massive penicillin G therapy in renal failure. Ann Intern Med 82:189, 1975.

49. Parry MF, Neu HC: Pharmacokinetics of ticarcillin in patients with abnormal renal function. J Infect Dis 133:46, 1976.

50. Latos DL, Bryan CS, Stone WJ: Carbenicillin therapy in patients with normal and impaired renal function. Clin Pharmacol Ther 17:692, 1975.

51. Jusko WJ, Lewis GP, Schmitt GW: Ampicillin and hetacillin pharmacokinetics in normal and anephric subjects. Clin Pharmacol Ther 14:90, 1973.

52. Diaz CR, Kane, JG, Parker RH, Pelsor FR: Pharmacokinetics of naficillin in patients with renal failure. Antimicrob Agents Chemother 12:98, 1977.

53. Drayer DE: Pharmacologically active drug metabolites: Therapeutic and toxic activities, plasma and urine data in man, accumulation in renal failure. Clin Pharmacokin 1:426, 1976.

54. O'Dea RF, Mirkin BL: Metabolic disposition of methyldopa in hypertensive and renal-insufficient children. Clin Pharmacol Ther 27:37, 1980.

55. Wilkinson GR, Shand DG: A physiological approach to hepatic drug clearance. Clin Pharmacol Ther 18:377, 1975.

56. Reidenberg MM: The binding of drugs to plasma proteins from patients with poor renal function. Clin Pharmacokin 1:121, 1976.

57. Kinniburgh DW, Boyd ND: Isolation of peptides from uremic plasma that inhibits phenytoin binding to normal plasma proteins. Clin Pharmacol Ther 30:276, 1981.

58. Olsen GD, Bennett WM, Porter GA: Morphine and phenytoin binding to plasma proteins in renal and hepatic failure. Clin Pharmacol Ther 17:677, 1975.

59. Gibaldi M: Drug distribution in renal failure. Am J Med 62:471, 1977.

60. Boston Collaborative Drug Surveillance Program. Diphenylhydantoin side effects and serum albumin levels. Clin Pharmacol Ther 14:529, 1973.

61. Pearson RM, Breckenridge AM: Renal function, protein binding and pharmacologic response to diazoxide. Br J Clin Pharmacol 3:169, 1976.

62. Levy G: Effect of plasma protein binding of drugs on duration and intensity of pharmacologic activity. J Pharmaceut Sci 65:1264, 1976.

63. Gwilt PR, Perrier D: Plasma protein building and distribution characteristics of drugs as indices of their hemodialyzability. Clin Pharmacol Ther 24:154, 1978.

64. Somani P, Shapiro RS, Stockard H, Higgins JT: Unidirectional absorption of gentamicin from the peritoneum during continuous ambulatory peritoneal dialysis. Clin Pharmacol Ther 32:113, 1982.

65. Keating MJ, Bodley GP, Valdivraso M, Rodriguez V: A randomized comparative trial of three aminoglycosides. Medicine 58:159, 1979.

66. Green TP, Mirkin BL: A method for the bedside application of first-order pharmacokinetics in therapeutic management. Ther Drug Monit 2:323, 1980.

# 29

# INFECTION IN THE CHILD RECEIVING THERAPY FOR ESRD

*Michael R. Leone, M.D.*
*Paul T. McEnery, M.D.*

Kidney transplantation and dialysis, despite vast technical advances and improved clinical expertise, remain an imperfect art for pediatric as well as adult patients with ESRD. Renal transplantation is the goal of all ESRD programs for children, but the course to a healthy child with a functioning kidney transplant is a delicate balance of immunosuppression and medical-surgical expertise to achieve that well-being. With this in mind it is imperative that the physician caring for the child with ESRD be continuously aware of and promote those principles of patient management which minimize inherent opportunistic and iatrogenic factors which lead to infection. This chapter reviews the various levels of altered immune responsiveness, types and frequency of infection, and the offending microbes found in patients receiving dialysis and transplantation.

## DEFECTS IN UREMIC HOST RESISTANCE

Infection is a frequent complication of acute and chronic renal insufficiency,[1-3] owing in large part to diminished immune responsiveness of affected patients. Alterations occur at various levels of the immune system in uremia, affecting both cellular and humoral immunity. Considering the extensive interaction between cellular immune mechanisms and humoral immune expression, the separation of the two is arbitrary. However, in order to facilitate discussion, cellular and

humoral immune alterations will be addressed individually.

**Cellular Immune System.** Delayed rejection of skin and kidney allografts by uremic patients and animals has been observed by several investigators.[4-6] Additional observations documenting impaired cellular immunity include an abnormally weak mixed lymphocyte culture (MLC) response, reduced production of lymphokines such as migration inhibitory factor (MIF), impaired phagocytosis by monocytes, and thymic atrophy unrelated to prior steroid therapy.[7-9] Also the number of circulating T lymphocytes, and their response to mitogenic agents, are depressed in uremia to a greater extent than that seen in patients receiving the usual immunosuppressive drugs after renal transplantation.[10]

Delayed cutaneous hypersensitivity is variably impaired in uremia, and studies report a later occurrence of the first kidney allograft rejection episode in patients who were anergic prior to transplantation.[7, 11] A polymorphonuclear leukocyte chemotactic defect, either intrinsic to the leukocyte[12] or arising from a serum inhibitor, has also been reported.[13]

**Humoral Immune System.** Although the alteration in cellular immunity associated with uremia is more clearly defined, there is unquestionably a significant impairment of humoral immunity as well. Hepatitis B infection in uremic patients fails to elicit a detectable antibody titer frequently.[14, 15] The response to hepatitis B virus vaccine has been found to be markedly reduced in patients on chronic hemodialysis, although this latter observation seemed to apply only to patients over 40 years of age.[16] The response to pneumococcal vaccine resulted in mean antibody titers which were felt to be adequate, but significantly lower than that reported for normal individuals.[17]

## INFECTIONS IN CHILDREN RECEIVING HEMODIALYSIS

**Hemodialysis Access Infection.** Most infectious complications of angioaccess are similar for children and adults receiving chronic hemodialysis. More than 90% of infections of arteriovenous (AV) shunts involve *Staphylococcus aureus*, with a remainder caused by pseudomonas and enterobacteriaceae. The incidence of local skin infection of shunts has been reported to range from one to three episodes per patient dialysis year[18-20] in adults and children. The incidence of local infections of internal AV fistulae is less, ranging from 0.15 or fewer episodes per patient dialysis year.[19-21]

Systemic bacteremia can occur if the access site infection does not immediately respond to treatment. The incidence of septicemia and type of bacteria in patients with shunts or fistulae are similar.[19] Experience with internal heterogenous AV materials suggests that sepsis occurred earlier and with greater frequency with bovine heterografts than with Brescia fistulas[20] and polytetrafluoroethylene material.[22, 23] Epidemiologic findings with phage typing and antibiotic sensitivity data suggest that autoinfection with skin bacteria is the primary cause of vascular access-site-related sepsis[19, 20] and not dialysis-related equipment or personnel.

Vascular access-site-related bacteremia or sepsis can often lead to metastatic complications with septic pulmonary emboli and endocarditis.[24] *Staphylococcus aureus* is most often the organism responsible for the infection, but streptococci and gram-negative organisms have also been reported.[20, 25] In recent years the use of percutaneous subclavian or internal jugular angioaccess catheters which remain in place between dialysis procedures has increased the incidence of bacteremia. Sepsis unrelated to the vascular access site is most often a complication of a surgical wound infection, nephrectomy site abscess, or urinary tract infection.

Improved detection and prompt initiation of antibiotic therapy in the treatment of dialysis-related infections has led to a marked decrease in the morbidity and mortality of both adults and children on dialysis in recent years. This emphasizes the absolute need for vigorous hygiene and thorough observation of the vascular access site by the patient and dialysis personnel prior to each dialysis procedure.

Common local signs of vascular access site infection include severe pain or tenderness, purulent discharge, skin necrosis, or abscesses. Erythema, warmth, and induration are signs normally present at the vascular access site and do not alone indicate local infection. Erosion and infection at the vascular access site of the shunt are signs that the shunt will not last long. Local infections rarely occur with internal AV fistulas, but may occur at the vessel anastomosis or a needle puncture site with abscess formation. Early postoperative infection of a grafted AV fistula is also rare. When infections occur they usually involve the entire length of the graft and sites of the arterial and venous anastomosis, necessitating early removal of the graft. Use of the grafted AV fistula during the initial two weeks post-surgery may lead to development of a hematoma at the needle puncture site and the hematoma's dissecting along the entire length of the graft tunnel.

Routine removal or ligation of a vascular access site associated with sepsis is not mandatory. Aggressive local and systemic antibiotic treatment in our experience and that of others[19, 20, 25] has allowed for resolution of infection and preservation of the vascular access.

Localizing signs of infection are the most common antecedent to bacteremia in the patient with an AV shunt, but localizing signs are rare in patients with internal grafts or fistulas. Fever and changes in a child's previously stable cardiac, pulmonary, or neurologic status should alert the observer to the need for a blood culture. Although sterile technique by dialysis personnel is not mandatory at the initiation of the dialysis procedure, it is important to note that clean and gloved techniques are necessary elements in the prevention of iatrogenic infections. Dialysis personnel should develop a systematic record of area of fistula entry so as to avoid repetitious cannulation at the same puncture site, which often leads to thrombosis and abscess formation.

**Hepatitis.** Hepatitis B virus (HBV) infection continues to be the most common infectious complication in long-term hemodialysis patients. Surveys have indicated that approximately 80% of the hemodialysis units in this country are contaminated with HBV[26] and that 57% of the patients studied have serologic evidence of present or prior HBV infection.[27] In comparison to an otherwise healthy population infected with HBV, dialysis patients suffer a more moderate illness, which is generally anicteric, and they often evolve into a chronic $HB_sAg$ carrier state, with a frequency reported as high as 75%.[28, 29]

Because of the frequency of the chronic carrier state in dialysis patients, and the frequency with which others are exposed to the vehicles of transmission of the HBV (blood, saliva, peritoneal fluid, semen, and urine), these patients represent a unique threat for transmission of the infection. It would appear that patients with $HB_sAg$ should be considered infectious, but the presence of $HB_sAg$ does not alone determine infectivity. Dialysis patients with $HB_sAg$ and $HB_eAg$ in their serum should be considered highly infectious because of the association of the e-antigen with Dane particle–associated DNA polymerase activity, indicating ongoing HBV replication.[30] Patients with antibody to $HB_cAg$ but without $HB_sAg$ or anti-$HB_sAg$ should likewise be considered infectious. Patients with antibody to $HB_eAg$, regardless of the presence or absence of $HB_sAg$, and patients with antibody to $HB_sAg$ can be considered noninfectious.[31, 32]

Despite the moderate nature of HBV infection in the dialysis patient, an alarmingly high mortality rate of 7% has been reported.[33] An additional risk factor is the potential for spread of the infection to hemodialysis staff members, family contacts directly participating in the dialysis procedure, and other dialysis patients.[32] With the advent of transfusion protocols to prepare prospective transplant recipients, the frequency of infection with non-A, non-B hepatitis in this patient population will undoubtedly increase, as this agent is responsible for approximately 90% of post-transfusion hepatitis.[34] A recent study reported an alarmingly high incidence of liver disease in several transplant recipients, which the investigators attributed to chronic hepatitis secondary to infection with the non-A, non-B hepatitis virus.[35]

Surveillance is essential if one is to avoid introduction of HBV into a dialysis unit. This includes careful screening of all new patients and staff for the presence of $HB_sAg$, anti-$HB_sAg$, anti-$HB_cAg$, and elevation of SGOT and SGPT levels. A complete medical history with attention to recent illnesses and exposures should be obtained. At regular intervals screening of patients and staff for the same three serologic markers of HBV infection should be undertaken. Patients additionally should be screened monthly for elevations of SGOT and SGPT levels to detect non-A, non-B hepatitis. Once HBV has been identified in a patient, established procedures for prevention of spread should be employed. These are carefully outlined in a Communicable Disease Center report of 1976.[36]

Because of the high prevalence and attack rates of HBV infection in hemodialysis units, immunoprophylaxis is often a consideration. The reader is referred to a set of recommendations concerning the use of immune serum globulins[37] and HBV vaccine[38] for a more complete discussion of this subject. The goal of active immunization is the production of antibody to $HB_sAg$, thereby conferring protection from infection with HBV. Considering the preliminary reports of shortened allograft survival in patients with anti-$HB_sAg$, and the reported low incidence of response of chronic dialysis patients to vaccination, the utility of the HBV vaccine in this high-risk population is uncertain at present.[38, 39]

**Cytomegalovirus.** Although cytomegalovirus (CMV) infection is much more clinically significant in the post-transplant population, epidemiologic considerations warrant discussion of CMV prevalence and transmission within hemodialysis units. Documentation of virus excretion, seroconversion from antibody-negative to antibody-positive (complement fixation or indirect hemagglutination), or a fourfold increase in antibody titer are the generally accepted means of ascertaining CMV acquisition or reactivation. The spectrum of clinical illness in the hemodialysis patient can vary from a mononucleosis-like illness to a more serious illness characterized by leukopenia, hepatitis, pneumonitis, and fever.[40] In addition, CMV has been implicated as the etiologic agent of pericarditis and pericardial effusion in hemodialysis patients.[41]

The risk of transmission of CMV via blood transfusions has long been recognized,[42] and it has been estimated that up to 12% of all blood donors are capable of transmitting CMV.[43] In these instances the virus can be isolated from the buffy coat of the donor blood, and transfusion of conventional (fresh whole) blood containing large numbers of viable leukocytes presents the greatest risk of virus transmission. Patients are most likely to acquire CMV when they receive multiple transfusions of conventional blood, whereas those who receive no blood transfusions or only frozen deglycerolized erythrocytes, which have been found to be devoid of viable leukocytes, are at minimal risk.[44]

## INFECTION IN CHILDREN FOLLOWING RENAL TRANSPLANTATION

**Immunosuppressive Therapy and Infection in the Transplant Recipient.** All the immunosuppressive agents affect primarily the cellular immune response of patients. Therefore, one would expect that those infectious agents which are handled by the cellular immune mechanism of the human host defense system would pose the most serious threat to those patients receiving one or a combination of immunosuppressive agents. T lymphocytes and the phagocyte system are critical for defense against the following microbial pathogens: bacteria (mycobacterium, salmonella, brucella, and listeria), fungi (candida, cryptococcus, and histoplasma), protozoa (toxoplasma, malaria, leishmania, and trypanosoma), and all viruses.[45] Clinical observations have shown that these "opportunistic" pathogens are indeed those which frequently complicate the post-transplant patient's medical course.

Histocompatibility differences between donor and recipient make pharmacologic alteration of the immune response a therapeutic goal in an effort to minimize immunologic rejection. These alterations are unavoidably nonspecific and affect many facets of the immune response, thereby rendering the host susceptible to infectious complications. The agents used in renal transplantation for their immunosuppressive properties are glucocorticoids, azathioprine, antilymphocyte globulin, and, recently, cyclosporin A. A brief discussion of the effects on the immune response of each of these agents follows.

*Glucocorticoids.* Glucocorticoids when administered in pharmacologic doses induce a characteristic shift in the pattern of circulating leukocytes: the number of neutrophils is increased markedly while there is a decrease in the absolute number of circulating lymphocytes. These observed changes are explained on the basis of cell redistribution.

The neutrophilia results from increased bone marrow release and decreased egress from the intravascular space, and the lymphopenia arises from increased deposition in lymphoid organs such as the bone marrow.[46] Cell lysis plays a minor role in the observed lymphopenia.

Cellular immunity is more clearly affected by glucocorticoid therapy than is humoral immunity. Monocyte chemotaxis and bactericidal activity, T-cell mitogenic responsiveness, and T-cell proliferative response to antigenic challenge are each diminished by steroid therapy.[47]

One of the major effects of steroid therapy is suppression of the inflammatory response. In this regard steroids interfere with macrophage access to sites of immunologic reactivity, and antagonize their interaction with soluble mediators of cellular immunity, such as macrophage migration inhibitory factor (MIF) and macrophage aggregating factor (MAF).[46]

*Azathioprine.* Azathioprine (Imuran) is a purine analog whose immunosuppressive potential lies with the action of its various metabolites, including 6-mercaptopurine. In experimental animals azathioprine inhibits primary antibody formation without affecting established antibody production. It was also found to be a potent inhibitor of the cellular immune mechanism, as evidenced by its ability to virtually eliminate delayed type hypersensitivity reaction.[48,49]

In renal transplant recipients with good allograft function receiving pharmacologic doses of azathioprine and low dose prednisone therapy, the cellular immune response was observed to be suppressed, whereas the primary and secondary humoral immune responses (antibody production) were found to be intact.[50]

*Antilymphocyte Globulin.* There have been few studies examining the effects of antilymphocyte globulin (ALG) on the immune system of humans, although ALG is generally conceded to be a potent inhibitor of the cellular immune system. ALG administered to humans has been found to deplete circulating T lymphocytes and abolish delayed hypersensitivity reactions. B lymphocytes are resistant to its effects, and in fact the percentage of circulating B lymphocytes increases after ALG treatment, while the total lymphocyte count is unchanged.[51]

*Cyclosporin A.* Cyclosporin A, a recently discovered fungal metabolite with potent immunosuppressive properties, is an attractive agent for use in organ grafting because of its steroid-sparing capability. As with the other immunosuppressives discussed, cellular immunity is primarily affected. More specifically, the T-helper cell subpopulation is suppressed with relative sparing of the B lymphocytes. There is little recorded bone marrow toxicity associated with its use.[52] In early clinical trials of organ grafting, cyclosporin A was used in conjunction with prednisone and cytotoxic drugs. The patients so treated were noted to be markedly immunosuppressed, with a number of deaths resulting from infection.[53]

**Type of Infection at Different Periods after Transplant Surgery.** Splenectomy, urologic and vascular surgical procedures in the uremic child, anemia, defects in coagulation, malnutrition, and pharmacologic immunosuppression are all factors which combine to make the transplant recipient susceptible to infection, especially during the initial post-transplant months. Even with these numerous variables one can, with good judgment, predict the type of infection and the offending agent at a given period post-transplantation (Fig. 29–1). During the first month post-transplant, opportunistic fungal and protozoal infections are almost nonexistent. Fever (38.3°C, or 101°F) is the most reliable sign of infection and should always be regarded with concern. The height and duration of fever, time of onset in the post-transplant period, associated symptoms, and results of diagnostic tests are all important factors which must be considered prior to alterations in immunosuppressive therapy or initiation of antibiotic therapy.

Viral infections have been reported to be responsible for greater than half of the post-transplant fevers,[54] but other microbes, pulmonary emboli, drug fever, malignancy, and, of course, rejection must be considered in the diagnostic work-up. Fevers of viral etiology tend to persist longer and may have daily exacerbations. The physical examination of the child with persistent fever of viral etiology is relatively negative, but occasionally there may be a rash or an annoying dry nonproductive cough. When a viral infection occurs

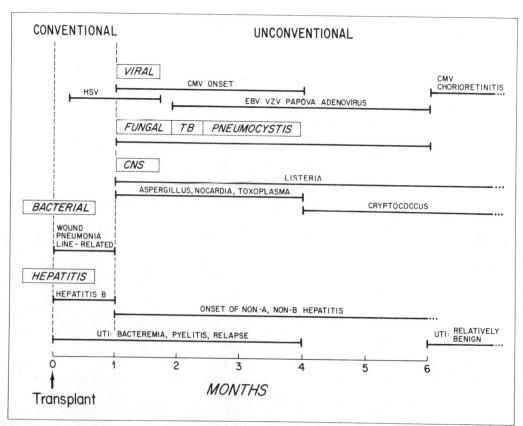

**Figure 29–1.** Timetable for the occurrence of infection in the renal transplant patient. (From Rubin RH, Wolfson JS, Losini AS, Tolkoff-Rubin NE: Infection in the renal transplant recipient. Am J Med70:405, 1981.)

in association with fungal, protozoan, or bacterial infection, the transplant recipient is most often more obviously ill. Bacterial infections, with few exceptions, respond rapidly with fever resolution once appropriate antibacterial therapy is instituted. In the compromised patient not responding to 48 hours of antibiotic therapy, the probability of opportunistic infection is likely. In such patients the dose of immunosuppressive drugs should be decreased, and in life-threatening situations discontinued.

Bacterial contamination of wounds, urinary tract, blood, and lungs, causing critical infection in the transplant recipient, may occur in the initial months post surgery and are described below.

*Wound Infection.* The proximity of the grafted organ to the incision site and the immunosuppressed state of the recipient are of immense significance in the management of a wound infection in the renal transplant recipient. The incidence of these infections and the attendant complications of bacterial sepsis and perinephric abscess formation resulting in graft loss have been reduced considerably in recent years. Broad-spectrum antibiotic administration at the time of transplantation and improved surgical technique have each contributed to the lowered incidence of wound infection.[55, 56] If one excludes the surgical complications of urinary fistulas and perinephric hematomas, the incidence and microbial etiology of wound infection in transplant patients is identical to that observed in non-immunosuppressed patients.[57, 58]

*Urinary Tract Infection.* The urinary tract continues to be the most frequent site of bacterial infection following transplantation, with a reported incidence of 58% in the pediatric population.[59, 60] The significance of infection in the urinary system depends in large part upon the time of onset: infections presenting within the first three months following transplantation are often associated with surgical complications such as ureteral leakage and deep wound infection[61] and frequently evolve into a clinical syndrome characterized by septicemia, pyelonephritis, and allograft dysfunction.[62] Without these complications, urinary tract infections presenting at any time after transplantation, but particularly those presenting after six months, are relatively benign, and may be handled in the usual fashion without fear of sepsis or allograft dysfunction.[60, 62, 63]

In those infections not associated with sur-

gical complications *Escherichia coli* has been isolated in 30 to 50% of first infections.[59, 60, 63, 64] Klebsiella, Pseudomonas, Proteus, and *Streptococcus faecalis* are found less frequently, but often they are involved in the more antibiotic-resistant infections and those with a high rate of relapse. *Streptococcus faecalis* urinary infection has been a common organism reported to occur in patients with unsuccessful grafts, but unsuccessful grafts do not have an increased incidence of infection.[60, 65]

*Septicemia.* Bacterial sepsis contributing to patient morbidity and mortality was reported with alarming frequency in the past,[66] but, as mentioned above, the avoidance of surgical complications, as well as antibiotic administration at the time of transplantation, has significantly reduced the incidence of septicemia. Predisposing factors which have not changed include bowel perforations associated with CMV infection or steroid therapy, leading to gram-negative septicemia,[54, 62, 64] and septicemia with encapsulated organisms seen in the asplenic transplant patient.[67, 68] In an individual suspected of sepsis but without an identifiable source, and who is more than one month post-transplant, the possibility of *Listeria monocytogenes* septicemia should be considered.[69] This organism has become one of the most frequent etiologic agents of bacterial septicemia in the transplant recipient, with a marked proclivity for CNS involvement.[56]

*Pneumonia.* Pulmonary infection in the renal transplant patient can occur at any time post-transplantation and is the most frequent infectious complication contributing to patient mortality.[64, 70] Because of the extensive list of etiologic agents, the following considerations are helpful in delineating the offending organism in the transplant patient with a fever and pulmonary infiltrate: the general health of the patient, the acuteness of the process, the time of onset of infection relative to transplantation, and the radiographic appearance. At times more aggressive diagnostic tools (biopsy) should be utilized to rapidly establish an etiology so that specific therapy may be employed.

*Bacterial pneumonia* (usually gram-negative rods, less often staphylococcus sp. or streptococcus) presents acutely in the early post-transplant period with a radiographic appearance of focal, multifocal, or lobar infiltrates. *Viral pneumonia*—CMV, rarely Epstein-Barr virus (EBV), herpes simplex virus (HSV), varicella-zoster virus (VZV)—presents subacutely one to four months after transplantation, with fever and diffuse pulmonary infiltrates. *Fungal pneumonia* (Aspergillus, Nocardia, Cryptococcus, less often Phycomycetes or Candida sp.) assumes a more indolent course, usually beginning more than one month after transplantation, with a radiographic appearance varying from small nodules to frank cavitation. The patient infected with a fungus historically experiences either progressive renal failure or graft rejection with increased immunosuppression. *Protozoan infection (Pneumocystis carinii*, rarely *Toxoplasma gondii)* presents in a fashion very similar to viral pneumonia, and often concurrent infection is observed.[62, 70, 71] These latter two infecting microbes reflect nosocomially acquired infection while the patient is receiving high dose immunosuppression and has leukopenia or other complications of a debilitating illness. Treatment of *Pneumocystis carinii* infection with trimethoprim-sulfa preparations is effective, and the prophylactic use of this antibiotic combination has resulted in a decreased incidence of infection with this agent in the allograft recipient.

***Central Nervous System (CNS) Infection.*** Acute infection of the CNS in the renal transplant recipient is in most cases a meningitis, with *Listeria monocytogenes* almost invariably the infectious agent.[56] Subacute or chronic CNS symptoms may be a manifestation of *cryptococcal* meningitis[72] or focal infection due usually to *Aspergillus* metastatic from a pulmonary focus.[62] Focal infection is also seen with *Listeria* and *Toxoplasma*, and up to 40% of cases of *Nocardia* pneumonitis disseminate, resulting in brain abscess formation.[73]

### Viral Infectious Syndromes

***Cytomegalovirus (CMV).*** CMV is the most frequent serious infectious complication following renal transplantation. CMV viruria ("infection") has been reported to occur in more than 90% of patients following transplantation,[74] whereas the incidence of an overt clinical syndrome ("disease") due to CMV viremia is reported with a much lower frequency, on the order of 30%.[75, 76] CMV infection may persist for months to years after onset. Although some investigators have related CMV viruria to the development of chorioretinitis,[77] its significance is largely unknown.

CMV viremia or disease presents as prolonged fever (> 7 days) usually between one and four months post-transplantation, and may progress to a severe clinical syndrome characterized by pneumonitis, gastrointestinal hemorrhage (with or without perforation), hepatitis, pancreatitis, and allograft dysfunction. Associated laboratory abnormalities include anemia, leukopenia, and thrombocytopenia. The reported mortality of CMV disease is 20%, and it is most often seen in patients with secondary bacterial or protozoan infections developing weeks after onset of CMV infection.[76]

CMV disease is most likely to develop in seronegative recipients of a seropositive donor, whereas infection or viruria is most often seen in seropositive recipients of a seropositive donor. Seronegative recipients and seronegative donors represent the combination least likely to result in either infection or disease.[75] Epidemiologically, CMV viremia results from primary CMV infection arising from the transplantation of a latently infected organ,[78] whereas CMV viruria and infection result from reactivation of dormant CMV via pharmacologic immunosuppression of a seropositive individual.[79, 80]

***Herpes Simplex (HSV), Varicella-Zoster (VZV) and Other Viruses.*** Infection with HSV in renal transplant patients has been reported to be as high as 70%, placing it second only to CMV as an infectious viral agent in this patient population. Features of HSV infection, which are different from comparable features of CMV infection, are as follows: (1) infection with HSV is seen within the first month following transplantation, at the time of peak immunosuppression; (2) the donor kidney appears to play little or no role in infection; (3) infection with HSV is usually symptomatic (oral mucocutaneous lesions); (4) dissemination is rarely observed, and (5) virus excretion does not persist once the clinical syndrome resolves.[74]

As in the normal population, infection with VZV in the transplant population is either primary (chickenpox) or secondary (shingles). Unlike the pattern in the normal population, however, a third pattern of infection has been documented: reinfection in a patient with a documented prior infection. In this latter instance, the disease spectrum is that of primary infection. The incidence of primary infection in the pediatric transplant population is reported to be 12%.[81]

Because primary infection in a transplant recipient can be virulent, passive immunization, using varicella-zoster immune globulin (VZIG) as soon as possible within 72 hours of known exposure, is recommended. If the patient is hospitalized, isolation should be instituted for up to 28 days following exposure.[82] The extent of the illness in the transplant patient is determined by the magnitude of immunosuppression. Therefore, once vesicle formation is documented, azathioprine should be discontinued and the prednisone dosage altered so as to minimize immunosuppression while simultaneously preventing addisonian crisis.[81]

Secondary VZV infections (herpes zoster or shingles) occur with a reported frequency of 8% in the transplant population. In contrast to primary VZV infection, dissemination has not been reported, and systemic symptoms are few.[82-84]

Epstein-Barr virus (EBV) excretion has been documented in up to 50% of transplant patients, and symptomatic infection is similar to that seen with CMV infection, with symptoms not unlike those manifested in the normal population. However, there has been reported in the transplant population a malignant lymphoproliferative disorder associated with EBV infection, and fatalities have resulted.[85, 86]

Adenovirus infections presenting as a respiratory illness or hemorrhagic cystitis occur in the transplant population with an incidence greater than that seen in the general population.[87] Papovaviruses have been implicated after transplantation as contributing to the development of ureteral stenosis, progressive multifocal leukoencephalopathy, diabetes mellitus, atherosclerosis, and malignancy.[88, 89]

**Fungal Infection.** Fungal infection occurs in renal transplant recipients with a reported incidence of 13%. The areas generally affected include the CNS, lungs, gastrointestinal system, and genitourinary system. Concurrent infections with bacteria, viruses, or protozoa are often present, which partially explains the frequent delay in diagnosis and the high case fatality rate.

*Cryptococcus* is the fungal organism which most often complicates the post-transplant course, with the CNS invariably affected. Symptoms suggesting the possibility of cryptococcal meningitis include headache and disorientation of a subacute nature, particularly in a patient with pulmonary infiltrates. Cerebrospinal fluid should be tested for cryptococcal antigen as well as examined with an India ink preparation.[90] *Nocardia*, although recently classified as a bacterium, is classically included in discussions of opportunistic infectious organisms. It presents usually in a chronic manner, frequently complicating an established infectious syndrome. Pulmonary infection progressing to frank cavitation is usually seen, with frequent concomitant focal CNS infection.[71, 73] *Coccidioidomycosis* is a prominent pulmonary pathogen, particularly in endemic areas such as Arizona.[91] Because of its propensity for dissemination and the associated high mortality rate, patients with known prior symptomatic coccidioidal infections may not be acceptable transplant recipients and recipients should be cautioned about visiting endemic areas. *Candida* infection, when limited to the gastrointestinal system (i.e., esophagitis), is usually not reported, so the true incidence of this infection, despite the debilitating nature, is unknown. However, in the immunosuppressed patient receiving broad-spectrum antibiotics who develops dysphagia, careful consideration should be given to this agent. When the genitourinary system is involved with symptomatic Candida infection, systemic therapy is indicated.[72] *Aspergillus* infects the pulmonary system, often invading blood vessels and resulting in thrombosis and distal pulmonary infarction. With diffuse involvement, the fatality rate is extraordinarily high.

## REFERENCES

1. Montgomerie JZ, Kalmanson GM, Guze LB: Renal failure and infection. Medicine 47:1, 1968.
2. Drukker, W, Moorhead JF, Cameron JS: Mortality during regular dialysis treatment (editorial). Lancet 2:968, 1970.
3. Dobbelstein H: Immune system in uremia. Nephron 17:409, 1976.
4. Dammin GJ, Couch NP, Murray JE: Prolonged survival of skin homografts in uremic patients. Ann NY Acad Sci 64:967, 1957.
5. Mannick JA, Powers JH, Mithoefer J, Ferreree JW: Renal transplantation in azotemic dogs. Surgery 47:340, 1960.
6. Souhami RL, Smith J, Bradfield JWB: The effect of uremia on organ graft survival in the rat. Br J Exp Pathol 54:183, 1973.
7. Huber H, Pastner D, Dittrich P, Braunsteiner H: "In vitro" reactivity of human lymphocytes in uremia—a comparison with the impairment of delayed hypersensitivity. Clin Exp Immunol 5:75, 1969.
8. Montgomerie JZ, Kalmanson GM, Guze LB: Leukocyte phagocytosis and serum bactericidal activity in chronic renal failure. Am J Med Sci 264:385, 1972.
9. Casciani CU, DeSimone C, Bonini S, et al: Immunological aspects of chronic uremia. Kidney Int 13:549, 1978.
10. Quadracci LJ, Ringden O, Krzymanski M: The effect of uremia and transplantation on lymphocyte subpopulations. Kidney Int 10:179, 1976.
11. Wilson WEC, Kirkpatrick CH, Talmage DW: Immunologic studies in human organ transplanta-

tion. III. The relationship of delayed hypersensitivity to the onset of attempted kidney allograft rejection. J Clin Invest 43:1881, 1964.

12. Salant DJ, Glover A, Anderson R, et al: Depressed neutrophil chemotaxis in patients with chronic renal failure and after renal transplantation. J Lab Clin Med 88:536, 1976.

13. Clark RA, Hamory BH, Ford GH, Kimball HR: Chemotaxis in acute renal failure. J Infect Dis 126:460, 1972.

14. Blumberg BS, Sutnik AI, London WT: Australia antigen as a hepatitis virus. Variation in host response. Am J Med 48:1, 1970.

15. Maynard JE: Viral hepatitis as an occupational hazard in the health care profession. In: Vyas GN, Cohen SN, Schmid R (eds): Viral Hepatitis. Philadelphia, Franklin Press, 1978, pp 321–331.

16. Maupas P, Goudeau A, Coursaget P, et al: Immunization against hepatitis B in man: A pilot study of two years duration. In: Vyas GN, Cohen SN, Schmid R (eds): Viral Hepatitis. Philadelphia, Franklin Press, 1978, pp 539–556.

17. Linnemann CC, First MR, Schiffman G: Response to pneumococcal vaccine in renal transplant and hemodialysis patients. Arch Intern Med 141:1637, 1981.

18. Potter D, Larsen D, Leumann E, et al: Treatment of chronic uremia in childhood. II. Hemodialysis. Pediatrics 46:678, 1970.

19. Ralston AJ, Harlow GR, Jones DM, Davis D: Infections of Scribner and Brescia arteriovenous shunts. Br Med J 3:408, 1971.

20. Dobkin JF, Miller MH, Stergbigel NH: Septicemia in patients on chronic hemodialysis. Ann Intern Med 88:28, 1978.

21. Lumley JSP, Cattell WR, Baker LRI: Access to the circulation for regular hemodialysis. Lancet 1:510, 1973.

22. Giacchino JL, Geis WP, Buckingham JM, et al: Vascular access: Long-term results, new techniques. Arch Surg 114:403, 1979.

23. Tellis VA, Kohlberg WI, Bhat DJ, et al: Expanded polytetrafluorethylene graft fistula for chronic hemodialysis. Ann Surg 189:101, 1979.

24. Leonard A, Raig L, Shapiro FL: Bacterial endocarditis in regularly dialyzed patients. Kidney Int 4:407, 1973.

25. Levi J, Robson M, Rosenfeld JB: Septicemia and pulmonary embolism complicating use of arteriovenous fistula in maintenance hemodialysis. Lancet 2:288, 1970.

26. Garibaldi RA, Forrest JN, Bryan JA, et al: Hemodialysis-associated hepatitis. JAMA 225:384, 1973.

27. Szmuness W, Prince AM, Grady GF, et al: Hepatitis B infection. A point prevalence study in 15 United States hemodialysis centers. JAMA 227:901, 1974.

28. Rashid A, Sengar D, McLeish W, et al: The effect of host immunity and hepatitis B antigen (HB$_s$Ag) infection in hemodialysis patients. Trans Am Soc Artif Intern Organs 21:483, 1975.

29. Snydman DR, Bryan JA, Hanson B: Hemodialysis-associated hepatitis in the United States—1972. J Infect Dis 132:109, 1975.

30. Hess G, Arnold W, Koesters W, Meyer Zum Buschenfelde KH: Tests for Dane particles in serum concentrates of HB$_s$Ag-positive hemodialysis patients. Clin Nephrol 11:18, 1979.

31. Gahl GM, Hess G, Arnold W, Grams G: Hepatitis B virus markers in 97 long-term hemodialysis patients. Nephron 24:58, 1979.

32. Gahl GM, Vogl E, Kraft D, et al: Hepatitis B virus markers among family contacts and medical personnel of 239 hemodialysis patients. Clin Nephrol 14:7, 1980.

33. Parsons FM, Brunner FP, Gurland HJ, Harlen H: Combined report of regular dialysis and transplantation in Europe. Proc Eur Dial Transplant Assoc 8:3, 1971.

34. Alter HJ, Purcell RH, Feinstone SM, et al: Non-A/Non-B hepatitis, a review and interim report on an ongoing prospective study. In: Vyas GN, Cohen SN, Schmid R (eds): Viral Hepatitis. Philadelphia, Franklin Press, 1978, pp 557–567.

35. Ware AJ, Luby JP, Hollinger B, et al: Etiology of liver disease in renal-transplant patients. Ann Intern Med 91:364, 1979.

36. Center for Disease Control: Perspectives on the control of viral hepatitis type B. Morbidity and Mortality Weekly Report 25:1, 1976.

37. Center for Disease Control: Immune globulins for protection against viral hepatitis. Recommendations of the immunization practices advisory committee. Ann Intern Med 96:193, 1982.

38. Jungers P, Delagneau JF, Prunet P, Crosnier J: Vaccination against hepatitis B in hemodialysis centers. Adv Nephrol. Year Book Medical Publishers, 1982, p 303.

39. London WT, Drew JS, Blumberg BS, et al: Association of graft survival with host response to hepatitis B infection in patients with kidney transplants. N Engl J Med 296:241, 1977.

40. Pabico RC, Hanshaw JB, Yakub YN, et al: Cytomegalovirus infections in chronic hemodialysis patients. I. Initial observations. Proc Clin Dial Transplant Forum 1:117, 1971.

41. Lazarus JM: Complications in hemodialysis: an overview. Kidney Int 18:783, 1980.

42. Kaariainen L, Klemola E, Paloheimo J: Rise of cytomegalovirus antibodies in an infectious mononucleosis–like syndrome after transfusion. Br Med J 1:1270, 1966.

43. Prince AM, Szmuness W, Millian SJ, David DS: A serologic study of cytomegalovirus infections associated with blood transfusions. N Engl J Med 284:1125, 1971.

44. Tolkoff-Rubin NE, Rubin RH, Keller EE, et al: Cytomegalovirus infection in dialysis patients and personnel. Ann Intern Med 89:625, 1978.

45. Benacerraf B, Unanue ER: Cellular immunity. In: Textbook of Immunology. Baltimore, Williams and Wilkins, 1979, pp 109–124.

46. Fauci AS, Dale DC, Balow JE: Glucocorticosteroid therapy: mechanisms of action and clinical considerations. Ann Intern Med 84:304, 1976.

47. Fauci AS, Dale DC: The effect of "in vivo" hydrocortisone on subpopulations of human lymphocytes. J Clin Invest 53:240, 1974.

48. Bach JF, Dardenne M: Serum immunosuppressive activity of azathioprine in normal subjects and patients with liver diseases. Proc R Soc Med 65:260, 1972.

49. Zweiman B: Immunosuppressive effects of specific classes of agents with special reference to organ transplantation. Immunosuppression by thiopurines. Transplant Proc 5:1197, 1973.

50. Ten Berge RJM, Schellekens PThA, Surachno S, et al: The influence of therapy with azathioprine and prednisone on the immune system of kidney transplant recipients. Clin Immunol Immunopath 21:20, 1981.

51. Heyworth MF: Effects of anti-lymphocyte globulin in human subjects. Immunology 43:793, 1981.

52. Morris PJ: Cyclosporin A. Transplantation 32:349, 1981.

53. Calne RY, Rolles K, White DJG, et al: Cyclosporin A initially as the only immunosuppressant in 34 recipients of cadaveric organs: 32 kidneys, 2 pancreases, and 2 livers. Lancet 2:1033, 1979.

54. Peterson PK, Balfour HH, Fryd DS, et al: Fever in renal transplant recipients: Causes, prognostic significance and changing patterns at the University of Minnesota Hospital. Am J Med 71:345, 1981.

55. Tilney NL, Strom TB, Vineyard GC, Merrill JP: Factors contributing to the declining mortality rate in renal transplantation. N Engl J Med 299:1321, 1978.

56. Strom TB: The improving utility of renal transplantation in the management of end-stage renal disease. Am J Med 73:105, 1982.

57. Kyriakides GK, Simmons RL, Najarian JS: Wound infection in renal transplant wounds: pathogenetic and prognostic factors. Ann Surg 182:770, 1975.

58. Ramos E, Karni S, Alongi SV, Dagher FJ: Infectious complications in renal transplant recipients. South Med J 73:751, 1980.

59. Ramsey DE, Finck WT, Britch AG: Urinary tract infections in kidney transplant recipients. Arch Surg 114:1022, 1979.

60. Krieger JN, Brem AS, Kaplan MR: Urinary tract infection in pediatric renal transplantation. Urology 15:362, 1980.

61. Myerowitz RL, Medeiros AA, O'Brien TF: Bacterial infection in renal homotransplant recipients. Am J Med 53:308, 1972.

62. Rubin RH, Wolfson JS, Cosini AS, Tolkoff-Rubin NE: Infection in the renal transplant recipient. Am J Med 70:405, 1981.

63. Frei D, Guttmann RD, Gorman P, et al: Incidence of early urinary tract infection and relationship to subsequent rejection episodes in renal allograft recipients. Am J Nephrol 1:37, 1981.

64. Murphy JF, McDonald FD, Dawson M, et al: Factors affecting the frequency of infection in renal transplant recipients. Arch Intern Med 136:670, 1976.

65. Byrd LH, Cheigh JS, Stenzel KH, et al: Association between *Streptococcus faecalis* urinary tract infections and graft rejection in kidney transplantation. Lancet 2:1167, 1978.

66. Eickhoff TC, Olin DB, Anderson RJ, Schafer LA: Current problems and approaches to diagnosis of infection in renal transplant recipients. Transplant Proc 4:693, 1972.

67. Schroter GPJ, West JC, Weill R: Acute bacteremia in asplenic renal transplant patients. JAMA 237:2207, 1977.

68. McEnery PT, Flanagan J: Fulminant sepsis in splenectomized children with renal allografts. Transplantation 24:154, 1977.

69. Schroter GPJ, Weill R: *Listeria monocytogenes* infection after renal transplantation. Arch Intern Med 137:1395, 1977.

70. Ramsey PG, Rubin RH, Tolkoff-Rubin NE, et al: The renal transplant patient with fever and pulmonary infiltrates: etiology, clinical manifestations and management. Medicine 59:206, 1980.

71. Ludmerer KM, Kissane JM: Cavitary lung disease following renal transplantation. Am J Med 72:145, 1982.

72. Gallis HA, Berman RA, Cate TR, et al: Fungal infection following renal transplantation. Arch Intern Med 135:1163, 1975.

73. Presant CA, Wiernick PH, Serpick AA: Factors affecting survival in Nocardiosis. Am Rev Respir Dis 108:1444, 1973.

74. Pass RF, Long WK, Whitley RJ, et al: Productive infection with cytomegalovirus and herpes simplex virus in renal transplant recipients: role of source of kidney. J Infect Dis 137:556, 1978.

75. Fryd DS, Peterson PK, Ferguson RM, et al: Cytomegalovirus as a risk factor in renal transplantation. Transplantation 30:436, 1980.

76. Peterson PK, Balfour HH, Marker SC, et al: Cytomegalovirus disease in renal allograft recipients: a prospective study of the clinical features, risk factors, and impact on renal transplantation. Medicine 59:283, 1980.

77. Fiala M, Payne JE, Berue TV, et al: Epidemiology of cytomegalovirus infection after transplantation and immunosuppression. J Infect Dis 132:421, 1975.

78. Suwansirikul S, Rao N, Dowling JN, Ho M: Primary and secondary cytomegalovirus infection: clinical manifestations after renal transplantation. Arch Intern Med 137:1026, 1977.

79. Ho M, Suwansirikul S, Dowling JN, et al: The transplanted kidney as a source of cytomegalovirus infection. N Engl J Med 293:1109, 1975.

80. Friedman HM: Cytomegalovirus: Subclinical infection or disease? Am J Med 70:215, 1981.

81. Feldhoff CM, Balfour HH, Simmons RL, et al: Varicella in children with renal transplants. J Pediatr 98:25, 1981.

82. Balfour HH, Groth KE, McCullough J, et al: Prevention or modification of varicella using zoster immune plasma. Am J Dis Child 131:693, 1977.

83. Rifkind D: The activation of varicella-zoster virus infection by immunosuppressive therapy. J Lac Clin Med 68:463, 1966.

84. Luby JP, Ramirez-Ronda C, Rinner S, et al: A longitudinal study of varicella-zoster virus infections in renal transplant recipients. J Infect Dis 135:659, 1977.

85. Marker SC, Ascher NL, Kalis JM, et al: Epstein-Barr virus antibody responses and clinical illness in renal transplant recipients. Surgery 85:443, 1979.

86. Cheeseman SH, Henle W, Rubin RH, et al: Epstein-Barr virus infection in renal transplant recipients. Effects of antithymocyte globulin and interferon. Ann Intern Med 93:39, 1980.

87. Ho M: Virus infections after transplantation in man; brief review. Arch Virol 55:1, 1977.

88. Coleman DV, Mackenzie EED, Gardner SD, et al: Human polyomavirus (BK) infection and ureteric stenosis in renal allograft recipients. J Clin Pathol 31:338, 1978.

89. Hogan TE, Borden EC, McBain JA: Human polyomavirus infections with JC virus and BK virus in renal transplant patients. Ann Intern Med 92:373, 1980.

90. Tipple M, Haywood H, Shadomy S: Cryptococcus in renal transplant patients. Proc Clin Dial Transplant Forum 6:13, 1976.

91. Cohen IM, Galgiani JN, Potter D, Ogden DA: Coccidioidomycosis in renal replacement therapy. Arch Intern Med 142:489, 1982.

# III

# Transplantation

# 30

# Immunology of Transplantation

*Dorit Gradus (Ben-Ezer), M.D.*
*Robert B. Ettenger, M.D.*

Despite significant advances in dialytic technology, successful renal transplantation remains the optimal form of therapy for children with ESRD. A well-functioning renal transplant brings about both physiologic and rehabilitative improvements in a child's quality of life, which cannot be attained with any current dialysis therapies. However, there are a number of immunologic barriers to successful renal transplantation. Allograft rejection is still the major impediment to successful renal transplantation. In this chapter, we will outline some of the important immunologic factors that play a role in avoiding or modulating the strength of the rejection process.

## HISTOCOMPATIBILITY

The success of kidney transplantation depends upon a number of factors. One of the most important is the immune response of the recipient to histocompatibility antigens present in the donor but absent in the recipient. Histocompatibility antigens are genetically determined cell surface molecules distinctive for each individual. The histocompatibility antigens of all species include a major system called the major histocompatibility complex (MHC) as well as a number of minor systems. Major and minor systems were originally designated in the mouse on the basis of the strength of rejection responses induced by skin and tumor grafts. The human major histocompatibility complex is called the HLA system (human leukocyte antigen) and the antigens of this system are present on virtually all nucleated cells to a greater or lesser degree. The minor histocompatibility systems in man are poorly defined but include several red cell antigen systems (e.g., Lewis) as well as a system of antigens on vascular endothelial cells.

### The HLA Genetic Region

The HLA system, which is one of the most polymorphic genetic systems yet defined in man, is situated on the short arm of chromosome 6 (Fig. 30–1). The phenotypic expression of HLA antigens follows a simple Mendelian codominant pattern, i.e., if an allele is present on the chromosome, it is always expressed on the cell surface. The antigens inherited from a given parent on a single chromosome are referred to as a haplotype.

The HLA genetic region includes three categories of genes: those inducing serologically defined (SD) antigens (class I antigens: HLA-A, B, and C); those inducing lymphocyte defined (LD) antigens (class II: HLA-D/DR), and a group of genes coding for $C_2$, $C_4$ and factor B ($C_3$ proactivator) of the complement system, as well as some enzymes. In addition, there are undoubtedly other genes coding for antigens important in transplant rejection which have not yet been defined.

**Class I, Serologically Defined (SD) Antigens: HLA-A, B, and C.** These classic HLA antigens (class I) are cell membrane molecules present on all nucleated cells and are known to consist of two noncovalently linked glycoproteins. One glycoprotein is a 44,000

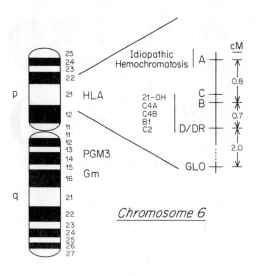

**Figure 30–1.** The major histocompatibility complex in man is located on the short arm of chromosome 6. This figure depicts the locations of genes coding for Class I and well-defined Class II (D/DR) antigens as well as those genes that govern the production of some complement components. In addition, closely linked genes are responsible for the development of several disease processes, including idiopathic hemochromatosis and congenital adrenal hyperplasia due to 21-hydroxylase deficiency (cM = centimorgan map unit). (From Strom TB: Am J Med 73:105, 1982.)

dalton heavy chain that carries the antigen specificity and is variable. The other glycoprotein molecule is an 11,500 dalton light chain $B_2$-microglobulin that is encoded by chromosome 15.[1] These SD antigens are detected by a standard microlymphocytotoxicity assay in which human serum containing a known HLA antibody is incubated in the presence of rabbit complement with lymphocytes from the individual being typed. The reaction mixture is placed into medium containing a vital dye. Cells bearing antigens recognized by the antibodies will undergo membrane damage, which will allow influx of the dye.[2, 3]

Each HLA gene locus is polymorphic to the extent that over 50 well defined HLA-antigen specificities have been established to date.[4] Virtually all the A and B antigens have

been detected (at least in Caucasoid races) since the total gene frequency at each locus is about 100%. At the C locus only about 60% of the genes have been detected.[5] The HLA antigens are termed by numbers, e.g., HLA-A1, A2, B5, Bw6, etc., where "w" stands for "workshop" and designates a specificity which is probably discrete but not yet well defined. Every individual has two HLA haplotypes, one inherited from each parent, and each haplotype codes for three antigenic structures, A, B, and C. Therefore, the typing of one given individual will reveal two HLA-A antigens, two HLA-B antigens, and two HLA-C antigens, although the latter are less routinely typed. An example of HLA haplotype distribution within a family is illustrated in Figure 30–2. By simple Mendelian inheritance any given sibling pair has a 25%

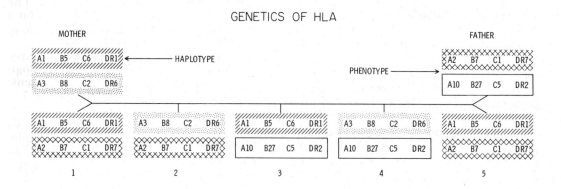

**Figure 30–2.** Genetics of HLA.

chance of having identical haplotypes; 50% will share one haplotype and the remaining 25% will be completely incompatible.

**Class II, Lymphocyte Defined (LD) Antigens: HLA-D/DR.** The class II HLA antigens consist of two noncovalently linked membrane glycoproteins, a 34,000 dalton Alpha chain and a 29,000 dalton Beta chain. These antigens are also highly polymorphic, carrying both "private" and "public" determinants. Public antigens are determinants common to several HLA molecules, each of which bears a distinctive, unique HLA private antigen as well. Class II (LD) antigens have a more restricted tissue distribution and can be found on B lymphocytes, macrophages, endothelial cells, activated T lymphocytes, and sperm, but not on platelets or quiescent T lymphocytes. Mismatching for the HLA-D antigens in a mixed lymphocyte culture (MLC) stimulates the in vitro proliferative response of the lymphocytes (see below).[6] One way to type the HLA-D antigens of an individual is to perform mixed lymphocyte reactions between a panel of HLA-D homozygous typing cells used as the stimulating cells (inactivated by x-irradiation or mitomycin C to make the reaction unidirectional) and the cells being typed. Cells lacking a specific HLA-D determinant will respond to this determinant on the typing cells with proliferation while cells possessing the determinant will not react. Twelve D specificities have been defined so far, termed HLA-Dw1 through Dw12.

A series of antigens closely related, if not identical to, the HLA-D antigens are the HLA-DR (for D-related) which have recently been described. These antigens are the targets of specific antibodies, and therefore can be serologically identified in a manner similar to the HLA-A, B, and C antigens.[7] The restricted cellular distribution of D-DR antigens makes it possible to use T-depleted, B-cell enriched lymphocyte preparations for typing. Platelets, which lack HLA-D/DR antigens, can be used to absorb anti-A, B, and C antibodies from antisera without removing anti-HLA-DR antibodies. Ten HLA-DR specificities have been described and termed DR1 through DR10.[8] DR1 is usually associated with Dw1, DR2 with Dw2, and so on. However, the precise relationship between HLA-D and DR is not yet clear. This association between D and DR determinants could represent either identity or a high degree of linkage between two closely located gene loci. There are reports of dissociation between a specific D and a corresponding DR antigen,[9, 10] supporting the second theory that the genes are separate but closely linked (so-called "linkage dysequilibrium").

**Endothelial-Monocyte System.** In the last few years the importance of a newly described antigen system has been recognized. This system is referred to as the endothelial-monocyte (E-M) system. These antigens are present on the plasma membrane of the endothelial cells[11] of peritubular capillaries and venules and are present to a lesser extent or are absent on the endothelial cells of arteries or arterioles.[11, 12] The endothelial antigens cross-react with peripheral monocytes but not with lymphocytes.[13–15]

E-M antigens appear to be important in graft rejection since: (1) pretransplant donor-specific antibodies against these antigens are associated with accelerated acute rejection in the absence of lymphocytotoxic antibodies[14] even in HLA identical living related transplants[16, 17]; (2) circulating anti E-M antibodies appear in close temporal association with irreversible vascular rejection in about 50% of the patients[18]; and (3) E-M antibodies can be eluted from rejected grafts.[14, 15, 18, 19]

Matching for E-M antigens is not yet practiced in transplant centers, but if these antigens prove to play an important role in kidney transplantation, prospective matching of donors and recipients for these antigens as well as crossmatching recipient serum with donor monocytes may become clinically desirable.

## THE ROLE OF HLA MATCHING IN TRANSPLANT OUTCOME

**The Effect of HLA-A and B (Class I) Matching.** HLA-A and B matching is of undeniable importance in intrafamilial living related transplantation. The survival of allografts from HLA identical siblings is far superior to the outcome of grafts from HLA haploidentical related donors. In reports detailing the results of intrafamilial HLA identical transplants, the 3-year graft survival rate ranges between 80 and 90%.[20, 21] In contrast, our data[22] and the data of others[20, 21] show a cumulative 3-year graft survival rate of 50 to 75% in intrafamilial haploidentical transplants. The importance of HLA matching in live related transplantation is probably due to the fact that matching for the known HLA determinants within a family virtually assures compatibility for all gene products encoded within the haplotype. This is not the case in cadaver HLA matching.

The value of HLA-A and B matching in cadaver renal transplantation is less clear. Some single center studies have demonstrated a correlation between HLA-A and B matching and improved cadaver renal allograft outcome.[23, 24] Broyer et al, for example, showed that in a group of 130 children the graft survival rate of 3 and 4 HLA-A and B antigen matched kidneys was 85% at 5 years while allografts matched for 0, 1, or 2 HLA antigens had a 5-year survival rate of only 59%.[24]

Recently the multicenter study from the Eurotransplant group reported their experience with HLA-A and B matching in 2522 transplants over a period of 5 years. They found that improved HLA-A and B matching conferred significant improvement in both patient and graft survival: at 5 years patient and graft survival rates with 4 antigen matched grafts were 72 and 51% respectively, while in grafts with no antigens matched patient and graft survival rates were 54 and 32% respectively (P = 0.0005).[25]

In contrast to these findings, however, the multicenter study of Opelz et al found no effect of HLA-A and B matching in 1697 transplants studied.[26] Other studies have also found little or no effect of HLA-A and B matching and graft outcome.[27-31] For example, in our experience with 178 first cadaver transplants in children, HLA-A and B matching had no effect on the allograft survival rate,[32] although a trend toward better outcome was noticed in the highly presensitized recipients. An important role of HLA-A and B (and also DR) matching in the graft survival of presensitized recipients has also been found by others.[33]

It seems reasonable to conclude that, although present, the overall effect of HLA-A and B matching on cadaver renal allograft survival is highly variable. In comparison to the effect of HLA-DR matching on graft survival, the effect of HLA-A and B matching appears to be minimal.

**The Effect of HLA-DR (Class II) Matching.** Matching for HLA-DR antigen in cadaver renal transplantation appears to correlate well with allograft outcome.[26, 34-39] A number of studies have shown that optimal DR matching is associated with significant improvement of graft outcome over that obtained with inferior degrees of matching. This is true whether one looks at DR matches[36, 38, 39] or mismatches.[35, 39] Taken to-

gether, these reports appear to show a 1-year graft survival rate of 75 to 92% with optimal (2-DR) matched kidneys, compared to 41 to 56% with a poor degree of DR matching (no DR antigen shared).

It is interesting to note that grafts mismatched for 1-DR antigen appear to do equally as poorly as those mismatched for 2-DR antigens.[35-38] Thus it would appear that the success of DR matching is an all-or-none phenomenon. The efficacy of DR matching is comprehensible on theoretical grounds. Class II antigens activate recipient helper lymphocytes, which in turn produce interleukin-2 and stimulate release of a macrophage stimulant and formation of interleukin-1 and interleukin-2 receptors which propagate the rejection process.[40] Matching for DR, therefore, would be expected to prevent this chain of events.

Optimal matching for DR antigens is feasible without significant prolongation of the waiting time on dialysis. Goeken et al found that the mean waiting time for a DR compatible kidney is approximately 4 months.[41]

**The Effect of HLA Antigen Matching on Multiple Transplants.** When multiple transplants are considered, most investigators have found no effect of HLA-A and B matching on graft survival.[26, 42-44] However, in our experience, there was a trend toward improved graft survival with better HLA-A and B matching.[32] This is particularly true for the highly presensitized patients.[32, 33, 42] HLA-DR matching was found to have a beneficial effect on the outcome of second cadaver kidney transplants.[26]

## IMMUNOLOGIC SELECTION OF THE DONOR (Tables 30–1, 30–2, 30–3)

Since graft loss is most frequently due to immunologic rejection, it follows that an important goal in clinical transplantation im-

**Table 30–1.** SUGGESTED INFORMATION DATA BASE NECESSARY WHEN CONSIDERING A RECIPIENT FOR RENAL TRANSPLANTATION

ABO, Rh blood typing

HLA-A, B, and DR tissue typing

Monthly sera for detection of lymphocytotoxic antibodies and storage for crossmatching

Number of transfusions (at least 5)

**Table 30-2.** SUGGESTED APPROACH TO THE EVALUATION OF LIVING RELATED DONORS

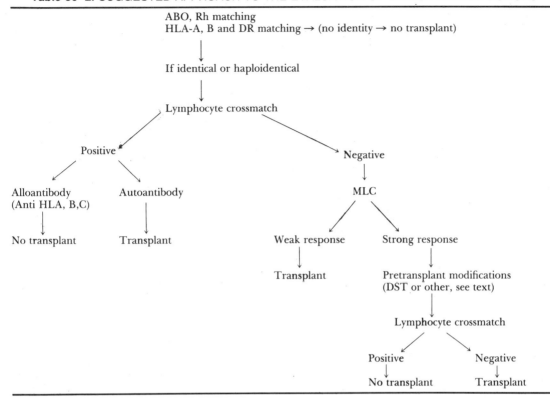

munology is to identify those immunologic dissimilarities that provoke an immunologic rejection response. At present, this selection process is largely empiric and based on a number of variables that have been shown to influence graft outcome. However, all the variables have not been identified. Therefore, even the best histocompatibility assessed by our present criteria will still have an appreciable failure rate. Some of the more important recognized variables will be considered.

**ABO Blood Group Antigens.** Compatibility between the ABO blood groups of donor and recipient as applied in clinical transfusion is considered an absolute requirement

**Table 30-3.** SUGGESTED APPROACH TO THE EVALUATION OF CADAVER DONORS

1. Typing for ABO, Rh, HLA-A, B, and DR of donor by CDC
2. Selection of recipient in order of importance
   A. ABO, Rh compatibility with donor
   B. HLA-DR match grade
   C. HLA-A and B match grade
3. T-lymphocyte crossmatching (must be negative; for other crossmatching, see text)
   A. Highest antibody serum
   B. Serum from day of transplant

for transplantation.[45-47] Almost all transplants done across this barrier have led to the destruction of the graft. Such ABO incompatibility between donor and recipient usually results in early vascular rejection,[48-50] suggesting that these antigens are important histocompatibility antigens. These rejections are probably due to the presence of A and B blood group antigens on the endothelial cell surface of the kidney[51,52] serving as targets to the naturally occurring anti-A and anti-B antibodies of the recipients.

**Rhesus (Rh) Antigens.** The role of Rh antigens in kidney transplantation is still debated. The presence of Rh antigens in kidney homogenates has been well documented.[53] However, a number of studies were unable to find a difference in graft survival between Rh-negative and Rh-positive recipients.[54,55] In fact, Huestis et al documented very good graft survival associated with the production of Rh antibodies following transplantation of Rh-positive kidneys to Rh-negative recipients.[56] Nevertheless, some reports have shown approximately a 13% poorer graft survival rate in Rh-negative compared to Rh-positive recipients.[57,58] We would conclude that if Rh antigens play a role in transplant immunology it is at most a minor one.

**Lewis Antigens.** Lewis a and b antigens have been identified on renal tubular epithelium.[59] Therefore, it is not surprising that a large retrospective study showed a significant effect of Lewis antigen matching on cadaver kidney graft survival.[60] Lewis-negative recipients had a graft survival rate that was 8% lower than that of Lewis-positive recipients. The difference was 18% when non-Caucasians in centers with less that 50% one-year overall graft survival were considered ("high risk" recipients). This study suffers from the shortcoming that donors were not typed for Lewis antigens. However, since 90% of the population are positive for the Lewis antigen system, it was assumed that a comparable percentage of Lewis-negative recipients had received a Lewis-positive kidney.

Currently, matching for Lewis antigens is not practiced in clinical transplantation. Recipients at "high risk" may benefit from prospective typing and matching for these antigens.

## Presensitization

Presensitization refers to the presence of preformed anti-HLA antibodies. These antibodies may arise after any of a number of stimuli: e.g., pregnancies, infections, blood transfusions, graft rejections. In the evaluation of the recipient before transplantation, two aspects of presensitization are considered; one is the presence of specific presensitization against the donor in question, and the other is the spectrum of presensitization against multiple HLA antigens (as represented by a lymphocyte panel).

**Humoral Donor-Specific Presensitization: Lymphocyte Crossmatching.** When a donor is considered for a specific recipient, it is of extreme importance to establish whether the recipient is specifically sensitized against the donor's histocompatibility antigens. Such presensitization, as manifested by preformed cytotoxic antibodies against donor's HLA-A and B antigens, is known to result in hyperacute rejection.[61–64] In practice, presensitization against a donor's antigens is tested by a lymphocyte crossmatch between the recipient serum and the donor lymphocytes (separated from donor's lymph nodes, peripheral blood, or spleen). The technique used in crossmatching is the standard complement-dependent microlymphocytotoxicity test (CDC).[2, 3]

Since preformed donor-specific cytotoxic antibodies are considered deleterious to graft outcome, a negative lymphocyte crossmatch has been considered an absolute prerequisite for transplantation. However, this requirement has undergone modification over the last few years. It has been shown that preformed antibodies against only donor B lymphocytes were not associated with hyperacute rejection or inferior graft outcome.[65–69] Occasionally, some studies have reported different results such as acute rejection or poorer graft survival rates in B-cell crossmatch positive transplants.[70–72] Some of these discrepant results can, in part, be traced to the fact that the B lymphocyte crossmatch may detect many different antibodies. When recipient serum is reactive against donor B lymphocytes but not T lymphocytes, the antibodies in this serum can be (1) anti-DR antibodies; (2) anti–HLA-A, B, or C antibodies that are too weak to react against T lymphocytes but will react with these antigens on the B lymphocytes[73, 74]; (3) autoreactive antibodies[75, 76]; or (4) others, including anti-Lewis antibodies.[77]

B lymphocyte antibodies have been divided by the temperature in which they react into (1) "cold" (5°C); and (2) "warm" (37°C) antibodies. Antibodies against B lymphocytes reactive in the cold frequently are autoantibodies[75, 76] and have been shown by some not to be harmful[78, 79] and even to be enhancing[80, 81] to graft survival. The significance of warm anti–B cell antibodies is not clear[82]; while some have reported graft failure following positive warm B cell crossmatches,[83–85] other groups have found no difference in graft outcome between recipients with negative, positive B cold, or positive B warm crossmatches.[26, 74] Thus, the issue of the significance of a positive anti–B cell crossmatch is not yet settled. A heterogeneity of antibodies may give rise to a B-cell–positive crossmatch, and although most of these antibodies are harmless, it does seem that some are damaging.[86] In this regard, the broadly presensitized dialysis patient presents a real challenge to the clinical transplant immunologist. On one hand, excluding all donors with positive B cell crossmatches would unduly limit the chances of expeditiously finding a suitable kidney for the highly presensitized patient.[66] On the other hand, indiscriminate transplantation in the face of positive crossmatches may lead to an increased rate of graft loss. Thus, whenever possible, efforts should be made to document that such positive crossmatches are due to autoreactive antibodies.

Despite adherence to the requirement for a negative pretransplant T lymphocyte crossmatch, antibody-mediated rejection episodes and graft failure do occur.[87, 88] One explanation for such episodes may be the presence of deleterious antibodies against antigenic systems not detected by lymphocyte crossmatching (e.g., the endothelial-monocyte system).[14] This may be overcome by developing a crossmatch technique utilizing appropriate targets such as monocytes, which cross-react with endothelial cell antigens (see above).

A second explanation for such a phenomenon is the existence of immunologic memory, allowing the secondary generation of donor-specific anti-HLA-A and B antibodies which were previously present and then receded. Anti-HLA antibodies are known to appear and disappear over time and so may not be present and detectable at the time of transplant. A solution to this problem may lie in performing pretransplant crossmatching with noncurrent sera samples collected at frequent intervals previously. However, it is still unclear whether a positive crossmatch using noncurrent sera is invariably predictive of graft rejection.[89]

A third possible cause of antibody-mediated rejection with a negative lymphocyte crossmatch may be the presence of low levels of anti-HLA-A and B antibodies below the sensitivity threshold of the CDC crossmatch technique.[90] This may be eliminated by improving the sensitivity of the crossmatch test. A number of such techniques have been employed; a few of the more frequently used include: (1) antibody-dependent cell-mediated cytotoxicity (ADCC), in which the presence of donor-specific IgG antibodies in the recipient's serum is detected in a non–complement-dependent reaction.[91, 92] The target cells (donor lymphocytes or PHA-induced blasts) with attached specific antibodies are lysed by a subpopulation of normal non-immune non-T, non-B lymphocytes called "K cells." Because of great variations in the techniques used in different centers, there is a great discrepancy in the results obtained, making the use of this crossmatch test difficult to interpret[46]; (2) complement-dependent cytotoxicity (CDC) using a radiolabeled chromium ($^{51}$Cr) release assay[93] which has been shown to detect anti–B cell antibodies undetected by CDC using the dye exclusion technique[87]; (3) antiglobulin-enhanced cytotoxicity[94] that was shown to be fourfold more sensitive than the NIH technique[74]; and (4) flow cytometry analysis, which is a recently described utilization of the flow cytometer to detect very low levels of anti-HLA antibodies not detected by other crossmatch techniques.[90, 95] In short, a crossmatch is performed and then fluorescein conjugated antihuman Ig is added. The presence of antiHLA antibodies attached to the donor lymphocytes causes a shift of the T cell peak on the histogram proportional to the level of antibodies.

**Donor-Specific Cellular Presensitization.** It is well known that renal allograft rejection can be cellularly mediated as well as antibody-mediated. A technique that can detect the presence of cellular immunity of the recipient against the donor is known as lymphocyte-mediated cytotoxicity (LMC). The LMC test is performed by incubating $^{51}$Cr-labeled target cells (donor lymphocytes or PHA blasts) with recipient effector cells in a ratio of 50 to 100 to 1 effector to target cells. After a 4-hour incubation period in 5% $CO_2$ at 37°C, $^{51}$Cr release is measured as a marker for cell lysis.[96] Almost all studies report a significant correlation between a positive LMC crossmatch and kidney graft loss from rejection.[97–99] It is of interest that there appears to be no relationship between fluctuations in antibodies to the lymphocyte panel and the waxing and waning of cytotoxic lymphocytes.[100] Also of interest is the fact that killer cells may have specificity to non-HLA antigens.[100] Although LMC is not used routinely in most renal transplant centers, it may ultimately become a standard pretransplant assay if these early studies are confirmed.

**Presensitization Against a Lymphocyte Panel.** Testing for presensitization against a lymphocyte panel serves as a pretransplant screen of the individual's anti-HLA antibody status. All histocompatibility laboratories examine at frequent intervals sera of patients awaiting transplantation for the presence of antibodies against HLA antigens represented by a lymphocyte panel. The tests are done by a standard complement dependent microlymphocytotoxicity assay.[2, 3] Patients' serum is added to a tray containing lymphocytes from a panel of normal donors, and cytotoxicity against each cell sample is measured after incubation with rabbit complement.[2, 3]

The type of information obtained from reactivity against a panel depends upon the method by which the panel is selected.[47] If the panel is randomly selected, the HLA antigens present will have approximately the same frequency as that found in the general population. Therefore, the percentage of positive reactions will yield information about the probability that a given recipient will have a positive crossmatch with a given donor.[47] For example, if a patient's serum is reactive against 90% of a random panel, only 10% of potential cadaver donors can be expected to be crossmatch-negative. If, on the other hand, the panel is selected to contain all HLA antigens, the specificities of the anti-HLA antibodies may be more precisely determined, but the percentage of reactivity is less relevant than with the random panel. Some centers use this all-HLA panel to identify all of the antibody specificities an individual has generated.[101] These data are then used to avoid transplanting kidneys that have antigens against which the recipient had previously made antibodies.

The significance in transplantation of broadly reactive lymphocytotoxic antibodies remains controversial. Does reactivity against a high percentage of a lymphocyte panel correlate with poor graft outcome despite a negative donor-specific crossmatch? Initial studies reported that sensitized patients, i.e., those reacting to more than 10% of a randomly selected panel, had a lower early graft survival rate than nonsensitized individuals.[47, 102, 103] Other centers found such a deleterious effect only among HLA-incompatible recipients.[46, 104, 105] Still others found no correlation between pretransplant panel cytotoxicity and graft survival.[106-109] The reason for the initial observations and the discrepancies among units appears to relate to (1) the more recent use of multiple high titer sera for lymphocyte crossmatches (as opposed to using only one current serum); and (2) more sensitive techniques to detect antibodies.[47] This prevents transplantation of patients specifically sensitized against the donor that, with the previous approach, would have been transplanted and done poorly.

It may be concluded that broad reactivity of multiple sera samples against a random lymphocyte panel is not necessarily predictive of graft survival. However, obtaining the results of such reactivity may serve to choose the most highly reactive sera for the crossmatch with the potential donor. It may also be of value in those centers where the cumulative list of specific antibodies produced

by the recipient is considered at the time of transplant (i.e., a patient who in the past had antibodies against HLA-A2 would not receive such a kidney, even when the crossmatch is negative).

## Live Related Donors
(See Table 30–2)

**Mixed Lymphocyte Culture (MLC).** In the evaluation of potential living related donors, the mixed lymphocyte culture (MLC, also known as mixed lymphocyte reaction—MLR) is an important tool. This test serves as a simplified in vitro model of an antiallogenic reaction and has a predictive value in renal transplant outcome.[110, 111] It has been shown that weak MLC reactivity between haploidentical living related donor-recipient pairs is associated with 90% one-year graft survival rates. This is strikingly better than the 50 to 60% one-year graft survival rate observed in such pairs in the presence of a vigorous MLC.[27]

The MLC test is based on the phenomenon first described by Bain et al[112] and Bach et al,[113] that contact between lymphocytes from two genetically different individuals in culture triggers blast transformation in the lymphocytes. The genetic control of the MLC is complex, and while the strongest control gene appears to be at the HLA-D complex, other MHC (e.g., SB) and non-MHC loci may play a role.[9]

In practice the amount of tritiated thymidine incorporated into the DNA of the transformed cells is used as a measure of the degree of stimulation.[113, 114] In the one-way MLC the potential donor's lymphocytes are used as stimulators and are therefore pretreated with irradiation or mitomycin to arrest their reaction. The donor's and recipient's lymphocytes are mixed and cultured together for five days at 37°C in a humidified 5% $CO_2$ atmosphere. The cultures are next pulsed with tritiated thymidine and incubated for an additional 18 hours at 37°C. The cells are then harvested and the radioactivity incorporated in the cells is determined by liquid scintillation counting. The results are expressed in counts per minute (cpm) (cpm of experimental culture minus cpm of background).[114]

**HLA-Identical Donors.** It is well established that the best graft survival rate can be obtained with live related HLA-identical transplants. Graft survival in such transplants has been reported to be from 85 to 93% at one year and 67 to 82% at five years.[115–118] Nevertheless, rejections do occur in HLA-identical transplants. Some of the rejection episodes have been associated with a reactive MLC,[118–120] while others have been accompanied by a negative MLC.[116, 119] Although the cause(s) for rejection in these "ideal" transplantations is not clear, some explanations have been offered: (1) patients with a negative MLC could have rejection secondary to donor-specific anti–E-M antibody[17]; and (2) some patients can be HLA-A,B,C,D–identical and still be MLC-positive, as reviewed by Carpenter.[119] Despite the possibility of graft loss to rejection in HLA-identical siblings, they are considered the first choice for transplantation, provided that they are ABO-compatible, have a low MLC, and are cross-match-negative. If the MLC is positive it is not clear at the present time whether one should avoid such a transplant or try donor-specific transfusions (see Chapter 31).

**HLA Haploidentical Donors.** Since the MHC is inherited in a classic Mendelian fashion, it follows that parents are obligatorily HLA haploidentical matches with their children, and each sibling has a 50% chance that another sibling is haploidentical (see Fig. 30–2). Overall, renal allograft survival rates in haploidentical donor-recipient pairs have been reported to be approximately 75%,[20–22] intermediate between that found in cadaver and HLA-identical living related donor-recipient pairs. From a practical point of view, it has been suggested that the MLC may be a useful way to evaluate the prognosis of transplantation in specific living related HLA haploidentical pairs. A number of laboratories have found a good correlation between pretransplant MLC reactivity and transplant outcome.[110, 111, 121] With low, albeit still weakly positive, MLC reactivity, these workers have found very good transplant outcome, in the range of 80 to 90% two year cumulative graft survival rates.[110, 111, 121] However, graft survival rates approaching that of cadaver donor transplants have been found in the presence of high reactivity in the MLC,[110] although one pediatric series reports outstanding results in such a situation.[122] The criteria for weak and strong responder status vary from laboratory to laboratory, so that the clinical decision as to whether to perform a given HLA haploidentical living related transplant should be made in consultation with the in-

dividual in charge of the laboratory performing the MLC. Recently the results of living related HLA haploidentical transplants with highly reactive MLC's have been greatly improved using either cyclosporin for immunosuppression[123] or pretransplant blood transfusions with third-party or donor-specific transfusions (see Chapter 31).

At most centers, siblings who are totally HLA mismatched are discouraged from being kidney donors, since from a theoretic point of view, their graft outcome should be no better than that achieved with cadaveric transplantation. However, at least one center has considered such donors preferable to parental donors.[124] The use of donor-specific transfusions to improve allograft survival in totally HLA-mismatched siblings has been promising in some recent studies.[125]

## IMMUNOLOGIC MONITORING AFTER TRANSPLANTATION
(See Table 30–4)

One of the major causes of kidney graft dysfunction in the early post-transplant period is acute immunologic rejection. Therefore, a number of assays have been employed to monitor the immunologic reaction of the host to the transplanted kidney (Table 30–4).

Rationales for performing immunologic monitoring in the post-transplant period include: (1) early detection of a rejection episode before it becomes clinically manifest; (2) separating renal failure episodes into those due to rejection and those resulting from

**Table 30–4. IMMUNOLOGIC MONITORING AFTER TRANSPLANTATION**

**Specific Anti-donor Immune Activity**
A. Humoral
  1. Complement-dependent cytotoxicity (CDC)
  2. Antibody-dependent cytotoxicity (ADCC)
  3. Anti–B cell antibodies
  4. Blocking factors in MLC
B. Cellular
  1. Lymphocyte-mediated cytotoxicity (LMC)
  2. Mixed lymphocyte culture (MLC)
  3. Migration inhibition factor (MIF)

**Nonspecific Immune Activity**
  1. Newly generated anti–B cell antibodies
  2. Spontaneous blastogenesis
  3. Enumeration of T lymphocytes
  4. Enumeration of T cell subsets (helper/suppressor-cytotoxic)

nonimmunologic causes; and (3) differentiating rejection episodes that are amenable to immunosuppressive therapy from those that are resistant.

The concept of immunologic monitoring suffers from some inherent problems. Chief among these is that in clinical transplantation today there are no pathognomonic criteria for rejection, either clinical, biologic, immunologic, or even pathologic. Clinicians usually utilize a rise in the serum creatinine level (or a fall in the creatinine clearance) as an indicator of rejection. But this defines only a "renal failure episode" rather than a rejection episode; it is well known that there are numerous nonimmunologic causes of "renal failure episodes." However, it is often the case that a nonimmunologic "renal failure episode" can be accompanied by evidence of immunologic reaction in the kidney biopsy which is not clinically relevant[126] and may bias the reference point of the immunologic monitoring tests. Moreover, some have found that about half of renal failure episodes thought to be rejection crises were in fact caused by previously unsuspected nonimmunologic factors,[127] a finding that can bias the validity of the immunologic monitoring assays still further.

Immunologic monitoring involves two basic types of assays, serially detecting either specific host anti-donor immune activity or nonspecific host immunologic activation (Table 30–4).

## Specific Anti-Donor Immunologic Activity

### Humoral Activity

1. Complement dependent cytotoxicity (CDC) in the recipient serum against donor peripheral blood lymphocytes has been shown by many authors to be associated with rejection.[128–130]

Although false positive results infrequently occur with this test,[128, 131] sensitivity has not always been good enough[128] to provide accurate diagnosis. Another problem is that CDC positivity persists for a long time after the rejection episode,[131] further limiting the utility of this test as a monitoring procedure.

2. Antibody-dependent cell-mediated cytotoxicity (ADCC) (see under *Presensitization*) is a sensitive test for IgG antibodies directed against donor cell antigens, both HLA and non-HLA.

The correlation between this test and acute rejection episodes is less universal than with the CDC, probably secondary to the technical differences between centers. While some have found a strong correlation between acute rejection episodes and positive ADCC,[27, 129, 132] others have found either a weak association[133] or no association at all.[131, 134] The latter studies may have detected enhancing antibodies or non-relevant non-HLA antibodies. The ADCC test may serve in predicting the prognosis of anti-rejection therapy; persistence of positive ADCC test despite high-dose steroid treatment for rejection has been associated with poor outcome.[129] Negativity by both assays, the CDC and the ADCC, may be useful in excluding rejection.[47]

3. Donor-specific anti–B cell antibodies may be of value in detecting rejection episodes. The presence of such antibodies, detected by CDC[136, 137] or by erythrocyte antibody (EA) rosette inhibition assay,[137, 138] has been shown to correlate quite well with the existence of acute rejection. However, others have found no correlation between the appearance of donor-specific anti–B cell antibodies and rejection,[139, 140] making the use of this test less valuable.

4. Mixed lymphocyte culture (MLC) inhibition by blocking factors (MLC-BFA). In this test, the MLC is performed with donor cells used either as stimulators or as responders; the recipient serum to be tested for the blocking factor activity (BFA) is added to the MLC. This test has been found to be sensitive but not selective in the diagnosis of rejection. The clinical significance of MLC-BFA is not clear, since its presence has been documented in the absence and at variable temporal relationships with the presence of rejection.[141, 142]

### Cellular Activity

1. Lymphocyte-mediated cytotoxicity (LMC) uses recipient lymphocytes as effector cells and donor lymphocytes as targets. A good correlation between LMC activity and clinical rejection has been reported.[130, 131] However, others have reported a 10 to 50% incidence of both false positive and false negative results.[129, 143, 144] These discrepancies may be accounted for by variations in technique, including incubation time and type of donor cells used as targets.

2. The mixed lymphocyte culture (MLC) has been shown by some to be decreased at

time of rejection.[145] However, as with other tests, others have not found it very specific, with nonreactivity occurring both during rejection and during quiescence.[146-148] Some of the diminution in MLC reactivity after transplantation may be due to immunosuppression therapy, since it has been shown that when immunosuppression is stopped, specific depression of recipient cell reactivity may be less evident. Therefore, the MLC does not seem to offer an effective tool for the diagnosis of rejection.

3. Migration inhibition factor (MIF) is released from recipient cells presensitized to donor cells when these two cell populations are mixed. MIF is assayed in vitro by its effect on macrophage migration.[149] Dormont et al have shown that the presence of MIF correlated well with rejection activity and may be useful in predicting rejection.[150] There have been occasional false positive and false negative results,[135] probably related to the lack of a standardized technique.

## Nonspecific Immune Activity

1. Newly generated anti–B cell antibodies directed against a lymphocyte panel[140] have been shown to be associated with poorer graft function[151] and rejection episodes.[140] However, the specificity of this test is not very high, since about 20% of the tests show either false postive or false negative results.

2. Spontaneous blastogenesis (SB) measures the spontaneous rate of DNA synthesis in recipient's lymphocytes in response to allogenic stimulation (the donor's kidney). A significant increase in DNA or RNA synthesis occurs either prior to or concomitant with clinical signs of early and late rejection.[152-155] This test suffers from a high frequency of false positive results secondary to a number of conditions commonly occurring after transplantation (e.g., surgical trauma, stress, steroid therapy, bacterial infection).[47] However, even with these limitations, it was possible to correlate three different levels of SB reactivity with clinical situations: (a) low level (680 cpm) reactivity, observed in pretransplant patients; (b) moderate elevation (2300–5300 cpm), seen post transplant during quiescent periods and following the onset of easily reversible rejection; and (c) marked elevations (greater than 10,000 cpm), frequently observed within 6 days prior to or during sustained rejection.[156] Thus, if the possible causes for false positive results are taken into account, monitoring the rate of spontaneous blastogenesis may offer a screening test for prediction and evaluation of rejection.

3. Enumeration of T lymphocytes. Observations in post-transplant patients treated with antithymocyte globulin (ATG) suggested that a low level of circulating T lymphocytes correlated well with the absence of rejection.[157, 158] It was expected that this relationship would also hold true in patients not treated with ATG. However, this was found not to be the case.[159] On the other hand, high "active" T cell levels (a subpopulation of T cells that posess high-affinity receptors for sheep red blood cells) may be useful in indicating rejection activity.[159, 160]

4. Enumeration of T lymphocytes subsets. Recently, it has become possible to identify functional T lymphocyte subsets by utilizing monoclonal antibodies to identify their membrane surface markers. Monoclonal antibodies have been developed for total T lymphocytes ($OKT_3$, Leu1), T helper/inducer cells (Th) ($OKT_4$, Leu3), T suppressor/cytotoxic cells (Tscy) ($OKT_8$, Leu2) and other cells with functions as yet less well defined. Cosimi et al initially reported a good corelation between normal or elevated Th/Tscy ratio and rejection, provided that the recipient did not have very low T cell levels ($< 150/mm^3$) or have an HLA identical donor.[161] This observation was confirmed by others.[162-165] Further extending these studies, Colvin et al found a strong overall correlation between the irreversibility of graft injury and a low ($\leq 1.0$) Th/Tscy ratio[164]; 78% of episodes with a low ratio were irreversible compared to only 6% of rejection episodes accompanied by a high Th/Tscy ratio ($\geq 1.0$). However, other reports have not confirmed as good a correlation or predictability between Th/Tscy ratio and rejection.[166, 167] A number of explanations can be offered for the discrepancy among the studies: (1) inclusion in the analysis of samples with too few total T lymphocytes to draw adequate conclusions[167]; (2) variation in Th/Tscy ratio secondary to superimposed infection, particularly CMV[168] infection, or to different immunosuppressive regimens; and (3) the appearance of circulating, immature T lymphocytes containing both Th and Tscy markers during severe immunologic stress,[161] interfering with meaningful results. Despite these limitations, the enumeration of T lymphocyte subsets is probably of value in the post transplant immunologic monitoring for rejection episodes and for prediction of their reversibility.

# REFERENCES

1. Carpenter CB, Strom TB: Transplantation: Immunogenetic and clinical aspects — part I. Hosp Pract 17:125, 1982.
2. Terasaki PI, Park MS: Microdroplet lymphocyte cytotoxicity test. In: Ray JG (Ed): NAIAD Manual of Tissue Typing Techniques. Bethesda, National Institute of Health, 1979. p 92.
3. Terasaki PI, Bernoco D, Park MS et al: Microdroplet testing for HLA-A, B, C, and D antigens. Am J Clin Pathol 69:103, 1978.
4. Garovoy MR: Immunogenetic associations in nephrotic states. In: Brenner BM, Stein JH (Eds): Contemporary Issues in Nephrology: Nephrotic Syndrome. New York, Chruchill Livingstone, 1982, p 259.
5. Fabre JW, Ting A: Immunobiology of transplantation. In: Morris PH: Kidney Transplantation, Principles and Practice. New York, Grune and Stratton, 1979, p 2.
6. Yunis EJ, Amos DB: Three closely linked genetic systems relevant to transplantation. Proc Natl Acad Sci USA 68:303l, 1971.
7. Van Rood JJ, van Leeuwen A, Keuning JJ, et al: The serological recognition of the human MLC determinants using a modified cytotoxicity technique. Tissue Antigens 5:73, 1975.
8. Hamburger J: The graft antigens. In: Hamburger J, Crosnier J, Bach JF, et al (Eds): Renal Transplantation, Theory and Practice. Baltimore, Williams and Wilkins, 1981, p 23.
9. Reinsmoen NL, Bach FH: HLA-D region complexity associated with HLA-DR, Dw, and SB phenotypes. Transplant Proc 15:76, 1983.
10. Suciu-Foca N, Godfrey M, Rohowsky C, et al: HLA-D-DR relationships. V. A crossover between HLA-D and DR. In: Terasaki PI (Ed): Histocompatibility Testing. UCLA Tissue Typing Laboratory, Los Angeles, California, 1980, p 881.
11. Paul LC, van Es LA, Fleuren G: Demonstration of transplantation antigens on the endothelium of peritubular capillaries in renal allografts by the immunoperoxidase method. Transplantation 28:72, 1979.
12. Paul LC, van Es LA, Kalf MW, et al: Intrarenal distribution of endothelial antigens recognized by antibodies from renal allograft recipients. Transplant Proc 11:427, 1979.
13. Moraes JR, Stastny P: A new antigen system expressed in human endothelial cells. J Clin Invest 60:449, 1977.
14. Paul LC, Cass FHJ, van Es LA, et al: Accelerated rejection of a renal allograft associated with pretransplantation antibodies directed against donor antigens on endothelium and monocytes. N Engl J Med 100:1258, 1979.
15. Class FHJ, Paul LC, van Es LA, et al: Antibodies against donor antigens on endothelial cells and monocytes in eluates of rejected kidney allografts. Tissue Antigens 15:19, 1980.
16. Cerilli GJ, Galouzis LB, De Francis ME: Clinical significance of antimonocyte antibody in kidney transplant recipients. Transplantation 32:495, 1981.
17. Etheredge EE, Bettonville P, Sicard GA, et al: Immunologic studes of rejection of HLA-identical renal allografts in sib pairs. Transplant Proc 15:1057, 1983.
18. Paul LC, van Es LA, van Rood JJ, et al: Antibodies directed against antigens on the endothelium of peritubular capillaries in patients with rejecting renal allografts. Transplantation 27:175, 1979.
19. Balldwein WM III, Soulillou JP, Class FHJ, et al: Antibodies to endothelial antigens in eluates of 88 human kidneys: Correlation with graft survival and presence of T- and B-cell antibodies. Transplant Proc 13:1547, 1981.
20. Opelz G, Mickey MR, Terasaki PI: Calculations on long term graft and patient survival in human kidney transplantation. Transplant Proc 9:27, 1977.
21. Solheim BG, Flatmark A, Halvorsen S, et al: Influence of HLA-A, B, C, and D matching and pretransplant blood transfusions on kidney graft survival. Transplant Proc 11:748, 1979.
22. Fine RN, Edelbrock HH, Riddell H, et al: Renal transplantation in children. Urology 9:61, 1977.
23. Richie RE, Johnson HK, Tallent MB, et al: The role of HLA tissue matching in cadaveric kidney transplantation. Ann Surg 189:581, 1979.
24. Broyer M, Gagnadoux MF, Buerton D, et al: Importance of HLA-A, B matching in kidney transplantation in children. Transplantation 30:310, 1980.
25. Persijn GG, Cohen B, Lansbergen Q, et al: Effect of HLA-A and HLA-B matching on survival of grafts and recipients after renal transplantation. N Engl J Med 307:905, 1982.
26. Opelz G, Terasaki PI: International study of histocompatibility in renal transplantation. Transplantation 33:87, 1982.
27. Strom TB: The improving utility of renal transplantation in the management of end-stage renal disease. Am J Med 73:105, 1982.
28. Berg B, Groth CG, Lundgren G, et al: Five-year experience with DR matching in cadaveric kidney transplantation. Transplant Proc 15:1132, 1983.
29. Albrechtsen D, Moen T, Thorsby E: HLA matching in clinical transplantation. Transplant Proc 15:1120, 1983.
30. Soulillou JP, Bignon JD, Hourmant M, et al: Effect of HLA-A, B, and DR typing, pregraft blood transfusions, and positive anti-B lymphocyte cross-matches on kidney graft survival — a one center prospective study. Transplant Proc 14:187, 1982.
31. Salvatierra O Jr, Perkins HA, Cochrum KC, et al: HLA typing and primary cadaver graft survival. Transplant Proc 9:495, 1977.
32. Ettenger RB, Jordan SC, Malekzadeh M, et al: Immunologic consideration in renal transplantation. In: Gruskin AB, Norman ME (Eds): Pediatric Nephrology. The Hague, Martinus Nijhoff, 1981, p 364.
33. Hors J, Busson M, Raffoux C, et al: Important role of HLA-A, B, DR matching on graft survival in 303 presensitized patients. Transplant Proc 15:134, 1983.
34. Svejgaard A: DR matching and cadaver kidney transplantation. Transplantation 33:1, 1982.
35. Moen T, Albrechtsen D, Flatmark A, et al: Importance of HLA-DR matching in cadaveric renal transplantation: A prospective one center study of 170 transplants. N Engl J Med 303:850, 1980.
36. Goeken NE, Thompson JS, Corry RJ: A 2-year trial of prospective HLA-DR matching: Effects on renal allograft survival and rate of transplantation. Transplantation 32:522, 1981.

37. Goeken NE, Thompson JS: Effect of prospective matching for HLA-DR on renal allograft survival in a single center. Transplantation 31:397, 1981.

38. Ayoub G, Terasaki PI: HLA-DR matching in multicenter, single-typing laboratory data. Transplantation 33:515, 1982.

39. Ting A, Morris PJ: Powerful effect of HLA-DR matching on survival of cadaveric renal allografts. Lancet 2:282, 1980.

40. Strom TR, Carpenter CB: Transplantation: Immunogenetic and clinical aspects — part II. Hosp Pract 18:135, 1983.

41. Goeken NE, Shulak JA, Nghiem DD, et al: Feasibility of optimal HLA-DR matching: A retrospective view. Transplantation 34:297, 1982.

42. Fine RN, Malekzadeh MH, Pennisi AJ, et al: Renal retransplantation in children. J Pediatr 95:244, 1979.

43. Husberg BS, Starzl TE: The outcome of kidney retransplantation. Arch Surg 108:584, 1974.

44. Casali R, Simmons RL, Ferguson RM, et al: Factors related to success or failure of second renal transplants. Ann Surg 184:145, 1976.

45. Dausset J, Rapaport FT: The role of blood group antigens in human histocompatibility. Ann Acad Sci 129:408, 1966.

46. Kreis H: Selection of a donor. In: Hamburger J, Crosnier J, Bach JF, et al (Eds): Renal Transplantation, Theory and Practice. Baltimore, Williams and Wilkins, 1981, p 36.

47. Carpenter CB, Strom TB, Garovoy MR: Renal transplantation: Immunobiology. In: Brenner BM, Rector FC (Eds): The Kidney, 2nd edition. Philadelphia, WB Saunders Company, 1981, p 2544.

48. Gleason RE, Murray JE: Report from kidney transplant registry: analysis of variables in the function of human kidney transplants. Transplantation 5:343, 1967.

49. Wilbrandt R, Tung KSK, Deodhar, SD, et al: ABO blood group incompatibility in human renal homotransplantation. Am J Clin Pathol 51:15, 1969.

50. Starzl TE, Marchioro TL, Holmes JH, et al: Renal homografts in patients with major donor-recipient blood group incompatibilities. Surgery 55:195, 1964.

51. Szulman AE: The histological distribution of blood group substances A and B in man. J Exp Med 111:785, 1960.

52. Bariety J, Oriol R, Hinglais N, et al: Distribution of blood group antigen A in normal and pathologic human kidneys. Kidney Int 17:820, 1980.

53. Boorman KE, Dodd BE: The group-specific substances A, B, M, N, and Rh: Their occurrence in tissues and body fluids. J Pathol 55:329, 1943.

54. van Hooff JP: Thesis, University of Leiden, 1976.

55. Annual Report, National Organ Matching Service, United Kingdom, 1974–1975.

56. Huestis DW, Zukoski CF: Secondary stimulation of Rh antibodies by kidney allografts from Rh-positive donors. Vox Sang 24:524, 1973.

57. Murrary S, Dewar PJ, Uldall PR, et al: Some important factors in cadaver-donor kidney transplantation. Tissue Antigen 4:548, 1974.

58. Opelz G, Terasaki PI: Cadaver kidney transplants in North America: Analysis 1978. Dial Transplant 8:167, 1979.

59. Oriol R, Cartron JP, Cartron J, et al: Biosynthesis of ABH and Lewis antigens in normal and transplanted kidneys. Transplantation 29:184, 1980.

60. Oriol R, Opelz G, Chun C, et al: The Lewis system and kidney transplantation. Transplantation 29:397, 1980.

61. Kissmeyer-Nielsen F, Olsen S, Peterson VP, et al: Hyperacute rejection of kidney allografts, associated with pre-existing humoral antibody. Lancet 2:662, 1966

62. Patel R, Mickey MR, Terasaki PI: Serotyping for homotransplantation. XVI. Analysis of kidney transplant from unrelated donors. N Engl J Med 279:501, 1968.

63. Williams GM, Hume DM, Hudson RP Jr, et al: Hyperacute renal-homograft rejection in man. N Engl J Med 279:611, 1968.

64. Patel R, Terasaki PI: Significance of the positive crossmatch test in kidney transplantation. N Engl J Med 280:735, 1969.

65. Ettenger RB, Terasaki PI, Opelz G, et al: Successful renal allografts across a positive crossmatch for donor B lymphocyte alloantigens. Lancet 2:56, 1976.

66. Ettenger RB, Uittenbogaart CH, Pennisi AJ, et al: Long term cadaver allograft survival in the recipient with a positive B lymphocyte crossmatch. Transplantation. 27:315, 1979.

67. Ettenger RB, Opelz G, Walker J, et al: Antibodies to donor B lymphocytes and mixed lymphocyte culture blocking in cadaveric renal transplantation. Transplantation 25:169, 1978.

68. Lobo PI, Westervelt FB, Rudolf LE: Kidney transplantability across a positive cross-match. Cross match assays and distribution of B lymphocyte in donor tissues. Lancet 1:925, 1977.

69. Morris PJ, Ting A, Oliver DO, et al: Renal transplantation and a positive serological crossmatch. Lancet 1:1288, 1977.

70. Albrechtsen D, Arnesen E, Solheim BG, et al: Significance of HLA-DR matching and of B cell crossmatch tests in vitro and in cadaver renal transplantation. Transplant Proc 9:743, 1979.

71. Dejelo CL, Williams TC: B cell cross-match in renal transplantation. Lancet 2:241, 1977.

72. Suthanthiran M, Gailiunas P, St Louis G, et al: Presensitization to donor B-cell ("Ia") antigens associated with early allograft failure. Transplant Proc 9:1807, 1977.

73. Richiardi P, Diotallevi T, Matejc T, et al: HLA antibodies cytotoxic only for B lymphocytes. Tissue Antigens 10:323, 1977.

74. Coxe-Gilliand R, Cross DE: A comparison of the sensitivities of T and B lymphocytes to HLA-A, B, C antibodies. The 8th International Workshop on Histocompatibility Testing, 1980, p 927.

75. Ettenger RB, Jordan SC, Fine RN: Autolymphocytotoxic antibodies in patients on dialysis awaiting renal transplantation. Transplantation 32:248, 1981.

76. Jeannet M, Vassali P, Hufschmid MF: Enhancement of human kidney allografts by cold B lymphocyte cytotoxins. Transplantation 29:174, 1980.

77. Hudelson B, Liu J, Ocariz J, et al: Lymphocytotoxic anti-Lewis[bH] antibody. Transplantation 31:449, 1981.

78. Iwaki Y, Terasaki PI, Weil R, et al: Retrospective tests of B cold lymphocytotoxins and transplant survival at a single center. Transplant Proc 11:941, 1979.

79. Iwaki Y, Terasaki PI, Park MS, et al: Enhancement of human kidney allografts and B-cold lymphocyte cytotoxins. Lancet 1:1228, 1978.

80. Ettenger RB, Jordan SC, Fine RN: Cadaver renal transplant outcome in recipients with auto-lymphocytotoxic antibodies. Transplantation 32:248, 1983.

81. Ayoub G, Park MS, Terasaki PI, et al: B cell antibodies and crossmatching. Transplantation 29:227, 1980.

82. Ettenger RB, Malekzadeh MH, Pennisi AJ, et al: B lymphocyte crossmatching: lack of effect on transplant outcome based on incubation temperature. Proc Dial Transplant Forum, 1979, p 197.

83. Salvatierra O, Vincenti F, Amend W, et al: Pretreatment with donor-specific blood transfusions in related recipients with high MLC. Transplant Proc 13:142, 1981.

84. Blank JL, Leo CM, Sollinger HW, et al: B-warm-positive crossmatch: a contraindication for transplantation in living related transplants undergoing donor-specific transfusion. Transplantation 33:212, 1982.

85. Ahern AT, Artruc SB, DellaPelle P, et al: Hyperacute rejection of HLA-AB-identical renal allografts associated with B lymphocyte and endothelial reactive antibodies. Transplantation 33:103, 1982.

86. Morris PJ, Ting A: The crossmatch in renal transplantation. Tissue Antigens 17:75, 1981.

87. Ettenger RB, Kerman R, Arnett J, et al: Sensitization following donor-specific transfusions for living related renal transplantation. Transplant Proc 15:943, 1983.

88. Carpenter CB: Deliberate transfusions of potential renal transplant recipients with specific donor blood. Am J Kidney Dis 1:116, 1981.

89. Cardella CJ, Falk JA, Peters P, et al: Do repeated blood transfusions prevent successful transplantation in highly sensitized potential transplant recipients? Transplant Proc 14:359, 1982.

90. Garovoy MR, Rheinschmidt MA, Bigor M, et al: Flow cytometry analysis (FCA): a high technology crossmatch. 15th Annual Meeting of the American Society of Nephrology, Chicago, Illinois, Dec. 1982, p 196A (Abstract).

91. Carpenter CB, d'Apice AJF, Abbas AK: The role of antibodies in the rejection and enhancement of organ allografts. Adv Immunol 22:1, 1976.

92. Descamps B, Gagnon R, Van DerGaag R, et al: Antibody-dependent cell-mediated cytotoxicity (ADCC) and complement-dependent cytotoxicity (CDC) in 229 sera from human renal allograft recipients. J Clin Lab Immunol 2:303, 1979.

93. Kerman RH, Kahan BD: Immunological evaluation of transplant rejection: pre and post operative indices detecting immune responsiveness. Ann Clin Res 13:244, 1981.

94. Johnson AH, Rossen RD, Butler WT: Detection of alloantibodies using a sensitive antiglobulin microcytotoxicity test: identification of low levels of preformed antibodies in accelerated allograft rejection. Tissue Antigens 2:215, 1972.

95. Scornick JC, Ireland JE, Howard RJ, et al: Evaluation by flow cytometry of the risk to produce leukocyte antibodies after blood transfusions. Second Annual Meeting of American Society of Transplant Physicians. Chicago, Illinois, June 1983 (Abstract).

96. Cerottini JC, Brunner KT: In vitro assay of target cell lysis by sensitized lymphocytes. In: Bloom B, Glade P (Eds): In Vitro Methods in Cell-Mediated Immunity. New York, Academic Press, 1971, p 369.

97. Myburgh JA, Smit JA: Pre-transplant lymphocyte mediated cytotoxicity (LMC) and antibody dependent cell-mediated cytotoxicity (ADCC) in kidney transplantation. Transplant Proc 10:425, 1978.

98. Stiller CR, Dossetor JB, Carpenter CB, et al: Immunologic monitoring of the transplant recipient. Transplant Proc 9:1245, 1977.

99. Carpenter CB, Morris PJ: The detection and measurement of pre-transplant sensitization. Transplant Proc 10:509, 1978.

100. Garovoy MR, Franco V, Zschaeck D, et al: Direct lymphocyte mediated cytotoxicity as an assay of presensitization. Lancet 1:573, 1973.

101. Garovoy MR, Myrburgh SJ, Cooper CM, et al: Computer analysis of presensitization and cross-reacting antibodies. Transplant Proc 9:1811, 1977.

102. Opelz G, Terasaki PI: Histocompatibility matching utilizing responsiveness as a new dimension. Transplant Proc 4:433, 1972.

103. Opelz G, Mickey MR, Terasaki PI: HLA and kidney transplant: re-examination. Transplantation 17:371, 1974.

104. Van Hoof JP, Schippers HMA, van der Steen GJ, et al: Efficacy of HL-A matching in Eurotransplant. Lancet 2:1385, 1972.

105. Descamps B, N'Guyen AT, Kreis H: New insights into immunologic selection of human cadaver renal allograft recipients based on immune response capacity criteria. Transplant Proc 10:497, 1978.

106. Thomas F, Thomas J, Mendez G, et al: Pretransplant immune monitoring of donor-recipient compatibility. Transplant Proc 10:429, 1978.

107. Ferguson RM, Yunis EJ, Simmons RL, et al: Does "responder"/"nonresponder" status influence renal allograft success? Transplant Proc 9:69, 1977.

108. Cross DE, Whittier FC, Weaver P, et al: A comparison of the antiglobulin versus extended incubation time crossmatch: results in 223 renal transplants. Transplant Proc 9:1803, 1977.

109. Fuller TC, Cosimi AB, Russel PS: Use of an antiglobulin-ATG reagent for detection of low levels of alloantibody-improvement of allograft survival in presensitized recipients. Transplant Proc 10:463, 1978.

110. Cochrum K, Salvatierra O, Belzer FO: Correlation between MLC stimulation and graft survival in living related and cadaver transplants. Ann Surg 180:617, 1974.

111. Garovoy MR, Person A, Carpenter CB: Correlation of mixed lymphocyte culture (MLC) reactivity and graft survival in 1 haplotype matched recipients. Proc Clin Dial Transplant Forum 8:209, 1978.

112. Bain B, Vas MR, Lowenstein L: The development of large immature mononuclear cells in mixed leukocyte cultures. Blood 23:108, 1964.

113. Bach FH, Voynow NK: One-way stimulation in mixed leukocyte cultures. Science 153:545, 1966.

114. Fournier C: Mixed lymphocyte reaction and cell-mediated lympholysis techniques. In: Hamburger J, Crosnier J, Bach JF, Kreis H (Eds): Renal Transplantation Theory and Practice, 2nd Ed. Baltimore, Williams and Wilkins, 1981, p 361.

115. Cheigh JS, Chami J, Stenzel KH, et al: Renal transplantation between HLA identical siblings: comparison with transplants from HLA semi-

identical related donors. N Engl J Med 296:1030, 1977.

116. Braun WE, Straffon RA: Long-term results in 35 HLA-identical siblings and 3 HLA-identical parent-child renal allograft recipients. Nephron 22:232, 1978.

117. Singal DP, Mickey MR, Terasaki PI: Serotyping for homotransplantation: analysis of kidney transplants from parental versus sibling donors. Transplantation 7:246, 1969.

118. Seigler HF, Ward FE, McCoy RE, et al: Longterm results with forty-five living related renal allograft recipients genotypically identical for HLA. Surgery, 81:274, 1977.

119. Carpenter CB: Transplant rejection in HLA-identical recipients. Kidney Int 14:283, 1978.

120. Etheredge EE, Shons AR, Schmidtke JR, et al: Mixed leukocyte culture reactivity and rejection in renal transplantation in HLA-identical siblings. Transplantation 17:538, 1974.

121. Rengdin O, Moller E, Lundgren G, et al: Role of MLC compatibility in intrafamilial kidney transplantation. Transplantation 22:9, 1976.

122. Papadopoulou ZL, Turner MA, Baird Helfrich G: Successful pediatric renal transplantation without donor specific transfusion (DST). 15th Annual Meeting of the American Society of Nephrology, Chicago, Illinois, 1982, p 201A (Abstract).

123. Flechner SM, Kerman RH, Van Buren CT, et al: The high risk haploidentical living related (HI-LRD) recipient: transplantation without blood transfusions and steroid withdrawal using cyclosporine (CyA). 2nd Annual Meeting of the American Society of Transplant Physicians, Chicago, Illinois, June 1, 1983 (Abstract).

124. Najarian JS: Immunologic aspects of organ transplantation. Hosp Pract 17:61, 1982.

125. Salvatierra O Jr, Iwaki Y, Vincenti F, et al: Update of the University of California at San Francisco experience with donor-specific blood transfusions. Transplant Proc 14:363, 1982.

126. Kreis H: Transplanted kidney: natural history. In: Hamburger J, Crosnier J, Bach JF, Kreis H (Eds): Renal Transplantation Theory and Practice, 2nd Ed. Baltimore, Williams and Wilkins, 1981, p 177.

127. Kreis H, Noel LH, Chailley J, et al: Kidney graft rejection: has the need for steroids to be re-evaluated? Lancet 11:1169, 1978.

128. Descamps B, Gagnon R, Debray-Sachs M, et al: Lymphocyte dependent and complement dependent antibodies in human renal allograft recipients. Transplant Proc 7:635, 1975.

129. Gailliunas P, Suthanthiran M, Person A, et al: Post-transplant immunologic monitoring of the renal allograft recipient. Transplant Proc 10:609, 1978.

130. Stiller CR, Sinclair NR, McGirr D, et al: Diagnostic and prognostic value of donor specific post-transplant immune responses: clinical correlates and in vivo variables. Transplant Proc 10:525, 1978.

131. Stiller CR, Sinclair NR, Abrahams S, et al: Anti-donor immune responses in prediction of transplant rejection. N Engl J Med 294:978, 1976.

132. Garovoy MR, Gailliunas P, Carpenter CB, et al: Immunologic monitoring of transplant rejection: correlation of in vitro assays with morphologic changes on transplant biopsy. Nephron 22:208, 1978.

133. Grunnet N, Kristensen T: Antibody and lymphocyte mediated immunological recipient versus donor reactions before and after human renal transplantation: a prospective study. Transplant Proc 10:531, 1978.

134. Descamps B, Gagnon R, Van DerGaag R, et al: Influence of azathioprine and prednisone in in vivo treatment of lymphocyte dependent antibody-mediated cytotoxicity (LDA) in 57 human renal allograft recipients. Transplant Proc 9:981, 1977.

135. Dossetor JB, Myburgh JA: Post-transplant immunologic monitoring summation. Transplant Proc 10:661, 1978.

136. Soulillou JP, Peyrat MA, Guenel J: Association between treatment resistant kidney allograft rejection and post-transplant antibodies to donor B-lymphocyte alloantigens. Lancet 1:354, 1978.

137. Suthanthiran M, Gailliunas P, Fagan G, et al: Detection of anti-donor "Ia" antibodies: a strong correlate of rejection. Transplant Proc 10:605, 1978.

138. Bakkaloglu A, Sandilands GP, Briggs JD, et al: Inhibition of Fc rosette formation by serum of patients with renal allograft rejection. Lancet 2:430, 1977.

139. Ting A, Morris PJ: Pre- and post-transplant B-cell antibodies in renal transplantation. Transplant Proc 11:393, 1979.

140. Ettenger RB, Terasaki PI, Ting A, et al: Anti B lymphocytotoxins in renal-allograft rejection. N Engl J Med 295:305, 1976.

141. Sengar DPS, Rashid A, Harris JE: Mixed leukocyte culture blocking factor activity in allograft recipients and its role in the clinical outcome of human cadaveric renal allografts. Clin Exp Immunol 22:409, 1975.

142. Suciu-Foca N, Herter FP, Buda J, et al: Comparison of lymphocyte reactivity in patients with cancer, systemic lupus erythematosus and renal allografts. Oncology 31:125, 1975.

143. Wolf JS, Fawley JC, Hume DM: In vitro quantitation of lymphocyte and serum cytotoxic activity following renal homograft rejection in man. Transplant Proc 3:449, 1971.

144. Kovithavongs T, Schlaut J, Pazderka V, et al: Lymphocyte mediated cytotoxicity (LMC) in post transplant monitoring: technical aspects and interpretation of results. Transplant Proc 10:547, 1978.

145. Miller J, Hattler BG: Reactivity of lymphocytes in mixed culture in response to human renal transplantation. Surgery 72:220, 1972.

146. Bach ML, Engstrom MA, Bach FH, et al: Specific tolerance in human kidney allograft recipients. Cell Immunol 3:161, 1972.

147. Hattler BG, Miller J: Changes in human mixed lymphocyte culture reactivity as an indicator of kidney rejection. Transplant Proc 4:655, 1972.

148. Woniquet K, Pichlmayr R: Post-transplant monitoring of donor-specific T-cell reactivity at the precursor cell level. Transplant Proc 10:563, 1978.

149. David JR, Al-Askari S, Lawrence HS, et al: The specificity of inhibition of cell migration by antigens. J Immunol 93:264, 1964.

150. Dormont J, Sobel A, Galanaud P, et al: Leukocyte migration inhibition with spleen extracts and other antigens in patients with renal allografts. Transplant Proc 4:265, 1972.

151. Silberman H, Terasaki PI, Berne T, et al: B cell

antibodies in patients rejecting transplants. Transplant Proc 10:603, 1978.

152. Anderson CB, Codd JE, Graff RJ, et al: Lymphocyte activation after renal transplantation. Transplantation 16:68, 1973.

153. Harris J, Bagai R, Rashid A, et al: Nucleic acid synthesis in peripheral blood lymphocytes as an indicator of rejection. Transplant Proc 4:659, 1972.

154. Hayry P, Pasternack A, Virolainen M: Cell proliferation within the graft and in blood during renal allograft rejection. Transplant Proc 4:195, 1972.

155. Hersch EM, Butler WT, Rossen RD, et al: In vitro studies of the human response to organ allografts: appearance and detection of circulating activation lymphocytes. J Immunol 107:571, 1971.

156. Vessella RL, Pierce GE, Barth RF, et al: Correlation of spontaneous leukocyte blastogenesis with human renal allograft rejection. Transplantation 23:277, 1977.

157. Thomas F, Lee HM, Wolf JS, et al: Monitoring and modulation of immune reactivity in human transplant recipients. Surgery 79:408, 1976.

158. Cosimi AB, Delmonico FL, Burdick JF, et al: Individualized management of immunosuppression according to serial monitoring of immunocompetence. Transplant Proc 10:647, 1978.

159. Kerman RH, Geis WP: Total and active T cell dynamics in renal allograft recipients. Surgery 79:398, 1976.

160. Kerman RH, Floyd M, Van Buren CT, et al: Correlation of non-specific immune monitoring with rejection or impaired function of renal allografts. Transplantation 32:16, 1981.

161. Cosimi AB, Colvin RB, Burton RC, et al: Use of monoclonal antibodies to T-cell subsets for immunologic monitoring and treatment in recipients of renal allografts. N Engl J Med 305:308, 1981.

162. Ellis TM, Lee HM, Mohanakumar T: Alterations in human regulatory T lymphocyte subpopulations after renal allografting. J Immunol 127:2199, 1981.

163. Binkley WF, Valenzuela R, Braun WE, et al: Flow cytometry quantitation of peripheral blood (PB) T-cell subsets in human renal allograft recipients. Transplant Proc 15:1163, 1983.

164. Colvin RB, Cosimi AB, Burton RC, et al: Circulating T-cell subsets in 72 human renal allograft recipients: the $OKT_4^+/OKT_8^+$ cell ratio correlates well with reversibility of graft injury and glomerulopathy. Transplant Proc 15:1166, 1983.

165. Nanni-Costa A, Vangelista A, Frasca GM, et al: T-cell subsets in renal allograft recipients. Transplant Proc 15:1176, 1983.

166. Carter NP, Cullen PR, Thompson JF, et al: Monitoring lymphocyte subpopulations in renal allograft recipients. Transplant Proc 15:1157, 1983.

167. Guttmann RD, Poulsen RS: Fluorescence activated cell sorter analysis of lymphocyte subsets after renal transplantation. Transplant Proc 15:1160, 1983.

168. Carney WB, Rubin RH, Hoffman RA, et al: Analysis of T lymphocyte subsets in cytomegalovirus mononucleosis. J Immunol 126:2114, 1981.

# 31

# The Role of Pretransplant Blood Transfusion in Renal Transplant Outcome

*Robert B. Ettenger, M.D.*
*Dorit Gradus (Ben-Ezer), M.D.*

In the early and mid-1970's, many dialysis units attempted to minimize the number of blood transfusions given to patients with ESRD awaiting transplantation in an effort to reduce the risk of adverse presensitization. However, Dossetor et al[1] and Opelz et al[2] suggested in early studies that, contrary to what had been expected, pretransplant blood transfusions were associated with improved cadaver allograft survival rates. A large body of evidence has now confirmed that pretransplant blood transfusions improve the outcome of subsequent renal transplantation.[3-6] The magnitude of the blood transfusion effect is quite remarkable. In one prospective study, untransfused transplant recipients had a one-year cadaveric transplant survival rate of 20% while recipients receiving 10 or more transfusions had a rate of 89%.[3] While the graft outcome statistics vary from study to study, virtually all studies have shown a beneficial effect of transfusions. A large retrospective series from Terasaki et al is shown graphically in Figure 31–1. This figure illustrates that transfusions have their greatest effect in the first months following transplantation by reducing the accelerated rejection occurring in this period.[5]

## CADAVERIC TRANSPLANTATION

Although the beneficial effect of transfusions has been amply confirmed, many ques-tions about the transfusion effect remain. At present, there is no consensus as to the optimal number of third-party transfusions in cadaveric renal transplantation. As shown in Figure 31–1, the studies of Terasaki, Opelz, and their co-workers indicate that the effect can be correlated with the number of pretransplant transfusions, i.e., graft survival is poorest in untransfused recipients and improves as more transfusions are given.[3-5] Their most recent data suggest that approximately half of the total effect is conferred by one transfusion.[3]

The value of a single transfusion had been stressed previously by the Leiden/Euro-transplant group; they showed maximal graft survival with only one leukocyte-poor transfusion.[6, 7] However, others have found only minimal effects with one[8] or two transfusions.[9] The recent multicenter study conducted by Terasaki et al showed that most of the beneficial effect was present after five transfusions.[5] The effect began to level off after this number and peaked at 14 transfusions.[10] Recommendations regarding the optimal elective pretransplant transfusion number vary from one,[7, 11] two,[12] or three,[9] to five[13] or ten.[14] At present, we utilize a minimum of five pretransplant transfusions in the preparation of children for cadaveric renal transplantation.

Another issue which must be considered is the type of blood product that will yield the optimal result. It is presently unclear which

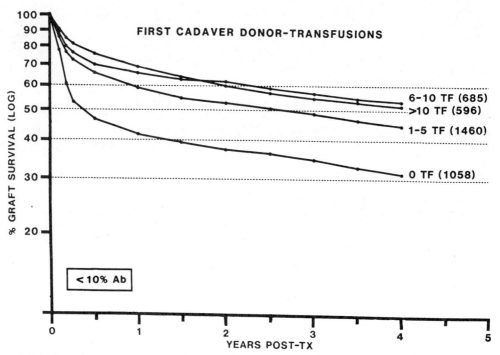

**Figure 31–1.** Actuarial graft survival in 3799 cadaver donor renal transplants grouped by number of pretransplant blood transfusions received. Note the poor graft survival in those patients receiving no transfusions. The majority of failures in this group occurred in the first 3 to 6 months.[5]

constituent of the transfusion is responsible for the effect. In mice, white blood cells are essential for skin graft prolongation,[15] but the requirement for white cells is less clear in rhesus monkeys receiving one transfusion.[16] In humans, leukocytes appear to be important, as leukocyte-poor blood (i.e., containing some leukocytes) is far superior to leukocyte-free blood for transfusion.[11] In fact, in limited studies, leukocytes have been successfully utilized as the only transfusion preparation.[17] However, it has also been suggested that transfused erythrocytes may result in immunologic unresponsiveness[18] and improved transplant outcome.[16] Even platelets have recently been reported to improve graft survival in rhesus monkeys.[19]

In a clinical setting, there is disagreement regarding the type of preparation to transfuse. When the relative effectiveness of packed red blood cells, frozen cells, and whole blood were compared in first cadaver grafts using the UCLA International Transplant Registry, whole blood was found to have the greatest enhancing potential.[4, 10] Packed red blood cell transfusions also showed an increase in graft survival rate with an increasing number of transfusions.[4, 10] Using the same registry, frozen cells have been

found to confer either no improvement with increasing number of transfusions,[4] or an effect after only four transfusions.[10] In another multicenter collaborative study, Spees and colleagues also found that packed cells, whole blood, or a mixture of preparations produced the most significant effect.[20] However, others have found that frozen blood,[21] and particularly frozen blood prepared by deglycerolization,[12, 23, 24] has a positive influence on graft survival equivalent to that found with other preparations. Considering the number of cell types and preparations which have shown transplant-enhancing capabilities, it seems reasonable to conclude that transfusions must work by a number of different mechanisms. Some of these are probably mediated by erythrocytes, while others may be mediated by leukocytes or platelets.

There are little data on the ideal amounts of blood and the timing of transfusion that will optimize transplant outcome while minimizing adverse presensitization. In immunosuppressed mice, minute amounts of blood are all that is necessary for skin graft prolongation.[15] These amounts of blood, equivalent to 10 to 20 cc in humans, are capable of generating histocompatibility antigen specific suppressor cells.[15, 25] In almost all the human studies so far conducted, transfusions have been given as "units," so there are little data on the effect of smaller aliquots of blood. Recently, Sirchia et al compared the immunologic and graft-enhancing effects of three random donor transfusions of 230 cc packed red cells with three 30 cc packed cell transfusions. They found that the aliquot transfusions sensitized the same number of recipients as the "standard" unit aliquots, but that the antibodies were transient and weak with the small aliquot, but persistent and strong with the standard transfusions. Preliminary graft outcome data showed a decreased six-month cadaver graft survival rate in patients treated with the small aliquot transfusions; however, this difference was not statistically significant.[26] Clearly, more data are needed on the pivotal question of the lowest dose of blood product that will improve graft survival without producing adverse presensitization (see below).

The optimal timing of transfusion therapy in relation to transplantation is also unclear. The UCLA International Transplant Registry found no evidence that the time interval between the last transfusion received by the recipient and the transplant operation had a significant influence on graft outcome.[4] This finding has been confirmed in single center studies as well.[27] However, other groups have presented data indicating that the best results were obtained when cadaveric transplantation was performed within three[8] or six months[28] of the last blood transfusion. It has been proposed that transfusions given in the perioperative period may have a beneficial effect on cadaver graft outcome.[29] In one study, previously untransfused recipients who received two units of blood at the time of transplantation surgery had a two-year cumulative graft survival rate of 76% compared to a 36% rate in the untransfused control group.[30] Other studies have compared untransfused recipients with those transfused either preoperatively or perioperatively. They have found that perioperative transfusions are associated with cadaver graft outcome that is intermediate between that seen with preoperative transfusions and no transfusions.[27, 31] Similarly, in the large UCLA multicenter study, perioperative blood transfusion reduced the frequency of accelerated rejection significantly only in recipients who had not received prior blood transfusions.[4, 5] Since preoperative transfusions confer some risk of adverse presensitization which may delay transplantation (see below), perioperative transfusions may have some application as a graft-enhancing modality. However, it appears from the above studies that the advantages of perioperative transfusions are not as great as those attained with preoperative transfusions.

**Sensitization Following Blood Transfusions.** A most important question surrounding the preparation of potential transplant recipients with blood transfusions is the incidence and significance of anti-HLA antibodies generated by the transfusions. The importance of this question evolves from the fact that, as noted above, preformed antibodies in the recipient directed against the HLA-A or B antigens of the kidney transplant donor can produce hyperacute rejection.[32] Such antibodies can be detected in the pretransplant T-cell crossmatch, and, when these antibodies are present, the recipient is prohibited from receiving the kidney in question. Thus, the question arises: Does a liberal transfusion policy lead to the generation of anti-HLA A and B antibodies often enough so that significant numbers of potential recipients will be rendered untransplantable? Cheigh et al found that 45% of their 140 prospective renal transplant recipients had lymphocytotoxic antibodies against 90% or more of a random panel of lymphocyte donors.[33] In a patient with 90% reactivity against a random donor test panel, only one of 10 potential cadaver donors will be crossmatch-negative. After examining the manner in which these patients developed their antibodies, these workers concluded that blood transfusions could increase the rate of sensitization to HLA antigens and deprive potential recipients of the opportunity of receiving future kidney transplants. Their data suggested that only those potential recipients not highly presensitized by blood transfusions could expeditiously receive kidney transplants. Data from other workers similarly showed a high rate of panel sensitization in response to blood transfusions.[34] Opelz et al, on the other hand, found that the formation of highly reactive lymphocytotoxins as a result of transfusions was relatively rare, and this was particularly so in patients without previous pregnancies.[35] They showed that with up to 20 pretransplant transfusions (usually given as packed red blood cells) highly reactive antilymphocyte antibodies (i.e., greater than 90% reactivity against a random T-cell panel) were not found in any prospectively studied males or females without previous pregnancies. Antibodies against a B-lymphocyte panel were found with greater frequency.[35]

In an attempt to address the question in another way, we studied the ability of uremic children to mount a post-transfusion antibody response against the lymphocytes of their unrelated blood donors.[36] We studied 10 patients who had received 42 blood transfusions, all with packed red blood cells. A new, definable and specific antibody response against blood-donor lymphocytes was identified after 14 of the 42 transfusions (33%). However, only 14% of the transfusions resulted in antilymphocyte antibodies against donor T cells at a 37° incubation temperature,[36] the conditions considered to be indicative of sensitization against HLA A, B, and C antigens. Antibody against transfusion-donor B lymphocytes was found after 11 of the 42 transfusions.[36]

Our data would tend to substantiate the position of Opelz et al[35] that significant post-transfusion sensitization against T lymphocytes does not occur often. Significant sensitization is far more frequent following a rejected renal transplant.[37] It therefore appears that the chances are minimal that a recipient will be rendered "untransplantable" because of prospective pretransplant transfusions only. While post-transfusion sensitization occurs more frequently against B lymphocytes, this is of less clinical import, since we[38] and others[39] have shown that positive crossmatches due to anti-B lymphocyte antibodies need not exclude a recipient from a given transplant.

Nevertheless, there is a strong correlation between the fraction of patients sensitized to lymphocyte antigens and the number of transfusions received.[40] With more than 10 transfusions, as many as 20% of recipients may develop some anti–T lymphocyte antibodies.[40] As noted above, this sensitization is rarely of such magnitude as to make individuals untransplantable. Still, the presence of such antibodies may sometimes delay cadaveric transplantation until a crossmatch-negative kidney can be found. A number of procedures have been advocated to reduce the sensitization while preserving the beneficial effect of transfusion. These are listed in Table 31–1.

Clearly, it would be ideal if we possessed some "immunobiologic laboratory endpoint"

**Table 31–1.** PROCEDURES WITH FAVORABLE TRANSFUSION EFFECT ON RENAL TRANSPLANT OUTCOME WITHOUT SENSITIZATION OF RECIPIENT

| Procedure | Reference |
|---|---|
| Transfusion of deglyceralized frozen blood | 22 |
| Transfusion of HLA A and B matched blood | 115 |
| Perioperative transfusions | 27, 29, 30, 31 |
| Platelet transfusion | 19 |
| Use of immunosuppression at time of transfusion | 41 |
| Storage of blood prior to transfusion | 42, 43 |

which would tell us when the beneficial effect(s) of transfusions were optimal. At present, we have no such endpoint because of our ignorance about the mechanism of the transfusion effect. We can, therefore, only monitor the possible adverse effects of transfusion. This is done by screening the post-transfusion sera against a panel of lymphocytes to detect the presence of cytotoxic antibodies. Such sera should also be stored and utilized for the pretransplant crossmatch.

Are patients who develop cytotoxic antibodies against a lymphocyte panel in response to transfusion at increased risk to reject their renal transplant, even if the pretransplant crossmatch is negative? Early observations suggested that sensitized patients reacting to more than 5% of a random lymphocyte panel had lower graft survival rates than "non-responder" patients; the poorest outcome was seen in patients with reactivity against more than 50% of the panel.[44] Nevertheless, these same authors note that patients sensitized by transfusions still had better cadaver allograft survival than unsensitized non-transfused recipients.[45] Other studies have confirmed that patients developing cytotoxic antibodies in response to transfusions have cadaver graft outcomes that are the same[46] or better[3, 13] than those of untransfused graft recipients.

Whether transfused patients develop preformed antibodies to all lymphocytes, B lymphocytes, or T lymphocytes, their one-year graft survival rate is still higher than that of nontransfused recipients.[40] In fact, many studies suggest that individuals who are highly presensitized by multiple transfusions have graft survival rates that are superior to[47] or, at the very least, almost equivalent to those of transfused patients who have remained unsensitized.[3, 48-51] Some studies, however, do show some diminution of graft survival with high levels of presensitization,[4, 45] although, as noted above, the percentage of well-functioning grafts is always superior to that of a comparable non-transfused group.

One group of transfused patients who appear to be at increased risk for poor graft outcome (approximately 18 to 25% at one year) is that group which develop broadly reactive antibodies in response to only two[9] to five[52] transfusions. On the other hand, those with broadly reactive antibodies in response to a higher number of transfusions appear to have one-year graft outcomes in the range of 50 to 75%.

**Relative Effect of Transfusions and Histocompatibility Matching.** Both transfusions and histocompatibility matching, particularly HLA-DR matching, appear to have a beneficial effect on cadaver graft outcome, but are these effects additive? Transfusions appear to have an additive effect to HLA A and B matching,[5, 50, 53] although, since the effect of HLA A and B matching is weak in first cadaver renal transplantations, the transfusion effect appears dominant.[5] Early studies suggested that the beneficial effect of transfusions and HLA DR matching were not additive.[54, 55] However, a number of recent studies showed that in both primates and humans, pretransplant transfusions improve graft survival rates in all match grades of HLA-DR matching.[56-58]

The positive effect of transfusions is more evident in transplants with a 0 or 1 HLA DR match;[54] with a 2 HLA DR match, the graft outcome is good enough so that additional improvement with transfusions may be more difficult to demonstrate statistically, particularly if the numbers of well-matched kidneys are small. However, there is some evidence that five or more transfusions in patients receiving a 2 DR–matched kidney may result in a one-year graft survival rate in excess of 85%, while those receiving fewer than five transfusions have a graft survival in the range of 75%.[58]

**Blood Transfusions and Second Cadaveric Renal Transplants.** While there is general agreement regarding the transfusion effect in first cadaver renal allografts, the effect, if any, of transfusions on the outcome of second cadaver grafts is less clear. Opelz and Terasaki, in a study of 247 second cadaver renal transplants, demonstrated no correlation of graft survival with blood transfusions.[4] They included all transfusions prior to the second allograft and could not evaluate separately the effectiveness of the number of transfusions given before the first transplant versus those given between first graft removal and the second graft.

Persijn and his colleagues were able to compare second cadaver renal allograft survival rates in 29 recipients who had not been transfused prior to their first renal transplant with 142 recipients who had received blood prior to their first transplant.[59] They found a one-year graft survival rate of 58% in the transfused group, but only a 38% survival rate in the non-transfused patients (p<0.05). On the other hand, a smaller study from Newcastle-upon-Tyne showed improved second cadaver allograft survival rates in recipients untransfused prior to their first renal allograft!ced[60] The reasons for these disparate results are not clear, but may be due at least in part to different transfusion protocols (e.g., transfusion while receiving immunosuppressive medications,[60] blood preparations, timing of transfusions, and sample size).[59]

## THE TRANSFUSION EFFECT IN LIVING RELATED TRANSPLANTATION

In contrast to the data in cadaveric transplantation, the efficacy of preoperative transfusions in living related transplantation has been less apparent. It may well be that, since graft outcome is generally much better than that in cadaveric transplantation, a transfusion effect may be more difficult to demonstrate statistically. This is almost certainly the case in renal transplantation between HLA-identical siblings.[61] With a two-year graft survival rate that exceeds 90% utilizing conventional therapy, it would be difficult to show a graft-enhancing effect of almost any adjunctive manipulation. For this reason, pretransplant transfusions are usually not recommended in this group unless clinically necessary.

The case for pretransplant transfusions in one-haplotype-matched living related transplants is stronger. While some reports have not shown a beneficial effect of transfusion,[24, 62, 63] the majority of such reports do show a clear-cut benefit.[61, 64-66] In one large series, third-party blood transfusions improved the two-year cumulative graft outcome in one-haplotype-matched transplants from 50% to 75%.[61] The number of transfusions did not appear to matter, in that a similar effect was seen whether the recipient had received less than five or more than five transfusions. It appears that third-party transfusions are of particular value in one-haplotype living related transplants in which the Mixed Lymphocyte Culture (MLC) between donor and recipient is highly reactive. Salvatierra and his colleagues found an overall one-year graft survival of 56% in 34 such transplants; however, the one-year graft survival was 74% in 23 recipients who had third-party transfusions and only 18% in the 11 recipients who had never received transfusions.[66]

As noted above, a number of laboratories have found that the results of living related one-haplotype-matched renal transplants correlated well with the results of the pretransplant MLC between donor and recipient.[67, 68] The one-year graft survival rate in these highly reactive recipients is similar to that obtained utilizing cadaver donors. In an attempt to improve graft outcome in these highly reactive donor-recipient pairs, investigators at the University of California, San Francisco, initiated a pretreatment transfusion protocol utilizing donor blood.[69] They drew upon both animal[70-73] and human[17] data showing prolonged graft outcome if recipients were pretreated with donor blood or lymphocytes. It has now been documented by this group[69] and others[74-76] that transfused recipients who do not respond to the donor-specific transfusions (DSTs) by developing deleterious anti-HLA antibodies can receive transplants with a graft outcome approaching that obtained when utilizing HLA-identical siblings as donors. One- and two-year graft survival rates of more than 90% have been reported in patients receiving DSTs and first living related one-haploidentical renal transplants. In addition, rejection episodes are said to be milder in DST recipients, although first rejection episodes tend to occur earlier than in patients not receiving DSTs.[77]

The DST procedure in adults involves the administration of 200 cc of fresh whole blood or its packed cell equivalent on three separate occasions at approximately two-week intervals.[78] We have modified the "dosage" schedule for children, so that the amount of each transfusion is 2.5 to 4 cc/kg body weight of packed red blood cells, to a maximum of 125 cc.[79] Some centers perform DST for all one-haplotype living related renal transplants[80] regardless of the MLC reactivity. However,

our group and most others[80] have continued to use MLC reactivity to discriminate between whether a recipient will or will not receive DST.

The major disadvantage of DST is the risk of developing deleterious antibodies against histocompatibility antigens of the potential donor. For this reason, weekly sera are assiduously obtained from the DST recipient and frozen for subsequent lymphocytotoxic crossmatching with T and B cells of the potential donor. Crossmatch testing is performed using the standard complement-dependent microlymphocytotoxicity test at 5°C, 20°C, and 37°C incubation temperatures;[81] in addition, we use the antiglobulin-enhanced crossmatch technique with donor T lymphocytes as targets.[82] In this way, we hope to be as complete as possible in excluding those donors against whom adverse presensitization has developed.

In our laboratory as in most others, criteria for transplantation are negative T and B cell crossmatches on all sera by standard microlymphocytotoxicity testing and negative antiglobulin crossmatches.[79] Utilizing these criteria, we have found that such adverse presensitization develops in 29% of children receiving DST; this sensitization rate is comparable to that reported in most studies[69] but higher than that reported in some centers.[74, 75] The transplant will be performed at our center if we can demonstrate that the positive crossmatch is due to an autolymphocytotoxic antibody, as such antibodies have been shown not to be deleterious in human renal transplantation.[75, 83, 84] Nevertheless, in spite of such rigorous screening protocols, immediate rejections have occurred, albeit rarely. These have been associated with negative crossmatches[79, 80] or positive B cell crossmatches at a 37°C incubation temperature.[69]

Hyperacute rejection in the presence of a totally negative crossmatch could be due to an antibody against an antigen system that is not easily detectable, such as the vascular endothelial antigen system;[85] alternatively, it could be due to the presence of anti-HLA antibody below the level detectable by standard tests.[86] The significance of antibody against donor B lymphocytes at 37°C is currently a major problem in DST therapy. Such positive "warm" B cell crossmatches may represent anti-HLA A or B antibody. This is suggested by the findings that (1) the warm anti-B cell activity which has been associated in at least one instance with hyperacute rejection was platelet absorbable[69] (platelets carry only HLA A and B antigen, not HLA-DR), and (2) a positive warm B cell cross-match often precedes the development of a positive T cell crossmatch.[87] However, even those warm B cell crossmatches that are not platelet absorbable may still represent deleterious antibody.[88]

A few patients have had successful kidney transplants following DST despite developing warm B cell crossmatches, but these antibodies have most often been transient, i.e., the antibody had disappeared by the time of transplant.[74, 75] At present, it seems prudent to disqualify a potential donor against whose cells a recipient has generated a consistent positive warm B cell crossmatch in response to DST.

The mechanisms of the DST effect is not understood. At least two possibilities have been suggested.[78] The first explanation is selection. The assumption is that the DSTs segregate a group of "high immunologic responders" from "nonresponders." The high responders are those who are very likely to reject the transplant in question, and they declare themselves by producing antibodies in response to DST. A number of lines of reasoning make it unlikely that selection is the only mechanism by which DST works: (1) all groups using DST have reported 85 to 95% success rates, yet sensitization rates vary from 0 to 40%. The use of stored (rather than fresh) blood[42, 43] and administration of azathioprine during DST[41] appear to reduce sensitization while giving equivalent graft outcomes; and (2) utilizing more sensitive radio-labeled chromium release assays, we have shown that the true incidence of post-DST sensitization, especially against B cells, is much more frequent than the 29% rate obtained with the standard lymphocytotoxicity testing.[79] In addition, after transplantation, DST recipients are able to make donor-specific complement-dependent antilymphocyte antibody, even though they did not make such antibody during transfusion.[79]

Taken altogether, these data indicate that it is unlikely that DST works solely by selection of the nonresponder. This would suggest that active processes play an important part in the beneficial DST effect. Such processes may include immunologic enhancement by small amounts of enhancing antibody or cellular immunologic mechanisms leading to recipient unresponsiveness. For example, decrements have been reported in the post-

DST donor-specific MLC[89] and cell-mediated lympholysis (an in vitro measure of cytotoxic T lymphocyte generation).[90]

Since its inception, the utilization of DST has been undergoing a number of modifications and refinements. Schweitzer et al have modified the procedure so that it can be used in donor-recipient combinations which are Rh-incompatible.[91] By sedimenting almost all the Rh + erythrocytes with Hetastarch, transfusing the resultant platelet and leukocyte-rich preparation, and treating the recipient with Rhogam, these workers administered 2 DST's with no significant Rh sensitization and resultant excellent graft outcome. As noted above, investigators have utilized pharmacologic[41] or storage[42, 43] modifications to diminish adverse presensitization. More sensitive methods are being developed to detect adverse presensitization.[70, 86]

Other investigators have suggested that very high MLC reactivity in the pretransfusion MLC may predict the development of a positive crossmatch in response to DST.[92] It is, therefore, possible that in the coming years we may be able to refine the DST procedure to the point where adverse presensitization can be uniformly predicted, detected, and avoided.

There are many important questions yet to be answered in regard to DST. Chief among these is the wisdom of performing a procedure which at present disqualifies almost one-third of living related donors. This would appear to be a particularly telling point in young children since they do so well with one-haplotype living related donors (usually parents).[93] Of 100 potential donors with highly reactive MLCs undergoing DST, only 70 will be eligible, using the current sensitization figure of 30%. If we assume a one-year success rate of 90%, this would mean that 63 of the original 100 donor kidneys would be functioning as allografts in the recipients at one year. In comparison, as noted above, 76% of patients receiving similar kidneys and third-party blood transfusions will have functioning kidneys at one year.[66] Of course, this type of argument against DST disregards the fact that with DST fewer living related donors will be giving up a kidney which is ultimately rejected. Nevertheless, the real future of DST, particularly for children, will be in these modifications which can lower the sensitization rate to below 10%.

## MECHANISMS OF THE TRANSFUSION EFFECT

The ultimate question with regard to transfusions is how they work to improve graft survival. Possible explanations for the transfusion effect include selection, antibody-mediated immunologic enhancement, and induction of immunologic unresponsiveness (either specifically or nonspecifically). It appears likely that no one of these mechanisms can account totally for the transfusion effect, and each may play a role.

**Selection.** This is perhaps the most readily postulated mechanism. It can be viewed in two ways: patient selection and donor selection.

*Patient Selection.* According to this hypothesis, it is assumed that, if all patients are exposed to transfusions, some will make broadly reactive anti-HLA antibodies (i.e., they are strong "immunologic responders"), while others will generate few or no antibodies (i.e., so-called "non-responders"). Transfusions then merely work by allowing 'responders" to be distinguished from 'non-responders."[94] Two further assumptions necessary for this hypothesis are (1) that strong immunologic responders are more likely to reject renal transplants than non-responders[45]; and (2) because of the generation of broadly specific antibodies by transfusions, the immunologic responders are more likely to be relegated to long-term dialysis while unsuccessfully awaiting the availability of a crossmatch negative transplant. By this reasoning, pretransplant transfusions do nothing more than serve as a discriminator which keeps high-risk potential recipients from receiving a transplant.[94] Graft outcome statistics are better in transfused patients, so the argment goes, because, in the main, only low-risk non-responders receive transplants.

Such a mechanism, if operative, can account for only a minor portion of the transfusion effect. As noted above, only a small minority of patients develop broadly reactive cytotoxic antibodies after multiple transfusions.[35] The large transfusion effect cannot be due merely to the exclusion of such a small percentage of "high responders." In addition, a number of studies show that first cadaver graft outcome in highly presensitized individuals (i.e., "responders") is as good[13, 47] or almost as good[3, 48-51] as in individuals who are not presensitized. While there is undoubtedly a group of "high responders" in whom graft outcome is poor (e.g., patients noted by

Glass et al[9] who make broadly reactive antibodies after fewer than two transfusions), the exclusion of this relatively small group will not account for the transfusion effect.

*Donor Selection.* This hypothesis is a variation of the one above. According to this proposed mechanism, it is assumed that individuals will react in different degrees to the various antigens presented to them in the transfusions. That is to say, an individual may make cytotoxic antibodies against some HLA antigens while not generating antibodies against others. It is reasonable to assume that grafts carrying antigens against which the patient would react vigorously are excluded because of the development of antibodies to these antigens after transfusion. Such exclusion would take place at the time of the crossmatch. Thus, if presented with a large enough panoply of antigens via transfusions prior to transplantation, the recipient is allowed to "select" his own donor by means of a negative crossmatch. This of course assumes that (1) enough transfusions (i.e., enough antigens) have been presented to the prospective recipient and (2) a crossmatch technique sensitive enough is carried out on all relevant post-transfusion sera.

Much of the data fit with such a mechanism. The finding that multiple transfusions have been shown by many to have the most pronounced effect agrees well with this selection mechanism. In addition, the demonstration that transfusions are most important in early (first three months) graft outcome[5] also favors this mechanism. On the other hand, the beneficial effect of perioperative transfusions and the well-documented finding that one transfusion can confer as much as 50%[3] to 100%[7] of the transfusion effect make it unlikely that selection is the sole mechanism by which pretransplant transfusion improves graft survival.

**Antibody-Mediated Immunologic Enhancement.** Antibodies in addition to classic anti–HLA A and B antibodies may be generated after blood transfusion.[38] While pretransplant donor-specific anti–HLA A and B antibodies may be deleterious to graft outcome,[32] other types of antibodies may have indifferent[38, 39] or even beneficial effects.[83, 96] There are adequate animal data to suggest that specific unresponsiveness may be induced by active immunization; in rat organ allograft models, such enhancement can be induced by administration of donor lymphocytes[97] or lymphocytes bearing antigens cross-reactive with the potential donor.[98]

Conclusive data for an active antibody-mediated enhancement mechanism in the clinical situation are presently still lacking.

Some antibodies whose presence favors improved graft outcome (e.g., cold lymphocytotoxins,[99] cold B lymphocytotoxins,[100] or autolymphocytotoxins[83]) do not appear to be primarily generated by blood transfusion.[35, 36, 99] It has been claimed that donor-specific anti–B lymphocyte antibodies may be graft-enhancing.[101] However, this has not been uniformly found.[38, 102] It is probable that post-transfusion anti–B cell antibodies are heterogeneous with regard to their targets and that better definition of such antibodies must precede the identification of a specific subset as mediators of a post-transfusion enhancing effect.

One area of considerable excitement is the possibility that transfusions engender the formation of anti-idiotypic antibodies. Variable regions of antibody molecules can be perceived by the immune system as antigenic substances. This form of antigenic potential is referred to as idiotype, and idiotypes are defined as the antigenic determinants on the variable regions of antibody molecules. It has been hypothesized that when antibodies are generated, e.g., anti-HLA antibody after transfusion, regulation of their synthesis is controlled in part by generation of anti-idiotypic antibody, in this example anti-anti-HLA antibody. The generation of such anti-idiotypic antibodies in response to transfusion may result in specific immunomodulation aimed against the transfused antigens.

It has been shown that the presence of antibodies against antigen combining sites in patients who received at least six blood transfusions was associated with a significantly better one-year graft survival rate than that seen in patients having a similar number of transfusions but no such antibody.[104] In addition, Singal and his co-workers have identified antibodies generated in response to transfusions which are associated with successful graft outcome and have some characteristics of anti-idiotypic antibodies.[105-107] It remains to be seen whether anti-idiotypic antibodies have a role in the transfusion effect, but this certainly appears to be a fruitful area for investigation.

**Induction of Immunologic Unresponsiveness by Cellular Mechanisms.** Recent studies support the hypothesis that repeated pretransplant blood transfusions induce suppressor cells, which may then regulate immune responsiveness and improve renal transplant outcome. Thomas et al showed that successful long-term human transplantation was associated with suppressor cell activity in over 50% of the cases studied.[108] Smith et al showed that two units of packed red blood cells induced increased suppressor cell function in humans between three and 20 weeks post-transfusion.[109] Lenhard and his colleagues observed that at least two different cell-mediated immunoregulatory mechanisms were induced by blood transfusions: (a) in the early post-transfusion period a nonspecific immunosuppression probably mediated by monocytes; and (b) in a later phase, increasing suppressor T cell activity.[110] Kerman et al were able to show that, although the number of suppressor T lymphocytes (as measured by the monoclonal antibody marked OKT 8) was not increased after five transfusions, there was a weakening of immunologic responsiveness concomitant with strong suppressor cell function in vitro.[111]

In contrast to these studies, however, others have found no increase in nonspecific suppressor cells[112] and, at best, an inconsistent increase in specific suppressor cell activity.[113] Some of these differences may be traceable to methodology in assaying for suppressor cells. However, while it is an attractive hypothesis that pretransplant blood transfusions improve graft survival by inducing an increase in the number or function of suppressor cells, more work is required to solidify this point and to more precisely elaborate the mechanism.

Even if cellular hyporesponsiveness is involved in the transfusion effect, there are other mechanisms by which this can occur. For example, there is evidence in humans to suggest that repeated antigenic stimulation may be associated with decreases in both spontaneous and mitogen-driven antigen-specific antibody-producing B lymphocytes. This effect can be correlated with a decreased precursor frequency of B lymphocytes as well as decreased B cell activity, but is not associated with excessive suppression mediated by T cells.[114] Alternatively, a direct immunosuppressive effect of erythrocytes on mononuclear phagocytic cell function has been postulated.[18]

# REFERENCES

1. Dossetor JB, MacKinnon KJ, Gault MH, et al: Cadaver kidney transplants. Transplantation 5:844, 1967.

2. Opelz G, Sengar DPS, Mickey MR, et al.: Effect of blood transfusions on subsequent kidney transplants. Transplant Proc 5:253, 1973.

3. Opelz G, Graver B, Terasaki PI: Induction of high kidney graft survival rate by multiple transfusions. Lancet 1:1223, 1981.

4. Opelz G, Terasaki PI: International study of histocompatibility in renal transplantation. Transplantation 33:87, 1982.

5. Terasaki PI, Perdue S, Ayoub G, et al: Reduction of accelerated failures by transfusion. Transplant Proc 14:251, 1982.

6. Van Hoof JP, Kalff MW, Van Poelgeest AE, et al: Blood transfusion and kidney transplantation. Transplantation 22:306, 1976.

7. Persijn GG, Van Hoof JP, Kalff MW, et al: Effect of blood transfusion and HLA matching on renal transplantation in the Netherlands. Transplant Proc 5:503, 1977.

8. Hourmant M, Soulillou JP, Bui-Quang D: Beneficial effect of blood transfusion. Transplantation 28:40, 1979.

9. Glass NR, Miller, DT, Sollinger HW, et al: Renal allograft prognosis as a function of pre-transplant parameters including transfusion history. Transplant Proc 14:290, 1982.

10. Mickey MR, Terasaki PI: Comparison of blood products for enhancing kidney graft survival. Ninth International Congress of the Transplantation Society. Brighton, England, 1982. p 11.8 (Abstr.).

11. Persijn GG, van Leeuwen A, Parlevliet J, et al: Two major factors influencing kidney graft survival in Euro-transplant: HLA DR matching and blood transfusion. Transplant Proc 13:150, 1981.

12. Frisk B, Brynger H, Sandberg C: Two random transfusions before primary renal transplantation—four years experience from a single center. Transplant Proc 14:386, 1982.

13. Feduska NJ, Vincenti F, Amend WJ, et al: Do blood transfusions enhance the possibility of a compatible transplant? Transplantation 27:35, 1979.

14. Strom TB: The improving utility of renal transplantation in the management of end-stage renal disease. Am J Med 73:105, 1982.

15. Wood P, Horsburgh T, Brent L: Specific unresponsiveness to skin allografts in mice. Graft survival in mice pretreated with blood. Transplantation 31:8, 1981.

16. Van Es AA, Marquet RL, Van Rood JJ, et al: Influence of a single blood transfusion on kidney allograft survival in unrelated rhesus monkeys. Transplantation 26:325, 1978.

17. Newton WT, Anderson CB: Attempted enhancement in patients undergoing renal allotransplantation. Arch Surg 114:1007, 1979.

18. Keown PA, Descamps B: Improved renal allograft survival after blood transfusion: a non-specific erythrocyte-mediated immunoregulatory process? Lancet 1:20, 1979.

19. Borleffs JCC, Neuhaus P, van Rood JJ, et al: Platelet transfusions have a positive effect on kidney allograft survival in rhesus monkeys and induce virtually no cytotoxic antibodies. Transplant Proc 15:985, 1983.

20. Spees EK, Vaughn WK, Williams GM, et al: Effects of blood transfusion on cadaver renal transplantation. Transplantation 30:455, 1980.

21. Green WF, Niblack GD, Johnson HK, et al: Multifactorial analysis of factors influencing graft survival in recipients of living-related renal allografts. Transplant Proc 14:282, 1982.

22. Fuller TC, Delmonico FL, Cosimi AB, et al: Impact of blood transfusion on renal transplantation. Ann Surg 187:211, 1978.

23. Fuller TC, Burroughs JC, Delmonico FL, et al: Influence of frozen blood transfusions on renal allograft survival. Transplant Proc 14:293, 1982.

24. Polesky, HF, McCullough JJ, Yunis EJ, et al: Reevaluation of the effects of blood transfusions on renal allografts survival. Transplantation 24:449, 1977.

25. Wood PJ, Horsburgh T, Brent L: Skin allograft survival in mice pretreated with blood. Transplant Proc 13:523, 1981.

26. Sirchia G, Mercuriali F, Pizzi C, et al: Blood transfusion and kidney transplantation: Effect of small doses of blood on kidney graft function and survival. Transplant Proc 14:263, 1982.

27. Corry RJ, West JC, Hunsicker LG, et al: Effect of timing of administration and quantity of blood transfusion on cadaver renal transplant survival. Transplantation 30:425, 1980.

28. Betuel H, Touraine JL, Malik MC, et al: Kidney transplantation in patients submitted to deliberate transfusions, to random transfusion and to thoracic duct drainage. Transplant Proc 14:276, 1982.

29. Stiller CR, Lockwood BL, Sinclair NR, et al: Beneficial effect of operation day blood transfusion on human renal allograft survival. Lancet 1:169, 1978.

30. Williams KA, Ting A, French ME, et al: Perioperative blood transfusion improves cadaveric renal allograft survival in non-transfused recipients. Lancet 1:1104, 1980.

31. Feduska NJ, Amend WJ, Vincenti F, et al: Blood transfusions before and on the day of transplantation: Effects on cadaver graft survival. Transplant Proc 14:302, 1982.

32. Patel R, Terasaki PI: Significance of the positive crossmatch test in kidney transplantation. N Eng J Med 280:735, 1969.

33. Cheigh JS, Fotino M, Stubenbord WT, et al: Declining transplantability of prospective kidney transplant recipients. JAMA 246:135, 1981.

34. Soulillou JP, Bignon JD, Peyrat MA, et al: Systematic transfusion in hemodialyzed patients awaiting grafts. Kinetics of anti-T and B lymphocyte immunization and its incidence on graft function. Transplantation 30:285, 1980.

35. Opelz G, Graver B, Mickey MR, et al: Lymphocytotoxic antibody responses to transfusion in potential kidney transplant recipients. Transplantation 32:177, 1981.

36. Ettenger RB, Jordan SC, Arnett J, et al: Specific anti-donor lymphocytotoxic antibodies following blood transfusion from non-related donors. Transplant Proc 14:347, 1982.

37. Morris PJ, Mickey MR, Singal DP, et al: Serotyping for homotransplantation. XXII. Specificity of cytotoxic antibodies developing after renal transplantation. Br Med J 1:758, 1969.

38. Ettenger RB, Uittenbogaart CH, Pennisi AJ, et al: Long-term cadaver allograft survival in the recipient with a positive B lymphocyte crossmatch. Transplantation 27:315, 1979.

39. Ting A, Morris PJ: Renal transplantation and B

cell crossmatches with autoantibodies and alloantibodies. Lancet 2:1095, 1977.

40. Iwaki Y, Terasaki PI, Heintz R, et al: Report of the pre-sensitization workshop. Transplant Proc 14:417, 1982.

41. Anderson CB, Sicard GA, Etheredge EE: Pretreatment of renal allograft recipients with azathioprine and donor-specific blood products. Surgery 92:315, 1982.

42. Whelchel JD, Shaw JF, Curtis JJ, et al: Effect of pretransplant stored donor-specific blood transfusions on early renal allograft survival in one-haplotype living related transplants. Transplantation 34:326, 1982.

43. Light JA, Metz S, Oddenino K, et al: Donor-specific transfusion with diminished sensitization. Transplantation 34:352, 1982.

44. Opelz G, Terasaki PI: Histocompatibility matching utilizing responsiveness as a new dimension. Transplant Proc 4:433, 1972.

45. Opelz G, Terasaki PI: Dominant effect of transfusions on kidney graft survival. Transplantation 39:153, 1980.

46. Sanfilippo F, Vaughn WK, Bollinger RR, et al: The relationship of transfusion and presensitization with graft and patient survival. Transplant Proc 14:287, 1982.

47. Kreis H: Selection of a donor. In: Renal Transplantation Theory and Practice, Hamburger J, Crosnier J, Back JF, Kreis H (Eds). Baltimore, Williams and Wilkins, 1981, p 36.

48. Werner-Favre C, Jeannet M, Harder F, et al: Blood transfusions, cytotoxic antibodies and kidney graft survival. Transplantation 28:343, 1979.

49. Vincenti F, Duca RM, Amend W, et al: Immunologic factors determining survival of cadaver kidney transplants: Effect of HLA serotyping, cytotoxic antibodies and blood transfusion on graft survivals. N Engl J Med 299:793, 1979.

50. Sirchia G, Mercuriali F, Scalamogna M, et al: Evaluation of the blood transfusion policy of the North Italy Transplant Program. Transplantation 31:388, 1981.

51. Sanfilippo F, Vaughn WK, Bollinger RR, et al: Comparative effects of pregnancy, transfusion and prior graft rejection on sensitization and renal transplant results. Transplantation 34:360, 1982.

52. Opelz G, Terasaki PI: Improvement of kidney-graft survival with increased numbers of blood transfusions. N Engl J Med 299:799, 1978.

53. Mahanakumar T, Ellis TM, Dayal H, et al: Potentiating effect of HLA matching and blood transfusion on renal allograft survival. Transplantation 32:244, 1981.

54. Moen T, Albrechtsen, D, Flatmark A, et al: Importance of HLA-DR matching in cadaveric renal transplantation: A prospective one-center study of 170 transplants. N Eng J Med 303:850, 1980.

55. Opelz G, Terasaki PI: International histocompatibility study on renal transplantation. In: Terasaki, PI (ed), Histocompatibility testing, 1980. Los Angeles, UCLA Tissue Typing Laboratory, 1980, p 592.

56. Borleffs JCC, Marquet RL, Neuhaus P: Effect of matching for DR antigens and pretransplant blood transfusion on kidney graft survival in rhesus monkeys. Transplant Proc 14:403, 1982.

57. Goeken NE, Thompson JS, Corry RJ: Effect of prospective matching for HLA-DR on renal allograft survival in a single center. Transplantation 31:397, 1981.

58. Ayoub G, Terasaki PI: HLA-DR matching in multicenter, single-typing laboratory data. Transplantation 33:515, 1982.

59. Persijn GG, Lansbergen Q, D'Amaro J, et al: Blood transfusion and second kidney allograft survival. Transplantation 32:392, 1981.

60. Dewar PJ, Murray S, Wilkinson R, et al: A new finding relating to transfusion and renal transplants. Transplantation 29:379, 1980.

61. Solheim BG, Flatmark A, Halvorsen S, et al: Effect of blood transfusions on renal transplantation: Study of 191 consecutive first transplants from living related donors. Transplantation 30:281, 1980.

62. Solheim BG, Flatmark A, Jervell J, et al: Influence of blood transfusions on kidney transplant and uremic patient survival. Scand J Urol Nephrol (Suppl) 42:65, 1977.

63. Fehrman I: Pretransplant blood transfusions and related kidney allograft survival. Transplantation 34:46, 1982.

64. Brynger H, Frisk B, Ahlmen J, et al: Blood transfusion and primary graft survival in male recipients. Scand J Urol Nephrol (Suppl) 42:76, 1977.

65. Opelz G, Terasaki PI, Graver B, et al: Correlation between number of pretransplant blood transfusions and between number of pretransplant blood transfusions and kidney graft survival. Transplant Proc 11:145, 1979.

66. Salvatierra O, Vincenti F, Amend W, et al: What about blood transfusions in living related transplantation? Am Soc Nephrol 1979, p 178A (Abstr).

67. Cochrum K, Salvatierra O, Belzer FO: Correlation between MLC stimulation and graft survival in living related and cadaver transplants. Ann Surg 180:617, 1974.

68. Ringdin O, Möller E, Lundgren G, et al: Role of MLC compatibility in intrafamilial kidney transplantation. Transplantation 22:9, 1976.

69. Salvatierra O, Vincenti F, Amend W, et al: Deliberate donor specific blood transfusions prior to living-related renal transplantation: A new approach. Ann Surg 192:543, 1980.

70. Halasz NA, Orloff MJ, Hirone F: Increased survival of renal homografts in dogs after injection of graft donor blood. Transplantation 2:453, 1964.

71. Marquet RL, Heystek GA, Tinbergen WJ: Specific inhibition of organ allograft rejection by donor blood. Transplant Proc 3:708, 1971.

72. Fabre JW, Morris PJ: The effect of donor strain blood pretreatment on renal allograft rejection in rats. Transplantation 14:608, 1972.

73. Okazaki H, Maki T, Wood ML, et al: Prolongation of skin allograft survival in $H_2K$ transfusion. Transplantation 32:111, 1981.

74. Mendez R, Iwaki Y, Mendez R, et al: Seventeen consecutive successful one-haplotype matched living related first renal transplants using donor-specific blood transfusion. Transplantation 33:621, 1982.

75. Schweizer R, Bow L, Generas D, et al: Serologic considerations in donor-specific transfusion therapy for kidney transplantation. Transplant Proc 14:374, 1982.

76. Takahashi I, Otsubo O, Nishimura M, et al: Pro-

longed graft survival by donor-specific blood transfusion. Transplant Proc 14:367, 1982.

77. Amend W, Vincenti F, Feduska N, et al: Unusual renal transplant rejections in recipients of pre-transplant, donor-specific transfusion. Am Soc Nephrol 1980, p 157A (Abstr).

78. Salvatierra O: Experiences and future considerations with donor-specific blood transfusions in living-related transplantation. Am J Kidney Dis 1:119, 1981.

79. Ettenger RB, Kerman R, Arnett J, et al: Sensitization following donor-specific transfusions for living-related renal transplantation. Transplant Proc 15:943, 1983.

80. Carpenter CB: Deliberate transfusions of potential renal transplant recipients with specific donor blood. Am J Kidney Dis 1:116, 1981.

81. Terasaki P, Bernoco D, Park MS, et al: Micro-droplet testing for HLA-A, -B, -C and -D antigens. Am J Clin Pathol 69:103, 1978.

82. Fuller TC, Phelan D, Gebel HM, et al: Antigenic specificity of antibody reactive in the antiglobulin-augmented lymphocytotoxicity test. Transplantation 34:24, 1982.

83. Ettenger RB, Jordan SC, Fine RN: Cadaver renal transplant outcome in recipients with autolymphocytotoxic antibodies. Transplantation 35:429, 1983.

84. Stastny P, Austin CL: Successful kidney transplant in patient with positive crossmatch due to auto-antibodies. Transplantation 21:399, 1976.

85. Paul LC, Claas FHJ, Van Es LA, et al: Accelerated rejection of a renal allograft associated with pretransplantation antibodies directed against donor antigens on endothelium and monocytes. N Engl J Med 300:1258, 1979.

86. Garovoy MR, Rheinschmidt MA, Bigor M, et al: Flow cytometry analysis: A high technolog cross-match. Am Soc Nephrol 1982, p 196A (Abstr).

87. Blank JL, Leo GM, Sollinger HW, et al: B-warm-positive crossmatch: A contraindication for transplantation in living related transplants undergoing donor-specific transfusion. Transplantation 33:212, 1982.

88. Ahern AT, Artruc SB, Della Pelle, P, et al: Hyperacute rejection of HLA-AB-identical renal allografts associated with B lymphocyte and endothelial reactive antibodies. Transplantation 33:103, 1982.

89. Cochrum K, Hanes D, Potter D, et al: Improved graft survival with donor-specific transfusion pretreatment. Transplant Proc 13:190, 1981.

90. Leivestad T, Flatmark A, Hirschberg H, et al: Effect of pre-transplant donor-specific transfusions in renal transplantation. Transplant Proc 14:370, 1982.

91. Schweizer RT, Bartus SA, Silver H, et al: Kidney transplantation using donor-specific blood transfusions despite Rh incompatibility. Transplantation 32:345, 1981.

92. Gailiunas P, Helderman JH, Atkins C, et al: A randomized prospective study of donor specific transfusion in 1-haplo disparate related renal transplants. Am Soc Nephrol 1982, p 196A (Abstr).

93. Miller LC, Bock GH, Lum CT, et al: Transplantation of the adult kidney into the very small

child: Long-term outcome. J Pediatr 100:675, 1982.

94. Solheim B: The role of pretransplant blood transfusion. Transplant Proc 11:138, 1979.

95. Kerman RH, Floyd M, Van Buren T, et al: Improved allograft survival of strong immune responder–high risk recipients with adjuvant antithymocyte globulin therapy. Transplantation 30:450, 1980.

96. Ting A: Leukocyte antibodies in renal transplantation. In: Zurukzoglu W, Papadimitriou M, Pyrpasopoulos M, et al (Eds), Proceedings, Eighth International Congress of Nephrology: Advances in Basis and Clinical Nephrology. Basel, Karger, 1981, p 506.

97. Lowry RP, Carpenter CB: Public B cell alloantigen determinants (Ia) and active enhancement of renal allografts in the rat. Transplantation 30:347, 1980.

98. Hendry WS, Tilney NL, Baldwin WM, et al: Transfer of specific unresponsiveness to organ allografts by thymocytes: Specific unresponsiveness by thymocyte transfer. J Exp Med 149:1042, 1979.

99. Jeannet M, Vassali P, Hufschmid MF: Enhancement of human kidney allografts by cold B lymphocyte cytotoxins. Transplantation 29:174, 1980.

100. Iwaki Y, Terasaki PI, Park MS, et al: Enhancement of human kidney allograft and B cold lymphocyte cytotoxins. Lancet 1:1228, 1978.

101. d'Apice AJF, Tait BD: Improved survival and functions of renal transplants with positive B cell crossmatches. Transplantation 27:324, 1979.

102. Suthanthiran M, Fotino M, Cheigh JS, et al: Adverse presensitization to renal transplants. Detection by utilization of a D locus antigen-defined lymphoblastoid cell panel as targets in antibody-dependent cell-mediated cytotoxicity assay. Transplantation 27:333, 1979.

103. d'Apice AJF, Tait BD: Most positive B cell crossmatches are not caused by anti-HLA-DR antibodies. Transplantation 30:382, 1980.

104. Chia D, Horimi T, Terasaki PI, et al: Association of anti-Fab and anti-IgG antibodies with high kidney transplant survival. Transplant Proc 14:322, 1982.

105. Singal DP, Joseph S, Szewczuk MR: Possible mechanisms of the beneficial effect of pretransplant blood transfusion on renal allograft survival in man. Transplant Proc 14:316, 1982.

106. Fagnilli L, Singal DP: Blood transfusion may induce anti-T cell receptor antibodies in renal patients. Transplant Proc 14:319, 1982.

107. Singal DP, Joseph S: Role of blood transfusion on the induction of antibodies against recognition sites on T lymphocytes in renal transplant patients. Hum Immunol 4:93, 1982.

108. Thomas J, Thomas F, Lee HM: Why do HLA-nonidentical renal allografts survive 10 years or more? Transplant Proc 9:85, 1977.

109. Smith MD, Williams JD, Coles GA, et al: The effect of blood transfusion on T-suppressor cells in renal dialysis patients. Transplant Proc 13:181, 1981.

110. Lenhard V, Massen G, Seifert P, et al: Characterization of transfusion-induced suppressor cells

in prospective kidney allograft recipients. Transplant Proc 14:329, 1982.

111. Kerman RH, Van Buren CT, Payne W, et al: Influence of blood transfusions on immune responsiveness. Transplant Proc 14:335, 1982.

112. Jeannet M, Neri-Legendre C, Descoeudres C, et al: Does blood transfusion induce a non-specific suppression of cell-mediated immunity? Transplant Proc 14:325, 1982.

113. Goeken NE, Flanigan MJ, Thomps JS, et al: Effects of blood transfusion on immune responses and their relationship to renal allograft survival. Transplant Proc 14:338, 1982.

114. Saxon A, Tamaroff MA, Morrow C, et al: Impaired generation of spontaneous and mitogen-reactive anti-tetanus toxoid antibody-producing B cells following repetitive in vivo booster immunization. Cell Immunol 59:82, 1981.

115. Nube MJ, Persijn GG, Kalff MW, et al: Kidney transplantation—transplant survival after planned HLA-A and -B matched blood transfusion. Tissue Antigen 17:449, 1981.

# 32

# Surgical Aspects of Transplantation: Technique and Complications

*Lester W. Martin, M.D.*
*John Noseworthy, M.D.*

Renal transplantation in children is a complex undertaking. It requires that the surgeon be a superb technician, have a thorough knowledge of the diseases and surgical complications peculiar to the pediatric patient, and also have a reasonable knowledge of immunology as well. Because of the complex course of the postoperative renal transplant patient, it is imperative that certain facilities be readily available: arteriography, nuclear scans, computed tomography, a laboratory for tissue typing, and a group of colleagues who can serve as consultants in the fields of hematology, immunology, nephrology, radiology, ultrasonography, nuclear medicine, and microbiology.[1] Successful transplantation extends beyond the technical maneuver of placing the kidney. Responsibility for the success of the endeavor must be shouldered by the surgeon until such time as the patient can be returned to the nephrologist for long-term follow-up care.[2]

In 1954, Murray et al, performed the first successful renal homotransplantation with an identical twin as the living donor.[3] This accomplishment confirmed the technical feasibility of renal transplantation in man. Subsequent discoveries of immunosuppressive agents, beginning with 6-mercaptopurine[4] and leading to azathioprine, steroids, antilymphocyte globulin, and cyclosporin-A, have made possible the transplantation of kidneys between unrelated donors.[5] Knowledge of the benefits as well as the complica-

tions of immunosuppressive agents has led to the widespread acceptance of renal transplantation as a highly successful endeavor. Transplantation is currently viewed as the keystone of the therapeutic armamentarium available for the treatment of ESRD in children.[6] The first kidney transplantation at the Children's Hospital in Cincinnati was performed in 1964 on an eight-year-old boy with ESRD due to hydronephrosis.[7] His mother was the donor. He received a second transplant 15 years later. It functions well after an additional four years—19 years following the first transplant. Our subsequent experience includes 156 kidney transplants in children.

## LIVING RELATED DONORS

In the first five years of our experience, 22 renal transplants were performed, 21 from living related donors. As knowledge of tissue typing and immunology has increased through the years, the importance of the living related donor has gradually decreased. At the present time, it is conjectural whether the advantages of the living related donor are sufficient to warrant the risks of the procedure to the donor. The recent advent of a program of preoperative donor-specific blood transfusions (Chapter 31) has resulted in a revival of enthusiasm for living related donor transplantation. As histocompatibility techniques improve, it is possible to visualize a time when cadaver donor selection may be far more specific. The living related donor does, however, offer certain other advantages to the recipient. The delay between renal failure and transplantation can be held to a minimum. The ischemia time during the actual transplant is shortened to the extent that renal function in the recipient is immediate, resulting in fewer postoperative surgical complications. It is important that the major blood group antigens be compatible. Crossing of the major blood type barriers may result in a violent hyperacute rejection, whereas the minor blood groups (Rh, Duffy, Kell, etc.,) do not appear to be histocompatibility antigens (Chapter 30).

Medical evaluation and selection of the living donor are important to minimize donor risk. It is also important to determine that the living donor is in excellent health, that the operation will cause no harm, and that renal function in the donor is normal. Table 32–1 lists the examinations routinely carried out on living related donors. It has been our routine practice to obtain and evaluate all other studies before subjecting the donor to an arteriogram. Multiple renal arteries are found in some individuals. It is preferable to use a kidney with a single renal artery, although kidneys with double renal arteries can be utilized.

The ethical problems in selection of a living related donor may at times assume significant

**Table 32–1.** RECOMMENDED EXAMINATIONS FOR LIVING RELATED KIDNEY DONORS

1. Complete history and physical examination
2. Hematology
   Complete blood count, hematocrit, differential, and platelet count
3. Coagulation
   Prothrombin time, partial thromboplastin time
4. Blood chemistry
   Serum sodium, potassium, $CO_2$, chloride; liver function tests; serum calcium, phosphorus, BUN, creatinine, fasting blood sugar level
5. Urine
   Routine urinalysis
   Clean, voided urine for culture
6. Immunology
   Blood type, tissue typing, leukocyte match for recipient and leukocyte antibodies, VDRL, HBs antigen
7. Radiology
   Anteroposterior and lateral chest x-ray, aortogram (demonstrating the renal arteries selectively if necessary), and follow-through excretory urogram
8. Electrocardiogram

proportions. There is a small risk to the donor, and the pain, anxiety, and loss of work time are serious considerations. Because of family pressures and a feeling of obligation on the part of a relative to donate a kidney, it is important that the physician resist the temptation to exert pressure to persuade a potential donor. Because of legal implications, donors below the age of consent are generally considered unacceptable. In our own practice, we have discouraged the use of unrelated living donors, although four such donors have been utilized in our series.

## CADAVER DONOR

The advent of histocompatibility typing and organ preservation techniques and high speed transportation facilities now make possible the transport and utilization of cadaveric kidneys around the world within a sufficient period of time to assure an acceptable success rate. We depend upon cadaveric kidneys in the majority of instances. In the past five years, 53 of 60 transplants have been from this source. Ideally, the donor should be young, healthy, normotensive, free of transmissible disease, and have died of a sudden death with brain damage, but with preservation of renal function until such time as the kidneys can be harvested while they are still functioning in a normal manner. The kidney can be removed with less than five minutes of warm ischemia time, cooled, transported, and utilized with dependable function within a period of 48 hours. While awaiting a final determination of brain death of the donor, histocompatibility typing and cross-matching with potential recipients can be performed. Computerization of a data base of recipients both nationally and internationally can provide immediate identification of potential recipients with a minimum expenditure of time.

## ORGAN HARVEST

**Living Donors.** To harvest a kidney from a living donor requires considerably more expertise and technical detail than a simple nephrectomy of a diseased kidney. It is important that during the operation the surgeon handle the kidney with the delicate care that he would an infant that is being delivered by cesarean section. There should be no traction or compression applied to the vascular pedicle of the organ during the process of its removal; otherwise, its subsequent function may be compromised. For this reason, it is important that the surgeon have adequate exposure with a reasonably lengthy incision. This generally involves resection of the twelfth rib. Urine output from the kidney is continuously monitored throughout the donor operation. The patient is well hydrated prior to operation. Mannitol and furosemide are administered shortly before the kidney is removed. Systemic heparinization is carried out five minutes prior to renal artery occlusion. The heparin effect may be neutralized with protamine following removal of the kidney.

The donor operation is generally carried out through a generous flank incision without entering the peritoneum or the pleura, even though the twelfth rib is resected subperiosteally. After gentle wide dissection, the ureter is divided below the pelvic brim. Care is taken to preserve the ureteral blood supply from the renal pedicle since the other elements of its segmental arterial supply will be interrupted. Leaving abundant periureteral tissue attached to the ureter aids in preserving anastomotic ureteral vessels. Both renal vein and renal artery are then mobilized and the kidney is observed to function for several minutes undisturbed prior to interrupting its blood supply. Care must be exercised in this dissection to clearly identify all venous tributaries to the renal vein. On the left side, these include the adrenal vein, gonadal vein, and occasionally a posteriorly entering lumbar vein. Following removal of the kidney, it is immediately flushed with ice-cold Sacks or Collins solution which is permitted to enter the renal artery by gravity from a height of 30 cm. This gentle flow of electrolyte solution to the kidney is continued until the return fluid is completely clear, and then the kidney is transported in sterile ice slush to the recipient in an adjacent operating room where reestablishment of the vascular supply should be immediately accomplished.

**Harvest of Cadaveric Kidneys.** In the harvesting of kidneys from a cadaver, it is preferable that the donor be declared "brain dead" but with intact circulation and urinary output. Nephrectomy can then be performed in an orderly manner by a transabdominal approach, with circulatory function maintained until the kidneys are actually removed. The kidneys are then flushed with ice cold Sacks or Collins solution and the kidneys preserved in a sterile container surrounded by ice or by one of the methods of pulsatile continuous perfusion until such time as they can be transported to the recipient.

## PREPARATION OF THE RECIPIENT FOR TRANSPLANTATION

Removal of the recipient's native kidneys is desirable if they have been recurrently or chronically infected, if they are hydronephrotic, if there is vesicoureteral reflux, if the patient has uncontrollable renal hypertension, or if there are other reasons to suspect that the native kidneys will result in infection or be otherwise detrimental to the recipient.

Recipient splenectomy was at one time recommended and indeed was carried out in all but seven of our first 60 patients prior to transplantation. It was believed that splenectomy reduced the risk of rejection. The risk of postsplenectomy sepsis, however, soon became apparent when four deaths from overwhelming sepsis occurred in the post-transplant period. In our subsequent transplants, we have not removed the spleen and have observed no further instances of overwhelming sepsis. It has been clearly demonstrated that splenectomy in children predisposes to this syndrome, and when combined with immunosuppression the risk of overwhelming sepsis is compounded. We therefore do not recommend routine splenectomy in conjunction with renal transplantation in children.

During the preparation for transplantation in the immediate pretransplant period, any possible source of sepsis must be carefully eliminated. Infected kidneys should be removed. Hemodialysis cannulas, urinary tract infections, skin infections, or pyocystis of a previously defunctionalized bladder can all lead to failure of the operation because of sepsis and must be assiduously avoided. All such potentially infectious foci must be dealt with prior to undertaking transplantation. Their presence may force postponement of a planned transplant.

## TECHNIQUE OF OPERATION— GENERAL PRINCIPLES

When the size of the donor and recipient are comparable, it is generally possible to place the kidney extraperitoneally in the right or left iliac fossa, attaching the donor vessels to the recipient's external or common iliac vessels. Ideally, the ends of the donor vessels are attached to the side of the recipient's iliac vessels. Use of the internal iliac artery was at one time recommended, but long-term follow-up of patients with a second graft, utilizing the second internal iliac artery, have demonstrated an alarming incidence of impotence resulting from compromised blood supply to the pelvic organs. We therefore are now hesitant to utilize even the first internal iliac artery.

The incision is made from the level of the twelfth rib in a gentle curve downward to the midline above the pubic symphysis. Muscles, including the recti, are divided in the direction of the incision. The spermatic cord is retracted and preserved. The deep inferior epigastric vessels are divided, providing easy access to the retroperitoneum. The peritoneum is then retracted medially and not opened. The iliac fossa is developed by blunt dissection. Care is taken to preserve the native ureter, if present and of normal size, for possible utilization in the event of compromised blood supply to the donor ureter. Iliac vessels are exposed and temporarily occluded. We take great care to ligate with fine ties the abundant perivascular lymphatics overlying the iliac vessels, to prevent the subsequent formation of a lymphocele. The internal iliac vessels are preserved and temporarily occluded if necessary. An end-to-side anastomosis is accomplished between the end of the donor renal vein and the recipient iliac vein, and between the end of the donor renal artery and the recipient iliac artery.

We attempt to locate the anastomoses at levels along the iliac artery and vein, a location which ensures a comfortable placement of the kidney in the iliac fossa with complete lack of tension on the vascular sutures lines. A few seconds of additional warm ischemia time may be tolerated at this point while the kidney is placed in the fossa and the arteriovenous relationships assessed to select the ideal location for the anastomoses. Any redundancy or other abnormality in the donor vessels can be carefully eliminated under cold conditions minimizing the warm-ischemic anastomotic time.

By spatulating the end of the renal artery, an anastomosis can be accomplished which is considerably longer than the diameter of the vessel itself (Fig. 32–1). It is important that, during the course of the anastomosis, all perivascular areolar tissue be freed from the vessels and that no adventitia be incorporated into the anastomosis because of the tendency of such tissue to initiate thrombosis. It is also important that any damaged or crushed end of the donor artery be carefully trimmed away and discarded in order to prevent the development of subsequent stenosis. Careful inspection, debridement, and angioplasty, if necessary, may be carried out at a side table while maintaining the donor kidney in an iced slush environment. These maneuvers allow meticulous preparation of the donor vessels and ensure a precise, problem-free anastomosis.

We currently use 5–0 and 6–0 polypropylene vascular suture for the vascular anasto-

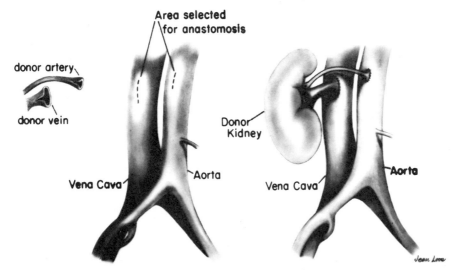

**Figure 32–1.** Technique of spatulation of the ends of the donor artery and vein in order to assure an anastomosis larger than the diameter of the donor vessel. This maneuver decreases the likelihood of postoperative occlusion of the anastomosis because of constriction.

moses. The venous side is performed first, making a longitudinal venotomy after appropriate occlusion, irrigating the lumen gently with heparinized sterile saline and flushing in ante- and retrograde directions. A running technique is preferred, and the sutures are initially placed at the apices of the venotomy before the kidney is brought from the iced environment to the fossa. When set up with precision, such an anastomosis can be accomplished swiftly with little mechanical trauma to the vessels. The same technique is used for the arterial anastomosis, except that if the donor artery is small, then interrupted horizontal mattress sutures provide more precise intimal approximation, less constriction of the new lumen, and greater potential for subsequent expansion with growth.

After completion of the vascular anastomosis, it is important that there be no deficit in the recipient's circulating blood volume, and that the vascular clamps be removed slowly. Otherwise, the loss of blood from circulation into the kidney can prove significant, particularly if a large kidney is placed into a small patient. The general rule is that an adult-sized kidney will hold approximately 300 cc of blood. If an adult kidney is placed into a small infant, this sudden loss of blood from the effective circulating volume of the recipient can result in hypovolemia, hypotension, and vascular thrombosis of the graft. Forethought and careful coordination with the anesthesiologist can permit avoidance of this dangerous sequence.

Methods available for establishing urinary tract continuity include ureteroneocystostomy, urethro-ureterostomy, and pyeloureterostomy. Following re-establishment of continuity of the urinary tract, the laparotomy incision is closed without drainage with nonabsorbable suture material, which is essential because of delayed healing caused by uremia, malnutrition, and immunosuppressive therapy.

## Specific Technical Variations— Size Considerations

When a small recipient (less than 20 kg) receives an adult-sized kidney, the kidney is generally placed on the right side of the retroperitoneum, with the colon being reflected medially. In this way, the kidney lies in an extraperitoneal position, but the vascular anastomoses are attached to the aorta and vena cava above their bifurcation.

When a small recipient receives a small kidney, essentially the same technique can be utilized as described in the section above, with the kidney being placed in the iliac fossa. The vascular anastomotic technique may require modification with additional spatulation of the vessels or preservation of a small cuff of aorta and vena cava in order to make the anastomosis sufficiently large to prevent the risk of thrombosis (Fig. 32–1). There is little question in our minds that a cuff of donor aorta and vena cava greatly facilitates the vascular union in this setting. Other modifications in anastomotic technique as noted above may also be employed. Interrupted sutures properly spaced ensure a secure, leak-proof anastomosis while simultaneously providing potential for nonconstricting growth of the lumen.

When a large recipient receives a small kidney, other modifications must be observed. In one of our 16-year-old recipients, the donor was a newborn. The size differential is difficult to comprehend prior to operation. The length of the ureter was barely sufficient to construct the submucosal tunnel into the bladder, and it was necessary to perform a psoas hitch, suturing the bladder to the surrounding tissues and thus keeping it adherent to the kidney itself. Otherwise, undue tension would result with emptying of the bladder and might lead to disruption of the ureteroneocystostomy or alternately place undue tension on the vascular anastomosis. A reasonable alternative is to attach the kidney to a pedicle consisting of internal iliac vessels, suturing the tiny kidney to the wall of the bladder itself so that it will rise and fall with filling and emptying of the bladder. It is in this setting that creative urinary tract reconstruction is most challenging. Native ureters may be utilized when length is needed. End-to-end ureteroureterostomy with spatulation and rotation of the pyeloureterostomy may be needed to solve these problems. Careful identification and dissection of recipient ureters early in the course of the operation is important for this group of patients.

## Technical Variations—Sequential Transplants

Technical modifications are also important aspects of second and third transplants in the same recipient. Thirty-six of our procedures have been performed in this category—29 second and 7 third grafts. It is our practice to use the opposite iliac fossa for second procedures. In most instances this has been the left side, where the iliac vein must be more extensively mobilized than on the right side, since its "retro-arterial" position forces it to a somewhat deeper pelvic position. Great care must be exercised in this dissection. The numerous deep pelvic tributaries, if disrupted, tend to retract irretrievably into the depths of the pelvis. Therefore, full upward mobility of the left iliac vein requires division of these vessels after double ligation in continuity.

Second grafts in the aortocaval position in small recipients are sometimes necessary, but the procedure is difficult because of scarring from the previous operation. If the first transplant has functioned long enough to permit recipient growth, it may be possible to utilize the iliac vessels in an area not previously mobilized. If a second graft to the aorta and vena cava is necessary, the dissection is more tedious, with the great vessels engulfed in fibrosis. Careful proximal and distal control of both vessels is essential prior to removal of the failed graft and/or performing the second graft anastomoses.

Third transplants are often additionally taxing, forcing further modification in placement and technique. As an illustration, a third transplant was required for a 32-month-old male, who was first transplanted at age 11 months for ESRD secondary to a solitary dysplastic kidney. He had received a cadaver graft from an 18-month-old drowning victim. It had been placed in the right iliac fossa, end-to-end to the internal iliac artery. Rejection ensued, leading to transplant nephrectomy a few months later. His second graft was performed at 20 months of age, implanting a pair of cadaver kidneys from an 18-month-old donor transabdominally to the distal aortocaval position, dissecting both proximal iliac vessels for control. Peritonitis with spontaneous ileal perforation complicated this second graft, necessitating laparotomy and transplant nephrectomy. His third graft (adult cadaver donor) was planned for a distal aortocaval position, but intense scarring made safe mobilization of recipient vessels impossible. In an effort to achieve an iliac fossa location, it was observed that the previously utilized right common iliac artery was now hypoplastic and constricted, eliminating its potential use. Finally,

after extensive mobilization of both iliac systems and the distal great vessels, the graft was placed high in the pelvis on the right side, partially straddling the vascular bifurcation. The graft arterial anastomosis was to the left common iliac artery, and the venous connection was to the right iliac vein. Two years later, the graft continues to function well, with normal renal function (Cr = 1.0 mg/dl). This sequence demonstrates the flexibility that subsequent transplants occasionally force the transplant surgeon to utilize and emphasizes that the outcome can be gratifying if such modifications are adapted to a given situation.

## Anencephalic Donors

Management of kidneys from the anencephalic donor presents a unique problem. The anencephalic infant may be pronounced dead at birth by the obstetrician or it may be pronounced at the time of the harvesting procedure. The infant is usually maintained on mechanical ventilation during transport and until such time as the kidneys can be harvested. If one is to use these donors, it is mandatory that the facilities of a Level III Neonatal Intensive Care Unit be available to allow full and careful physiologic resuscitation and care of the infant donor. Under ideal circumstances, however, the kidneys can be utilized and transplanted the same as other kidneys and can prove a valuable source of donor material.[8]

Six such donors have been used in our series. The first graft was performed in 1968,[9] as the initial transplant to a 4½-year-old male with Eagle-Barrett (abdominal muscular deficiency) syndrome and severe renal dysplasia (Fig. 32–2). The patient is now 19 years of age. His serum creatinine level is 1.3 mg/dl. Three of the six anencephalic donor grafts were lost within two months post-transplant from rejection. One functioned well for three years, but was ultimately lost to chronic rejection. Two continue to function long-term. In addition to the patient above, another child received an anencephalic donor organ nine years ago as a third transplant and currently has a serum creatinine level of 1.4 mg/dl. It should be pointed out that in none of these patients has the vascular anastomosis, although small in size and technically demanding, been a limiting factor in graft survival.

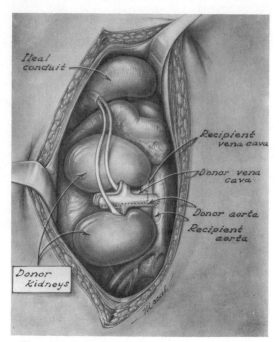

**Figure 32–2.** Placement of a pair of neonatal kidneys in a 17-pound recipient with ileal conduit. (From Martin LW et al: Homotransplantation of both kidneys from an anencephalic monster to a 17-pound boy with Eagle-Barrett syndrome. Surgery 66:603, 1969.)

## POST-TRANSPLANT CARE

Management of the kidney transplant patient in the early post-transplant period may present significant problems in regard to fluid replacement. It is imperative that the patient be monitored carefully with measurements of central venous pressure, blood pressure, and urinary output, particularly if the kidney is functioning adequately, and especially if the patient was significantly uremic prior to transplantation. The urine output is measured at least every hour and the volume replaced with intravenous fluids consisting of one-half normal saline with 5% dextrose in water and 10 mEq of sodium bicarbonate per liter. Half-hourly readjustments may be necessary if a diuretic phase is present. Potassium replacement will be required on an individual basis. Initial urinary output during the first few hours may be enormous, even in the patient who is well dialyzed prior to operation. This may be especially true in the living related transplant where intraoperative treatment of the donor with mannitol and furosemide can potentiate a continuing post-transplant diuresis. If not replaced, the high output results in hypovolemia with the potential for renal vascular thrombosis. Foley cath-

eter drainage of the bladder is utilized to protect the urinary reconstruction during the postoperative period and antibiotic coverage is maintained as long as the Foley catheter is in the bladder. We make every effort to remove the urinary catheter as soon as possible. We generally wait until the urine is clear and the volumes are sufficiently small to permit relatively normal spontaneous voiding, and the risk of leakage from the cystotomy has passed. This usually requires four to seven days.

Ambulation is generally advisable on the first postoperative day, and relatively standard postoperative pulmonary prophylaxis is instituted. Other items of general careful postoperative care must be attended. Hematocrit determinations are obtained at frequent intervals during the periods of excessive diuresis, and occasionally transfusion with packed red blood cells may be necessary in order to maintain adequate oxygen-carrying capacity, since many of the recipients are moderately anemic on a chronic basis. Moderate postoperative hypertension frequently occurs in the early post-transplant period, and antihypertensive medication is advisable.

We routinely obtain an isotope renal scan and/or excretory urogram in the early postoperative period in order to establish a baseline picture of the transplanted kidney and ureter. More recently, we have excluded excretory urography except in specific circumstances, relying on a combination of the renal scan and ultrasound to provide this early post-transplant information. BUN and serum creatinine determinations are carried out every 12 hours. Serum electrolyte determinations are performed daily until the period of diuresis has abated. Blood glucose levels during the period of diuresis are advisable in order to detect a possible rare case of steroid-related diabetes. An occasional patient with large volume urine output replaced cc for cc with 5% dextrose solutions may become hyperglycemic from the intravenous glucose load. This must be detected early or anticipated and dealt with by adjusting the composition of replacement fluids to decrease or eliminate its glucose content. Daily CBC and platelet counts are obtained in order to evaluate the state of bone marrow activity, and serum calcium and phosphorus levels are obtained at regular intervals until discharge from the hospital.

Immunosuppressive therapy regimens vary from one institution to another. Our policy throughout our entire experience has

**Table 32–2.** POST RENAL TRANSPLANT IMMUNOSUPPRESSION THERAPY*

Date of transplant surgery = _____ 0 day P.O.

*Imuran* (azathioprine)                 Patient Weight = _____ kg
    Pretransplant 3.0 mg/kg = dose _____ mg     Date _____
    Day 0–4 post op 3.0 mg/kg = dose _____ mg     Date _____ to _____
    Day 5–15 post op 2.0 mg/kg = dose _____ mg     Date _____ to _____
    Day 15+ post op 1.5–1.0 mg/kg = dose _____ mg     Date _____

*Prednisone* (methylprednisolone)
    Pretransplant 2.0 mg/kg (min 50; max 100 mg) = dose _____     Date _____
    Day 0–4th wk      Pt wt <30 kg = 7.5 mg Tid,     Date _____ to _____
                    Pt wt >30 kg = 10.0 mg Tid,
    5th–8th wk       Pt wt <30 kg = 12.5 mg Bid,     Date _____ to _____
                    Pt wt >30 kg = 15 mg Bid,
    9th–12th wk      Pt wt <30 kg = 15 mg Qam     Date _____ to _____
                    Pt wt >30 kg = 20 mg Qam
    13th wk +        Switch Qod 2 mg/kg (min 30; max 80 mg) Date _____
                    Q3 mo decrease 5 or 10 mg to final dose
                    15–20 mg Qod

Rejection Therapy
    Imuran—no change (if patient azotemic possible ↓ dose)
    Prednisone (methylprednisolone)— patient will receive 3 daily intravenous doses of
      Solumedrol 500 mg/dose. The patient will then return to above outlined schedule of
      oral prednisone with no alteration in total dose regimen.

*Children's Hospital Medical Center, Cincinnati, Ohio, 7/82 Revision

been to begin systemic azathioprine and prednisone therapy prior to operation and continue it through the post-transplant period. Table 32–2 lists the routine dosage scheme which we utilize. Antilymphocyte globulin as an immunosuppressive agent is utilized in many centers, but in our hands the results have been somewhat disappointing. Immunosuppressive therapy is discussed in more detail elsewhere (Chapter 35).

## COMPLICATIONS

A multitude of serious and life-threatening complications may be associated with renal transplantation.[10] The surgeon's efforts are directed at prevention of complications by meticulous attention to detail and careful observation of basic surgical principles. Nevertheless, in the best of hands and with the most conscientious efforts, the following complications may be observed:

1. rejection
2. nonfunction from causes other than rejection
3. acute tubular necrosis with delayed function
4. renal vein thrombosis
5. renal artery stenosis
6. lymphocele
7. urinary tract infection
8. sepsis
9. nonbacterial infections
10. steroid-related complications
    a. peptic ulceration
    b. pancreatitis
    c. diabetes
11. wound complications
12. hypertension
13. recurrence of disease
14. malignancy
15. intestinal ischemia

## Rejection

Immunologic rejection may be hyperacute, acute or chronic (see Chapter 34). The hyperacute rejection occurs immediately and is recognized at the operating table by the surgeon on the basis of the gross appearance of the graft, which fails to regain its normal turgor and healthy pink color following completion of the vascular anastomosis despite demonstrable patency of the anastomosis. The hyperacute rejection is mediated by humoral antibody with subsequent participation of the complement, coagulation, and kinin cascade systems. It occurs most frequently in patients who have demonstrable cytotoxic antibody directed against donor histocompatibility antigens. Unfortunately, the current state of the art is such that a certain number of patients will develop hyperacute rejection in the absence of demonstrable cytotoxic antibody.

Biopsy of the kidney and histologic examination by frozen section will generally confirm the diagnosis of hyperacute rejection, necessitating removal of the graft. If left in place, the acutely rejected organ will sometimes cause intravascular coagulation and consumptive coagulopathy, with a bleeding diathesis of life-threatening proportions. It is important that the surgeon recognize the complication of hyperacute rejection and perform an immediate nephrectomy. Of 156 kidney transplants, we have experienced a hyperacute rejection in one instance. The living related donor had been determined to be a perfect HLA antigen match for the recipient, her brother. The diagnosis of hyperacute rejection was confirmed by immediate biopsy and frozen section and the transplanted kidney was removed prior to closure of the laparotomy incision created for the transplant.

In a few instances we have observed kidneys which manifested a transient appearance akin to hyperacute rejection in the face of perfectly full vascular perfusion. Within 10 or 15 minutes of reinstituting flow to the graft, the transplant kidney, which is initially pink and normally firm will suddenly become dusky and lose its turgor. Direct hilar inspection demonstrates excellent pulsatile flow in the pedicle. Biopsy on two occasions has failed to demonstrate the changes of hyperacute rejection, and the kidney has gradually returned to a normal appearance. Whether such changes are reflections of transient immunologically mediated intrarenal vascular constriction or shunting is not clear. Such transient gross changes should not, however, lead to immediate nephrectomy since both of our patients currently have functioning grafts.

A less severe acute rejection may occur after a day or two of function. In these patients, the isotope renogram will show poor uptake of the isotope. Subsequent complete rejection results in complete intrarenal vascular thrombosis, which, on occasion, is difficult to differentiate from technical complications of vascular anastomoses. If the graft is removed early, the histologic changes will demonstrate immunopathological evidence of rejection. If nephrectomy is delayed, it is often impossible for the exact cause of the rejection to be determined by histologic examination. In our experience, acute rejection of this sort has developed on two occasions.

In one instance, a completely normal excretory urogram one week following transplantation was later followed by gradually diminishing renal function and subsequent graft necrosis, with diffuse small vessel thrombosis throughout the graft. Nephrectomy was performed following confirmation of complete rejection.

Chronic rejection may occur over a period of weeks, months, or years, with a gradually deteriorating renal function leading once again to chronic renal failure in spite of what would appear to be adequate immunosuppressive therapy. Compliance with medication, particularly in the teen-aged patient, is often a major problem. In our experience, one patient lost a functioning kidney because of surreptitious refusal to take the prescribed immunosuppressive medication. This is a particular problem when daily doses of steroids are required for the teenager who is particularly conscious about his or her appearance. These self-image concerns often assume a priority greater than the awareness of the need for the medication to preserve renal function.

Documentation of rejection, whether acute or chronic, has generally rested on clinical criteria rather than on direct histologic confirmation. We have not practiced percutaneous needle biopsy of transplanted kidneys in an effort to document rejection in the acute phase. In small children with infant grafts, the risk of these manipulations is too great to justify their use. If histologic documentation is necessary in order to plan appropriate changes in immunosuppressive therapy or to decide if transplant nephrectomy is warranted, an open surgical biopsy of the graft is recommended.

## Nonfunction of the Graft for Reasons Other Than Rejection

On three occasions, we have transplanted cadaveric kidneys which failed to ever function because of unknown reasons. The problem was felt not to be one of rejection. Since the kidneys had been harvested elsewhere, one can conjecture that adverse factors related to harvesting or the condition of the donor may not have been fully appreciated by the harvesting team. Unappreciated periods of warm ischemia, spasm of the vessels at the time of harvesting under adverse circumstances, unappreciated shock of the donor prior to organ retrieval, and unknown factors involved in organ preservation are considerations which are sometimes impossible to define when investigated retrospectively.

## Acute Tubular Necrosis

The term "acute tubular necrosis" (ATN) is a misnomer since histologic examination of the tubules of the kidney does not actually demonstrate necrosis but merely hydropic changes. The term has, however, been utilized to define a clinical state in which delayed renal function occurs, probably secondary to ischemic or other nonspecific changes related to organ retrieval, perfusion, or preservation. ATN, therefore, is observed almost exclusively following transplantation of kidneys from cadaver donors, although we occasionally have noted it following living related transplants. Return of function following a period of ATN may be a matter of days or even weeks. In one of our patients the graft failed to function for six weeks. At exploration for transplant nephrectomy, the kidney was viable, its blood supply fully patent, and the collecting system unobstructed. The transplant renal pelvis was filled with urine and began a steady output intraoperatively. The kidney continues to function now seven years later.

Other presentations of post-transplant ATN may be seen. Occasionally after an initial, reasonable volume of urine flow has been established, there may ensue a failure of the graft to clear blood urea nitrogen and serum creatinine. The radioisotope renogram may show a good vascular phase but poor excretion and may be interpreted as consistent with rejection. It is important that ATN not be confused with rejection in this setting. Since it appears that ATN is completely reversible and that, even after long periods of initial poor function, complete recovery will generally ensue, a period of ATN following transplantation must not prompt early nephrectomy. These episodes of ATN appear completely unrelated to subsequent long-term outcome with regard to success or failure of the graft.

## Renal Vein Thrombosis

Renal vein thrombosis within the first 48 hours following transplantation must be regarded as a technical complication. It is first recognized by persistence of gross hematuria, enlargement of the graft, and gradually diminishing renal function. Occasionally, kinking of the iliac-renal venous anastomosis or clot within the iliac vein itself will impair iliac vein drainage, leading to engorgement or edema of the lower extremity. The thrombosis may be initiated by adventitia inadvertently included in the anastomosis, an irregular intimal surface at the anastomosis, intimal damage during harvesting or transplantation, postoperative hypotension, or it is sometimes due to causes which cannot be determined. Some surgeons recommend routine heparinization of the recipient postoperatively, although this is not uniformly practiced. If recognized early, re-exploration with revision of the anastomosis could theoretically result in graft preservation. In our experience, however, this has not proved feasible. One such episode has been identified in our series and, at exploration, was found to be due to kinking and mechanical occlusion of the donor vein. It appeared that the donor vein had not been sufficiently shortened prior to anastomosis to prevent redundancy. This redundancy led to gross mechanical distortion of the pedicle. Shortening, reperfusion of the graft, and reanastomosis failed to salvage the kidney.[11]

An alternative form of therapy is systemic heparinization at the earliest suspicion of renal vein thrombosis. Unfortunately, our diagnostic methods are not sufficiently sophisticated to allow confirmation of the diagnosis at a stage early enough to be practical. Renal vein thrombosis generally results in loss of the graft and is treated by nephrectomy.

## Renal Artery Stenosis

Stenosis of the transplanted renal artery (Fig. 32–3) may occur secondary to the anastomosis being made too small, kinking of the renal artery, torsion of the artery, or intimal damage related to harvesting, preservation, or transplantation. When kidneys are maintained on pulsatile perfusion, it is customary for a constricting band to be placed about the artery at its junction with the perfusion cannula. We consider it important to excise and discard the segment of the artery which has been included in this constricting band. We also feel it important to spatulate the end of the artery in order to provide an anastomosis somewhat larger in diameter than the

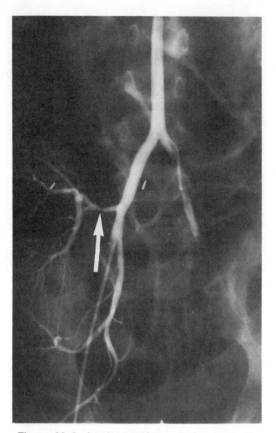

**Figure 32–3.** Arteriogram demonstrating renal artery stenosis. Six-year-old female recipient of a single pediatric cadaver kidney developed progressive severe hypertension four months after uncomplicated transplant. This focal high-grade segmental stenosis with poststenotic dilatation lies well beyond the widely patent iliorenal anastomosis. It is probable that injury to the intima of the artery may have unknowingly occurred during the process of harvesting, transporting, or transplanting the kidney.

diameter of the artery itself. The surgeon is careful to prevent kinking or torsion of the artery, and it is important to inspect the anastomosis following its completion in order to lyse any constricting bands of adventitial tissue which may subsequently contract, constricting the lumen. Clinically, renal artery stenosis may present as unexplained hypertension or inadequate renal function and may be demonstrated radiographically by poor concentration of the radioisotope in the renogram and confirmed by digital subtraction imaging angiography or arteriography.

Renal artery stenosis is a correctable condition best treated by re-exploration, resection, and reanastomosis of the vessels. This has been required in two patients in our series. Enthusiasm has recently been expressed for transluminal balloon dilatation of the stenotic vessel when stenosis is demon-

strated several months or years following transplantation.[12] We are reluctant to apply this maneuver to the post-transplant patient since the etiology appears to be considerably different from those in which transluminal angioplasty has had uniformly demonstrable success. Our experience with this treatment modality has been limited to one patient who presented with malignant hypertension some months after cadaveric transplantation and was shown by angiography to have developed a segmental stenosis at the takeoff of the posterior division of the main renal artery. This lesion was treated by balloon dilatation which was followed by marked improvement of the hypertension for more than a year after the dilatation was performed.

## Lymphocele

The development of fluid accumulations about the kidney following renal transplantation may be due to either urinary extravasation or the development of a lymphocele in the area of dissection. The diagnosis of urinary extravasation can generally be best confirmed by the radioisotope renogram which leads to concentration of isotope in the area of extravasation. The collection will be free of nuclide emission if the diagnosis is that of lymphocele.

Lymphoceles result from accumulation of lymph from the severed ends of small lymphatic vessels in the area of the dissection. The lymphatics travel in the area immediately surrounding the great vessels. To prevent the formation of a lymphocele, it is important at the time of operation to ligate all lymphatic vessels located in the perivascular tissue which surrounds the recipient vessels.[13]

Small lymphoceles will generally resorb spontaneously. If they persist or are of large volume, an endothelial layer will grow about the fluid accumulation. This restricted mass effect can eventually constrict the renal vessels or the ureter, resulting in late vascular compromise or hydronephrosis. If the lymphocele persists for longer than three weeks without demonstrable decrease in size, surgical evacuation and drainage is recommended. Some surgeons prefer to decompress the lymphocele by constructing a lymphocele-peritoneal window, believing that simple external drainage will not resolve the leak and will only lead to persistence of a lymphocutaneous fistula. If large distal lymphatic vessels communicate with the interstices of the lymphocele, such a consequence is possible.

## Sepsis

The post-transplant patient is particularly susceptible to infections of various types. The patient's resistance is reduced because of his chronic illness and perhaps exacerbated by the accompanying poor nutritional state.[14] Susceptibility to infection is increased because of uremia. Furthermore, the immunosuppressive agents directed at combating rejection result in suppression of the immunologic defenses against infection. In addition, the clinical evidence of sepsis may be masked by the steroid therapy. Prevention of these potentially lethal infectious complications is of paramount importance. The donor must be free of infection. The transplanted organ must not be bacterially contaminated during the process of harvesting, preservation, or transplantation. The recipient should be completely free of any infection elsewhere in the body. Careful complete physical examination is imperative to exclude any source of infection in the ears, throat, dialysis catheter, access sites, remote skin lesions, or the urinary tract. The presence of active clinical infection in any of these areas must be cleared prior to transplantation.

Meticulous surgical technique must be practiced during the course of the operation. Gentle handling of tissue and precise anatomic reconstruction are mandatory. Surgical judgment must be equally pristine. Additional "incidental" surgical maneuvers should be kept to an absolute minimum at the time of transplantation. Conventional appendectomy is generally not recommended because of the fear of contamination of the wound. We have occasionally performed inversion appendectomy when the area of the cecum is exposed during the course of the operative procedure. This permits inversion of the ligated appendix, which subsequently sloughs into the lumen of the cecum and is passed in the stool without opening the lumen of the appendix. This is sometimes helpful, particularly when the kidney lies in the right side of the abdomen behind the cecum. The diagnosis of appendicitis following transplantation can be confused with that of acute rejection. The consequences of this confusion with delay in appendectomy leading to subsequent perforation could be disastrous. Furthermore, wound infections in the area of the transplanted kidney are equally dangerous, particularly if anaerobic organisms are involved. Their ability to destroy normal tissues could result in erosion of a major vessel with sudden fatal hemorrhage.

Although some authors have suggested that the routine use of antibiotics following renal transplantation is not necessary,[15] we have continued to employ prophylactic perioperative antibiotics and prefer the combination of penicillin and an aminoglycoside.[16] Postoperative cultures of urine from the catheter for both aerobic and anaerobic organisms is important. Antibiotics are continued as long as a catheter remains in the bladder. We have seen no impairment of renal function attributable to the aminoglycosides. Every effort is made to monitor the blood levels (peak and trough) and to calculate the drug half-life for each patient on the basis of renal function.

## Urinary Tract Infection

Postoperative urinary tract infection in the transplant patient, in our experience, has been uncommon. It is important that hydronephrotic kidneys or refluxing ureters be completely removed flush with the mucosal lining of the bladder prior to or at the time of transplantation, that urinary drainage be provided in the immediate post-transplant period, and that the method of re-establishment of continuity of the urinary tract be one which completely avoids vesicoureteral reflux or urine stasis. Some form of chemotherapeutic prophylaxis is recommended for a period of several days following removal of the bladder catheter.

## Nonbacterial Infections

The transplant recipient is an immunocompromised host, particularly susceptible to various types of nonbacterial infections such as with *Pneumocystis carinii*, viremias, fungemias, and others. These may develop at any time in the post-transplant period, but particularly within the first six months. It is appropriate that these complications be recognized and immediate therapy instituted. When the post-transplant patient develops diffuse interstitial pneumonitis in the first few months, and when routine cultures fail to identify an etiologic agent in the face of clinical progression of the disease, open lung biopsy for histologic examination and appropriate culture are recommended. We have obtained lung biopsy material on five patients, and one death was attributed to fungemia.

## Peptic Ulcer

Duodenal ulcer as a complication following renal transplantation is probably more common in the adult than it is in the pediatric patient. Nevertheless, five of our patients developed demonstrable duodenal ulcers, which presented with pain, perforation, or hemorrhage. Some authorities recommend the routine use of prophylactic cimetidine or antacid therapy in the transplant patient. If there is a history of peptic ulcer or if the patient's illness has been particularly prolonged or complicated, we employ simple titration of gastric pH with antacids by mouth or per nasogastric tube but do not routinely institute ulcer therapy prophylactically. Minimal signs may follow perforation because of masking of the physical findings related to massive steroid therapy. The diagnosis must be considered in any instance of unexpected or unusual abdominal complaints in the post-transplant patient. Treatment is generally by nonsurgical means, except in the event of perforation or massive hemorrhage. One of our patients required operation for perforation and one for hemorrhage; both patients survived. In the event of life-threatening complications of this proportion, it is probably advisable to sacrifice the kidney, save the patient, and plan for another transplant at a later date.

## Pancreatitis

Steroid-related pancreatitis is a rare but possible complication, experienced in our series in only one instance in a preterminal patient with numerous additional complications and receiving massive steroid therapy. Pancreatitis is a grave complication in this setting and is probably best managed by discontinuation of immunosuppressive therapy and sacrifice of the graft in the hope of preserving the life of the patient.

## Delayed Wound Healing

Wound healing is delayed in the immunosuppressed patient who is chronically ill,

uremic, and receiving large doses of steroids. This is taken into consideration at the time of operative wound closure, which is accomplished with a meticulous anatomic reconstruction of the wound by layers with interrupted nonabsorbable sutures. Skin sutures are generally left in place for at least three weeks, or else the skin is supported with Steri-strips following their removal, if they are removed at an earlier time. We have not encountered any instance of wound dehiscence, although this has been reported by others as a significant complication.

## Hypertension

Some degree of hypertension has occurred in practically all postoperative patients in our experience, necessitating antihypertensive medication at least for a temporary period. The exact nature of this phenomenon is poorly understood. Many of our patients were hypertensive prior to operation, but the phenomenon observed following operation seems to be of a different etiology. It may be related to a combination of steroids and a failure to regulate the normal salt and water balance in the early post-transplant period. Some authorities have attributed this phenomenon to elaboration of renin from the immediately transplanted kidney. Others have attributed hypertension to rejection, but in our own experience there seems to have been no association between the level of blood pressure and the presence or absence of rejection. The degree of post-transplant hypertension is often mild and often controlled with a single drug.

Arterial stenosis is rare, but must be considered in any instance of hypertension, particularly if it is refractory to conventional therapy. Assessment of renal artery flow is important where significant, progressive, or refractory hypertension is noted. Although vascular pulsations are routinely observed in the grafts by ultrasound and flow assayed by the renal scan, angiography is mandatory for this group of patients. The detailed anatomy of the graft anastomosis and its branches must be clearly demonstrated. Digital imaging venous angiography has not been used in our series because of concern that the detail in the pediatric transplant patient does not appear to be adequate to define potential stenosis, particularly in branch vessels, as was seen in one of our patients. However, other centers have used this technique.

## Recurrence of the Disease

Recurrence of the original renal disease in a transplanted kidney has been given considerable attention by some authorities and is undoubtedly a definite risk in conditions such as glomerulonephritis and focal glomerulosclerosis. Differentiation from chronic rejection, however, has been difficult in our experience (Chapter 37).

## Malignancy

An increased incidence of malignant disease has been reported in patients following renal transplantation.[17] Inadvertent transplantation of a small tumor within the kidney has been reported,[18] and other distant malignancies have been reported with increased frequency. The mechanisms of stimulation of these de novo tumors is not defined. It appears to be more than simple depression of the inherent host immune surveillance, although this must certainly play some role.[19] Activation of latent tumorigenic viruses as well as chronic graft-versus-host disease have been proposed.

In our experience with 156 transplants, none of our patients has subsequently developed malignancy. The period of observation has extended as long as 18 years. At the University of Colorado the rate of development of malignancy in patients surviving renal transplantation was reported as 6%.[17] The rate of development of tumors has been estimated at 58 per 100,000 patients. The majority of these tumors, however, were skin lesions, and even when Penn et al corrected for skin tumors, the corrected incidence of malignancy was 3.8%.[17] Therefore, it seems clear that the incidence of malignancy is increased within the first two or three years following transplantation, but beyond this time such tumors are much less likely to develop.

## Intestinal Ischemia

Ischemic colitis after transplantation is not common, but has been reported to occur and carries a high mortality.[20] The mechanism of its occurrence is unclear, but some evidence suggests that uremia is able to potentiate other ischemic insults, at least in laboratory animals.[21] To our knowledge, ischemic colitis has not been reported in a pediatric transplant patient, supporting the view that atheromatous mesenteric vascular disease is the primary culprit.

One child in our series did develop spontaneous perforation of the distal ileum. It occurred 16 days after transplantation. A focal antimesenteric perforation some two feet from the ileocecal valve was present at exploration. No congenital abnormality of the bowel, such as Meckel's diverticulum or duplication, was present. No other areas of intestinal abnormality were noted, and no adjacent mucosal ulceration was seen. Whether this represents an area of very focal ischemia remains in question.

## SUMMARY

In summary, renal transplantation in children is a demanding and frustrating, yet a challenging and gratifying, experience. The initial graft survival for up to 19 years for 122 patients has been 50% for living donors and 52% for cadaver donors. The overall patient survival of 81% is gratifying when one considers that without transplantation or chronic dialysis there would have been no survivors. Assiduous follow-up care for the remainder of the patient's lifetime by a nephrologist and a surgeon experienced in transplantation is absolutely essential for every patient undergoing renal transplantation.

## REFERENCES

1. Fine RN, Korsch RM, Stiles Q, et al: Renal homotransplantation in children. J Pediatr 76:347, 1970.
2. Gonzales LL, Martin LW, West CD, et al: Renal homotransplantation in children. Arch Surg 101:232, 1970.
3. Murray JE, Merrill JP, Harrison JH: Renal homotransplantation in identical twins. Surg Forum 6:432, 1955.
4. Calne RY: The rejection of renal homografts: Inhibition in dogs by 6-mercaptopurine. Lancet 1:417, 1960.
5. Medawar PB: The behavior and fate of skin autografts and skin homografts in rabbits. J Anat 78:176, 1944.
6. Starzl TE, Marchioro TL, Zuhlke V, Brettschneider L: Transplantation of the kidney. Med Times 95:196, 1967.
7. Martin LW, McEnery PT, Rosenkrantz JG, et al: Renal homotransplantation in children. J Pediatr Surg 14:571, 1979.
8. Itaka K, Martin LW, Cox JA, et al: Transplantation of cadaver kidneys from anencephalic donors. J Pediatr 93:216, 1978.

9. Martin LW, Gonzales LL, West CD, et al: Homo-transplantation of both kidneys from an anence-phalic monster to a seventeen pound boy with Eagle-Barrett syndrome. Surgery 66:603, 1969.

10. Martin LW, Gonzales LL, West CD, et al: Clinical problems encountered in renal homotransplan-tation in children. J Pediatr Surg 5:207, 1970.

11. Duncan RE, Evans AE, Martin LW: Natural history and treatment of renal vein thrombosis in chil-dren. J Pediatr Surg 12:639, 1977.

12. Starzl TE, Marchioro TL, Zuhlke V, Brettschneider L: Transplantation of the kidney. Med Times 95:196, 1967.

13. Burleson RL, Marbarger PD: Prevention of lympho-cele formation following renal allotransplanta-tion. J Urol 127:18, 1982.

14. Schubert WK, Fowler R Jr, Martin LW, West CD: Studies of homograft survival in children with inborn errors of protein metabolism associated with increased susceptibility to infection. Am J Dis Child 100:474, 1960.

15. Novick AC: The value of intraoperative antibiotics

16. Tilney NL, Strom TB, Vineyard GC, Merrill JP: Factors contributing to the declining mortality rate in renal transplantation. N Engl J Med 299:1321, 1978.

17. Penn I, Halgrimson CG, Starzl TE: De novo malig-nant tumors in organ transplant recipients. Trans-plant Proc 3:773, 1971.

18. McIntosh DA, McPhaul JJ Jr, Peterson EW, et al: Homotransplantation of a cadaver neoplasm and a renal homograft. JAMA 192:1171, 1965.

19. Schwartz RW, Beldotti L: Malignant lymphomas following allogenic disease: Transition from an immunological to a neoplastic disorder. Science 149:1511, 1965.

20. Archibald SD, Jirsch DW, Bear RA: Gastrointestinal complications of renal transplantation. 2. The Colon. Can Med Assoc J 119:1301, 1978.

21. Gehrken GA, Flanigan RC, Madison JB, et al: Is-chemic colitis in uremic rats. Surg Forum 33:640, 1982.

in preventing renal transplant wound infections. J Urol 125:151, 1981.

# 33

# Urologic Aspects of Transplantation in Children

*Casimir F. Firlit, M.D., Ph.D.*

Renal transplantation has become the best form of therapy for children with end stage renal disease (ESRD). It offers the greatest opportunity for rehabilitation to a near normal life. The educational and psychosocial retardation and physical limitations of ESRD are dramatically altered. The technical aspects of renal transplantation have improved enormously during the past 20 years, owing, in large part, to technical refinements in organ procurement and preservation, donor and recipient evaluation, surgical technique and diagnostic modalities, and the skills associated with the proper selection and interpretation of these techniques. Herein, we present the urologic aspects in the art and practice of renal transplantation in children.

## PATIENT SELECTION AND ASSESSMENT

Notions regarding the appropriateness of transplantation during the early 60's prejudiced early and aggressive application of this form of treatment in childhood. Hemodialysis was in its infancy and limited in its availability and skillful application to children. Further, presumptions regarding the immunologic responsiveness in this group suggested that children would be hyperreactive, and consequently tolerance and acceptance of the homograft would be poor. Hemodialysis, peritoneal dialysis, and dietary and metabolic management skills have evolved concomitantly in quality and sophistication. This evolution has resulted in better patient selection and preparedness. In addi-

tion, psychosocial and educational deficits are better appreciated and managed. The totality of care rendered by medical and paraprofessional interest groups produces gratifying results.

Theoretically, renal transplantation as a form of therapy for ESRD can be applied to any age group.[1] The reality of this is limited only by dialytic skills and immunotherapeutic experience of the dialysis/transplant team in the management of the neonate, infant, and young child. Bold and pioneering attempts continue to be made in the younger child (1 to 2 years).[2] Neonatal and infant transplantation, although possible, has not been practiced frequently or very successfully (Chapter 3). Doubt exists in regard to the appropriateness of transplantation in this young age group. This is founded on the basis that metabolic and dietary management by skilled pediatric nephrologists will allow for near normal growth, with the achievement of normal developmental landmarks. Specific disorders such as bilateral cystic dysplasia can be managed well with skillful nephrologic and dietary support. This management will allow for sufficient growth with "quality" for 1 to 2 years or more before dialysis or transplantation is offered. Hemodialysis is technically difficult in the infant and prolonged hemodialysis is usually accompanied by retarded growth and development. Peritoneal dialysis (continuous ambulatory peritoneal dialysis) appears to offer an improved outlook in this young age group. Even though technical and infection problems do occur, sometimes at an alarming rate, the beneficial effects appear to be well worth the efforts.

**473**

Treatment with renal transplantation may be applied after appropriate patient and family preparedness has occurred. The majority of younger children present with congenital renal and urologic pathology, culminating in renal failure.

Prior to transplantation a complete urologic assessment is necessary to define clearly the entire urinary transport and storage systems, and to institute whatever treatments are necessary to prepare each child as an appropriate recipient. All available excretory urograms, cystourethrograms and cystoretrograde pyeloureterograms are evaluated. Every centimeter of the urinary storage and transport system must be delineated and reviewed by the transplant surgeon. Careful attention to the underlying renal disease and its cause is necessary to exclude and prevent obstructive phenomena. Extirpative and corrective urologic surgery must be performed prior to transplantation if one is to maximize patient and graft survival.

Nephrectomy is appropriate but only under specific circumstances. In children aged 0 to 5 years with congenital uropathy and 6 to 10 years with obstructive uropathy resulting in ESRD, nephrectomy is frequently performed.[3] Its rationale is based on the feeling that cryptic infectious foci in failed kidneys of children with obstructive or infectious uropathy represent a realistic threat post transplantation. Atropic hydronephrosis, chronic pyelonephritis, or kidneys which mediate hypertension are removed.

Renal ultrasonography is used frequently to evaluate renal and ureteral morphology and size. This is helpful in planning the surgical approach. Posterior vertical lumbotomy has become a preferable approach to small atropic kidneys where an extensive ureterectomy is not necessary. This approach offers minimal postoperative morbidity, improved patient comfort, and diminished hospital stay, and preserves body image.

Nephroureterectomy, because of massive vesicoureteral reflux, is best achieved by an anterior midline transperitoneal or preperitoneal approach. Under usual circumstances recipient ureteral preservation is preferred. Future homograft complications may occur wherein a defunctionalized recipient ureter is usable in a salvage procedure. Where cutaneous urinary diversion exists, a selective decision is made in regard to the extent of ureteral preservation and/or excision.

Bladder assessment is necessary to exclude obstructive posterior urethral valves and diverticula, and to determine capacity and function. Generally speaking, the vast majority of urinary bladders may be used as reservoirs following transplantation.[4, 5] Long-term supravesical urinary diversion was once believed to cause bladder involution and fibrosis. Consequently, use of these bladders in transplantation was shunned. Early and continued use of defunctionalized bladders has demonstrated that the majority regain normal vesicoelastic properties, function as good urinary reservoirs, and empty efficiently. There are, however, noteworthy exceptions to identify. A bladder which has been the object of repeated surgical assaults may be so fibrotic and contracted that recoverability is poor or impossible. A heavily trabeculated, thickened, diverticulated bladder may prove to be more of a liability than an asset. Further, neuropathic vesical disease may, under certain circumstances (hyperreflexia and dysreflexia), disqualify the use of a bladder in transplantation. These conditions may demand dynamic bladder testing prior to transplantation.

Bladder "cycling," using a suprapubic catheter, may be applied to dynamically assess bladder recoverability and function.[6] Bladder capacity, proprioceptive, sensory, and motor function, resting (filling) bladder pressure, uroflowmetry, and continence are provocatively tested. Cycling may be used for days to weeks to be assured of vesical function. Further, it serves as a training technique, restores confidence, and eliminates doubts in the minds of all concerned. Scarred, thickened urinary bladders result in a higher incidence of post-transplant urinary extravasation.[7-11] Defunctionalized, nonscarred bladders will regain vesicoelastic function. Children with a history of posterior urethral valves must be evaluated to be assured of the adequacy of valvular ablation. These children usually have dysplastic bladders, many times a thickened detrusor and/or fixed contracted, tight bladder neck and dilated prostatic urethra. Urinary continence in these children with "bad bladders" may be inadequate.

Some children with ileal conduit urinary diversions may present for transplantation. As indicated above, these children also require a thorough assessment of their urinary tract. A careful assessment of all medical records is necessary to determine the rationale employed at the time of urinary diversion. Diagnoses such as "neuropathic bladder," failed ureteroneocystostomies, and hydronephrosis may be documented. Each of these bladders, if retained, should be assessed to determine their use in renal transplantation.[12, 13]

Myelodysplasia with urinary diversion does not in itself disqualify the use of a "neuropathic bladder" for transplantation. Patients with low level myelomeningocele lesions with leg sparing typically have arreflexic large-capacity bladders with normal urethral sphincter function. These can serve as urinary reservoirs, provided intermittent clean catheterization is accepted as the mode of bladder emptying.[14]

Chronic cystitis occurs secondary to intermittent clean catheterization in over 50% (40–93%).[15] Although asymptomatic chronic cystitis is acceptable and tolerable in the non-immunosuppressed host, its benefit-versus-risk ratio in the transplant recipient has yet to be defined. This form of urinary drainage management was met with considerable prejudice when introduced to the urologic community in the early 1960's. However, gradual acceptance and now liberal application in the field of urology has boosted urologic awareness. This technique is now freely employed as the primary mode of management in children with dysfunctional voiding secondary to spina bifida[16] and other related congenital or acquired neuropathic disease. Preservation of renal function in this group has allowed for a more normal growth and development. The probability that more children with neuropathic vesical dysfunction will be considered for renal transplantation because of intermittent clean catheterization has increased.

Cystoscopy is useful in the assessment of defunctionalized urinary bladders or in situations in which urethral or vesical anatomy is unclear and where an obstructive lesion is suspected. Urethral stricture disease is usually acquired from previous instrumentation. Urethral surgery, such as employed for hypospadias, urethral diverticula, or Cowper's gland duct cyst, may result in stricture. Identification and surgical treatment of the lesions is mandatory before transplantation. If unrecognized, high-grade bladder outlet resistance occurs, which may provoke urinary extravasation in the early postoperative period or late, silent hydroureteronephrosis.

A small number of defunctionalized urinary bladders may be rejected as appropriate urinary reservoirs because of inelasticity (a failure to regain compliance) due to fibrosis resulting from previous surgical procedures. Further, an occasional patient may be devoid

of a bladder because of a previous cystectomy. Alternate and creative forms of urinary storage and conveyance are possible. These include preservation of a previous cutaneous ureterostomy with its proximal ureteral segment, retention and relocation of an ileal or colonic conduit, or creation of a retroperitoneal ileal conduit. The possibility of augmentation cystoplasty to increase storage capacity in a fibrotic, inelastic bladder is highly attractive in situations in which patient acceptance of intermittent clean catheterization would be applied for "bladder" emptying. Experience with cutaneous ureteral diversion, either primary or through the reuse of defunctionalized segments, and ileal conduits has proved highly successful and acceptable in select individuals.[17–18] Interestingly, stoma stenosis, epithelialization, fissuring, and bleeding do not occur in the renal transplant recipient.

The protective (inhibition) role of prednisone is most intriguing. Retrograde urinary infections also occur but at a lesser incidence in this select population. Improved personal hygiene or the decreased incidence of obstructive gradients may be contributory factors. Proper-fitting, newly improved urinary collection devices and appropriate emptying schedules further lessen the incidence of ascending infection and pyelonephritis. When a "new" ileal conduit is selected for a patient's urinary conveyance, the "new conduit" must be created and properly positioned weeks before the contemplated renal transplant. If combined with renal transplantation, poor healing in the postoperative period may result in dehiscence, urinary extravasation, infection, and death. Proper planning, with an appreciation of the poor healing characteristics of the chronically debilitated patient, is paramount.

## THE DONOR URETER

Studies of ureteral vascular anatomy clearly identify three sources of vascular supply to the intact, orthotopic ureter. These include descending vessels from the renal artery/renal hilum, segmental ureteral branches from lumbar and penetrating psoas vessels, and finally retrograde arteries originating from the superior vesical, hypogastric, and presacral pelvic arteries. Donor nephrectomy demands a full knowledge and, above all, an appreciation of this vascular anatomy, if one is to preserve ureteral vascularity and ultimately ureteral viability. Many postoperative urinary complications can be attributed directly to a loss of ureteral vascularity. Many reports have clearly identified this as a major cause of ureteral complications and have offered suggestions for improvement.[19, 20] Anatomically, the entire ureter cannot sustain viability even if the best of surgical techniques are employed. However, 50 to 60% of ureteral length with viability is possible if one preserves most of the renal hilar fat and periureteral fibroadipose ureteral sheath. Careful manipulation and tissue handling techniques are critical in preserving distal ureteral viability.

Upper and lower polar vessels are extremely important to preserve because of their influence on ureteral and calyceal viability.[21] Upper polar infarcts secondary to disruption of polar arteries may result in focal parenchymal necrosis, which may impair the viability of a renal calyx. A blow-out (calyceal) leak is the product of this vascular insult. It usually takes days to suspect and considerable effort to diagnose. Lower polar arteries are highly involved in the antegrade pelviureteric vascular plexus which nourishes the renal pelvis, but more importantly the ureter. In some kidneys the ureteral blood supply is predominantly dependent on this anatomy. Aggressive dissection (cleaning) of this peripelvic tissue can prove disastrous. As a consequence, a quality donor kidney is dependent on a skillful, knowledgeable surgeon who possesses a true appreciation of, and a respect for, this delicate vascular anatomy. Further, during the donor nephrectomy and ureterectomy procedure, a careful observation of the transected ureter for antegrade ureteral bleeding will aid in the dissection and document ureteral vascular preservation.

Once core and surface cooling occurs, only minimal perinephric capsular fat excision should be allowed, with complete avoidance of the perihilar renal pelvic ureteral areas. If pulsatile preservation is used, a respectful caring for the ureter should exist at all times. Ureteral desiccation must be prevented by close vigilance and proper manipulation.

## SURGICAL TECHNIQUE

The technical aspects of renal transplantation require a detailed appreciation of pelvic anatomy and surgical physiology.

Throughout the operative period a considerable amount of attention is focused upon vascular anastomosis, preservation of pelvic lymphatics, and, where appropriate, proper ligation of bridging lymphatics. Through this first phase of the operative period the ureter seems to "come along for the ride." Frequently, little attention is paid to it. As a consequence, trauma from finger compression or tissue squeeze occurs. Further, and on a continual basis, desiccation occurs unless measures are employed to prevent it.

After the vascular anastomosis is complete and vascularization occurs, the ureter is carefully inspected. Color, motility, bleeding from the distal end, and urinary efflux should be observed. Surveillance of the ureter for viability and integrity of the ureteral sleeve are critical observations. A pale, denuded distal ureteral segment, which is not bleeding from its end, must be amputated proximally at a level where viability is assured. The amount of functional and viable ureteral length is dependent on these observations and practices. Enough viable ureter must be salvaged to "bridge the gap" to the bladder. The amount of usable ureteral length is a judgment made at surgery. There should be enough length to reach the bladder comfortably without tension at the vascular or ureterovesical anastomosis. Redundant ureteral length may contribute to obstruction and hydroureteronephrosis.

## Ureteral Implantation Technique

**Ureteroneocystostomy.** The principles of correct ureterovesical implantation demand maintenance of ureteral intravesical length-to-diameter ratio to ensure a proper and functional ureterovesical juncture. The intravesical (submucosal) length must be four to five times the ureteral diameter to prevent reflux. Further, a longer length may serve only to obstruct the ureter. The terminal end of the ureter must be fixed on a relatively rigid portion of the posterior inferior bladder wall, in such a way that would allow for low pressure filling without "J-hook" obstruction of the distal ureteral segment.[22] The distal ureter should be manipulated with care and sutured with fine (5–0 chromic) suture to the trigone. A precise, mucosa-to-mucosa anastomosis of the ureter to bladder is necessary to prevent a fistula or urinary leak. Further, if a hiatal mucosal incision is employed, this

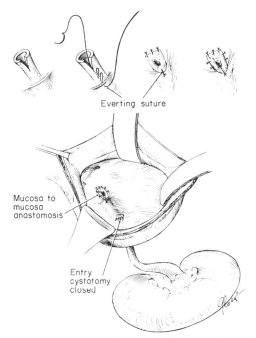

**Figure 33–1.** The precise mucosal to mucosal anastomosis critical to proper healing and prevention of urinary extravasation. Note the careful placement of the 5–0 chromic sutures on the spatulated ureter and at the entry cystotomy. Proper placement of the terminal ureter on the trigone and a long submucosal tunnel will prevent vesicoureteral reflux. (From Martin DC, Mimms MM, Kaufman JJ, Goodwin WE: The ureter in renal transplantation. J Urol 101:680, 1969.)

must also be closed with precision.[23] Ureteral stents are rarely employed in transplantation.[20] Postoperative edema occurs but fails to produce significant obstruction to urine efflux (Fig. 33–1).

Closure of the cystotomy also requires proper tissue layer approximation and a "watertight" meticulous closure.[23, 24] The typical cystotomy closure is closed in three layers, with absorbable sutures (Fig. 33–2). A urethral catheter is necessary to allow free urinary drainage while affording total bladder decompression. Bladders that exhibit thickened detrusor or small capacities (< 60 ml) or that have undergone previous surgery are predictably more at risk because of poor healing with resultant urinary leakage.

**Pyeloureterostomy.** An alternate form of urinary tract reconstruction in the transplant recipient is the pyeloureterostomy.[25, 26] Although this technique is less popular than the ureteroneocystostomy, it has nevertheless gained a level of acceptance in the transplant surgical community. This technique boasts freedom from early and late ureteral obstruc-

tion, ureteral slough, prolonged bladder drainage, and leakage from the ureteroneocystostomy site or the anterior cystotomy. Because the surgery is performed at a higher level than the bladder, these complications can be avoided. As in all techniques, adherence to meticulous surgical technique may explain the relative freedom from complications. This technique stresses the need to leave the recipient ureter long enough to avoid tension on the anastomosis. Excessive ureteral length may lead to kinking and obstruction.

Before the anastomosis the donor ureter is amputated at a level for comfortable anastomosis. This is typically at the homograft pelvis but on occasion may be more distal. Hence, a ureteroureterostomy is an alternate procedure. The homograft pelvis is spatulated as well as the recipient proximal ureter.[27] This spatulation establishes a basis upon which an anastomosis of considerable caliber can be created. Usually two running 5–0 chromic sutures are used, although some reports have favored 6–0 chromic and/or

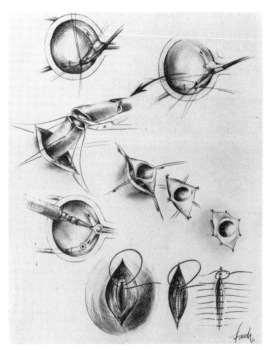

**Figure 33–2.** Spatulation and fixation of ureter, with bladder closure. The layered closure of the cystotomy is clearly defined. Three-layer closure with precise mucosa-to-mucosa approximation is critical. Each "layer" is closed in an overlapping manner. These steps help prevent urinary extravasation. (From Weil R III, Simmons RL, Tallent MB, Lillehei RC, Kjellstrand CM, Najarian JS et al: Prevention of urological complications after kidney transplantation. Ann Surg 174:154, 1971.)

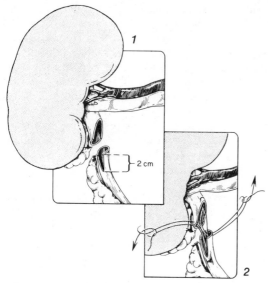

**Figure 33–3.** The precise steps involved in pyeloureterostomy. (1) Spatulation of the donor pelvis and recipient ureter. (2) Placement of the mattress sutures at the apices of the anastomosis. Proper pelvic and ureteral spatulation with preservation of peripelvic and ureteral adventitia permits proper healing without stenosis. (From Whelchel JD, Cosimi AB, Young HH, Russell PS: Pyeloureterostomy reconstruction in human renal transplantation. Ann Surg 181:61, 1975.)

interrupted sutures. Rarely, nonabsorbable, fine 7–0 Tevdek suture has been used because of presumed increased tension strength. However, in general, nonabsorbable sutures are not encouraged for urinary tract reconstruction because of late intraluminal migration, infection, and calculus formation.

Following the anastomosis, reapproximation of the peripelvic and periureteric fibrovascular sheet with interrupted 5–0 or 6–0 chromic suture adds further insurance. When this procedure is performed with a religious respect for tissue manipulation, excellent healing will result frequently (Figs. 33–3 and 33–4).

The use of nephrostomy tube drainage or an indwelling ureteral stent is not recommended. These favor retrograde inoculation of bacteria and infection, which place the anastomosis in jeopardy. A pyelotomy incision, common in the urologic community as a vent, favors urinary extravasation and infection. This is to be condemned. Penrose drainage of a pyeloureterostomy should be avoided and may on occasion favor urine leakage by "wick" action.

**Extravesical Ureteroplasty (Lich-Gregoir).** The extravesical ureteroplasty has been gaining more and more interest and enthusiasm in the transplant community.[28–30] This technique, although described many years ago, has never gained much popularity in this country. In contrast, this technique is very popular in European countries. It offers the advantages of ease in performance, precise mucosa-to-mucosa "watertight" anastomosis, and appropriate submucosal intravesical ureteral length with a good detrusor buttress (Fig. 33–5).[31] Further, all this can be achieved with a single bladder incision. Bladder drainage postoperatively may be limited to 12–24 hours. Urinary urgency, dysuria, and hematuria with or without clot retention

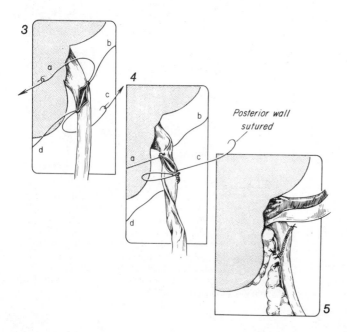

**Figure 33–4.** Individual steps in the anchoring of the spatulated ureter to the renal pelvis. (3) Direction of rotation of the pelvis and ureter to expose the back wall of the anastomosis. (4) Initial suture placement in the back wall of the anastomosis. Note torsion of the ureter to allow for a running closure of the posterior wall. (5) The completed, watertight anastomosis without proximal venting. (From Whelchel JD, Cosimi AB, Young HH, Russell PS: Pyeloureterostomy reconstruction in human renal transplantation. Ann Surg 181:61, 1975.)

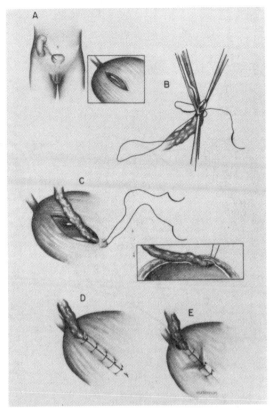

**Figure 33–5.** Extravesical ureteroneocystostomy depicted in detail. This technique requires a detrusor myotomy (A) down to the mucosa. A mucosal fenestration is made and the distal end of the ureter is anastomosed mucosa to mucosa with fine suture (B and C). The detrusor is then reconstructed over the submucosally placed ureter (D and E). (From Wasnick RJ, Butt KMH, Laungani G, Shirani K, Hong JH, Adamsons RJ, and Waterhouse K: Evaluation of anterior extravesical ureteroneocystostomy in kidney transplantation. J Urol 126:306, 1981.)

can be eliminated. Complications appear extremely minimal. Ureteral stenting is not necessary.

**Use of Intestinal Conduits.** The use of intestinal conduits to facilitate the transport of urine to the skin in pediatric renal transplantation is an extremely valuable tool in the surgeon's armamentarium.[5, 18, 23, 32] Clinically, it is used infrequently. The child who has had a cystectomy and the child with myelodysplasia, where vesical augmentation and/or intermittent catheterization are not useful alternatives, serve as examples. Past notions in the urologic community enforced the concept that once a urinary bladder was defunctionalized it would fibrose, shrink, and be permanently unusable. This notion proved fallacious within the early years of renal transplantation, and the transplantation of ureters into defunctionalized bladders

proved to be a viable answer to urine storage and evacuation.[5, 11, 13] As a consequence, fewer and fewer defunctionalized bladders were found to be unusable. Careful bladder assessment, as described earlier, is the key in identifying when to use an intestinal conduit.

The technique of renal transplantation into intestinal conduits ideally requires the placement or restoration of the intestinal conduit into the retroperitoneal space, with the proximal end secured to the sacrum, weeks prior to the renal transplant procedure. This relocation is usually a transperitoneal procedure,[11] carefully avoiding the inferolateral substomal position. Later, the transplant operative procedure is undertaken in the customary fashion, with the conduit distended via a Foley catheter for ease in dissection. When the iliac fossa is prepared, the conduit is easily identified, attached to the peritoneum, and reflected superomedially. The kidney is anastomosed, with the pelvis dissected superiorly, to the hypogastric artery and common iliac vein. The ureter is amputated at the renal pelvis. A fenestration of 2 to 3 centimeters is created in the proximal inferior end of the intestinal conduit. The renal pelvis is spatulated to accommodate the intestinal fenestration. A closure of two running, 5–0 chromic sutures is accomplished. Further, interval interrupted 5–0 chromic sutures bolster the anastomosis. When completed, the kidney assumes a transverse lie in the bony pelvis, with the renal pelvis dissected superiorly and anastomosed to the intestinal conduit (Fig. 33–6). The intestinal stoma is left catheterized for 24 hours. Occasionally, the ureter may be utilized for an intestinal anastomosis. This technique has a much higher incidence of complications when compared with the pyelointestinal anastomosis.[17, 18]

## POST-TRANSPLANT UROLOGIC COMPLICATIONS

A present-day review of the surgical and urologic literature has demonstrated a decrease in the number of reports describing urinary leakage in transplant recipients. Further, these reports have substantiated the fact, which is consistent with our experience, that urinary complications have been decreasing. Hopefully, this indicates that we have learned and are applying preventive techniques. In addition, reported complications are recognized early and prompt treat-

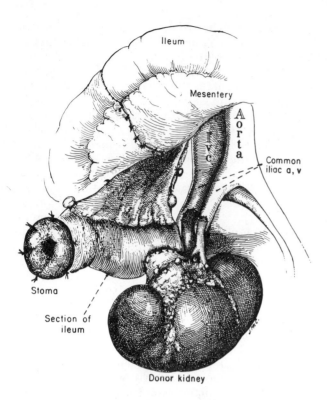

**Figure 33–6.** Intestinal conduit as a form of urinary conveyance in renal transplantation. Note the inverted posture of the renal allograft with the pelvis situated superiorly. The ureter is amputated at the pelvis, leaving a large fenestration for anastomosis to the antimesenteric proximal end of the retroperitonealized ileal segment. No catheter or stent drainage is employed. (From Firlit CF, Merkel FK: The application of ileal conduits in pediatric renal transplantations. J Urol 118:647, 1977.)

ment initiated. This has resulted in greater patient survival, reduction in morbidity, and a greater salvage of renal homografts.

Urologic complications may be divided into major and minor groups. The major complications include urinary leaks from ureteral obstruction, necrosis, fistula, and bladder extravasation,[2, 7, 10, 31, 33–40] disruption, and ureteropelvic junction obstruction. The minor complications include ureteral reflux.

The major complications pose a serious threat to patient and graft survival. The recognition of a urinary complication demands critical suspicion with prompt and appropriately directed diagnostic studies followed by the immediate implementation of specific treatment.

Urinary extravasation has been reported to range from 0.5% to 35%. The higher incidences were reported during the infancy of renal transplantation; the lower incidence is occurring now, during the adolescence of renal transplantation.[39] Urinary extravasation occurs as a consequence of surgical reconstruction of the urinary transport system and the inherent problems of vascular integrity and tissue healing. Available techniques include ureteroneocystostomy, ureteropyelostomy (ureteroureterostomy), extravesical ureteroplasty, and anterior cystotomy. Each will be discussed separately.

Ureteroneocystostomy involves the deliberate implantation of the homograft ureter into the bladder in a modified Politano-Leadbetter technique.[22] This requires an anterior cystotomy to expose the interior of the bladder, to identify the position for homograft ureteral fixation (meatus) and the point of ureteral entry into the bladder (hiatus).[19] The hiatal-meatal distance is known as the submucosal segment or length. This length is critical when taken in relation to the ureteral diameter to achieve a competent antireflux segment. The submucosal dissection (tunnel) is usually more liberal in its lateral and medial dissection to prevent encroachment on the ureter.[20] A precise mucosa-to-mucosa anastomosis with fine suturing technique is necessary to prevent extravasation. A tight hiatus and a narrow submucosal tunnel will compromise distal ureteric blood flow. Ischemia, stenosis, or necrosis may occur. Ischemic stenosis results in obstructive hydronephrosis, while necrosis results in perivesical and retroperitoneal urinary extravasation.

The critical aspect of the ureteroneocystostomy is the distal ureteral blood supply. The ureter must exhibit peristalsis, appear pink, and demonstrate capillary bleeding from the transected end at the time of homograft revascularization. A successful ureteroneocystostomy demands vascular integrity, a strict adherence to the technical principles described, and reasonably good healing qualities of the host. A properly performed donor nephrectomy with preservation of ureteric blood supply is critical.[20] Salvatierra et al described an incidence of primary urinary leakage to be 0.5% in 540 renal homografts.[19]

Urinary extravasation at the neocystotomy site may be suspected when oliguria or anuria occurs in association with abdominal distension, particularly when there are no signs of clinical rejection. A cystogram may confirm leakage if the ureterovesical anastomosis was disrupted. However, the isotopic renogram with delayed images with catheter drainage will demonstrate the extravasation.[41] Real-time abdominal ultrasonography has added a new dimension in the evaluation of renal transplant recipients for extravesical fluid accumulations. These can be identified easily, painlessly, and without invasive morbidity.

These diagnostic techniques can only demonstrate an extravasation or fluid collection.[42] Surgical exploration is urgently necessary to identify the specific cause of the extravasa-tion. Treatment will depend on ureteral viability. If a disruption or a distal necrosis has occurred, debridement of the distal ureteral segment and a repeat ureteroneocystostomy will suffice in most instances. It is on these occasions that a ureteral stent is of value. However, if the ureter has sloughed[33] in its entirety or if the ureteral length is insufficient to bridge to the bladder comfortably, a pye-loureterostomy or ureteroureterostomy employing the recipient's ipsilateral or contra-lateral ureter will suffice.[20]

Under rare circumstances, a recipient ureter or ureters may not be present—as a consequence of a previous nephroureterec-tomy. Here, a large, posteriorly based bladder flap[43] may be developed to "bridge the distance to the renal pelvis." This technique re-establishes the continuity and integrity of the urinary tract; vesicoureteral reflux will result (Fig. 33–7). A bladder flap vesicoure-teroplasty requires prolonged drainage of the bladder to allow for proper healing. Urinary leakage secondary to poor or retarded healing is common.

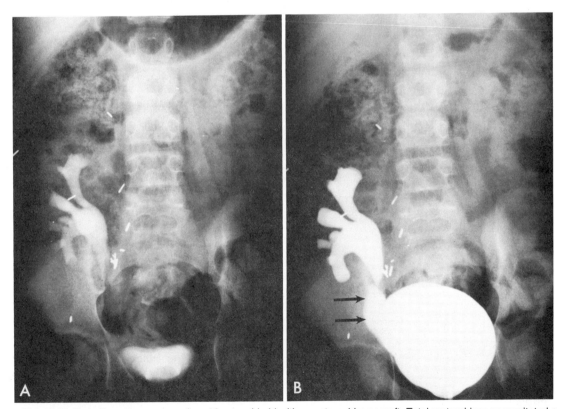

**Figure 33–7.** *A*, Excretory urogram in a 12-year-old girl with a maternal homograft. Total ureteral loss necessitated a "vesical flap" (Boari) ureteroplasty as a form of urinary conveyance. Ureteral (tubularized bladder flap) stents were used for four weeks. Postoperative cystogram *(B)* four weeks post surgery demonstrates vesicoureteral reflux without extravasation. Reflux was managed by long-term prophylactic antibacterial therapy. (From Firlit CF: Unique urinary diversions in transplantation. J Urol 118:1043, 1977.)

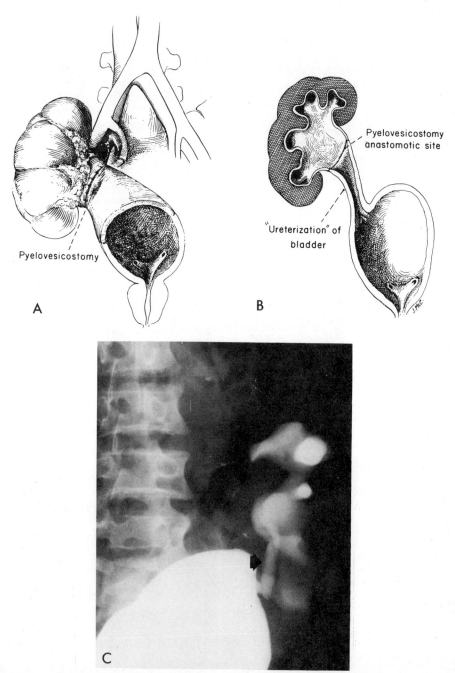

**Figure 33–8.** Pyelovesicostomy. An alternate "bail-out" procedure in situations of total ureteral loss where recipient ureters are absent and the bladder is large enough to bridge the distance to the renal pelvis. *A,* Large single-layer anastomosis of bladder and renal pelvis. *B,* Long-term surveillance demonstrates "ureterization" of the bladder. *C,* Contrast cystography demonstrates reflux up the ureterized bladder two years following pyelovesicostomy. Voiding pressures do not appear to adversely affect renal function or promote urinary infection. (From Firlit CF: Unique urinary diversions in transplantation. J Urol 118:1043, 1977.)

An additional alternative to re-establish continuity of the urinary tract is the pyelovesicostomy. This technique is extremely valuable as a "bail-out" when no ureteral material is available in the recipient. It incorporates the establishment of a large spatulated renal pelvis and a large cystotomy site into a fistula. This large fistula is created with running and interrupted 4–0 chromic suture. The integrity of the anastomosis is good. This technique can be used only if the bladder and renal pelvis are large enough to reach each other without tension (Fig. 33–8).[30] Vesicoureteral reflux will exist in this anatomic relationship. Urinary reflux, particularly if the patient remains uninfected, is believed to be of negligible consequence.

## Calyceal Urinary Fistula

Calyceal fistulae are recognized as a subtle cause for urinary extravasation. Clinically, the child may exhibit pain over the homograft, increasing abdominal girth, declining renal function, and oliguria. The diagnosis may be suspected on excretory urography, but is further defined with $^{131}$I hippuran homograft scanning with delayed images. These studies will document a urinary fistula, but the diagnosis is confirmed only by a retrograde pyeloureterogram.[44] A cystogram is extremely useful to exclude a bladder fistula and to define bladder displacement.

The treatment of a calyceal fistula depends upon the magnitude of the extravasation and general health of the recipient. Present-day treatment includes the placement of a double-ended "J" stent to facilitate a drop in intrapelvic pressure. If this is ineffective or if the leak is extremely large, then a formal exploration and drainage is necessary. A nephrostomy tube and stent can be employed as an alternate measure.[33]

A calyceal fistula is the result of polar infarction and subsequent necrosis of the renal parenchyma and underlying calyceal tissue. This infarct is related to the inadvertent sacrifice of a polar vessel during organ retrieval. Upper polar infarcts do not impair ureteral viability but are associated with calyceal ischemia or necrosis.[21] Fortunately, the incidence of significant or recognizable calyceal urinary leaks is low. This is particularly startling when one considers the frequency of polar infarcts.

## Pyeloureterostomy Urinary Fistula

Urinary extravasation has been reported to occur in 5 to 14% of pyeloureteral anastomoses.[25] Although it is technically easier to perform than ureteroneocystostomy, the minute and critical aspects of renal pelvic and proximal ureteral preparation and anastomotic surgery stress that pyeloureterostomy should be performed only by surgeons with experience and instruction.[25] As a primary choice for reconstruction it is easier and quicker to perform. There is no need for a cystotomy, which itself may encourage a urinary leak. If a fistula develops, exploration and reconstruction may be necessary. Since a pyeloureterostomy has already been performed, an alternate procedure is necessary if debridement and a repeat anastomosis cannot be performed.[26] If ureteral length is insufficient, contralateral ureteral transposition could be accomplished.[11] Otherwise, a bladder flap or nephrostomy tube and stent may be the only alternative. Occasionally, nephrectomy may be advisable.[36]

Re-exploration of homografts because of urinary extravasation has been associated with a high rate of morbidity and mortality.[7] Consequently, several transplant centers have advocated a conservative, nonoperative management of urinary fistulae.[40, 44, 45] Cystotomy leaks and ureteroneocystostomy tunnel extravasation may be managed with minimal morbidity under select conditions by prolonged urethral catheter drainage. The patient's physiologic status is the predominant criterion upon which a nonoperative approach can be based. Ureteroureterostomy or calyceal extravasations may respond to transurethral placement of a ureteral stent and bladder drainage. These patients require vigilant observation. Any evidence of increasing morbidity would mandate exploration and possible transplant nephrectomy.

## Ureteral Obstruction

Ureteral obstruction has been reported as a post-transplant complication in 3.1 to 12.5% of cases.[34] However, recent reports have documented a reduction in incidence to 1.8%.[35] The literature is replete with reports demonstrating significant technological refinement and improvement in technical success. Ureteral strictures appear to occur at approximately equal incidence in ureterovesical (0.4%) and pyeloureteral (0.6%) areas. It is interesting to note that ureterovesical strictures are recognized in the early postoperative period (1–3 months), whereas strictures at the pyeloureteral junction tend to be recognized later (12–72 months). This tendency toward later recognition may be characteristic of the larger anastomosis.[35]

## Bladder Extravasation

Urinary extravasation from the anterior cystotomy has been reported to account for 1.5 to 40% of reported urologic complications.[20, 46] Cystotomy closure requires a precise mucosa-to-mucosa anastomosis. Further, a multiple layered approach is mandatory for early and precise healing.[10] This is especially desirable since early removal of the urethral catheter is important to reduce infection. Each layer of closure must be precise and closed in a "watertight" fashion with running chromic suture. The detrusor layer should overlap the mucosal layer at the superior and inferior ends. This further aids in leak prevention. The outer layer of the detrusor and perivesical tissue is closed with a running chromic or interrupted technique.

A problem of extravasation becomes evident once the urethral catheter has been removed. Suspicion may arise days following removal of the catheter because of declining urine output, pain in the lower abdomen, cutaneous urine drainage, flow, and occasionally extreme urgency. Cystography will confirm the diagnosis, and treatment is initiated by allowing the urethral catheter to remain indwelling. If there is wound drainage, a sampling of this drainage as well as of urine for electrolytes, urea nitrogen, and creatinine will be helpful. Large extravasations of urine need exploration and drainage. The majority of vesical extravasations tend to respond well to bladder drainage alone.[38]

The usual cause of a bladder leak is a combination of surgical repair and healing. However, on occasion these leaks are a result of high intravesical pressure gradients secondary to outflow obstruction or resistance. Further, noncompliant (scarred or thickened), cystic, neurogenic bladders are also responsible. Proper preoperative bladder and urethral assessment helps avoid these as a cause of bladder leaks. Urinary fistulae heal within 4 to 8 weeks while bladder drainage

continues. Prior to removal of the catheter, cystography is necessary to document complete healing.

## Vesicoureteral Reflux

The occurrence of vesicoureteral reflux following successful renal transplantation varies from less than 1% to 37.6%. The clinical significance of vesicoureteral reflux appears moot. Debate exists as to whether it causes or promotes homograft rejection episodes.[35] Although statistical correlation implicates reflux with this phenomenon, proof is lacking. Vesicoureteral reflux in the renal transplant recipient is recognized typically following routine postoperative cystography. It may be associated with residual urine volumes and infection. However, the clinical reality of this event is rare. The majority of transplant centers do not consider the occurrence of reflux a major urologic complication. The need to interfere surgically in these patients appears to be limited to those in whom severe urinary infections occur. A repeat ureteroneocystostomy corrects the problem.

In summary, the urologic aspects of renal transplantation in children continue to evolve. Proper patient selection and evaluation identify those most at risk for urologic complications. Improved knowledge of bladder function, avoidance of cutaneous diversions, and the ability to rehabilitate defunctionalized bladders have served to improve the quality of life and rehabilitative potential of children with end stage renal disease.

## REFERENCES

1. Kwun YA, Butt KMH, Kim KH, et al: Successful renal transplantation in a 3 month old infant. J Pediatr 92:426, 1978.
2. Hodson EM, Najarian JS, Kjelstrand CM, et al: Renal transplantation in children ages 1 to 5 years. Pediatrics 61:458, 1978.
3. Barnes BA, Bergan JJ, Braum WE, et al: The 12th report of the human renal transplant registry. JAMA 233:787, 1975.
4. Cerilli J, Anderson GW, Evans WE, Smith JP: Renal transplantation in patients with urinary tract abnormalities. Surgery 79:248, 1976.
5. Firlit CF: Use of defunctionalized bladders in pediatric renal transplantation. J Urol 116:634, 1976.
6. Schmaelzle JF, Cass AS, Hinman F Jr: Effect of disuse and restoration of function on vesical capacity. J Urol 101:700, 1969.

7. Kiser WS, Hewitt CB, Montie JE: The surgical complications of renal transplantation. Surg Clin North Am 51:1133, 1971.

8. Starzl TE, Groth CG, Putman CW, et al: Urological complications in 216 human recipients of renal transplants. Ann Surg 172:1, 1970.

9. Tunner WS, Whitsell JC II, Rubin AL, et al: Renal transplantation in children with corrected abnormalities of the lower urinary tract. J Urol 106:133, 1971.

10. Weil R III, Simmons RL, Tallent MB, et al: Prevention of urological complications after kidney transplantation. Ann Surg 174:154, 1971.

11. Edelbrock HH, Riddell H, Mickelson JC, et al: Urologic aspects of renal transplantation in children. J Urol 106:934, 1971.

12. Warshaw BL, Edelbrock HH, Ettenger RB, et al: Renal transplantation in children with obstructive uropathy. J Urol 123:737, 1980.

13. Fine RN, Edelbrock HH, Riddell H, et al: Renal transplantation in children. Urology 9:61, 1977.

14. Marshall FF, Smolev JK, Spees EK, et al: The urological evaluation and management of patients with congenital lower urinary tract anomalies prior to renal transplantation. J Urol 127:1078, 1982.

15. Lapides J, Diokno AC, Gould FR: Further observations on self-catheterization. J Urol 116:169, 1976.

16. Lapides J, Diokno AC, Silber ST: Clean intermittent self-catheterization in the treatment of urinary tract disease. J Urol 107:458, 1972.

17. Stenzel KH, Stubenbord WT, Whitsell JC, et al: Kidney transplantation: use of intestinal conduits. JAMA 229:534, 1974.

18. Firlit CF, Merkel FK: The application of ileal conduits in pediatric renal transplantation. J Urol 118:647, 1977.

19. Salvatierra O Jr, Kountz SL, Belzer FO: Prevention of ureteral fistula after renal transplantation. J Urol 112:445, 1974.

20. Belzer FO, Kountz SL, Najarian JS, et al: Prevention of urological complications after renal allotransplantation. Arch Surg 101:449, 1970.

21. Hricko GM, Birtch AG, Bennett AH, Wilson RE: Factors responsible for urinary fistula in the renal transplant recipient. Ann Surg 178:609, 1973.

22. Politano VA, Leadbetter WF: An operative technique for the correction of vesicoureteral reflux. J Urol 79:932, 1958.

23. Merkel FK, Ing TS, Ahmadian Y, et al: Transplantation in and of the young. J Urol 111:679, 1974.

24. Shenasky JH II: Renal transplantation in patients with urologic abnormalities. J Urol 115:490, 1976.

25. Whelchel JD, Cosimi AB, Young HH II, Russell PS: Pyeloureterostomy reconstruction in human renal transplantation. Ann Surg 181:61, 1975.

26. Leiter E, Kim KH, Glabman SH, et al: Urinary reconstruction by pyeloureteral anastomosis in human renal transplants. J Urol 109:28, 1973.

27. Starzl TE, Groth CG, Putnam CW, et al: Urologic complication in 216 human recipients of renal transplants. Ann Surg 172:1, 1970.

28. Lich R Jr, Howerton LW, Davis LA: Recurrent urosepsis in children. J Urol 86:554, 1961.

29. Wasnick RJ, Butt KMH, Laungani G, et al: Evaluation of anterior extravesical ureteroneocystostomy in kidney transplantation. J Urol 126:306, 1981.

30. Konnak JW, Herwig KR, Finkbeiner A, et al: Extravesical ureteroneocystostomy in 170 renal transplant recipients. J Urol 113:299, 1975.

40. Palmer JM, Kountz SL, Swenson RS, et al: Urinary tract morbidity in renal transplantation. Arch Surg 98:352, 1969.

31. Barry JM, Lawson RK, Strong D, Hodges CV: Urologic complications in 173 kidney transplants. J Urol 112:567, 1974.

32. Kelly WD, Merkel FK, Markland C: Ileal urinary division in conjunction with renal homotransplantation. Lancet 1:222, 1966.

33. Martin DC, Mims MM, Kaufman JJ, Goodwin WE: The ureter in renal transplantation. J Urol 101:680, 1969.

34. Holden S, O'Brian DP III, Lewis EL, et al: Urologic complications in renal transplantation. Urology 5:182, 1975.

35. Williams G, Birtch AG, Wilson RE, et al: Urological complications of renal transplantation. Br J Urol 43:21, 1970.

36. Dreikorn K, Rohl L, Rossler W: Urologic complications in renal transplantation. Transplant Proc 14:77, 1982.

37. Bewick M, Collins REC, Saxton HM, et al: The surgery and problems of the ureter in human renal transplantation. Br J Urol 46:493, 1974.

38. Marx WL, Halaz NA, McLaughlin AP, Gittes RF: Urological complications in renal transplantation. J Urol 112:561, 1974.

39. Colfry AJ Jr, Schlegerl JV, Lindsey ES, McDonald JC: Urological complications in renal transplantation. J Urol 112:564, 1974.

40. Palmer JM, Kountz SL, Swenson RS, et al: Urinary tract morbidity in renal transplantation. Arch Surg 98:352, 1969.

41. Morehouse DD, Macramalla EF, Guttmann RD, et al: The conservative management of urinary fistulas following renal allografts. J Urol 110:502, 1973.

42. Shkolnik A: Gray scale ultrasound of the pediatric abdomen and pelvis. *In* Current problems in diagnostic radiology. Vol 7, No 4, Jul/Aug 1977, Chicago, Year Book Publishers.

43. Conger K, Rouse PV: Ureteroplasty by the bladder flap technique. J Urol 74:485, 1955.

44. Hoch WH, Kest L, Cohen S, et al: Supravesical urinary fistulas after transplantation. Surg Gynecol Obstet 139:82, 1974.

45. Desai SG, McRoberts JW, Hellebusch AA, Luke RG: Conservative non-operative management of ureteral fistulas following renal allografts. J Urol 112:572, 1974.

46. Smolev JK, McLaughlin MG, Rolley R, et al: The surgical approach to urological complications in renal allotransplant recipients. J Urol 117:10, 1977.

# 34

# Allograft Rejection: Types, Mechanisms, and Diagnosis

*Stanley C. Jordan, M.D.*
*Jacques M. Lemire, M.D., FRCP (C)*

Successful renal transplantation is considered the optimal therapy for ESRD in children. Although impressive advances in tissue typing and efforts to transplant a histocompatible kidney have occurred, allograft rejection continues to be the major cause of allograft failure.

Therapeutic approaches to allograft rejection have changed little in recent years and rejection continues to be a significant cause of patient morbidity. Despite the identification of over 60 antigens associated with the human leukocyte antigen (HLA) A and B loci, the survival of cadaveric HLA-identical matched kidneys is only 10 to 30% better than in recipients who receive a complete HLA-histoincompatible allograft.[1] It is also known that approximately 40% of cadaver HLA-histoincompatible kidneys will survive more than five years.[1] Recently, typing for the newly defined HLA-DR antigen system has provided more encouraging data: up to 85% one-year survival rates in some studies when cadaver donor/recipient pairs are matched only for the first eight DR antigens.[2] These revelations and other recent developments have led to a rethinking of the immunologic mechanism responsible for allograft rejection.

## IMMUNOLOGIC MECHANISMS OF ALLOGRAFT REJECTION

Renal allografts are known to be rejected by the host immunologic mechanisms. Allograft rejection involves both cellular and humoral immune mechanisms. The primary mechanism(s) involved in a particular individual and the specific characteristic of an allograft rejection event (i.e., time of onset, intensity of clinical and laboratory manifestations, and specific morphology) appear to be genetically controlled.[3] Unmodified allograft rejections do not occur in humans because all patients are treated with specific immunosuppressive protocols. Most centers use prednisone and azathioprine; other centers have explored the use of antithymocyte globulin (ATG) and ionizing radiation.[3] Presently, clinical trials are under way to evaluate the efficacy of cyclosporin A in preventing allograft rejection. Initial results are encouraging, but the nephrotoxicity and hepatotoxicity of cyclosporin A may limit its widespread use.[4] The use of immunosuppression, technical factors, and the possibility of recurrent original disease in allografts have made interpretation of histopathologic data derived from renal allografts difficult. However, some general principles can be agreed upon: if a significant histoincompatibility exists between the donor and recipient, a more intense and rapid rejection process will occur. This can be seen best in the living-related donor transplant situation. Renal isografts between identical twins are not rejected. Alteration in allograft function usually represents technical problems and not immunologically mediated events, although recurrence of the original disease has been reported.[74] Renal allografts between HLA-identical sibs are rejected mildly, if at all. This is in contrast to the data from more remotely related donor (less HLA-identical) and cadaver donor allografts, which are rejected more aggressively.[5]

Although cellular mechanisms have been assigned a central role in the classic concepts of allograft rejection, there is now strong evidence that antibody-mediated mechanisms are also important as mediators of certain types of allograft rejection.[6]

The types of allograft rejection can be classified according to immunopathology, time of onset, and duration of symptoms. Clinically, four well-defined types of allograft rejection have been described: hyperacute (HR), accelerated acute (AAR), acute (AR), and chronic rejection (CR).[7]

Once the allograft is revascularized, it becomes both a target and antigenic source for response of the host immune system. The type of immunologic response (primarily cellular or humoral) depends, in large part, upon the immune response characteristic of the host, prior sensitization to transplantation antigens, and the competence of immunologic effector mechanisms.[3, 8] The nature of the immunologic contact that is required to elicit a cellular immune response is not completely understood; however, cytotoxic "killer" lymphocytes may react with histoincompatible allograft-specific antigens in situ or may be exposed to solubilized antigens in the circulation. In the latter situation, sensitized T lymphocytes would recirculate to the allograft and react with the antigenic determinants.[9]

A more recent characterization of the cellular immune mechanisms involved in allograft rejection has been presented by Drevyanko et al.[10] These investigators examined renal biopsy material from allograft recipients who had: (a) no rejection (NR), (b) acute cellular rejection (AR), (c) hyperacute rejection (HR), or (d) chronic rejection (CR). Cellular infiltrates were characterized utilizing OKT3 (Pan-T-cell), OKT4 (Helper-Inducer), OKT8 (Suppressor-Cytotoxic), and OKM1 (Macrophage-Monocyte) monoclonal antibodies (Ortho-Clone), which are specific for the lymphocyte subsets mentioned. Infiltrating cells were increased during all types of rejection when compared to NR. The ratio of OKT4$^+$/OKT8$^+$ in NR was the same as that of peripheral blood. In AR, OKT3$^+$ and OKT8$^+$ cells were increased over OKT4$^+$ and OKM1$^+$ cells. The cells involved in CR were found to be B cells, plasma cells, fibroblasts,

and OKM1$^+$ cells. Cells involved in HR were granulocytes and OKM1$^+$ cells. These data indicate that characterization of cellular infiltrates by monoclonal antibodies may be useful in diagnosing the nature of the rejection episodes. The relative increase in OKT8$^+$ cells in AR suggests that the cytotoxic (rather than suppressor) cell population is involved in direct cell-mediated injury of the allograft. Further confirmation of this fact awaits application of monoclonal antibodies that distinguish cytotoxic OKT8$^+$ from suppressor OKT8$^+$ populations.

Primary antibody-mediated allograft rejection many be mediated by preformed antibodies that react with allograft-specific antigens,[3] with subsequent activation of the effector mechanism (i.e., complement, polymorphonuclear leukocytes (PMNs), and the kinin-coagulation systems). This type of antibody-mediated allograft injury is most likely responsible for the hyperacute and accelerated acute types of allograft rejection. Antibody-producing cells can also be stimulated to form antibodies reactive with allograft-specific antigens in previously unsensitized individuals, or anamnestic responses may result in vigorous and avid antibody generation with subsequent allograft injury.

Immune complex injury to the allograft may occur when allograft-specific antigens are released into the circulation and react with specific antibody to form circulating immune complexes (CICs).[2, 20, 21] Although initial reports described the association of vascular acute rejection with CICs,[32] subsequent studies have failed to confirm these observations. Investigations conducted in our laboratory have shown that selected patients developed CICs with allograft rejection episodes,[20, 21] but statistical analysis of the data showed no significant relationship of CICs with allograft rejection. Johny et al have also reported similar findings.[33]

## TYPES OF ALLOGRAFT REJECTION

Although allograft rejection is a common occurrence post transplant, efforts to classify allograft rejection episodes are often very difficult. One of the most useful classifications has been that based on clinical criteria. However, one must also take into account the immunopathology of the rejection episode (primarily cellular or humoral) as well as the intensity of the rejection reaction.

Classification of allograft rejection is also complicated by the occurrence of more than one specific type of rejection in a single allograft. Despite these considerations we will present a classification of types of allograft rejection episodes which will encompass all the above considerations.

## Hyperacute Rejection (HR)

HR occurs immediately after allograft revascularization and is associated with the presence of preformed lymphocytotoxic antibodies (LCA) to either HLA-A and -B antigens or to ABO blood group antigens.[1] This fulminant rejection reaction usually occurs in highly sensitized individuals (multiparous women or multiply transplanted individuals). The graft characteristically fails within minutes of vascular perfusion. Clinically, the graft becomes swollen, mottled, and a loss of pulsation is noted. The process is irreversible and, if left in place for several days, significant cortical necrosis will be noted[11] (Fig. 34–1.

Histologic changes seen within the first hour after vascular anastomosis include marked dilation of the glomeruli, which are

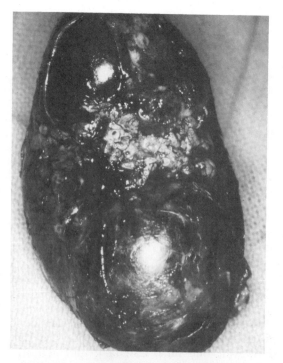

**Figure 34–1.** Hyperacute rejection. An extremely swollen, mottled, and hemorrhagic allograft removed 48 hours after transplantation.

also engorged with red blood cells (RBCs) and polymorphonuclear white blood cells (PMNs) (Fig. 34–2). There is endothelial cell swelling with fibrin deposition and occasional necrosis. The endothelial cells of the peritubular capillaries often demonstrate the same finding.[3] The peritubular capillaries are often dilated and engorged with PMNs. Cortical arterioles and interlobular arteries are also dilated and engorged with RBCs. If the graft is allowed to be perfused for several hours to days, extensive vascular thrombosis with fibrin deposition and cortical necrosis will be seen. Mononuclear cells may also play a role in HR.[10]

The mechanism of HR is predominantly humoral. Donor-specific antibodies react with ABO or HLA-A and -B alloantigens in or on the vascular endothelial cells of the allograft.[1] As with classic antigens-antibody reactions, this "in situ" immune complex formation results in the activation of specific effector mechanisms (complement activation, release of vasoactive amines, activation of kinin and coagulation systems). Release of complement-derived chemotactic factors ($C_3e$ and $C_5a$) results in PMN infiltration, with subsequent damage to the endothelial cells. Once endothelial damage has occurred, the endothelial cells retract and the glomerular basement membrane (GBM) is exposed. The GBM activates platelets, which activate the coagulation system, and fibrin deposits appear in the glomeruli. PMNs, which are recruited by complement activation to the area of inflammation, adhere to the GBM and release proteolytic enzymes, which further potentiate glomerular injury and dysfunction.

Since HR is primarily an antibody-mediated event, one would expect to see immunoglobulins and complement as well as other inflammatory proteins deposited in the glomerular or vascular structures. Direct immunofluorescence of hyperacutely rejected allografts taken early in the course show linear glomerular deposition of host IgG. Complement, which is also seen, is more discontinuous in the glomeruli but increased significantly in the peritubular capillaries.[3, 12] If biopsies are taken at 12 to 24 hours post transplant, no immunoreactive proteins may be found. This is most likely due to the denudation of endothelial cells after acute injury has occurred.[3, 12] Since antibodies and complement bind to alloantigens located in or on the renal endothelial cells and not to the GBM, there is no persistence of these inflammatory proteins in the allograft.[3, 12]

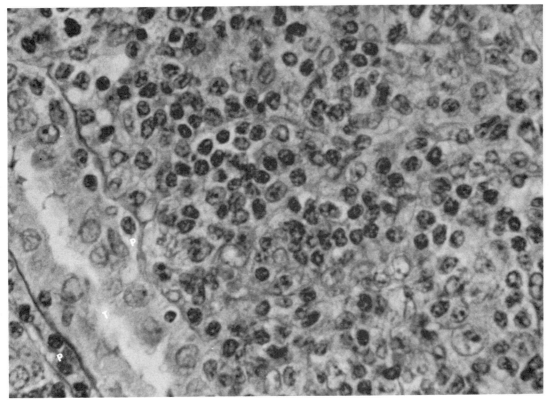

**Figure 34–2.** Hyperacute rejection. The peritubular capillaries (P) and intertubular spaces are dilated and filled with PMNs. The tubules (T) are also necrotic.

Although most investigators feel that HR is antibody mediated,[12, 13] Starzl et al have offered an alternative explanation.[14] These investigators proposed that a Shwartzman-like reaction may occur in presensitized individuals, causing a localized intravascular coagulopathy involving the allograft. This view is supported by the extensive deposition of fibrin-fibrinogen, platelet thrombi, and other coagulation proteins in the allograft. The pathology of HR (acute allograft failure, ischemia, and cortical necrosis) is also consistent with this view. Schiff et al reported a case of HR occurring in the second post-transplant week associated with gram-negative sepsis.[15] Since endotoxin is responsible for the Shwartzman reaction in rabbits, these data lend further support to a Shwartzman-like reaction mediating HR.

## Accelerated Acute Rejection (AAR)

Recently, a distinct clinical type of allograft rejection has been described under several different names: early severe rejection, AAR, and early acute rejection.[7] The clinical char-

acteristics of AAR appear to be similar for each group of patients reported. AAR typically occurs within the first post-transplant week. Clinical symptoms such as fever, hypertension, graft swelling and tenderness, and length of rejection episodes are prolonged when compared to acute rejection episodes.[7] Our data[7] and that of others[16, 17] have shown that all allografts eventually fail despite intense antirejection therapy. However, Anderson and Newton reported a 58% recovery rate after antirejection therapy.[18] The reason(s) for these discrepancies are unresolved since the antirejection protocols were similar for all groups.

The renal pathological examination of AAR allografts usually shows hemorrhagic infarction and necrosis of the renal cortex. Inflammatory angiitis of the medium and large arteries and fibrinoid necrosis of smaller vessels are present (Fig. 34–3). In our study 7 of 10 patients experiencing AAR had mild to moderate lymphocytic infiltrates. Immunofluorescence studies are inconsistent, especially if the biopsy is not performed shortly after onset of the rejection reaction. Since AAR is most likely an antibody-me-

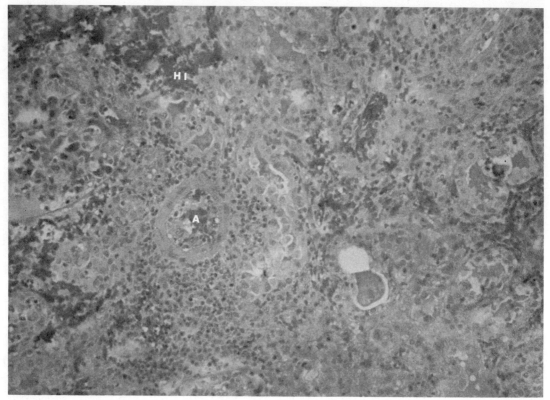

**Figure 34–3.** Accelerated acute rejection. Hemorrhagic infarction (HI) is noted in the renal cortex. A proliferative vasculitis of a small artery (A) with concomitant cellular infiltrate is also apparent. Diffuse tubular necrosis is prominent throughout the biopsy specimen.

diated event, one would expect to see IgG and complement in the allograft shortly after onset of the rejection episode. Paul et al reported a case of AAR in which antibodies to donor-specific endothelial-monocyte antigen were demonstrated in the allograft shortly after transplant.[17] These investigators have presented subsequent data confirming an important role for antibodies to endothelial cell–specific antigens in the mediation of AAR.[7]

Lucas et al[19] demonstrated lymphocytotoxic antibodies (LCA) in the sera and kidney eluates of allograft recipients who had undergone AAR. Our studies and those of others[7, 16-18] tend not to support these data. The role of other nephritogenic substances (CICs, anti-Lewis antibodies and antibodies to glomerular or tubular basement membrane antigens) in the mediation of AAR is minimal.[17, 20, 21] Baldwin et al have reported that the most commonly detected antibodies associated with AAR are those which react with renal vascular endothelial antigen (anti-E antibodies) and those reacting with HLA-DR antigens.[1, 22] A more detailed discussion

of the anti-E antibody system and its mediation of rejection episodes appears later in this chapter.

Finally, the consistent demonstration of hemorrhagic infarction and intra- as well as extraglomerular deposition of fibrin may indicate dysfunctional coagulation similar to that seen in experimental situations (Shwartzman reaction) or in certain cases of hyperacute rejection[14, 15] (Fig. 34–4).

## Acute Rejection (AR)

AR is found commonly during the first three to four months post transplant, although it may occur at any time. AR episodes are uncommon after the first post-transplant year. Clinically, AR episodes are characterized by graft swelling and tenderness, fever, hypertension, weight gain, leukocytosis, and proteinuria. Although the above signs and symptoms may be present with varying frequency, the most consistent features of AR are decreased urine output and decreasing renal function. The histopathologic picture

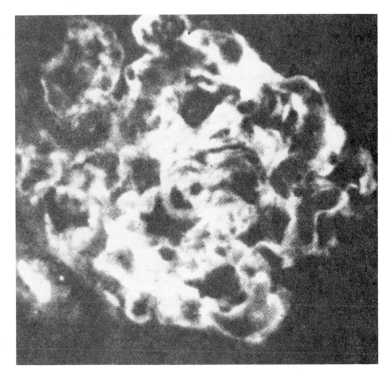

**Figure 34–4.** Accelerated acute rejection. Glomeruli showing fibrin deposits. (×400.)

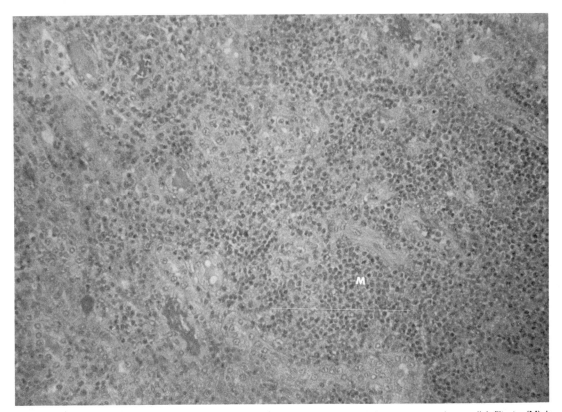

**Figure 34–5.** Acute cellular rejection. Diffuse interstitial edema with a prominent mononuclear cell infiltrate (M) is evident, which can be seen to invade the tubular walls.

of AR is either predominantly cellular or humoral (antibody-mediated). Overlap between the two types is common and may make specific diagnosis difficult.

**Lymphocyte-Mediated AR.** Acute cellular rejection is primarily a tubulointerstitial nephritis[3] manifested by diffuse interstitial edema with mononuclear cell infiltrates which invade the tubular wall (Fig. 34–5). The infiltrate is primarily mononuclear in nature with small and medium-sized lymphocytes admixed with transformed lymphocytes (immunoblasts).[23] Plasma cells are seen when the process has proceeded beyond one week. In more severe cases of acute cellular rejection, lymphocytic infiltrates can be seen in the walls of arteries and arterioles.[3, 23] The recent use of monoclonal antibodies to characterize lymphocytic infiltrates during AR has been accomplished.[10] The most common cell type infiltrating during AR is the OKT8[+] cell. These cells represent lymphocytes with suppressor-cytotoxic functions. Since monoclonal antisera are just becoming available to distinguish the cytotoxic OKT8[+] cells from the OKT8[+] suppressor cells, resolution of the specific cell type (suppressor or cytotoxic) that predominates awaits further investigation.

**Antibody-Mediated AR.** Antibody-mediated AR is characterized by generalized damage to the vascular endothelium. The capillaries, arteries, arterioles, and veins of the allograft are involved,[24] with a conspicuous absence of cell-mediated rejection (i.e., no evidence of tubulointerstitial damage) (Fig. 34–6). The vessels involved in antibody-mediated acute rejection show vacuolization, lytic necrosis, and swelling of the vascular endothelial cells.[3, 24] In severe cases, fibrinoid necrosis of the vessel is associated with extravasation of red blood cells into areas around the damaged vessels. The presence of cortical necrosis is associated with early failure of the allograft.[24, 25] The glomeruli are usually shrunken and appear hypoperfused. PAS staining usually demonstrates a mild to moderate increase in mesangial matrix with normal GBM thickness.[3, 25] Glomerular thrombi may be present and variable numbers of PMNs can be seen in many glomeruli.[25] In many cases the histopathology is identical to that observed in either HR or AAR. The most consistent electron microscopic finding is an expansion of the subendothelial space, most likely due to a collection of cellular debris, fibrin, or fibrin-related material, and platelets[3, 24, 25] (Fig. 34–7). The glomerular

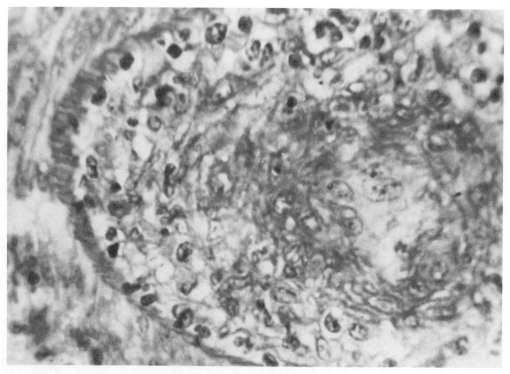

**Figure 34–6.** Acute vascular rejection. Fibrinoid necrosis of the arterial wall with obliteration is noted. Little interstitial infiltrate is found in this form of rejection.

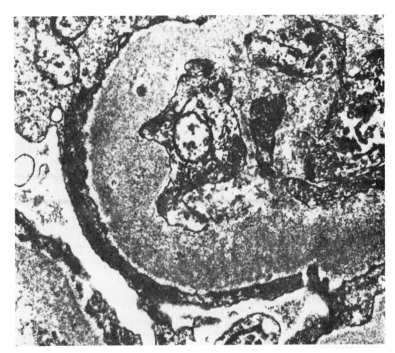

**Figure 34–7.** Acute vascular rejection. Widening of the subendothelial zone (S) of the GBM has occurred, with deposition of lamina densa–like material.

changes seen in the vascular type of AR are identical to those observed in other systemic diseases which affect the renal arteries (scleroderma, malignant hypertension, and hemolytic-uremic syndrome).[26]

## Chronic Rejection (CR)

CR usually becomes apparent after the sixth post-transplant month and is manifested by a slowly progressive deterioration of allograft function with no definable AR episodes. The histologic features and clinical manifestations of CR can be divided into two distinct types: (1) chronic vascular rejection, not as fulminant as acute vascular rejection but associated with ischemic damage to the allograft interstitium, and (2) chronic glomerular transplant disease, in which a spectrum of glomerular lesions is seen.[3]

**Chronic Vascular Rejection.** The proliferative vascular lesion which primarily involves the cortical interlobular and arcuate arteries may be seen in as many as 50% (Fig. 34–8) of allografts surviving more than three months.[27] The lesions initially are focal but become more widespread as the process progresses. Progression of the vascular lesions is felt to be the most common cause of allograft failure in long-term survivors.[3] Lipid vacuoles and foamy macrophages can be seen in the intima of involved vessels. Fibrin thrombi

are not as frequent as in acute vascular rejection.[3] A focal disruption of the internal elastic lamina is characteristic. The obliterative vasculitis results in glomerular and interstitial damage (tubular atrophy) (Fig. 34–9). In severe cases, as many as 50% of the glomeruli may be involved.[3, 27]

**Glomerular Transplant Disease (GTD).** GTD is characterized by the onset of a slowly progressive deterioration in allograft function six months to several years post transplant, with significant proteinuria.[28] The time relationship between deterioration of allograft function after the onset of proteinuria is variable, but most allografts survive only a few months when this sequence of events is recognized.[3, 28] The incidence of GTD varies from study to study, but when the definition of GTD is restricted to include only patients with severe proteinuria and functional deterioration of the allograft, most studies report an incidence of approximately 20% in allografts surviving longer than six months.[28, 29]

The histologic characteristics of GTD do not conform to any known type of de novo glomerulonephritis but can be described in characteristic categories. These changes include glomerular atrophy, which is usually associated with fibrin deposition and obliteration of the glomerular tuft; focal mesangial proliferation, which may be segmental in nature and is occasionally associated with small cellular epithelial crescents; membra-

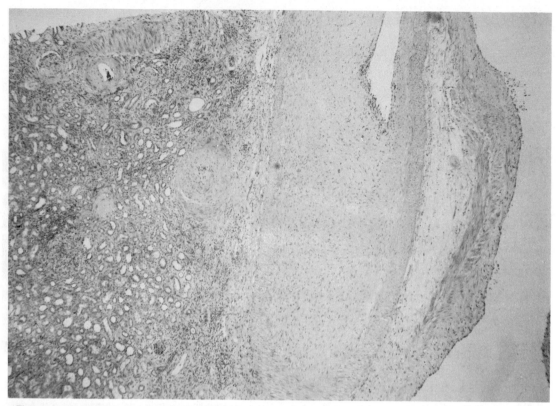

**Figure 34–8.** Chronic vascular rejection. This is a medium-sized artery which shows significant compromise of the lumen due to proliferation of connective tissue in the subendothelial area.

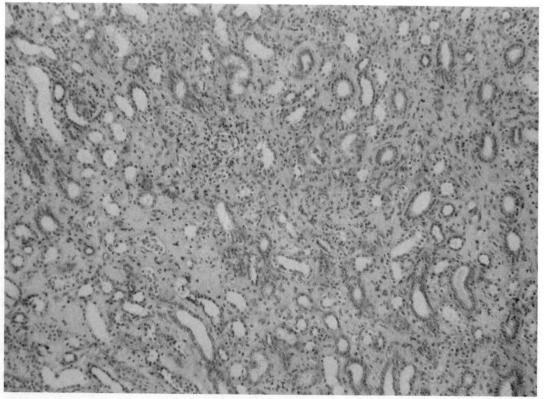

**Figure 34–9.** Chronic vascular rejection. Tubular atrophy and fibrosis secondary to ischemia from chronic obliterative vasculitis has occurred.

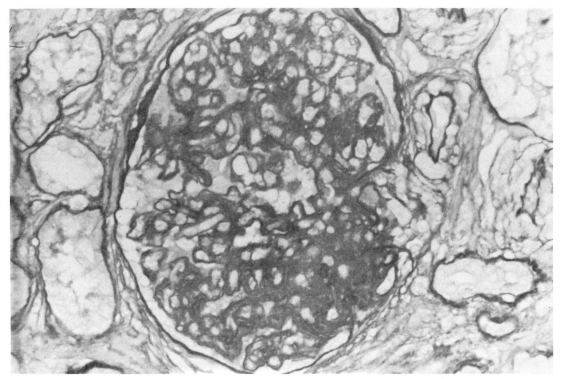

**Figure 34–10.** Glomerular transplant disease. There is an increased mesangial matrix associated with thickening of the GBM. Diffuse tubular atrophy is also noted (PAS ×400.)

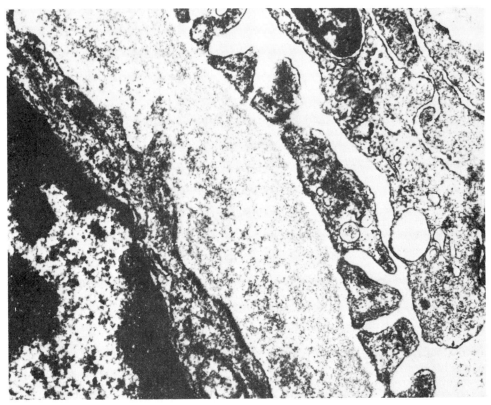

**Figure 34–11.** Glomerular transplant disease. Electron micrograph showing expanded subendothelial zone (S). Replication of lamina densa–like material with fibrin deposits and cellular debris probably account for this finding.

nous thickening of the glomerular capillary walls, and membranous changes associated with mesangial hyperplasia (membranoproliferative changes) (Fig. 34–10).

The membranoproliferative variety of GTD is associated with peripheral capillary wall thickening with diffuse splitting of the GBM noted on PAS stains, which is due to mesangial interpositioning along the GBM. It is of interest that these lesions are often indistinguishable from the membranoproliferative glomerulonephritis seen in native kidneys.[3, 28] In many cases, GTD coexists with chronic vascular rejection. The worst prognostic sign for allograft survival is the presence of the mesangiocapillary changes.[30] The most significant electron microscopic finding in GTD is the presence of a subendothelial collection of an "abnormal basement membrane substance."[3, 31] Characteristically, the subendothelial zone of the capillary loop is expanded with cellular debris or fibrin deposited in this zone. Replication of lamina densa-like material may also occur in this area.[3, 31] (Fig. 34–11).

## Antigen Determinants in or of the Kidney Responsible for Allograft Rejection

Recent developments in monoclonal antibody technology have allowed investigators to specifically define the antigenic anatomy of the human kidney.[1] Baldwin et al described kidney-specific antigens that were unrelated to those of the major histocompatibility locus (HLA-A, B, C, and DR).[1, 22] These allograft-specific antigens were also shown to be important in allograft rejection. Some of the antigenic determinants in or of the kidney, such as those of the glomerular basement membrane (GBM), tubular basement membrane (TBM), or tubular brush border, have poor immunogenicity in relation to renal allograft rejection. The reason for this is most likely the weak immunogenicity of these antigens or the fact that they are sequestered from the individual's immunoreactive cells and antibodies.[1] However, exceptions do exist, as recent studies have shown that de novo antiglomerular basement membrane (anti-GBM) glomerulonephritis develops in renal allografts given to patients with ESRD secondary to Alport's syndrome.[38] Since patients with Alport's syndrome do not have serologically definable GBM antigens in

their native kidneys, the GBM(+) allograft would then represent a new antigen to which antibody responses would be engendered.

Another group of non-HLA antigens that are expressed on the renal vascular endothelial cells (E antigens) are immunogenic and have been demonstrated to be responsible for certain types of allograft rejection.[1, 17, 22, 34, 36] Although antibodies to E antigens are not formed in patients with good allograft function, they have been repeatedly demonstrated in the circulation of approximately 50% of patients undergoing irreversible acute rejection[1] and have also been demonstrated in the eluates of rejected kidneys.[17, 34] Since the E antigen system is not expressed on unstimulated lymphocytes, platelets, or red blood cells, antibodies to E antigens would not be detected by standard tissue typing techniques.[1, 17, 35]

Although E antigens are also expressed on both monocytes and granulocytes[1, 17, 35] not all monocyte or granulocyte antigens are expressed on the renal endothelial cell.[1] It is therefore understandable that crossmatching for monocyte- or granulocyte-specific antigens does not always correlate with the presence or absence of antibodies specific for E-antigen determinants expressed only on renal vascular endothelial cells. It seems that the most optimal method to detect E-antigen–specific antibodies would be the use of indirect immunofluorescent techniques on allograft biopsy material from the specific donor.[1, 17] Antibodies which react with ABO and HLA-A, -B, and -C determinants expressed on arterial and glomerular endothelial cells most often mediate HR. In contrast, those antibodies which react with E antigens and HLA-DR antigens (expressed primarily on venous, peritubular capillary, and glomerular endothelial cells) most commonly mediate irreversible AR.[22]

### Elution Studies

Elution studies of renal allografts have been reported by relatively few investigators. One of the better studies of rejected allografts is that of Baldwin et al who recently presented data on a double blind study performed on the IgG eluted from 88 rejected allografts.[22] Approximately 40% of the eluates contained antibodies reactive with E antigens, data which were also confirmed by study of serum samples from the same patients. The most important observations were that the antibodies specific for E antigen were most commonly seen in second allografts, in acutely rejecting first grafts, and in recipients who received allografts without pretransplant blood transfusions.[1, 22] IgG eluted for the rejected allografts also showed a high reactivity (33%) with B-cell–specific antigens (presumably DR), while only 10% of the eluates had reactivity against T cells (presumably HLA, A, B, and C) antigens. Similar studies which were performed on rejected allografts are available.[34, 36]

The higher incidence of B-cell rather than T-cell–specific antibodies in eluates of rejected allografts is more likely explained by the higher density of HLA-DR antigenic determinants in human kidneys.[35] Since many B-cell–positive eluates also contained anti-E-antibody activity, it was felt that the strong immunogenicity of the E antigen may be related to its co-expression with DR on the peritubular capillary endothelial cells.[7, 35] DR-antigens are thought to stimulate helper T cells (OKT4[+]), which subsequently participate in the generation of antibody-producing cells.[7] Thus, the DR antigens may stimulate helper T cells, which participate in anti-E-antigen antibody generation.

In contrast to the studies of Baldwin et al,[1, 22] Moy and Rosenau presented data on eluates of acutely rejected renal allografts that showed only minimal endothelial or vascular injury, but contained large quantities of infiltrating lymphoid cells, which produced prominent tubular injury.[37] These investigators demonstrated alpha-lymphotoxin in the eluates of several acutely rejected allografts (primarily cellular). The mechanism by which one cell kills another, as in lymphocyte-mediated cytolysis, is still controversial. However, these investigators have proposed cytotoxic lymphokines (lymphotoxins) as mediators of this reaction.[37] In this experiment, Moy and Rosenau demonstrated the presence of alpha-lymphotoxin in the eluates of rejected allografts, which contained heavy lymphocytic infiltrates. Although the precise role for alpha-lymphotoxin in allograft rejection is not clear, the presence of this substance in rejecting allografts where cellular mechanisms predominate is suggestive of its participation in the process. Further investigation will be necessary before the precise mechanism of cell-mediated tissue injury is demonstrated.

## Clinical Implication of Antibody to E Antigen

In a study of 20 patients who acutely rejected their allografts, Baldwin et al found that virtually all individuals who acutely rejected second or third transplants formed antibodies to E antigen.[1, 22] Approximately 30% of patients rejecting first allografts developed circulating anti–E antibodies (all DR-mismatched) and virtually all patients who rejected a second or third transplant and who had not had blood transfusions prior to their first transplant. The conclusions drawn were: (a) pretransplant blood transfusions not only prolong the survival of the first allograft but blunt antibody responses to subsequent blood transfusions and transplants; (b) DR matching appears to be important in reducing the development of anti-E antibodies since a good DR antigen match would presumably reduce the "helper" effect engendered by DR antigens; and (c) circulating anti-E antibodies not only injure existing allografts but can mediate rejection in subsequent allografts.[17] Baldwin et al have shown that 50 to 75% of patients with anti-E antibodies will demonstrate positive indirect immunofluorescence when tested against a panel of normal renal tissue.[1] It is, therefore, conceivable that anti-E antibodies in the sera of potential transplant recipients may be more deleterious to allograft survival than preformed antibodies to specific HLA-A or -B antigens.[1, 17, 34, 36]

In summary, a better understanding of immunogenic antigens in or of the human kidney will allow a more accurate prediction of allograft rejection. In addition, the data presented by Baldwin et al[1] suggest that pretransplant blood transfusions and good DR antigen matching inhibits antibody responses to E antigens and presumably enhances allograft survival.

## REJECTION DIAGNOSIS (TABLE 34–1)

Rejection of the allograft is essentially a clinical diagnosis. Most often, the association of clinical symptoms and signs of rejection and the time of onset of the clinical manifestations after transplantation will define the nature of rejection. However, in some instances the expression of the rejection process may be obscured by pathophysiological

**Table 34–1.**  DIAGNOSIS OF REJECTION

| Type | Nature | Time Interval from Transplantation | Clinical Manifestations | | | | Renal Scintiscan | Outcome |
|---|---|---|---|---|---|---|---|---|
| | | | Fever | Allograft Tenderness | Reduction in Renal Function | Hypertension | | |
| Hyperacute | Humoral | Immediate | N.A. | N.A. | No function | N.A. | No uptake | Nil |
| Accelerated Acute | Humoral & cellular(?) | 2–7 days | ++ | ++ | ++ | ++ | Normal at 24 hours—no uptake at onset of rejection | Poor |
| Acute | Mainly cellular & humoral (vascular) | 1st: 7–10 days Then: anytime | + | + | + | + | Decreased uptake and excretion | Good (if cellular), poor (if vascular) |
| Chronic | Humoral | Few months to years | – | – | + (Insidious) | ± | Variable | Poor |

N.A.: Not applicable.

insults to the transplanted kidney (e.g., acute tubular necrosis or acute ureteral obstruction). In addition, AR can occur in allografts undergoing CR. Histologic and immunologic techniques have contributed to our understanding of the mechanisms of allograft rejection. In the majority of instances, however, the need for biopsy can be alleviated by the evaluation of a constellation of clinical, biochemical, and radiologic manifestations characteristic of a specific type of rejection.

The transplanted kidney can potentially be affected by the four types of rejection previously described.

## Hyperacute Rejection

The onset of HR is often dramatic. Immediately after revascularization of the renal allograft, the organ becomes cyanotic and flaccid with loss of pulsations rather than being pink and firm. Occasionally, function established initially rapidly deteriorates within the first 12 to 48 hours following surgery. Left in place, the allograft suffers from ischemia, and extensive cortical necrosis rapidly follows.

When performed, the renogram will reveal a poor or even an absent vascular phase,[39] and arteriography will demonstrate a severe vasculitis with infarction and cortical necrosis.

The routine use of pretransplant crossmatching has dramatically reduced the incidence of HR. A classic example of HR would be encountered either in an ABO-incompatible donor-recipient situation or when the recipient has preformed LCA to donor HLA antigens.

Biopsy of the allograft has the potential to induce hemorrhage and laceration of the kidney. Because of the irreversibility of the insult, allograft nephrectomy is the treatment of choice.

## Accelerated Acute Rejection

Also described as delayed hyperacute rejection, AAR usually occurs after an initial 48 hours or more of normal allograft function, with onset within the first post-transplant week. After establishment of an initial diuresis with subsequent improvement of allograft function, urine output decreases and the patient experiences fever and localized pain at the allograft site. Hypertension, allograft swelling, and anuria may also be noted. When compared to typical AR, these symptoms and signs are more severe and the length of the episode is more prolonged.[7] The renal scintiphotoscan using both hippuric acid and technetium may be completely normal when performed within 24 hours of transplantation (Fig. 34–12). However, at the onset of rejection, a repeat study will reveal the characteristic findings of AAR[40] (Fig. 34–13); when performed after the development of anuria, the perfusion phase may be significantly reduced. Arteriography shows slowing of renal blood flow and patchy filling defects in the outer cortex and arterioles, with irregularities and tapering of distal branches of the arcuate, interlobular, and intralobular arteries, referred to as the "dead tree" image.

AAR carries a poor prognosis; irreversibility is the rule in a majority of cases despite aggressive antirejection therapy.[7, 41] Allograft nephrectomy is usually required.

## Acute Rejection

AR episodes complicate the clinical course of the majority of transplanted kidneys. The first episode of AR usually occurs within the first two months and can occur as early as seven to 10 days post transplant. Fever, allograft tenderness, swelling, and declining

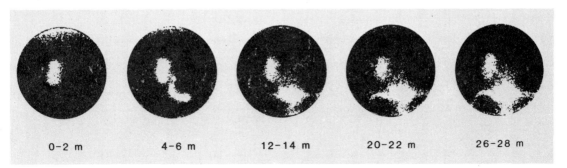

0–2 m        4–6 m        12–14 m        20–22 m        26–28 m

**Figure 34–12.** [123]I-orthoiodohippurate renal scintiphotoscan of a normal functioning allograft transplanted into an ileal loop.

renal function with reduction in urine volume are the classic clinical manifestations. Weight gain is a consequence of reduced renal function and avid sodium reabsorption. Hypertension, which frequently accompanies the various signs, may occasionally be the sole manifestation of the rejection episode. Treatment with steroids will reverse the hypertension occurring with the rejection episode while other forms of hypertension will be aggravated by similar therapy. The alterations of renal function observed reflect the ischemia present in the renal allograft.[42] If initial allograft function was present, this decline in function will be reflected by an elevation of the serum creatinine level. The development of oliguria after a period of adequate diuresis, decreased urinary sodium excretion, and increased urinary osmolality in the absence of hypertension suggest rejection.[43] Proteinuria is almost always present in AR; however, nephrotic-range proteinuria is rarely encountered. Recently, Jaber et al reported that the degree of protein excretion post transplant was helpful in identifying AR episodes, and lack of response of proteinuria to antirejection treatment predicted poor graft outcome.[44]

Various tubular abnormalities have been reported in association with AR.[45] The development of renal tubular acidosis may either accompany or precede the rejection episode by one to two weeks. It usually does not bear any correlation with prognosis, but the finding of complement deposition ($C_3$) in the tubules of the allograft has been suggested as a poor prognostic sign.[46] Other findings, such as lysozymuria or urinary fibrin fragments, only reflect tubular impairment. In rare instances, the complete expression of the Fanconi syndrome has been reported.[47] Ultrasonography may be useful in differentiating AR from obstruction of the allograft. In AR, the medullary pyramids are enlarged, followed by a heightened cortical echogenicity resulting in an increased thickness of the renal cortex with an overall increase in renal size. The enlargement of renal cortex of the graft may precede the rise in the serum creatinine level.[48]

The renal scintiphotoscan with [123]I-orthoiodohippurate appears to be particularly useful in detecting AR. The study is usually performed on the first postoperative day for early assessment of allograft function and as a baseline for subsequent studies when indicated. In AR (Fig. 34–13), comparison with the original study will reveal: (1) reduced rate of uptake of the hippurate; (2) frequent irregular uptake of the hippurate in the allograft cortex; (3) delay in intrarenal transit of hippurate; and (4) decreased excretion of the tracer into the renal collecting structures.[40]

With the availability of the renal scintiphotoscan in most centers, and because of the particular sensitivity of the allograft to contrast nephropathy, renal arteriography of the allograft is now rarely indicated for the diagnosis of AR. When performed, it will reveal a prolongation of the arterial washout time, with enlargement of the kidney due to interstitial edema, hemorrhage, and inflammation. According to the severity or the stage of rejection, the arteriogram will show various degrees of stretching of the intrarenal arterial branches, with poor filling of the cortical vessels and an ill-defined non-uniform or striated cortical nephrogram and corticomedullary junction with poor or no visualization of the renal vein.[49, 50]

Biopsy of the allograft is rarely indicated with AR, since the diagnosis of AR can usually be made on the basis of clinical and laboratory presentation or by noninvasive techniques (e.g., renal ultrasound and renal scintiphotoscan). However, a biopsy should be considered in recipients unresponsive to

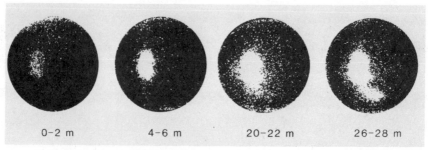

0–2 m          4–6 m          20–22 m          26–28 m

**Figure 34–13.** [123]I-orthoiodohippurate renal scintiphotoscan during an acute rejection episode of the allograft. Note the delayed uptake, transit, and excretion of the tracer.

antirejection therapy or where other factors (e.g., cytomegalovirus glomerulopathy or recurrence of original disease) are suspected. Routine biopsies performed in patients with normal and stable allograft function have revealed latent rejection episodes.[51] Whether treatment is indicated or not in these instances remains unclear, but in some patients treated with steroid therapy subsequent biopsies showed improvement. The correlation of the biopsy findings with long-term allograft survival has not been well established.

Allograft biopsies may provide useful information when multiple rejection episodes are encountered, since the demonstration of a predominantly vascular rejection would predict poor allograft outcome.[52] At the present time, the role of routine post-transplant biopsy in predicting AR is minimal;[53] however, using routine immunofluorescence on the one-hour post-transplant biopsy, Paul et al were able to predict AAR by demonstrating anti-E antibody fixation to vascular endothelial cells.[36] The allograft ceased to function 72 hours later. Therefore, routine allograft biopsy may be useful in predicting AR or AAR in certain allograft recipients.

## Chronic Rejection

While the expression of other types of rejection is usually abrupt and restricted to a definite period of time, the development of CR is more insidious and occurs in the absence of obvious physical symptoms and signs. There is a slow and progressive rise in the serum creatinine level. Hypertension may complicate the rejection progress. Significant proteinuria may occur, particularly when glomerular lesions are well developed. The spectrum of pathologic manifestations is variable, as described earlier and is unresponsive to antirejection therapy. In the majority of cases, there is a progressive reduction of allograft function that leads to reinstitution of dialysis therapy. However, in some instances, stabilization of allograft function may occur for a prolonged period of time before any further deterioration occurs.

## DIFFERENTIAL DIAGNOSIS OF REJECTION (TABLE 34–2)

There are several conditions that may simulate rejection episodes in both the early and late post-transplant period. A consideration of these conditions follows.

## Early Post-Transplant Period

**Hypovolemia.** Reduction of allograft function in the post-transplant period may be a consequence of inadequate hydration of the recipient, particularly if the diuresis is well established and the urinary losses not adequately replaced. Fluid therapy will reverse the fluid deficit, but prolonged hypovolemia is associated with the development of acute tubular necrosis (ATN).

**Acute Tubular Necrosis.** ATN represents the most common cause of renal failure in the immediate post-transplantation period. Its frequency is often related to the increased duration of the warm ischemic time with agonal hypotension in the donor.[54] Oliguria is the rule, but, as in AAR, a brief period of diuresis occasionally occurs. In other instances, nonoliguric renal failure is present. In recipients with their native kidneys in place, the assessment of urine output may be unreliable.

The renal scintiphotoscan with [123]I-orthoiodohippurate provides helpful information in the presence of ATN. The allograft demonstrates uniformity of tracer uptake without evidence of excretion (Fig. 34–14). It should be emphasized, however, that the first scintiphotoscan should not be performed until 24 hours post transplantation since the renal damage produced by anoxia in ATN tends to reach its maximum after 24 hours.[40] Further deterioration due to the tubular insult is not seen after that period. Allograft rejection occurring in patients with ATN is difficult to detect clinically, since one cannot monitor urine output, serum creatinine level, elevated blood pressure, and weight gain as indicators of the rejection episode. However, the renal scintiphotoscan can be used to differentiate ATN from rejection. In continuing uncomplicated ATN, there is no change in uptake of [123]I-hippuran by the allograft. Deterioration of radiopharmaceutical uptake and reduced excretion compared to the baseline study 24 hours post transplantation is diagnostic of rejection.

In some recipients with ATN, in the absence of other signs of rejection, the onset of persistent or recurrent fever may suggest superimposed AR.

**Obstruction.** In the immediate post-transplant period, abrupt cessation of diuresis may indicate catheter obstruction by a blood clot, particularly if macroscopic hematuria is present. Irrigation or replacement of the catheter is curative.

**Table 34-2.** DIFFERENTIAL DIAGNOSIS OF REJECTION

| Early Post-Transplantation Period | | Late Post-Transplantation Period |
|---|---|---|
| Hypovolemia | | Superimposed acute rejection |
| Acute tubular necrosis | | Recurrence of original disease |
| Obstruction: Extrinsic: | Urinary catheter obstruction (blood clot) | Obstruction |
| | Ureteral obstruction (hematoma, lymphocele) | Renal artery stenosis |
| Intrinsic: | Ureteral or vesical obstruction (swelling or infarction of ureter | Nephrotoxic agents |
| | tip, edema of bladder with compression of intramural ureter) | Infection |
| Extravasation of urine | | |
| Arterial complications: | Thrombosis | |
| | Stenosis | |
| Venous complications: | Thrombosis | |
| | Venous embolism | |
| Infection | | |

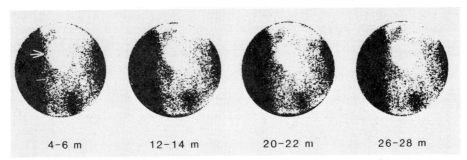

**Figure 34–14.** [123]I-orthoiodohippurate renal scintiphotoscan showing adequate tracer uptake (arrow) by the allograft undergoing acute tubular necrosis but no evidence of excretion.

Ureteral obstruction may be difficult to detect because it may be completely asymptomatic. Oliguria and reduction in renal function are often present, but a partial obstruction may be accompanied by adequate diuresis.

Many factors contribute to ureteral obstruction. An extrinsic compression of the ureter may be due to a hematoma or a large lymphocele. Occasionally, obstruction at the ureterovesical junction may be due to swelling or infarction of the ureteral tip or to edema of the bladder with external pressure on the intramural portion of the ureter. Ultrasonography of the allograft and the adjacent urinary structures is useful, even in the case of partial obstruction. The study will often reveal minimal to moderate dilation of the renal pelvis. However, mild dilation is often present in the normal functioning allograft. The renal scintiphotoscan with [123]I-orthoiodohippurate is helpful in moderate to severe obstruction when oliguria or anuria is present (Fig. 34–15). The scintiphotoscan reveals the presence of a large hilar defect in the allograft corresponding to the absence of radioisotope in an enlarged renal pelvis. In a patient with a slowly rising serum creatinine level, moderate ureteral obstruction can be

differentiated from rejection by the accumulation and persistence of radioisotope in an enlarged renal pelvis.

**Extravasation of Urine.** Urinary extravasation which may mimic rejection is manifested clinically by a reduction in urine output, progressive allograft tenderness, unexplained fever, impaired allograft function, and swelling at the operative site. In addition, edema of the scrotum, labia, or thigh ipsilateral to the allograft may be present with drainage from the wound. The diagnosis can be confirmed by ultrasonography, intravenous urography, or occasionally by renal scintiphotoscan. In some instances, the intravenous injection of 5 ml of indigo carmine or methylene blue is diagnostic when these substances are rapidly detected in the extravasated urine.[55]

Interruption of the arterial supply to the allograft ureter due to damage by close dissection of the allograft or the possibility of rejection of the ureter[56, 57] has been proposed as potential causes for the urinary extravasation.

Urinary leakage is occasionally seen secondary to bladder fistulae with manifestations similar to those of ureteral disruption. Rapid detection of the defect is mandatory

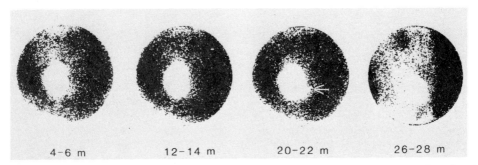

**Figure 34–15.** [123]I-orthoiodohippurate renal scintiphotoscan in the presence of obstruction of the allograft at the renal pelvis (arrow).

as it is associated with serious complications, such as wound infection, perirenal abscess, septicemia, or progressive and irreversible deterioration of allograft function.

**Vascular Complications.** *Thrombosis.* Allograft artery thrombosis may develop immediately post transplant or up to several weeks following surgery. It is heralded by sudden oliguria or anuria, macroscopic hematuria and edema, or retroperitoneal bleeding. The diagnosis should also be suspected if the paired kidney in another recipient has satisfactory function. The renal scintiphotoscan shows virtually no uptake of the tracer because of the lack of renal perfusion[40] (Fig. 34–16). Immediate surgical exploration is mandatory; however, recovery of allograft function is minimal. Renal venous thrombosis occurs infrequently.

*Stenosis.* Stenotic lesions of the renal artery may mimic AR as early as three to four weeks post transplantation.[57]

*Infection.* The immunosuppressive therapy used in allograft recipients results in an increased risk of infection, particularly viral infection. Herpesviruses (cytomegalovirus [CMV], herpes simplex, and herpes zoster) have been frequently isolated. The clinical presentation of fever and reduction of renal function associated with these infections (particularly CMV) may suggest AR. Not infrequently, allograft function deteriorates with CMV infection. It is not clear whether the virus initiates a rejection episode or if the decreased allograft function is due to CMV glomerulopathy.[61]

Certain clinical findings may suggest a viral origin to explain the nature of the febrile episode.[62] The fever is frequently recurrent, and, despite significant elevation of temperature, the patient may be in no particular distress. In addition, the determination of the white blood cell count will often reveal a leukopenia (total peripheral leukocyte count less than 5000/mm³ for two or more consecutive days), and seroconversion is frequent. CMV can be isolated from blood (buffy coat), urine, and bone marrow, but the incubation period for viral growth may be 10 days to two weeks. The diagnosis of CMV or other viral infections is important, since alteration in immunosuppressive therapy is indicated and because other opportunistic pathogens (i.e., *Pneumocystis carinii* and Legionella) commonly complicate the course of CMV infection.

### Late Post-Transplant Period

CR is the commonest cause of late allograft failure. Its development may be seen as early as a few weeks after transplantation or years after a long period of good allograft function.

The occurrence of AR is significantly reduced with time, but AR may be superimposed on an allograft undergoing CR.

**Recurrence of Original Disease.** The glomerular lesions associated with CR described earlier in this chapter vary from mesangial proliferation to alterations of the GBM with deposits. Diseases such as focal and segmental glomerulosclerosis (FGS), membranoproliferative glomerulonephritis (MPGN), and rapidly progressive glomerulonephritis (with or without glomerular basement membrane antibodies) have reappeared in the transplanted kidney.[63-68] As for FGS, significant proteinuria may occur, but the recurrence of the disease is frequently seen soon after transplantation, and reduction of renal function may not appear despite marked proteinuria. MPGN, particularly associated with dense deposit disease, may reappear late in the posttransplant period and be responsible for allograft failure.[69, 70] In these circumstances, recurrence of the original disease can be differentiated from glomerular lesions of CR only by allograft biopsy.

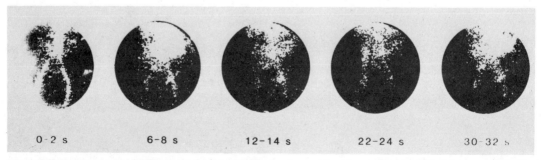

| 0–2 s | 6–8 s | 12–14 s | 22–24 s | 30–32 s |

**Figure 34–16.** ⁹⁹Technetium-DTPA renal scintiphotoscan showing no blood flow to the allograft. Subsequent pathologic examination of the allograft revealed renal artery thrombosis.

**Obstruction.** The development of ureteral obstruction may be insidious and may be expressed by slowly deteriorating allograft function as in CR. The obstruction is frequently at the site of the uretero-neocystostomy, and ultrasonography may once again be diagnostic. Occasionally, ureteral obstruction may be due to surrounding fibrosis, lymphocele, local host immunologic responses, or the development of lithiasis, especially in patients with persistent hyperparathyoidism following transplantation.

**Renal Artery Stenosis.** Renal artery stenosis is a not infrequent complication seen in the late post-transplant period and may present with hypertension and a reduction in renal function. The development of an audible bruit over the allograft suggests stenosis, but its absence does not exclude this diagnosis. Digital vascular imaging (DVI-scan), a venous substraction study, will often reveal the stenosis, which can be confirmed by renal arteriography. Transluminal dilatation of the stenotic segment may correct the hypertension, improve allograft function, and eliminate or delay the need for surgical correction.[71, 72]

**Nephrotoxic Agents.** Occasionally, reduction of allograft function has been seen after administration of antibiotic therapy, particularly with gentamycin.[73] It appears that the renal allograft is more sensitive to all nephrotoxins (contrast material, aminoglycosides, etc.) and nonsteroidal anti-inflammatory agents.[76, 77]

**Infection.** The viral agents implicated in the alteration of renal function in the early post-transplant period may be operative after establishment of normal allograft function in spite of reduced antirejection therapy. CMV remains an ominous pathogen and its presentation is similar to that described earlier.

Occasionally, ureteral obstruction associated with hydronephrosis, stasis, and bacterial infection is associated with fever and reduction in allograft function. Ultrasonography and appropriate cultures may delineate the problem.

Bacterial infection of the urinary tract in allograft recipients often results in fever and reduction in allograft function. Appropriate diagnosis and therapy usually results in improved allograft function. If recurrent infection occurs, evaluation of the urinary tract (both native and allograft) is essential to rule out obstruction, reflux, and occult abscess.

# REFERENCES

1. Baldwin WM, Claas FHJ, van Es LA, et al: Renal graft rejection and the antigenic anatomy of the kidney. Transplant Clin Immunol 13:140, 1981.
2. Ting A, Morris PJ: Powerful effect of HLA-DR matching on survival of cadaveric renal allografts. Lancet 2:282, 1980.
3. McPhaul JJ Jr, Mauk R, Mullins JD: Renal transplantation: Some contemporary problems. *In:* Wilson CB (ed), Immunologic Mechanisms of Renal Disease. New York, Churchill-Livingstone, 1979, p 323.
4. Stiller C: Cyclosporin A treatment of the renal transplant recipient. Symposia presented at the 15th annual meeting of The American Society of Nephrology, Chicago, Ill., December 14, 1982.
5. Dausset J, Hons J, Busson, M., et al: Serologically defined HL-A antigens and long-term survival of cadaver kidney transplants. A joint analysis of 918 cases performed by the France transplant and the London Transplant Group. N Engl J Med 290:979, 1974.
6. Carpenter CB, D'Apice AJF, Abbas AK: Role of antibodies in the rejection and enhancement of organ allografts. Adv Immunol 22:1, 1976.
7. Jordan SC, Malekzadeh MH, Pennisi AJ, et al: Accelerated acute rejection of primary renal allograft in pediatric patients. Transplantation 30:5, 1980.
8. Strober S, Gowans JL: The role of lymphocytes in the sensitization of rats to renal homografts. J Exp Med 122:347, 1965.
9. Balch CM, Wilson CB, Lee S, Feldman JD: Thymus-dependent lymphocytes in tissue sections of rejecting rat renal allografts. J Exp Med 138:1584, 1973.
10. Drevyanko T, Encolanil L: Evaluation of cellular infiltrates in human renal allografts with monoclonal anibodies and heteroantisera. Presented, American Society of Nephrology, Chicago, Illinois, December 12–14, 1982 (Abstr), p 195a.
11. Kissmeyer-Nielsen F, Olsen S, Petersen VP, Fieldbong O: Hyperacute rejection of kidney allografts, associated with preexisting humoral antibodies against donor cells. Lancet 2:662, 1966.
12. Williams GM, Hume DM, Hudson RP, et al: "Hyperacute" renal-homograft rejection in man. N Engl J Med 279:611, 1968.
13. Patel R, Terasaki PI: Significance of the positive cross-match test in kidney transplantation. N Engl J Med 280:735, 1969.
14. Starzl TE, Lerner RA, Dixon FJ, et al: Shwartzman reaction after human renal homotransplantation. N Engl J Med 278:642, 1968.
15. Schiff M Jr, Goffinet JA, Hendler E, et al: Shwartzman reaction in an HL-A identical renal allograft. Transplantation 17:580, 1974.
16. Berne TV, Gustafsson LA, Chatterjee SN: Early severe renal allograft rejection. Arch Surg 111:758, 1976.
17. Paul LC, Claas FH, van Es L, et al: Accelerated rejection of renal allograft associated with pre-transplant antibodies directed against donor antigens on endothelium and monocytes. N Engl J Med 300:1258, 1979.
18. Anderson CB, Newton WT: Accelerated human

renal allograft rejection. Arch Surg 110:1230, 1975.

19. Lucas ZJ, Coplon N, Kempson R, et al: Early renal transplant failure associated with subliminal sensitization. Transplantation 10:522, 1970.

20. Jordan SC, Sakai RS, Malekzadeh M, et al: Circulating immune complexes in pediatric renal allograft rejection. Transplantation 31:190, 1981.

21. Jordan SC, Sakai RS, Ettenger RB, Fine RN: Circulating immune complexes during various forms of allograft rejection episodes. Nephron 31:141, 1982.

22. Baldwin M, Souillou JP, Claas FHJ, et al: Antibodies to endothelial antigens in eluates of 88 human kidneys: Correlation with graft survival and presence of T- and B-cell antibodies. Transplant Proc 13:1547, 1981.

23. Dammin GJ: The pathology of human renal transplantation. In: Human Transplantation, Rapaport FT, Dausset J (Eds) New York, Grune & Stratton, 1977, p 170.

24. Busch GJ, Reynolds ES, Galvanek EG, et al: Human renal allografts: the role of vascular injury in early graft failure. Medicine 50:29, 1974.

25. Corson JM: The pathologist and the kidney transplant. Pathol Annual 7:251, 1972.

26. Sinclair RA, Antonovych TT, Mostofi FK: Renal proliferative arteriopathies and associated glomerular changes: a light and electron microscopic study. Hum Pathol 7:565, 1976.

27. Lindquist RR, Guttmann RD, Merrill JP, Dammin GJ: Human renal allografts. Interpretation of morphologic and immunohistochemical observations. Am J Pathol 53:851, 1968.

28. Petersen VP, Elsen TS, Kissmeyer-Nielsen F, et al: Late failure of renal transplants. An analysis of transplant disease and graft failure among 125 recipients surviving for 1–8 years. Medicine 54:45, 1975.

29. Mathew TH, Mathews DC, Hobbs JB, Kincaid-Smith P: Glomerular lesions after renal transplantation. Am J Med 59:177, 1975.

30. Hulme BP, Andres GA, Porter KA, Ogden DA: Human renal transplants. IV. Glomerular ultrastructure, macromolecular permeability and hemodynamics. Lab Invest 26:2, 1972.

31. Olsen S, Bohman S-O, Petersen VP: Ultrastructure of the glomerular basement membrane in long term renal allografts with transplant glomerular disease. Lab Invest 30:176, 1974.

32. Ooi YM, Ooi BS, Vallota EH, et al: Circulating immune complexes after transplantation. J Clin Invest 60:611, 1977.

33. Johny KV, Dasgupta MK, Kovithavorgs T, Dossetor JB: Serial studies of circulating immune complexes before and after renal transplantation. Kidney Int 19:322, 1981.

34. Souillou JP, deMouzon-Camlbon A, Dubois M, et al: Immunological studies of eluates of 83 rejected kidneys. Transplantation 32:368, 1981.

35. Baldwin WM, Claas FHJ, van Es LA, van Rood JJ: Distribution of endothelial-monocyte and HLA antigens on renal vascular endothelium. Transplant Proc 3:103, 1980.

36. Paul LC, van Es LA, van Rood JJ, et al: Antibodies directed against antigens on the endothelium of peritubular capillaries in patients with rejecting allografts. Transplantation 27:175, 1979.

37. Moy J, Rosenau W: Demonstration of alpha-lym-

photoxin in human rejected renal allografts. Clin Immunol Immunopathol 20:49, 1981.

38. Milliner DS, Pierides DS, Holley KE: Renal transplantation in Alport's syndrome. Mayo Clin Proc 57:35, 1982.

39. Collins JJ, Wilson RE: Functional evaluation of human kidney transplant with renograms. Ann Surg 161:428, 1965.

40. Salvatierra O, Powell MR, Price DC, et al: The advantages of [131]I-orthoiodohippurate scintiphotography in the management of patients after renal transplantation. Ann Surg 180:336, 1974.

41. Baltzman MA, Baltzman RB, Pastershank S, et al: Early acute rejection of renal homografts: a characteristic clinical syndrome. Can Med Assoc J 109:101, 1973.

42. Lee DBN, Prompt CA, Upham AT, Kleeman CR: Medical complications of renal transplantation. I. Graft and infectious complications in recipient. Urology (Suppl) 9:7, 1977.

43. Merrill JP: Diagnosis and management of rejection in allografted kidneys. Transplant Proc 3:387, 1971.

44. Jaber P, Davidson E, Lau K: Proteinuria as an early marker of renal transplant rejection and poor steroid response. Abstract presented at American Society of Nephrology Annual Meeting 198A, 1982.

45. Mookerjee B, Gault MH, Dossetor JB: Hyperchloremic acidosis in early diagnosis of renal allograft rejection. Ann Intern Med 71:47, 1969.

46. Battle DC, Mozes MF, Manaligod J, et al: The pathogenesis of hyperchloremic metabolic acidosis associated with kidney transplantation. Am J Med 70:786, 1981.

47. Leonard L, Vertuno MC, Preuss HG, et al: Fanconi syndrome following homotransplantation. Arch Intern Med 133:302, 1974.

48. Hricak H, Toiedo-Pereyra LH, Eyler WR, et al: The role of ultrasound in the diagnosis of kidney allograft rejection. Radiology 132:667, 1979.

49. Pool, R: Angiographic aspects in kidney transplantation. Radiol Clin 47:22, 1978.

50. Michel JR, Moreau J, Japhet Y: L'arteriographic dans la transplantation renale. Ann Radiol 16:361, 1973.

51. Hamburger J, Crosnier J, Back JF, Kreis H: Renal Transplantation: Theory and Practice. London, Williams & Wilkins, 1981, pp 205, 240.

52. Banfi G, Imbasciati C, Tarantino A, et al: Prognostic value of renal biopsy in acute rejection of kidney transplantation. Nephron 28:222, 1981.

53. Matas AJ, Sibley R, Mauer SM, et al: Pre-discharge, post-transplant kidney biopsy does not predict rejection. J Surg Res 32:269, 1982.

54. Simmons RL, Kjellstrand CM, Najarian JS: Technique, complications and results. In: Najarian JS, Simmons RL (Eds), Transplantation. Philadelphia, Lea and Febiger, 1972, p 465.

55. Williams GM: Clinical course following renal transplantation. In: Kidney Transplantation: Principles and Practice, Morris PH (Ed). London, Academic Press, 1979.

56. Haber MH, Putong PB: Ureteral vascular rejection in human renal transplants. JAMA 192:417, 1965.

57. Simmons RL, Jallent MB, Kjellstrand CM, et al: Renal allograft rejection simulated by arterial stenosis. Surgery 68:800, 1970.

58. Rao KV, Smith EJ, Alexander JW, et al: Throm-

boembolic disease in renal allograft recipients. Arch Surg 111:1086, 1976.

59. Arruda JAL, Gutierrez LF, Jonasson O, et al: Renal vein thrombosis in kidney allografts. Lancet 2:585, 1973.

60. Golden J, Stone RA, Goldberger L: Immune-related vein thrombosis in a renal allograft. Ann Intern Med 85:612, 1976.

61. Richardson WP, Colvin RB, Cheeseman SH, et al: Glomerulopathy associated with cytomegalovirus viremia in renal allografts. N Engl J Med 305:57, 1981.

62. Lopez C, Simmons RL, Mauer SM, et al: Association of renal allograft rejection with virus infections. Am J Med 56:280, 1974.

63. Dixon FJ, McPhaul JJ Jr, Lerner RA: Recurrence of glomerulonephritis in the transplanted kidney. Arch Intern Med 123:554, 1969.

64. Galle P, Hinglais N, Crosnier J: Recurrence of an original glomerular lesion in three renal allografts. Transplant Proc, 3:368, 1971.

65. Hume DM, Bryan CP: The development of recurrent glomerulonephritis. Transplant Proc 4:673, 1972.

66. Hoyer JR, Raij L, Vernier RL, et al: Recurrence of idiopathic nephrotic syndrome after renal transplantation. Lancet 2:343, 1972.

67. Beleil OM, Coburn JW, Shinaberger JH, Glassock AJ: Recurrent glomerulonephritis due to anti-glomerula basement membrane antibodies in two successive allografts. Clin Nephrol 1:377, 1973.

68. Droz D, Zanetti M, Noel LH, Leibowitch J: Dense deposits disease. Nephron 19:1, 1977.

69. Turner DR, Cameron JS, Bewick M, et al: Transplantation in mesangiocapillary glomerulonephritis with intramembranous dense "deposits." Recurrence of disease. Kidney Int 9:439, 1976.

70. Eddy A, Sibley R, Kim Y: Renal allograft failure due to recurrent dense intramembranous deposit disease (DIDD). Abstract presented at American Society of Nephrol of Annual Meeting, 1982, p 29A.

71. Grossman RA, Dafoe DC, Shoenfeld RB, et al: Percutaneous transluminal angioplasty treatment of renal transplant artery stenosis. Transplantation 34:339, 1982.

72. Barth KH, Brusilow SW, Kaufman SL, Ferry FT: Percutaneous transluminal angioplasty of homograft renal artery stenosis in a 10-year-old girl. Pediatrics 67:675, 1981.

73. Wellwood JM, Simpson PM, Tighe JR, Thompson GE: Evidence of gentamycin nephrotoxicity in patients with renal allografts. Br Med J 3:278, 1975.

74. Dixon FJ, McPhaul JJ Jr, Lerner R: Recurrence of glomerulonephritis in the transplanted kidney. Arch Intern Med 123:554, 1969.

75. Van Caugh PV, Ehrlich RM, Smith RB: Renal rupture after transplantation. Urology 9:8, 1977.

76. Neidman M, Claes G, Nilson AE: The risk of renal allograft rejection following angiography. Transplantation 21:289, 1976.

77. Mudge GH: Nephrotoxicity of urographic radiocontrast drugs. Kidney Int 18:540, 1980.

# 35

# Immunosuppressive Therapy for Pediatric Renal Allograft Recipients

*Gerald S. Arbus, M.D., F.R.C.P. (C)*
*Brian E. Hardy, M.B., Ch.B., F.R.A.C.S.*

## PRINCIPLES OF REJECTION WITH POSSIBLE AVENUES FOR TREATING WITH MEDICATION

An immunologically mature animal presented with a non-self antigen mounts an immune response. For this reason tissue allografting must be accompanied by attempted immunosuppression if the allograft is to survive over the long term. There are two basic components to the immune response—humoral and cellular. The humoral response is mediated by macrophages, thymus-dependent (T) lymphocytes and thymus-independent bone-marrow-derived (B) lymphocytes working together. In this interaction B cells are directly responsible for the synthesis and secretion of the antigen-specific antibody, while T cells provide the essential regulatory signals. The cell-mediated immune response is not dependent upon secreted antibodies but rather works through the direct contact of antigen-specific effector lymphocytes (T cells) and target cells.[1]

To understand the developing trends in immunosuppression, this simplified view of the immune system needs some amplification. There are functionally distinct populations of T cells which participate in different aspects of the immune response. Helper and suppressor T cells contribute to the regulation of humoral immunity while cytotoxic T cells and T-cell mediators of delayed-type hypersensitivity are the effectors of cell-mediated immunity.

The antigen encountered in the humoral response is responsible for first expanding the appropriate B-cell clone and then inducing the maturation of those lymphocytes into plasma cells capable of delivering secreted antibody into the serum. Except for T-independent antigens it appears that two kinds of signals are necessary to trigger both proliferation and differentiation. One signal can induce proliferation in a population of mature B cells without aid from helper T cells or macrophages, but antibody synthesis cannot be induced by this single signal alone. Much of the negative regulation (suppression) of the immune response is mediated by suppressor T lymphocytes. Suppressor T cells appear to work largely by targeting on helper T cells, but they may also interfere with B cells directly.

Whereas suppressor T cells can bind free antigen, helper T cells and cytolytic T cells can only recognize antigen which is associated with major histocompatibility center gene products. Macrophages take up antigen and, having made this association, present the antigen in a form which is immunogenic to helper T cells and cytolytic T cells. If macrophages fail to process and present the antigen in its original form, the organism is unable to mount an immune response against that antigen. Furthermore, a subsequent state of antigen-specific unresponsiveness develops. (This is probably mediated by suppressor T cells.)

If tolerance is defined as the failure of an animal to mount an immune response against a specific antigen (self or non-self in origin), the subject is clearly of major importance to anyone attempting immunosuppression. It appears that immaturity of the lymphocytes, not of the animal, is the essential ingredient of the ability to induce tolerance. The mechanisms involved in inducing tolerance are as yet unclear but could include deletion or inactivation of specific lymphocyte clones, suppression of reactive B or T lymphocytes by suppressor T cells, and inactivation of the receptors by antigen. Such a state of tolerance can be maintained through either the B- or the T-cell population.

Finally, it has been postulated that the immune system regulates itself via an immune response. As lymphocytes proliferate in response to an antigen, the receptors on those lymphocytes can themselves act as antigens (idiotype). Anti-idiotypic lymphocytes then exert an inhibitory influence on the initial population. Clearly, this would be only step one in a succession of similar events. To date the theory is neither proved nor disproved. Its integration into immunologic theory is far from complete.

## IMMUNOSUPPRESSIVE THERAPY IN RENAL TRANSPLANT RECIPIENTS

Medication is the major form of immunosuppressive therapy in renal transplant recipients. During the past 15 years there has been little change in the drugs used, since few new drugs have been developed. Glucocorticoids (steroids) and azathioprine remain the medications of choice for preventive therapy. Various early types of therapy, such as actinomycin, are now seldom used while others, for example, splenectomy, continue to be used in some centers but remain controversial. The validity of recently developed therapies (plasmapheresis and monoclonal antibodies) has not been tested sufficiently to be considered scientifically established.

Confirming the validity of new approaches is difficult. During the past several years, many reports have compared results in early and later years within a single program in which a new therapy has been introduced at a particular stage. Unfortunately, such comparisons are often invalid since programs may undergo many changes over a few years, for example, in blood transfusion protocol, use of less selective admission procedures, involvement of more experienced personnel, or use of better monitoring procedures. A new treatment which is expected to provide a small but significant improvement (about 10%) is not easily validated. Very large numbers of patients are required for control trials and few centers are prepared to undertake them. As a result, new treatments are often used routinely in some centers before their efficacy is established.

## Glucocorticoids (Steroids)

Glucocorticosteroid therapy has been part of host immunosuppression since the first successful human renal allograft.[2] Corticosteroids alter the circulation of lymphocytes and cause lymphocytopenia. However, they also reduce the number of macrophages and cause decreased phagocytosis. Steroid-induced suppression of cell-mediated immune responses appears to be achieved largely via its effects on macrophages.[3]

Glucocorticoids (steroids), usually in the form of prednisone, prednisolone, or methylprednisolone, are still the mainstay for patients with renal transplants. Steroids are used for both preventive therapy and treatment of acute rejection episodes. In isolated cases, however, prophylactic steroids have not been given.[4] One study compared the outcome in two groups: 54 patients who were given steroids only at the onset of their first renal failure episode and 53 patients who received prophylactic steroid treatment. The incidence of reversible and irreversible renal failure episodes was identical in the two groups.[5] Nevertheless, prophylactic steroids continue to be generally accepted as a necessary form of treatment for renal transplant recipients.

Most programs begin post-transplant maintenance with relatively high doses of prednisone (1 to 3 mg/kg body weight per day). Recently McGeown et al,[6, 7] Buckels et al,[8] and Morris et al[9] reported giving 20 to 30 mg prednisone (prednisolone) per day from day one post-transplant with no untoward problems. We have not employed this treatment regimen.

**Glucocorticoids as Maintenance Therapy at The Hospital for Sick Children, Toronto.** Since our first renal transplant in 1969, we have used oral prednisone or intravenous methylprednisolone. We start with a single dose of 3 mg/kg body weight (maximum 120 mg) daily for one week, with an additional dose initially given pretransplant.[10] The prednisone is reduced to about 1.5 mg/kg body weight per day by the end of the second or third week post-transplant, then gradually tapered to about 20 to 30 mg/day (less than this in very small children), and finally switched to alternate days. At discharge five or six weeks after transplant most of our patients are on alternate-day therapy, although an occasional patient is still in the transition period to such therapy. Only nine of our first 200 renal transplants involved living donors and, except for two days of azathioprine and prednisone pretransplant, the medication regimen was identical in these patients to that in recipients of cadaveric renal transplants.

Immunosuppressive therapy in hospitalized patients is usually given in the afternoon, after the morning serum creatinine values have been reviewed. At home, this medication is given each morning.[11] Gradually the alternate-day prednisone is reduced so that by three to six months post-transplant the number of mg of prednisone the patient is taking every second day is approximately equal to the patient's age in years; thus children less than three years old take approximately 2.5 mg, four- to seven-year-olds take 5 mg, and eight- to 12-year-olds take 10 mg every second day.

Patients returning to our transplant clinic for follow-up arrive before 1100 hours to have blood drawn and are seen from 1300 hours when blood test results are known. About half the children live a distance from Toronto; having the serum creatinine values available for the clinic is therefore helpful in allowing us to act (e.g., do a repeat blood test, start anti-rejection treatment in clinic), if necessary, before the patient returns home.

If patients are stable while the every-second-day medication is being reduced, they attend the clinic once every two weeks. They are advised to reduce the medication one week preceding the next clinic visit so that any problems arising with the new dose can be detected within one week of change in therapy. By one year post-transplant, children are seen monthly and, eventually, long-term patients are seen about every six weeks.

**Alternate-Day Glucocorticoid Therapy.** Initially, switching to alternate-day steroids was undertaken only after the patient was stable on daily steroids for upward of two to three years[12–14] and the actual switch was usually done very gradually.[15] Early reports of this procedure were from adult centers and included only the occasional child.[12, 13, 15] The few controlled studies[16–18] have shown no appreciable risk in switching patients to alternate-day prednisone therapy. All programs have reported stability and, in many cases, a lessening of the steroid side effects in patients maintained on alternate-day therapy. Recently, a dose of 15 mg prednisone every second day has been shown to be as effective in adults as 15 mg daily.[16]

A trial of alternate-day steroid therapy became warranted in our pediatric transplant patients and in 1971 every transplanted patient was switched to alternate-day therapy. As expected, a few rejection episodes ensued, but all were readily reversed. Since then, no patient in our program who is still growing has been maintained on daily prednisone. The switch to alternate-day prednisone is usually accomplished within four to six weeks post-transplant. In older patients, daily prednisone is continued in the few patients who have repeated minor rejection episodes, which are more of a nuisance than anything else; in these instances, the daily dose is equivalent to what would have been given as an alternate-day dose (e.g., 10 mg prednisone every day rather than 20 mg every second day).

**Diagnosis of an Acute Rejection and Treatment with Glucocorticoids.** At present no single test can precisely diagnose when renal allografts are undergoing an acute rejection. We tend to assign a narrow 0.3 mg/dl unit range for serum creatinine values to a patient. For example, a child may be expected to keep his serum creatinine levels between 1.0 and 1.2 mg/dl. If a value of 1.3 mg/dl occurs occasionally within a period of a year or so, we are not too concerned, provided the patient is otherwise stable, since growth with increases in muscle mass may naturally cause elevated serum creatinine values. However, if such a rise in serum creatinine occurs in the first month post-transplant, the child undergoes a full assessment including physical examination (looking particularly for fever, graft tenderness, signs of extrarenal infection, vascular volume), urinalysis, renal scan, and so on to rule out causes not related to rejection that might be responsible for the rise in serum creatinine. Still, at times the diagnosis of rejection is one of exclusion, with steroid therapy given because no other cause is found.

If a patient continues to maintain an elevated serum creatinine level despite high-dose glucocorticoid therapy or if other treatment is being contemplated, a renal biopsy is usually performed. The problems in interpreting the pathology seen from doing a renal biopsy are manifold. What pathologic picture is usually seen in a non-rejecting kidney after weeks, months, or years of being in place? Can a biopsy predict whether (and what type of) medication will be useful in reversing the rejection?[19] How often is sampling error introduced when a closed biopsy is taken? This last problem is reduced if an open biopsy is done and the surgeon can take a representative sample.

To compound the confusion, it has been shown recently that infections such as cytomegalovirus have given clinical and renal pathologic pictures similar to that of rejection;[20] in view of this, additional anti-rejection medication may be contraindicated.

When rejection is "diagnosed," most programs give an increased dose of steroids orally or intravenously. This treatment is given daily or every second day for a total of three or four doses and then either abruptly or gradually reduced to the previous maintenance dosage. Although very high amounts of steroids were used some years ago, equally good success has been shown more recently with much lower doses;[21, 22] one pediatric center reported that low-dose oral medication seemed as efficacious as high-dose intravenous therapy.[23]

In the early 1970's we employed two forms of therapy for an acute rejection.[10] In one, oral prednisone was given, starting with 500 mg and decreasing by 100 mg per day to 100 mg and thereafter by 10 to 25 mg per day back to the previous prednisone dose. In the other, patients were given a gram of methylprednisolone intravenously every second day for three or four doses. As young patients have entered the program, the dose of methylprednisolone has been changed to 10 mg/kg body weight. At present, a rejection episode occurring early post-transplant or a severe rejection at any time is treated with oral or intravenous prednisone, 10 mg/kg body weight daily, whereas milder rejections are treated with 2 to 5 mg prednisone (or methylprednisolone) per kg body weight per day; in either case a total of three or four doses is given.

Our switch to intravenous therapy was prompted by the apparent good success one could achieve with three or four doses of medication rather than one to two weeks of treatment.[24, 25] We were also impressed that for an equivalent dose there appeared to be fewer cushingoid features with the intravenous medication.[24–26] At times we feel more confident giving a medication intravenously in the clinic rather than sending a patient home and relying on the patient to take oral medication.[27, 28]

Since low-dose prednisone therapy has been reported to be successful, we now use such a regimen on occasion. Although taking this treatment orally may present a compliance problem, we hope giving a lower dose of medication will, in the long run, account for appreciably fewer side effects.[22, 29, 30]

**Growth and Glucocorticoid Therapy.** One early report dealing solely with children suggested that growth following transplantation was not spectacular in patients on alternate-day therapy.[31] However, the study of Potter et al involved what would now be considered high doses of prednisone (1 to 2 mg/kg body weight every 48 hours). To date there are few reports on suggested maximum doses of steroids that will allow for optimal growth. Values for prednisone include less than 8.5 mg prednisone/m² per day and less than 15 mg/day.[32] Patients receiving 0.2 to 0.3 mg/kg body weight per day appeared to grow better than those receiving 0.50 mg/kg body weight per day.[33] Growth also appears to be better when prednisone is given as a single dose on alternate days than when it is given daily in divided doses.[33]

Until recently we used one of the lowest doses of prednisone in any pediatric program,[33, 34] and we have now had an opportunity to assess growth under these circumstances. In 67 children who were still growing and had a functioning graft at least one year post-transplant we found that low-dose alternate-day prednisone therapy allowed normal or "catch-up" growth (i.e., at least 5 cm/yr in preadolescents) in all but 16 children.[35] In all but two of the 16, periods of poor growth were accompanied by serum creatinine levels ≥1.5 mg/dl; of patients with serum creatinine levels ≥1.5 mg/dl, only three grew normally. Although it is tempting to suggest that patients with the higher serum creatinine values received more steroids and for this reason did not grow, in fact many such patients have maintained a relatively constant serum creatinine value >1.5 mg/dl for years without additional steroids being given. Thus, it appears that the level of renal function is critical in maintaining a normal growth pattern.

Unfortunately, despite impressive improvements in growth with low-dose alternate-day prednisone therapy following successful transplantation, 55 (83%) of the 67 children were below the 10th percentile at transplant and 50 (75%) had continued at this level when last assessed. Apparently when severe growth retardation is evident by the time of transplantation, it is unlikely that the patient's final height will reach the 25th to 50th percentile for normal children.

**Drugs Interfering with Glucocorticoids.** A few drugs have been shown to adversely affect the therapeutic usefulness of steroids.[36–41] Phenobarbital,[36] phenytoin,[39] and rifampin[38] have been shown to cause the induction of hepatic microsomal enzymes, resulting in increased catabolism of glucocorticoids. In assessing the disappearance of prednisone in patients treated with phenobarbital, Wolff suggested two alternative treatment schedules (personal communication): either to give ten times the single dose of prednisone or to double the dose of prednisone normally given, and administer it in divided doses. Buffington et al[38] suggested that when rifampin therapy is initiated, the daily dose of glucocorticoid should be doubled.

Although a number of our patients were on phenobarbital and/or phenytoin early in our program, no apparent detrimental effect was detected. Nevertheless, with time, we have more readily discontinued anticonvulsant therapy post-transplant, switched to another anticonvulsant therapy when feasible such as carbamazepine (Tegretol), or in the case of one child taking rifampin· doubled the daily dose of steroids.

## Azathioprine and Cyclophosphamide

Azathioprine is an $S$-substituted 6-mercaptopurine (6-MP). Many, but not all, of the biological and biochemical effects of azathioprine are attributable to its cleavage to 6-MP, which is a competitive inhibitor of purine synthesis.[42] The primary lymphocytotoxic effects of azathioprine are directed against actively replicating cells. There is a reduction in the number of large lymphocytes, which are believed to be transformed cells that have entered a proliferative cycle following antigen exposure.[43]

The cytotoxicity of cyclophosphamide, which only becomes manifest once the drug has been metabolized by the liver, is due to its ability to cross-link DNA. Affected cells may recover completely or, with more extensive nuclear damage, die immediately or during subsequent mitosis. B cells are more susceptible to this alkylating agent than T cells because they apparently have a slower rate of recovery from nuclear damage.[43]

Apart from prednisone, azathioprine is the most widely used medication in renal transplant recipients. Adults appear to be more sensitive to the leukopenic effect of azathioprine than children[44] and adults are thus given doses of approximately 1 to 2 mg/kg body weight per day.[45] In our pediatric patients we usually give 3 mg azathioprine per kg body weight per day as a single daily posttransplant dose as well as an initial pretransplant dose. During the hospital stay, the patients' white blood cell counts are monitored daily to assess individual response to azathioprine since the use of antithymocyte globulin and other factors might also lower the white cell count. Usually by discharge a long-term regimen for azathioprine can be employed. Since the medication comes in 50 mg tablets, a dose to the nearest 25 mg/day is used in older children. With very young children the pharmacist will crush the tablet and add the amount required (e.g., 20 mg) to lactose to make a final weight of 200 mg. Individual packets of powder in this form are prescribed.

Side effects such as macrocytosis,[46] pure red cell anemia,[47, 48] pancytopenia,[49] pancreatitis,[50, 51] and liver disease[52] have been reported but are unusual. A few years ago a random screen of liver enzymes was done in our renal transplant patients, all of whom were receiving close to 3 mg azathioprine per kg body weight per day, to determine whether any had evidence of long-term azathioprine liver toxicity. One patient had a temporary rise in liver enzymes but this did not appear to be related to the azathioprine. Furthermore, reports suggest that if chronic liver disease is seen in a renal transplant recipient it is not likely to be related to azathioprine.[52, 53]

Azathioprine is preferred to the alternative drug, cyclophosphamide. As early as 1971, Starzl et al. compared the immunosuppressant effects of cyclophosphamide and azathioprine and found no appreciable differences in renal transplant recipients.[54] At that time they had been using azathioprine for 10 years. In view of their satisfactory experience with the drug and its low incidence of side effects, they recommended that azathioprine be continued as the main immunosuppressant along with glucocorticoid and that cyclophosphamide be substituted only if indicated, for example, in cases of liver malfunction. When cyclophosphamide is given, the usual dose is approximately 1 mg/kg body weight per day.

Our procedure when medication must be adjusted is to reduce or temporarily stop azathioprine rather than substitute cyclophosphamide. No patient in our program has been switched to cyclophosphamide for prolonged periods. Early in our experience one patient had azathioprine discontinued because of jaundice from hepatitis B virus infection; cyclophosphamide was subsequently substituted but the patient nevertheless underwent a severe rejection and lost his graft.

Can azathioprine be discontinued indefinitely? In one study, in which a number of patients had azathioprine discontinued by the physician's choice at least two years after transplantation, there was no significant increase in loss of graft function.[55] The authors felt that if azathioprine had to be stopped there seemed no good reason for restarting it. Subsequent reports have confirmed that in some instances azathioprine therapy has been stopped for two to 109 months with no accompanying increase in rejection episodes or loss of graft function.[56, 57] Although in some cases, azathioprine has been discontinued or greatly reduced during periods of sepsis and restarted a month later without apparent detrimental effect (Fine, personal communication), others have found that a significant loss of graft function resulted from such a procedure.[58]

## Antithymocyte/Antilymphocyte Globulin (ATG)

Heterologous sera have been raised in a variety of species (e.g., horses, goats, rabbits), using immunizing human lymphocytes from a number of sites (e.g., circulating blood, lymph nodes, thoracic duct, thymus, spleen, lymphocyte culture). When such sera were first used to protect allografts they were seen simply as a method of achieving chronic lymphocyte depletion.[59] The mode of beneficial action was soon questioned,[60] and, by the time the use of a heterologous antilymphoid agent was first reported in human renal allografting, the authors felt that the immunosuppressive effect was not necessarily contingent upon either lymphopenia or lymphoid depletion.[61]

Fifteen years later the immunosuppressive mechanisms of these sera are still being debated. While several mechanisms may be involved, the main effect seems to be closely related to the deletion of T cells from the peripheral blood and from the lymphoid centers of treated recipients.[62] Both individual patient response and the potency of each batch of serum vary widely. Potency appears to depend on the response of the animal to produce a T-cell antibody, and the effectiveness of the purification technique appears largely responsible for untoward side effects.[63, 64] Monitoring T-cell counts during therapy seems to assist in achieving a safe yet therapeutic level of antithymocyte globulin administration.[65, 66]

The ability to reduce the number of cells forming rosettes with sheep red cells, i.e., the number of T lymphocyte cells, is the major in vitro test of ATG potency. Unfortunately, clinical experience has shown that this test does not necessarily correlate to transplant anti-rejection potency. More recently, prolongation of a skin graft in a monkey has been suggested as a reliable means of predicting anti-rejection potency in man.[63, 67]

To date, no treatment for renal transplant recipients has been as expensive to produce, available for as long a period, and, until recently, as little accepted as an essential part of the everyday armamentarium in a renal transplant program as ATG. The only accurate assessment of a batch is obtained after it has been used in vivo and analyzed for its ability to reverse or prevent rejection.[63, 64] By that time the same donor cells and the animal in which the antibody was produced are no longer available for reuse. Despite all these problems, many centers are totally committed to using ATG, at times without ever considering controlled trials.

Usually a skin test is performed initially for "horse" sensitivity. ATG has been given intramuscularly[68] and subcutaneously[69] but is more routinely given intravenously, in which case each dose is infused over several hours up to a full 24-hour day.

ATG has been used for both prevention of graft rejection and treatment of acute rejection. Although preventive treatment is often given for two to four weeks (until a patient is discharged from the hospital),[66, 70] it is sometimes continued for up to four months.[71] Several studies have reported a beneficial effect on graft survival,[65–67, 70, 72] while other controlled trials have shown no significant advantage in using ATG to either prevent or treat an acute rejection.[64, 73, 74]

At The Hospital for Sick Children we have had an ATG product available at various times from Upjohn (AtGam, Upjohn, Kalamazoo, Michigan), from Levey et al,[75] and an ATG used in the Canadian trial.[76] In the past three years we have used a product manufactured at The Toronto Western Hospital, Toronto.[77] This ATG product alone or in conjunction with plasmapheresis has been the mainstay of our treatment for early acute (first three to six months post-transplant) rejections unresponsive to high-dose steroids, and has all but replaced our earlier routines of graft irradiation, actinomycin D, and the very rare use of a heparin infusion.[9]

The group at The Toronto Western Hospital evaluated the effectiveness of their rabbit ATG in treating resistant rejection episodes by comparing results in 81 patients from 1976 to 1978, when ATG was not available, to results in 61 patients from 1979 to 1980, when ATG was used.[77] Overall one-year graft survival was better in the ATG group (81% vs 60%). When only those who received pretransplant transfusions were compared in the two periods, a significant improvement in one-year graft survival was still seen in the ATG group (85% vs 67%).

In our program when ATG is given, the amount used is intended to reduce the absolute lymphocyte count quickly and keep it below 250/mm³. If there is no therapeutic response after one week, the treatment is usually discontinued. In some cases the treatment may be extended for two weeks and is given daily or every second day; occasionally it is continued up to one month. We commonly use ATG for early preventive therapy in patients who have had at least one delayed hyperacute rejection. In these cases treatment is begun immediately after transplant or at the first sign of a possible rejection.

We have found that neither ATG nor plasmapheresis significantly reverses acute rejections beyond the first three to six months post-transplant. Furthermore, we have noted recently that patients in whom ATG and/or plasmapheresis appears effective in reversing severe, acute, early rejections often return in the second year post-transplant with a progressive severe rejection that is unresponsive to any therapy.

In our program there have been three deaths from sepsis following successful transplant when ATG has been used in conjunction with steroids and azathioprine. Thus, as more potent immunosuppression is used to save a renal graft from rejecting, susceptibility to infection from virus, bacteria, and fungus can be expected to increase.[76, 78]

Many of the side effects (serum sickness and anaphylaxis) of ATG are secondary to a foreign protein being injected into a patient.[79] Thrombocytopenia occurs when an antibody against platelets has been produced in the animal (horse, rabbit) and not effectively removed in the processing of the animal's serum.[79] Other possible side effects include a bradykinin reaction,[69] nephrotic syndrome,[76] and thrombosis of veins at the site where the ATG was injected.[79]

## Monoclonal Antibodies

The monoclonal antibodies used so far in clinical renal allografting are made by hybridizing mouse cells. First, mice are immunized with suspensions of human T cells. Antibody-producing cells are then separated from the spleens of these mice and fused in vitro with cells from a mouse myeloma. Such hybrid cells can reproduce indefinitely in culture. Each cell will produce the specific antibody made by the antibody-producing parent cell. If such hybrid cells are cultured individually a monoclonal antibody results. In this way a panel of monoclonal antibodies specifically reactive with the human leukocyte subpopulations is produced.[80]

Recently, antibodies against certain T-cell (and monocyte) subsets have been developed to detect these cells in the sera of renal transplant recipients (Table 35–1). Each antibody has been shown to react with distinct antigenic determinants on the surfaces of the human leukocyte. By detecting these subsets

**Table 35–1. CELLS DETECTED BY VARIOUS MONOCLONAL ANTIBODIES**

| Monoclonal Antibody | Cell Detected |
|---|---|
| OKT3 | All T cells |
| OKT4 | Helper/inducer T cells |
| OKT6 | Thymocytes |
| OKT8 | Suppressor/cytotoxic T cells |
| OKT10 | Immature/activated cells |
| OKM1 | Monocytes/granulocytes/natural killer cells |

and monitoring their number and ratio, a Boston group concluded that it is possible to monitor the efficacy of immunosuppressive therapy.[81, 82] In evaluating the patients with rejection episodes, they found that the number of OKT3 cells and the ratio of OKT4/OKT8 were useful in identifying patients with a high probability of rejection. During the first six weeks post-transplant, an acute rejection occurred in nine of 11 patients in whom the OKT4/OKT8 ratio was >1.3. Rejection episodes were rather unlikely when the ratio was <1.3 unless the OKT3 count was >150/mm³.

The ratio may also have potential as a diagnostic tool in the post-transplant patient with diminishing renal function. In such a patient a high ratio indicates rejection, whereas a low ratio suggests virus-induced allograft damage.[20] These same authors have used the pan-T-cell reagent OKT3 as a clinical immunosuppressive agent. All 11 patients with biopsy-proven renal allograft rejection whom they have so treated have responded and seven have recovered satisfactory renal function. Although this procedure is potentially more encouraging than just infusing ATG, further studies in additional patients are needed to assess the efficacy of such an approach in renal transplant recipients.

## Plasmapheresis

Plasma exchange is used in treating renal allograft rejection in the hope that it will remove any humoral antibodies which are contributing to graft destruction.[83] On a theoretical basis, this technique can assist only in those situations where there is a major humoral component to the rejection episode.

By the mid 1970's our group was not satisfied with any of the conventional forms of therapy (actinomycin, graft irradiation) for acute rejection. We were impressed with the preliminary results of Cardella et al,[84] and embarked on a plasmapheresis program whereby acute rejection episodes unresponsive to high-dose prednisone therapy are treated with a minimum of five plasma exchanges (usually daily), and then the patient's condition is reassessed. Usually each treatment involves the removal of an equivalent of one plasma volume from the child; this is replaced with an albumin/saline solution or fresh frozen plasma. If the patient's condition improves with plasmapheresis and there is

another acute rejection in the first three to six months post-transplant a repeat five treatment course is occasionally employed.

Cardella et al are conducting a controlled trial in which half of their patients who have their first rejection episode during the first three months post-transplant receive intensive plasma exchange for five consecutive days.[84] Patients in both groups receive graft irradiation and bolus methylprednisolone for three consecutive days. To date, one-year actuarial graft survival has improved by 13% in patients receiving plasmapheresis over those in the controlled group. The future of plasmapheresis in the treatment of renal transplant rejection episodes is still controversial;[85] interestingly, a potential role for leukopheresis has also been suggested.[86, 87]

## POSSIBLE NEW THERAPIES FOR PATIENTS WITH HIGH CYTOTOXIC ANTIBODIES

Cytotoxic antibodies develop in about 10% of patients with ESRD to the point that it is difficult or impossible to obtain a donor kidney which, on direct cross match, is likely not to be rejected very soon after transplant. Over the past few years the group at The Toronto Western Hospital[88] and to a lesser extent our group have transplanted a few patients with a positive T-cell cross match to donor cells on back panels of sera, but with the recent sample giving a negative cross match. Receiving ATG therapy and occasionally plasmapheresis, such patients have been given transplants with a one-year graft survival of 60%.[88] Starzl et al have also been successful with transplants in such individuals;[89] however, their patients were given cyclosporin instead of ATG.

## Cyclosporin

The in vitro and in vivo immunosuppressive properties of the fungus metabolite, cyclosporin, were first described by Borel in 1976.[90] The first report of cyclosporin A (CyA) use in clinical renal transplantation followed two years later.[91]

CyA is known to act specifically against T cells at an early stage in their differentiation.[92, 93] It has been shown to exhibit a far greater toxicity toward a subpopulation of T-cells (T helper) than toward either B lymphocyte or hematopoietic precursor cells.[91]

The use of monoclonal antibodies has made it possible to examine the T-lymphocyte subpopulations of human renal allograft recipients being treated with CyA. There does not appear to be any major change in the number of T lymphocytes or in the ratio of OKT4 to OKT8 lymphocytes in such patients.[94]

CyA is the major new addition to treatment for renal transplant patients in the past decade. It may be useful either as the only form of preventive immunosuppressive therapy[95] or as a steroid-sparing drug.[96] CyA does not appear to be effective in treating an acute rejection episode, especially if humoral in nature.

Initially, nephrotoxicity appeared to be a major problem with this drug. Although early papers questioned CyA nephrotoxicity and suggested that the lesions which occured merely reflected rejection episodes, later studies showed evidence of CyA nephrotoxicity in patients receiving bone marrow or liver transplants.[97, 98] The toxicity appears dose-related;[91, 99] less nephrotoxicity and adequate immunosuppression are observed if serum CyA trough concentrations are maintained between 0.1 and 0.4 μg/ml.[100] Renal lesions associated with CyA include interstitial nephritis, and a direct toxic effect has been noted on renal tubules or their blood supply, possibly as a result of a haptene interaction.[91] It appears that the nephrotoxicity can be reversed if the CyA dosage is decreased or stopped.[97, 100] Because of the potential for hepatotoxicity, usually seen when CyA serum trough levels in the two hours after dose administration are greater than 0.4 to 1.0 μg/ml,[101] it has been recommended that azathioprine not be used concomitantly.[91] Other side effects from CyA include facial and limb hirsutism; gum hypertrophy, which tends to resolve with time; and lymphomas.[96]

Recently it has been suggested that patients on CyA may be lacking in effective cytotoxic T cells. This may enable EB virus–infected B cells to persist and proliferate in vivo, resulting in lymphoma development.[102] Lowering the dose of CyA appears to allow normal elimination of EB virus–infected B cells and may explain why no lymphomas to date have been detected in patients receiving low doses.[102] At present the efficacy of CyA is being assessed in a randomized controlled trial of over 200 patients from across Canada who have received cadaveric allografts. Comparing CyA plus low-dose prednisone with each center's standard therapy has shown the one-year cumulative graft survival estimate to be about 15% better in the CyA group (Stiller, personal communication). If the impressive graft survival associated with CyA continues, there may well be a role for its use in children. With closer monitoring of the CyA blood level to avert nephrotoxicity and an elevated serum creatinine level, CyA might even be used in children who are still growing. Starzl et al[89] have already reported that it has been used effectively as an immunosuppressant in three children under 14 years of age. However, after noting some degree of renal impairment in all 36 of their bone marrow patients who were given the drug, Joss et al[99] have suggested that younger patients may be more susceptible to the toxic effects of CyA. Complications in these patients included fluid retention from the renal impairment, leading to hypertension with convulsions, and were directly related to the CyA blood levels.

## OTHER THERAPIES

**Irradiation of Graft, Actinomycin, and Extracorporeal Irradiation of Blood.** In addition to the major current treatment regimens already discussed, various other procedures have been used in an attempt to treat acute rejection. In the early 1970's severe rejection or rejection that did not respond to high-dose prednisone was usually treated by irradiating renal grafts, using 150 rads daily or every second day for a total of 450 rads. However, like others,[70, 103] we did not find this procedure particularly effective. We also used actinomycin C or D (3 mg/kg body weight for three doses) as did many other centers.[79, 103] Both therapies have been discontinued for some time in our center in favor of ATG and/or plasmapheresis therapy.

Other centers have reported using prophylactic graft irradiation[104] and extracorporeal irradiation.[105, 106] Although it was once thought that prophylactic graft irradiation had a beneficial effect on the course of cadaveric transplantation,[107] this now seems unlikely.[108] If such therapy is at all immunosuppressive, it may be as a result of either impaired macrophage activity or reduced potency of effector lymphocytes within the graft.

## SPLENECTOMY, THYMECTOMY, THORACIC DUCT DRAINAGE

Many procedures have been employed to rid the transplant recipient of cells that could be potentially detrimental to the renal allograft. These include splenectomy, thymectomy, thoracic duct drainage, and total lymphatic irradiation. One Minnesota group still routinely splenectomizes children.[109] Such children are usually maintained indefinitely on prophylactic antimicrobials.

It has been shown that splenectomy allows larger doses of azathioprine to be given.[110] Furthermore, some studies have reported better graft survival in patients who have undergone pretransplant splenectomy than in those who have not.[111-113] However, other studies have shown no definite role for splenectomy and have reported an increased incidence of death from sepsis in splenectomized children.[114-116] For these reasons plus the lack of any persuasive theory as to how splenectomy might achieve a beneficial effect, we have not used the procedure as an adjunct to immunosuppression.

Thymectomy[71] has not gained any prominence as a form of immunosuppressive therapy.

Thoracic duct drainage[70, 117, 118] and total lymphatic irradiation[105] are somewhat cumbersome methods of achieving immunosuppression, but several groups[118-121] have shown improved renal graft survival and fewer rejection episodes when these methods have been used. Butt et al[70] feel that similar advantages are noted when ATG is given and this can be done more simply.

Thoracic duct cannulation and lymph drainage result in a reduction in circulating lymphocytes, the depletion being mainly in the T-cell fraction. There is a concomitant diminution of cells in the T-cell areas of lymphoid tissue. In addition to being reduced in number, the T-lymphocyte population is modified. Immunocompetent T cells are replaced by comparatively immature T lymphocytes. Whether or not the replacing cells are predominantly suppressor T cells is not yet clear.[118, 120]

## ANTICOAGULANT/ANTIPLATELET AGENTS

Histologically, many rejecting renal allografts show some thrombosis of intrarenal vessels. The presumed chain of events in these instances is immunologically mediated endothelial damage, resulting in platelet aggregation, which then initiates the thrombotic cascade. Anticoagulant or antiplatelet agents have been used in the hope that they would prevent or reduce the severity of the final steps in this postulated sequence.

A few centers have presented preliminary results suggesting that heparin and/or dipyridamole might be useful in treating hyperacute[122] or acute rejection.[123] However, the results of one controlled trial with heparin[124] and another with dipyridamole plus an oral anticoagulant[125] showed no significant difference in mean serum creatinine level or graft survival rate despite a beneficial effect in the histologic appearance of glomeruli and blood vessels. Another study using prophylactic dipyridamole for two years reported no beneficial effect pathologically, clinically, or radiologically to the renal graft.[126]

## NO THERAPY

Weil et al reported a successful outcome in a few cases when isografts were performed and no immunosuppressive therapy was given.[127] In a nationwide survey Zoller et al identified 48 patients who had discontinued all immunosuppressive therapy.[128] After reviewing the status of the patients, these authors concluded that if therapy had been stopped for one to three years medication should be reinstituted. However, in patients who had done well without immunosuppressive therapy for more than three years, reinstitution of therapy did not appear to be necessary to maintain good graft function. Nevertheless, elective stopping of all antirejection medication should not be encouraged until we have a greater understanding of the probable implications.

## DONOR PRETREATMENT

The concept of reducing the immunogenicity of a foreign graft by treating the graft rather than the recipient tissue has obvious appeal because of the limitations and inherent dangers of host immunosuppression. There have been several approaches directed at altering graft antigenicity.

Transplantation antigens are most highly immunogenic when presented to recipient T cells on the surface of donor stimulator cells of lymphoreticular origin. Tissue parenchymal cells are not as immunogenic as leukocytes.[129] Reducing the number of donor leukocytes passed with a renal allograft might reduce the immunogenic stimulus and hence lessen the severity of rejection. This hypothesis has been substantiated in animals. Irradiating intact donors has resulted in prolonged renal allograft survival in both rats and dogs but only if the irradiation preceded transplantation by the 48 to 96 hours required to achieve profound peripheral leukopenia.[130] The interval required to achieve this leukopenia prevents whole body donor irradiation from being applicable to clinical renal allografting. Washing out graft passenger leukocytes before grafting animals has been said to improve renal allograft success.[131] However, in human renal transplantation prolonging graft perfusion beyond an initial flush out has not increased graft survival.[132]

Donor pretreatment with cyclophosphamide and methylprednisolone has caused a significant prolongation of renal allograft survival time in dogs.[133] The effect of this donor pretreatment was mediated by cyclophosphamide and its metabolites residing in the graft after surgery. This increased graft survival is not fully explained by an effect on passenger leukocytes. Having entered such a drug-laden graft, the viability of host cells would also be reduced, affecting their subsequent ability both to sensitize and to proliferate. In human renal transplantation earlier encouraging results using donor pretreatment with cyclophosphamide[134, 135] have not been substantiated recently.[136, 137] To date, none of the attempts to reduce graft antigenicity has been successful enough to win widespread clinical acceptance.

# REFERENCES

1. Sato VL, Gefter ML (Eds): Cellular Immunology: Selected Readings and Critical Commentary. Reading, Massachusetts, Addison-Wesley Publishing Co, 1981.
2. Merrill JP, Murray JE, Harrison JH, et al: Successful homotransplantation of the kidney between nonidentical twins. N Engl J Med 262:1251, 1960.
3. Fauci AS, Dale DC, Balow JE: Glucocorticosteroid therapy: mechanisms of action and clinical considerations. Ann Intern Med 84:304, 1976.
4. Rosenfeld JB, Levi J, De Vries A, Levy M: Prolonged survival after kidney transplantation without the use of corticosteroids. Isr J Med Sci 7:589, 1971.
5. Kreis H, Lacombe M, Noel LH, et al: Kidney-graft rejection: has the need for steroids to be re-evaluated? Lancet 2:1169, 1978.
6. McGeown MG, Douglas JF, Brown WA, et al: Advantages of low dose steroid from the day after renal transplantation. Transplantation 29:287,1980.
7. McGeown MG, Douglas JF, Brown WA, et al: Low dose steroid from the day following renal transplantation. Proc Eur Dial Transplant Assoc 16:395, 1979.
8. Buckels JAC, Mackintosh P, Barnes AD: Controlled trial of low versus high dose oral steroid therapy in 100 cadaveric renal transplants. Proc Eur Dial Transplant Assoc 18:394, 1981.
9. Morris PJ, Chan L, French ME, Ting A: Low dose oral prednisolone in renal transplantation. Lancet 1:525, 1982.
10. Arbus GS, Galiwango J, DeMaria JE, Churchill BM: Transplantation and complications of chronic renal failure. Can Med Assoc J 122:659, 1980.
11. Knapp MS, Byrom NP, Pownall R, Mayor P: Time of day of taking immunosuppressive agents after renal transplantation: a possible influence on graft survival. Br Med J 281:1382, 1980.
12. Reed WP, Lucas ZJ, Cohn R: Alternate-day prednisone therapy after renal transplantation. Lancet 1:747, 1970.
13. Sampson D, Albert DJ: Alternate-day therapy with methylprednisolone after renal transplantation. J Urol 109:345, 1973.
14. Burleson RL, Scruggs BF, Brennan A: Successful immunosuppression of renal allograft recipients with alternate day steroid therapy. Clin Nephrol 10:87, 1978.
15. Diethelm AG, Sterling WA, Hartley MW, Morgan JM: Alternate-day prednisone therapy in recipients of renal allografts. Arch Surg 111:867, 1976.
16. Rao V, Andersen R, O'Brien T, et al: Is 15 mg of prednisone every other day a safe, tolerable dose in the late post-transplant period? Experience with a large number of adults over a prolonged period of time. The American Society of Nephrology 11th Annual Meeting, November 19–21, 1978, New Orleans, La, p 162A (Abstract).
17. McDonald FD, Horensten ML, Mayor GB, et al: Effect of alternate-day steroids on renal transplant function: a controlled study. Nephron 17:415, 1976.
18. Breitenfield RV, Hebert LA, Lemann J Jr, et al: Stability of renal transplant function on alternate day steroid therapy. The American Society of Nephrology, 10th Annual Meeting, November 20–22, 1977, Washington DC, p 128A (Abstract).
19. Hsu AC, Arbus GS, Noriega E, Huber J: Renal allograft biopsy: a satisfactory adjunct for predicting renal function after graft rejection. Clin Nephrol 5:260, 1976.
20. Richardson WP, Colvin RB, Cheeseman SH, et al: Glomerulopathy associated with cytomegalovirus viremia in renal allografts. N Engl J Med 305:57, 1981.
21. Touraine JL, Traeger J: Mode of administration of steroids in treatment of renal-allograft rejection. Lancet 1:607, 1978.
22. Kauffman HM Jr, Stromstad SA, Sampson D,

Stawicki AT: Randomized steroid therapy of human kidney transplant rejection. Transplant Proc 11:36, 1979.

23. Orta-Sibu N, Haycock GB, Chantler C, Bewick M: High dose intravenous methylprednisolone (IVMP) versus low dose oral prednisolone (OP) in acute renal allograft rejection in children. Pediatr Res 14:992, 1980 (Abstract).

24. Mussche MM, Ringoir SMG, Lameire NN: High intravenous doses of methylprednisolone for acute cadaveric renal allograft rejection. Nephron 16:287, 1976.

25. Bell PRF, Briggs JD, Calman KC, et al: Reversal of acute clinical and experimental organ rejection using large doses of intravenous prednisolone. Lancet 1:876, 1971.

26. Feduska NJ, Turcotte JG, Gikas PW, et al: Reversal of renal allograft rejection with intravenous methylprednisolone "pulse" therapy. J Surg Res 12:208, 1972.

27. Beck DE, Fennell RS, Yost RL, et al: Evaluation of an educational program on compliance with medication regimens in pediatric patients with renal transplants. J Pediatr 96:1094, 1980.

28. Korsch BM, Fine RN, Negrete VF: Noncompliance in children with renal transplants. Pediatrics 61:872, 1978.

29. Harrington KD, Murray WR, Kountz SL, Belzer FO: Avascular necrosis of bone after renal transplantation. J Bone Joint Surg 53-A:203, 1971.

30. Walman GB, Chisholm L, Arbus GS: Cataracts in pediatric renal transplant recipients. Can Med Assoc J 117:1257, 1977.

31. Potter DE, Kaye J, Belzer FO, et al: Growth following renal transplantation: daily vs alternate day steroid therapy. Abstracts of papers presented at Fifth International Congress of Nephrology, Mexico, October 3–13, 1972, p 155.

32. Reimold EW: Intermittent prednisone therapy in children and adolescents after renal transplantation. Pediatrics 52:235, 1973.

33. Travis LB, Chesney R, McEnery P, et al: Growth and glucocorticoids in children with kidney disease. Kidney Int 14:365, 1978.

34. Hoda Q, Hasinoff DJ, Arbus GS: Growth following renal transplantation in children and adolescents. Clin Nephrol 3:6, 1975.

35. Bell MJ, Martin LW, Gonzales LL, et al: Alternate-day single-dose prednisone therapy: a method of reducing steroid toxicity. J Pediatr Surg 7:223, 1972.

36. Levin W, Welch RM, Conney AH: Effect of chronic phenobarbital treatment on the liver microsomal metabolism and uterotropic action of 17-estradiol. Endocrinology 80:135, 1967.

37. Brooks SM, Werk EE, Ackerman SJ, et al: Adverse effects of phenobarbital on corticosteroid metabolism in patients with bronchial asthma. N Engl J Med 286:1125, 1972.

38. Buffington GA, Dominguez JH, Piering WF, et al: Interaction of rifampin and glucocorticoids: adverse effect on renal allograft function. JAMA 236:1958, 1976.

39. Wassner SJ, Pennisi AJ, Malekzadeh MH, Fine RN: The adverse effect of anticonvulsant therapy on renal allograft survival. J Pediatr 88:134, 1976.

40. McEnery PT, Stempel DA: Commentary: anticonvulsant therapy and renal allograft survival. J Pediatr 88:138, 1976.

41. Wolff ED, deJong FH, Schalm SW: The acceler-

ated metabolism of prednisolone in transplant recipients using barbiturates or phenytoin. Eur Soc Pediatr Nephrol, Capri, 1979.

42. Elion GB, Hitchings GH: Azathioprine. Handbook of Experimental Pharmacology 38:404, 1975.

43. Skinner MD, Schwartz RS: Immunosuppressive therapy. N Engl J Med 287:221, 1972.

44. Pollak R, Nishikawa RA, Mozes MF, Jonasson O: Azathioprine-induced leukopenia—clinical significance in renal transplantation. J Surg Res 29:258, 1980.

45. Oesterwitz H, Horpacsy G, May G, Mebel M: Frequency of leukopenia incidents following azathioprine therapy after kidney transplantation. Eur Urol 4:167, 1978.

46. Wickramasinghe SN, Dodsworth H, Rault RMJ, Hulme B: Observations on the incidence and cause of macrocytosis in patients on azathioprine therapy following renal transplantation. Transplantation 18:443, 1974.

47. DeClerck YA, Ettenger RB, Ortega JA, Pennisi AJ: Macrocytosis and pure RBC anemia caused by azathioprine. Am J Dis Child 134:377, 1980.

48. Old CW, Flannery EP, Grogan TM, et al: Azathioprine-induced pure red blood cell aplasia. JAMA 240:552, 1978.

49. Bacon BR, Treuhaft WH, Goodman AM: Azathioprine-induced pancytopenia: occurrence in two patients with connective-tissue diseases. Arch Intern Med 141:223, 1981.

50. Isenberg JN: Pancreatitis, amylase clearance, and azathioprine. J Pediatr 93:1043, 1978.

51. Paloyan D, Levin B, Simonowitz D: Azathioprine-associated acute pancreatitis. Dig Dis 22:839, 1977.

52. Ireland P, Rashid A, von Lichtenberg F, et al: Liver disease in kidney transplant patients receiving azathioprine. Arch Intern Med 132:29, 1973.

53. Ware, AJ, Luby JP, Hollinger B, et al: Etiology of liver disease in renal-transplant patients. Ann Intern Med 91:364, 1979.

54. Starzl TE, Putnam CW, Halgrimson CG, et al: Cyclophosphamide and whole organ transplantation in human beings. Surg Gynecol Obstet 133:981, 1971.

55. Sheriff MHR, Yayha T, Lee HA: Is azathioprine necessary in renal transplantation? Lancet 1:118, 1978.

56. Pirson Y, van Ypersele de Strihou C, Alexandre GP: Is azathioprine necessary in renal transplantation? Lancet 1:506, 1978.

57. Schmidt P, Kopsa H, Balcke P, et al: Cadaveric renal graft acceptance without azathioprine. Proc Eur Dial Transplant Assoc 16:388, 1981.

58. Hurley JK, Greenslade T, Lewy PR, et al: Varicella zoster infections in pediatric renal transplant recipients. Arch Surg 115:751, 1980.

59. Woodruff MFA, Anderson NA: Effect of lymphocyte depletion by thoracic duct fistula and administration of antilymphocyte serum on the survival of skin homografts in rats. Nature 200:702, 1963.

60. Levey RH, Medawar PB: Some experiments on the action of antilymphoid antisera. Ann NY Acad Sci 129:164, 1966.

61. Starzl TE, Marchioro TL, Porter KA, et al: The use of heterologous antilymphoid agents in canine renal and liver homotransplantation and in human renal homotransplantation. Surg Gynecol Obstet 124:301, 1967.

62. Russell PS: Monoclonal antibodies in renal transplantation: preliminary results. Kidney Int 20:530, 1981.

63. Tagnon A: Antilymphocyte globulin and renal transplantation. Postgrad Med J 52:64, 1976.

64. Wechter WJ, Brodie JA, Morrell RM, et al: Antithymocyte globulin (ATGAM) in renal allograft recipients. Transplantation 28:294, 1979.

65. Cosimi AB, Wortis HH, Delmonico FL, Russell PS: Randomized clinical trial of antithymocyte globulin in cadaver renal allograft recipients: importance of T cell monitoring. Surgery 80:155, 1976.

66. Kreis H, Mansouri R, Descamps J, et al: Antithymocyte globulin in cadaver kidney transplantation: a randomized trial based on T-cell monitoring. Kidney Int 19:438, 1981.

67. Thomas F, Mendez-Picon G, Thomas J, et al: Effect of antilymphocyte-globulin potency on survival of cadaver renal transplants: prospective randomised double-blind trial. Lancet 2:671, 1977.

68. Putnam, CW, Bell RH Jr, Beart RW Jr, et al: Past experience and future studies with antilymphocyte globulin in recipients of kidney homografts. Postgrad Med J 52(Suppl):59, 1976.

69. Barnes AD, Sansom JR: The clinical problems of dosage and the route of administration of antilymphocyte globulin. Postgrad Med J 52(Suppl):39:1976.

70. Butt KMH, Zielinski CM, Parsa I, et al: Trends in immunosuppression for kidney transplantation. Kidney Int 13(Suppl 8):S-95, 1978.

71. Starzl TE, Porter KA, Andres G, et al: Long-term survival after renal transplantation in humans: (with special reference to histocompatibility matching, thymectomy, homograft glomerulonephritis, heterologous ALG, and recipient malignancy). Ann Surg 172:437, 1970.

72. Filo RS, Smith EJ, Leapman SB: Therapy of acute cadaveric renal allograft rejection with adjunctive antithymocyte globulin. Transplantation 30:445, 1980.

73. Birkeland SA: Session IIb. Renal transplantation. Treatment of rejection. The use of antilymphocyte globulin in renal allograft rejection. A controlled study. Postgrad Med J 52(Suppl 5):82, 1976.

74. Jakobsen A, Flatmark A, Sødal G, Thorsby E: Controlled trial of antilymphocyte globulin in cadaveric transplantation. Postgrad Med J 52(Suppl 5):72, 1976.

75. Levey RH, Ingelfinger J, Grupe WE, et al: Unique surgical and immunologic features of renal transplantation in children. J Pediatr Surg 13:576, 1978.

76. Michel RP, Guttmann RD, Knaack J, et al: Antilymphocyte globulin in renal transplantation: nephrotic syndrome and infection as possible complications. Arch Surg 110:90, 1975.

77. Pierratos A, Tam P, Cook GT, Cardella CJ: Improved graft survival due to rabbit antithymocyte sera (RATS) and pretransplant transfusions (T). Royal College Meeting, September, 1982 (in press).

78. Sansom JR, Barnes AD, Hall CL: A randomized prospective clinical trial of antilymphocyte globulin in 100 cadaveric renal transplants. Postgrad Med J 52(Suppl 5):75, 1976.

79. Mee AD, Evans DB: Antilymphocyte-serum preparations in treatment of renal-allograft rejection. Lancet 2:16, 1970.

80. Kung PC, Talle MA, DeMaria ME, et al: Strategies for generating monoclonal antibodies defining human T-lymphocyte differentiation antigens. Transplant Proc 12(Suppl 1):141, 1980.

81. Cosimi AB, Colvin RB, Burton RC, et al: Use of monoclonal antibodies to T-cell subsets for immunologic monitoring and treatment in recipients of renal allografts. N Engl J Med 305:308, 1981.

82. Russell PS: New approaches to the use of antibodies for immunosuppression. Transplant Proc 14:506, 1982.

83. Cardella CJ, Sutton D, Uldall PR, deVeber GA: Intensive plasma exchange and renal transplant rejection. Lancet 1:264, 1977.

84. Cardella CJ, Sutton DMC, Katz A, et al: Plasma exchange in renal transplantation. Proceedings of the 8th International Congress of Nephrology, Athens, 1981, p. 45.

85. Cardella CJ: Does plasma exchange have a role in renal transplant rejection? Plasma Ther Transfus Technol 3:153, 1982.

86. Strauss F, Kleinman S, Goldfinger D: Use of pheresis in the management of acute renal allograft rejection. Am Soc Nephrol 27:172A, 1981.

87. Collett PV, Stiller CR, Ulan RA, Lockwood JFB: Treatment of renal transplant rejection with leukopheresis. Am Soc Nephrol 154A, 1978.

88. Cardella CJ, Falk JA: Graft outcome in patients with T cell reactivity (TCR) to donor cells (abstract). Clin Res (in press).

89. Starzl TE, Iwatsuki S, Malatack JJ, et al: Liver and kidney transplantation in children receiving cyclosporin A and steroids. J Pediatr 100:681, 1982.

90. Borel JF: Comparative study of in vitro and in vivo drug effects on cell-mediated cytotoxicity. Immunology 31:631, 1976.

91. Calne RY, White DJG, Thiru S, et al: Cyclosporin A in patients receiving renal allografts from cadaver donors. Lancet 2:1323, 1978.

92. Borel JF, Feurer C, Magnée C, Stähelin H: Effects of the new anti-lymphocytic peptide cyclosporin A in animals. Immunology 32:1017, 1977.

93. White DJG, Plumb AM, Pawelec G, Brons G: Cyclosporin A: An immunosuppressive agent preferentially active against proliferating T-cells. Transplantation 27:55, 1979.

94. Morris PJ: Some experimental and clinical studies of cyclosporin A in renal transplantation. Transplant Proc 14:525, 1982.

95. Calne RY, Rolles K, White DKG, et al: Cyclosporin A initially as the only immunosuppressant in 34 recipients of cadaveric organs: 32 kidneys, 2 pancreases, and 2 livers. Lancet 2:1033, 1979.

96. Calne RY: Cyclosporin. Nephron 26:57, 1980.

97. Gratwohl A, Müller M, Osterwalder B, Nissen C, Speck B: Nephrotoxicity of cyclosporin A in bone marrow transplant recipients. Lancet 2:635, 1981.

98. Klintmalm GBG, Iwatsuki S, Starzl TE: Nephrotoxicity of cyclosporin A in liver and kidney transplant patients. Lancet 1:470, 1981.

99. Joss DV, Barrett AJ, Kendra JR, Lucas CF, Desai S: Hypertension and convulsions in children receiving cyclosporin A. Lancet 1:902, 1982.

100. Keown PA, Stiller CR, Ulan RA, et al: Immuno-

logical and pharmacological monitoring in the clinical use of cyclosporin A. Lancet 1:686, 1981.

101. Laupacis A, Keown PA, Ulan RA, Sinclair NR, Stiller CR: Hyperbilirubinaemia and cyclosporin A levels. Lancet 2:1426, 1981.

102. Crawford DH, Edwards JMB: Immunity to Epstein-Barr virus in cyclosporin A–treated renal allograft recipients. Lancet 1:1469, 1982.

103. Myburgh JA, Goldberg B, Meyers AM, et al: Tissue typing, anti-lymphocyte globulin, and prophylactic graft irradiation in cadaver kidney transplantation. Br Med J 3:670, 1970.

104. Popowniak KL, Nakamoto S: Immunosuppressive therapy in renal transplantation. Surg Clin North Am 51:1191, 1971.

105. Wolf JS: Extracorporeal irradiation of blood as an immunosuppressive agent. Transplant Proc 9:469, 1972.

106. Weeke E, Thaysen JH: Extracorporeal irradiation of the blood. Acta Med Scand 193:181, 1973.

107. Murray JE, Barnes BA, Atkinson J: Transplantation: fifth report of the Human Kidney Transplant Registry. Transplantation 5:752, 1967.

108. Advisory Committee of the Human Kidney Transplant Registry: An analysis of the incidence of early transplant failure data from the Human Kidney Transplant Registry. Transplant Proc 1:197, 1969.

109. Miller LC, Bock GH, Lum CT, Najarian JS, Mauer SM: Transplantation of the adult kidney into the very small child: long-term outcome. J Pediatr 100:675, 1982.

110. Woods JE, DeWeerd JH, Johnson WJ, Anderson CF: Splenectomy in renal transplantation: influence on azathioprine sensitivity. JAMA 218:1430, 1971.

111. Vertuno LL, Bansal VK, Hano JE, Giacchino JL, Geis WP: The role of splenectomy in cadaveric renal transplantation. Nephron 27:273, 1981.

112. Kauffman HM, Swanson MK, McGregor WR, Rodgers RE, Fox PS: Splenectomy in renal transplantation. Surg Gynecol Obstet 139:33, 1974.

113. Schulak JA, Hill JL, Reckard CR, Simonian SJ, Stuart FP: Infectious and functional consequences of splenectomy in adult renal transplant recipients. J Surg Res 25:404, 1978.

114. Eraklis AJ, Kevy SV, Diamond LK, Gross RE: Hazard of overwhelming infection after splenectomy in childhood. N Engl J Med 276:1225, 1967.

115. Cerilli J, Jones L: A reappraisal of the role of splenectomy in children receiving renal allografts. Surgery 82:510, 1977.

116. Rai GS, Wilkinson R, Taylor RMR, Uldall PR, Kerr DNS: Adverse effect of splenectomy in renal transplantation. Clin Nephrol 9:194, 1978.

117. Sarles HE, Remmers AR Jr, Fish JC, et al: Depletion of lymphocytes for the protection of renal allografts. Arch Intern Med 125:443, 1970.

118. Traeger J, Touraine JL, Archimbaud JP, Malik MC, Dubernard JM: Thoracic duct drainage and antilymphocyte globulin for renal transplantation in man. Kidney Int 13 [Suppl 8]:103, 1978.

119. Franksson C, Lundgren G, Magnusson G, Ringden O: Drainage of thoracic duct lymph in renal transplant patients. Transplantation 21:133, 1976.

120. Fish JC, Sarles HE, Remmers A Jr, Townsend CM Jr, Bell JD, Flye MW: Renal transplantation after thoracic duct drainage. Ann Surg 193:752, 1981.

121. Starzl TE, Weil R III, Koep LJ, Iwaki Y, Terasaki PI, Schröter GPJ: Thoracic duct drainage before and after cadaveric kidney transplantation. Surg Gynecol Obstet 149:815, 1979.

122. Beleil OM, Lecky JW, Stanley TM, Mittal KK, Olmsted WW, Kaufman JJ: Protective value of heparin in hyperacute rejection of renal allografts in presensitized dogs. Invest Urol 10:318, 1973.

123. Kincaid-Smith P: Modification of the vascular lesions of rejection in cadaveric renal allografts by dipyridamole and anticoagulants. Lancet 2:920, 1969.

124. Griffin PJA, Salaman JR: A controlled trial of heparin in renal transplant rejection. Transplantation 32:306, 1981.

125. Mathew TH, Kincaid-Smith P, Clyne DH, et al: A controlled trial of oral anticoagulants and dipyridamol in cadaveric renal allografts. Lancet 1:1307, 1974.

126. Anderson M, Dewar P, Fleming LB, et al: A controlled trial of dipyridamole in human renal transplantation and an assessment of platelet function studies in rejection. Clin Nephrol 2:93, 1974.

127. Weil R III, Starzl TE, Porter KA, Kershaw M, Schröter GPJ, Koep LJ: Renal isotransplantation without immunosuppression. Ann Surg 192:108, 1980.

128. Zoller KM, Cho SI, Cohen JJ, Harrington JT: Cessation of immunosuppressive therapy after successful transplantation: a national survey. Kidney Int 18:110, 1980.

129. Lafferty KJ, Woolnough J: The origin and mechanism of the allograft reaction. Immunol Rev 35:231, 1977.

130. Stuart FP, Garrick T, Holter A, Bastien E: Delayed rejection of renal allografts in the rat and dog by reduction of passenger leukocytes. Surgery 70:128, 1971.

131. Brede HD: The impact of transplantation surgery on the development of immunology. In Steinberg CM, Lefkovits I (Eds): The Immune System, Vol 1, Basel, Karger, pp 234–237.

132. Opelz G, Terasaki PI: Advantage of cold storage over machine perfusion for preservation of cadaver kidneys. Transplantation 33:64, 1982.

133. Brom HLF, van Breda Vriesman PJC, Terpstra JL: Prolongation of canine allograft survival with donor pretreatment. Kidney Int 21:323, 1982.

134. Zinche H, Woods JE: Donor pretreatment in cadaver renal transplantation. Surg Gynecol Obstet 145:183, 1977.

135. Guttmann RD, Morehouse DD, Meakins JL, Klassen J, Knaack J, Beaudoin JG: Donor pretreatment in an unselected series of cadaver renal allografts. Kidney Int 13 [Suppl 8]:S99, 1978.

136. Soulillou JP, Baron D, Rouxel A, Guenel J: Steroid-cyclophosphamide pretreatment of kidney allograft donors: a control study. Nephron 24:193, 1979.

137. Chatterjee SN, Smith R, Fine S, Schulman B, Fine RN: A prospective randomized double-blind controlled study of cadaver donor pretreatment with cyclophosphamide in human renal transplantation. Transplant Proc 13:709, 1981.

# 36

# The Clinical Nurse Specialist in Renal Transplantation

*Shawney E. Fine, R.N.*

The major goal in treating the pediatric patient with ESRD is a successful renal transplant and full rehabilitation. The modality of renal transplantation in the pediatric and adolescent patient is perceived with a full range of emotions, including hope for a normal life, fear of rejection and return to dialysis, fear of death, dependency, isolation, and, for the infant, disruption of their trust relationship with parents.

In a study by Sebastian and Webb, patients with a good understanding about their condition and patient care plan showed a positive correlation with optimal social adjustment. However, the longer a patient received a particular therapy, the *less* likely the patient was to have a *positive* health adjustment score. Given these findings, it is obvious that early and continuous education, which is constantly redesigned to meet the ever-changing needs of the patient and family, is imperative to ensure optimal physical and psychological success of transplantation.[1]

The clinical nurse specialist (CNS) who is involved in the care of the pediatric and adolescent patient undergoing renal transplantation is in a unique position to ameliorate some of the above anxieties. The CNS should be cognizant of the fact that increased knowledge and understanding reduces patient and family anxiety. Maximal comprehension of the clinical situation by the patient and family facilitates a feeling of control of their destiny. The CNS must recognize that the patient and family have a *right* to this basic knowledge. As the CNS develops an effective relationship with patient and family, education in the preparatory, preoperative, postoperative, and outpatient phases of care is facilitated.

The CNS uses basic methodology for interfacing with the patient and family, including assessment, planning, intervention, and evaluation. The modality of education will vary and is dependent upon the CNS and the particular patient and family. Audiovisual aids and written material are essential for reinforcing the information given. Equipment similar to that utilized for the various procedures and dolls such as "Kelly"[2] may be used not only for instruction but also in a play therapy situation for the younger child. This allows the patient to act out performing the procedures, thereby minimizing anxieties.

The patient and family require a tremendous amount of psychological support in addition to education. Topor states that "three-quarters of nurses' time on the transplant unit involves psychologic care."[3] The CNS is involved in the psychological support of the patient and family and provides psychological support for the health care team as well.

Jones noted that primary nursing had a beneficial effect on the transplant patient by providing a "highly satisfactory communication experience for the patient."[4] The ability of the patient and family to cope with the multiple stresses of transplantation was enhanced by such communication. Not all institutions provide for primary nursing care, and therefore the CNS may be the primary individual accessible to the patient and family, thereby providing a vehicle for communication with the patient.

## PREPARATION FOR RENAL TRANSPLANT

The pediatric patient with ESRD and his family interact with many members of the health care team in preparation for the renal transplant. The CNS, as the most accessible member of the team, uses the initial conferences to build rapport with the patient and family. The methods used to establish an effective therapeutic relationship vary with the patient population. It is important to recognize that every patient is an individual with special needs and rights, and that every family presents a unique situation. The CNS frequently is the primary source of information for the patient and family before, during, and after the transplant. Because the CNS is consistently available and easily approachable, she may become the primary person upon whom families may release their anxieties and frustrations.[5] Speaking with the family in their native language whenever possible is desirable. If this is not feasible, a good translator, some member of the family or close friend whom the family can trust, is preferable.

The CNS utilizes the initial patient-family conference prior to the initial team conference to assess the patient and family's readiness to learn. Without readiness, learning will not occur.[6] If the patient and family have not accepted the diagnosis of irreversible renal failure and the patient is on dialysis, but the patient and family hold out the hope that renal function will return, they will not be ready to discuss the concept of transplantation. It is important to realize that every family unit differs in their readiness to learn.

Prior to the initial team conference the CNS must assess the level of knowledge of the patient and family concerning renal transplantation. The patient with ESRD receives information from many sources. It is important in planning the initial team conference to document the knowledge base, to ascertain the correctness of the information and to determine what the patient wants to know and what the patient needs to know.[6]

The composition of the initial team conference with the patient and family regarding renal transplantation includes the primary physician (pediatric nephrologist or transplant surgeon), the CNS, and the social worker. The primary goal of the initial team conference is to give the family an adequate *knowledge base* about renal transplantation in order to enable the patient and family to feel some control and to share in the decision-making process regarding their destiny.[7] When parents are anxious about transplantation, this is transmitted to the child; if the parents are well-informed and their anxieties thus reduced, the attitude of the child will be positively affected.[8] The content of the initial team conference provides a basic concept of renal transplantation. Topics covered include transplantation as a therapy and not a cure; living related versus cadaver donor transplantation; histocompatibility testing; the surgical procedure; the preoperative care of the patient; the immunosuppressive medications and their side effects; postoperative risks, including rejection; and delineation of the potential benefits. Obviously, the CNS must have precise knowledge of all these various areas. It can be anticipated that the CNS will be requested to explain in detail and to redefine on many subsequent occasions most of the information given to the family in the initial conference.

Following the initial conference, the CNS arranges for the family to meet and to speak with other patients and their families who have received both successful and unsuccessful renal transplants. An effort is made to pair families as to cultural and socioeconomic background and to patient age. The opportunity to discuss transplantation openly with other patients and families helps families in several ways: unique support can be given by one who has experienced the same situation; a peer's understanding of the transplantation experience is provided; a safe haven is offered to discuss troubling issues; and finally, issues requiring further discussion with the transplant team can be identified.

Subsequently, the CNS assures that blood samples for histocompatability testing and antibody screening are obtained from the patient. If there is a potential live related donor, the CNS coordinates the initial histocompatability testing between potential donor(s) and recipient.

All patients awaiting renal transplantation are seen on a monthly basis by the CNS following initiation of dialysis. During these visits, education continues, with the orientation changing to meet the patient and family's needs. If the patient is awaiting a cadaveric transplant, the CNS provides psychological support for the patient and family during the sometimes long, anxiety-producing wait.

Frequently, parents offer to become a donor for their child. Mothers consider organ donation as part of their obligation to their children and sustain enhanced self-esteem subsequent to the donation.[9]

In the potential live related donor situation, the CNS plays a critical role not only in coordinating the physical and psychological evaluation of the donor but also as a source of continuing education. Such education encompasses outcome statistics, risks to the donor, pre- and postoperative care, and rehabilitation. In addition, the CNS plays a vital role in offering psychological support to the entire family, all of whom are affected in various ways by the potential organ donation.

## PREOPERATIVE MANAGEMENT

As indicated previously the level of patient-family education is highly correlated with compliance with therapeutic regimens,[10, 11] and thus it is incumbent upon the CNS to assure appropriate preoperative education. Despite the fact that the patient may have had previous surgery, even a previous transplant, it is important that all patients and their families receive education which is designed to meet the current clinical situation. As the child matures, he develops new kinds of learning needs and the CNS must not assume that the patient and family with previous transplant experience is necessarily completely knowledgeable and free of anxiety.

As in the preparatory phase of education regarding renal transplantation, it is important to assess the patient's readiness to learn. If the patient and family are highly stressed, comprehension will be minimal. With the highly stressed family, it is important to initially relieve some anxieties by allowing them to express their anxieties and ask questions. By offering psychological support, the CNS can frequently create a milieu which facilitates and fosters learning.

The teaching of the family should be individualized to meet the particular level of comprehension of the family. The methods of teaching the child should be appropriate for developmental age.

In the case of the potential living related donor, the initial preoperative teaching of the recipient may occur on an outpatient basis not more than two weeks before surgery. In the case of a cadaver donor transplant, teaching begins upon the patient's admission to the hospital for the transplant. If the preoperative teaching is initiated too early, there is too much time to stimulate unconscious fantasies and fears. On the other hand, if the time interval between initiation of teaching and the transplantation is too short, the patient's ego may be unable to prepare the necessary psychological defenses.[12]

For the infant or very young child, the most traumatic aspect of transplantation is parental separation. The parents should be encouraged to remain with the child as much as possible; if they are unable to remain with the child, a significant other person should be identified to be with the child when the parents are absent.[13]

Luciano states that the value of preoperative teaching in the two- to three-year-old child is controversial.[14] However, some ESRD patients of this age who have had multiple procedures and previous hospitalizations have a sophistication beyond their chronologic age; therefore, such children deserve simple explanations of the preoperative procedures. Separation anxiety is significant in this age group and must be addressed by the staff and family.

For the young child three to six years of age, even if a live related donor transplant is contemplated, the preoperative teaching should not begin prior to one week before transplantation. The child of this age is characteristically egocentric,[15] and thus information given should focus on feelings and encourage participation in the procedures. The child over the age of seven years may receive preoperative teaching up to two weeks prior to surgery.[14] The child in this age group is most interested in the reason for the procedures. He wants to know what is going to be done and why it is going to be done to him.[16]

Adolescents have much greater anxieties than younger children[13] and need to feel they have some control over their destiny. In the instance of a live related donor transplant, this can be accomplished by allowing the adolescent to schedule the transplantation on a date which presents the least conflict with his or her social and school schedule. In the preoperative teaching of the adolescent, allowing for questions and permitting as much decision making as possible will tend to relieve some anxieties. The adolescent requires a great deal of reassurance during the preoperative teaching period.

All preoperative teaching should be simple, accurate, and in language the child understands. The basic information to be imparted includes: where the incision will be made; how long the surgery will take; and where the patient can expect to wake up. The patient needs to know that he will have an IV, a Foley catheter, perhaps a nasogastric tube, and will be placed on a cardiac monitor in the ICU; that he will have some pain and that he will be given medication to relieve the pain; that he may have a very large amount of urinary ouput or a small amount or none at all and that none of these eventualities is alarming; that dialysis may be necessary postoperatively. In addition, the patient needs to know what is expected of him postoperatively, including remaining flat in bed or slightly elevated for the first 24 hours. Deep breathing and coughing should be demonstrated and practiced. It is important not to give too much information. One should focus on what to expect in the first 24 to 48 hours following surgery.

The preoperative period is filled with anxiety for the patient and family. The CNS is in a unique position to help alleviate some anxiety not only by educating the family but also by giving psychological support and encouraging them to ask questions and express their fears, while offering them realistic and honest reassurance.

An additional role of the CNS in the preoperative period is to consult with the ICU nursing staff and, if necessary, to review the postoperative patient care plan. This includes frequent monitoring of vital signs (every hour for the first 24 hours); accurate measurement of intake and output and replacement therapy; assuring patency of the Foley catheter; observing the incision for bleeding; weighing the patient daily; frequent blood chemical determinations and urine testing; aseptic care of the wound, Foley catheter, and IV tubing; care of the fistula, shunt, or peritoneal catheter; encouraging pulmonary toilet; observing for signs of infection and rejection; administering appropriate immunosuppressive drugs; and finally, delineating the psychological needs of the post-transplant patient. The ICU nurse should be given pertinent data regarding the special physical and psychosocial needs of the patient and family, thus allowing the nurse to deliver optimal individualized care. Information regarding the patient's daily urinary output prior to transplant, baseline laboratory values, and range of vital signs and previous medications will assist the ICU nurse in assessing the patient optimally postoperatively. Information regarding the patient's level of cooperation, interactions with family members, and availability of family members maximizes the ability of the ICU nurse to give optimal support to the patient. The ICU nurse should be reassured that the CNS is available for consultation concerning any physical or psychological problems which arise with the patient or his family.[17]

## POSTOPERATIVE MANAGEMENT

In the immediate postoperative period, the patient is occupied with multiple activities of the ICU nurse, who must monitor kidney function, prevent infection, and observe for clinical evidence of rejection and other potential complications. The CNS offers reassurance to the patient and family by explaining the basis for these routine activities. The CNS can support the patient and ICU nursing staff by encouraging the patient to deep-breathe and cough. Because of the special rapport with the CNS, the patient is frequently more responsive to her suggestions in the early postoperative period when the patient is physically uncomfortable and emotionally labile.

During the early postoperative period both the patient and family are overly concerned about the level of kidney function. The family is concerned about immediate rejection and the longevity of kidney function. The CNS can reassure them that rejection episodes are almost always anticipated and that these episodes do not portend ominously for kidney survival. The anxieties and frustrations of the patient and family may be expressed as hostility toward the transplant team and ICU nursing staff. If this occurs, the CNS offers support, encouragement, and specific information that is reassuring, and encourages the patient and family to verbalize their fears.

Prior to the transfer of the patient from the ICU to a regular hospital floor care, the CNS interfaces with the floor nursing staff by reviewing the standards of care with them including accurate intake and output records, daily weights, immunosuppressive therapy regimen, observation for infection and rejection, assessment of daily laboratory results,[17] and appropriate dietary allowances. The CNS apprises the floor staff nurse of the special physical and psychological needs of the patient, thus facilitating delivery of individualized patient care. The CNS is available for participation in patient care conferences.

Postoperative teaching begins on the third postoperative day or at a time when the patient is clinically stable and mentally alert. The indications that the patient is ready to learn are similar to those described earlier.

The goal of postoperative education is to assure that, by the time of discharge, the patient and family are familiar with the prescribed medications, and knowledgeable about the side effects of these medications. The patient and parents, depending upon patient age, should demonstrate the ability to count the number of pills prescribed and also show the ability to take them. The patient and parents are taught to count the number of pills remaining prior to coming to the clinic so that appropriate prescriptions can be obtained to assure that sufficient medication is available to last until the next clinic visit. The importance of taking the immunosuppressive drugs as long as the kidney functions is stressed. The patient and family are taught the signs and symptoms of rejection. They are taught the meaning of the laboratory tests used to evaluate renal function and the effectiveness of the immunosuppressive therapy in maintaining kidney function. The CNS arranges for the patient and family to receive dietary instruction from the renal dietitian. At this time the need for good general health habits is emphasized. If age permits the patient is encouraged to be an active participant in his care. Information is given regarding resumption of activities and the importance of follow-up visits to the transplant clinic.

The CNS participates in the discharge planning of the patient, including focusing on the special needs of the transplant patient, reassuring him or her concerning medications by devising a medication calendar detailing the daily dosage schedule, planning a follow-up transplant clinic appointment and making sure the family has the names and telephone numbers of the members of the transplant team. If any transportation problems to the transplant clinic are identified, the CNS consults with the social worker to facilitate appropriate transportation.

Leaving the security of the hospital is associated with anxiety for the patient and family. Reassurance that a physician or nurse is available on a 24-hour basis is helpful in reducing some of the anxiety.

## OUTPATIENT MANAGEMENT

Effective long-term close follow-up care is essential to ensure the success of renal transplantation in the pediatric allograft recipient. The CNS participates in the outpatient care by continuing patient-family assessment, education, and support. The CNS is responsible for orienting the new post-transplant patient to the transplant clinic format, including routine laboratory work and routine consultation at each visit with the CNS, physician (pediatric nephrologist and/or transplant surgeon), social worker, and renal dietitian. The CNS undertakes a nursing assessment during each clinic visit, which facilitates identification of problems requiring immediate intervention. The assessment is holistic, focusing on both the physical and psychological aspects of care. Physical evaluation includes obtaining vital signs, voiding characteristics, bowel habits, adverse symptoms, and activity level. The patient or parent is asked to list the current medications, the dosage schedule, and the purpose for each medication. Any difficulties encountered in taking the medications are elicited. Reviewing the medication at each clinic visit reinforces the knowledge about the therapy and the need to comply with it.

Psychosocial assessment includes observation of the patient and family mood, detection of anxieties regarding rejection episodes, information regarding patient-family interactions, determination of current level of activity, and detection of problems inhibiting compliance with the post-transplant outpatient regimen. The CNS uses the clinic visit as an opportunity to give emotional support to the family, allowing them to express any anxieties or frustrations.

Irwin,[18] Rees,[19] and Sachs and Hargrove[20] have developed good nursing assessment tools for the renal transplant recipient. Other methods of docmentation include the use of SOAP (subjective objective assessment plan) or POR (problem oriented record) charting. It is incumbent upon the CNS to document findings as a method of communication with the transplant team, and this will enhance total patient care.

The patient-family education is less formalized in the outpatient setting but is of no less importance. Areas of need for education are identified during assessment of the patient. The most frequent areas requiring re-education include type of medications, their purpose and dosage schedule; signs and symptoms of rejection; permitted level of activity; and laboratory results and their meaning.

If changes in medication are made by the physician at the time of the clinic visit, the CNS re-educates the patient and family regarding these changes. The patient and family are told that the CNS will call them with the results of the laboratory studies or any medication changes following the clinic visit. The CNS assures that the transplant team has the current telephone number and address of the patient so that any follow-up information can be transmitted easily.

Rejection episodes are extremely anxiety-producing for both the patient and family. The CNS frequently is the individual who calls the patient or family when additional laboratory studies are required. The CNS supports the family in this situation by being honest and giving concrete information regarding the reason for additional studies. At such times the CNS solicits and allows for expression of fear and frustration. During treatment of rejection episodes the CNS sees the patient daily and in some institutions administers the therapy.

## OTHER ROLES OF THE CNS IN PEDIATRIC RENAL TRANSPLANTATION

The role of the CNS in pediatric renal transplantation varies from one institution to another but may include any of the following responsibilities:

1. Develop administrative and nursing policies and procedures for care of the pediatric transplant patient.
2. Assure the implementation of policies and procedures required by the federal regulations pertaining to transplantation.
3. Complete state and federal ESRD medical information systems questionnaire required by federal regulations.
4. Participate in organ procurement activities.
5. Collate patient data.
6. Participate in the transplant team patient review conferences.
7. Schedule transplants with surgeon, inpatient nursing staff, and ICU nursing staff.
8. Update list of patients awaiting cadaveric transplant.
9. Coordinate patient care activities of the transplant team.
10. Provide inservice education for pediatric nursing staff and pediatric house staff.

## CONCLUSION

The CNS working with the pediatric renal transplant patient must have a high level of technical, intellectual, and interpersonal skills. These patients and their families are highly stressed and in need of care, education, and reassurance. Through education and support, the CNS may ameliorate some of the stress and promote a successful outcome.

## REFERENCES

1. Sebastian J, Webb D: Relationship between knowledge about condition and care and adjustment by renal dialysis and transplant patients. Proc Am Assoc Nephrol Nurses Tech 5:45, 1978.
2. Dory J: Teaching the young child nephrology care. Nephrol Nurse 4:50, 1982.
3. Topor MA: Nursing the renal transplantation patient. Nurs Clin North Am 4:461, 1969.
4. Jones K: Study documents effect of primary nursing of renal transplant patients. Hospitals, JAHA 49:85, 1975.
5. Ayer, AH: Is partnership with patients really possible? J Mat Child Health Nurs 3:107, 1978.
6. Arsianian J: The need for patient education. Proc Am Assoc Nephrol Nurses Tech 5:71, 1978.
7. Kodadek S: Family-centered care for the chronically ill child. J Am Operating Rm Nurses 30:635, 1979.
8. Smitherman CH: Parents of hospitalized children have needs, too. Am J Nurs 79:1423, 1979.
9. Fellner CH, Marshall JR: Twelve kidney donors. JAMA 206:2703, 1968.
10. Hecht AB: Improving medication compliance by teaching outpatients. Nurs Forum 13:112, 1974.
11. Weintraub, M: Promoting patient complicance. NY State J Med 75:2263, 1975.
12. Freud A: The role of bodily illness in the mental life of children. In Psychoanalytic Study of the Child. New York, International Universities Press, 8:69, 1952.
13. Mellish RWP: Preparation of a child for hospitalization and surgery. Pediatr Clin North Am 16:543, 1969.
14. Luciano K: The who, when, where, what and how of preparing children for surgery. Nursing '74 4:64, 1974.
15. Piaget J: Judgement and reasoning in the child. Patterson, NJ, Littlefield, Adams and Co, 1959, p 256.
16. Wu R: Explaining treatments to young children. Am J Nurs 65:71, 1965.
17. American Association of Nephrology Nurses and Technicians: Standards of Clinical Practice II: Transplantation. Pitman, NJ, AANNT, revised, 1976.
18. Irwin BC: An expanded role for nurses: Systematic assessment of renal transplant recipients. J Am Assoc Nephrol Nurses Tech 6:109, 1979.
19. Rees PL: Nursing assessment in follow-up care of the renal transplant recipient. Nephrol Nurse 2:49, 1980.
20. Sachs BL, Hargrove JC: Patient outcome criteria: a tool for quality assurance. J Am Assoc Nephrol Nurses Tech 5:41, 1978.

# 37

# Recurrence of the Primary Disease in the Transplanted Kidney

*Ernst P. Leumann, M.D.*
*Jakob Briner, M.D.*

Recurrence of the original disease in the transplanted kidney was noted in the early experience with renal transplantation of both isografts and allografts.[1-3] Subsequently a large number of additional cases have been published. Several review articles on recurrence of primary glomerular disease are available.[4, 5, 5a]

Recurrence is defined as the reappearance of a lesion in the renal transplant that is due to the persistence of the pathogenic process which led to the original renal disease. The diagnosis of recurrence is often difficult to establish because the precise pathogenic mechanism of the original disease is only rarely known and, also, only a few renal lesions are truly specific. If a pathologic marker is present, examination by electron microscopy or by immunofluorescence will permit diagnosis of recurrence in a high percentage of cases despite the absence of light microscopic abnormalities or clinical evidence of recurrence. In many instances, it is difficult to differentiate recurrence from *de novo* glomerulonephritis, glomerulonephritis associated with rejection, transplant glomerulopathy, or donor glomerulonephritis.[4, 6-9]

The rate of recurrence depends primarily on the original disease (Table 37–1). Immunosuppression, disease activity, and length of the observation period may also be important factors. The overall incidence as judged from large individual series ranges from 5.6% to 9.3%.[4, 7, 10] The clinical significance of recurrence is modest or even absent in most conditions, but occasionally it is of great importance. Recurrence may become a more important determining factor in transplantation once the problem of rejection is overcome.

The study of recurrence has contributed considerably to a better understanding of the natural history of many renal diseases. Furthermore, it has helped to establish the specificity of certain diseases (e.g., dense deposit disease) as well as to suggest heterogeneity (e.g., focal segmental glomerulosclerosis). It has also led to questioning the validity of certain pathogenetic concepts, e.g., the role of circulating immune complexes in systemic lupus erythematosus, where recurrence is minimal.[11]

In this chapter, special attention will be given to those diseases in which recurrence has major clinical implications in the pediatric age group, i.e., primary hyperoxaluria, focal segmental glomerulosclerosis, and membranoproliferative glomerulonephritis types I and II. Diseases which rarely lead to renal failure in childhood will only be briefly considered.

We would like to thank Dr. J. S. Cameron, Guy's Hospital, London, and Dr. R. Habib and Dr. M. Broyer, Hôpital des Enfants Malades, Paris, for access to their data prior to publication.

**Table 37–1.** INCIDENCE AND CLINICAL SIGNIFICANCE OF RECURRENCE

| Disease | Number of Patients with Recurrence Reported[a] | Rate of Recurrence[b] | Clinical Significance of Recurrence[c] |
|---|---|---|---|
| *Primary Glomerular Diseases* | | | |
| Focal segmental glomerulosclerosis | 59 | 26% | often severe |
| Membranoproliferative GN type I | 50 | 33% | often severe |
| Dense deposit disease | 54 | 90% | often minor |
| Membranous nephropathy | 14 | 29%[d] | often severe |
| IgA nephropathy | 15 | 58%[e] | minor |
| Crescentic GN (idiopathic) | 6 | 33%[f] | — |
| Hereditary nephritis | 1 | 1% | — |
| *Systemic Diseases* | | | |
| Henoch-Schönlein purpura | 12 | 40%[g] | often minor |
| Systemic lupus erythematosus | 3 | 1% | — |
| Anti-GBM nephritis | 20 | 5% | minor |
| Wegener's granulomatosis/Polyarteritis nodosa | 3 | (low) | — |
| Amyloidosis | 1[h] | low[h] | — |
| Hemolytic-uremic syndrome | 4 | low | — |
| Progressive systemic sclerosis | 4 | (33%) | — |
| *Metabolic Diseases* | | | |
| Primary hyperoxaluria | 36 | 100% | usually severe |
| Diabetes mellitus | 1[i] | rare[i] | — |
| Cystinosis | 0 | 0% | — |

[a]Several patients have been reported more than once; hence the numbers given are only approximate.
[b]These are probably maximum figures, as nonrecurrent cases are rarely reported.
[c]Indicated only in diseases with more than 10 recurrent cases reported.
[d]5 of 17 grafts reported in four series.[5, 5a, 6, 10]
[e]14 of 24 cases.[70]
[f]Data from Cameron.[5]
[g]6 of 15 cases.[5, 83]
[h]For glomerular lesions. Vascular lesions recurred in 14%.
[i]For diabetic glomerulosclerosis. Diabetic microangiopathy recurred in 12 of 12 cases.[144]

# RECURRENCE IN PRIMARY GLOMERULAR DISEASES

## Focal Segmental Glomerulosclerosis (FSGS)

Idiopathic nephrotic syndrome with FSGS is an important cause of terminal renal failure in childhood. Recurrence of FSGS was first reported by Hoyer et al in 1972[12] and has since been described in almost 60 patients.[5a, 7, 10, 13–32] It has become evident, however, that FSGS recurs only in a minority of patients.

Recurrent FSGS usually presents as heavy proteinuria within the first days or weeks, or even within the first hours of transplantation.[5, 21] However, it must be noted that significant proteinuria at this early stage is not an uncommon finding after renal transplantation, but heavy protein excretion (over 2 gm per 24 hours) at two weeks is suggestive of recurrence.[24] Heavy proteinuria may decrease after several months, but in most cases, a full-blown nephrotic syndrome is observed, which usually is associated with progressive deterioration of renal function. In a survey conducted in 1982 by the pediatric registry of the European Dialysis and Transplant Association,[33] 11 of the 21 grafts with recurrent FSGS were lost owing to recurrence within 30 months following transplantation; however, one patient did maintain adequate function for nine years despite recurrence.

Although the presence of recurrence may be strongly suspected on clinical grounds, a transplant biopsy is required for definitive diagnosis. Characteristic findings of FSGS have been noted six to eight weeks after transplantation,[10, 24, 27] but are usually noted only later. FSGS, however, is not a specific finding and can be seen as a superimposed feature in various other conditions.

Neither bilateral nephrectomy nor prolonged dialysis prior to renal transplantation prevent recurrence. If present in the first graft, recurrent FSGS is likely to occur in subsequent transplants as well.[5a, 10, 15, 16, 17, 22, 25, 26, 27] However, the clinical course in subsequent grafts may not be identical to that of the initial graft. The following *risk factors* have been implicated:

**1. Duration of the Original Disease.** Three reports on large groups of patients have noted that a short duration of the original disease (less than two to three years from diagnosis until ESRD) is associated with a higher risk of developing recurrence.[20, 22, 27] In the Paris series, the mean duration of the original disease was 2.8 years in the recurrent group compared to 5.3 years in the nonrecurrent group.[20] In our collected data (mainly from pediatric series), the duration of the original disease was less than three years in 24 of 33 recurrent cases (73%) (Fig. 37–1). However, not all patients with a rapid course will show recurrent FSGS: 26 of 50 patients had no recurrence (Fig. 37–1). These data may be biased; therefore, the estimated risk of recurrence in FSGS is probably less than 50% in cases with a rapid course (duration of the original disease less than three years), and only 10 to 20% in those with a longer duration of the original disease.

**2. Mesangial Proliferation.** The presence of mesangial proliferation in the native kidney, which is frequently associated with a rapid, malignant course,[34, 35] has been noted in a number of patients whose disease subsequently recurred (in 11 of 19 of one series).[33]

**3. Age.** Older children are at a greater risk of developing recurrence than younger ones. Mean age at onset was 8.9 years in the recurrent group compared to 3.9 years in the nonrecurrent groups.[20] In the EDTA survey, 11 of 21 patients (52%) whose age at onset was 6 years or more had recurrence, whereas only 6 of 38 patients (16%, $p < 0.01$) who were younger than 6 years of age manifested recurrence.[33] Nine of the patients in this survey had the two risk factors "mesangial proliferation" and "age $\geq$ 6 years" combined, and 8 of these (89%) demonstrated recurrence. Adult patients over the age of 20 years have a low incidence of recurrence.[27]

**4. Tissue Matching.** A distressingly high recurrence rate for 4-antigen matched transplants from sibling donors was noted by Zimmerman;[31] however, this observation has not been verified.[5, 24]

The *etiology* of the idiopathic nephrotic syndrome with FSGS remains unknown. Recurrent FSGS might constitute a specific subgroup of patients. Hoyer et al postulated the existence of a circulating humoral substance.[12] Attempts directed to induce proteinuria by injecting plasma from affected patients into animals have not been successful.[12, 32] Plasmapheresis directed toward re-

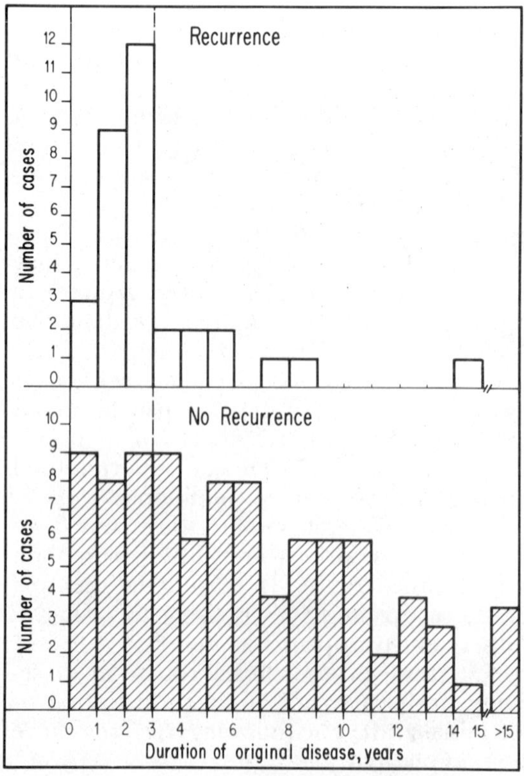

**Figure 37–1.** Focal segmental glomerulosclerosis: Risk of recurrence in relation to duration of original disease (from apparent onset until dialysis). Duration was less than 3 years in 24 of 33 patients (73%) *with* recurrence (upper panel) and in 26 of 93 patients (28%) *without* recurrence. Data is taken from the literature[13, 18, 20, 22, 25–27] and our own observations (6 patients).

moval of this postulated substance has been tried with no[27] or only minimal[30, 32] success. The risk of recurrence is probably not increased in patients with familial FSGS.

*Steroid-responsive* idiopathic nephrotic syndrome with minimal changes on light microscopy rarely leads to progressive renal failure. One unusual case was reported of a five-year-old child with frequently relapsing nephrotic syndrome who developed renal failure secondary to severe interstitial nephritis.[36] Severe proteinuria three years post transplantation responded to increased prednisone administration in this patient.

# Membranoproliferative Glomerulonephritis Type I (Mesangiocapillary Glomerulonephritis with Subendothelial Deposits) (MPGN I)

One hundred and fifty patients with MPGN I who received 157 grafts have been reported up to 1982.* These data include 23 pediatric patients, of whom seven (30%) had recurrent MPGN I.[14, 39, 43, 45, 48] The recurrence rate for the entire group of patients was similar (33%).

Recurrent MPGN I is the most difficult type of glomerulonephritis to delineate in a transplant biopsy because of the close resemblance to glomerular lesions associated with rejection. Marked proliferation, clear-cut double contouring of the glomerular basement membrane, and the presence of electron-dense subendothelial deposits allow distinction from transplant glomerulopathy. Since transplant glomerulonephritis closely resembles recurrent MPGN I, the diagnosis of the latter can be made with confidence only in the absence of rejection. The rate of recurrence therefore may have been overestimated in the past. Serum complement levels are of no diagnostic value.

Subdivision of MPGN I into three types could be important, in that recurrence was present in only two of 23 patients with "pure" MPGN I, in two of 13 with the lobular variant, and in three of the four patients with isolated C3 deposits.[5a]

Recurrence is thus observed in a minority of patients with MPGN I, but the clinical impact on those affected is potentially serious. Half of the 53 patients in whom suffi-

cient clinical data was given had severe impairment of renal function (serum creatinine above 5 mg/100 ml), and only one fourth of the patients had a serum creatinine level of less than 2 mg/100 ml.[6] Recurrent MPGN I was considered a major factor leading to graft failure in 12 of 49 grafts.[6]

# Membranoproliferative Glomerulonephritis Type II: Dense Deposit Disease (DDD)

Recurrence is seen in a very high percentage of patients with DDD. Since children and young adults are primarily affected by this disease,[49] recurrent DDD is important in pediatric kidney recipients, even though clinical signs of recurrence are often minor.

To date, information on 84 allografts transplanted into 69 recipients is available.† Unlike the situation in most other conditions, diagnosis of recurrence can definitely be established by electron microscopic examination of the graft biopsy, since the intramembranous "deposits"—which correspond to an alteration of the basement membrane[53]—are specific for this disease. Dense "deposits" were observed in 54 of 60 grafts (90%). Without electron microscopic examination, diagnosis of recurrence would have been missed in more than half of the patients. Glomerular proliferation was seen in only 19 of 45 grafts (42%).[6, 38, 52]

Clinical signs of recurrence (hematuria and proteinuria or the nephrotic syndrome) were noted in one third of cases (in 21 of 57 patients), and often became evident only after several years. Graft failure was attributed to recurrence in 14 instances, whereas 22 grafts were lost for other reasons, primarily rejection.[6, 10, 14, 52] Extensive crescent formation with rapid deterioration of graft function was observed in one of our patients 20 months after transplantation.[57]

Deposition of electron-dense material starts shortly after transplantation. Such deposition can be seen as early as three weeks after transplantation and was present by six months in all patients who ultimately showed recurrence.[51] In contrast, fixation of C3 and glomerular proliferation, if present, are noted later. The serum complement profile predicts neither recurrence nor prognosis. Persistent hypocomplementemia was always

---

*References 5a, 6, 7, 10, 14, 37–48, 140, and 157.

†References 5a, 6, 7, 10, 14, 37, 39, 40, 45, 49–59.

associated with recurrence, but the presence of normal levels of C3 does not exclude recurrence.[56] Recurrence is not prevented by bilateral nephrectomy[57–59] and may occur in subsequent transplants.[39, 45, 55, 58, 59]

## Membranous Nephropathy

Membranous nephropathy (MN), although a common type of glomerulonephritis, infrequently causes ESRD in children. Considered previously to be very rare, recurrent MN has now been reported in 14 (all adult) patients.[8–10, 60–68] Recurrent MN is rare in most series except in that reported by Morzycka et al in which it recurred in 4 of 7 grafts.[10] The low recurrence rate is unexpected since MN is considered to represent a typical example of immune complex nephritis (with in situ immune complex formation). In fact, *de novo* MN is twice as frequent as recurrent MN in renal allografts and has been observed in 37 instances to date.[5] One case of recurrent *de novo* MN has been reported.[61]

Recurrent MN usually presents as massive proteinuria leading to the nephrotic syndrome. Proteinuria may become evident only after several years[8, 10, 65] or during the first year,[62] or even within the first week after transplantation.[66, 67] Graft loss due to recurrent MN has been reported only once,[65] in a case with superimposed extracapillary proliferation.

## IgA Nephropathy

Mesangial proliferative glomerulonephritis with IgA deposits is a chronic and usually benign disease which often begins in childhood. Renal transplantation has been reported in 35 patients.[5a, 6, 7, 10, 69, 70] In 14 patients, the age was indicated[6, 7, 69] and five of the recipients were under 16 years of age.

IgA nephropathy frequently recurs in the graft. The largest series reported by Berger in 1982 records recurrence in 14 of 24 cases (58%).[70] The recurrence rate would certainly be underestimated if such an easily recognized marker of the disease—mesangial deposits of IgA—were unavailable.

Recurrent IgA nephropathy follows a relatively benign course comparable to that of the original disease. Graft failure was attributed to recurrence in only one of 20 trans-

plants.[6, 7] The high recurrence rate should therefore not contraindicate renal transplantation.

## Crescentic Glomerulonephritis

Extracapillary proliferation represents an easily recognized, albeit nonspecific, marker. This feature may explain the fact that extracapillary proliferative (crescentic) glomerulonephritis was among the first types of recurrences to be described in isografts[1] and allografts.[3, 71, 72] Extracapillary proliferation can be seen in various types of renal disease, some of which are not even immunologic in nature. It is a heterogeneous lesion which may occur without a recognizable basic pattern; however, in most instances, an underlying primary lesion can be detected. Recurrence of crescentic glomerulonephritis has been described in membranoproliferative glomerulonephritis type I,[6, 44] in dense deposit disease,[6, 57] in anti-GBM nephritis,[73, 74] in Henoch-Schönlein syndrome,[75] and in membranous nephropathy.[65] In a number of cases of recurrent crescentic glomerulonephritis the underlying disease was not identified.[10, 72]

## Hereditary Nephritis (Alport's Syndrome)

Renal transplantation has been performed in a large number of patients with hereditary nephritis (EDTA report, 1979:[76] 127 patients; ASC/NIH report, 1975:[77] 73 patients). Recurrent glomerular lesions have been described in only one patient, whose graft was lost due to rejection.[7]

A few patients developed *de novo* anti-GBM nephritis in their transplant.[78, 79] This observation is extremely interesting in view of recent findings which suggest that the basic abnormality in Alport's syndrome may consist of the presence of a glomerular basement membrane that is deficient in the non-collagen portion and lacks an antigen present in normal kidneys. After transplantation the newly introduced glomerular basement membrane of the donor kidney may induce the production of antibodies, which in turn might fix to the graft and lead to *de novo* anti-GBM antibody nephritis.

A case with possible recurrence of an unusual form of familial glomerulonephritis has recently been reported.[80]

## RECURRENT GLOMERULAR LESIONS IN SYSTEMIC DISEASES

### Anaphylactoid Purpura (Henoch-Schönlein Purpura) (HSP)

Results of renal transplantation have been reported in 41 patients with HSP, 18 of whom were children.[5, 5a, 43, 75, 81–85] Mesangial deposition of IgA without glomerular proliferation and without clinical manifestations of recurrence was the only evidence of recurrent HSP in a number of patients. Mesangial deposits of IgA in the transplant biopsy were present in six of eight patients studied by Levy et al,[83] but were absent in all seven patients reported by Cameron.[5] In one case, IgA deposits were demonstrated at three years, but were not present in the first biopsy at five months post transplant.[83]

Clinical evidence of recurrent HSP, manifested by proteinuria and hematuria, was present in five cases.[75, 81, 83–85] Graft loss due to recurrence was observed in three patients, whose transplant biopsies showed proliferative glomerulonephritis with occasional crescents.[75, 81, 84]

Recurrent HSP is seen primarily in patients whose initial course had been characterized by rapid progression and a short time interval between the onset of disease and transplantation.[75, 84] Therefore, it is advisable to wait until purpura has subsided for at least 12 months before contemplating transplantation.[83]

Extrarenal manifestations of recurrent HSP after renal transplantation were reported in only one patient.[75] In the remaining cases recurrence was confined to the glomerular lesions, which were identical to those in IgA nephropathy, further underscoring the close relationship between HSP and IgA nephropathy.

### Systemic Lupus Erythematosus (SLE)

Recurrence of SLE in the graft is exceptional. Only three cases have been reported,[11, 86] while there are probably more than 400 functional grafts in the world in patients with SLE.[5] The three reported cases presented with extrarenal clinical manifestations of SLE despite quiescent clinical features during dialysis. The rarity of recurrence is surprising in view of the hypothesis that SLE represents a classic example of soluble immune complex nephritis. Several explanations have been put forward for the paucity of recurrence: (1) immunosuppressive therapy may prevent recurrence; (2) pathogenic mechanisms of SLE are burnt out once patients come to renal transplantation; and (3) current theories on the pathogenesis of lupus nephritis need to be revised.

### Anti-Glomerular Basement Membrane Nephritis (Anti-GBM Nephritis) and Goodpasture Syndrome

Anti-GBM nephritis occurs alone or in combination with pulmonary hemorrhage (Goodpasture syndrome) and is almost exclusively seen in adults. Recurrence in this disease has been intensely studied.[5, 6, 10, 73, 74, 87–92] The risk of recurrence has become low (less than 5%)[5] since renal transplants are no longer performed when the antibody titer is elevated. The results of earlier publications are therefore not representative of the current situation. In the series published in 1973 by Wilson and Dixon,[92] three of nine patients with typical Goodpasture syndrome had recurrence, as evidenced by linear IgG deposition on immunofluorescence; however, only one patient had glomerulonephritis on light microscopic examination and lost the graft owing to recurrence. Five of 15 patients with isolated anti-GBM nephritis received 18 grafts and developed mild clinical signs of recurrence with positive staining by immunofluorescence. Only one patient developed heavy proteinuria. It should be noted, however, that linear IgG immunofluorescence is a relatively common and nonspecific finding in the early phase of renal transplantation. There are no reports of renal transplantation in children with anti-GBM nephritis.

Cameron advocates delaying renal transplantation until six to 12 months after anti-GBM antibodies have become negative and has not observed recurrence in four patients with five grafts.[5] Recurrence was noted in one patient only two weeks after transplantation, even though grafting was delayed for one year.[88] On the other hand, successful transplantation was achieved in a patient despite the presence of a high antibody titer following plasmapheresis and immunosuppression.[90] Recurrence of the pulmonary lesions of Goodpasture syndrome after renal transplantation has been mentioned only once.[91]

## Wegener's Granulomatosis

The number of patients transplanted with Wegener's disease is small. Detailed information is available on only 10 patients.[93-98] All the recipients were young adults (25 to 43 years; average 33 years).

Recurrence of extrarenal manifestations of Wegener's disease was reported in two cases. In the first one, recurrent pulmonary manifestations developed three years after transplantation.[96] In the second patient, Wegener's granulomatosis recurred in the upper airways four years after transplantation.[93, 97] Microscopic hematuria suggested recurrent glomerulonephritis, but no biopsy of the graft was performed. Renal function was not impaired. Substitution of cyclophosphamide for azathioprine resulted in rapid remission of the clinical manifestations of Wegener's granulomatosis.[96, 97]

## Polyarteritis Nodosa (PAN)

Experience with renal transplantation in PAN is limited and confined to adult patients.[3, 5, 99] Recurrent PAN was believed to have been responsible for an early graft failure in a patient reported by Hume et al in 1955.[3] No evidence of recurrence was noted in a recently reported patient five years after renal transplantation.[99] Cameron mentions three patients, of whom one had recurrent extrarenal disease after transplantation, but without recurrence in the allograft.[5]

## Amyloidosis

Primary and secondary amyloidosis are slowly evolving diseases. Renal failure due to amyloidosis is rarely seen in childhood. Kidney transplantation has been reported only once in a pediatric patient with renal failure due to amyloidosis, which was secondary to familial Mediterranean fever.[100] Amyloid deposition in the allograft has been noted in 14 of 70 patients transplanted for amyloidosis.[77, 101-111] The rate of recurrence can be calculated from the three largest series.[104, 106, 108] Recurrence was observed in six of 41 patients who had received 44 grafts.

Deposition of amyloid in the transplant was noted mainly in arterioles and interlobular arteries, and less frequently in the interstitial tissue. Glomerular amyloid deposition in the mesangium and subendothelial space has been recorded only once.[103] This pattern of deposition differs from that in the native kidney, where the glomeruli are primarily affected.

Recurrence of amyloidosis did not affect the longevity of the graft,[106] and clinical findings were usually minimal or absent. Systemic amyloidosis nevertheless proceeded and adversely influenced patient and graft survival.[102, 103, 109]

## Hemolytic-Uremic Syndrome (HUS)

Recurrence of HUS is exceptional. Indeed, the paucity of reports on recurrent HUS[112-116] contrasts with the relative frequency of HUS as a cause of ESRD in childhood. Recurrent HUS has been described in detail in only two pediatric patients, an eight-year-old girl who developed recurrence 12 hours after transplantation in a second graft,[113] and a four-year-old boy who manifested recurrence four months after transplantation in both a second and fourth graft.[114] It must be admitted, however, that the diagnosis of recurrence is very difficult or sometimes impossible to substantiate, since vascular rejection with thrombosis can mimic HUS, both clinically and histologically.[114]

In one instance of familial HUS, the sister (adult) of the recipient developed a severe episode of HUS three weeks after kidney donation.[117] HUS may also occur in association with pregnancy or in women using oral contraceptives. In one adult female patient recurrent HUS was triggered by oral estrogens and occurred eight years after the initial episode of HUS and five years after cadaver kidney transplantation.[115]

Since the course of HUS is often characterized by repeated clinical episodes, it is advisable to delay renal transplantation for several months to assure quiescence.[14]

## Progressive Systemic Sclerosis

Thirty-four patients with progressive systemic sclerosis (scleroderma) were treated for ESRD in Europe by the end of 1979; only two patients received a renal allograft.[118] Although a few recipients have done well after renal transplantation,[119] four patients lost their grafts within three months, possibly to recurrent disease.[10, 119–121] Distinction of recurrence from rejection is exceedingly difficult.[119, 120]

## RECURRENCE IN METABOLIC DISEASES

### Primary Hyperoxaluria (PH)

PH type I is a rare inborn error of metabolism which usually leads to ESRD before the age of 20 years. The term oxalosis refers to generalized deposition of calcium oxalate and is not confined to PH. Some reports on renal transplantation in oxalosis include patients with secondary oxalosis.[77, 122]

Therapy of ESRD in young patients with primary hyperoxaluria is controversial, because recurrence uniformly occurs after renal transplantation and usually severely affects graft function. Therapy by either hemodialysis or CAPD removes insufficient amounts of oxalic acid and thus does not prevent progressive deposition of calcium oxalate with severe vascular and bone disease.[123] Theoretically, a renal transplant should be expected to be able to cope with the increased load of oxalate, even though slowly progressive deposition of calcium oxalate might not be avoided. However, clinical results have so far been rather poor. Data on 36 patients who received 44 grafts have been published.[14, 77, 122, 124–141] Ten of these grafts had been functioning for more than two years, and four for more than five years at the time of publication. However, half the patients for whom the age was given were older than 20 years and presumably had a milder form of the disease. By the end of 1979, only nine pediatric patients with PH had received a transplant in Europe, and five of the 10 grafts were still functioning.[123] Altogether, 29 pediatric and adult patients with PH have undergone renal transplantation in Europe by the end of 1980, and eight recipients were alive with a functioning graft. The two-year patient survival rate was 51%.[142] Disabling bone disease, sometimes accompanied by complete growth arrest,[124, 132] is a serious problem in most pediatric patients despite renal transplantation.[123, 124, 126] Only four pediatric patients with grafts functioning for more than five years are known[123, 124, 132, 143] and dialysis had to be re-lj

sumed at 62 months in the last patient.[132] How are these disappointing results explained? Any temporary decrease of renal function, e.g., by acute tubular necrosis or rejection, leads to rapid accumulation of oxalate and to permanent and often progressive loss of function. Cadaver renal transplantation should nevertheless still be considered in older children and adults, as it provides a better alternative to dialysis. However, in very young patients, it is still debatable if any ESRD therapy should be undertaken.

We would recommend the following guidelines for renal transplantation in PH: (1) Administration of high doses of pyridoxine (0.6 to 1.2 gm per day); (2) selection of a cadaver kidney with a short ischemia time; (3) daily dialysis in the case of temporary graft dysfunction. This is especially important during the first days after transplantation because of the large oxalate pool; (4) regular intake of *very* large quantities of fluid to enhance the solubility of oxalate. Administration of orthophosphate and of thiamine (400 mg/day) may be of additional value, probably more so than magnesium peroxide or methylene blue; (5) avoiding oxalate-rich food and high doses of ascorbic acid, a known precursor of oxalic acid.

No kidney-transplanted patient with *PH type II* (L-glyceric aciduria) has been reported to date.

### Diabetes Mellitus

The largest single experience with renal transplantation in diabetics is that reported from Minnesota, where 305 type I diabetic patients had undergone renal transplantation between 1968 and 1978.[144] Recurrence of diabetic microangiopathy was noted in all 12 patients whose grafts had been examined by biopsy at an average interval of 32 months after transplantation.[144] Diabetic nodular glomerulosclerosis was observed only once.[145] Despite this 100% recurrence rate of diabetic microangiography on light microscopy, graft function was not affected, and in no single case was proteinuria attributed to recurrence.

### Cystinosis/Fanconi Syndrome

Recurrence of the Fanconi syndrome after renal transplantation has *never* been noted in patients with cystinosis. Although deposition of cystine crystals has been observed in the interstitium, and occasionally in mesangial cells,[146, 147] it was never observed in tubular cells (except in one patient observed by Langlois et al[148]) or in glomerular epithelial cells, as occurs in the native cystinotic kidneys.[146, 147] The interstitial deposition of cystine is undoubtedly due to migrating recipient cells which infiltrate the graft. The concentration of cystine in the allograft increases with time and approaches levels found in the native kidneys.[146] Nevertheless, first graft survival rate in patients with cystinosis is significantly higher than that observed in recipients with other renal diseases (79% at three years for 47 grafts versus 56% in all other diseases).[148a] However, renal transplantation does not correct the primary metabolic defect, and extrarenal clinical manifestations, such as photophobia and hypothyroidism, persist.

In contrast to cystinosis, the florid Fanconi syndrome recurred several months after transplantation in a 14-year-old boy with *idiopathic Fanconi syndrome*.[149]

Severe hypophosphatemia after renal transplantation in a 47-year-old male patient with *X-linked hypophosphatemic rickets* and ESRD due to chronic glomerulonephritis was attributed to recurrent disease.[150] However, persisting hypophosphatemia in the absence of hyperparathyroidism is not uncommon after renal transplantation.

## Fabry's Disease

Renal failure in Fabry's disease occurs only in the third or fourth decade of life. Initial reports claiming that renal transplantation may also correct the metabolic defect in sphingolipid metabolism[151–153] have not been supported by later observations.[154–157] Recurrence of the renal lesion has *not* been reported. In one allograft typical multilamellar bodies were found only within infiltrating mononuclear cells from the host and not in the donor renal epithelial cells.[154] Striking clinical improvement of extrarenal manifestations has sometimes been noted after renal transplantation;[154, 155, 157] however, the vascular involvement persists, and the risk of cardiac complications progresses.[156]

## NONRECURRENT DISEASES

No recurrence to date has been reported in nephronophthisis (medullary cystic dis-ease), nail-patella syndrome,[14] the congenital nephrotic syndrome of Finnish type,[158, 159] gout,[77] cystinuria,[160] Bartter's syndrome,[14] cystinosis, and Fabry's disease.

## REFERENCES

1. Glassock RJ, Feldman D, Reynolds ES, et al: Human renal isografts: a clinical and pathologic analysis. Medicine (Baltimore) 47:411, 1968.
2. Hamburger J, Crosnier J, Dormont JA: Observations in patients with a well tolerated homotransplanted kidney. Ann NY Acad Sci 120:558, 1964.
3. Hume DM, Merrill JP, Miller BF, Thorn GW: Experiences with renal homotransplantation in the human: Report of nine cases. J Clin Invest 34:327, 1955.
4. Cameron JS, Turner DR: Recurrent glomerulonephritis in allografted kidneys. Clin Nephrol 7:47, 1977.
5. Cameron JS: Glomerulonephritis in renal transplants. Transplantation 34:237, 1982.
5a. Hamburger J, Crosnier J, Noël LH: Recurrent glomerulonephritis after renal transplantation. Ann Rev Med 29:67, 1978.
6. Briner J: Glomerular lesions in renal allografts. Adv Int Med Pediatr 49:1, 1982.
7. Mathew TH, Mathews DC, Hobbs JB, Kincaid-Smith P: Glomerular lesions after renal transplantation. Am J Med 59:177, 1975.
8. Olsen S, Bohman SO, Petersen VP: Ultrastructure of the glomerular basement membrane in long-term renal allografts with transplant glomerular disease. Lab Invest 30:176, 1974.
9. Petersen VP, Olsen TS, Kissmeyer-Nielsen F, et al: Late failure of human renal transplants. An analysis of transplant disease and graft failure among 125 recipients surviving for one to eight years. Medicine (Baltimore) 54:45, 1975.
10. Morzycka M, Croker BP, Seigler HF, Tisher CC: Evaluation of recurrent glomerulonephritis in kidney allografts. Am J Med 72:588, 1982.
11. Amend WJ, Vincenti F, Feduska NJ, et al: Recurrent systemic lupus erythematosus involving renal allografts. Ann Intern Med 94:444, 1981.
12. Hoyer JR, Raij L, Vernier RL, et al: Recurrence of idiopathic nephrotic syndrome after renal transplantation. Lancet 2:343, 1972.
13. Brown CB, Cameron JS, Turner DR, et al: Focal segmental glomerulosclerosis with rapid decline in renal function (malignant FSGS). Clin Nephrol 10:51, 1978.
14. Broyer M, Gagnadoux MF, Beurton D, et al: Transplantation in children: technical aspects, drug therapy and problems related to primary renal disease. Proc Eur Dial Transplant Assoc 18:313, 1981.
15. Case Records of the Massachusetts General Hospital: Case No. 20–1976. N Engl J Med 294:1108, 1976.
16. Chandra M, Lewy JE, Mouadian J, et al: Recurrent nephrotic syndrome with three successive renal allografts. Am J Nephrol 1:110, 1981.
17. Cheigh JS, Soliman M, Mouradian L, et al: Focal segmental glomerulosclerosis in kidney transplants. Transplant Proc 13:125, 1981.
18. Currier CB, Papadopoulou Z, Helfrich B, et al: Successful renal transplantation in focal segmen-

tal glomerulosclerosis. Transplant Proc 11:49, 1979.

19. Ettenger RB, Heuser ET, Malekzadeh MH, et al: Focal glomerulosclerosis in renal allografts. Association with the nephrotic syndrome and chronic rejection. Am J Dis Child 131:1347, 1977.

20. Habib R, Hebert D, Gagnadoux MF, Broyer M: Transplantation in idiopathic nephrosis. Transplant Proc 14:489, 1982.

21. Hamburger J, Berger J, Hinglais N, Descamps B: New insights into the pathogenesis of glomerulonephritis afforded by the study of renal allografts. Clin Nephrol 1:3, 1973.

22. Leumann EP, Briner J, Donckerwolcke RA, et al: Recurrence of focal segmental glomerulosclerosis in the transplanted kidney. Nephron 25:65, 1980.

23. Lewis EJ: Recurrent focal sclerosis after renal transplantation. Kidney Int 22:315, 1982.

24. Maizel SE, Sibley RK, Horstman JP, et al: Incidence and significance of recurrent focal segmental glomerulosclerosis in renal allograft recipients. Transplantation 32:512, 1981.

25. Malekzadeh MH, Heuser ET, Ettenger RB, et al: Focal glomerulosclerosis and renal transplantation. J Pediatr 95:249, 1979.

26. Papadopoulou Z, Helfrich GB, Turner ME, et al: Recurrence of focal segmental glomerulosclerosis in children following renal transplantation. Am Soc Artif Intern Organs 27:325, 1981.

27. Pinto J, Lacerda G, Cameron JS, et al: Recurrence of focal segmental glomerulosclerosis in renal allografts. Transplantation 32:83, 1981.

28. Saint-Hillier Y, Morel-Maroger L, Woodrow D, Richet G: Focal and segmental hyalinosis. Adv Nephrol 5:67, 1975.

29. Velosa JA, Donadio JV, Holley KE: Focal sclerosing glomerulopathy. A clinicopathologic study. Mayo Clin Proc 50:121, 1975.

30. Willassen Y: Reduction of proteinuria following plasma exchange in recurrent renal allograft focal glomerulosclerosis. Kidney Int 21:669, 1982 (Abstract).

31. Zimmerman CE: Renal transplantation for focal segmental glomerulosclerosis. Transplantation 29:172, 1980.

32. Zimmerman SW: Study of a patient with recurrent focal glomerular sclerosis in two renal allografts. Kidney Int 23:298, 1983 (Abstract).

33. Broyer M, Donckerwolcke RA, Brunner FP, et al: Combined report on regular dialysis and transplantation of children in Europe, 1981. Proc Eur Dial Transplant Assoc 19:60, 1982.

34. Schoeneman MJ, Bennett B, Greifer I: The natural history of focal segmental glomerulosclerosis with and without mesangial hypercellularity in children. Clin Nephrol 9:45, 1978.

35. Waldherr R, Gubler MC, Levy M, et al: The significance of pure diffuse mesangial proliferation in idiopathic nephrotic syndrome. Clin Nephrol 10:171, 1978.

36. Mauer SM, Hellerstein S, Cohn RA, et al: Recurrence of steroid-responsive nephrotic syndrome after renal transplantation. J Pediatr 95:261, 1979.

37. Berthoux FC, Ducret F, Colon S, et al: Renal transplantation in mesangioproliferative glomerulonephritis (MPGN): Relationship between the high frequency of recurrent glomerulonephritis and hypocomplementaemia. Kidney Int 7(Suppl 3):323, 1975.

38. Cameron JS, Turner DR, Heaton J, et al: Idiopathic mesangiocapillary glomerulonephritis: comparison of types I and II in children and adults, and long term prognosis. Am J Med 74:175, 1983.

39. Curtis JJ, Wyatt RJ, Bhathena D, et al: Renal transplantation for patients with type I and type II membranoproliferative glomerulonephritis. Serial complement and nephritic factor measurements and the problem of recurrence of disease. Am J Med 66:216, 1979.

40. Davis AE, Schneeberger EE, Grupe WE, McCluskey RT: Membranoproliferative glomerulonephritis (MPGN type I) and dense deposit disease (DDD) in children. Clin Nephrol 9:184, 1978.

41. Fine RN, Grushkin CM: Hemodialysis and renal transplantation in children. Clin Nephrol 1:243, 1973.

42. Gonzales LL, Martin L, West CD: Renal homotransplantation in children. Arch Surg 101:232, 1970.

43. Levy M, Arsan A: Récidive de la maladie originale sur le rein transplanté. Seminaire de Néphrologie Pédiatrique, March 6–7, Paris, 1978.

44. McCoy RC, Clapp J, Seigler HF: Membranoproliferative glomerulonephritis. Progression from the pure form to the crescentic form with recurrence after transplantation. Am J Med 59:288, 1975.

45. McLean RH, Geiger H, Burke B, et al: Recurrence of membranoproliferative glomerulonephritis following kidney transplantation. Serum complement component studies. Am J Med 60:60, 1976.

46. Mönninghoff W, Intorp HW, Themann H, Losse H: Recurrent antibasement membrane nephritis after renal homotransplantation. Beitr Pathol 160:274, 1977.

47. Schürch W, Leski M, Hinglais N: Evolution of recurrent lobular glomerulonephritis in a human kidney allotransplant. Virchows Arch (Pathol Anat) 355:66, 1972.

48. Zimmermann SW, Hyman LR, Uehling DT, Burkholder PM: Recurrent membranoproliferative glomerulonephritis with glomerular properdin deposition in allografts. Ann Intern Med 80:169, 1974.

49. Habib R, Gubler C, Loirat C, et al: Dense deposit disease: a variant of membranoproliferative glomerulonephritis. Kidney Int 7:204, 1975.

50. Beaufils H, Gubler MC, Karam J, et al: Dense deposit disease: Long-term follow-up of three cases of recurrence after transplantation. Clin Nephrol 7:31, 1977.

51. Droz D, Nabarra B, Noël LH, et al: Recurrence of dense deposits in transplanted kidneys: I. Sequential survey of the lesions. Kidney Int 15:386, 1979.

52. Eddy A, Sibley R, Kim Y: Renal allograft failure due to recurrent dense intramembranous deposit disease. Kidney Int 23:122, 1983 (Abstract).

53. Galle P, Mathieu P: Electron dense alteration of kidney basement membranes. Am J Med 58:749, 1975.

54. Jukkola AF, Mantaring T, Roy S, Murphy WM: Recurrent dense deposit disease in renal allograft. Urology 11:395, 1978.

55. Lamb V, Tisher CC, McCoy RC, Robinson RR: Membranoproliferative glomerulonephritis with dense intramembranous alterations: A clinicopathologic study. Lab Invest 36:607, 1977.

56. Leibowitch J, Halbwachs L, Wattel S, et al: Recur-

rence of dense deposits in transplanted kidney: II. Serum complement and nephritic factor profiles. Kidney Int 15:396, 1979.

57. Leumann EP, Briner J, Fierz W, Largiadèr F: Verlust zweier Nierentransplantate infolge Rezidivs einer membranoproliferativen Glomerulonephritis Typ II. Schweiz Med Wschr 110:408, 1980.

58. Schmidt P, Kerjaschki D, Syré G, et al: Rezidiv einer intramembranösen Glomerulonephritis in zwei konsekutiven homologen Nierentransplantaten. Schweiz Med Wschr 108:781, 1978.

59. Turner DR, Cameron JS, Bewick M, et al: Transplantation in mesangiocapillary glomerulonephritis with intramembranous dense "deposits": Recurrence of disease. Kidney Int 9:439, 1976.

60. Briner J, Binswanger U, Largiadèr F: Recurrent and de novo membranous glomerulonephritis in renal cadaver allotransplants. Clin Nephrol 13:189, 1980.

61. Cosyns JP, Pierson Y, van Ypersele de Strihou C, Alexandre GP: Recurrence of de novo graft membranous glomerulonephritis. Nephron 29:142, 1981.

62. Crosson JT, Wathen RL, Raij L, et al: Recurrence of idiopathic membranous nephropathy in a renal allograft. Arch Intern Med 135:1101, 1975.

63. Dische FE, Herbertson BM, Melcher DH, Morley AR: Membranous glomerulonephritis in transplant kidneys: recurrent or de novo disease in four patients. Clin Nephrol 15:154, 1981.

64. Gaffney E: Allograft membranous glomerulonephritis. Arch Pathol Lab Med 105:559, 1981 (letter).

65. Hill GS, Robertson J, Grossman R, et al: An unusual variant of membranous nephropathy with abundant crescent formation and recurrence in the transplanted kidney. Clin Nephrol 10:114, 1978.

66. Iskandar SS, Jennette JC: Recurrence of membranous glomerulopathy in an allograft. Case report and review of the literature. Nephron 29:270, 1981.

67. Lieberthal W, Bernard DB, Donohoe JF, et al: Rapid recurrence of membranous nephropathy in a related renal allograft. Clin Nephrol 12:222, 1979.

68. Rubin RJ, Pinn VW, Barnes BA, Harrington JT: Recurrent idiopathic membranous glomerulonephritis. Transplantation 24:4, 1977.

69. Berger J, Yaneva H, Nabarra B, Barbanel C: Recurrence of mesangial deposition of IgA after renal transplantation. Kidney Int 7:232, 1975.

70. Berger J: Mesangial IgA glomerulonephritis. Sixteenth Meeting of the European Society for Paediatric Nephrology, Stockholm, 1982 (cited by Cameron[5]).

71. Petersen VP, Olsen S, Kissmeyer-Nielsen F, Fjeldborg O: Transmission of glomerulonephritis from host to human kidney allotransplant. N Engl J Med 275:1269, 1966.

72. Porter KA, Dossetor JB, Marchioro TL, et al: Human renal transplants. I. Glomerular changes. Lab Invest 16:153, 1967.

73. Arias M, de Francisco AM, Cotorruelo JG, et al: Recidiva de glomerulonefritis extracapilar por anticuerpos antimembrana basal en dos trasplantes sucesivos. Rev Clin Espanola 160:417, 1981.

74. Beleil OM, Coburn JW, Shinaberger JH, Glassock RJ: Recurrent glomerulonephritis due to antiglomerular basement membrane-antibodies in two successive allografts. Clin Nephrol 1:377, 1973.

75. Baliah, T, Kim KH, Anthone S, et al: Recurrence of Henoch-Schönlein purpura glomerulonephritis in transplanted kidneys. Transplantation 18:343, 1974.

76. Brunner FP, Brynger H, Chantler C, et al: Combined report on regular dialysis and transplantation in Europe, IX, 1978. Proc Eur Dial Transplant Assoc 16:2, 1979.

77. Advisory Committee to the Renal Transplant Registry: Renal transplantation in congenital and metabolic disease. A report from the ASC/NIH renal transplant registry. JAMA 232:148, 1975.

78. McCoy RC, Johnson HK, Stone WJ, Wilson CB: Absence of nephritogenic GBM antigen(s) in some patients with hereditary nephritis. Kidney Int 21:642, 1982.

79. Milliner DS, Pierides AM, Holley, KE: Renal transplantation in Alport's syndrome. Anti-glomerular basement membrane glomerulonephritis in the allograft. Mayo Clin Proc 57:35, 1982.

80. Kourilsky O, Gubler MC, Morel-Maroger L, et al: A new form of familial glomerulonephritis. Nephron 30:97, 1982.

81. Bar-On H, Rosenmann E: Schönlein-Henoch syndrome in adults. A clinical and histological study of renal involvement. Isr J Med Sci 8:1702, 1972.

82. Crumb CK: Renal involvement in Schönlein-Henoch syndrome. In: Suki WN, Eknoyan G: The Kidney in Systemic Disease, 2nd ed. New York, J Wiley, 1981, p 99.

83. Levy M, Ami Moussa R, Habib R, Gagnadoux MF, Broyer M: Anaphylactoid purpura nephritis and transplantation. Kidney Int 22:326, 1982 (Abstract).

84. Sakai T, Tanaka T, Kasai N, et al: Recurrence of Henoch-Schönlein purpura glomerulonephritis in transplanted kidney. International Congress of Nephrology, 1975, Florence (Abstract 1023).

85. Weiss JH, Bhathena DB, Curtis JJ, et al: A possible relationship between Henoch-Schönlein syndrome and IgA nephropathy (Berger's disease). An illustrative case. Nephron 22:582, 1978.

86. Yakub YN, Freeman RB, Pabico RC: Renal transplantation in systemic lupus erythematosus. Nephron 27:197, 1981.

87. Almkuist RD, Buckalew VM, Hirszel P, et al: Recurrence of anti-glomerular basement membrane antibody mediated glomerulonephritis in an isograft. Clin Immun Immunopathol 18:54, 1981.

88. Bergrem H, Jervell J, Brodwall EK, et al: Goodpasture's syndrome. A report of seven patients including long-term follow-up of three who received a kidney transplant. Am J Med 68:54, 1980.

89. Couser WG, Wallace A, Monaco AP, Lewis EJ: Successful renal transplantation in patients with circulating antibody to glomerular basement membrane: Report of two cases. Clin Nephrol 1:381, 1973.

90. Cove-Smith JR, McLeod AA, Blamey RW, et al: Transplantation, immunosuppression and plasmapheresis in Goodpasture's syndrome. Clin Nephrol 9:126, 1978.

91. Houde M, Dandavino R, Laplante L, et al: Recidive

du syndrome de Goodpasture après transplantation rénale. Union Med Canada 110:236, 1981.

92. Wilson CB, Dixon FJ: Anti-glomerular basement membrane antibody-induced glomerulonephritis. Kidney Int 3:74, 1973.

93. Fauci AS, Balow JE, Brown R, et al: Successful renal transplantation in Wegener's granulomatosis. Am J Med 60:437, 1976.

94. Kuross S, Davin T, Kjellstrand CM: Wegener's granulomatosis with severe failure: clinical course and results of dialysis and transplantation. Clin Nephrol 16:172, 1981.

95. Lyons GW, Lindsay WG: Renal transplantation in a patient with Wegener's granulomatosis. Am J Surg 124:104, 1972.

96. Salaman R, Coles GA, Saltissi D: Haemodialysis and transplantation in Wegener's granulomatosis. Br Med J 1:254, 1980 (letter).

97. Steinman TI, Jaffe BF, Monaco AP, et al: Recurrence of Wegener's granulomatosis after kidney transplantation. Successful re-induction of remission with cyclophosphamide. Am J Med 68:458, 1980.

98. van Ypersele de Strihou C, Pirson Y, Vandenbroucke JM, Alexandre GP: Haemodialysis and transplantation in Wegener's granulomatosis. Br Med J 2:93, 1979.

99. Montalbert C, Carvallo A, Broumand B, et al: Successful renal transplantation in polyarteritis nodosa. Clin Nephrol 14:206, 1980.

100. Touraine JL, Vital-Durand D, Malik MC, et al: Récidive amyloide sur le transplant rénal malgré la colchicine au cours d'une maladie périodique. Ann Med Int (Paris) 132:511, 1981.

101. Benson MD, Skinner M, Cohen AS: Amyloid deposition in a renal transplant in familial-Mediterranean fever. Ann Intern Med 87:31, 1977.

102. Cohen AS, Bricetti AB, Harrington JT, et al: Renal transplantation in two cases of amyloidosis. Lancet 2:513, 1971.

103. Dorman SA, Gamelli RL, Benziger JR, et al: Systemic amyloidosis involving two renal transplants. Hum Pathol 12:735, 1981.

104. Helin H, Pasternack A, Falck H, Kuhlbäck B: Recurrence of renal amyloid and de novo membranous glomerulonephritis after transplantation. Transplantation 32:6, 1981.

105. Jacob ET, Bar-Nathan N, Shapira Z, Gafni J: Renal transplantation in the amyloidosis of familial Mediterranean fever. Arch Intern Med 139:1135, 1979.

106. Jacob ET, Siegal B, Bar-Nathan N, Gafni J: Improving outlook for renal transplantation in amyloid nephropathy. Transplant Proc 14:41, 1982.

107. Jones MB, Adams JM, Passer JA: Amyloidosis in a renal allograft in familial Mediterranean fever. Ann Inter Med 87:579, 1977.

108. Jones NF: Renal amyloidosis: pathogenesis and therapy. Clin Nephrol 6:459, 1976.

109. Kennedy CL, Castro JE: Transplantation for renal amyloidosis. Transplantation 24:382, 1977.

110. Kuhlbäck B, Falck H, Törnroth T, et al: Renal transplantation in amyloidosis. Acta Med Scand 205:169, 1979.

111. Light PD, Hall-Craggs M: Amyloid deposition in a renal allograft in a case of amyloidosis secondary to rheumatoid arthritis. Am J Med 66:532, 1979.

112. Campion JP, Ramee MP, Marsili E, et al: Recurrent nephritis in allografted diseases: Prognosis reappraisement. Abstracts 19th Congress Eur Dial Transplant Assoc Madrid, 1982, p 26.

113. Cerilli GJ, Nelsen C, Dorfmann L: Renal homotransplantation in infants and children with the hemolytic-uremic syndrome. Surgery 71:66, 1972.

114. Folman R, Arbus GS, Churchill B, et al: Recurrence of the hemolytic uremic syndrome in a 3½-year-old child, 4 months after second renal transplantation. Clin Nephrol 10:121, 1978.

115. Hauglustaine D, Van Damme B, Vanrenterghem Y, Michielsen P: Recurrent hemolytic uremic syndrome during oral contraception. Clin Nephrol 15:148, 1981.

116. Stevenson JA, Dumke A, Glassock RJ, et al: Thrombotic microangiopathy. Recurrence following renal transplant and response to plasma infusion. Am J Nephrol 2:227, 1982.

117. Bergstein J, Michael A, Kjellstrand C, et al: Hemolytic-uremic syndrome in adult sisters. Transplantation 17:487, 1974.

118. Brynger H, Brunner FP, Chantler C, et al: Combined report on regular dialysis and transplantation in Europe, X, 1979. Proc Eur Dial Transplant Assoc 17:2, 1980.

119. Merino GE, Sutherland DE, Kjellstrand CM, et al: Renal transplantation for progressive systemic sclerosis with renal failure. Case report and review of previous experience. Am J Surg 133:245, 1977.

120. McCoy RC, Tisher CC, Pepe PF, Cleveland LA: The kidney in progressive systemic sclerosis. Immunohistochemical and antibody elution studies. Lab Invest 35:124, 1976.

121. Woodhall PB, McCoy RC, Gunnels JC, Seigler HF: Apparent recurrence of progressive systemic sclerosis in a renal allograft. JAMA 236:1032, 1976.

122. Jacobs C, Rottembourgh J, Reach I, Legrain M: Terminal renal failure due to oxalosis in 14 patients. Proc Eur Dial Transplant Assoc 11:359, 1974.

123. Donckerwolcke RA, Chantler C, Broyer M, et al: Combined report on regular dialysis and transplantation of children in Europe, 1979. Proc Eur Dial Transplant Assoc 17:87, 1980.

124. Breed A, Chesney R, Friedman A, et al: Oxalosis-induced bone disease: a complication of transplantation and prolonged survival in primary hyperoxaluria. J Bone Joint Surg 63A:310, 1981.

125. Deodhar SD, Tung KSK, Zühlke V, Nakamoto S: Renal homotransplantation in a patient with primary familial oxalosis. Arch Pathol 87:118, 1969.

126. Donckerwolcke RA, Kuijten RH, van Gool JD, Kramer PP: The treatment of primary hyperoxaluria with intermittent dialysis and transplantation. In Bulla M: Renal Insufficiency in Children, Berlin, Springer, 1982, p 42.

127. Frei D, Binswanger U, Keusch G, et al: Intakte Nierentransplantatfunktion 3 Jahre nach Organübertragung bei primärer Oxalose. Schweiz med Wschr 109:979, 1979.

128. Halverstadt DB, Wenzl JE: Primary hyperoxaluria and renal transplantation. J Urol 111:398, 1974.

129. Jacobsen E, Mosbaek N: Primary hyperoxaluria, treated with haemodialysis and kidney transplantation. Dan Med Bull 21:72, 1974.

130. Klauwers J, Wolf PL, Cohn R: Failure of renal transplantation in primary oxalosis. JAMA 209:551, 1969.

131. Koch B, Irvine AH, Barr JR, Poznanski WJ: Three kidney transplantations in a patient with primary hereditary hyperoxaluria. Canad Med Assoc J 106:1323, 1972.

132. Leumann EP, Wegmann W, Largiadèr F: Prolonged survival after renal transplantation in primary hyperoxaluria of childhood. Clin Nephrol 9:29, 1978.

133. Mahoney JP, Storey BG, McCarthy SW, Stewart JH: Treatment of oxaluric renal failure. N Engl J Med 287:1252, 1972 (letter).

134. McKenna RW, Dehner LP: Oxalosis. An unusual cause of myelophthisis in childhood. Am J Clin Pathol 66:991, 1976.

135. Morgan JM, Hartley MW, Miller AC, Diethelm AG: Successful renal transplantation in hyperoxaluria. Arch Surg 109:430, 1974.

136. O'Regan P, Constable AR, Joekes AM, et al: Successful renal transplantation in primary hyperoxaluria. Postgrad Med J 56:288, 1980.

137. Rosier JGMC, Baadenhuijsen H, Koene RAP: Long-term survival of a renal allograft in a patient with primary hyperoxaluria (type I). Neth J Med 24:179, 1981.

138. Saxon A, Busch GJ, Merrill JP, et al: Renal transplantation in primary hyperoxaluria: report of a case and review of the literature. Arch Intern Med 133:464, 1974.

139. Solomons CC, Goodman SI, Riley CM: Calcium carbimide in the treatment of primary hyperoxaluria. N Engl J Med 276:207, 1967.

140. Stacy TM: Renal oxalosis. South Med J 69:1206, 1976.

141. Toussaint C, Goffin Y, Potvliege P, et al: Kidney transplantation in primary oxalosis. Clin Nephrol 5:239, 1976.

142. Jacobs C, Broyer M, Brunner FP, et al: Combined report on regular dialysis and transplantation in Europe, XI, 1980. Proc Eur Dial Transplant Assoc 18:4, 1981.

143. David DS: Personal communication.

144. Najarian JS, Sutherland DE, Simmons RL, et al: Ten year experience with renal transplantation in juvenile onset diabetics. Ann Surg 190:487, 1979.

145. Mauer SM, Barbosa J, Vernier RL, et al: Development of diabetic vascular lesions in normal kidneys transplanted into patients with diabetes mellitus. N Engl J Med 295:916, 1976.

146. Mahoney CP, Strike GE, Hickman RO, et al: Renal transplantation for childhood cystinosis. N Engl J Med 283:397, 1970.

147. Malekzadeh MH, Neustein HB, Schneider JA, et al: Cadaver renal transplantation in children with cystinosis. Am J Med 63:525, 1977.

148. Langlois RP, O'Regan S, Pelletier M, Robitaille P: Kidney transplantation in uremic children with cystinosis. Nephron 28:273, 1981.

148a. Broyer M, Donckerwolcke RA, Brunner FP, et al: Combined report on regular dialysis and transplantation of children in Europe, 1980. Proc Eur Dial Transplant Assoc 19:60, 1982.

149. Briggs WA, Kominami N, Wilson RE, Merrill JP: Kidney transplantation in Fanconi syndrome. N Engl J Med 286:25, 1972.

150. Morgan JM, Hawley WL, Chenoweth AI, et al: Renal transplantation in hypophosphatemia with vitamin D-resistant rickets. Arch Intern Med 134:549, 1974.

151. Bühler FR, Thiel G, Dubach UC, et al: Kidney transplantation in Fabry's disease. Br Med J 3:28, 1973.

152. Desnick RJ, Simmons RL, Allen KY, et al: Correction of enzymatic deficiencies by renal transplantation: Fabry's disease. Surgery 72:203, 1972.

153. Philippart M, Franklin SS, Gordon A: Reversal of an inborn sphingolipidosis (Fabry's disease) by kidney transplantation. Ann Intern Med 77:195, 1972.

154. Clarke JT, Guttmann RD, Wolfe LS, et al: Enzyme replacement therapy by renal allotransplantation in Fabry's Disease. N Engl J Med 287:1215, 1972.

155. Clement M, McGonigle RJ, Monkhouse PM, et al: Renal transplantation in Anderson-Fabry disease. J Roy Soc Med 75:557, 1982.

156. Maizel SE, Simmons RL, Kjellstrand C, Fryd DS: Ten-year experience in renal transplantation for Fabry's disease. Transplant Proc 13:57, 1981.

157. Spence MW, MacKinnon KE, Burgess JK, et al: Failure to correct the metabolic defect by renal allotransplantation in Fabry's disease. Ann Intern Med 84:13, 1976.

158. Broyer M, Gagnadoux MF, Niaudet P, Habib R: Kidney transplantation in congenital nephrotic syndrome of Finnish type. Int J Pediatr Nephrol 3:111, 1982 (Abstract).

159. Hoyer JR, Mauer SM, Kjellstrand CM, et al: Successful renal transplantation in 3 children with congenital nephrotic syndrome. Lancet 1:1410, 1973.

160. Kelly S: Postscript on excretion rates in posttransplant cystinuric patient. JAMA 243:1897, 1980 (letter).

# 38

# Survival on Renal Replacement Therapy

*R. A. Donckerwolcke, M.D.*

The assessment of morbidity in patients receiving renal replacement therapy is an extremely important aspect of patient care. Mortality and survival data are essential for the evaluation of various factors affecting the outcome of treatment. These factors can be assessed only by analyses based upon data from a large number of patients. Data on more than 3000 pediatric patients collected by the Registry of the European Dialysis and Transplant Association (EDTA) form the basis for this review.[1-5]

## SURVIVAL ON RENAL REPLACEMENT THERAPY

Although renal transplantation is the preferred treatment for children with end stage renal disease (ESRD), dialysis and transplantation are integrated treatment modalities, and most patients experience both methods of therapy. Evaluation of the benefit of a particular treatment modality should address both survival and rehabilitation of these patients. Survival data can be compared with the outcome of treatment of other life-threat-

ening diseases. A comparison of the results of treatment of pediatric patients with lymphocytic leukemia and ESRD is shown in Table 38–1.[4, 6] The outcome of the treatment of acute lymphocytic leukemia has been recognized as a remarkable achievement.[6] However, the cumulative survival achieved by dialysis and transplantation is superior to that of acute lymphocytic leukemia at four years following initiation of treatment. The long-term survival may ultimately be superior in patients treated for leukemia.

Long-term survival data are unavailable for both disease entities owing to the small number of children treated for more than ten years. However, the available data indicate that at least half the children accepted for renal replacement therapy are alive ten years after initiation of treatment.[7-9] Life expectancy of the child with ESRD is influenced by many variables related to patient and treatment. The relationship of these factors to outcome will be discussed subsequently.

## SURVIVAL ON DIALYSIS

Several factors influence the outcome of dialysis in children. These include age of the patient, mode of treatment, primary renal disease, health status at the initiation of dialysis, and the expertise in pediatric dialysis of the unit providing treatment. Data on patient survival collected at the end of 1979 by the Registry of the EDTA are summarized in Table 38–2.[2]

Patient survival on hospital hemodialysis at one, two, and five years was 87.7%, 79.5%,

**Table 38–1.** RESULTS OF TREATMENT OF CHILDHOOD LYMPHOCYTIC LEUKEMIA AND ESRD

| | Patient Survival (%) | | | |
| | 12 mo | 24 mo | 36 mo | 48 mo |
|---|---|---|---|---|
| Acute lymphocytic leukemia[6] | 85.0 | 75.0 | 70.0 | 64.0 |
| End stage renal disease (ESRD)[4] | 89.0 | 82.8 | 78.2 | 74.4 |

**Table 38–2.** PATIENT SURVIVAL RATES (%) ACCORDING TO AGE, PERIOD OF TREATMENT, AND MODES OF TREATMENT (EDTA—1979)

| | Age (yr) | Period of Treatment | Sample Size | 1 Year | 2 Years | 3 Years | 4 Years | 5 Years |
|---|---|---|---|---|---|---|---|---|
| First hospital hemodialysis | All | All | 1886 | 87.7 ± 0.9 | 79.5 ± 1.3 | 75.7 ± 1.5 | 72.1 ± 1.8 | 66.3 ± 2.4 |
| | 0–4 | | 109 | 84.3 ± 4.1 | 73.1 ± 5.9 | | | |
| | 5–9 | | 482 | 87.1 ± 1.9 | 74.3 ± 3.0 | 69.9 ± 3.8 | 64.9 ± 4.3 | (57.7 ± 5.5) |
| | 10–15 | | 1285 | 88.3 ± 1.1 | 81.8 ± 1.5 | 77.9 ± 1.8 | 75.1 ± 2.0 | 69.3 ± 2.7 |
| | All | | 737 | 90.2 ± 1.4 | 81.5 ± 2.4 | 77.3 ± 3.7 | | |
| Home hemodialysis | All | All | 252 | 95.5 ± 1.4 | 92.9 ± 1.9 | 90.8 ± 2.3 | 84.6 ± 3.7 | 84.6 ± 3.7 |
| | All | Last 3 years | 97 | 100.0 ± 0.0 | 100.0 ± 0.0 | | | |

Data on numbers less than 25 have been omitted; data on numbers less than 35 in parentheses.

**Table 38–3.** CAUSES OF DEATH IN PATIENTS ON RENAL REPLACEMENT THERAPY (PERCENTAGE OF ALL CAUSES OF DEATH, EDTA—1979)

| Causes of Death | Hospital Hemodialysis | Home Hemodialysis | Transplantation | | | |
|---|---|---|---|---|---|---|
| | | | Live Donor | | Cadaver | |
| | | | Functioning | Failed | Functioning | Failed |
| Cardiac failure | 28.3 | 44.4 | 6.7 | 16.2 | 23.1 | 22.3 |
| Hypertension | 9.5 | 5.6 | 6.7 | 5.4 | 0.0 | 5.4 |
| Hyperkalemia | 18.7 | 11.1 | 0.0 | 2.7 | 0.0 | 3.1 |
| Cerebrovascular accident | 14.1 | 0.0 | 33.3 | 8.1 | 10.3 | 8.5 |
| Hemorrhage | 1.5 | 0.0 | 13.4 | 2.7 | 7.7 | 4.6 |
| Infections | 8.4 | 22.3 | 20.1 | 18.9 | 43.6 | 24.6 |
| Liver disease | 1.6 | 0.0 | 0.0 | 0.0 | 0.0 | 1.6 |
| Therapy ceased | 1.5 | 0.0 | 0.0 | 0.0 | 0.0 | 1.5 |
| Uremia (graft failure) | | | 6.7 | 24.3 | 2.6 | 10.8 |
| Cachexia | 3.4 | 0.0 | 0.0 | 0.0 | 0.0 | 1.5 |
| Other | 13.0 | 16.6 | 13.1 | 21.7 | 12.7 | 16.1 |
| Number of patients | 262 | 18 | 15 | 37 | 39 | 130 |

and 66.3% respectively for all pediatric patients. In children less than five years of age the survival rate on hospital hemodialysis was poorer, with one- and two-year survival rates of 84.3% and 73.1% respectively. Patient survival was superior in children in the age group 10 to 15 years as compared with those aged five to nine years. Patient survival rates for hospital and home hemodialysis show significant differences. Patient survival on home hemodialysis at one, two, and five years was 95.5%, 92.9%, and 84.6% respectively, for all pediatric patients less than 15 years old at the initiation of treatment.

Selection of the patients appears to be the most important factor for the better results observed in home dialysis patients. Selection criteria for home hemodialysis include the health status at the start of treatment, the age of the patient, and the motivation of the parents. Children weighing less than 20 kg are usually not considered candidates for home dialysis because of the technical skill required to perform dialysis in such small children.[10] High-risk patients commence treatment on hospital dialysis, and only after improvement of health status is home dialysis training considered.

In 1981, 10% of all pediatric patients undergoing regular dialysis in Europe were on continuous ambulatory peroneal dialysis (CAPD). Patient survival at one and two years was 85% and 80% respectively.[4]

The annual mortality rate of children undergoing hemodialysis as reported by the EDTA in 1978 was 92 per 1000. The most frequent causes of death were cardiac failure, hypertension, hyperkalemia, and cerebrovas-cular accident (Table 38–3). In the age group less than five years old, 25% of the deaths were related to infection.[1] Mortality is also related to the nature of the primary renal disease. High-risk diseases are steroid-resistant nephrotic syndrome due to focal sclerosis, Wilms' tumor, and lupus erythematosus.[4, 8]

In the 1978 analysis of the EDTA, the European centers treating children were divided into specialized and nonspecialized centers. A specialized center was defined as one with a pediatrician, pediatric dietitian, hospital school, social worker, availability of a child psychiatrist, pediatric ward, and at least three children on treatment during the year.[1] Patient survival on hospital hemodialysis was significantly better in specialized centers for children starting treatment during the years 1976 to 1978, as shown in Figure 38–1. In specialized pediatric centers the death rate was 34 per 1000. In these centers fewer children died as a result of hyperkalemia, cerebrovascular accidents, and cachexia.

The expertise of these centers is related not only to facilities available for the treatment of children but also to the years of experience of the center. Most pediatric centers experienced higher mortality rates at the beginning of the treatment program. This is illustrated by a large pediatric center at the Hôpital des Enfants Malades in Paris. During the first ten years of the treatment program, 13 of 138 children undergoing long-term hemodialysis died; nine of those 13 deaths occurred during the first five years.[11] Similarly, the 1979 EDTA data indicated improved survival rates over the years. Patient

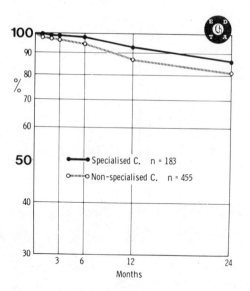

**Figure 38–1.** Patient survival on hospital hemodialysis in specialized and nonspecialized centers during the years 1976 to 1978 (EDTA 1978).[1]

survival was better during the last three years as compared with data of all patients in the Registry (Table 38–2).

## TRANSPLANTATION: PATIENT AND GRAFT SURVIVAL

Separate survival rates are available for patients and grafts. The cumulative survival rates for patients and grafts, as recorded by the EDTA Registry in 1981, for children less than 15 years old at the start of treatment are shown in Tables 38–4 and 38–5.[4] Determinants of patient and graft survival rates include donor age, donor source, primary renal disease, age of the recipient, HLA matching, pretransplant blood transfusions, previous transplantation, immunosuppressive therapy, and experience of the transplant center.

Conflicting data have been reported regarding the impact of donor age on the outcome of cadaveric kidney transplantation.[12–15] Patient survival is not related to cadaver donor age, and several reports have indicated that the use of pediatric cadaver donors does not adversely affect graft survival.[12, 15] A recent study based upon the Eurotransplant data has shown a difference in the graft survival rate in the pediatric donor group (age less than 11 years) as compared with that of the adult donor group (age between 11 and 50 years); the two-year graft survival rates were 51.8% and 56.9% respectively. The Eurotransplant data also indicated superior graft survival rates in pediatric recipients receiving an adult donor graft as compared to those receiving a pediatric donor graft; the two-year survival rates were 69% and 52% respectively.[13] The use of kidneys from infants and newborns may result in a high incidence of primary nonfunctioning grafts and decreased graft survival rates.[14] En bloc transplantation of both kidneys from pediatric donors less than three years old has no beneficial effect on graft survival or function. The one-year graft survival rates of en bloc grafts and single grafts from these young pediatric donors were 50.5% and 56.2% respectively.[13, 15]

Discouraging results have been obtained utilizing kidneys from anencephalic donors. Rapid clinical deterioration of the donor and a high incidence of urinary tract abnormalities result in only a fraction of anencephalic donor kidneys being utilized.[16] If successfully transplanted, anencephalic kidneys rapidly increase in size and provide adequate function.[13, 16]

Patient survival rates following live-related donor kidney transplantation are not different from those of recipients of cadaver donor grafts. However, graft survival rates of live-related donor grafts are significantly better than those of cadaver donor grafts (Table 38–4). Most large series of kidney transplantation in children include a large number of live-related donor grafts.[8, 17–19] In the majority of instances a parent of the child is the donor. The 1979 EDTA Registry recorded that 279 of 295 live-related donors were parents. In single center reports the five-year graft survival rates ranged between 71 and 85% following live-related donor transplantation. Graft survival rates with cadaver donors from the same centers were poorer, and at five years ranged between 39 and 65%.[17–19]

The improved outcome of live-related kidney transplantation is primarily the result of better graft tolerance, with the recipients experiencing fewer rejection episodes.[19] In addition, better preparation of the recipient and less ischemic damage of the donor kidney contribute to the improved outcome of live-related kidney transplantation. Data from transplantation in adult recipients have shown that the best graft survival rates are obtained with kidney transplantation between monozygotic twins and HLA-identical siblings; however, only a few children have received such grafts.[17]

The specific primary renal disease may impact upon both patient and graft survival. In a survey conducted by the EDTA Registry in 1982 on recipients with focal segmental glomerulosclerosis, recurrence was reported in 17 of 59 recipients (29%), of which four received second grafts. Recurrence was associated with graft failure in 11 of these 21 grafts within 30 months following transplantation, and four of the recipients with recurrence died.[4] Recurrence universally occurs in patients with primary hyperoxaluria type I, ultimately leading to graft failure; however, some recipients may have a functioning graft for several years.[2] Cardiac involvement with oxalate is an important cause of death in these patients. In contrast, superior patient and graft survival rates in children with cystinosis have been reported in comparison to those reported in patients with other primary renal diseases.[3] The mortality rate is high in children with Wilms' tumor who undergo

**Table 38–4.** PATIENT SURVIVAL RATES (%) FOLLOWING TRANSPLANTATION ACCORDING TO AGE GROUPS (EDTA—1981)

| | Age (years) | Sample Size | 1 Year | 2 Years | 3 Years | 4 Years | 5 Years | 6 Years | 7 Years | 8 Years |
|---|---|---|---|---|---|---|---|---|---|---|
| Patient Survival (1st cadaver graft) | 0–5 | 36 | (72.1 ± 11.1) | | | | | | | |
| | 5–10 | 274 | 89.1 ± 3.9 | 81.0 ± 5.1 | 75.9 ± 5.6 | 71.6 ± 5.9 | 67.9 ± 6.1 | 67.9 ± 6.1 | 62.1 ± 6.9 | |
| | 10–15 | 617 | 90.1 ± 2.8 | 88.0 ± 3.0 | 84.9 ± 3.3 | 81.7 ± 3.6 | 77.7 ± 4.1 | 74.6 ± 4.4 | 70.4 ± 4.8 | 69.5 ± 4.9 |
| Patient Survival (1st living donor) | 0–5 | 15 | | | | | | | | |
| | 5–10 | 97 | 90.3 ± 4.5 | 90.3 ± 4.5 | 84.7 ± 5.9 | (82.2 ± 6.2) | | | | |
| | 10–15 | 261 | 96.0 ± 1.8 | 91.5 ± 3.0 | 87.6 ± 3.7 | 86.2 ± 3.8 | 83.6 ± 4.1 | 78.5 ± 5.1 | 76.1 ± 5.3 | 71.9 ± 5.9 |
| Patient Survival (2nd cadaver graft) | 0–15 | 105 | 78.7 ± 7.3 | 74.0 ± 7.6 | 71.3 ± 7.6 | 63.2 ± 8.4 | (57.2 ± 8.7) | | | |
| | >15 | 106 | 84.7 ± 6.3 | 77.0 ± 7.3 | 73.8 ± 7.5 | (71.5 ± 7.6) | | | | |

Data on numbers at risk of less than 25 have been omitted; data on numbers less than 35 in parentheses.

**Table 38–5.** GRAFT SURVIVAL RATE ACCORDING TO AGE (EDTA—1981)

| | Age Group (years) | Sample Size | 1 Year | 2 Years | 3 Years | 4 Years | 5 Years |
|---|---|---|---|---|---|---|---|
| Graft Survival (1st living donor) | 0–5 | 15 | | | | | |
| | 5–10 | 97 | 80.8 ± 7.1 | 73.9 ± 7.8 | 64.4 ± 8.9 | | |
| | 10–15 | 261 | 80.7 ± 5.5 | 71.3 ± 6.3 | 65.8 ± 6.5 | 57.3 ± 7.0 | 50.8 ± 7.1 |
| Graft Survival (1st cadaver graft) | 0–5 | 36 | | 56.0 ± 7.3 | 49.5 ± 7.2 | 48.1 ± 7.1 | 47.1 ± 7.0 |
| | 5–10 | 274 | 65.6 ± 7.2 | 63.0 ± 5.7 | 57.9 ± 5.7 | 54.1 ± 5.6 | 50.8 ± 5.6 |
| | 10–15 | | 63.3 ± 5.6 | | | | |
| Graft Survival (2nd cadaver graft) | All | 143 | 51.0 ± 10.4 | 39.0 ± 9.7 | (35.0 ± 9.1) | | |

Data on numbers at risk less than 25 have been omitted; data on numbers less than 35 are in parentheses.

renal transplantation within two years following completion of treatment of renal malignancies. The principal causes of death in these children are metastasis and sepsis.[20]

Patient and graft survival rates are superior in children 10 to 15 years of age compared with those five to nine years of age. Patient and graft survival rates in children less than five years old are lower than those of older children.[21, 22] Analysis of published data shows that the success rate in infants less than one year of age is very low. In children one to five years old divergent results have been reported. Following cadaver donor transplantation, patient and graft survival rates at two years were 75% and 31% respectively.[22] However, the success rate of live-related donor transplantation does not differ from that of older children, with patient and graft survival rates at two years of 94% and 72% respectively.[21]

Eurotransplant data for adult and pediatric recipients have shown improved cadaver graft survival rates with better HLA-A and -B antigen matching. A 20% difference in the graft survival rate was found at two years between grafts identical for HLA-A and -B antigens compared with those with three or four mismatches.[23] In pediatric recipients of first cadaver donor grafts a significant effect on graft survival of HLA matching was demonstrated. The graft survival rate at four years post transplant of well-matched grafts was 85%, whereas the graft survival rate of poorly matched grafts was only 59%.[24] The survival rate of multiple cadaver donor grafts was also improved in well-matched grafts. The survival rate at four years of multiple grafts with one or two mismatches was 69%, whereas the survival rate of poorly matched grafts was 32%.[25] This effect of matching was demonstrated only in highly presensitized patients.[25] The influence of HLA-A and -B matching on the survival rate of all cadaver grafts in children recorded by Eurotransplant is shown in Table 38–6. Graft survival rates are progressively worse with increasing numbers of mismatches (G. Persijn, personal communication).

Graft survival rates improve when donor and recipient share two DR antigens. Recipients with no HLA-DR incompatibilities have a graft survival rate of 85% at one year, whereas patients with one and two incompatibilities have graft survival rates of 64% and 56% respectively.[26] Grafts which are identical for both HLA-DR and -AB have a 92% survival rate at one year.[23] Similar results have been obtained in children. HLA-DR identical grafts had a 64% survival rate, whereas grafts with one or two DR incompatibilities had a 32% one-year graft survival rate.[25]

The beneficial effect on graft survival of blood transfusions given to recipients of cadaver donor grafts is well documented. Con-

**Table 38–6.** HLA-A AND -B MATCHING AND GRAFT SURVIVAL IN CHILDREN (EUROTRANSPLANT—1982)

| No. of Mismatches | Sample Size | Graft Survival (%) at | | | |
|---|---|---|---|---|---|
| | | 1 Year | 2 Years | 3 Years | 5 Years |
| 0 | 67 | 77 | 73 | 69 | 65 |
| 1 | 177 | 77 | 69 | 65 | 62 |
| 2 | 165 | 70 | 66 | 60 | 53 |
| 3 | 54 | 58 | 56 | 50 | 45 |
| 4 | 13 | | | | |

flicting results have been reported regarding the number of blood transfusions required, the administration of perioperative transfusions, the time interval between the last transfusion and transplantation, and the specific blood component administered. HLA matching and the duration of dialysis modify the effect of transfusions on graft survival.[27] The pertinent factors concerning the effect of blood transfusions on graft survival rates in first cadaver donor recipients can be summarized as follows:

- Graft survival rates of nontransfused patients are poor. The one-year graft survival rate of such recipients varies between 20% and 40%.[27, 28]

- Graft survival rates are superior in multitransfused patients compared to patients receiving less than five transfusions. Opelz et al reported a one-year graft survival rate in recipients receiving fewer than five transfusions of 57% compared to 87% in multitransfused patients.[28]

- Patients receiving transfusions only perioperatively have a graft survival rate comparable to that of nontransfused recipients.

- Most studies have failed to show an effect on graft survival of the time interval between last transfusion and transplantation.[27]

- Leukocytes should be present in the blood component. Survival of the graft is not improved if the recipients receive frozen or filtered blood.[28, 29]

In live-related donor transplantation the effect of pretransplant blood transfusions is less pronounced. Only multitransfused recipients have a significantly improved graft survival rate when compared to nontransfused recipients.[27] Donor-specific blood transfusions appear to improve the graft survival rate of one-haplotype-matched live-related donor recipients with a reactive mixed lymphocyte culture.[30] Recipients of donor-specific blood transfusions have a 98% one-year graft survival rate.[30] Preliminary results of donor-specific transfusions in pediatric recipients are encouraging.[31, 32] Blood transfusion to the donor before nephrectomy also improves the graft survival rate.[33-35]

The graft survival rates for second cadaver donor grafts are considerably less than those for first cadaver donor grafts (EDTA, 1981) (Table 38–5). However, conflicting data have been reported from a single pediatric center. Fine et al reported a five-year graft survival rate for second cadaver donor grafts of 59% compared to a 38% graft survival rate for first cadaver donor grafts.[17] The outcome of the second graft is strongly related to the presence of lymphocytotoxic antibodies; however, in highly presensitized recipients the graft survival rate can be improved by better HLA-A and -B matching.[25] The survival rates of third and fourth cadaver donor grafts are poor.[17]

Infections are a major cause of death occurring during the early months after transplantation. These deaths may be related to the high steroid doses given during the first months after transplantation. Reduction of steroid dosage has resulted in a lower incidence of infections as well as a significant improvement in patient survival in centers with high post-transplant mortality rates.[36] Lower doses of oral prednisone provide as efficient immunosuppression as do high doses.[37] No difference in the graft survival rate was found in a prospective randomized

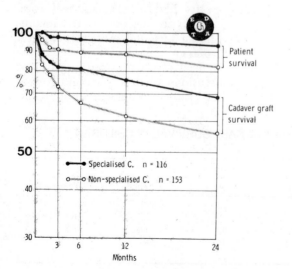

**Figure 38–2.** Patient and graft survival following transplantation in specialized and nonspecialized centers during the years 1976 to 1978 (EDTA 1978).[1]

trial comparing high- and low-dose steroid regimens.[38] Other measures designed to decrease the incidence of infections have also contributed to a decline in mortality among transplant recipients.[39] In pediatric recipients infection is an important cause of death (Table 38–3). Steroid doses recommended for immunosuppression in children during the early months after transplantation are high.[8, 18, 19, 40] No data are available comparing low- and high-dose regimens in children.

The causes of death in pediatric recipients as reported in 1979 by the EDTA are shown in Table 38–3. Infection was the principal cause of death in all pediatric recipients, but was more important in recipients of cadaver donor grafts. Analysis of mortality and causes of death collected from the reports of six large centers showed that 167 of 737 pediatric transplant recipients died.[7, 8, 18, 19, 40, 41] Of these deaths 56 were related to infection. Other important causes of death were cerebrovascular accident in 12, hemorrhage in four, malignancies in four, and cessation of therapy after graft failure in four recipients. This analysis shows that further improvement of survival is largely dependent on reduction of mortality related to infection.

Patient and graft survival rates are reported to improve with increasing center size.[5, 42] However, the results of kidney transplantation are more dependent upon experience of the physicians and upon the facilities available than upon the absolute number of transplants performed annually.[1, 41] Using the previous formulated definition of a specialized pediatric center, the 1978 EDTA data have shown that patient and graft survival rates are better in specialized pediatric centers as compared to nonspecialized centers (Fig. 38–2). The improved graft survival rates at one and two years are due primarily to a lower graft loss from rejection and other causes during the first year following transplantation.[1]

# REFERENCES

1. Chantler C, Donckerwolcke RA, Brunner FP, et al: Combined report on regular dialysis and transplantation of children in Europe, 1978. Proc Eur Dial Transplant Assoc 16:74, 1979.
2. Donckerwolcke RA, Chantler C, Broyer M, et al: Combined report on regular dialysis and transplantation in Europe, 1979. Proc Eur Dial Transplant Assoc 17:87, 1980.
3. Broyer M, Donckerwolcke RA, Brunner FP, et al: Combined report on regular dialysis and transplantation of children in Europe, 1980. Proc Eur Dial Transplant Assoc 18:60, 1981.
4. Donckerwolcke RA, Broyer M, Brunner FP et al: Combined report on regular dialysis and transplantation of children in Europe, 1981. Proc Eur Dial Transplant Assoc 19:60, 1982.
5. Jacobs C, Broyer M, Brunner FP, et al: Combined report on regular dialysis and transplantation in Europe, XI, 1980. Proc Eur Dial Transplant Assoc 18:4, 1981.
6. Kobrinsky NL, Robinson LL, Nesbit ME: Acute nonlymphocytic leukemia. Pediatr Clin North Am 27:345, 1980.
7. Chantler C, Broyer M, Donckerwolcke RA, et al: Growth and rehabilitation of long-term survivors of treatment for end stage renal failure in childhood. Proc Eur Dial Transplant Assoc 18:329, 1981.
8. Potter DE, Holliday MA, Piel CF, et al: Treatment of end-stage renal disease in children: A 15 year experience. Kidney Int 18:103, 1980.
9. Fine RN, Malekzadeh MH, Pennisi A, et al: Long-term results of renal transplantation in children. Pediatrics 61:641, 1978.
10. Baillod RA: Home dialysis. In: Replacement of Renal Function by Dialysis, 1st Edition, Drukker W, Parsons FM, Maker JF (Eds).The Hague, Martinus Nijhoff, 1978, p 462.
11. Broyer M, Gagnadoux MF, Bacri JL, Laborde K; Problems of long-term dialysis in children. In: Pediatric Nephrology, Gruskin AB, Norman ME (Eds). The Hague, Martinus Nijhoff, 1981, p 185.
12. Boczko S, Tellis V, Veith FJ: Transplantation of children's kidneys into adult recipients. Surg Gynaecol Obstet 146:387, 1978.
13. Cohen B: The influence of pediatric donor age and pediatric recipient age on kidney graft survival in Eurotransplant, 1982. (Personal communication.)
14. Hong JH, Shirani K, Arshad A, et al: Influence of cadaver donor age on the success of kidney transplants. Transplantation 32:532, 1981.
15. Van der Vliet JA, Persijn GG, Cohen B, et al: Influence of donor age on outcome of cadaveric renal transplantation. Dial Transplant 11:122, 1982.
16. Iitaka K, Martin LW, Cox JA, et al: Transplantation of cadaveric kidneys from anencephalic donors. J Pediatr 93:216, 1978.
17. Fine RN: Renal transplantation in children. Proc Eur Dial Transplant Assoc 18:321, 1981.
18. Chantler C, Carter JE, Bewick M, et al: 10 years' experience with regular haemodialysis and renal transplantation. Arch Dis Child 155:435, 1980.
19. Squifflet JP, Pirson Y, van Gangh P, et al: Renal transplantation in children. Transplantation 32:278, 1981.
20. Penn I: Renal transplantation for Wilms tumor: Report of 20 cases. J Urol 122:793, 1979.
21. Hodson EM, Najarian JS, Kjellstrand CM, et al: Renal transplantation in children ages 1 to 5 years, Pediatrics 61:458, 1978.
22. Rizzoni G, Malekzadeh MH, Pennisi AJ, et al: Renal transplantation in children less than 5 years of age. Arch Dis Child 55:532, 1980.
23. Van Rood JJ, Persijn GG, Cohen B, et al: Hierarchy of factors influencing kidney graft survival. Dial Transplant 12:111, 1982.
24. Broyer M, Gagnadoux MF, Beurton D, et al: Importance of HLA-A, B matching in kidney trans-

plantation in children. Transplantation 30:310, 1980.

25. Ettenger RB, Jordan S, Malekzadeh M, et al: Immunologic considerations in renal transplantation. *In:* Pediatric Nephrology, Gruskin AB, Norman ME (Eds). The Hague, Martinus Nijhoff, 1981, p. 364.

26. Ting, A, Morris PJ: Powerful effect of HL-DR matching on survival of cadaveric renal allograft. Lancet 1:282, 1980.

27. Fehrman I: Pretransplant blood transfusions and kidney allograft survival. Scand J Urol Nephrol (Suppl) 65, 1981.

28. Opelz G, Terasaki PJ, Graver B: Induction of high kidney graft survival rate by multiple transfusion. Lancet 1:1223, 1981.

29. Persijn GG, Cohen B, Lansbergen G, van Rood JJ: Eurotransplant 1979. Dial Transplant 9:176, 1980.

30. Salvatierra O: Experiences and future considerations with donor specific blood transfusions in living related transplantation. Am J Kidney Dis 1:119, 1981.

31. Broyer M, Gagnadoux MF, Beurton D, et al: Transplantation in children: Technical aspects, drug therapy, and problems related to primary renal disease. Proc Eur Dial Transplant Assoc 18:313, 1981.

32. Niaudet P, Beaurain G, Gagnadoux MF, et al: Pretreatment with donor specific blood transfusions before living related renal transplantation in children. Int J Pediatr Nephrol 3:137, 1982.

33. Frisk B, Berglin E, Brynger H: Positive effect on graft survival of transfusions to the cadaveric kidney donor. Transplantation 32:252, 1981.

34. Jeckel J, Hersche O, Marquet R, et al: Effect of blood transfusions to the donor on kidney graft survival in man. Transplantation 32:453, 1981.

35. Persijn GG, Landsbergen G, d'Amaro J, van Rood JJ: Blood transfusions and second kidney allograft survival.Transplantation 32:392, 1981.

36. Vincenti F, Amend W, Feduska NJ, et al: Improved outcome following renal transplantation with reduction in the immunosuppression therapy for rejection episodes. Am J Med 69:107, 1980.

37. McGeown MG, Douglas JF, Brown WA, et al: Advantages of low dose steroid from the day after renal transplantation. Transplantation 29:287, 1980.

38. Morris PJ, Frenck ME, Chan L, Ting A: Low dose oral prednisolone in renal transplantation. Lancet 1:525, 1982.

39. Tilney NL, Strom TB, Vineyard GC, Merrill JP: Factors contributing to the declining mortality rate in renal transplantation. N Engl J Med 299:1321, 1978.

40. Broyer M, Gagnadoux MF, Arsan A, et al: Transplantation renale chez l'enfant. Rev Pediatr 15:377, 1979.

41. Avner ED, Harmon WE, Grupe WE, et al: Mortality of chronic hemodialysis and renal transplantation in pediatric end stage renal disease. Pediatrics 67:412, 1981.

42. Banowsky LH, Chauvenet PA, Nicastro-Lutton JJ, et al: Patient survival in cadaveric renal transplantation: Report from a small centre. J Urol 127:867, 1982.

# IV

# Psychosocial Considerations

# 39

# Psychosocial Adaptation of Children with ESRD: Factors Affecting Rehabilitation

*Barbara M. Korsch, M.D.*
*Vida Francis Negrete, P.H.N., M.S.*

Before the second half of the twentieth century there was no definitive treatment for children and adolescents whose renal function was insufficient to support life and growth. Conservative treatment, consisting primarily of dietary modifications and certain medications to help control hypertension, accumulation of body waste, and the resulting metabolic imbalances, was the only known approach to the prolongation of life in these children. Support for child and family in adapting to the illness and in accepting the uniformly negative prognosis constituted the only tasks for the psychosocial staff during these times. These tasks were not essentially different from those appropriate in other chronic and fatal illnesses.

In the 1950's, with the introduction of dramatic techniques such as dialysis and renal transplantation and with a quantum leap in life expectancy for these patients, a host of new challenges were faced by patient, family, community, and treatment team. When dialysis and transplantation were offered to children, the essential question was, Is the tremendous cost, not only in dollars but also in terms of pain and suffering involved in these treatments, justified on the basis of the resulting prolongation and *quality of life*? It was with the aim of answering this question that Fine, when establishing his pioneering dialysis and transplant program for children at Childrens Hospital of Los Angeles in 1967, included a psychosocial team to study the impact of the illness and treatment on patient, family, and transplant team.[1]

This discussion is based on the systematic observations made by the Childrens Hospital of Los Angeles group,[2-4] reports from other selected treatment programs in Europe[5-7] and the United States,[8-12] and on clinical observations of children with chronic illnesses.[13-16] The focus is on adaptation and rehabilitation of the "normal" spectrum of children and families and not on gross social problems or psychopathology. Normal is an ambiguous term and most ESRD teams informally report that their caseloads seem to include very few "normal" families. However, for the purpose of this report, this term is used to exclude clinical pathology, diagnosed and treated by psychiatric specialists.

## NONSPECIFIC IMPACT OF CHRONIC DISEASE

It has been documented repeatedly that the psychosocial impact of chronic illness on child and family is determined in large measure by factors not intrinsic to any particular diagnostic category. Funding for health care is frequently allocated on a categorical basis and many clinical services are so organized, based on technologic considerations and mostly for the physician's convenience. However, evidence has accumulated that there are more commonalities between the attributes of chronically ill children across diagnostic categories than within any one specific diagnosis[17, 18] and that the determinants for ultimate function are to a large degree demographic, psychosocial, and developmental.[4]

These considerations are relevant to program planning, especially in treatment centers where there is not the critical mass of patients present which would be required to justify adequate psychosocial support systems within any one diagnostic category. In such centers a support team could be provided if chronically ill children were considered as a group noncategorically and treated on the basis of their common needs.

In pediatric medicine the chronologic age and the developmental stage of the sick child as he or she experiences illness and treatment are two uniquely important considerations. The developmental tasks characteristic for a specific time in the child's life span will be the ones most vulnerable to the stress of the illness. In the first year of life, separation from the mother or caretaker will be one of the most stressful experiences. Also in the first year, the feeding experience for mother and infant may be so altered as to influence the child's attitude about food as well as the mother's self-esteem for a long time to come.

In the second year inadequate outlets for development of autonomy and limitation of the opportunity for big muscle activities such as walking, running, and climbing will constitute a major deprivation. Also, in the second year habit training and the achievement of sphincter control are a central task for mother and child which will be uniquely distorted, for instance, in the case of the child with major anomalies of the genitourinary tract. During the preschool years, socialization within the family, progressive identification with the parent of the same sex, learning the roles within the family, socialization outside the family, and development of increasing independence may all be prejudiced by the need for repeated hospitalization and by periods of enforced inactivity and malaise.

Although an exhaustive inventory of stage specific developmental tasks and their distortion by illness and treatment is beyond the scope of this discussion, a few other generalizations are worthy of mention in this context. Education and acculturation, the main accomplishments of the school age child, are especially important for the child with physical illness who may later have to substitute

brains for brawn. Clearly, sick children are at a great disadvantage in this respect. Not only may physical limitations, hospital visits, and treatment interfere with school attendance and study but, unfortunately, the school system is not sufficiently educated, prepared, or funded to deal appropriately with these children's needs. In many cultures competitive sports are an important feature of the educational experience. The sick child's inadequacies in this respect may also greatly depress his or her already vulnerable self-esteem and socialization.

Separate emphasis needs to be devoted to the many sources of special anguish for the adolescent patient suffering from a physical illness. Maturing physically, rebelling against childhood dependency and family control, developing the adult sexual role, and planning a career are difficult even for many adolescents in our society who do enjoy robust physical health. When the strain of illness and treatment is experienced during these crucial years, the patient may not be able to adapt and compensate. The most severe failures in adaptation and the least satisfactory rehabilitation have been observed in patients whose disease manifested itself in adolescence.[4] Unfortunately, ESRD frequently declares itself during the growth spurt of the adolescent period, which makes these considerations especially relevant to the discussion of ESRD in young patients.

Family function is another basic consideration in assessing the outcome of physical illness in childhood. Related to family function are the personality attributes of the child/parent which will influence adaptation to illness and treatment. There are many observations[16] that a child who thinks well of himself and has experienced affection and respect in his early years from family members and others and who does not have an unusually vulnerable temperament may withstand even catastrophic illness and traumatic prolonged treatment without personality distortion. Looking at the genesis of these resilient personality profiles, one confronts certain basic temperamental attributes and also becomes aware that family function, including availability of supportive parents, siblings, and others, is most important. *Good communication* within the family, generally, and about the illness in particular, is one attribute of family function that has been found helpful to the child in his response to illness and handicap.[4, 19]

Not all determinants of child and family response to illness are in the psychologic sphere. Certain reality factors, such as financial and other resources within the family, distance from the treatment facility, availability of transportation, ethnic, cultural, religious, and educational background, community resources and support, all play important parts in structuring the illness experience for child and family. Single-parent families, disorganized families, and dislocated and isolated families are least likely to be able to muster the needed support for the sick child, although there are exceptions.

In considering noncategorical, nondisease specific features of chronic illness, another important determinant may be the contribution of the treatment team. It is generally accepted that support, sensitivity, continuity, and a comprehensive family-centered approach will make for a better outcome than fragmented, technologically oriented care. These assumptions have face validity, but the only evidence derives from studies by Pless indicating that a community worker, by supporting families, can contribute to the sick child's adaptation.[14, 20] It is difficult to assess how much impact the health professional's contribution, beyond his technical competence and appropriate interventions, has on child and family adaptation to illness and on the ultimate level of function. Yet, a host of clinical, anecdotal, and humanitarian information justifies attempts at ameliorating the illness experience for child and family from day to day, even when the ultimate outcome has not been documented to be altered.

## PSYCHOSOCIAL FEATURES SPECIFIC TO RENAL DISEASE IN CHILDHOOD

While all the general considerations for child and family faced with catastrophic illness are dramatically illustrated and validated in the patient with ESRD, specific features of renal disease and its treatment are also germane. Adolescence—the most vulnerable time in the child's growth and development—is the time when renal function is frequently no longer sufficient to maintain life. This timing constitutes a specifically stressful feature of renal disease. Some other specific features of renal disease constitute threats to the growing individual. Those patients with congenital anomalies of the genitourinary tract, obstructive uropathy, extrophy of the bladder, prune belly syndrome, grossly abnormal collecting systems, and other major defects are burdened with visible and functional abnormalities in respect to excretory and, later, sexual function which will ultimately have special significance in personality development.

Uremia in the first year of life interferes with normal growth and development of the central nervous system, which means that a number of ESRD patients will have the additional burden of developmental delay or limited intellect.[21] Compromised renal function hinders somatic growth and at times causes grotesque osseous abnormalities—a combination which impairs the child's physical prowess and self-esteem as well as his potential for socialization. Poor appetite and the occurrence of nausea and vomiting, the need for varied diet restrictions, and danger of malnutrition all tend to place unusual emphasis on eating, feeding, and diet. Noncompliance with dietary restrictions in dialysis, noncompliance with immunosuppressive medication, obesity after renal transplantation, and generally low self-esteem are probably in part related to emotionally charged features of the illness and treatment.

There are also aspects of diagnostic procedures and treatment for ESRD which constitute threats to the growing personality. In the children whose renal disease begins with nephrotic syndrome, an additional threat to self-esteem lies in the waxing and waning of edema, leading to dramatic differences between episodes of grotesque swelling and shrinking to pathetic bodily dimensions, accompanied by diffuse uncertainty and anxiety about bodily proportions and the factors that determine it.

## PSYCHOLOGIC IMPLICATIONS OF RENAL TRANSPLANTATION

Without delving into the unconscious processes and fantasies that may be elicited or exaggerated by the dramatic process of having another's kidney placed into one's own body, one can make certain observations on the basis of practical experience with these patients.[22, 23] In the case of the cadaveric kidney, the source of the kidney is the focus of unending speculation by patient, friends, and family. Efforts to keep the origin of the kidney a carefully guarded secret in a large institution are rarely successful. The main preoccupations relate to sex, age, personality, and sometimes race of the donor. Continuing relationship between the family of the donor and the recipient should probably not be encouraged: it has often led to unhealthy future reactions, to allograft rejection, and to other complications.

Live related donation involves dramatic psychologic reactions for accepted donor, rejected donor, and recipient, whether the kidney functions or is rejected. There is a whole literature on the psychology of giving and receiving gifts even without reference to the unusual situation involved in giving a part of one's own body to another. It seems of great importance not to add to the existing pressures on the live related donor. Community, family, the patient, and the donor's conscience combine into a tremendous force impelling the suitable potential donor to proceed with the donation. If he tries to resist, this bespeaks anxiety or other emotional turmoil which should not be ignored. Likewise, the recipient should not be coerced to accept a live related allograft from a donor whom he deems unacceptable. This may lead to undesirable emotional reactions, failure to cooperate with the medical regimen after transplantation, and even rejection of the allograft. Relationship between donor and recipient, which at best is burdened, at worst can be seriously threatened after the actual transplant has taken place.

However, obviously, judging a donor "unworthy" carries a severe emotional impact. Also, the risk of continued dialysis or cadaveric transplantation may be so great for a particular patient that some of the psychologic considerations alluded to above must be regarded in the context of health and welfare of child and family.

It appears that, at the least, careful consideration, assessment and continued support are needed for responsible decision making in this area. In certain cases continued exploration and support for donor and recipient may be indicated. In some cases, psychiatric input may be required.

## RESULTS FOR PATIENT AND FAMILY

The psychosocial team at Childrens Hospital of Los Angeles was originally destined to assess the psychosocial impact of illness and treatment on patient and family. Although service needs encroached increasingly on this research effort, it was possible to carry out systematic psychosocial assessment of all patients and families at the time of intake as well as regularly for follow-up. The aim was to utilize methods of assessment which were easily administered and interpreted by the regular members of the health care team. These did not require the expertise of psychologists and psychiatrists. Simple semistructured interviews to explore family function, communication patterns, sources of support, and family value systems from the point of view of the family and the patient were utilized. Also, a few short pen and pencil tests were administered to provide a uniform format for evaluation of individual personality profiles.[1] Questions relating to the patient's activities, to his self-esteem, and to his social and personal adjustment appeared to elicit the most helpful information in predicting rehabilitation and in planning appropriate intervention. There is reason to believe that the child's sense of mastery of his own fate and his own bodily functions ("internal" vs. "external" controls) also are worth exploring as part of the basic assessment. Using this simple battery of tests, the results of which are suitable for computer processing, served as a helpful foundation in the provision of comprehensive care. In certain instances extremely low test results yielded a formula that seemed to be predictive of poor adaptation and noncompliant behavior.

The results of this psychosocial assessment based on follow-up data collected for 13 years on 238 patients with 322 renal transplants have been published.[4] These are not dramatically different from those obtained elsewhere, except for the differences explicable by the higher percentage of cadaveric transplantations and by very eclectic intake criteria for this program. Some general conclusions from these studies relating to patients and families will be summarized here.

There was a strong correlation between the number and the extent of biological complications of dialysis and transplantation and the psychosocial outcome. In this context it can be understood why live related allografts led to better outcomes psychosocially as well as medically. For many children successful renal transplantation made for a better quality of life than did existence on any other type of treatment. For a smaller number, who by choice or for medical reasons remained on dialysis, especially those more recently treated by CAPD, acceptable adaptation was achieved without allograft. This was also the case in some who, following allograft rejection, returned to dialysis. It was observed that the majority of the children in the sample enjoyed an adequate level of rehabilitation and adaptation one or more years post renal transplantation. This included essentially normal physical activities, education, or vocational placement, and the assumption of appropriate roles in society, including marriage and procreation.[3, 4] Family life also in most instances returned to pre-illness equilibrium one or more years post transplantation.

These encouraging conclusions must be tempered by the following considerations: In general the patients' adaptation reflected the pre-illness personality attributes and functional level, which were not necessarily "normal" or desirable. Similarly, in many of the more troubled families "return to pre-illness equilibrium" did not represent a very desirable level of family function. A significant proportion of children and families developed major psychologic or emotional problems at some point in their illness experience. This was especially true in the adolescent patients. Since there are few reliable prevalence statistics or even good descriptive data on comparable populations without renal disease, it is difficult to infer to what extent ESRD and its treatment contributed to these problems.

The vulnerability to poor outcome seemed strongly increased for those patients put at risk by the following factors: (1) poor family support, (2) poor family function including family disorganization, (3) vulnerable personality before illness, including high anxiety and poor self-esteem, (4) complex medical course, (5) low income and other practical problems such as dislocation and poor community support systems, and (6) the experience of renal failure and treatment for ESRD occurring during adolescence.

One form of maladaptation documented in the Childrens Hospital Program was noncompliance with the immunosuppressive medication following transplantation, leading in some cases to decreased renal function and in some cases to allograft loss.[2] The risk factors for noncompliance were essentially the same as those for generally poor overall adaptations outlined above.

Support and intervention in the usual mental health model offered by the team to patients individually and in groups, as well as to families, did not predictably prevent maladaptation, although it was thought to improve the patients' and families' experi-

ence with the illness and treatment and made for better cooperation. Limited effectiveness seemed to relate in part to the failure of the most stressed patients and families to participate in psychotherapeutic ventures for practical and psychologic reasons.

At this time more recent rehabilitation data are available only in respect to a portion of the original sample. Of 209 patients who came to Childrens Hospital of Los Angeles for treatment of ESRD between 1967 and 1977 some data were obtained in respect to 203. Of these, 62 are no longer living. Of the 141 who were alive at the time of the survey in 1982, 104 had functioning transplants and 37 were on dialysis, 21 of these on hemodialysis and 15 on CAPD.

Among the 203 patients from whom data concerning occupation and education were obtained, the distribution of activities on inspection seemed similar to what one might expect from a similar population without special medical problems. Personal and social adaptation as assessed was also distributed in what seemed to be a normal pattern. For most of the sample self-esteem measurements were within the normal range. Their personal adaptation by their own reports was also normal in most instances. Their ambitions, life plans, and expectations from their children, as well as their perceived problems and dissatisfaction with daily life, were generally not attributed to their experience with the illness and treatment. Almost all had formulated career goals even though all were not in active pursuit of these. Most of them stated that their current adaptation was not specifically influenced by the experience with ESRD.

It must be emphasized that this level of adaptation was reported by patients whose experience with the disease and its treatment was essentially in the past. This time interval also helps explain why some of the patients about whose ultimate adjustment the psychosocial team had been very pessimistic turned out surprisingly well. Among the 94 patients who had reached the age of 18, 17 were married, and there were 30 healthy offspring reported.

## ETHICAL DILEMMAS

One of the very complex issues which may have to be faced by the health care team for children with ESRD relates to families in which the parents' choices and decisions are at variance with those of the medical team and at times even with the standards of the medical establishment. Occasionally a family will opt for "conservative" treatment and refuse to accept either dialysis or transplantation. In such situations there is need for very careful assessment of the families' motivations, strengths, and weaknesses. In the experience at Childrens Hospital of Los Angeles it was usually in the case of a severely retarded or disabled child that the problem surfaced.

If the family's decision seems well thought out, and the child's rehabilitation potential is minimal (in that there is little hope for education, training, or independent living), the family should be supported through the decision process and helped with their feelings of self-blame and with the negative reactions they may encounter from others.

If the decision seems poorly thought out and based on denial of the seriousness of the condition, misconceptions of the treatment, or short-term anxieties or resentment, the family needs to be worked with intensively, educated, counseled, and supported in the hope that they will become capable of more rational appropriate decision making.

If in the judgment of the responsible physician (in concert with any resident ethics committee or available consultant) the decision seems unjustified, he has to make some difficult choices. Invoking legal counsel is not always as helpful as is hoped and may lead to decisions which have medical or human consequences that are unwelcome to the health care team. There have been instances in which the legal decision was to support the parents in their opposition to the medical recommendations, which meant that the medical team could only sit by and support the family while the disease ran its inexorable course. More often, there have been decisions to remove the child from the parents' guardianship and to insist on treatment even when this meant removing the child from his home and placement in a foster family. Since such dislocations may be more traumatic to the child than the disease or the treatment process, one embarks upon this step with a heavy heart.

There are two other contingencies with grave ethical implications that need to be anticipated. There are situations in the care of older children when the child and the parents disagree as to the desirability of continuing treatment. In such a conflict careful assessment, including psychiatric appraisal of the entire family group, is needed to arrive at the best possible understanding of the whole complex situation.[24] Also, there needs to be someone to speak for the child in the family, although it is not easy to decide who should serve as such a child's advocate. In general it is difficult to imagine a situation where a child who is sufficiently mature to make a decision to continue treatment should not be honored in his decision. If the child decides against treatment, decision making becomes more difficult.

The last of the series of ethical dilemmas relates to the family who seems unable to support the child in the treatment program, i.e., parents who do not help their young child with his dietary restrictions or support his taking the essential medications. Even this kind of destructive behavior of the family at times compels the health care team to seek legal assistance in removing the child from the parents' jurisdiction and to place the child at least temporarily in an atmosphere where the treatment program can be appropriately supported. Here again the separation and dislocation is very painful for all involved and should be resorted to only when all attempts at supporting and helping the family have been explored and have proved unsuccessful.

## RESULTS FOR THE TREATMENT TEAM

The availability and utilization of new knowledge and technology and treatment modalities for children with ESRD have increased therapeutic options for patient and health care team. An adjunct to this development has been the psychosocial stresses on the health professionals as well as on the patients and families. Dealing with multiproblem families and children with catastrophic illnesses is always burdensome to the caretakers. When treatment is centralized, the specialists seeing these families are exposed to a very concentrated, continuous stressful experience.[25] Also, the treatment offered to these patients is both very traumatic yet limited in scope. This contributes to the frustrations of the caretakers. Dramatic interventions such as transplantation involve decision making, often in the face of insufficient knowledge and uncertainty. Psychologic considerations about which many health professionals feel less confident must be included. The nature and implications of these psychologic considerations may be intrinsically disturbing to the health professionals involved.

It has been observed that these responsibilities, when they are not taken into account explicitly, take a heavy toll on the effectiveness of the medical care offered. Approaches to lessening the burden lie in providing associated health professionals with expertise in psychosocial aspects of illness and treatment, in having support personnel share in patient-care activities, and in providing the opportunity for the biological-medical-surgical treatment team to communicate with the psychosocial team members about patients' problems and about their own concerns in caring for these difficult patients.

# REFERENCES

1. Korsch BM, Fine RN, Grushkin CM, Negrete VF: Experiences with children and their families during extended hemodialysis and kidney transplantation. Pediatr Clin North Am 18:625, 1971.
2. Korsch BM, Fine RN, Negrete VF: Noncompliance in children with renal transplants. Pediatrics 61:876, 1978.
3. Korsch BM, Klein JD, Negrete VF, et al: Physical and psychological follow-up on offspring of renal allograft recipients. Pediatrics 65:275, 1980.
4. Korsch BM, Negrete VF, Gardner JE, et al: Kidney transplantation in children: Psychosocial followup study on child and family. J Pediatr 83:399, 1973.
5. Debre M, Dulong O, Raimbalt G: Etude psychologique d'enfants en hemodialyse chronique. Arch Fr Pediatr 30, 163, 1973.
6. Scharer K, Chantler C, Brunner FP, et al: Combined report on regular dialysis and transplantation in children in Europe. Proc Eur Dial Transplant Assoc 13:59, 1976.
7. Schuler HS, Rohl L, Asbach HW, Möhring K, et al: Experiences in pediatric hemodialysis. Proc Eur Dial Transplant Assoc 9:325, 1972.
8. Abram HS: Survival by machine: The psychological stress of chronic hemodialysis. Psychiatr Med 1:37, 1970.
9. Bernstein DM: After transplantation—The child's emotional reactions. Am J Psychiatry 127:109, 1971.
10. Kahn AU, Herdon MA, Ahmandian SY: Social and emotional adaptations of children with transplanted kidneys. Am J Psychiatry 127:1194, 1971.
11. Sampson TF: The child in renal failure: Emotional impact of treatment on the child and his family. J Child Psychiatry 14:462, 1975.
12. Van Leeuwen JJ, Matthews DE: Comprehensive mental health care in a pediatric dialysis-transplantation program. Can Med Assoc J 113:959, 1975.
13. Grave GD, Pless IB: Chronic Childhood Illness: Assessment of Outcome. DHEW Publication, Vol 3, 76, 1974 (NIH Monograph).
14. Haggerty RJ, Roghmann KJ, Pless IB: Child Health and the Community. New York, John Wiley & Sons, 1975, p 388.
15. Talbot NB, Howell MC: Social and Behavioral Causes and Consequences of Diseases Among Children. In: Behavioral Science in Pediatric Medicine. Philadelphia. WB Saunders Company, 1971, p. 1.
16. Travis G: Chronic Illness in Children: Its Impact on Child and Family. Stanford, California. Stanford University Press, 1976, p 556.
17. Stein REK, Jessup DJ: A noncategorical approach to chronic illness. PH Reports 97:354, 1982.
18. Pless IB, Pinkerton P: Chronic Childhood Disorders: Promoting Patterns of Adjustment. Henry Kimpton, London, 1975, p 58.
19. Pless IB, Satterwhite B: A measure of family functioning and its application. Soc Sci Med 7:613, 1973.
20. Pless IB, Satterwhite B: Chronic illness in childhood: Selection, activities and evaluation of non-professional family counselors. Clin Pediatr 11:403, 1972.
21. Rotundo A, Nevins TE, Lipton M, et al: Progressive encephalopathy in children with chronic renal insufficiency in infancy. Kidney Int 21:486, 1982.
22. Fox RC: A sociological perspective on organ transplantation and hemodialysis. (New Dimensions in Legal and Ethical Concepts for Human Research.) Ann NY Acad Sci 169:406, 1970.
23. Korsch BM: Moral and Ethical Considerations. In: Edelmann CM, Barnett HL, Bernstein S, et al (Eds). Pediatric Kidney Disease. Boston, Little, Brown and Company, 1978, p 531.
24. Schowalter JE, Ferholt JB, Mann NM: The adolescent patient's decision to die. Pediatrics 51:97, 1973.
25. Kaplin De-Nour a, Czaczkes JW: Emotional problems and reactions of the medical team in a chronic hemodialysis unit. Lancet 2:987, 1968.

# 40

# The Role of the Social Worker in the Management of the Child with ESRD

*Robin S. Johnson, M.A., M.S.S., A.C.S.W.*

Enacted in 1972, Public Law 92–603, Section 2991 (known as HR1), amended the Social Security Act to provide Medicare coverage to persons with ESRD. Provision of social work services was specifically mandated in this legislation, formally recognizing the psychosocial component of chronic renal disease, and placing firm emphasis on the social worker's contribution to comprehensive care of the patient. The role of the social worker in ESRD was first addressed in 1973 in a position paper of the National Council of Nephrology Social Workers, which included the following statement:

Psychosocial factors affect all persons with chronic renal disease who must (1) confront the possibility of death; (2) select and incorporate a machine or a new kidney into one's system of self as a basis for living; (3) deal with a different and more restricted life style; (4) find meaningful roles for the family and society; (5) cope with continual social, emotional, and financial pressures . . . (6) reassess one's quality of life on dialysis or with a transplant, and the physical and psychic energy demanded by chronic renal disease. The social worker in the nephrology field has a special responsibility and a unique contribution to make in dealing with these psychosocial factors. Although physicians and other members of the nephrology team are, of course, concerned with psychosocial factors, the social worker is the only one with a consistent and central focus on social functioning. The major contributions of nephrology social workers can be described as two related activities: (1) to develop awareness of the significance and importance of the psychosocial components which

are a constant element in chronic renal disease; (2) to participate actively in the provision of adequate services to meet these social needs, either by giving direct services to patients or by influencing the development of specific programs and of social policy as a basis for future programs.[1]

These concepts have since been developed in a growing body of literature on the role of the social worker in adult nephrology.[2–5] Yet review of the literature reveals no clear picture of the role of the social worker in pediatric nephrology.[6, 7]* This chapter describes the social work role in a regional dialysis and transplantation program as it has evolved over its 13-year history. As a foundation for future theory building and research,[8] the chapter is divided as follows: (1) the role of the social worker is briefly summarized; (2) conceptual models are introduced upon which practice is established; and (3) clinical practice is described as it relates to each major stage of management of the child with ESRD.

## ROLE OF THE SOCIAL WORKER

The Clinical Social Worker facilitates all stages of treatment and care of the ESRD patient and family through provision of diagnostic and consultancy services, including psychosocial evaluation, advocacy, education,

---

*Travis provides an excellent overview of social work and pediatric nephrology.

team building, and psychotherapeutic support to patient, family, and staff. He or she provides continuity of contact from initial diagnosis through dialysis, transplant, and follow-up, including the terminal phase and beyond.[9]

## CONCEPTUAL MODELS FOR SOCIAL WORK PRACTICE

**Background.** The medical model is an impressive achievement of modern civilization. Grounded in accepted standards of health, it depicts deviations from those standards in terms of individual pathology. Assumptions of underlying malfunction and its observable symptoms lead in turn to diagnosis, and the individual is prescribed appropriate therapy. The child with ESRD benefits medically from this conceptual framework, and is introduced to the variety of professional languages and frames of reference that express it.

Whether in an integrated regional center or in a setting where pediatrics, nephrology, surgery, and dialysis staffs work separately, this model of individual pathology is not adequate to conceptualize the complex psychosocial dimensions of management of the child with ESRD. While often deemed adequate to assess the child suffering from disease and his age-appropriate coping and adaptational responses, this model lacks the power to reveal or explain the child within his family of origin, his social/cultural context outside the hospital, his impact upon caregivers at every level, and, of course, their impact upon him. Many have struggled with a unitary approach to mind and body, and have concluded that the individual is best viewed as a biopsychosocial entity,[7, 10] yet it is often difficult for those working within the medical model, and dealing with acute medical issues, to switch perceptual gears and see the child as more than his disease. While intellectually aware of the need to see the patient as a whole person, health professionals are accustomed to perceiving symptomatic distress as arising from physiological or biological causes, and are socialized by education and experience to do so. Such professionals can sometimes find it emotionally difficult to deal with the psychosocial components of chronic disorders. Professional training too often fails to focus on the therapeutic significance of total patient care with its complex interrelationship of medical and psychosocial factors.

Misconceptualization of a situation or event can in itself produce problems. Under certain circumstances, problems will arise purely as a result of wrong attempts at changing existing difficulties: a difficulty may be defined as "an undesirable life situation for which there exists no known solution, and, which at least for the time being, must simply be lived with."[11] ESRD may aptly be described as an undesirable life event for which there exists, presently, no predictable solution. The unpredictability of ESRD can lead to painful physical and/or emotional difficulties on the part of child and family whose reactions or coping responses may be misinterpreted or mislabeled (diagnosed), often by equally distraught staff. At this point, action is taken (prescribed). Then problems occur. These are not semantic niceties. Primary prevention is a basic tenet of pediatric practice, and while primary prevention has yet to become a medical reality for ESRD, the simple and rarely asked question, "Are we conceptualizing this situation in the right way?" can facilitate solution and prevent further occurrence of psychosocial problems that may substantially interfere with appropriate medical management of the child.

**The Interactional Approach.** Recognizing the long-term biopsychosocial complexity of ESRD, our group has adopted a systems-oriented or interactional model as the essential complement and extension to the medical model.[12, 13] Grounded in the epistemologic cornucopia of family systems theory,[12] the interactional model assumes that symptomatic distress in the child can arise from a variety of causes: physiological, biological, familial, and societal. It recognizes and attempts to deal with the impact of a child's illness *and of the response of others to it.* It reminds us that the child, the family, the therapeutic regimen, and the effect of the program providing the regimen each deserve equal attention.

This model is process-oriented, concerning itself with movement and change over time, and systematically redefining its goals to reflect ongoing interactions and their effects. Unlike the medical model, the interactional model emphasizes care and not cure: ongoing adaptation to chronic illness is its goal. While it acknowledges the necessity of professional control, it respects the values and fosters the inputs of *all* parties to the therapeutic endeavor—child, family social system, and professional social system—and recognizes

A.

PROGRAM ⟶ CHILD

B.

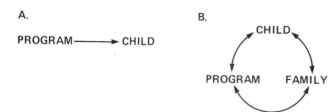

Figure 40–1. *A*, The linear medical model of individual pathology. *B*, The circular interactional model of child, family, and program.

and deals with the conflicts that arise from their mutual interaction.

The interactional model stresses concepts of normal coping and adaptation to chronic disease and its management: in this regard, it considers the reactions of the caregiver to the child and family to be just as significant as the child's reaction to disease and its management.[14] Such a model of care requires more input of time and emotional energy (especially during the initiation of treatment) than the medical model. In our experience, the outcome has been that children, families, and professionals work together better, and that the net result may be less time spent overall, better compliance, more meaningful life experience, less hospitalization, fewer dialysis complications, and reduced morbidity. In addition, the interactional model obliges all members of the team to constantly evaluate their concepts of success and failure. There are times, for example, when the price of prolonging life is too high in terms of patient suffering. "Medical failure" may be more accurately labeled "responsible medical practice" when the patient is allowed a dignified and relatively pain-free death. This model allows for continual personal growth and an opportunity for the refinement of ethical practice.

**Normal Coping and Adaptation.** Much of the literature on the behavior of people dealing with illness has been drawn from a psychodynamic base, itself grounded in a model of individual pathology. Responses of pa-

tients and families to chronic disease have been described in the language of defense mechanisms such as regression, denial, and dependency—mechanisms related to an assumed premorbid personality. This language can be of value to explain behavior, or to predict response to hospitalization or medical intervention. It is important to recognize regression, dependency, denial, and other defenses as attempts to protect the self from ego disorganization in the face of life-threatening illness and the rigors of its management. Yet this perspective is limited in its lack of the more flexible, operational terms of coping and mastery.[10] The interactional model reminds us that recognition of defensive structures should not exclude recognition of healthy patterns of adaptation: appropriate family efforts to deal with the total therapeutic environment, and to restructure the life style of the child in the family[10] as best suits their need. Child and family can be expected to mix defensive and coping mechanisms.[15] Since problem definition can affect type of treatment offered, excessive attention to individual psychopathology, premorbid behavior, and personality defects often prevents caregivers from recognizing, utilizing, and encouraging the unique coping capacities of each child and family. Apparently noncompliant or deviant behaviors often reflect idiosyncratic attempts to master or cope with the feelings of helplessness engendered by chronic disease.

Social and emotional factors exert a deci-

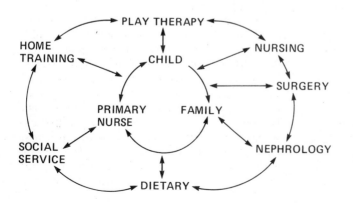

Figure 40–2. Expansion of the interactional model to demonstrate the central place of child and family within the treatment team.

sive effect on the way ESRD is managed, and affect the degree of social impairment in child and family, and the ways in which child, family, and caregivers adjust. Various conceptual models have emphasized that individual and family face a series of adaptive tasks necessitated by illness.[16–18] Failure to recognize and encourage mastery of these adaptive tasks is to rob patient and family of their own best coping strategies. Assumptions about family behavior and response to the medical regimen often reflect attitudes and values that belong to the caregiver and not to the child and family.

Much of medical training consists of learning to cope with pervasive uncertainty and with the limits of medical knowledge.[20] Nowhere is that more true than in management of the child with ESRD. We know that stresses upon child and family may at times become intolerable. The caregiver, too, suffers in a personal way despite the excellence of the care provided. Sometimes, it can be more tolerable for a much feared thing to happen because of something one has done than it is to be at the mercy of chance.[21] On occasion, medical action is taken (with the best of intention) to meet the needs of those taking it, and with less judgment as to its total impact upon a child and family. This may explain why attempts to change child and family behaviors are often unsuccessful. Understanding the coping and adaptational style of each child and family is essential. Recognition of similar dynamics in the caregiver is of equal importance.

**Loss and the Significance of Time.** Models of normal process, coping, and adaptation are available in the literature of griefwork, mourning, loss, and bereavement.[22–25] Dialysis and transplantation are often conceptualized by the caregiver in terms of gain of life, relative health, and future potential. While this may be valid, it is essential also to address the many losses involved in ESRD and its management: of vital organs and one's sense of personal wholeness, of the hopes and assumed predictability and control of a normal life, and potentially of life itself. Failure to recognize these losses and address them with child and family can be expected to cause problems.

Fundamental to coping with loss is time for successful problem resolution; normal adaptation to *any* change demands recognition of the unique personal time frame of child and family. Management of ESRD often demands quick and unpredictable changes in the medical regimen that can leave child, family, and caregivers with a surplus of unfinished emotional business. Our team has learned that the ultimate outcome is improved by allowing as much time as medically possible between each phase of treatment to facilitate adjustment, and to provide a sound emotional foundation for the next necessary intervention. This also establishes a firm base for dealing with medical setbacks should they occur.

**The Child in the Family.** Pediatric medicine has long recognized that to treat the child outside the context of the family is to do a grave disservice to each. As the sick child is a member of a family, it follows that meaningful involvement of the whole family, including grandparents, uncles and aunts, is vital to the therapeutic regimen. Extended families are an important source of support to patient and parents.[26] The family is a powerful system. What happens to the child resonates throughout the family system: less obvious, but just as significant, is the reverse—what happens in the family resonates back through the child.[27] The interactional view allows us to watch children rehearse, accept, or reject the coping mechanisms of their parents as they attempt to evolve their own strategies for managing their disease. It also allows us to discriminate between the child's response to ESRD and the child's response to the ups and downs of life within the family and the program.

**Separation and Individuation.** A major function of living with chronic illness is to accept all possible control over its management. Nowhere is this more true than in the pediatric setting. Fostering the normal process of separation and individuation[28] under the strain of chronic disease is one of the greatest challenges to the ESRD program, and it is upon this growth-oriented principle that the true success of a program is based. The most obvious practical manifestation is dialysis self-care, with the close support of primary nursing regimens that enable it. To teach the child to "own" his disease by encouraging active participation wherever possible is to foster that mastery, personal autonomy, and resulting sense of self-worth so vital to child development. It returns to the child the confidence to continue education, maintain contacts with peer groups beyond the hospital or dialysis unit, and, above all, continue the age-appropriate tasks of growing up and away from frequently anxious parents. The interactional approach may reveal a relationship between parental anxiety and decreased competence in the child; similarly, increased competence in the child leads to decreased parental anxiety—which leads to increased competence in the child, and so on. Taking control is the best antidote to the helplessness, loss of hopes, health, and potentials, and the unpredictability of ESRD.

**Significance of Socialization.** Children learn from their families and from all those around them, especially those with whom they spend considerable amounts of time. This has implications for the ways in which children and families conceptualize their illness and its putative course. Regardless of what we tell our patients, they will learn the full significance of their condition and what the future holds for each one of them by a process of careful observation and exposure to other patients and families. As they pass from clinic to hospital, to dialysis unit to hospital to clinic and so on, child and family gain an education that is more eloquent than any we can give.[29] Recognition of this dynamic argues the need for a program philosophy shared and implemented by all members of the treatment team. Confidence in both caregivers and medical regimen is undermined, and anxiety with its attendant mood or behavior problems is engendered when child and family hear information from team members that is contradicted by their empirical observation.

**Autonomy and Information.** It is important to recognize that the concept of autonomy is closely related to the way people regulate information. Each one of us regulates the information we receive. Some things we "hear," other things we do not—often in proportion to perceived threatening content. This adaptive mechanism demands careful recognition and respect so that child and family may move between denial and acceptance as part of normal adjustment, and so that both concrete and adaptive learning tasks may be performed.[30] Complex ethical issues arise—whose responsibility is it to regulate information—patient, family, or caregiver? If people have the right to know, do they also have the right not to know? Should the parent be told and not the child? As stated above, the adjustment process will be mediated by an exposure to other patients and their individual scenarios.[28] While there are no clear answers to these questions, all possible freedom and personal autonomy should be supported in child and family, and to this end, they must have the necessary

amount of information for informed decision making. But how much can be comprehended by the uremic child and stressed family?[31]

**Therapeutic Value of Education.** One answer to the above dilemma lies in a thorough introduction to ESRD and its treatment modalities through formal meetings designed for that purpose alone. These meetings should begin quite soon after diagnosis and precede each major therapeutic stage. Major topics should include an overview of ESRD, the program's approach to ESRD, dialysis modalities, transplant success and failure, and mortality risks. Verbal and visual presentations to family and child should be couched in simple language that they can understand; early introduction to the dialysis unit and staff as well as to the medical and surgical floors in the hospital is vital.[32] Time for education should be set aside quite separately from visits for medical reasons, when anxiety is usually at a peak. Opportunities should be given for child and family to check back in person or by phone to clarify concerns and raise questions over time. Verification of knowledge gained from individual team members is essential to ensure that information is both heard and understood. Each treatment team member is involved in this education process at one time or another to reinforce the impression given. Individual areas of expertise complement each other to present unified information on ESRD and its management.

**Conceptualization of ESRD.** There is, at present, no known cure for ESRD. Definitions of "a successful transplant" may vary. While the goal of pediatric ESRD programs is to obtain a "good working transplant" for each child, a good working transplant does not happen for everyone. Rejection, dialysis, transplant nephrectomy, transplant, rejection, dialysis, can follow hard upon one another for the less fortunate patient in a vicious debilitating cycle. Some young people have had as many as four transplants before they come of age to vote.

Realistic conceptualization of the disease management continuum can in itself reduce that bitter sense of failure when a desired dialysis modality fails, or when a transplant moves to irreversible rejection. The linear "cure" model of dialysis and transplant is what we aim for, but it fails us every time a child loses a transplant. The interactional model makes the treatment team aware of the circular repetitive pattern of ESRD. Such

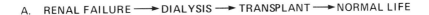

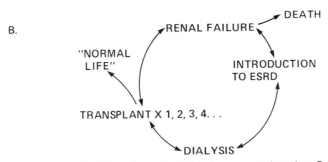

**Figure 40–3.** *A*, The linear medical *"cure"* model of dialysis and transplantation. *B*, The circular interactional *"care"* model.

awareness may, over time, reduce staff, patient, and family anxiety, provide relief from feelings of personal failure, and optimize the therapeutic regimens appropriate to each stage of the chronic disease process. Dialysis and transplantation together reflect the therapeutic continuum.[33] Making this clear to children and families at or around the time of diagnosis avoids problems of who has failed whom, and in what way.

**Quality of Life.** It is incumbent upon the treatment team to ascertain what quality of life means to each child and family, and to reassess this meaning as time goes by. Therapeutic action should be recommended with this concept in mind. It must be addressed from the beginning of treatment. The value of so doing when the medical regimen is relatively trouble-free becomes most apparent later in the course when complex life and death decisions may have to be made. Degrees of suffering and disability mean different things to different people, as does death itself. Sensitivity to these issues in others demands prior scrutiny of their meaning for each member of the treatment team. Personal meaning is a fundamental dimension of each individual, and there can be no real understanding of human illness or suffering without taking it into account.[21]

Close involvement with children and their families over time, coupled with a greater availability of organs for transplantation than in the adult field, can lead professionals to believe that there is always another therapeutic answer for the child with ESRD. Sadly, experience has shown this not yet to be the case. Although we may be sophisticated in knowing when to initiate treatment and how to manipulate technological advances, such sophistication often deserts us as we approach the terminal phase of the child chronically ill with ESRD. Quality of life should be a major criterion to determine specific treatments for ESRD as the medical circumstances of the child allow.[34]

## CLINICAL SOCIAL WORK PRACTICE

**Diagnosis.** The diagnosis of ESRD in a child precipitates a major crisis for both child and family. Depending upon the individual facts of the case, the child may already have been seen by local pediatricians, and perhaps evaluated at a local hospital before referral to the regional dialysis and transplant center. The family senses they have a major problem on their hands before they walk into the renal clinic. In many cases, they may have traveled several hours, leaving home early in the morning to reach the center. In addition to the possible culture shock of entering a big city, they may have trouble locating the center, parking, and finding the clinic. Perhaps the clinic is typically busy and they have to wait. Blood samples are drawn, urine samples taken, and a medical history and physical examination follow. In a teaching hospital, more than one physician may be involved. Perhaps there is then another wait of hours or days. At the end of this simplified scenario, the family and child sit down with the nephrologist and discuss medical realities. The nephrologist has spent a major portion of his professional career on kidney disease; he is in his familiar workplace, surrounded by one of the most sophisticated support systems mankind has developed. Often preoccupied with the many complex cases he is carrying, pressured to finish a backlog of outpatients before rushing to rounds, a teaching conference, or to deal with another medical crisis, he makes time to try to calm the family and begin to explain to them, in the limited time available, a situation which is to radically change their lives. Even with years of practice simplifying complex facts, the nephrologist is at best using words and frames of reference that can be totally foreign to family and child.

This interaction is the prototype of similar scenarios that will occur despite increasing increments of lay knowledge throughout the course of the child's management: fearful, anxious, disoriented child and family receive complex technical advice in unfamiliar language from an authority who, in effect, holds life and death in his hands. At this stage, it is the role of the social worker to support not only the child and family but also the physician, with whom, over time, total management of the child with ESRD will be shared. Interpreting the affective response of the family to the treatment team is as important as helping family and child to temper anxiety and cope with their fears, correct distortions, and clarify facts.[35] If this phase is handled by recognizing the value of early crisis intervention, which holds that the outcome of crisis depends more on external intervention during the crisis than upon the personality or past life experiences of the individual,[35] many future problems simply do not arise. Family theory confirms that the interactional patterns of child, parents, and extended family are so closely interwoven that it is productive to assess family rather than individual reaction.[27] During any crisis, the family is most susceptible to influence by others. Crisis provides unique opportunities for caregivers to influence the mental health of parents and child[35] in either a positive or negative way.

We are all impaired by the selective myopia of our professional training and our professional tasks. Despite sometimes considerable awareness of psychosocial issues, the nephrologist, too, is limited by his or her own expected agenda, namely, to present significant medical facts in a hopefully comprehensive way. Recognizing the value of social service intervention and ensuring that it is provided at this time can be difficult for the busy physician whose assumptions about service needs may rest upon conceptual blind spots.[36] In the absence of a differential social/emotional assessment,[37] strengths and coping abilities which may not be readily identified in certain races and cultures are often ascribed to families of elevated educational or economic status. Yet such families, because of

their particular privilege and life success, are often most in need of help at times of powerlessness and enforced helplessness brought on by major illness and injury.[38] Social service needs are independent of socioeconomic status, culture, and race. It has been our experience that inclusion of the social worker in significant meetings with the family does much to address the issues raised above. The role of the social worker is to ensure that all families receive necessary support at the time of diagnosis.

**Psychosocial Evaluation.** Properly performed, a social/emotional assessment should be one of the cornerstones upon which the health care team builds its relationship with child and family over time. The purpose of the assessment is to generate information that will facilitate long-term medical management. Conceptually, it should operate along at least two dimensions: (1) to assess child and family, and (2) to do it in such a way that it becomes a resource for the team. It should also complement the various consultations from other disciplines that contribute to the full patient work-up, especially the psychometric and developmental data generated by the consulting child psychologist.

A family systems model is useful for evaluation. Developmental history, coping patterns, individual psychodynamics, and educational history of the child should be noted. However, assessment of parental cohesion and marital stability, degree of parental enmeshment with child, degree of respect for personal autonomy in the family system, quality of involvement of grandparents or significant others, and degree of total family cohesion all may be valuable predictors of how child and family will manage the therapeutic regimen, and can explain apparently idiosyncratic reactions to it. A better understanding is obtained, for example, of the child who initially fights treatment, if we know that his father has an extreme fear of needles and speaks of having once himself left a hospital to avoid a feared procedure.

As many members of the family as possible are asked to participate in the evaluation. Who presents, how they arrange themselves in the interview room, what issues are raised and by whom can all provide the perceptive social worker with clues to family functioning. Depending on the medical realities of the case, this meeting should take place fairly soon after diagnosis and, again, should be timed not to coincide with medical interventions. Of course it must be emphasized that assessment is an ongoing process as the social worker joins with the child and family, observes their coping strategies, and works with them over time. It is the role of the social worker to update the team as relevant information is gained, coping strategies change, and family dynamics alter with the adjustment process.

Confidentiality in the medical setting falls within an ethical no man's land.[39] The social worker guarantees confidentiality to child and parents while reserving the right to discuss with either, or both, material that would help the treatment team come to decisions that will further the medical management of the child. The summary of the evaluation that goes on the chart satisfies administrative documentation needs, but clearly does not provide detail. The social worker uses professional judgment in deciding what is relevant to the medical management, and must maintain an ethical relationship with child and family. A responsible relationship with the treatment team, and especially with the primary nurse, allows certain kinds of confidential material to be screened from full team discussion and dealt with between selected team members. Consideration of this issue is crucial to maintain privacy and trust on the one hand, and to tactfully manage human situations, such as paternity issues and organ donorship, as they arise.

While the social worker should be available to counsel about financial matters, to obtain financial aid from patient support groups or other organizations when needed, and to help the family with transportation, accommodations, and other material services, it is the role of the hospital financial consultant to advise the family on the specifics of insurance coverages, applications for Medicare, state renal programs, and the interlocking coverage net. The role of the social worker is primarily clinical. Although financial evaluation is appropriate, the social worker should be available to help the family discriminate between truly financial and primarily symbolic issues. The connection between money and more general narcissistic supplies is common theoretical knowledge.[40] Many families are able to talk openly about fears for their financial future, yet cannot address the feared loss of a child. While the therapeutic value of obtaining concrete services should not be underestimated, nor the subtle ways in which it allows for "joining" a

guarded family, these services can be provided by other professionals trained for that purpose. The role of the social worker is to ensure that child and family have free access to these services, and that they are being delivered as they should be.

The unsophisticated administrative eye has sometimes perceived the social work role as focused primarily upon concrete services. Certainly, need and provision of such services are easier to measure than the necessary psychotherapeutic functions performed by the trained clinical social worker. In the team experience consistent early social work intervention not only facilitates and enhances the medical regimen but is cost-effective in doing so. Early intervention can diminish patient/family/staff problems that result in costly expenditure of time, emotional energy, and resources. High social work caseloads inhibit adequate provision of preventive care, but there is little agreement at present as to what an appropriate social-worker-to-patient ratio should be. In this regard, the interactional approach, using the clinical social worker as consultant to the treatment team, guarantees that service needs are comprehensively provided.

**Modalities and Management Meetings.** It is the role of the social worker to arrange and facilitate meetings with child, parents, and other family members and friends, the nephrologist, the primary nurse, and other members of the team at major turning points in the management continuum: especially (1) to review the alternative dialysis modalities prior to initiation of dialysis; (2) to explore and explain transplantation, graft failure, and nephrectomy where indicated; (3) to explore possible changes in dialysis modality; (4) at any time that the physician or family demands, to explore, clarify, or resolve medical or psychosocial issues. These meetings are held preferably in a neutral environment, and are designed to educate while lowering anxiety, to promote mutual understanding, and to facilitate the medical regimen. Intervention by the physician at the bedside or in the outpatient clinic should not be minimized; however, neither environment is conducive to the clear exchange and assimilation of information.

Following each meeting, the social worker remains with the family, as at diagnosis, to allow for expression of affect, to clarify fact and correct misperception, and to explore feelings. The fear and anxiety generated by management meetings are commonly translated to anger at specific caregivers or the timing of medical interventions. The social worker is a safe person upon whom to displace these feelings, and is someone who will help child and family uncover real fears, and interpret and work through needs or fantasies, or explore and place in context regressive primitive thought processes of early childhood. The consistent presence of the social worker at each meeting, with what may be different team physicians at different times, reduces stress and provides a common link for the family. It is the role of the social worker to document and bring to the team his or her perception of the family and child's understanding of the current situation and their adjustment to it. This can provide other caregivers with insight or information that will facilitate their own roles.

These meetings function also to provide families with a model for participation that fosters their own necessary autonomy, and demonstrates more eloquently than words that a team effort between child, family, and program is based in practice. It has been said that the relationship between family and treatment team is like a marriage from which there is no divorce.[41] If that is true, it is the role of the social worker to provide sufficient counseling to each party such that the marriage remains as functional and as harmonious as circumstances allow.

**First Hospital Admission.** The foundation of introductory meetings, prior familiarization with staff and hospital (as age-appropriate[32]), and suitable crisis intervention at diagnosis and follow-up usually ensures that hospitalization for vascular access or catheter insertion is less troublesome than it might otherwise be. Emergency admissions, however, still demand intensive crisis intervention.

If parent and child are adequately prepared and trust the treatment team, hospitalization can go as smoothly as one might expect of any new and unfamiliar experience. While we recognize the need for detailed and painstaking psychological preparation of the child for the stress of painful medical and surgical procedures[32] (including an age-appropriate explanation of what is to be expected both pre- and postoperatively), preparation of the parents and siblings is equally important. In many pediatric institutions, separation anxiety is precluded by offering the **parent** an opportunity to stay with the

child while hospitalized. The psychosocial evaluation, especially the impression of family coping strategies, may be selectively shared with inpatient nurses and resident staff to help prepare them to care for the child and family. Hospitalization provides an opportunity to observe parents and child together under stress, and in some families, to encourage sufficient separation (if need be) so that the child will be prepared to participate in self-care in the dialysis unit or at home. This is especially difficult for a parent with separation anxieties of his or her own. Tactful exploration of loss of those significant to them, and their coping strategies, including patterns of mourning and grief resolution, may give clues to how parents will tolerate the process of allowing a child to accept appropriate responsibility for participating in treatment. Divorce or parental separation is often a clue that parent or child will have difficulty with a hospitalization.[42] These issues should be addressed discreetly but directly by the social worker.

Typical reactions to hospitalization may be minimized by directly recognizing them, and reframing them within a context of normal behavior; the elegant paradoxical strategy of "symptom prescription" can also be a potent tool for problem resolution.[11] Patient and family may be informed about what "most people" experience in their particular situation; pain may be "prescribed," allowing that "it" will sting/throb/ache/hurt, that "most people" are very scared/angry/frightened/upset, and that this is the natural healthy response to being in hospital. The family is assured they will be depressed/down/out of sorts/at each other's throats "for a while," that they will probably be angry with team members, and that it's all a normal response to ESRD and its management. The family and child are told that now is the right time to "practice" all these feelings, and to get really good at them. This normalizing of an abnormal situation is of significant psychotherapeutic benefit. Because ESRD is an extreme condition, prescribing extreme reactions can be appropriate where pre-existing psychopathology is absent.

It is not uncommon to be called to "do something" for a depressed child mourning a significant loss: a predictable future, a kidney, a body image, or, perhaps, separation from home and friends. Although a close eye must be kept upon the course of the depression, mistimed intervention can interfere with vital mourning and adjustment processes. Sometimes it is a staff member's over-identification with patient or family that requires therapeutic intervention.

**The Initiation of Dialysis.** One of the main functions of the social worker is to know what *not* to do, and when not to do it. If preparation of child and family has been successful as above, the role of the social worker, when the child begins dialysis, is to help support the staff, and especially the primary nurse or home training nurse, as they carry out their tasks. Pertinent psychosocial information should be provided as required, and the primary nurse encouraged to further know the family and child so they can begin to establish their relationship in their own way. Consulting with the nursing staff on child and family dynamics, normal problems of compliance and adjustment, and management of the unique stresses of dialysis work, perhaps through weekly support group experience, is part of the social worker's role. Judicious support of the primary nurse through development of his or her psychosocial skills is a vital contribution to the well-being of the child on dialysis and his family.

**The Health Care Team in ESRD.** Research on health care teams in the adult hemodialysis setting suggests that team agreement and common philosophy result from shared values, and that these are essential to the optimal functioning of the ESRD team.[43] Fundamental to agreement is recognition of difference: different roles, functions, professional languages, and styles of intervention. Conflict can arise simply from misunderstanding or misdefinition of professional roles. While an obvious role is to define his or her own role clearly and unequivocally, the social worker is in a strong position to facilitate the team's work and encourage team strengths through judicious use of group and process skills. It has been suggested that discrepancies in expectations between team members can explain discrepancies in reports of adult patients' adjustments to dialysis, and that this may be one of the major reasons for poor patient compliance with the medical regimen.[43] Experience in the pediatric setting supports this suggestion, but the concept may be expanded further. The interactional model supports the conclusion that the team gains its own satisfactions from both medical *and* psychosocial response of the child and family to service provided. When quality service meets with a negative response—for example, patient noncompliance or clearly expressed dissatisfaction or deviant behavior—team members may need to defend themselves from feelings of guilt at inadequate performance. The role of the social worker is to interpret patient and family response to the medical regimen in a way that clearly recognizes the unique qualities and abilities of each team member, and that also allows patient and family issues to be addressed undefensively by the team. While failure of medical interventions often has to be accepted, this rarely results from personal failure on the part of the professional. The interactional model can provide a successful framework for the team to understand its reciprocal interaction with child and family.

A team value base evolves from the mutual respect of team members for each other. Such respect can be more readily gained when members recognize the professional strengths and talents of each other and have appropriate expectations for both their colleagues and themselves. The social worker can aid the team in clarifying these expectations. Promoting open and trusting communication must, in the first instance, be modeled by the secure social worker as he or she establishes professional relationships with colleagues on the treatment team.

**Transplantation.** It is commonly accepted that the most effective long-term therapy for ESRD in children is a good working transplant. The social worker facilitates the family/physician/primary nurse meetings to discuss transplant and possible complications, and to address the medications, their side effects, and the post-transplant management. It is the social worker's role to help the child and family understand the full implications of transplantation, to see it as the possible key to an unknown number of years of relative normality, but also to keep in mind that it may not be a total solution. Often at diagnosis, families with no knowledge of ESRD have been led to believe, or need to believe, that transplantation is, or will be, the cure for their child's disease. They wish to rush immediately to transplant and will brook no delay. Even the most experienced professional is hard pressed not to tell the family those success stories they long to hear. In consideration of the problems of growth, renal osteodystrophy, and nutrition in keeping the child for lengthy periods of time on dialysis, recommendations are made always in full knowledge of the medical condition of the individual patient. It has, however, been our impression that a period of two to three months between major procedures ensures the physical and psychological consolidation necessary to fully optimize transplant and prepare for possible failure. It is the social worker's role to advise the team on the adjustment of child and family to dialysis as the foundation for transplant.

Preparation for the possibility of ultimate failure of a transplant is as vital as preparation for the successful transplant. This is especially true of a transplant from a live related donor. When speaking of the relative success of live related versus cadaveric transplant, it is tempting to use the successful rather than unsuccessful case as a model. This is well and good: we must, however, be careful of putting donor and recipient in the category of medical failures when a live related transplant is rejected. Unbiased interpretation of allograft function statistics to the neophyte ESRD family can severely tax the conscientious nephrologist and treatment team. Detailed presentation of all aspects of live related and cadaveric transplant, if necessary on more than one occasion, prepares child and family to make an informed transplant choice and to successfully manage the post-transplant course—whatever that may be.

We believe that *planning each stage of therapy as the foundation for the next* is the therapeutic strategy best fitted to the needs of child and family. It is tempting to think that receiving a transplant, itself such an astonishing feat of medical/surgical ingenuity, is *ipso facto* an end to many problems child and family face. This is simply not true. Sadly, even a successful transplant does not guarantee an easy adjustment to life. While earlier studies focused upon the effects of live related transplant on child and donor,[44-46] a more recent study explores its potential for total family stability or disequilibrium over time.[47] For this reason, the social worker must help both the family and the health care team steer a course between positive, hopeful involvement in the transplant phase and a realistic appraisal of all possible outcomes. Close collaboration and a shared conceptualization and treatment philosophy of ESRD between transplant surgeon and nephrologist are vital in this regard. Close liaison between social worker and team can help prevent long-term problems for child, family, and team caused by well-intentioned but poorly communicating professionals in the busy acute care hospital setting.

This is essentially a preventive approach designed to stress the reality of any chronic illness. Strictly speaking, nothing that happens to the child with ESRD should be seen as failure—for without kidney function, life is very brief. Any existence bought with dialysis and transplantation would not otherwise have been.

In considering the uncertainty of outcome in transplantation, it is vital to defend the parental right *not* to donate a kidney as well as to donate one. Motives for donating a kidney are complex and varied;[48] working single parents with other children may wish to think twice before running the risk of donating a kidney. Other potential donors may be at occupational or psychological risk. It is the role of the social worker to ensure that considerations like these are fully explored prior to transplant, and that true informed consent is obtained. Team evaluation of child and donor must be thorough and should occur over time. This also protects the physician from the consequences of speedy decision making grounded in brief sessions with child and family.

The social worker explores fantasies and fears with all potential transplant recipients, and child and donor are assessed for their interactional patterns and psychological fit. Marked fear or ambivalence (if it has not been apparent before) may indicate the need for counseling before transplant plans are finalized. Consultation with the liaison psychiatrist may be useful at this time. The social worker keeps the treatment team informed of relevant child and family dynamics, and helps the team deal with their own feelings about families, and the treatment choices they make. With the best of intentions, professionals may at times make false assumptions about who is, and who is not, suitable for transplant or different dialysis modalities.

Even with a good working kidney, the post-transplant course poses many problems for the child (and especially for the adolescent patient whose specialized problems are beyond the scope of this brief summary). High-dose steroids and relief from dietary restrictions bring yet another change in body image. Infections occur. The specter of rejection hovers menacingly over child and family. Idiosyncratic reactions to medications occur. Renal dwarfism (where present) does not miraculously disappear. The social worker may work even more closely than usual at this time with the renal dietitian. Family and child should be advised to delay assessment of effects of transplantation until at least a year after the transplant date. Once medical opinion indicates that prognosis for graft function is positive, emphasis is placed on readjustment to a normal life style while facing the uncertainty inherent in the post-transplant course.

Should chronic rejection and transplant nephrectomy occur, there is sometimes an urgency to proceed again to transplant on the part of parents or staff. The child is often less keen. Again, we would stress the significance of models of grief, loss, and mourning.[18-20] Time must be allowed for appropriate emotional and physical adjustment. A long fight with rejection—with its adjunctive high-steroid doses and perhaps antihypertensive medication—can leave the child bereft of physical and emotional reserves. Depressive sadness and psychosis are documented side effects of some of these medications.[49] Saddled with the heavy losses of hopes, time, normal social contacts, body image, approval as a "successful" patient, and, of course, the kidney, it is little wonder it takes the child some time to become excited about being alive. It is the role of the social worker to facilitate this adjustment period, and allow it to be experienced as a foundation for the next transplant attempt. In order to evaluate the child and discriminate between the interactional, characterological, and iatrogenic aspects of care, the social worker must gain some understanding of medicine, and nephrology in particular. It must be the personal responsibility of the social worker to ensure that he or she achieves reasonable fluency in the professional languages of the treatment team.

It is worth remarking that each loss of a kidney is, as it were, rehearsal for the child's death. Though there is no need for this to be raised, or indeed brought to consciousness, in child, family, or team, its recognition may explain some of the extreme emotional reactions of all parties, including the child, at the time of rejection. Increased support and acceptance of child and family at this time is crucial despite the caregivers' own helplessness. Sensitive handling of this phase will considerably ease the terminal phase should it occur.

**The Terminal Phase.** Despite the best ef-forts of all concerned, there comes a time when some children will die. How and when this occurs hinges upon highly involved moral, ethical, and medical considerations. Each terminal scenario, however it is managed, brings into play issues that are complex, and emotionally charged. It is the role of the social worker to join with both the family and the health care team to support them as they cope with loss, and as they try to put into some coherent personal framework their own response. Why, after such expense of medical and surgical expertise, time, and energy, after such mobilization of resources and personnel, after such love and attention has been given, such fights made for decreasing gains, in short, why, after such heroic efforts have been made, did death have to come? And was it really worth it? These are, in the end, intensely personal questions demanding personal answers. It is the social worker's role to support expressions of feeling around these and the other issues that arise at this time, and to sanction and help work through the variety of emotional responses that inevitably arise for everyone involved. At such a time, a private space in which to grieve and the presence of someone who will listen to and tolerate emotional pain should be available to all.

The need to control external reality is strong in all of us. When a child dies, professionals feel guilty or, in some way, responsible despite the excellent professional work they have done. Clinical attention has been drawn to the concept that guilt may perhaps be a way of defending oneself against feelings of helplessness: that it is an unconscious process whereby people can choose to blame themselves rather than admit to the inevitability of an illness that finally nothing can be done to control.[50] This is an especially delicate area with both parents and caregivers alike. The social worker should be sensitive to this dynamic in the terminal phase: attempts to diminish or remove feelings of guilt can result in their replacement with yet more threatening alternatives.

The child's perception of death has been the topic of a variety of literature.[51-53] The terminal child will rarely address death until the parents have indicated, by their own openness, that it is safe to do so.[29] Parents will find their child's terminal state harder to deal with when there is disagreement within the health care team as to the child's terminal management. It is, therefore, incumbent upon the social worker to help the team in coming to a consensus on this difficult issue. Working closely to support both the attending nephrologist and the family, should the team recommend conservative management, is one of the most challenging roles of the social worker. It is our experience that once all parties have agreed that the child will die, management, paradoxically, becomes much easier despite the natural anticipatory grief of all concerned.

## POST-TERMINAL CARE

While the work of the health care team draws to an end when a child dies, it remains for the social worker to facilitate family termination from the ESRD program. It is ironic that personal and professional relationships and the massive supportive resources of the program are necessarily withdrawn from the family at their time of greatest loss, when all parties are at their most vulnerable. Caregivers may be forgiven for subtly withdrawing from the family at such a time: they must replenish their psychic reservoirs to continue with their professional tasks. Some, feeling guilt and responsibility for the loss, may compensate by attending the funeral, or by communicating with the bereaved family in ways that may compound their grief. Team members should be free to express their feelings as their needs dictate, but it is the role of the social worker to formally represent the team in maintaining contact with the family to support the grief process as required. In the early weeks, regular telephone contact is offered, with a home visit several weeks after the child's death. As time goes by, telephone contact may be made at the social worker's discretion. Experience has shown this follow-up to be of inestimable value to the mourning process for family and team alike. Team grief can be mitigated by knowledge that the family is coming to terms with its loss. In turn, the family benefits from the knowledge that they and the memory of their child are not forgotten.

## SUMMARY

Little has been written on the role of the social worker in pediatric nephrology. This chapter has outlined some of the conceptual premises upon which social work practice may be built, and has examined some aspects of practice against the continuum of ESRD in the child. It has postulated the practical value of an interactional model of care that addresses the needs of child, family, and program and the relationship between these three parties to the therapeutic endeavor. This is an elegant and powerful complement to the medical model.

It is the author's hope that the concepts and practice described here can be subjected to more rigorous critical research scrutiny in the future, and that this will be to the benefit of children with ESRD, their families, and the professionals who care for them.

## REFERENCES

1. Kari J, Kyle E, Vivalda E: Position of the nephrology social worker. Ad Hoc Committee on PL 92-603, May, 1973. Dial Transplant, December-January, 1974.
2. Cain LP: Casework with kidney patients. Social Work 8:76, 1973.
3. Landsman M: Renal social worker in a satellite. Dial Transplant, 5:25, 1976.
4. Bare M: Confronting a life-threatening disease: Renal dialysis and transplant program. In: Kerson TS (Ed): Social Work in Health Settings. New York, Longman, 1982, pp 71–88.
5. Fortner-Frazier CL: Social Work and Dialysis. Berkeley, University of California Press, 1981.
6. Medline Search revealed no references relating the role of the social worker to pediatric dialysis and transplantation.
7. Travis G: Chronic Illness in Children. Stanford, Stanford University Press, 1976.
8. Dickoff J, James P, Wiedenbach E: Theory in a practice discipline. Nurs Res, 5:415, 1968.
9. Job Description of Clinical Social Worker ESRD, Personnel Policies and Procedures, St. Christopher's Hospital for Children, Philadelphia, Pa, 1980.
10. Mailick M: The impact of severe illness on the individual and family: an overview. Social Work in Health Care, 2:117, 1979.
11. Watzlawick P, Weakland JH, Fisch R: Change. New York, WW Norton & Co, Inc, 1974.
12. Hoffman L: Foundations of Family Therapy. New York, Basic Books, Inc, 1981.
13. Minuchin S, Rosman BL, Baker L: Psychosomatic Families. Cambridge, Harvard University Press, 1978.
14. Engel GL: The clinical application of the biopsychosocial model. Am J Psychiatry, 5:535, 1980.
15. Adams J, Lindemann E: Coping with long term disability. In: Coelho G, Hamburg D, Adams J (Eds): Coping and Adaptation. New York, Basic Books, 1974, p 127.
16. Perlman HH: Persona, Social Role and Personality. Chicago, University of Chicago Press, 1968.
17. Parad HJ: Crisis Intervention: Selected Readings. New York, Family Service Association of America, 1965.
18. Kaplan DM: A concept of acute situational disorders. Social Work, 2:15, 1962.
19. Germain CB: An ecological perspective on social

work practice in health care. Social Work in Health Care. 1:67, 1977.

20. McCue JD: The effects of stress on physicians and their medical practice. N Engl J Med 304:458, 1982.

21. Cassel EJ: The nature of suffering and the goals of medicine. N Engl J Med 306:638, 1982.

22. Bowlby J: Attachment and Loss (Vol II: Separation, Anxiety and Anger). New York, Basic Books, 1973.

23. Pincus L: Death and the Family: The Importance of Mourning. New York, Pantheon Books, 1974.

24. Parkes CM: Bereavement. New York, International Universities Press, 1972.

25. Bowlby J: Attachment and Loss (Vol 3: Loss, Sadness and Depression). New York, Basic Books, 1980.

26. Stack CB: All Our Kin. New York, Harper and Row, 1974.

27. Minuchin S: Families and Family Therapy. Cambridge, Harvard University Press, 1974.

28. Mahler M, Pine F, Bergman A: The Psychological Birth of the Human Infant. New York, Basic Books, 1975.

29. Langner MB: The Private Worlds of Dying Children. Princeton, NJ, Princeton University Press, 1978.

30. Weisman A: On Dying and Denying. New York, Behavioral Publications, 1972.

31. Schreiner GE, Tartaglia C: Uremia: soma or psyche. Kidney Int (Suppl) 8:32, 1978.

32. Eckhardt LO, Prugh DG: Preparing children psychologically for painful medical and surgical procedures. In: Gellert E (Ed): Psychosocial Aspects of Pediatric Care. New York, Grune & Stratton, 1978, pp 75–83.

33. Muller-Wiefel DE: Dialysis or transplantation. Monatsschr Kinderheilkd, 11:692, 1980.

34. Calland CH: Iatrogenic problems in end stage renal failure. N Engl J Med 287:334, 1972.

35. Caplan G: Principles of Preventive Psychiatry. New York, Basic Books, 1964.

36. Berkman BG, Rehr H: Early social service casefinding for hospitalized patients: an experiment. The Social Service Review, 2:264, 1973.

37. Williams M: Crisis intervention: a social work method. Social Work and Health Care, 1:23, 1979.

38. Rapoport RN: Notes on deprivation of the privileged. Am J Orthopsychiatry, 3:656, 1958.

39. Promislo E: Confidentiality and privileged communication. Social Work, 1:10, 1979.

40. Fenichel O: The Psychoanalytic Theory of Neurosis. New York, WW Norton & Co, 1972.

41. Gruskin AB: Meeting with families to introduce them to ESRD. St. Christopher's Hospital for Children, Philadelphia, Pa.

42. Ahrons CR, Arnn S: When children from divorced families are hospitalized: issues for staff. Health and Social Work, 3:21, 1981.

43. Kaplan De-Nour A, Czaczkes JW, Lilos P: A study of chronic hemodialysis teams—differences in opinions and expectations. J Chronic Dis 25:441, 1972.

44. Bernstein DM: After transplantation—the child's emotional reactions. Am J Psychiatry, 127:1189, 1971.

45. Kahn AU, Herndon CH, Ahmadian SY: Social and emotional adaptation of children with transplanted kidneys and chronic hemodialysis. Am J Psychiatry, 127:1194, 1971.

46. Korsch BM, Fine RN, Grushkin CM, Negrete BF: Experiences with children and their families during extended hemodialysis and kidney transplantations. Pediatr Clin North Am 18:625, 1971.

47. de Parra MLV: Changes in family structure after a renal transplant. Family Process, 2:195, 1982.

48. Fost M: Children as renal donors. N Engl J Med, 296:363, 1977.

49. Hall RCW, Stickney SK, Gardner ER: Behavioral toxicity of nonpsychiatric drugs. In: Hall CW (Ed): Psychiatric Presentations of Medical Illness. New York, SP Medical and Scientific Books, 1980, pp 311–336.

50. Gardner R: The guilt reactions of parents of children with severe physical diseases. Am J Psychiatry 126:636, 1969.

51. Chapman JA, Goodall J: Helping a child to live whilst dying. Lancet, April 5:753, 1980.

52. Spinetta JJ, Rigler D, Karon M: Anxiety in the dying child. Pediatrics, 6:841, 1973.

53. Singher LJ: The slowly dying child. Clin Pediatr, 13:861, 1974.

# Index

**575**